Community Health Nursing

Promoting the Health of Aggregates

Community Health Nursing

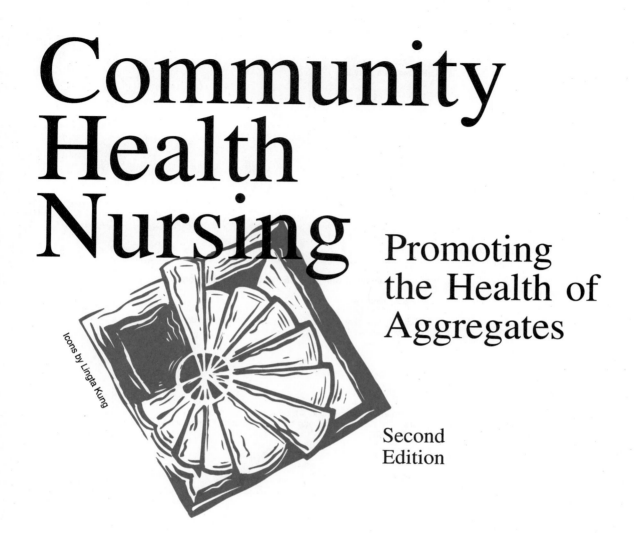

Icons by Lingta Kung

Promoting the Health of Aggregates

Second Edition

Janice M. Swanson, PhD, RN, FAAN
Professor
Department of Nursing
Samuel Merritt College
Oakland, California

Mary A. Nies, PhD, RN, FAAN
Associate Professor
Community Health Systems
School of Nursing
Vanderbilt University
Nashville, Tennessee

W.B. SAUNDERS COMPANY
A Division of Harcourt Brace & Company

Philadelphia   London   Toronto
Montreal   Sydney   Tokyo

W.B. SAUNDERS COMPANY
A Division of
Harcourt Brace & Company

The Curtis Center
Independence Square West
Philadelphia, Pennsylvania 19106

Library of Congress Cataloging-in-Publication Data

Swanson, Janice M.

Community health nursing: promoting the health of aggregates/
Janice M. Swanson, Mary A. Nies.—2nd ed.

p.   cm.

Includes bibliographical references and index.

ISBN 0–7216–6167–X

1. Community health nursing.   I. Nies, Mary A.   II. Title.
  [DNLM: 1. Community Health Nursing. 2. Health Promotion.   WY 106
  S972c 1997]

RT98.S9   1997   610.73′43—dc20

DNLM/DLC   96–31896

COMMUNITY HEALTH NURSING:
Promoting the Health of Aggregates   ISBN 0–7216–6167–X

Printed in the United States of America.

Last digit is the print number: 9   8   7   6   5   4   3   2   1

This book is dedicated to all community health nurses, educators, and students who raise questions and search for answers to improve the health of the community, and to my family for their support and endurance— Richard, Karen, and Betsy Swanson.

JANICE M. SWANSON

I dedicate this book to Phil Yankovich, my husband, companion, and best friend whose love, caring, and true support are always there for me. He provides me with the energy I need to pursue my dreams.

To Earl and Lois Nies, my parents, for their never-ending encouragement and lifelong support, and who helped me develop a foundation for creative thinking and new ideas.

To all my teachers and mentors, especially Judith Sullivan, PhD, RN, FAAN, Jean Goeppinger, PhD, RN, FAAN, and Nola Pender, PhD, RN, FAAN, who have influenced my thinking and vision about health of the community and who taught me the value of critical inquiry and spirited debate.

MARY A. NIES

AUTHORS

Janice M. Swanson

Janice M. Swanson, PhD, RN, FAAN, is Professor, Department of Nursing, Samuel Merritt College, Oakland, California. Dr. Swanson received her diploma from Emanuel Hospital School of Nursing in Portland, Oregon; her baccalaureate in nursing from Wayne State University in Detroit, Michigan; and her master of science degree in community health nursing and doctorate in education from the University of Maryland. She completed a postdoctoral fellowship in medical sociology and nursing with the late Anselm Strauss at the University of California, San Francisco. Dr. Swanson has coauthored two other books: *Men's Reproductive Health,* with Katherine Forrest, and *From Practice to Grounded Theory: Qualitative Research in Nursing,* with the late Carole Chenitz. Her research interests focus on reproductive and sexual health issues in the community. She has just completed a study of condom use decision-making in Latinas, funded by the National Institutes of Health. She has served as a member of the Nursing Research Study Section, Division of Research Grants, National Institutes of Health. She also serves as a consultant to research teams studying HIV prevention/AIDS in high risk populations.

Mary A. Nies

Mary A. Nies (formerly Albrecht), PhD, RN, FAAN, is Associate Professor, Community Health Systems, School of Nursing, Vanderbilt University Medical Center. Dr. Nies received her diploma from Bellin School of Nursing in Green Bay, Wisconsin; her BSN from University of Wisconsin, Madison; her MSN from Loyola University, Chicago; and her PhD in Public Health Nursing, Health Services, and Health Promotion Research at the University of Illinois, Chicago. She completed a postdoctoral research fellowship in health promotion and community health with Dr. Nola Pender at the University of Michigan, Ann Arbor. She has been a Fellow of the American Academy of Nursing since 1994. Dr. Nies co-edited *Community Health Nursing: Promoting the Health of Aggregates,* which received the 1993 Book of the Year award from the American Journal of Nursing, with Jan Swanson. Her program of research focuses on outcomes of health promotion interventions for minority and non-minority women as well as low-income women in the community. Dr. Nies is principal investigator on a research grant funded by the National Institutes of Health, National Institute of Nursing Research (NIH, NINR). This five-year study tests a nursing intervention targeted at sedentary women in the community to increase their physical activity levels. Her research is involved with energy metabolism, particularly in areas of fitness, physical activity, and obesity prevention for populations, especially women. Dr. Nies is a Co-investigator on a NIH-funded P30 program grant, entitled Development of a Clinical Nutrition Research Unit. Her work also includes consulting in the areas of public/community health and health promotion education, practice, and research.

CONTRIBUTORS

Mary E. Allen, PhD, RN
Associate Professor and Division Director, Psychiatric/Mental Health and Community Health Nursing, College of Nursing University of Oklahoma Oklahoma City, Oklahoma
Mental Health

Margaret M. Andrews, PhD, RN
Chairperson and Professor, Department of Nursing, Nazareth College of Rochester; Adjunct Faculty, School of Nursing, University of Rochester, Rochester, New York
Cultural Diversity and Community Health Nursing

Constance M. Baker, EdD, MA, RN
Professor, Nursing Administration, Department of Environments for Health, Indiana University, School of Nursing, Indianapolis, Indiana
School Health

Lucretia A. Bolin, DNS, RN
Assistant Professor of Nursing, Samuel Merritt College, Oakland; Family NARC Practitioner, Chemical Dependency Program, Kaiser Permanente Medical Center, San Francisco, California
The African-American Community; Substance Abuse

Christine DiMartile Bolla, DNS, RN
Assistant Professor, Nursing, Samuel Merritt College, Oakland, California
The Home Visit and Home Health Care

Deborah Godfrey Brown, MS, RN
Undergraduate Director, Assistant Professor, College of Nursing, University of Rhode Island, Kingston, Rhode Island
Community Health Planning and Evaluation

Patricia M. Burbank, DNSc, RN
Associate Professor, College of Nursing, University of Rhode Island, Kingston, Rhode Island
Community Health Planning and Evaluation

Patricia G. Butterfield, PhD, RN
Associate Professor, College of Medicine, Montana State University–Bozeman, Bozeman, Montana
Thinking Upstream: Conceptualizing Health from a Population Perspective; Rural Health

Mary Brecht Carpenter, MPH, RN
Project Director/Research Instructor, Georgetown University, Washington, D.C.
Child and Adolescent Health

Holly B. Cassells, PhD, MPH
Associate Professor, University of
Incarnate Word, San Antonio,
Texas
*Community Assessment and
Epidemiology*

Kathleen Chafey, PhD, RN
Associate Professor of Community
Health Nursing, College of
Nursing, Montana State
University–Bozeman, Bozeman,
Montana
Rural Health

Della J. Dash, MPH, BSN, RN
Project Officer,
c/o UNICEF–Ethiopia,
New York, New York
Communicable Disease

Nellie S. Droes, DNSc, RNC, CS
Assistant Professor, East Carolina
University, Greenville, North
Carolina
The Homeless

Nancy Edwards, PhD, RN
Associate Professor,
University of Ottawa,
Faculty of Health Sciences,
School of Nursing,
Ottawa, Ontario, Canada
*Model 2: Primary Health Care in
Canada (World Health)*

Susan Rumsey Givens, BSN,
MPH, RN
Childbirth Educator, ASPO
Certified Lamaze Instructor, St.
Ann's Hospital, Westerville, Ohio
Child and Adolescent Health

Joanne M. Hall, PhD, RN
Associate Professor, School of
Nursing, University of
Wisconsin–Milwaukee,
Milwaukee, Wisconsin
*Substance Abuse; Environmental
Health*

Diane C. Hatton, DNSc, RN, CS
Associate Professor, Hahn School
of Nursing, University of San
Diego, San Diego, California
The Homeless

Doris Henson, MS, MPH, RN
Assistant Professor, Community
Health Nursing, College of
Nursing, Montana State
University–Bozeman, Missoula
Campus, Missoula, Montana
Rural Health

Peggy Hickman, EdD, RN
Associate Professor, College of
Nursing, University of Kentucky,
Lexington, Kentucky
*Community Organization: Building
Partnerships for Health*

Barbara J. Horn, PhD, RN
Professor Emeritus, University of
Washington, Seattle, Washington
The Health Care System

Beverly M. Horn, PhD, RN
Associate Professor, School of
Nursing, University of
Washington, Seattle, Washington
The Health Care System

Vera Labat, MPH, PNP, RN
Adjunct Faculty Member, Western
Institute for Social Research,
Berkeley, California; Public Health
Nurse, Immunization Assistance
Program, City of Berkeley, Health
and Human Services Department,
Berkeley, California
Communicable Disease

Jean Cozad Lyon, PhD, FNP, RN
Family Nurse Practitioner, The
Medical Group of Northern
Nevada, Reno, Nevada
*The Home Visit and Home Health
Care; Models of Nursing Care
Delivery and Case Management:
Clarification of Terms*

Erika Madrid, DNSc, RN, CS
Assistant Professor, Department of
Nursing, Holy Names College,
Oakland, California
Substance Abuse

Ricardo Martinez, PhD, MPH, RN
Principal Healthcare and
Medicolegal Consultant,
Medicolegal Consultants, San
Antonio, Texas
*The Mexican-American
Community*

Cherryl E. McDougall, BSN, RN,
COHN
Worldwide Health Services
Manager, Digital Equipment
Corporation, Maynard,
Massachusetts
*Occupational Health Nurse: Roles
and Responsibilities, Current and
Future Trends*

Cathy D. Meade, PhD, RN
Associate Professor, College of
Medicine, University of South
Florida, Tampa; Director,
Education Program, H. Lee Moffitt
Cancer Center and Research
Institute, Tampa, Florida
Community Health Education

Barbara S. Morgan, PhD, RN
Visiting Professor, School of
Nursing, University of Miami,
Coral Gables, Florida
*Community Health Planning and
Evaluation*

Mary A. Nies, PhD, RN, FAAN
Associate Professor, Community
Health Systems, School of
Nursing, Vanderbilt University,
Nashville, Tennessee
*Health: A Community View; The
Home Visit and Home Health
Care; Community Health Nursing:
Making a Difference*

Olive T. Roen, MSN, MPH,
RNC, NP
Senior Research Assistant, Center
for Health Policy Studies, School
of Public Health, University of
Texas Houston Health Science
Center, San Antonio, Texas
Senior Health

Patricia E. Stevens, PhD, RN
Associate Professor, School of
Nursing, University of
Wisconsin–Milwaukee,
Milwaukee, Wisconsin
Environmental Health

Ruth F. Stewart, MS
Associate Professor (Retired),
University of Texas Health
Science Center School of Nursing,
San Antonio; Member, Texas
Board of Health, Texas
Department of Health, Austin,
Texas
*Policy, Politics, Legislation, and
Public Health Nursing*

Janice M. Swanson, PhD, RN,
FAAN
Professor, Department of Nursing,
Samuel Merritt College, Oakland,
California
*Health: A Community View;
Historical Factors: Community
Health Nursing in Context; Men's
Health; Addressing the Needs of
Families; Cultural Influences in
the Community: Other Popula-
tions; World Health; Community
Health Nursing: Making a
Difference*

Karen A. Swanson, MS, BA
Research Analyst, California
Department of Health Services,
Berkeley, California
World Health

Donna Neal Thomas, PhD, RNC
Chief Executive Officer,
Community Health Centers Inc.,
Mary Mahoney Memorial Health
Center, Healing Hands Health
Care Services, Oklahoma City,
Oklahoma
Women's Health

Jack Thompson, MSW
Lecturer, Department of Health
Services, School of Public Health
and Community Medicine,
University of Washington, Seattle,
Washington
The Health Care System

Patricia Hyland Travers, ScM, MS,
RN, COHN-S
Visiting Lecturer, Harvard School
of Public Health, Boston; Program
Manager, Worldwide Health
Strategy, Digital Equipment
Corporation, Maynard,
Massachusetts
*Occupational Health Nurse: Roles
and Responsibilities, Current and
Future Trends*

Ann C. Watkins, MSN, CNM, RN
Health Program Specialists, State
of California, Department of
Health Services, Maternal and
Child Health Branch, Sacramento,
California
Violence in the Community

Roma D. Williams, PhD, CRNP
Associate Professor, Graduate
Programs in Nursing, School of
Nursing, University of Alabama at
Birmingham, Birmingham,
Alabama
Women's Health

More money is spent per capita for health care in the United States than in any other country ($3,510 in 1994), yet many countries have far better indices of health, including traditional indicators such as infant mortality and longevity for both men and women, than does the United States. The United States is the only western country with the exception of South Africa that lacks a program of national health service or national health insurance. Although the United States spent 13.7% of its gross domestic product on health care expenditures in 1994—a record high of $949 billion—15.2% of the population had no health care coverage. While some progress toward the objectives set for the health of the nation in **Healthy People 2000** has been made, the **Midcourse Review and 1995 Revisions** (see Appendix VII) shows that we are far from our goals, particularly for those in the greatest need—high risk populations.

The greater the proportion of money put into health care expenditures in the United States, the less money there is to improve education, jobs, housing, nutrition, etc. Over the years, the greatest improvements in the health of the population have come about through advances in public health, using organized community efforts, such as improvements in sanitation, immunizations, and pasteurization of food. The greatest determinants of health are still equated with factors in the community, such as education, employment, housing, and nutrition. Although access to health care services and individual behavioral change are important, they are but components of the larger determinants of health, such as one's social and physical environments.

The traditional focus of many health care professionals has been to deliver health care services to ill persons and to evolve needed behavioral change at the individual level, known as a *downstream focus*. The focus of community health nursing has traditionally been on health promotion and illness prevention by working with individuals and families within the community. Needed is a shift to an *upstream focus*. An upstream focus is a shift in focus to include working with aggregates and communities in activities such as organizing and setting health policy, which will help aggregates and communities work to create options for healthier environments that include essential components of health. These components include adequate education, housing, employment, and nutrition, as well as possible choices that allow all people to make behavioral changes, to live and work in safe environments, and to access equitable and comprehensive health care.

Grounded in the tenets of public health nursing and the practice of public health nurses such as Lillian Wald, this second edition of **Community Health Nursing: Promoting the Health of Aggregates** builds on the earlier work by highlighting an aggregate focus in addition to the traditional areas of family and community health and thus promotes upstream thinking. The primary focus is on the promotion of the health of aggregates. Including the family as an aggregate, yet going beyond the traditional home visit to the family, this text also addresses the needs of other aggregates or population subgroups. It conceptualizes the individual not only as a member of a family, but individuals and families as members of other aggregates, including organizations and institutions; and individuals as a part of a population within an environment, that is, within a community.

The aggregate is made up of a collective of individuals be it family or other group that, with others, make up a community. In this book, the aggregate as a unit of focus is emphasized; how aggregates that make up communities promote their own health is also emphasized. The aggregate is presented within the social context of the community, and the opportunity is given to students to define and analyze environmental, economic, political, and legal constraints to the health of aggregates.

Community health nurses have traditionally addressed the needs of aggregates, such as families and school, worksite, clinic, and community groups. Community health nursing texts, however, have traditionally defined the unit of care of the community health nurse generalist, with undergraduate preparation, as limited primarily to the individual and family. These texts have defined the unit of care of the specialist, with graduate preparation, as primarily to other aggregates, the community, or population. If community health nursing is truly a synthesis of nursing and public health practice in order to promote and preserve the health of populations, then all community health nurses carry out this mandate. The "diagnosis and treatment of human responses to actual or potential health problems" (American Nurses' Association Social Policy Statement, 1980) is from the nursing component. The ability to prevent disease, prolong life, and promote health through organized community effort is from the public health component. Community health nursing practice is responsible to the population as a whole; nursing efforts to promote health and prevent disease are applied to the public, which includes all units in the community, be they individual or collective, be they a person, family, other aggregate, community, or population. The generalist is competent to practice such at a minimum safe level, while the specialist is expected to have expert competence, through practice over time, and knowledge and a higher level of autonomy and freedom. Community health nurses at both generalist and specialist levels of practice need to claim their right to the full synthesis of nursing and public health practice and to increase their alliance with public health to promote and preserve the health of populations.

In this text, the student is encouraged to become a student of the community, to learn from families and other aggregates in the community how they define and promote their own health, and to learn how to become an advocate of the community by working with the community to initiate change. The student is exposed to the view that the complexity and rich diversity of the community and evidence of how the community organizes to meet change are strengths. For example, the use of language or terminology varies in different parts of the country by clients and by agencies, and it may vary from that used by government officials. The contributors of this textbook are a diverse group from various parts of the country. Their terms vary from chapter to chapter, as well as those in use in local communities. For example, some authors refer to African-Americans, some to blacks, some to Euro-Americans, some to whites. It is important for the student to be familiar with a range of terms and, most important, to know what is used in his or her local community.

Outstanding features of this second edition include its provocative nature as it raises consciousness regarding the social injustices that exist in America and how these injustices, embodied in our market-driven health care system, prevent the realization of health as a right for all. With a focus on an ethic of social justice, this text emphasizes society's rather than the individual's responsibility for the protection of all human life to ensure that all persons have their basic needs met, such as adequate health protection and income. Shifts in reimbursement and the growth of managed care have revitalized the notion of the need for population-focused care, or care that covers all persons residing within geographic boundaries, rather than only those populations enrolled in systems of managed care. Working toward providing health promotion and population-focused care to all requires a dramatic shift in thinking from individual-focused care for the practitioners of the future. It is clear that the future paradigm for health care is demanding that the focus of nursing move toward community health promotion if we are to forge toward a health-promoting and wellness-achieving nation.

This text is designed **to stimulate critical thinking and challenge students to question and debate issues.** Because complex problems demand complex answers, the student *is expected to synthesize prior biophysical, psychosocial, cultural, and ethical arenas of knowledge.* But experiential knowledge is also necessary, and the student is challenged to *enter new environments within the community* and to gain, firsthand, new sensory, cognitive, and affective experiences. We have integrated the concept of **upstream thinking,** introduced in the first edition, throughout this second edition, as an important conceptual basis for nursing practice of aggregates and the community. The student is introduced to both the individual and aggregate roles of community health nurses as they are engaged collectively and interdisciplinarily, working **upstream,** to facilitate the community's promotion of its own health. Students using this text will be better prepared to work with aggregates and communities in health promotion as well as to work with individuals and families in illness. Students using this text will also be better prepared to see the need to take responsibility for participation in organized community action targeting inequalities in arenas such as education, jobs, and housing as well as to participate in targeting individual health-behavioral change. These are important shifts in thinking for future practitioners who must be prepared to function in a community-focused health care system.

The text is also designed to increase the **cultural awareness and competency** of future community health nurses as they prepare to address the needs of culturally diverse populations. Students must be prepared to work with these growing populations, as participation in the nursing work force by ethnically and racially diverse persons continues to lag. An expanded section in this edition focuses on sociocultural diversity and the needs of these and other special aggregates. Various models are introduced to assist students to understand the growing link between social problems and health status, experienced disproportionately by diverse populations in the United States, and to methods of assessment and intervention used to meet the special needs of these populations.

The goals of the text are (1) to provide the student with the ability to assess the complex of factors in the community that affect individual, family, and other aggregate responses to health states and actual or potential health problems; and (2) to use this ability to plan, implement, and evaluate community health nursing interventions to increase contributions to the promotion of the health of populations.

MAJOR THEMES RELATED TO PROMOTING THE HEALTH OF THE AGGREGATE

This text is built on the following major themes:

- A social justice ethic of health care in contrast to a market justice ethic of health care in keeping with the philosophy of public health, as "health for all."
- A population-focused model of community health nursing as necessary to achieve equity in health for the entire population.
- Integration of the concept of *upstream thinking* throughout the text and other appropriate theoretical frameworks related to chapter topics.
- The use of population-focused and other community data to develop an assessment, or profile of health, and potential and actual health needs and capabilities of aggregates.
- The application of all steps in the nursing process at the individual, family, and aggregate levels.
- A focus on identifying needs of the aggregate from common interactions with individuals, families, and communities in traditional environments.
- An orientation toward the application of all three levels of prevention at the individual, family, and aggregate levels.
- The experience of the underserved aggregate, particularly the economically disenfranchised, including those cultural and ethnic groups disproportionately at risk of developing health problems.

Themes were developed and related to promoting the health of the aggregate in the following ways:

- The commitment of community health nursing is to an equity model, and as such, community health nurses work toward the provision of the unmet health needs of the population, including aggregates, in a system that allows access to care only for those who can pay (Chapters 1, 2, and 3).
- The development of a population-focused model is necessary to close the gap between unmet health care needs and health resources on a geographic basis to the entire population. The contributions of intervention at the aggregate level work toward the realization of such a model (Chapters 4 and 9).
- Contemporary theories provide frameworks for holistic community health nursing practice that help the students conceptualize the reciprocal impact of various components within the community on the health of aggregates and the population (Chapter 4 and throughout).
- The ability to gather population-focused and other community data in developing an assessment of health is a crucial initial step that precedes the identification of nursing diagnoses and plans to meet aggregate responses to potential and actual health problems (Chapter 5).
- The nursing process includes, in each step, a focus on the aggregate: assessment of the aggregate; nursing diagnosis of the aggregate; planning for the aggregate; and intervention and evaluation at the aggregate level (Chapter 5, Unit 3, and Unit 4).

- The development of the ability to gather cues about the needs of aggregates from complex environments such as with a home visit, with parents in a waiting room of a well-baby clinic, or with elders receiving hypertension screening, and to promote individual, collective, and political action that addresses the health of aggregates (Units 2, 3, 4, 5, and 6).
- Primary, secondary, and tertiary prevention strategies include a major focus at the aggregate level (Units 1, 2, 3, 4, 5, and 6).
- In addition to offering an extended chapter sequence on cultural influences in the community, the text includes data on and the experience of the underserved aggregates at high risk of developing health problems, groups most often in need of community health nursing services: low and marginal income, cultural, and ethnic groups (Chapters 17 through 20 and throughout).

The book is divided into seven units. Unit 1 presents an overview of the concept of health, a perspective of health as evolving and as defined by the community, and the concept of community health nursing as the nursing of aggregates from both historical and contemporary mandates. Health is viewed as an individual and collective right, brought about through individual and collective/political action. The definitions of public health and community health nursing and their foci are presented. Current crises in public health and in the medical care system and consequences for the health of the public frame implications for community health nursing. The historical evolution of public health, the health care system, and community health nursing is presented. The evolution of humans from wanderers and food gatherers to those who live in larger groups and the impact of the group on health contrasts with the evolution of a health care system built around the individual person, increasingly fractured into many parts. Community health nurses bring awareness to their practice of the social context; of economic, political and legal constraints from the larger community; and knowledge of the current health care system and its structural constraints and limitations on the care of populations.

Unit 2 presents the art and science of community health nursing. The theoretical foundations for the book, with a focus on the concept of *upstream thinking,* and the rationale for an aggregate approach to community health nursing are presented. The application of the nursing process—assessment, planning, intervention, and evaluation—to aggregates in the community using selected theory bases is presented. The unit addresses the need for a population-focus that includes the public health sciences of biostatistics and epidemiology as key in community assessment and the application of the nursing process to aggregates in order to promote the health of populations. Application of both art and the science of community health nursing to meeting the needs of aggregates is evident in chapters that focus on community health planning and evaluation; community organization; community health education; and policy, politics, and legislation.

Unit 3 presents the application of the community health nursing process to aggregates in community health: children and adolescents, women, men, families, seniors, the homeless, and those living in rural areas. The focus is on the major indicators of health (longevity, mortality, and morbidity), types of common health problems, utilization of health services, pertinent legislation, health services and resources, selected applications of the community health nursing process to a case study, application of the levels of prevention, selected roles of the community health nurse, and relevant research.

Unit 4 addresses the application of the community health nursing process to the special needs of aggregates of diverse cultural backgrounds, including the African-American community and the Mexican-American community. Reprinted articles have been selected for inclusion to introduce readers to information about the health status of diverse populations that may be found living in the United States and to focus on various approaches to community assessment and/or prevention to stimulate critical thinking and problem-solving in application of concepts to diverse cultural groups living within the reader's local community. Examples presented focus on the following groups: Southeast Asian immigrants, urban American Indians, Alaska natives, Asian Americans and Pacific Islanders, and Arab-American women. In addition, the concept "marginalization" is presented in a reprinted article to expand the concept of diversity to other groups and to guide the reader in the development of nursing knowledge regarding vulnerable populations that value diversity.

Unit 5 addresses the application of the community health nursing process to special needs of aggregates of increasing importance in the community: needs related to violence in the community, mental health, and substance abuse. Basic community health nursing strategies are applied to promoting the health of these vulnerable high-risk aggregates.

Unit 6 has a focus of special services needs in community health nursing, including communicable disease, school health, environmental health, and occupational health. A final chapter within this unit focuses on the process of carrying out a home visit and the growing field of home health care.

Unit 7 presents an overview of the future of community health nursing. The chapter on world health presents the features of the health care systems in both a developing country, Cuba, and a developed country, Canada. The final chapter emphasizes the need for community health nursing to show that it "makes a difference," which calls for an accountability-creativity link from community health nurses in all settings.

Seven appendices present information about current standards of community health nursing and home health nursing, the Declaration of Alma-Ata, population-focused care and case management, recommendations of the U.S. Preventive Services Task Force 1996, and a midcourse review of Healthy People 2000 and 1995 revisions.

FEATURES

The following features are presented to enhance student learning:

- Learning Objectives
    Learning objectives set the framework for the content of each individual chapter.
- Theoretical Frameworks
    The use of theoretical frameworks common to nursing and public health will aid the student in application of both familiar and new theory bases to problems and challenges in the community.
- Case Studies/Application of Nursing Process at Individual, Family, and Aggregate Levels
    The use of case studies and anecdotal material throughout the text is

designed to ground the theory, concepts, and the application of the nursing process in practical and manageable examples for the student.

- Nursing Research

   The introduction of students to the growing bodies of community health nursing and public health research literature will be enhanced by highlighting boxed references to relevant research at the end of each chapter.

- Boxed Information

   Summaries of content by section, examples, research, and other pertinent information will be presented as "boxed information" to aid the student's learning by focusing on major points, illustrating concepts, and breaking up sections of "heavy" content.

- Learning Activities

   Selected learning activities are listed at the end of each chapter to enable students to have affective learning experiences in the community as well as cognitive experiences.

- Photo-novellas

   Stories in photograph form of community health nurses (a) making a home visit to a well family, (b) making a home visit to a family caring for a member with a chronic illness, and (c) giving clinic-based community services to a well family.

The following features are new to this edition:

- The theoretical construct, *upstream thinking,* is integrated into chapters throughout the text.
- The chapter on *Community Assessment and Epidemiology* expands the concepts of *screening* and *surveillance*—concepts important to upstream thinking.
- A new *Community Health Education* chapter includes a focus on practical strategies such as assessment of *health literacy* and *reading level.*
- A new chapter addresses *The Homeless,* a high risk population that is becoming increasingly visible in our communities throughout the nation.
- A new chapter addresses *Cultural Influences in the Community: Other Populations.* Five reprinted current publications describe varied models of assessment and/or intervention used with diverse populations. Students are challenged to develop approaches to meeting the needs of diverse populations within their own communities by accessing and synthesizing data bases and other information available at the national, state, and/or local levels, and/or, if need be, by creating their own.
- A new chapter on *School Health* uses a critical theory framework to approach the practice of nursing in schools.
- The chapter on *World Health* includes two models of primary care: (1) a reprint of an updated article on Cuba (developing world), and (2) an original contribution on Canada (developed world).
- The appendices include reprints of two articles which will augment students' knowledge relevant to current changes in the health care system: (1) "Models of Nursing Care Delivery and Case Management: Clarification of Terms," and (2) "Population Management in an HMO: New Roles for Nursing." Included also are updates on the Recommendations of the U.S. Preventive Services Task Force, 1996, and Healthy People 2000, Midcourse Review and 1995 Revisions.

ACKNOWLEDGMENTS

Community Health Nursing: Promoting the Health of Aggregates could not have been written without the sharing of experiences, thoughtful critique, and support of many people—individuals, families, groups, and communities. Special thanks go to everyone who made significant contributions to this book.

We are indebted to our contributing authors whose inspiration, untiring hours of work, and persistence have continued to build a new era of community health nursing practice with a focus on the aggregate level. We thank the many community health nursing faculty who welcomed the first edition of the text and who responded to our inquiries with comments and suggestions for the second edition. We also thank our colleagues in our respective work settings for their understanding and support during the writing and editing of this edition.

To Melanie McEwen, PhD, RN, CS, Assistant Professor, Baylor University School of Nursing, Dallas, goes special recognition and thanks for writing and revising the Instructor's Manual, examination questions, and transparency masters to accompany the text.

We especially thank the following authors whose articles are reprinted in this text: Moon S. Chen, Jr., Betty Lee Hawks, Afaf I. Meleis, Patricia A. Omidian, Juliene G. Lipson, David C. Grossman, James W. Krieger, Jonathan R. Sugarman, Ralph A. Forquera, Joanne M. Hall, Patricia E. Stevens, Marjorie A. Muecke, Jean Cozad Lyon, Wendy L. Graff, Wendy Bensussen-Walls, Eileen Cody, Joanne Williamson, Karen A. Swanson, Ayesha E. Gill, and Chris Walter.

DETAILED CONTENTS

UNIT 3   *Aggregates in the Community*   215

Chapter 10   ***Child and Adolescent Health***   **217**

Mary Brecht Carpenter
Susan Rumsey Givens

Chapter 11   ***Women's Health***   **237**

Roma D. Williams
Donna Neal Thomas

Chapter 12   ***Men's Health***   **269**

Janice M. Swanson

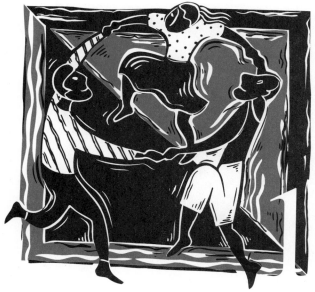

Introduction to Community Health Nursing

Health:
A Community View

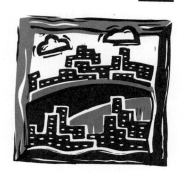

Upon completion of this chapter, the reader will be able to:

1. **Compare and contrast definitions of health as used in public health nursing.**

2. **Define and discuss the focus of public health.**

3. **List the three levels of prevention and give one example of each.**

4. **Differentiate between the conceptual models of community health nursing, as defined by the American Nurses Association, and public health nursing, as defined by the Public Health Nursing Section of the American Public Health Association.**

Mary A. Nies
Janice M. Swanson

Public health nurses are in a position to assist the U.S. health care system in a transition from a system that is disease oriented to one that is health oriented. Current costs of caring for the sick account for the majority of the escalating health care dollars, which increased from 5.9% of the gross domestic product in 1965 to 13.9% in 1993 (National Center for Health Statistics, 1995). National annual health care expenditures reached $884.2 billion in 1993, or $3299 per person. U.S. health expenditures reflect a focus on care of the sick. In 1993, $.37 of each health care dollar was spent on hospital care, and $.19 was spent on physician services, mostly for care of the sick. In contrast, only $.03 of every health care dollar was spent on preventive government public health activities. Despite hospital and physician expenditures, U.S. health indexes rate far below the health indexes of many other countries, a consequence that reflects the severe disproportion of funding for preventive services and social and economic opportunities. Furthermore, the health status of the population within the United States varies markedly among areas of the country and among groups (e.g., the economically disadvantaged and many cultural and ethnic groups).

Nurses constitute the largest group of health care workers and are instrumental in the evolution of a health care delivery system that will meet the health-oriented needs of the people. According to the National Sample Survey of Registered Nurses conducted by the Division of Nursing, Bureau of Health Professions, Health Resources and Services Administration, in 1992 about 66.5% of the approximately 1.85 million employed registered nurses in the United States worked in hospitals and about 15% (approximately 250,000) worked in community, school, or occupational health settings (U.S. Department of Health and Human Services, 1994).

The number of nurses employed in hospitals in 1992 represents an increase of more than 100,000 in the number employed in hospitals in 1988 (1,232,717 vs. 1,104,978), whereas the number of nurses employed in community health areas increased 38% between 1988 and 1992. However, it has been predicted that there will be a marked decline in hospital employment of nurses and an increase in the number of nurses working in community settings that focus on health promotion and preventive care. More nurses will be employed by alternative delivery systems that provide ambulatory care to meet cost-containment mandates as well as fulfill a growing proportion of health care needs.

Community health nursing is the synthesis of nursing practice and public health practice. The major goal of community health nursing is the preservation of the health of the community and populations through a focus on health promotion and health maintenance of individuals, families, and groups within the community. Thus, community health nursing is oriented toward health and the identification of populations at risk rather than toward an episodic response to patient demand.

The mission of public health is social justice, which entitles all persons to basic necessities such as adequate income and health protection and accepts collective burdens to make such possible. Public health, with its egalitarian tradition and vision, conflicts with the predominant U.S. model of justice: market justice, or the entitlement of people to only what they have gained through individual efforts. Although individual rights are respected, collective action and obligations are minimal. An overinvestment in technology and curative medical services has cut short the evolution of a health ethic to protect and preserve the health of the population.

Current U.S. health policy calls for individuals to change behavior that might predispose them to chronic disease or accident. People are asked to exercise, eat healthfully, and give up smoking or alcohol use. However, to ask the individual to overcome the effects of unhealthy social and physical environments negates the collective behavior necessary to change the many determinants of health stemming from those environments such as air and water pollution and work place hazards. Because both lifestyle and disease are a result of the environment in which we live, public health policy seeks to bring about not only lifestyle change but also social and environmental changes.

Community health nurses work within the larger health care system and so probably are influenced to accept a narrow view of public health as activities addressing health problems that are unresolvable by the market model of health care or call for collective action at the community level. With the predicted changes in the health care system and increasing employment of nurses in the community setting, greater demands will be made on community health nursing to broaden its view of public health. As nurses leave the hospital setting, they bring to the community expertise in working with individuals and families as well as the mandate in the American Nurses Association's (ANA) Social Policy Statement to carry out prevention and health promotion. With the move into the community, then, comes a growing responsibility for community health nurses to claim their right to the full synthesis of nursing and public health practice and to increase their alliance with public health to promote and preserve the health of populations.

In this chapter, we establish a perspective of health from a community viewpoint. To do so requires definition of how people identify and describe the focus of health and related concepts. Four major ideas are explored:

- Definitions of health
- Definition and focus of public and community health
- What constitutes a preventive approach to health
- Definition and focus of public health and community health nursing

DEFINITIONS OF HEALTH
World Health Organization

In many disciplines, the definition of health is evolving. A trend to define health in social rather than medical terms is reflected in the World Health Organization's (WHO) classic definition of health (1947, p. 1) as "a state of complete physical, mental, and social well-being and not merely the absence of disease or infirmity."

Why define health in social terms? *Social* means "of or having to do with human beings living together as a group in a situation requiring that they have dealings with one another" (*Webster,* 1979, p. 1094). Social, then, refers to units of persons in communities who interact with each other. Social health is a result of positive interaction among groups within the community, such as sponsoring food banks in churches and civic organizations. Social health promotes community vitality, hence the need to define health in social terms. Social health is negatively affected by interaction that results in poverty, violence, and other problems stemming from lack of opportunity for groups within the community.

WHO has now expanded the definition of health to include a socialized conceptualization of health; thus, health is defined as follows:

The extent to which an individual or group is able, on the one hand, to realize aspirations and satisfy needs; and, on the other hand, to change or cope with the environment. Health is, therefore, seen as a resource for everyday life, not the objective of living; it is a positive concept emphasizing social and personal resources, as well as physical capacities.

(WHO, 1986, p. 73)

Public Health Nursing

Health has been defined as an "optimal level of functioning" by the client (Archer and Fleshman, 1979); "community competence" (Goeppinger et al., 1980); a "purposeful and integrated method of functioning within an environment" (Hall and Weaver, 1977); "fitness as a result of individual adaptation to stress" (Leahy et al., 1982); and "an orientation toward wellness focusing on the maintenance and promotion of the health of the entire population being served" (Stanhope and Lancaster, 1984). Although this variety of definitions illustrates that health is not easy to define, the major problem involves the unit of analysis. For these authors except Archer and Fleshman, Goeppinger and colleagues, and Lancaster, the unit of analysis is the individual, and the community is excluded. Many authors include the concepts of stress, adaptation, and environment in definitions of health. Environment is presented as a given to which one must adapt rather than as something that is changing, something that humans have affected and can affect, change, or modify in the future.

For many years, nurses have used Dunn's (1961) classic concept of wellness, in which family, community, society, and environment are interrelated and have an impact on health. Illness, health, and peak wellness are considered as being on a continuum; the goals are individual performance at a potential consistent with age and other factors and overall goals set for not only the individual but also the family, the community, and society. Health, then, is seen as a fluid and changing state. The state of health depends on the goals and potentials of individuals, families, communities, and societies within an environment affected by the performance of social units; its purpose is to enhance the potential development of such units.

Community

Social units achieve health in multiple, complex ways to meet the demands of rapidly changing conditions. For example, in a social unit of a couple, the elderly woman who has become the caretaker of her ill husband notes that she has less energy than when her husband first became bedfast; because caring for his incontinence takes so much of her energy, she now withholds a portion of his diuretic to conserve energy she needs to care for him in other ways.

Another example of a social unit is the Sierra Club, whose members lobby for preservation of natural resource lands, or a group of disabled persons who take over an office building to obtain equal access to not only public buildings but also education, jobs, and transportation.

Each of these social units is striving to realize a level of potential "health" beyond that of past states, which, in turn, will provide the impetus for future changes.

It is important for the community health nurse to recognize how the community defines its health, and definitions should be obtained from families, organizations, various groups, and other aggregates (subgroups) within the community.

Communities have a wide range of values. For some, protection of their economic interests is a primary factor in achieving health; for others, human needs and family closeness are primary factors. From the rich cultural diversity within a community, the community health nurse learns many different definitions and views of health.

DEFINITION AND FOCUS OF PUBLIC HEALTH AND COMMUNITY HEALTH

C. E. Winslow is known for his classic definition of public health:

Public health is the Science and Art of (1) preventing disease, (2) prolonging life, and (3) promoting health and efficiency through organized community effort for
(a) the sanitation of the environment,
(b) the control of communicable infections,
(c) the education of the individual in personal hygiene,
(d) the organization of medical and nursing services for the early diagnosis and preventive treatment of disease, and
(e) the development of the social machinery to ensure everyone a standard of living adequate for the maintenance of health, so organizing these benefits as to enable every citizen to realize his birthright of health and longevity

(HANLON, 1960, P. 23).

The key phrase in this definition of public health is "through organized community effort." The term *public health* connotes organized efforts made through governmental agencies such as health departments, which are authorized by legislation, serve all people, and are supported by taxes.

The newer term *community health* extends the realm of public health to include organized efforts for health at the community level through both government and private efforts, including private agencies supported by private funds, such as the American Heart Association. A mosaic of private and public structures serves community health efforts.

Public health efforts are aimed at prevention and promotion of the health of populations at federal, state, and local levels. Public health efforts at federal and state levels focus on providing supportive and advisory services to public health structures at the local level. Public health structures at the local level provide direct services to communities through two avenues:

- Community health services to protect the public from hazards such as polluted water or air, tainted food, or unsafe housing
- Personal health care services such as immunization, well-infant care, family planning services, or care for persons with sexually transmitted diseases

Personal health services are a part of public health efforts and are targeted to populations most at risk or most in need of services.

Public health efforts are multidisciplinary because they require people with many different skills. Community health nurses work with a diverse team of public health professionals, including epidemiologists, local health officers, and health educators. Special public health sciences are used to assess the needs of populations, and biostatistics provide a method of measuring characteristics and health indexes within a community.

PREVENTIVE APPROACH TO HEALTH

Health Promotion and Levels of Prevention

Health promotion and disease prevention are the focus of public health efforts. Health promotion activities enhance resources aimed at improving well-being, whereas disease prevention activities protect persons from disease and its consequences. There are three levels of prevention (Leavell and Clark, 1958) (Fig. 1–1 and Table 1–1):

Level 1.	**Primary Prevention Activities**
	Prevention of problems before they occur
	Example: Immunizations

Level 2.	**Secondary Prevention Activities**
	Early detection and intervention
	Example: Screening for sexually transmitted disease

Level 3.	**Tertiary Prevention Activities**
	Correction and prevention of deterioration of a disease state
	Example: Teaching insulin administration in the home

Figure 1–1
The three levels of prevention.

- Primary prevention activities prevent a problem before it occurs (e.g., immunizations to prevent disease);
- Secondary prevention activities provide early detection and intervention (e.g., screening for sexually transmitted diseases); and
- Tertiary prevention activities correct a disease state and prevent it from further deteriorating (e.g., teaching insulin administration in the home).

Unfortunately, society resists public funding of preventive health care measures. According to Beauchamp (1986), this resistance is due to a mistaken concept of individual responsibility for health, one that is modeled on the ethics of market justice, which gives people only what they are entitled to through their own efforts. Beauchamp called for an ethic of social justice, which emphasizes society's rather than the individual's responsibility for the protection of all human life to ensure that all persons have their basic needs met, such as adequate health protection and income. Market justice, claimed Beauchamp, ignores socially determined preconditions that strongly influence behavior, particularly those involving health.

The nature of the private sector, however, has been to vie for more of the health care dollar. The private sector has pulled money into the corporate health care world, which has tended to emphasize expensive equipment and supplies, buildings, and pharmaceuticals and to polarize the domains of prevention and cure. In fact, health services have little or nothing to do with health. Currently, needed resources and services such as education, housing, nutrition, clear air and water, and safe work places are not given financial support.

Prevention Versus Cure: Can We Afford One Over the Other?

The question is asked, "Can we continue to resist public funding of prevention?" In fact, spending money on cure (additional dollars for health care services) does not improve the health of a population, whereas spending money on prevention does. As stated by Lamarche (1995) and others (Evans et al., 1994), there is no convincing evidence that the amount of money expended for health care improves the health of a population. The real determinants of health are prevention efforts such as the provision of education, housing, food, a minimum decent income, and a safe social and physical environment. The large proportion of wealth—close to one seventh—spent on health care or "cure" for individuals by the United States may well divert money away from these needed resources and services that *do* determine our health (Evans and Stoddart, 1994; National Center for Health Statistics 1995). Yet the United States has lacked a commitment to achieve these important health outcomes for the poor, vulnerable, and uninsured populations. The common person has always known that "an ounce of prevention is worth a pound of cure." With a limited health work force and monetary resources, we can no

Table 1–1
Examples of Levels of Prevention and Clients Served in the Community

| Definition of Client Served* | Level of Prevention | | |
	Primary (Health Promotion and Specific Prevention)	Secondary (Early Diagnosis and Treatment)	Tertiary (Limitation of Disability and Rehabilitation)
Individual	Dietary teaching during pregnancy Immunizations	HIV testing Screening for cervical cancer	Teaching new client with diabetes how to administer insulin Exercise therapy after stroke Skin care for incontinent patient
Family (two or more individuals bound by kinship, law, or living arrangement and with common emotional ties and obligations [see Chapter 13])	Education regarding smoking, dental care, or nutritional counseling Adequate housing	Dental examinations Tuberculin testing for family at risk	Mental health counseling or referral for family in crisis (e.g., grieving, experiencing a divorce) Dietary instructions and monitoring for family with overweight members
Group or aggregate (interacting persons with a common purpose or purposes)	Birthing classes for pregnant teenage mothers AIDS and other sexually transmitted disease education for high school students	Vision screening of first grade class Mammography van for screening of women in a low-income neighborhood Hearing tests at a senior center	Group counseling for grade school children with asthma Swim therapy for physically disabled elders at a senior center Alcoholics Anonymous and other self-help groups Mental health services for military veterans
Community and populations (aggregate of people sharing space over time within a social system [see Chapter 5]; population groups or aggregates with power relations and common needs or purposes)	Fluoride water supplementation Environmental sanitation Removal of environmental hazards	Organized screening programs for communities, such as health fairs VDRL screening for marriage license applicants in a city Lead screening for children by school district	Shelter and relocation centers for fire or earthquake victims Emergency medical services Community mental health services for chronically mentally ill Home care services for chronically ill

HIV = human immunodeficiency virus; AIDS = acquired immunodeficiency syndrome; VDRL = Venereal Disease Research Laboratories.

*Note that terms are used differently in literature of various disciplines. There are no clear-cut definitions; for example, families may be referred to as an aggregate, and a population and subpopulations may exist within a community.

longer continue to spend "pounds" on health care services when the monies spent no longer improve health outcomes. For example, in industrialized countries, life expectancy at birth is not related to the level of expenditures for health care; in developing countries, longevity is closely related to the level of economic development and education of the population of a country (Lamarche, 1995).

Continuing overexpansion of health care could be detrimental to the health of a population by preventing a large proportion of the wealth of a country from investing in education and other development efforts

The concepts of prevention and population-focused care figure prominently in a conceptual orientation to nursing practice referred to as "thinking upstream." This orientation is derived from an analogy of patients falling into a river upstream and being rescued downstream by health providers overwhelmed with the struggle of responding to disease and illness. The river as an analogy for the natural history of illness was first coined by McKinlay (1979), with a charge to health providers to refocus their efforts toward preventive and "upstream" activities. In a description to the daily challenges of providers to address health from a preventive versus curative focus, McKinlay contrasts the consequences of illness (downstream endeavors) from its precursors (upstream endeavors). The author then charges health providers to critically examine the relative weight of their activities toward illness response versus the prevention of illness.

Butterfield (1990) adapted McKinlay's upstream analogy to nursing practice by examining preventive health efforts in nursing from a historical and theoretical perspective. In this context, a population-based perspective on health and health determinants is critical to understanding and formulating nursing actions to prevent the development of chronic disease. By examining the origins of disease, nurses identify social, political, environmental, and economic factors that often lead to poor health options for both individuals and populations. The call to refocus the efforts of nurses "upstream, where the real problems lie," (McKinlay, 1979) has been welcomed by community health nurses in a variety of practice settings. For these nurses, this theme provides affirmation of their daily efforts to prevent disease in populations at risk in schools, worksites, and clinics throughout their local communities and in the larger world. —P. Butterfield

There is a need for an ethic of social justice, for society's rather than the individual's responsibility for meeting the basic needs of all persons. There is a need for public funding of prevention to ensure the health of our population.

that do impact health. Managed care organizations focus on prevention and have begun to show that the rate of health care cost increases has begun to slow among employees of large firms receiving their services (Shine, 1995). Prevention programs for enrolled populations may make a difference in costs, but who will provide these services for the uninsured, the poor, and other vulnerable populations? In addition, who will provide education, housing, food, a minimum decent income, and a safe social and physical environment for these vulnerable populations? Reductions in health care spending would allow investments in adequate housing, jobs, nutrition, and safe work places and other environments to decrease the effects of economic disparities.

DEFINITION AND FOCUS OF PUBLIC AND COMMUNITY HEALTH NURSING

Public Health Nursing

Freeman (1963) provided a classic definition of public health nursing:

Public health nursing may be defined as a field of professional practice in nursing and in public health in which technical nursing, interpersonal, analytical, and organizational skills are applied to problems of health as they affect the community. These skills are applied in concert with those of other persons engaged in health care, through comprehensive nursing care of families and other groups and through measures for evaluation or control of threats to health, for health education of the public, and for mobilization of the public for health action. (p. 34)

Public health nursing is a synthesis of public health and nursing practice, as reflected in two contemporary definitions that provide similar yet distinctive ideologies, or visions of reality. The first definition is from the American Public Health Association (APHA) Ad Hoc Committee on Public Health Nursing (1981):

Public health nursing synthesizes the body of knowledge from the public health sciences and professional nursing theories for the purpose of improving the health of the entire community. This goal lies at the heart of primary prevention and health promotion and is the foundation for public health nursing practice. To accomplish this goal, public health nurses work with groups, families, and individuals as well as in multidisciplinary teams and programs. Identifying subgroups (aggregates) within the population which are at high risk of illness, disability, or premature death, and directing resources toward these groups, is the most effective approach for accomplishing the goal of [public health nursing]. Success in reducing the risks and in improving the health of the community depends on the involvement of consumers, especially groups experiencing health risks, and others in the community, in health planning, and in self-help activities. (p. 10)

The second definition is from the ANA (1980 p. 2):

Community health nursing is a synthesis of nursing practice and public health practice applied to promoting and preserving the health of populations. The practice is general and comprehensive. It is not limited to a particular age group or diagnosis and is continuing, not episodic. The dominant responsibility is to the population as a whole; nursing directed to individuals, families, or groups contributes to the health of the total population. Health promotion, health maintenance, health education and management, coordination, and continuity of care are utilized in a holistic approach to the management of the health care of individuals, families, and groups in a community.

A common theme of these definitions is the provision of nursing service to the community or population as a whole. Muecke (1984) noted that whereas the ANA definition focuses on care to individuals, families, and groups within a community, the APHA definition focuses on care to the community as a whole and considers the individual or family *only* when viewed as members of groups at risk. Both definitions are important for addressing the health of aggregates. Individual health and family health in the community are necessary building blocks to the health of populations, but they represent only one facet of health care provision at the aggregate level.

Historically, the public health nursing tradition, begun in the late 1800s by Lillian Wald and her associates, clearly portrays this important distinction (Wald, 1971) (see Chapter 2). After moving into the immigrant community to provide care to individuals and families, these nurses saw that the true determinants of health were not solely combated by bedside clinical nursing or even by teaching care of the sick to family members in the home. They saw that the social and environmental determinants of health—child labor, pollution, and poverty—had to be addressed through collective political activity aimed at improving the health of aggregates by improving social and environmental conditions. Organizing the community, establishing school nursing, and taking impoverished mothers to testify in Washington, D.C., were the types of activities engaged in by Wald and her colleagues that impacted the health of the community (Wald, 1971).

Today interventions with families and individuals in the community, although important, are incomplete unless they are extended to intervention at the aggregate level. Aggregate care encompasses care based on the ANA definition of community health nursing as well as care extended to aggregates identified by the APHA.

The distinction between actions based on the two definitions is made clearly by Muecke (1984) in an example involving provision of prenatal care to adolescents. According to Muecke, a nurse subscribing to the ANA definition would focus on each family in the case load and address the problem of low-birth-weight infants among this population through individual family assessment of nutritional factors, health education related to nutrition and fetal development, and referral to community resources for nutritional services.

The nurse who subscribes to the APHA definition would focus on characteristics of the community as a whole. The nurse would determine the proportion of teenagers in the community and rates of teenage pregnancy, intervene at the community level by assessing teenagers' sources of nutrition, and work politically to make nutritious foods available to teenagers in settings such as in food vending machines in schools. Alternatively, the nurse would lobby for nutritional supplements to be provided to low-income pregnant women in the community. Thus, aggregate care extends the concept of individual and family care to care of the population as a whole.

Community and Public Health Advanced Practice Nursing

The need for advanced skills in community and public health nursing is evidenced in the Association of Community Health Nursing Educators working document on the community and public health nursing practice in the community. New directions in community and public health nursing indicate that more than just direct care is needed. Today the need is aggregate- and population-focused care.

The following is from the working document of the Community/Public Health Advanced Practice Nurse (C/PHAPN) Position statement published in the *Association of Community Health Nursing Educators [ACHNE] Newsletter* (1995).

Community/public health advanced practice nursing (C/PHAPN) is the practice of nursing and public health to achieve specific health outcomes for the community. While additional advanced nursing specialties may deliver health care within communities, the definitions here refer to the community/public health advanced practice nurse.

C/PHAPN is one type of clinical nursing specialization. The generic term, clinical nurse specialist in community and public health, may be used to describe this specialty. C/PHAPN is provided by registered nurses with a minimum of a master's degree that includes content and practice in nursing and the public health sciences. The C/PHAPN nurse functions in administrative and clinical roles, with titles such as director, bureau chief, clinical specialist, consultant, and coordinator. C/PHAPN practice is focused on a community or a population. It includes promotion, maintenance, protection, and restoration of health and prevention of disease and disability of communities or aggregates, groups of individuals who share common characteristics (ACHNE, 1991).

The C/PHAPN nurse defines and implements the nursing aspects of the core public health functions of assessment, policy development, and assurance (Quad Council on Public Health/Community Health Nursing, 1993). These functions are based on an understanding of the community as the setting, the unit, and the target of practice (Sills & Goeppinger, 1985). C/PHAPN activities are performed in collaboration with generalist public and community health nurses, interdisciplinary professionals, community leaders, and consumers. Assessing needs for services and developing teams to address the needs are large components of C/PHAPN. Although care may be ultimately implemented at the individual and family levels, the impact is on the total community's health through community development, community empowerment, and policy formulation.

C/PHAPN is practiced within two major types of settings: (1) settings with a public health mandate to provide services to the entire community or a significant segment thereof and (2) settings that serve only a segment of the community (American Public Health Association [APHA] 1980). Within both settings, the C/PHAPN nurse, "in collaboration with other disciplines" (APHA, 1980) and with consumers, assesses the health needs of the population, identifies aggregates with specific health needs, and sets priorities for health services. Regardless of practice setting, C/PHAPN nurses endeavor to extend the scope of service to the population within the community who meet the program criteria but who are not actually receiving service (APHA, 1980).

Population-Focused Practice

Williams (1992) has stated that community health nurses must use a population-focused approach to move beyond the orientation of providing direct care to individuals and families. Although individuals and organizations may be responsible for a specific subpopulation in the community (e.g., a school may be responsible for its pregnant teenagers), population-focused practice ultimately is concerned with many community subpopulations, both distinct and overlapping. That is, population-focused community health nurses would not limit their interest to one or two subpopulations but rather would focus on the many subpopulations that make up the entire community. A population focus involves concern for those who do not receive health services as well as for those who do. A population focus also involves a scientific approach to community health nursing in that an assessment of the community or population is necessary and basic to planning, intervention, and evaluation at the individual, family, aggregate, and population levels.

We propose that the difference between the generalist and the specialist application of a population focus is that the generalist community health nurse with baccalaureate preparation is able to plan and intervene with individual groups, aggregates, and subpopulations, whereas the specialist community health nurse with graduate preparation is able to plan and intervene with multiple and overlapping subpopulations within the community (Fig. 1–2). Regardless of the level of practice, however, both generalist and specialist community health nurses must be aware of and use a population focus to aid in assessment, planning, intervention, and evaluation with larger units. A population focus also is needed to plan care required by groups of individuals and groups of families with needs that are not addressed within a community.

According to Williams (1992), a population focus bases assessment and management decisions on the status of a subpopulation. The subpopulation may be made up of a group of individuals (e.g., unmarried, pregnant teenagers), a group of families (e.g., families

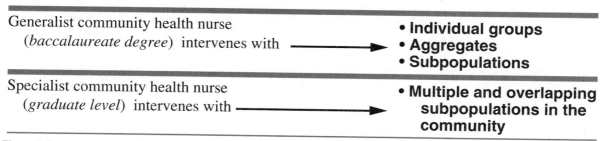

Figure 1–2
Differences in generalist and specialist applications of population focus.

with high-risk infants younger than 1 year), or a group of "groups" (e.g., children in several age groups or classes in a school).

A scientific approach to, or population focus on, community health nursing practice requires two types of data: (1) the epidemiology, or body of knowledge, of a particular problem and its solution, and (2) information about the community (Williams, 1984). Each type of knowledge as well as its source is presented in Table 1–2.

Data collection for assessment and management decisions should be ongoing, not episodic, within a community, to best determine the overall patterns of health in a population. Many of the data that are needed for surveillance of a community are gathered inadequately or are nonexistent (Miller et al., 1986).

Aggregate-Focused Practice

Community health nurses focus on the care of not only individuals but also aggregates in many settings, including homes, clinics, and schools. In addition to interviewing clients and assessing individual and family health, community health nurses must be able to assess an aggregate's health needs and resources, identify its values, work with the community to identify and implement programs that meet health needs, and evaluate the effectiveness of programs after their implementation. School nurses, for example, no

longer only run first aid stations but also are actively involved in assessing the needs of their population and in defining programs to meet those needs through activities such as health screening and group health education and promotion. Activities of school nurses may be as varied as designing health curricula with a school and community advisory group, leading support groups for elementary school children with chronic illness, and monitoring the health status of teenage mothers.

Similarly, occupational health nurses are no longer tied to an office or dispensary but are involved in monitoring records of workers' complaints resulting from excessive exposure to physical or chemical risks or in classes for workers with health-related problems such as alcoholism.

Community health nurses also are employed in private associations such as the American Diabetes Association, in which their organizational abilities as well as their health-related skills are used. Other community health nurses work with multidisciplinary groups of professionals, serve on boards of voluntary health associations such as the American Heart Association, are members of health planning agencies and councils, and form and work with nursing organizations directed at major public health problems, such as the Nurses' Environmental Health Watch. Education of nurses regarding environmental conditions and threats to the health of populations,

Table 1–2			
Data Required for Population Focus			
Body of Knowledge About Problem		**Information About the Community**	
Definition	Sources	Definition	Sources
Cause or etiology	Epidemiologic research	Demographic data	Demographics such as age, sex, and socioeconomic and racial distributions
Groups at high risk	Community health nursing research	Health status of the sub-populations	
Treatment methods	Clinical research in nursing and medicine	Services given to various subpopulations	Vital statistics such as mortality and morbidity
Effectiveness of treatment methods	Research in other fields	Measure of effectiveness of services	Annual reports of health care organizations
			Services provided by health planning agencies
			Computerized information systems for monitoring high-risk population

Data from Williams CA. Population-focused practice. *In* Stanhope M, Lancaster J (eds). Community Health Nursing: Process and Practice for Promoting Health. St. Louis: CV Mosby, 1984, p. 809.

such as nuclear armament, is carried out to involve nurses in collective activity aimed at improving environmental conditions at national, state, and local levels (McCarty and Pratt, 1986; Pope et al., 1995).

Community health nurses are also involved in the Public Health Nursing Section of the APHA and the Division of Community Health Nursing of the ANA and perform activities such as updating the definition and role of community health nursing. Community health nurses involved in state nurses associations perform activities such as promoting health-related legislation, promoting the use of safety infant car seats, and serving on state task forces that address health issues.

PUBLIC HEALTH NURSING AND MANAGED CARE

Shifts in reimbursement and the growth of managed care have revitalized the notion of population-based care. The foundation for managed care is the organization and management of health care for an enrolled group of individuals (Baker et al., 1994). This group of enrollees becomes the population of interest.

Most managed care players have become sophisticated in identifying key subgroups within the population of enrollees. An understanding of the enrolled populations and their health care patterns is essential to managing health care services and resources effectively. Thus, within managed care systems, subgroups are typically targeted according to characteristics associated with risk or expensive service use such as selected clinical conditions, functional status, and past patterns of service use (Baker et al., 1994).

Although comprehensive national health reform has not occurred, the dialogue about health care reform continues. Many experts believe that health care reform is occurring at the state level. The trend toward managed care is occurring in part because of market forces and cost-containment efforts (Mechanic, 1994). In many states, Medicaid populations are increasingly part of managed care plans. Nationally, about 50 million people are part of health maintenance organizations (HMOs), and the number of people enrolled in HMOs and other types of managed care arrangements continues to grow (Mechanic, 1994). A reformed health care system will include principles of managed care and a population-based approach to public health practice (Baker et al., 1994).

The purpose of public health is to improve the health of the public by promoting healthy lifestyles, preventing disease and injury, and protecting the health of communities (Berkowitz, 1995). In the past, shrinking public health resources have been increasingly applied to personal health services rather than to community health. In public health practice, the population of interest is the community itself. In managed care settings, the individuals belonging to the health care organization and specific groups of its clients may be viewed as the population served. As public health practice continues to focus on the public's health and the community, and as managed care focuses on service delivery, the personal health care system will be under increasing pressure to provide certain services previously provided by health departments. The most vulnerable and hard-to-reach populations (the groups traditionally served by public health) will pose tremendous challenges to managed care providers. It will be public health's responsibility to work as partners and assist managed care providers in providing service to these populations.

Nurses in community and public health have an opportunity to share their expertise regarding population-based approaches to health care services for groups of individuals across health care settings. Health care practitioners today require additional skills in assessment, policy development, and assurance to provide both public health practice at the community level and population based services. A Pew Health Professions Commission report (1994) identified key competencies that health care practitioners will need in the year 2005. Competencies pertinent to practitioners in managed care include promoting healthy lifestyles, providing preventive and primary care, expanding and ensuring access to cost-effective and technologically appropriate care, participating in coordinated and interdisciplinary care, and involving patients and families in the decision-making processes. Public health nurses must work in partnership with colleagues in managed care settings to improve the community's health. Information management, the role of the physical environment in health, cultural values, and improving health care systems may be addressed by partnerships. Partnerships may require complex negotiations in order for data to be shared across boundaries. New community assessment strategies may need to be developed to augment epidemiologic methods that often mask the context or meaning of the human experience of vulnerable populations.

Providing population-based care requires a dramatic shift in thinking from individual-based care. Some of the practical demands of population-based care as described by Hegyvary (1994) and Greenlick (1991) include (1) recognition that populations are not homogeneous (the needs of special subpopulations within populations must be addressed); (2) high-risk and vulnerable subpopulations need to be identified early in the care delivery cycle; (3) nonusers of services often become high-cost users (outreach strategies are essential); and (4) quality and cost of all health care services are linked across the health care continuum.

Health care reform provides rich opportunities for collaboration between service and academia (Barker et al., 1994). Health professional schools can take an active leadership role in the preparation of public health nurses for the 21st century and in shaping the values and directions of the health care system. If the reformed health care system is to enhance community health, all health professionals, including students, must be challenged to use new skills and knowledge in creating, monitoring, implementing, and evaluating systems of care from a population perspective. It is our hope that we are preparing students to manage the care of communities and preparing communities to effectively build and maintain healthy environments.

SUMMARY

Community health nurses have knowledge and skills that enable them to work in diverse community settings, ranging from the isolated rural area to the crowded urban ghetto. To meet the health needs of the population, the community health nurse must work with many individuals and groups within the community. A sensitivity to these groups and a respect for the community and its established method of managing its problems will enable the community health nurse to become more proficient in helping the community improve its health.

Learning Activities

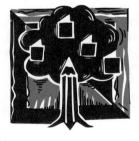

1. Interview several community health nurses and several clients regarding their definitions of health. Share the results with your classmates. Do you agree with their definitions? Why or why not?

2. Interview several community health nurses regarding their opinions on the focus of community health nursing. Do you agree?

3. Ask several neighbors or consumers of health care about their views of the role of public health and community health nursing. Share your results with your classmates.

REFERENCES

American Nurses Association. A Conceptual Model of Community Health Nursing (ANA Publication No. CH-10). Kansas City, MO, 1980.

American Public Health Association (APHA). The definition and role of public health nursing in the delivery of health care: A statement of the public health nursing section. Washington, DC. Author, 1980.

American Public Health Association, Ad Hoc Committee on Public Health Nursing. The definition and role of public health nursing practice in the delivery of health care. The Nation's Health, September, 1981.

Archer SE, Fleshman EP. Community Health Nursing Patterns and Practice, 2nd ed. North Scituate, MA, Duxbury Press, 1979.

Association of Community Health Nursing Educators (ACHNE). Essentials of Master's Level Nursing Education for Advanced Community Health Nursing Practice. Lexington, KY. Author, 1991.

Baker E, Melton R, Stange P, et al. Health reform and the health of the public. JAMA, 272:1276–1282, 1994.

Barker JB, Bayne T, Higgs ZR, et al. Community analysis: A collaborative practice project. Public Health Nurs, 11:113–118, 1994.

Beauchamp DE. Public health as social justice. In Mappes T, Zembaty J (eds). Biomedical Ethics, 2nd ed. New York, McGraw-Hill, pp. 585–593, 1986.

Berkowitz B. Health system reform: A blueprint for the future of public health. J Public Health Pract, 1:1–6, 1995.

Butterfield, PG. Thinking upstream: Nurturing a conceptual understanding of the societal context of health behavior. Adv Nurs Sci 12:1–8, 1990.

Community/Public Health Advanced Practice Nurse. Position statement. Assoc Community Health Nurs Educators (Newsletter) 13(2):3–5, 1995.

Dunn HL. High Level Wellness. Arlington, VA, R. W. Beatty, Ltd, 1961.

Evans RG, Baver ML, Marmor TR (eds). Why Are Some People Healthy and Others Not? The Determinants of Health of Populations. Hawthorne, NY, Aldine de Gruyter, 1994.

Evans RG, Stoddart GL. Providing health, consuming health care. In Evans RG, Baver ML, Marmor TR (eds). Why Are Some People Healthy and Others Not? The Determinants of Health of Populations. Hawthorne, NY, Aldine de Gruyter, pp. 27–64. 1994.

Freeman RB. Public Health Nursing Practice, 3rd ed. Philadelphia, WB Saunders, 1963.

Goeppinger J, Lassiter PG, Wilcox B. Community health is community competence. Nurs Outlook 30:464–467, 1980.

Greenlick M. Educating physicians for population-based clinical practice. JAMA 267:1645–1648, 1991.

Hall JE, Weaver BR. Distributive Nursing Practice: A Systems Approach to Community Health. Philadelphia, JB Lippincott, 1977.

Hanlon JJ. Principles of Public Health Administration, 3rd ed. St. Louis, CV Mosby, 1960.

Hegyvary S. The shift in focus from provider processes to population outcomes. Nurs Administration Q 17:viii–ix, 1994.

Lamarche PA. Our health paradigm in peril. Public Health Rep, 110:556–560, 1995.

Leahy KM, Cobb MM, Jones MC. Community Health Nursing, 4th ed. New York, McGraw-Hill, 1982.

Leavell HR, Clark EG. Preventive Medicine for the Doctor in His Community. New York, McGraw-Hill, 1958.

McCarty TL, Pratt MA. Nuclear freeze and disarmament: A mandate for community health nursing. Public Health Nurs 3:71–79, 1986.

McKinlay, JB. A case for refocusing upstream: The political economy of illness. *In* Jaco, EG (ed). Patients, Physicians, and Illness. 3rd ed. New York, The Free Press, pp. 9–25, 1979.

Mechanic D. Managed care: Rhetoric and realities. Inquiry, 31, 124–138, 1994.

Miller CA, Fine A, Adams-Taylor S, Schorr LB. Monitoring Children's Health: Key Indicators. Washington, DC, American Public Health Association Publications Department, 1986.

Muecke MA. Community health diagnosis in nursing. Public Health Nurs, 1:23–35, 1984.

National Center for Health Statistics. Health, United States, 1994. Hyattsville, MD, Public Health Service, 1995.

Pew Health Professions Commission. Current Issues in Health Professions: Education and Workforce Reform. University of California, San Francisco, 1994.

Pope AM, Snyder MA, Mood LH. (eds). Nursing Health and the Environment: Strengthening the Relationship to Improve the Public Health. Institute of Medicine. Washington, DC, National Academy Press, 1995.

Quad Council on Public Health/Community Health Nursing. Public health nursing in a revitalized health care agenda, 1993.

Shine KI. Informed joint decision-making. Public Health Rep 110:555, 1995.

Shortell SM, Gillies RR, Anderson DA, et al. Creating organized delivery systems: The barriers and facilitators. Hosp Health Service Administration 38:447–466, 1993.

Sills GM, Goeppinger J. The community as a field of inquiry in nursing. Annu Rev Nurs Res 3:3–24, 1985.

Stanhope M, Lancaster J (eds). Community Health Nursing: Process and Practice for Promoting Health. St. Louis, CV Mosby, 1984.

U.S. Department of Health and Human Services, Health Resources and Services Administration, Bureau of Health Professions, Division of Nursing. The Registered Nurse Population: Findings from the National Sample Survey of Registered Nurses, March, 1992. Rockville, MD, 1994. Author.

Wald LD. The House on Henry Street. New York, Dover Publications, 1971.

Webster N. Webster's Deluxe Unabridged Dictionary. New York, Simon & Shuster, 1979.

Williams CA. Population-focused practice. *In* Stanhope M, Lancaster J (eds). Community Health Nursing: Process and Practice for Promoting Health. St. Louis, CV Mosby, pp. 805–815, 1984.

Williams CA. Community-based population-focused practice: The foundation of specialization in public health nursing. *In* Stanhope M, Lancaster J (eds). Community Health Nursing: Process and Practice for Promoting Health, 3rd ed. St. Louis, CV Mosby, pp. 244–252, 1992.

World Health Organization. Chronicle of WHO 1:1–2, 1958.

World Health Organization. A discussion document on the concept and principles of health promotion. Health Promotion, 1:73–78, 1986.

Historical Factors: Community Health Nursing in Context

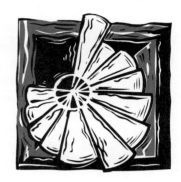

Upon completion of this chapter, the reader will be able to:

1. Describe the impact of the aggregate on the health of populations from the hunting and gathering stage to the present.

2. Trace approaches to the health of aggregates from prehistoric times to the present.

3. Analyze three historical events that have influenced a holistic approach to the health of populations.

4. Compare the application of the principles of public health to the nation's major health problems at the turn of the century (infectious disease) with that in the 1990s (chronic disease).

5. Describe two leaders in nursing who had a profound impact on addressing the health of aggregates.

6. Discuss two major contemporary issues facing community health nursing, and trace their historical roots to the present.

Janice M. Swanson

This chapter presents an overview of selected historical factors that influenced the evolution of community health nursing and help explain present-day challenges. Areas examined are (1) evolution of the state of health of Western populations from prehistoric to recent times; (2) the evolution of modern health care, including public health nursing; (3) consequences for the health of aggregates; and (4) challenges for community health nursing.

EVOLUTION OF THE STATE OF HEALTH OF WESTERN POPULATIONS

The study of the evolution of humankind has seldom taken into consideration the interrelationship of an individual's environment and health and the nature and size of the aggregate of which the individual is a member. Medical anthropologists use paleontological records and accounts of disease in primitive societies on which to base their speculations of the interrelationship among early humans, probable diseases, and environment (Armelagos and Dewey, 1978). Historians have also documented the existence since prehistoric times of public health activity (i.e., an organized community effort to prevent disease, prolong life, and promote health). The impact on the health of Western populations resulting from the aggregate and early public health efforts is presented.

Aggregate Impact on Health

Polgar (1964) defined five stages in the disease history of humankind: (1) hunting and gathering, (2) settled villages, (3) preindustrial cities, (4) industrial cities, and (5) the present (Fig. 2–1). In these stages, changes in cultural adaptation occurred as consequences of increased population, increased population density, and the ecological imbalance that results when humans tamper with their environment to accommodate group living. Human tampering, in turn, had a marked consequence on health. Although these stages often have been used to portray the evolution of civilization, it is important to note that they have limitations. First, the stages depict the evolution of Western civilization as chronicled from the perspective of the Western world. Second, the stages are not discrete historical time periods but instead overlap; the time periods often associated with the stages are widely debated in the field of anthropology. The stages do provide, however, a frame of reference to aid in determination of the

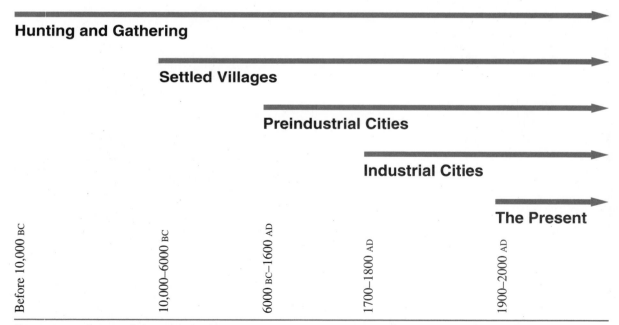

Stages overlap and time periods are widely debated in the field of anthropology. Some form of each stage remains evident in the world today.

Figure 2–1
Stages in the disease history of humankind.

relationship among humans, disease, and environment since before recorded history to the present day. Although the stages chronicle the initiation of each stage in the Western world, it is important to realize that each stage exists in civilization today. For example, Australian aborigines still hunt and gather food, and settled villages are common in many countries, especially third world countries.

Of importance to the community nurse is aware-ness that populations from each stage represent a great variety of persons who have distinct cultural traditions and a broad range of health care practices and beliefs. For example, a nurse in an American community may have to plan care for immigrants or refugees from a settled village or preindustrial city. It is important for nurses in the community to recognize not only the health risks faced by each aggregate but also the strengths and contributions made by the host culture and environment to the health status of each particular aggregate. Data from the Hispanic Health and Nutrition Examination Sur-vey (HHANES) (conducted from 1982 to 1984) show that perinatal outcomes among Mexican-born women worsen corresponding to the length of time lived in the United States (Guendelman et al., 1990). The "cultural orientation" of Mexico is accredited with protecting these mothers compared with United States–born mothers of Mexican descent, in whom the risk-associated behaviors of drinking and smok-ing increased. Similarly, the HHANES data showed that acculturation into U.S. society by Mexican-Americans, Puerto Ricans, and Cuban-Americans was associated with an increase in illicit drug use (Amaro et al., 1990). An increase in risk-associated behaviors was attributed to influences of the norms and practices of the dominant U.S. culture.

HUNTING AND GATHERING STAGE

During the Paleolithic period (Old Stone Age), nomadic and semi-nomadic people lived by hunting and gathering food. For 2 million years, small groups (aggregates) wandered in search of food. Armelagos and Dewey (1978) reviewed how the health of hunters and gatherers probably was affected by their size, density, and relationship to the environment. For example, a wide range of foods was eaten, which probably provided a diverse selection of nutrients. Hunters and gatherers are thought to have suffered from wounds and from diseases caused by parasites such as lice and pinworms; by insect bites (e.g.,

sleeping sickness and relapsing fever), and by the consumption of infected meat (e.g., trichinosis and tularemia). These people are thought to have had few contagious diseases because the scattered aggregates were not sufficiently large, were not stationary, and were not in contact with other aggregates often enough to sustain the diseases. The disposal of human feces and waste was not perceived of as a great problem because the people were nomadic; caves probably were abandoned as waste accumulated.

SETTLED VILLAGE STAGE

Small settlements are characteristic of the Mesolithic (Middle Stone Age) and Neolithic (New Stone Age) periods. As wandering peoples became sedentary, small encampments and villages were formed. The concentration of people in small areas brought differ-ent kinds of problems. For example, the domestication of animals led to living close to herds, which probably transmitted diseases such as salmonella, anthrax, Q fever, and tuberculosis (Polgar, 1964). The domesti-cation of plants probably reduced the range of nutrients compared with that available from gathering days and may have led to diseases of deficiency. Water had to be secured, and wastes had to be disposed of. With the evolution of the agricultural societies, other diseases probably appeared; scrub typhus, for ex-ample, increases with cultivation of new ground, and malaria appears with the creation of new mosquito breeding areas. With irrigation, schistosomiasis in-creases; medical anthropologists have found refer-ences to such a parasite in ancient Chinese and Mesopotamian literature (Brothwell, 1978).

PREINDUSTRIAL CITIES STAGE

With expanding populations, large urban centers formed in preindustrial times. Preexisting problems increased with even larger populations living in small areas. For example, food and water had to be supplied to a larger population, and greater amounts of waste products had to be removed. Elaborate water systems were developed in some cultures. For example, in Mexico City, the Aztec king Ahuitzutl had a stone pipeline built to transport spring water to the inhab-itants (Duran, 1964). However, removal of wastes via the water supply led to diseases such as cholera. With the development of towns, rodent infestation increased and facilitated the spread of plague. Because more people had more frequent contact with each other, the transmission of disease by contact increased, and endemics occurred, such as mumps, measles, influenza, and smallpox (Polgar, 1964). A population must reach a certain size for it to maintain a disease in endemic proportions; for example, approximately 1 million persons are needed to sustain measles at an endemic level (Cockburn, 1967). Different forms of disease also appeared. Syphilis, originally a nonvenereal disease, became a venereal disease because of changes in population density, the family, and sexuality (Hudson, 1965). This and other diseases were carried to other countries by explorers. Occupational threats to health resulted from handling of poisons in mining and metal processing, handling of pottery glazes, and using poisons directly in fishing and hunting (Brothwell, 1978).

INDUSTRIAL CITIES STAGE

With industrialization, urban areas became more dense and heavily populated, and the slum areas expanded. Increased industrial wastes, increased air and water pollution, and harsh working conditions took their toll on health. For example, there was an increase in respiratory diseases such as tuberculosis, pneumonia, and bronchitis; common during the 18th and 19th centuries were epidemics of infectious diseases such as diphtheria, smallpox, typhoid fever, typhus, measles, malaria, and yellow fever (Armelagos and Dewey, 1978). Enactment of imperialism spread epidemics to populations that had no immunity.

DISEASE DEFINITIONS

Endemic: Diseases that are always present in a population. (Examples: colds, pneumonia)
Epidemic: Diseases that are not always present in a population but flare up on occasion. (Examples: diphtheria, malaria)
Pandemic: The existence of disease in a large proportion of the population. (Example: outbreaks of annual influenza type A)

PRESENT STAGE

Although infectious diseases no longer account for a majority of mortalities in the Western world, they remain prevalent in the West among low-income populations and in some racial and ethnic groups and account for many mortalities in the non-Western world. Diseases characteristic of Western populations are almost unknown in traditional communities and appear with adaptation to Western customs (Burkitt,

1978). These diseases include large bowel diseases such as cancer, diverticulitis, and ulcerative colitis; venous disorders, including varicose veins, thrombosis, pulmonary embolism, and hemorrhoids; heart disease; obesity; diabetes; and gallstones. These diseases occurred infrequently in the Western world until the past 100 years and have increased significantly during the past 50 years. Changes from traditional patterns of life to urban environments appear to be associated with the appearance of these diseases. Epidemiological studies suggest that common factors are changes in diet, especially increases in refined sugar and fats, and lack of fiber; environmental and occupational hazards are also increasingly being identified. An increase in population and density of population also increases mental and behavioral disorders (Garn, 1963).

As wandering, hunting, and gathering aggregates became sedentary and grew into large populations, the disease patterns as well as demands on environment changed. Humans fit reasonably well into the natural world but have had to adapt to an overpopulated, largely urban existence with marked consequences for health (i.e., mortalities that have changed in nature from infectious to chronic). Public health efforts traditionally have been viewed as 18th- and 19th-century activities associated with the Sanitary Revolution. Historians have shown, however, that organized community efforts toward preventing disease, prolonging life, and promoting health have also occurred since prehistoric times.

Evolution of Early Public Health Efforts

Public health efforts have evolved slowly over time. The evolution of organized public health efforts is traced briefly here, highlighting the periods of (1) prehistoric times (before 5000 BC); (2) classical times (3000 to 200 BC); (3) Middle Ages (500 to 1500 AD); (4) Renaissance (15th, 16th, and 17th centuries); (5) 18th century; and (6) 19th century. It is important to note, however, that, as with the disease history of humankind, public health efforts exist in various stages of development throughout the world. A brief history encapsulates organized public health efforts as viewed by the Western world.

PREHISTORIC TIMES

Early nomadic humans became domesticated and tended to live in ever larger groups. Episodes of life, health, sickness, and death are inevitably shared by members of aggregates ranging from family to community. Health practices, whether based on superstition or sanitation, evolved as a way for many aggregates to ensure survival. For example, from earliest records, it has been documented that primitive societies have used elements of psychosomatic medicine (e.g., voodoo), isolation (e.g., banishment), and fumigation (e.g., smoke) to manage disease and thus protect the community (Hanlon and Pickett, 1984).

CLASSICAL TIMES

As early as 3000 to 1400 BC, the Minoans devised ways to flush water and construct drainage systems. Circa 1000 BC, the Egyptians constructed elaborate drainage systems, developed pharmaceutical preparations, and embalmed the dead. Pollution has long been a problem; in *Exodus,* it was reported that "all the waters that were in the river stank," and *Leviticus* contains the first written hygiene code, formulated by the Hebrews, which dealt with laws governing both personal and community hygiene, such as contagion, disinfection, and sanitation through the protection of water and food.

Greece. Greek literature contains accounts of communicable diseases such as diphtheria, mumps, and malaria (Rosen, 1958). The Hippocratic book *Airs, Waters and Places,* a treatise on the balance between humans and their environment, is said to have been the only such volume on this topic until the development of bacteriology in the late 19th century (Rosen, 1958). Diseases that were always present in a population, such as colds and pneumonia, were called *endemic.* Those that were not always present but flared up on occasion, such as diphtheria and malaria, were called *epidemic.* Another important distinction made by the Greeks was their emphasis on the preservation of health, as personified by the goddess Hygeia, or good living, as well as on curative medicine, as personified by the goddess Panacea. Life had to be in balance with the demands of environment, and the importance of factors such as exercise, rest, and nutrition was weighed according to factors such as age, sex, constitution, and climate (Rosen, 1958). However, only the aristocracy could afford to be concerned with maintaining a healthful lifestyle, and the masses, in particular, the slaves who supported the economy, could not afford to maintain "health" (Rosen, 1958).

Rome. The Romans readily adopted Greek culture but far surpassed the Greeks in engineering ability, as evidenced by massive aqueducts, bathhouses, and sewer systems. For example, records show that at the height of the rule of the Roman Empire, Rome provided 40 gallons of water per person per day to its 1 million inhabitants, which is comparable with modern rates of consumption (Rosen, 1958). Inhabitants of the overcrowded Roman slums, however, did not share in such public health amenities as sewer systems and latrines.

The Romans also made mention of occupational health, in particular referring to the pallor of the miners, the danger of suffocation, and "vitriolic fumes" (Rosen, 1958, p. 46). Safeguards were devised and used by the miners in the form of bags, sacks, and masks made of membranes and bladder skins.

Priests dispensed medicine in the early years of the Roman Republic; Greek physicians migrated to Rome. Medical care benefited the aristocracy rather than the poor, who used folk medicine. Public physicians were appointed to towns and were paid to care for the poor. In addition, they were allowed to charge a fee for service to those patients who could pay. As a prototype of a health maintenance organization or group practice, several families paid a set fee for yearly services. Hospitals, surgeries, and infirmaries (for slaves) as well as nursing home–type structures appeared. A hospital for the sick poor was established by Fabiola, a Christian woman who lived in the fourth century; this model was repeated throughout medieval times.

ROMANS PROVIDED PUBLIC HEALTH SERVICES

The Romans provided public health services that included the following (Rosen, 1958):

- A water board to maintain the aqueducts
- A supervisor of the public baths
- Street cleaners
- Supervision of the sale of food

MIDDLE AGES

The decline of Rome, circa 500 AD, led to the Middle Ages, during which magic and religion were applied to health problems. Collective activity on behalf of health occurred largely through the monasteries. Measures to protect the public were reflected in reports of wells and fountains, street cleaning, and disposal of refuse. Communicable diseases occurred and included measles, smallpox, diphtheria, leprosy, and bubonic plague. Physicians had little to offer, and the management of leprosy, in particular, was taken over by the church, which used hygienic codes from *Leviticus* and established isolation and leper houses, or leprosaria (Rosen, 1958). Response to the plague (Black Death) of the 14th century, which claimed close to half the world's population at that time, led to the establishment of public health practices, such as quarantine of ships, isolation, and disinfection, that are still carried out today (Hanlon and Pickett, 1984). Ships without crews were reported drifting about the Mediterranean Sea, infecting ports with which they came into contact. *Pandemic* (the existence of disease in a large proportion of the population) waves of plague and other communicable diseases swept over Europe well into the 18th century. Although bubonic plague ravaged the population and quarantine was used to protect people, the role of fleas and rodents in its existence was not known for centuries.

HUMAN PLAGUE CASE DOCUMENTED IN THE UNITED STATES

The human plague is endemic and, on occasion, epidemic in Africa, Asia, and South America. There were reports of 770 cases from 11 countries in 1989. A low frequency of human plague occurs in the United States owing to the usual control of plague in most parts of the world and the immunization of persons at high risk (e.g., military personnel and Peace Corps volunteers). A recorded case of plague in the United States occurred in Washington, D.C., in 1990, in a 47-year-old mammologist from the United States who had been collecting small rats for study in La Paz, Bolivia. She had not received a booster immunization for plague since 1971 (Wolfe et al., 1990).

During the Middle Ages, physicians usually were clergymen and treated mostly kings and noblemen. Hospitals were largely small houses in which nursing care was provided by monks and nuns. Hygiene was written about in medieval tracts and addressed such topics as housing, diet, personal cleanliness, and sleep (Rosen, 1958).

THE RENAISSANCE

The Renaissance began in the 14th and 15th centuries and marked an era of expanding trade, population growth, and migration. Interest in human dignity,

human rights, and scientific truth was awakening, as seen in discourses by Galileo, Spinoza, and Descartes.

LIFE IN AN ENGLISH HOUSEHOLD IN THE 16TH CENTURY

The way life was lived in the 16th century as described in the following account by Erasmus must have affected health; such accounts continued to appear in the literature into the 19th century (Hanlon and Pickett, 1984, p. 26):

As to floors, they are usually made with clay, covered with rushes that grow in the fens and which are so seldom removed that the lower parts remain sometimes for twenty years and has in it a collection of spittle, vomit, urine of dogs and humans, beer, scraps of fish and other filthiness not to be named.

The cause of infectious disease was yet to be discovered. Two events important to public health occurred during this time. In 1546, Girolamo Fracastoro presented a theory of infection as a cause and epidemic a consequence of "seeds of disease." In 1676, Anton van Leeuwenhoek described microscopic organisms but did not associate them with disease (Rosen, 1958).

Measures taken to deal with poverty resulted in the Elizabethan Poor Law, which was enacted in England in 1601 and put the responsibility of providing relief for the poor upon the parishes. This law governed care for the poor for more than two centuries and served as a prototype for later U.S. laws.

18TH CENTURY

Great Britain. The 18th century was marked by imperialism and industrialization. Sanitary conditions remained a great problem:

The roads around London were neither very attractive nor very safe. The land adjoining them was watered with drains and thickly sprinkled by laystalls and refuse heaps. Hogs were kept in large numbers on the outskirts and fed on the garbage of the town . . . . In 1706 it was said of the highways, though they are mended every summer, yet everybody knows that for a mile or two about this City, the same and the ditches hard by are commonly so full of nastiness and stinking dirt, that oftentimes many persons who have occasion to go in or come out of town, are forced to stop their noses to avoid the ill-smell occasioned by it.

(GEORGE, 1925, CITED IN HANLON AND PICKETT, 1984, P. 27.)

During the Industrial Revolution, in which a gradual change in production occurred, lives were sacrificed for profit, particularly those of poor children, who were forced into labor. The parishes, which were responsible for providing relief for the poor under the Elizabethan Poor Law, established workhouses to employ the poor. Orphaned and poor children, who were wards of the parishes, were placed in parish workhouses, where they were forced to labor for long hours at an early age (George, 1925). Those apprenticed to chimney sweeps were reported to suffer the worst fate; they were forced into chimneys at the risk of being burned and suffocated and made to beg and steal. At 12 to 14 years of age, children were apprenticed to a master, a worse fate for most, as stated by a writer on the Poor Laws in 1738:

The master may be a tiger in cruelty, he may beat, abuse, strip naked, starve, or do what he will with the innocent lad, few people take much notice, and the officers who put him out the least of anybody.

(HANLON AND PICKETT, 1984, P. 24.)

A major discovery of the times was inoculation. In 1796, Edward Jenner observed that persons who worked around cattle were less likely to have smallpox. He discovered that immunity to smallpox resulted from inoculation with cowpox virus. Jenner's contribution was significant because, during the 18th century, approximately 95% of the population suffered from smallpox, as evidenced by a pocked face, and approximately 10% of the population died of it.

Although liberal views of human nature were being expounded by men such as Hume, Voltaire, and Rousseau in Europe and Adams, Jefferson, and Franklin in America, public health reforms culminating in the Sanitary Revolution were beginning to take place throughout Europe and especially in England. The study of community health problems using the survey method, which dates from Hippocrates, was further developed in the 18th century (Rosen, 1958). Geographic factors related to health and the diseases by region were mapped as "medical topographies." A health education movement provided books and pamphlets on health to the middle and upper classes; it was said to neglect "economic factors" and did not concern the working classes (Rosen, 1958).

19TH CENTURY

Communicable diseases ravaged the population who lived in unsanitary conditions. Each year in the mid-1800s, typhus and typhoid fever claimed twice as many lives as did the battle of Waterloo (Hanlon and Pickett, 1984).

Edwin Chadwick called attention to the cost of the unsanitary conditions, which shortened the life span of the laboring class in particular, from whence came the wealth of the nation. The first sanitary legislation was passed in 1837, establishing a National Vaccination Board. However, in 1842, according to Chadwick, death rates were high in large industrial cities such as Liverpool; more than half of all children of working class parents died by 5 years of age. Laborers lived an average of 16 years compared with 22 years for tradesmen and 36 for the upper classes (Richardson, 1887). In 1842, Chadwick published his famous *Report on an Inquiry into the Sanitary Conditions of the Laboring Population of Great Britain.* One consequence of the report was the establishment of the General Board of Health for England in 1848. Legislation for social reform followed and was concerned with child welfare, care of elders, the sick, mentally ill, factory management, and education. The appearance of a water supply, sewers, fireplugs, and sidewalks marked the new changes.

PUBLIC HEALTH INTERVENTIONS USED IN THE THIRD WORLD NEEDED IN THE UNITED STATES

In 1991, a conference sponsored by the National Council on International Health and public health organizations in San Francisco, California, urged public health professionals to consider using technology from the third world to handle third world health conditions that exist in the United States. For example, each year in the United States about 500 infants die of dehydration, a common problem in the third world, and about 200,000 are hospitalized for this condition, at a cost of approximately $500 million per year. Use of a United Nations Children's Fund device to help parents treat dehydration was recommended. The device is a block of wood into which are bored wells that hold the appropriate amounts of sugar and salt to be mixed with water to create a solution to rehydrate the baby. In addition, the conference recommended that funds be shifted from high-technology interventions to hiring more public health nurses to work in needy communities to introduce methods of care that are inexpensive.

Data from State Studies Third World Solutions. (1991). Nurseweek, Northern California Edition, March 18, p. 5.

Social action—bettering the lives of the people through improving economic, social, and environmental conditions—to attack the root social causes of disease was argued for in 1849 by Rudolf Virchow, a pathologist. He proposed "a theory of epidemic disease as a manifestation of social and cultural maladjustment" (Rosen, 1958, p. 86). He further argued that the health of the people was the responsibility of the public, that health and disease were heavily affected by social and economic conditions, that efforts to promote health and fight disease must be social and economic as well as medical, and that the social and economic determinants of health and disease must be studied to yield knowledge to guide appropriate action. These principles were best embodied in a draft for a public health law to the Berlin Society of Physicians and Surgeons in 1849 by Neumann (Rosen, 1958 p. 225):

According to this document, public health has as its objectives (1) the healthy mental and physical development of the citizen; (2) the prevention of all dangers to health; and (3) the control of disease. Public health must care for society as a whole by considering the general physical and social conditions that may adversely affect health, such as soil, industry, food, and housing, and it must protect each individual by considering those conditions that prevent him from caring for his health.

"Conditions" may be considered to be in one of two major categories: conditions in which the individual has the right to request assistance from the state (e.g., poverty and infirmity) and conditions in which the state has the right and the obligation to interfere with the personal liberty of the individual (e.g., transmissible diseases and mental illness).

In 1854, John Snow, an English physician, anesthetist, and epidemiologist, made another major contribution. By removing the pump handle to a well that served as a water resource to a large population afflicted with cholera and by keeping track of the decreasing number of new cases, he demonstrated that cholera was transmissible (Rosen, 1958).

United States. In the United States during the 19th century, waves of epidemics continued and included yellow fever, smallpox, cholera, typhoid fever, and typhus. As cities grew, the poor crowded into inadequate housing with unsanitary conditions, causing deadly illness. Lemuel Shattuck, a Boston bookseller and publisher with a keen interest in public health and welfare, organized the American Statistical Society in 1839 and issued a *Census of Boston* in 1845. The census showed high overall mortality rates and very high infant and maternal mortality rates. Living conditions of the poor were inadequate, and communicable diseases were widely prevalent (Rosen, 1958). Shattuck's 1850 *Report of the Massachusetts Sanitary Commission* outlined the findings and recommended modern public health reforms that included keeping vital statistics and providing environmental, food, drug, and communicable disease control information. Well-infant and well-child care, school-age child health, vaccination, mental health, health education, and planning were called for. However, the report fell on deaf ears; the recommendation, for example, for a state board of health was not implemented until 19 years later. The newly formed American Medical Association (1847) was asked by the National Institute, a Washington, D.C., scientific organization, to form a committee to uniformly collect vital statistics, which it began in 1848.

The evolution of early public health efforts was making some progress in the mid-19th century in terms of administrative efforts, initial legislation, and debate regarding the determinants and thus approaches to health, whether social, economic, or medical. The advent of what we call "modern" health care occurred about this time, to which nursing made a large contribution. Discussed are the areas of the evolution of modern nursing, the evolution of modern medical care and public health practice, the evolution of the community caregiver, and the establishment of public health nursing.

ADVENT OF MODERN HEALTH CARE

Evolution of Modern Nursing

During the mid-19th century, Florence Nightingale, the woman credited with establishing "modern nursing," began her work. Florence Nightingale is usually remembered by historians for her contributions to the health of British soldiers during the Crimean War and the establishment of nursing education. Her remarkable use of public health principles and distinguished scientific contributions to health care reforms have gone unrecognized with few exceptions (Cohen, 1984; Grier and Grier, 1978). This review of Nightingale's work emphasizes her concern for environmental determinants of health; her focus on the aggregate of British soldiers through emphasis on sanitation, community assessment, and analysis; the development of the use of graphically depicted statistics; and the gathering of comparable census data and political advocacy on behalf of the aggregate.

Nightingale was from an established English family and was well educated. Her father tutored her in many subjects, including mathematics. She later studied with and was profoundly influenced by Adolphe Quetelet, a Belgian statistician, from whom she learned the discipline of social inquiry (Goodnow, 1933). She also had a passion for hygiene and health. A proper Englishwoman, she traveled extensively and was allowed finally in 1851 at the age of 31 years to enter a period of training in nursing at Kaiserswerth Hospital in Germany with Pastor Fliedner. She also studied the organization and discipline of the Sisters of Charity in Paris. She wrote extensively and published her analyses of the many nursing systems she studied in France, Austria, Italy, and Germany (Dock and Stewart, 1925).

In 1854, Nightingale responded to the outbreak of the Crimean War by going to Scutari, which at the time was part of the Ottoman Empire but later became part of Albania, with 40 nurses, Roman Catholic and Anglican sisters, and lay nurses in response to distressing accounts of the lack of care for wounded soldiers. She was sponsored by government officials but not officially backed by the army. Her greatest achievement was the overthrow of the British army management method, which had created a horror of horrors and allowed conditions that produced extraordinarily high death rates to persist. Scathing letters of criticism accompanied by constructive recommendations were sent to Secretary of War Sidney Herbert.

Nightingale faced an assignment in The Barrack Hospital, which had been built for 1700 patients. She found 3000 to 4000 patients in 4 miles of beds only 18 inches apart (Goodnow, 1933, pp. 55–56).

The beds were mostly of straw, and many were laid directly on the floor. The few sheets to be had were of canvas, and so rough that the men begged not to have them used. Practically no laundry was being done; there was no hospital clothing, and the patients were still in their uniforms, stiff with blood and covered with filth. There was no soap, no towels, nor basins, very few utensils of any sort. Every place swarmed with vermin. Men ate half-cooked food with their fingers as utensils did not exist.

Cholera and "contagious fever" were rampant. As many men died from the diseases as they did from battlefield injuries (Cohen, 1984). Nightingale found that supplies had been allocated but were tied up owing to bureaucratic red tape. For example, supplies were "sent to the wrong ports or were buried under munitions and could not be got" (Goodnow, 1933, p. 86).

Problems were caused by having to work through eight departments of the army concerned with military affairs related to her assignment. For example, Nightingale sent to London reports of the conditions of the buildings. "A committee had been appointed to investigate the buildings. Miss Nightingale had them repaired before the committee's report was even in" (Goodnow, 1933, p. 87). Nightingale immediately set up a laundry and diet kitchens and provided food, clothing, dressings, and equipment for a laboratory with government money and donated funds given her (Dock and Stewart, 1925). Her nurses provided care only to patients of sympathetic physicians.

Major reforms occurred during the first 2 months. Aware of the emerging interest in keeping social statistics, Nightingale realized that her most forceful argument would be statistical in nature. She reorganized the inept methods of keeping statistics. Through the use of careful never-before-used Coxcomb graphs of wedges, circles, and squares, shaded and in varying colors, she illustrated the preventable deaths of soldiers in the hospitals during the Crimean War versus the average annual mortality in Manchester and of soldiers in military hospitals in and near London at the time (Fig. 2–2). She also showed through her reforms that, by the end of the war, the death rate among ill soldiers during the Crimean War was no higher than that among well soldiers in Britain (Cohen, 1984). Keeping careful statistics, she showed that the death rate for those treated decreased from 42 to 2%. She then established community services and activities to improve the quality of life of the soldiers; these included rest and recreation facilities, a savings fund, an opportunity for study, and a post office. She also organized care for the families of the soldiers (Dock and Stewart, 1925).

Returning to London at the close of the war in 1856 and ill herself, she devoted her efforts to making compelling arguments on behalf of sanitary reform; this probably was her greatest contribution. However, she showed no interest in the emerging germ theory of disease (Cohen, 1984). At home, she surmised that if the sanitary neglect of the army of soldiers existed in the battle area, it probably existed at home in London

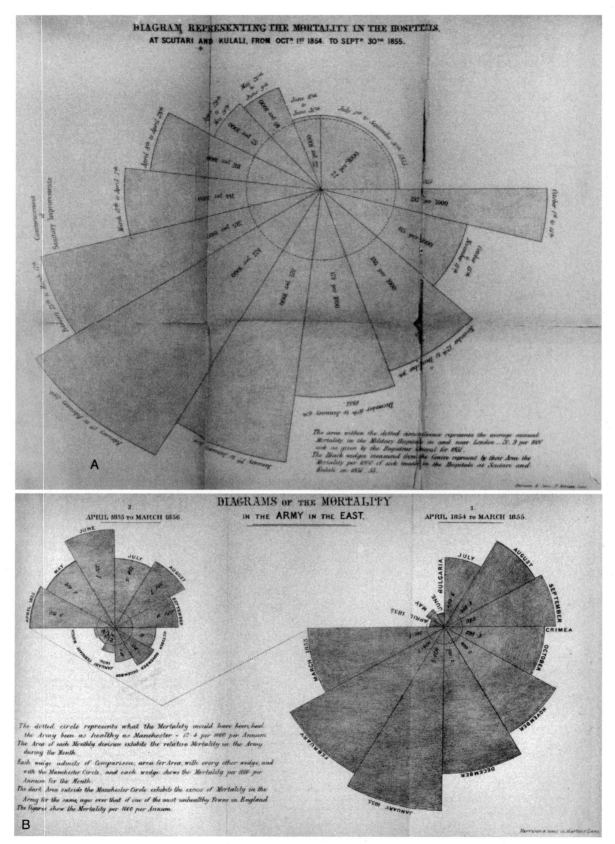

Figure 2–2
A and *B,* Coxcomb charts by Florence Nightingale from her publication *Notes on Matters Affecting the Health, Efficiency and Hospitalization of the British Army.* London, Harrison and Sons, 1858. These photographs of the large, fold-out charts are from an original preserved at the University of Chicago Library (public domain; courtesy of University of Chicago Library).

as well. She prepared statistical tables that backed up her suspicions (Table 2–1).

In one study comparing the mortality of men aged 25 to 35 years in the army barracks in England with that of men the same age in civilian life, Nightingale found the mortality of the soldiers to be nearly twice that of the civilians. In one of her reports, she stated that she believed it was as criminal to allow the young soldier to die needlessly from unsanitary conditions as to take him out, line him up, and shoot him (Kopf, 1978). "Our soldiers enlist to death in the barracks," she reiterated (Kopf, 1978, p. 95). She was not content to keep her community assessment and analysis to herself and was very political; from her sick bed, she distributed her reports to army medical and commanding officers and to members of Parliament (Kopf, 1978). Her reports were challenged by prominent male leaders

of the time; undaunted, she rewrote them in greater depth and redistributed them.

Through her earlier comparative work of hospital systems in European countries, she showed that data kept from each hospital were not comparable and that the names and classification of diseases varied among hospitals. This difference prevented collection of similar statistics from larger geographical areas that would create a health-illness profile of a region and allow comparison with other regions. She printed common statistical forms that were adopted by some hospitals in London experimentally. A study of the tabulated results revealed the promise of this strategy (Kopf, 1978).

Her development and application of statistical procedures continued, and recognition was won. She was elected a fellow by the Royal Statistical Society in 1858; in 1874, she was made an honorary

Table 2–1
Nightingale's Crimean War Mortality Statistics: Nursing Research That Made a Difference

Year	Deaths That Would Have Occurred in Healthy Districts Among Males of the Soldiers' Ages*	Actual Deaths of Noncommissioned Officers and Men	Excess of Deaths Among Noncommissioned Officers and Men
1839	763	2,914	2,151
1840	829	3,300	2,471
1841	857	4,167	3,310
1842	888	5,052	4,164
1843	914	5,270	4,356
1844	920	3,867	2,947
1845	911	4,587	3,676
1846	930	5,125	4,195
1847	981	4,232	3,251
1848	987	3,213	2,226
1849	954	4,052	3,098
1850	919	3,119	2,200
1851	901	2,729	1,828
1852	915	3,120	2,205
1853	920	3,392	2,472
Total	13,589	58,139	44,550

Number of deaths of noncommissioned officers and men shows also the number of deaths that would have occurred if the mortality were 7.7 per 1000, such as it was among Englishmen of the soldiers' age in healthy districts, in the years 1849 to 1853, which fairly represent the average mortality.

*The exact mortality in the healthy districts is 0.0077122, the logarithm of which (3.8871801) has been used in making this calculation.

From Grier B, Grier M: Contributions of the passionate statistician. Res Nurs Health 1:103–109, 1978. Copyright © 1978 by John Wiley & Sons, Inc. Reprinted by permission of John Wiley & Sons, Inc.

member of the American Statistical Association (Kopf, 1978).

NIGHTINGALE USED STATISTICAL METHODS IN COMMUNITY ASSESSMENT

An example of Nightingale's application of her statistical method to the health needs of the community is related to Southeastern Railway's plans to remove St. Thomas' Hospital to increase the railway's right-of-way between London Bridge and Charing Cross. Nightingale conducted a *community assessment,* plotting the cases served by the hospital, analyzing the proportion by distance, and calculating the probable impact on the community should the hospital be relocated to the proposed sites. In her view, hospitals were but a part of the wider community that together served the needs of humanity. This means of health planning, matching resources to the needs of the population, was visionary and, as noted by Kopf (1978), was not reapplied until the 20th century.

In 1861, Nightingale prevailed on the census officials to add two areas to census taking, as had been done earlier in Ireland: the number of sick and infirm in the population and data depicting the housing of the population (Kopf, 1978, p. 98). She stated the following:

The connection between the *health* and the *dwellings* of the population is one of the most important that exists. The "diseases" can be approximated also. In all the more important—such as smallpox, fevers, measles, heart disease, etc., all those which affect the *national* health, there will be very little error. Where there *is* error, in these things, the error is uniform . . . and corrects itself.

Although they were not adopted, Nightingale's suggestions were, again, visionary. According to Kopf (1978), only a few countries currently gather census data on sickness and housing.

Another of her concerns dealt with the need to make use of statistics at the administrative and political levels to direct health policy. Noting the ignorance of politicians and those who set policy regarding the interpretation and use of statistics, she stressed the need to teach national leaders to use statistical facts.

In addition to her contributions to nursing and the development of nursing education, Nightingale has been credited with using statistics to replace the individual case method to provide a grasp of the total

environmental situation (Kopf, 1978). An often-neglected contribution, it has marked implications for the development of public health and, later, public health nursing. Grier and Grier (1978) said of Nightingale's contributions to statistics, "Her name occurs in the index of many texts on the history of probability and statistics . . . in the history of quantitative graphics . . . and in texts on the history of science and mathematics." To be more precise, these authors pointed out that Nightingale's research occurred *before* later works that defined correlation in 1880, the *t* test in 1908, and chi-square, contingency table analysis, and analysis of variance, which were also developed about this time. These tests were later developed to aid in judging the relevance of data when the numbers were few and the effects small, neither of which was the case in Nightingale's research. It may be asked why her contributions to current nursing education did not include and build on the need to determine the social and environmental determinants of the health of aggregates by using a sound research base and statistics to determine the need for and effects of nursing practice, as she so aptly demonstrated in her own short but significant period of practice.

Establishment of Modern Medical Care and Public Health Practice

After Nightingale's birth in 1820, other important scientists were born: Louis Pasteur in 1822, Joseph Lister in 1827, and Robert Koch in 1843. Their research also had profound impacts on health care, medicine, and nursing. To place Nightingale's work in perspective, the development of medical care must be considered in light of common education and practice during the late 19th and early 20th centuries. Goodnow (1933) called this time a "dark age." Few medical schools existed at the time, so apprenticeship was the route to a medical education. Medical sciences were underdeveloped, and bacteriology was unknown. The majority of physicians believed in the "spontaneous generation" theory of disease causation (Najman, 1980) (i.e., that disease organisms grew from nothing). Typical medical treatment included bloodletting, starving, the use of leeches, and large doses of metals such as mercury and antimony (Goodnow, 1933). Even the clinical thermometer was not used until 1850. Nightingale's uniform classification of hospital statistics noted the need not only to tabulate the classification of diseases of patients in the hospital but also to note diseases contracted by patients while under treatment during hospitalization; these diseases, such as gangrene and septicemia, were later called *iatrogenic* diseases (Kopf, 1978). That infection was rampant is not surprising, as Goodnow (1933, pp. 471–472) related:

Before an operation the surgeon turned up the sleeves of his coat to save the coat, and would often not trouble to wash his hands, knowing how soiled they soon would be! The area of the operation would sometimes be washed with soap and water, but not always, for the inevitability of corruption made it seem useless. The silk or thread used for stitches or ligatures was hung over a button of the surgeon's coat, and during the operation a convenient place for the knife to rest was between his lips. Instruments . . . used for . . . lancing abscesses were kept in the vest pocket and often only wiped with a piece of rag as the surgeon went from one patient to another.

Pasteur was a chemist, not a physician. While experimenting with wine production in 1854, he proposed the theory of the existence of germs. He was ridiculed, and acknowledgment of his work came later; Koch later applied his theories and developed methods for handling and studying bacteria.

Lister, whose father perfected the microscope, noted the healing processes of compound fractures. When the bone was broken but the skin was not, he noted that recovery was uneventful. When both the bone and the skin were broken, however, fever, infection, and even death were frequent. Only through the work of Pasteur did he find the proposed answer to his observation: that something from outside got into the wound through the broken skin (Goodnow, 1933). His surgical successes eventually improved with the soaking of dressings and instruments in mixtures of carbolic acid (phenol) and oil.

Koch's discovery of cholera and the tubercle bacillus (1882) and Pasteur's discovery of immunization (1881) and rabies vaccine (1885) were of significance to the development of public health and medicine. In general, however, such discoveries were slow to be accepted (Rosen, 1958). For example, in late-19th-century America, tuberculosis was a major cause of death and often plagued its victims with chronic illness and disability. It was a highly stigmatized disease; most physicians of the time thought it was a hereditary, constitutional disease associated with poor environmental conditions. Family members with the disease were hidden, which increased the communicability of the disease, and hospitalization for tuberculosis was rare. Common treatment was a change of climate (Rosen, 1958). Although Koch had

announced the discovery of the tubercle bacillus in 1882, it was 10 years before the first organized community campaign against the disease began.

Another example of slow innovation stemming from scientific discoveries is seen in laboratory work by Pasteur that showed that *Streptococcus* caused puerperal (childbirth) fever. It was years before his discovery was accepted, however, and medical practice changed and physicians no longer delivered infants without washing their hands after the performance of autopsies on puerperal fever cases (Goodnow, 1933).

The causes of disease were questioned and debated throughout the 19th century; scientific discoveries of organisms during the latter part of the century supported the theory of specific contagious entities that caused disease and challenged an earlier, miasmic theory that environment and atmospheric conditions caused disease (Greifinger and Sidel, 1981). The new scientific discoveries had a major impact on the development of both public health and medical practice. The birth of the germ theory of disease encouraged a focus on the individual organism and the individual disease in diagnosis and treatment. The birth of allopathism (treatment of the part) rather than holism (considering the social, economic, and environmental context as a whole as contributing to disease) influenced the direction of public health as well as medical care practitioners of the time.

With new discoveries, state and local governments felt increasingly responsible for controlling the spread of bacteria and other microorganisms. They also were forced to heed a community outcry for social reform of deplorable living conditions in the cities—overcrowding, filth in the street, no provision for the poor, and inadequate food, water, and housing, as voiced by the populace in the New York City riots of 1863. Local boards of health were formed and charged with safeguarding water and food and managing sewage and quarantine of victims of contagious diseases (Greifinger and Sidel, 1981). The New York Metropolitan Board of Health was established in 1866. Later state health departments were formed. States built large public hospitals and treated both tuberculosis and mental disease with rest, diet, and quarantine. In 1889, the New York City Health Department recommended surveillance of tuberculosis and health education regarding tuberculosis, although neither recommendation was well received by physicians (Rosen, 1958). In 1894, the New York City Health Department required reporting of cases of tuberculosis by institutions and, in 1897, by physicians. Although sanitation was largely accomplished in the later part of the 19th century by organized community effort, this marked the first application of such effort to a disease. The National Tuberculosis Association was formed to control tuberculosis by "enlisting community support and action through a systematic and organized campaign of public health education" (Rosen, 1958, p. 390). Many voluntary health organizations were to follow, and many were organized efforts to "further community health through education, demonstrating ways of improving health services, advancing related research or legislation, as well as guarding and representing the public interest in this field" (Rosen, 1958, p. 384). Rosen further noted the subsequent organization of these agencies largely on behalf of diseases and organs:

Despite the great multiplicity and variety of such agencies, the voluntary health organizations tend generally to fall into four categories: (1) those concerned with specific diseases, such as tuberculosis, cancer, poliomyelitis, diabetes, and multiple sclerosis; (2) those concerned with disorders of certain organs of the body, such as the heart, defects of vision or hearing, dental defects, and diseases of the locomotor and skeletal systems; (3) those concerned with the health and welfare of special groups in the community such as mothers and children, the aged, or the Negro; and (4) those that dealt with health problems that affect the community as a whole, such as accident prevention, mental health, or planned parenthood.

Although environmental control was bringing about remarkable changes in health on the one hand, the increased use of anesthetics and the increasing awareness of pathology led to the establishment of many medical schools and a focus on one-to-one practice. Greifinger and Sidel (1981, p. 130) stated the following:

During the late nineteenth century, as many as 400 medical schools were founded in the United States; most lasted only a short time, but at least 147 medical schools were operating near the end of the century. These were privately owned institutions, and, lacking standardized graduation requirements, they produced physicians and surgeons who had inconsistent and often inadequate education.

In 1883, The Johns Hopkins University Medical School was established in Baltimore, Maryland, on the German model that espoused medical education on principles of scientific discovery after the great breakthroughs in identifying disease organisms. In the United States, the Carnegie Commission appointed Abraham Flexner to visit medical schools throughout the country and to evaluate them on the basis of the German model. In 1910, the Flexner Report outlined the shortcomings of U.S. medical schools not using this model and, within a few years, successfully brought about withdrawal of funding of these schools by philanthropic organizations such as the Rockefeller and Carnegie Foundations. Thus, the closure of scientifically "inadequate" medical schools occurred (Greifinger and Sidel, 1981). A "new breed" of physicians was promulgated, physicians who adhered to the germ theory of disease causation and the consequences included closing schools of midwifery and medical schools for women and blacks. Further consequences are outlined by Greifinger and Sidel (1981, p. 132).

> The emphasis on the utilization of scientific theory in medical care, especially in a society wedded to the "single agent theory" of the genesis of illness, developed into a focus on disease and symptoms rather than on therapy, prevention of disability, and caring for the "whole person." The old-fashioned family doctor had viewed patients in relation to their families and communities and had apparently been able to help people cope with problems of personal life, family, and society; the vigor with which American medicine adopted science left many of these qualities in the lurch. Science allowed the physician to deal with tissues and organs, which were much easier to comprehend than were the dynamics of human relationships, being propounded by Sigmund Freud and Carl Jung, or the complexities of disease prevention. Many physicians made efforts to integrate the various roles; however, the main thrust within society was toward academic science.

Aggregates with special needs for physicians and midwives who were female, nonwhite, or poor were forced to do without these practitioners (Ehrenreich and English, 1973).

Philanthropic foundations continued to influence health care efforts. For example, the Rockefeller Sanitary Commission for the Eradication of Hookworm was established in 1909 in conjunction with discovering that preventive efforts to eradicate hookworm, which was an occupational hazard among southern workers, kept the workers healthy and, therefore, greatly benefited industry. The model was so successful that the Rockefeller Foundation established The Johns Hopkins School of Hygiene and Public Health, the first school of public health, in 1916. The focus was on the preservation and improvement of health of individuals and the community and the prevention of disease through multidisciplinary efforts. The faculty came from a broad range of sciences: biological, physical, social, and behavioral. Additional efforts by foundations resulted in an International Health Commission, schools of tropical medicine, and medical research institutes in foreign ports to raise the level of health and, thus, production of the workers who loaded cargo bound for American shores.

Although community caregivers or traditional healers continue to exist, they often have been overlooked in holistic approaches to the provision of health care in the community.

Community Caregiver

Little has been preserved of the traditional role of the community caregiver or the traditional healer. Inferences are made, however, by medical and nurse anthropologists who have studied primitive and Western cultures (Leininger, 1976; Logan and Hunt, 1978).

The traditional healer is common in non-Western, ancient, and primitive societies (Hughes, 1978). The healer may have been manifest in various forms (e.g., shaman, midwife, herbalist, curandero, or priest). Traditional healers have, however, always existed, even in industrialized societies, although they may have a less visible role or their role may be overlooked by professionals as well as by selected parts of the community. The role of the healer often is integrated with other institutions of society: religion, medicine, and morality, for example. The notion that there is "one" person who serves as healer may be foreign to many societies; healers can be individuals, kin, or even entire societies (Hughes, 1978).

Societies have theories of disease and of the relationship of disease to other aspects of group life. Disease often is considered an expression of one's relationship to the environment (disharmony) rather than as a condition that is caused by a specific "germ."

Both supernatural and empirical theories of disease exist. Many practices are empirically efficacious by public health standards (e.g., the practice of reheating food that has been left overnight to do away with "coldness" also destroys pathogens) (Hughes, 1978).

A "THEORY OF DISEASE"

In common with a great many other people, Tiv do not regard "illness" or "disease" as a completely separate category distinct from misfortunes to compound and farm, from relationship among kin, and from more complicated matters relating to the control of land. However, it would be completely erroneous to say that Tiv are not able, in a cognitive sense, to recognize disease. As Bohannan stated, "The concept of a disease is not foreign to the Tiv: mumps, smallpox . . . yaws and gonorrhea are all common and each has a name" (p. 125). What is meant is that disease is seldom viewed in isolation (Price-Williams, 1962).

With repeated success, folk practices are kept by the society. Many therapeutic and preventive practices exist, and most cultures have a pharmacopoeia. From one fourth to one half of folk medicines are "empirically effective," and many modern drugs are based on the experience of primitive cultures (e.g., eucalyptus, coca, and opium) (Hughes, 1978).

Results of folk healing practices not only may benefit the "patient" but also may be socially cohesive; healing rituals and sessions frequently involve not only the patient but also the patient's family and neighbors. A chance to participate in one's own treatment and to involve one's fellows may result in the application of the "treatment" to a whole group, or aggregate (Hughes, 1978).

Other cultural practices affecting the health of the people have occurred since ancient times and include isolation of those who are "unclean" (lepers) and treatment of food, water, and even housing.

An example of the taking of "healing" from the people by modern medicine is provided by midwifery as practiced during the late 19th and early 20th centuries (Ehrenreich and English, 1973; Smith, 1979). Traditional midwifery practices of getting women up within 24 hours of delivery to help "clear" the lochia stood in sharp contrast to medical recommendations of keeping women in bed (Smith, 1979).

Modern nursing also developed from caregiving tasks carried out by men and women in the community. Richards' account of village women in America before the Industrial Revolution who gave community and family services is given by Baer (1985).

> *Linda Richards called certain of these women "born nurses . . . one or more of whom could be found in every village or community." Identified as a woman's role, the nurse needed to have kindness of heart, give cheerful service, and have "a love for the work and a strong desire to alleviate suffering." Trained by "experience . . . the instruction of older women and of the family doctors," these nurses "were always subject to call."*
>
> (RICHARDS, 1911, PP. 3–4)

Both the consumer movement in health, which arose in the 1830s, and the self-help movement have evolved to meet the needs of the community and society for health care and a safe environment.

Another holistic approach that was developing in the late 19th and early 20th centuries was public health nursing. Public health nursing and, later, community health nursing evolved from practice in the home, known as home health care, community organization, and political intervention on behalf of aggregates.

Establishment of Public Health Nursing and Focus

ENGLAND

Public health nursing developed from two traditions that stem from the Enlightenment: providing nursing care to the sick poor and helping the poor by providing information and channels of community organization that enable them to improve their health status.

District Nursing. District nursing, based on the first tradition, first developed in England. The Epidemiological Society of London developed a plan between 1854 and 1856 to train selected poor women to provide nursing care to the sick poor in the community. It was theorized that nurses of the same social class as their patients would be more effective and that, overall, more nurses would be available in the community (Rosen, 1958). Although this particular plan failed, a later plan was carried out in Liverpool in 1859 to provide nursing care to the sick poor.

After experiencing the excellent care given his sick wife by a nurse in his home, William Rathbone, a Quaker, believed strongly that such a plan was needed. He then divided the community into 18 districts, each to be assigned a nurse and a social worker to meet the needs of their communities for nursing, social work, and health education. Because the plan was accepted widely in the community, Rathbone needed education for these nurses and consulted Nightingale. She assisted him by providing for the training of the district nurses, referring to them as "health nurses." The model was successful and widely adopted, eventually on the national level under voluntary agencies (Rosen, 1958).

Health Visiting. A parallel service—health visiting—was originated in Manchester in 1862 by the Ladies Section of the Manchester and Salford Sanitary Association. Because the distribution of health pamphlets alone had little effect, the purpose of this service was to establish home visitors to give health information to the poor. In 1893, Nightingale pointed out that the district nurse should be a health teacher as well as a nurse for the sick in the home and that "health missioners" should be educated for this purpose. The model that was adopted, however, was that of the district nurse who provided care to the sick in the home and the health visitor who provided health information in the home. Eventually, health visitors were placed under the auspices of government agencies, supervised by the medical health officer, and paid by the municipality. Thus, a collaborative model existed between government and voluntary agencies, which largely exists today in the United States.

UNITED STATES

In the United States, public health nursing similarly developed from district nursing and home nursing. In 1877, the Women's Board of the New York City Mission sent Francis Root, a graduate nurse, into the home to provide care to the sick. The innovation spread, with nursing associations, later called visiting nurse associations, set up in Buffalo (1885) and then in Boston and Philadelphia (1886).

In 1893, nurses Lillian Wald and Mary Brewster established a district nursing service known as the House on Henry Street on the Lower East Side of New York City, a crowded area teeming with immigrants with minimal resources such as jobs, housing, and health care. This organization, later to become the Visiting Nurse Association of New York City, played an important role in the establishment of public health nursing in the United States. Wald provided a compelling account of her early exposure to the community where she identified public health nursing needs.

LILLIAN WALD: THE HOUSE ON HENRY STREET

Highlights from *The House on Henry Street*, published in 1915, bring Lillian Wald's experience to life:

A sick woman in a squalid rear tenement, so wretched and so pitiful that, in all the years since, I have not seen anything more appealing, determined me, within half an hour, to live on the East Side.

I had spent two years in a New York training-school for nurses. . . . After graduation, I supplemented the theoretical instruction, which was casual and inconsequential in the hospital classes twenty-five years ago, by a period of study at a medical college. It was while at the college that a great opportunity came to me.

While there, the long hours "on duty" and the exhausting demands of the ward work scarcely admitted freedom for keeping informed as to what was happening in the world outside. The nurses had no time for general reading; visits to and from friends were brief; we were out of the current and saw little of life save as it flowed into the hospital wards. It is not strange, therefore, that I should have been ignorant of the various movements which reflected the awakening of the social conscience at the time.

Remembering the families who came to visit patients in the wards, I outlined a course of instruction in home nursing adapted to their needs, and gave it in an old building in Henry Street, then used as a technical school and now part of the settlement. Henry Street then as now was the center of a dense industrial population.

From the schoolroom where I had been giving a lesson in bedmaking, a little girl led me one drizzling March morning. She had told me of her sick mother, and gathering from her incoherent account that a child had been born, I caught up the paraphernalia of the bedmaking lesson and carried it with me.

The child led me over broken roadways—there was no asphalt, although its use was well established in other parts of the city,—over dirty mattresses and heaps of refuse,—it was before Colonel Waring had shown the possibility of clean streets even in that quarter,—between tall, reeking houses whose laden fire-escapes, useless for their appointed purpose, bulged with household goods of every description. The rain added to the dismal appearance of the streets and to the discomfort of the crowds which thronged them, intensifying the odors which assailed me from every side. Through

Hester and Division street we went to the end of Ludlow; past odorous fishstands, for the streets were a market-place, unregulated, unsupervised, unclean; past evil-smelling, uncovered garbage-cans; and—perhaps worst of all, where so many little children played—past the trucks brought down from more fastidious quarters and stalled on these already overcrowded streets, lending themselves inevitably to many forms of indecency.

The child led me on through a tenement hallway, across a court where open and unscreened closets were promiscuously used by men and women, up into a rear tenement, by slimy steps whose accumulated dirt was augmented that day by the mud of the streets, and finally into the sickroom.

All the maladjustments of our social and economic relations seemed epitomized in this brief journey and what was found at the end of it. The family to which the child led me was neither criminal nor vicious. Although the husband was a cripple, one of those who stand on street corners exhibiting deformities to enlist compassion, and masking the begging of alms by a pretense at selling; although the family of seven shared their two rooms with boarders—who were literally boarders, since a piece of timber was placed over the floor for them to sleep on—and although the sick woman lay on a wretched, unclean bed, soiled with a hemorrhage two days old, they were not degraded human beings, judged by any measure of moral values.

In fact, it was very plain that they were sensitive to their condition, and when, at the end of my ministrations, they kissed my hands (those who have undergone similar experiences will, I am sure, understand), it would have been some solace if by any conviction of the moral unworthiness of the family I could have defended myself as a part of a society which permitted such conditions to exist. Indeed, my subsequent acquaintance with them revealed the fact that, miserable as their state was, they were not without ideals for the family life, and for society, of which they were so unloved and unlovely a part.

That morning's experience was a baptism of fire. Deserted were the laboratory and the academic work of the college. I never returned to them. On my way from the sickroom to my comfortable student quarters my mind was intent on my own responsibility. To my inexperience it seemed certain that conditions such as these

Box continued on following page

were allowed because people did not know, and for me there was a challenge to know and to tell. When early morning found me still awake, my naive conviction remained that, if people knew things—and "things" meant everything implied in the condition of this family—such horrors would cease to exist, and I rejoiced that I had had a training in the care of the sick that in itself would give me an organic relationship to the neighborhood in which this awakening had come.

To the first sympathetic friend to whom I poured forth my story, I found myself presenting a plan which had been developing almost without conscious mental direction on my part.

Within a day or two a comrade from the training-school, Mary Brewster, agreed to share in the venture. We were to live in the neighborhood as nurses, identify ourselves with it socially, and, in brief, contribute to it our citizenship.

I should like to make it clear that from the beginning we were most profoundly moved by the wretched industrial conditions which were constantly forced upon us. . . . I hope to tell of the constructive programmes that the people themselves have evolved out of their own hard lives, of the ameliorative measures, ripened out of sympathetic comprehension, and finally, of the social legislation that expresses the new compunction of the community. (pp. 1–9)

From Wald L: The House on Henry Street. New York, Henry Holt, 1915; reprinted by Dover Publications, New York, 1971.

Wald described a range of services that evolved from Henry Street. Home visiting was provided by nurses, and patients paid carfare for the nurses or a cursory fee. Physicians were consultants to Henry Street, and families could initiate a visit by calling the nurse directly or nurses could respond to a call by a physician. The philosophy was one of meeting the health needs of aggregates, broadly defined to include the many evident social, economic, and environmental determinants of health. This, by necessity, involved an aggregate approach, one that empowered people of the community.

Helen Hall, a later director of the House at Henry Street, wrote of the settlement's role as "one of helping people to help themselves" (Wald, 1971) through the development of centers of social action aimed at meeting the needs of the community as well as the individual. Community organizing led to the formation of a great variety of programs such as youth clubs, a program for juveniles, sex education for local school teachers, and support programs for immigrants. A community studies department carried out systematic community assessments (surveys) "so that we could tell our neighbors' story where it would do the most good" (Wald, 1971, p. vi). Mothers from the settlement went to Washington, D.C., and testified regarding the experience of bringing up children in "decaying tenements." Whether it was the need for traffic lights, schools, garbage collection, unemployment insurance, or health care, neighbors of the settlement were drawn into a democratic process that took them from the steps of city hall to the nation's capital to speak out on behalf of the needs of the aggregate that was affected by the condition. Legislation resulting from these efforts and those of others led to the formation of the Children's Bureau and the Social Security Act. As late as 1963, elders' testimonies had an impact on the formation of Medicare.

On the basis of individual observations and interventions, programs were planned for aggregates. One example is that of school nursing. Wald reported an incident that preceded her later successful trial of school nursing (1971, pp. 46–47):

I had been downtown only a short time when I met Louis. An open door in a rear tenement revealed a woman standing over a washtub, a fretting baby on her left arm, while with her right she rubbed at the butcher's aprons which she washed for a living.

"Louis," she explained, "was 'bad.' He did not 'cure his head,' and what would become of him, for they would not take him into the school because of it?" Louis, hanging the offending head, said he had been to the dispensary many times. He knew it was awful for a twelve-year-old boy not to know how to read the names of the streets on the lamp-posts, but "every time I go to school Teacher tells me to go home."

It needed only intelligent application of the dispensary ointments to cure the affected area, and in September, I had the joy of securing the boy's admittance to school for the first time in his life. The next day, at the noon recess, he fairly rushed up our five flights of stairs in the Jefferson Street tenement to spell the elementary words he had acquired that morning.

Overcrowded schools, an uninformed and uninterested public, and an unaware department of health all contributed to this neglect. Wald and the nursing staff at the settlement kept anecdotal notes of children they encountered who had been excluded from school owing to illness. One nurse found a boy in school whose skin was desquamating from scarlet fever and took him to the president of the Department of Health in an attempt to have physicians placed in the schools. A later program in which physicians screened children in school for 1 hour a day suffered from lack of comprehensiveness.

In 1902, Wald talked Dr. Lederle, Commissioner of Health in New York City, into trying a school nursing experiment. A public health nurse, Linda Rogers, from Henry Street was loaned to the New York City Health Department to work in a school (Dock and Stewart, 1925). School nursing was adopted on a widespread basis; school nurses were sometimes hired by the Board of Health and sometimes by the Board of Education. School nurses performed physical assessments, treated minor infections, and carried out health teaching with pupils and with parents.

HISTORICAL NURSING RESEARCH

In 1909, the Metropolitan Life Insurance Company adopted a program of home visiting by nurses to lower mortality rates and improve the company's image. Originally associated with the Henry Street settlement house, the Metropolitan Visiting Nurse Service (MVNS) created a system of more than 650 Visiting Nurse Associations throughout the United States. Nurses promoted the health of the policyholders, many of whom were immigrants, by teaching them health habits, including the importance of immunizations, and caring for them at times of illness in their homes. The nurses also carried out projects in selected communities (e.g., a treatment-of-tuberculosis demonstration project in Framingham, an infant mortality study in the Thetford mines, and a study to decrease high rates of mortality in Kingsport, a railroad town). In these projects, "nurses collected baseline health data, initiated health clinics, gave immunizations, established home visits, and taught health to policyholders." Statistics kept by Metropolitan Life documented the lowered mortality rates and increased health of the citizens as an outcome of the nurses' public health and clinical expertise. The MVNS continued to operate until 1953, when rising costs, unquestioned by the nurses, supported the company's decision to close.

Data from Hamilton D: Clinical excellence, but too high a cost: The Metropolitan Life Insurance Company Visiting Nurse Service (1909–1953). Public Health Nurs 5:235–240 1988.

In 1909, Wald mentioned the efficacy of home nursing to one of the officials of the Metropolitan Life Insurance Company. The company decided to provide home nursing to its industrial policyholders; the program proved very successful and was used throughout the United States and Canada (Wald, 1971).

The demand for public health nursing increased and was hard to meet. In 1910, the Department of Nursing and Health was started at the Teachers College of Columbia University in New York City. A course in visiting nursing was offered that placed nurses at the Henry Street settlement for fieldwork. In 1912, the National Organization of Public Health Nursing was formed, and Lillian Wald was elected president. This organization was open to public health nurses and to others in the community who were interested in public health nursing. In 1913, the Los Angeles Department of Health formed the first Bureau of Public Health Nursing (Rosen, 1958). That same year, the first public health nurse was appointed to the U.S. Public Health Service to perform fieldwork in trachoma.

At first, many public health nursing programs used nurses in specialized areas such as school nursing, tuberculosis nursing, maternal-child health nursing, and communicable disease nursing. A more generalized program has come to be acceptable in which a nurse hired by an official agency covers the entire population of one district and, with the exception of occupational health, provides prevention, health promotion, and health maintenance care. Collaboratively, visiting nurses in voluntary home health agencies such as the Visiting Nurse Association provide care to the homebound ill who are referred by a physician. Combination agencies providing both services also exist but are less available in urban areas.

With the current focus on cost containment and the provision of health care services under managed care, change is taking place in the traditional models of public health nursing and visiting nurses in voluntary home health agencies. Because the focus of care will increasingly be in the community, new models to contain costs using nursing in the community are appearing and may vary among states and areas within a state. Models are varied and may range, for example, from a focus on nurses providing care to populations who subscribe to health care services provided by health maintenance organizations (HMOs) (Graff et al., 1995; Shamansky, 1995) to a focus once again on specialized areas such as communicable disease nursing by public health nurses as in Alameda County, California (J. Strauss, personal communication, July

1995). Many concerns related to this historical shift exist and are addressed in this text; one concern, in particular, is the lack of access to and continuity of care for all members of a community, particularly those persons, families, and aggregates who are not members of an HMO (e.g., the unemployed and new immigrant or refugee populations).

Conclusions and implications for community health nursing from history cannot be made without considering the consequences of the evolution of health for the health of aggregates.

CONSEQUENCES FOR THE HEALTH OF AGGREGATES

Implications for the health of aggregates are explored in relation to new causes of mortality, Hygeia versus Panacea, and additional theories of disease causation.

New Causes of Mortality

The causes of mortality in Western societies have changed since the turn of the century from infectious diseases largely to chronic diseases. The decline in the rate of deaths from infectious diseases has been attributed mainly to increased food production and better nutrition during the 18th and 19th centuries; other factors include better sanitation through purification of water, sewage disposal, improved care of food, and pasteurization of milk. According to such authors as McKeown (1981) and Evans, Barer, and Marmor (1994), "modern" medicine (such as antibiotics) and immunization had little effect on health until well into the 20th century. Improved vaccination programs were begun in the 1920s; powerful antibiotics came into use after 1935.

The advent of modern chronic disease in Western populations places selected aggregates at risk. Aggregates at risk for chronic disease need, for example, health education, screening, and programs to ensure occupational and environmental safety. Because of the pursuit of the germ theory of disease, however, health services have focused expenditures on treatment of the acutely ill and have treated the chronically ill with an acute care approach. Yet preventive care, health promotion, and restorative care are necessary to combat escalating rates of chronic disease. This focus may change under new systems of cost containment such as managed care, which, theoretically, should focus on health promotion, prevention, and restorative care.

Hygeia Versus Panacea

The "healthful living" (Hygeia) versus "cure" (Panacea) dichotomy, which originates from Greek times, is still seen today. The change in the nature of health "problems" is identifiable, yet the roles of individual and collective activities in the prevention of illness and premature death are slow to evolve. The focus of medical technology and academic science on the disease organism has created more than 85 medical subspecialties. A consequence is that "complex life-threatening disorders are better understood; on the other hand, few professionals have been trained to specialize in the treatment of the common, uncomplicated health problems that account for 90 percent of visits to doctors" (Lee et al., 1981, p. 197). In 1993, two thirds of the 591,000 active physicians in the United States were specialists (National Center for Health Statistics, 1995). With a trend toward managed care, the interest in and need for providing primary care services has generated considerable attention to the utilization of nurse practitioners as a point of entry into primary care (Thibodeau and Hawkins, 1994). Medical education will be increasingly called on to focus on the training of primary care physicians (e.g., internal medicine, obstetrics-gynecology, family medicine, pediatrics) to meet the growing need for primary care.

To achieve "healthful living," in addition to primary care, a coordinated system that addresses the problem holistically, using multiple approaches and planning outcomes for aggregates and populations, is needed. A redistribution of interest and resources to address the major determinants of health, such as food, housing, education, and a healthy social and physical environment, is necessary (Evans et al., 1994; Lamarche, 1995; McKeown, 1981).

Additional Theories of Disease Causation

The germ theory of disease causation, which evolved in the late 19th century, is a unicausal model. Challenges to the germ theory of disease include that made by Max von Pettenkofer, a German physician and hygienist. In the late 19th century, von Pettenkofer, with his students, defiantly swallowed a large number of cholera bacteria and did not die as a result (Hume, 1927). McKeown's research (1981) also refutes this model. For example, although Koch named the tubercle bacillus in 1882, no treatments were

VIEWING IMMIGRANTS AS ASSETS: A GLIMPSE INTO AUSTRALIA'S PUBLIC HEALTH HISTORY

Australia, like the United States and Canada, is a land of immigration with its own unique public health history. Eighteen years after Captain Cook claimed the continent for Britain, Australia was used as a land to settle England's convicts (1788–1825) and later its excess population (1826–1850). (After 1850, the living conditions in England had improved significantly enough that the level of British immigration dropped dramatically.) Given the difficult and long journey of 6 to 8 months at sea, populating the Australian colony turned into a public health disaster for England.

The first few convict fleets barely survived the journey. By the time these immigrants arrived in Australia, they were plagued with disease and unable to work and build a settlement. British historical records show that the second fleet from England contained 1260 convicts. By the time the fleet reached Australia, 267 (21%) had died. Shortly after arrival, 124 of the survivors died in the Sydney hospital. For the next 25 years, the convicts who survived the arduous journey were of limited ability to help England build a settlement as a result of their arrival as starved and diseased immigrants. The journey was difficult to survive given the poor travel conditions such as overcrowding to increase space for cargo and the reduced rations of food and water for its passengers. (Both these conditions were related to the overall negligence and corruption of the private contractors.)

The British authorities realized that something had to be done to make sure that the convicts arrived alive. On counsel from William Redfern, the assistant surgeon of New South Wales (and a former convict), Governor Macquarie established regulations to control the shipping contractors and supervise the health of the convicts. Assistant surgeon Redfern recommended that a convict surgeon be placed aboard each ship to improve traveling conditions. More specifically, he recommended that the cabins and bedding of the passengers be aired out daily, that more drinking water be made available, that no rations or articles of comfort be withheld, that bathing and cleaning facilities be installed, and that the ship be regularly fumigated with nitric or muriatic acid. After the installment of these regulations, from 1788 to 1868, the death rate among convicts on ships to Australia plummeted compared with those among passengers on similar private fleets from Europe to North America, which is a much shorter trip.

Because the Australian government believed that it was even more important that settlers, rather than convicts, arrive healthy and ready to work, these public health standards were extended to ships that carried assisted immigrants. Assisted immigrants were those whose fares were prepaid by the Australian government. Regulations from London mandated that surgeons and matrons be responsible for the hygiene, medical care, welfare, and discipline of each ship's passengers. Basically, this measure, called the Passenger Acts, created a marked improvement in the health of young children and all immigrants by placing a doctor and nurse aboard each ship. By bringing the health conditions on all passenger ships under its control, the British Board of Trade made the passage to Australia "so safe that it was looked upon as a holiday by many immigrants, who arrived healthier than when they had left England" (Jupp, 1990).

This glimpse into Australia's immigration policy exemplifies one development in the history of public health. Be it through coercing the convicts or assisting passage to settlers, the Australian government populated its country by believing that immigrants are assets and by proving that the health of immigrants is a public responsibility.

Based on data from Jupp J: Two hundred years of immigration. In Reid J, Trompf P (eds): The Health of Immigrant Australia. Sydney: Harcourt Brace Jovanovich, pp. 1–38, 1990. Summarized by K. Swanson.

effective until the appearance of streptomycin in 1947. By 1947, however, mortality from tuberculosis was a fraction of what it was in the 19th century because of improved food, nutrition, sanitation, and other environmental factors.

Najman (1980) reviewed two additional theories of disease causation: the multicausal view, which considers environment to have many contributing causes, and the general susceptibility view, which takes into account stress and lifestyle factors. Najman contended that each theory accounts for some disease under some conditions, but no theory can account for largely unexplained phenomena in modern illness patterns and contradictory findings commonly found in research. The continued concentration by medicine and research on specific diseases is a consequence of the laboratory science approach to medical care that has existed since the time of Koch. Classic studies by Scrimshaw (1969) and McDermott (1972) and their colleagues questioned the efficacy of public health measures as well as medical measures in non-Western countries beset with infectious diseases. As pointed out by Najman (1980), literacy (Stewart, 1971) and nutrition (Scrimshaw et al., 1969) "may reduce the level of infectious disease morbidity and mortality to a greater extent than do 'medical' interventions" (p. 231). A rethinking of "intervention" at the aggregate level aimed at these larger needs is past due.

CHALLENGES FOR COMMUNITY HEALTH NURSING

Community health nurses face the challenge of promoting the health of populations with the new causes of mortality and underserved populations, who are more likely to experience both infectious and chronic diseases in our society. The specialization of medicine has affected the way in which nursing care as well as medical care is delivered. Nurses must be aware of the increased technological advances spawned by the many medical specialties that have existed. Nurses have been called on to seek increasing specialization to care for the "specialist's" patients. The number of nurses seeking specialized clinical preparation increased with medical specialization. For example, the proportion of master's prepared nurses choosing an advanced clinical specialty over teaching, administration, supervision, or other functional purpose of curricula increased from 59% in 1976 to 69% in 1984 to 1985 (American Nurses Association, 1987). The proportion of master's prepared nurses choosing a clinical practice specialty over others in 1992 was 43.4%, considerably less than in 1985 (U.S. Department of Health and Human Services, 1994). The percentage of nurses employed in public or community health settings accounted for 15% of employed registered nurses, up from 11% in 1988 (U.S. Department of Health and Human Services, 1990, 1994). About 8% worked in ambulatory care settings, HMOs, and physician- and nurse-based practices.

In the National Sample Survey of Registered Nurses (U.S. Department of Health and Human Services, 1994), 28% of the nurses who worked in a community or public health setting reported a diploma as their highest educational preparation, 27.5% reported an associate degree, 35.4% reported a baccalaureate degree, and 8.9% reported a master's degree as their highest nursing-related educational preparation. These statistics and trends reflect a phenomenon of concern to community health nursing: the need for a baccalaureate education as entry level to practice in community health nursing.

The need for a bimodal focus on prevention and health promotion and on home care of the ill within the community may become more widespread with changing patterns of reimbursement in managed care models. Holistic care, which requires both dimensions, has suffered and must receive attention in the future. This phenomenon has been affected by a long-standing ideology that has favored service in pursuit of the alleviation of illness, which has been in keeping with the germ theory of disease causation. An ethnohistorical study of public health nursing in rural New England from the turn of the century examined the cost-benefit ratios of the population-based district nurse that have persisted since 1900 in parts of New England (Dreher, 1984). The district nurse provided preventive, curative, and health maintenance services. Such a model, proposed Dreher, may better address the nation's health problems.

The need for education in community health nursing raises questions as to the pull from the HMOs for primary care versus a broader population approach that would prepare students to meet the needs of aggregates via strategies such as community organizing (e.g., to promote literacy, nutrition programs, decent housing and income, education, and safe social and physical environments). Determining the point at which to intervene along the health-illness continuum and the method of comprehensive intervention is, as Dreher suggested, a challenge.

Care and cure have been taken from the hands of many of the people. Medicine has "medicalized" social problems and normal life events, from childbirth to death. Medicine cannot solve today's health problems; nurses must work with and on behalf of aggregates, helping them build a constituency for issues facing them as consumers.

A focus on aggregates will mean many approaches, including the careful gathering of anecdotes (the experience of the people or organization) and statistics, known as a population focus, which addresses the health of all in the population (Williams, 1984). A population focus will better enable community health nurses to contribute to the ethic of social justice by emphasizing society's rather than the individual's responsibility for health (Beauchamp, 1986). Helping aggregates—with the goal being all of them in a community—to help themselves will empower the people and create with the people ways of carrying their concerns forward to help redress the balance.

A TIMELY MODEL OF DISTRICT NURSING

In an ethnohistorical study of the development of public health nursing in rural New England, a model of population-based nursing was found, unexpectedly, that holds promise for meeting the nation's current and even future health concerns (Dreher, 1984). Data were collected from public records, the census, interviews with town residents, public officials, medical care providers, active and retired public health nurses, and direct observations. The use of a district nurse, or "town hall" nurse, a health model from the 1920s, was found to exist today. The district nurse described in the findings provided health education and services to persons in four neighboring towns. The district nurse's activities were administered locally and paid for by property tax revenues, not by patients or third-party reimbursement. The district nurse provided a full range of community nursing services to persons in need regardless of ability to pay or insurance coverage. The nurse carried out responsibilities in the following areas: school nursing, health promotion and prevention, and home health care. She held office hours weekly in the town halls of the four communities, where she performed blood pressure screening and gave routine parenteral medications and health counseling. Mobility was not an issue because patients who were confined to their homes received home visits from the district nurse. The district nurse conducted routine screening in the schools and planned and carried out programs that addressed identified needs. The annual cost per visit of health services provided by the district nurse was far less than that provided by nurses in a nearby home health agency. The model is recommended as a way of addressing the nation's needy health problems through prevention, promotion, and maintenance care.

A knowledge of our history provides insight into the dilemmas faced in contemporary times, which in many ways are not so different from the past. As Duffus (1938) stated of Wald's work:

The "case" element in these early reports of [Wald] got less and less emphasis; she instinctively went behind the symptoms to appraise the whole individual, saw that one could not understand the individual without understanding the family, saw that the family was in the grip of larger social and economic forces which it could not control. (p. 51)

The historians of health care have reconstructed the past from written fragments of "the facts" carefully sifted and weighed and thought to be worthy of mention. Values and theories held by the historian influence the writing of our past. Versluysen (1980) pointed out the consequences of the inevitable selectivity of the reconstruction of the history of health care: the history of health care has been written largely from the viewpoint of men, and the history of health care has been narrowly interpreted as the history of medicine.

Nonphysician healers, especially women, traditionally have been viewed by historians as inauthentic "amateurs" who were marginal to "the maintenance of the physical health and well-being of society" (Versluysen, 1980, p. 176). However, throughout history until the late 19th century, healing took place largely in the home by healers, who were invisible yet representative of an extensive system of care delivery. Sources of accounts of home care by healers, such as diaries, health manuals, and letters, have been overlooked by male historians and are only now being researched by female historians and, often, feminists (Newbern, 1994). Davies (1980) stated that Versluysen (1980) implied we should ask whether the study of nursing's history is even appropriate and contended that the history of healers, who usually were women, might be more appropriate.

According to Versluysen (1980), another historical trend is for historians to mention a few heroines in typical feminine stereotypes. For example, Nightingale's lifelong intellectual endeavors and marked achievements expand considerably the profile of this remarkable woman beyond the typical focus on only her limited time (2 years) in the Crimea and the founding of modern nursing education. These achievements include being a health statistician, a prolific writer and scientist, a radical environmental sanitarian, and a reformer of both the British Army medical care system and sanitary policy in India.

In addition, historians have also neglected to a large extent the social and environmental contexts of health and medical care, dimensions that are necessary to place health care in a broader context. Such a context is necessary to grasp the state of the health of the public and public health efforts during specific periods.

SUMMARY

As Western civilization evolved from the Paleolithic Period to the present and people began to live in increasingly closer proximity to each other, the nature of the health problems they experienced also changed.

In the mid-19th and early 20th centuries, public health efforts, including the precursors of modern nursing and public health nursing, began to make progress in improving societal health. Nursing pioneers such as Nightingale in England and Wald in the United States focused on the collection and analysis of statistical data, health care reforms, home nursing, community empowerment, and nursing education and laid the groundwork for the establishment of community health nursing as it exists today.

Modern community health nurses must grapple with an array of philosophical controversies that affect the way they practice. These include differences of opinion about what "intervention" means, a focus on both the individual and the aggregate, and the steps that should be taken to best solve the problem of runaway health care costs.

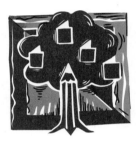

**L e a r n i n g
A c t i v i t i e s**

1. Research the history of the health department or Visiting Nurse Association in your city or county.

2. Find two recent articles about Florence Nightingale. After reading the articles, analyze and list the contributions made by Nightingale to public health and public health nursing and, later, community health nursing according to the accounts given by the authors.

3. Read Henrik Ibsen's play *The Enemy of the People.* Write a summary of the main points of the play, and list the implications of the play for health professionals who want to bring about similar changes in a contemporary community.

RECOMMENDED READINGS

Nursing Research

Buhler-Wilkerson K: Bringing care to the people: Lillian Wald's legacy to public health nursing. Am J Public Health 83:1778–1786, 1993.

Burgess W: The Great White Plague and other epidemics: Lessons from early visiting nursing. J Home Health Care Pract 6:12–17, 1993.

Dennis KE, Prescott PA: Florence Nightingale: Yesterday, today, and tomorrow. Adv Nurs Sci 7:66–81, 1985.

Erickson GP: One hundred years of powerful women: A conversation with Sylvia R. Peabody. Public Health Nurs 10:146–150, 1993.

Grier B, Grier M: Contributions of the passionate statistician. Res Nurs Health 1:103–109, 1978.

Hawkins JE, Hayes ER, Corliss CP: School nursing in America—1902–1994: A return to public health nursing. Public Health Nurs 11:416–425, 1994.

Mayer SL: Amelia Greenwald: Pioneer in international public health nursing. Nurs Health Care 15:74–78, 1994.

Mosley M: Jessie Sleet Scales: First black public health nurse. Asso Black Nurs Faculty, J 5:45–51, 1994.

Newbern VB: Women as caregivers in the South, 1900–1945. Public Health Nurs 11:247–254, 1994.

Roberts ER, Reeb RM: Mississippi public health nurses and midwives: A partnership that worked. Public Health Nurs 11:57–63, 1994.

Shore HL: Frances Redmond: A pioneer in community health in Vancouver. Can J Public Health 84:13, 1993.

Silverstein NG: Lillian Wald at Henry Street, 1893–1895. Adv Nurs Sci 7:1–12, 1985.

REFERENCES

Amaro H, Whitaker R, Coffman G, Heeren T: Acculturation and marijuana and cocaine use: Findings from HHANES 1982–84. Am J Public Health 80 (suppl):54–60, 1990.

American Nurses Association: Facts About Nursing 86–87. Kansas City, MO, American Nurses Association, 1987.

Armelagos GK, Dewey JR: Evolutionary response to human infectious diseases. *In* Logan MH, Hunt EE (eds): Health and the Human Condition. North Scituate, MA, Duxbury Press, pp. 101–107, 1978.

Baer ED: Nursing's divided house—An historical view. Nurs Res 34:32–38, 1985.

Beauchamp DE: Public health as social justice. *In* Mappes T, Zembaty J eds: Biomedical Ethics, 2nd ed. New York, McGraw-Hill, pp. 585–593, 1986.

Brothwell D: The question of pollution in earlier and less developed societies. *In* Logan MH, Hunt EE (eds): Health and the Human

Condition. North Scituate, MA, Duxbury Press, pp. 129–136, 1978.

Burkitt DP: Some diseases characteristic of modern western civilization. *In* Logan MH, Hunt EE (eds): Health and the Human Condition. North Scituate, MA, Duxbury Press, pp. 137–147, 1978.

Cockburn TA: The evolution of human infectious diseases. *In* Cockburn T (ed): Infectious Diseases: Their Evolution and Eradication. Springfield, IL, Charles C Thomas, pp. 34–107, 1967.

Cohen IB: Florence Nightingale. Sci Am 250:128–137, 1984.

Davies C: Rewriting Nursing History. Totowa, NJ, Barnes and Noble, 1980.

Dock LL, Stewart IM: A Short History of Nursing: From the Earliest Times to the Present Day. New York, Putnam, 1925.

Dreher M: District nursing: The cost benefits of a population-based practice. Am J Public Health 74:1107–1111, 1984.

Duffus RL: Lillian Wald—Neighbor and Crusader. New York, Macmillan, 1938.

Duran FD: The Aztecs: The History of the Indies of New Spain (translated, with notes, by Heyden D, Horcasitas F). New York, Orion Press, 1964.

Ehrenreich B, English D: Witches, Midwives, and Nurses: A History of Women Healers. Old Westbury, NY, The Feminist Press, 1973.

Evans RG, Barer ML, Marmor TR: Why are some people healthy and others not? The determinants of health of populations. Hawthorne, NY, Aldine de Gruyter, 1994.

Garn SM: Culture and the direction of human evolution. Hum Biol 35:221–236, 1963.

George MD: London Life in the XVIIIth Century. New York, Knopf, 1925.

Goodnow M: Outlines of Nursing History. Philadelphia, WB Saunders, 1933.

Graff WL, Bensussen-Walls W, Cody E, Williamson J: Population management in an HMO: New roles for nursing. Public Health Nurs 12:213–221, 1995.

Greifinger RB, Sidel VW: American medicine: Charity begins at home. *In* Lee P, Brown N, Red I (eds): The Nation's Health. San Francisco, Boyd and Fraser, pp. 124–134, 1981.

Grier B, Grier M: Contributions of the passionate statistician. Res Nurs Health 1:103–109, 1978.

Guendelman S, Gould J, Hudes M, Eskenazi B: Generational differences in perinatal health among the Mexican American population: Findings from HHANES 1982–84. Am J Public Health 80 (suppl):61–65, 1990.

Hanlon JJ, Pickett GE: Public Health Administration and Practice, 8th ed. St. Louis, MO, Times Mirror/Mosby, 1984.

Hudson EH: Treponematosis and man's social evolution. Am Anthropologist 67:885–901, 1965.

Hughes CC: Medical care: Ethnomedicine. *In* Logan MH, Hunt EE (eds): Health and the Human Condition. North Scituate, MA, Duxbury Press, pp. 150–158, 1978.

Hume EE: Max von Pettenkofer. New York, Hoeber, 1927.

Jupp J: Two hundred years of immigration. *In* Reid J, Trompf R (eds): The Health of Immigrant Australia. Orlando, Harcourt Brace & Co, pp. 1–38, 1990.

Kopf EW: Florence Nightingale as statistician. Res Nurs Health 1:93–102, 1978.

Lamarche PA: Our health paradigm in peril. Public Health Rep 110:556–560, 1995.

Lee PR, Brown N, Red I (eds): The Nation's Health. San Francisco, Boyd and Fraser, 1981.

Leininger M: Transcultural Health Care Issues and Conditions. Philadelphia: FA Davis, 1976.

Logan MH, Hunt EE (eds): Health and the Human Condition. North Scituate, MA, Duxbury Press, 1978.

McDermott W, Deuschle KW, Barnett CR: Health care experiment at Many Farms. Science 175:23–31, 1972.

McKeown T: Determinants of health. *In* Lee P, Brown N, Red I (eds): The Nation's Health. San Francisco, Boyd and Fraser, pp. 49–57, 1981.

Najman JM: Theories of disease causation and the concept of a general susceptibility: A review. Soc Sci Med 14A:231–237, 1990.

National Center for Health Statistics: Health, United States, 1994. Hyattsville, MD, Public Health Service, 1995.

Newbern VB: Women as caregivers in the South, 1900–1945. Public Health Nurs 11:247–254, 1994.

Polgar S: Evolution and the ills of mankind. *In* Tax S (ed): Horizons of Anthropology. Chicago, Aldine, pp. 200–211, 1964.

Price-Williams DR: A case study of ideas concerning disease among the Tiv. Africa 32:123–131, 1962.

Richards L: Reminiscences of Linda Richards: America's First Trained Nurse. Boston, Whitcomb and Barrows, 1911.

Richardson BW: The Health of Nations: A Review of the Works of Edwin Chadwick, vol. 2. London, Longmans, Green, 1887.

Rosen G: A History of Public Health. New York, MD Publications, 1958.

Scrimshaw NS, Béhar M, Guzmán MA, et al: Nutrition and infection field study in Guatemalan villages, 1959–64. Arch Environ Health 18:51–62, 1969.

Shamansky SL: A longer-than-usual editorial about population-based managed care (editorial). Public Health Nurs 12:211–212, 1995.

Smith FB: The People's Health 1830–1910. London, Croom Helm, 1979.

Stewart CT: Allocation of resources to health. J Hum Res 6:103–122, 1971.

Thibodeau JA, Hawkins JW: Moving toward a nursing model in advanced practice. West J Nurs Res 16:205–218, 1994.

U.S. Department of Health and Human Services, Health Resources and Services Administration, Bureau of Health Professions, Division of Nursing: The Registered Nurse Population: Findings from the National Sample Survey of Registered Nurses. Springfield, VA, National Technical Information Service, 1990.

U.S. Department of Health and Human Services, Health Resources and Services Administration, Bureau of Health Professions, Division of Nursing: The Registered Nurse Population: Findings from the National Sample Survey of Registered Nurses, March, 1992. Rockville, MD, Division of Nursing, 1994.

Versluysen MC: Old wives' tales? Women healers in English history. *In* Davies C (ed): Rewriting Nursing History. Totowa, NJ, Barnes and Noble, pp. 175–199, 1980.

Wald L: The House on Henry Street. New York, Dover Publications (original work published 1915), 1971.

Williams CA: Population-focused practice. *In* Stanhope M, Lancaster J (eds): Community Health Nursing: Process and Practice for Promoting Health. St. Louis, CV Mosby, pp. 805–815, 1984.

Wolfe M, Tuazon C, Schultz M: Imported bubonic plague—District of Columbia. MMWR Morb Mortal Wkly Rep 39:895, 901, 1990.

The Health Care System

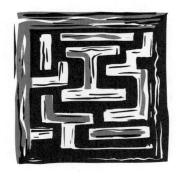

Upon completion of this chapter, the reader will be able to:

1. Describe the private health care subsystem and the public health subsystem.

2. Analyze landmark health care legislation and its impact on the delivery system.

3. Describe the organization of the public health care subsystem at the national, state, and local levels.

4. Describe the scope of the public health care subsystem at all levels.

5. Describe the goals for health care in the future.

Barbara J. Horn
Beverly M. Horn
Jack Thompson

OVERVIEW OF THE HEALTH SYSTEM

The health care system of the United States is dynamic, multifaceted, and not comparable to any other health care system in the world. It is often praised for its technological breakthroughs, frequently criticized for its high costs, and difficult to access by those most in need. What is this system, how did it come to be, and how is its viability maintained? In this chapter, we describe landmark health care legislation, the organization of the private health care subsystem and the public health subsystem, and present a futuristic perspective.

Major Legislation and the Health Care System

To understand the evolution of the health care system in the United States, it is critical to know the major legislative actions that have been taken by the federal government that influence health and health care. The Congress of the United States enacted bills, particularly in the 20th century, that had a major impact on both the personal and private health care services subsystem and the public health subsystem. Legislation pertaining to health increased in each decade of the 20th century and aimed at improving the health of populations. Some of the landmark federal acts that influenced health services include the following:

Although not exhaustive of all the legislation enacted, the pattern of increased involvement in health issues by the federal government is clear. The 1906 Pure Food and Drugs Act (Hanlon and Pickett, 1984) reflected an early concern for prevention of morbidity and mortality resulting from environmental influences. In 1912, the Children's Bureau was founded to protect children from the unhealthy child labor practices of the time and to enact programs that had a positive effect on children's health. In 1921 the Sheppard-Towner Act aimed specifically at providing funds for the health and welfare of infants.

The Social Security Act (SSA) of 1935 and its subsequent amendments of 1965 and 1972 (Hanlon and Pickett, 1984) had a far-reaching effect by providing welfare for high-risk mothers and children. Benefits were later expanded to include health care provisions for the elderly and handicapped.

Services expanded in the areas of health, education, and welfare after World War I, the Great Depression, and the post-World War II years. The Hill-Burton Act (1946) authorized federal assistance in the construction of hospitals and health centers with stipulations about services for the uninsured. As a result, large numbers of hospitals with obligations to care for the uninsured were built in towns and cities across America. Although health care became available on a wide basis, the high cost of health care today has forced the closure of many of the hospitals built with Hill-Burton funds.

Date	Legislation
1906	Pure Food and Drugs Act
1912	Children's Bureau
1921	Shepard-Towner Act
1935	Social Security Act
1946	Hill-Burton Act
1953	Department of Health, Education and Welfare as a cabinet-status agency
1964	Nurse Training Act
1964	Economic Opportunity Act
1965	Social Security Act amendments: Title XVIII Medicare Title XIX Medicaid
1970	Occupational Safety and Health Act
1972	Social Security Act amendments: Professional Standards Review Organization Further benefits under Medicare, Medicaid including dialysis
1973	Health Maintenance Organization
1974	National Health Planning and Resources Act
1981	Omnibus Budget Reconciliation Act
1987	Omnibus Budget Reconciliation Act
1989	Omnibus Budget Reconciliation Act
1990	Omnibus Budget Reconciliation Act
1983	Tax Equity and Fiscal Responsibility Act (established prospective payment fees)
1988	Family Support Act
1990	Health Objectives Planning Act

Coordination of services under several agencies culminated in the establishment of the Department of Health Education and Welfare under President Eisenhower in 1953. In 1979, this department was separated into the Departments of (1) Education and (2) Health and Human Services (DHHS). Today, the DHHS is the second largest department of the federal government. Only the Department of Defense is larger.

The Health Amendments Act of 1956, Title II, authorized monies to aid registered nurses in full-time study of administration, supervision, or teaching. In 1963, the Surgeon General's Consultant Group on Nursing noted that there were still too few nursing schools, that nursing personnel were not well utilized, and that limited research was being done in nursing. In 1964 the Nurse Training Act provided money for loans and scholarships for full-time study for nurses as well as money for nursing school construction.

A major governmental action was the enactment of legislation for Medicare and Medicaid. Medicare, Title XVIII Social Security Amendment (1965), is a federal program that pays specified health care services for all persons older than 65 years who are eligible (approximately 90%) to receive Social Security benefits (Robert Wood Johnson Foundation, 1994). Persons with permanent total disabilities are also covered. The objective of Medicare is to protect older adults against large medical outlays. The program is funded through payroll tax for all working citizens. Thus, private monies in the form of payroll taxes go to the federal government. Individuals or providers may submit payment requests for health care services and are paid according to Medicare regulations, or a flat fee may be paid to a health maintenance organization (HMO) for each member on Medicare. The manner in which this flat fee is determined is described later.

Medicare, Part A, pays for institutional care (hospital and nursing home and skilled home health services). The benefits are the same for all recipients. There is no monthly premium; however, copayments and limitations on type and duration of services are in place.

Medicare, Part B, pays for noninstitutional care (physician, outpatient, home health and ambulatory care); Part B requires a monthly fee and is voluntary (individuals do not have to subscribe). The majority of dollars are spent for illness care (more than 70% to hospitals and 20% to physicians). Medicare does not cover prescription drugs, preventive services, long-term care, or dental care.

Medicaid, Title XIX Social Security Amendment (1965), is a federal and state program (Robert Wood Johnson Foundation, 1994). The program provides access to care for the poor and medically needy of all ages. Each state is allocated federal dollars on a matching basis (50% of costs are paid with federal dollars). Each state has the responsibility and right to determine services to be provided and the dollar amount allocated to the program. Basic services (inpatient and outpatient hospital care, physical therapy, laboratory, radiography, skilled nursing, and home health care) are required to be eligible for matching federal dollars. States may choose from a wide range of optional services. These include drugs, eyeglasses, intermediate care, inpatient psychiatric care, and dental care. Limits can and are placed on the amount and duration of service. Unlike Medicare, Medicaid provides long-term care services (nursing home and home health) and personal care services (e.g., chores and homemaking). In addition, Medicaid has eligibility criteria based on level of income.

There is great variability in both services and dollars provided by each state. In addition to the required services for matching of federal dollars, some states and three territories provide fewer than 10 additional services: Georgia, Guam, Mississippi, Puerto Rico, Virgin Islands, and Wyoming. In contrast, Minnesota and California offer 29 additional services, and Michigan, New York State, and Wisconsin offer 26 additional services (Health Care Financing Administration, 1988). In 1993, the states with the lowest ratios of Medicaid recipients to persons below the poverty level (less than 65.8 per 100 persons) were located predominantly in the South and mountain states (National Center for Health Statistics, 1995). Also average payments per Medicaid recipient varied more than 12-fold among the states from a low of $524 in Arizona to a high of $6,402 in New York State (National Center for Health Statistics, 1995). Ten states with the highest Medicaid payments per recipient in 1993 were located predominantly in the Northeast, and 10 states with the lowest payments were predominantly in the South and West (National Center for Health Statistics, 1995).

The National Health Planning and Resources Act (1974) established Health Service Areas and was the strongest piece of legislation that enhanced the roles of citizens in the development of state and local health policy (Zimmerman, 1990). The Omnibus Budget

Reconciliation Acts (1981, 1987, 1989, 1990) were responses to the huge federal deficit, and each act further reduced eligibility of poor women and children for welfare and health care. The Family Support Act (1988) expanded coverage for poor women and children and required states to extend Medicaid coverage for 12 months to families with increased earnings but no longer receiving cash assistance. This act also required states to expand Aid to Families with Dependent Children coverage to two-parent families when the principal wage earner was unemployed (Cohen, 1990).

The thrust of legislation was either prevention of illness through influencing the environment (Occupational Safety and Health Administration [OSHA], 1970) or provision of funding to support programs that had a direct impact on health care provision (SSA, 1935). Beginning with the Shepard-Towner Act of 1921 and continuing to the present time, federal grants increased the involvement of state and local governments in health care. The involvement of the federal government through funding of money to state and local governments provided money for programs not previously available to state and local areas. Similar services became available in all states. Monies supporting these services were accompanied by regulations that applied to all recipients. Many state and local government programs were developed based on availability of funds. Thus, the involvement of the federal government through funding tended to standardize public health policy in the United States (Pickett and Hanlon, 1990).

As health care costs escalated in the 1970s and 1980s, efforts to control costs ensued. In 1973 HMOs were thought to be a potential answer to ever rising costs (Robert Wood Johnson Foundation, 1994). The Tax Equity and Fiscal Responsibility Act (TEFRA, 1982) was enacted in response to HMO proliferation and as health care costs continued to escalate. A Medicare prospective payment system (1983) was introduced and replaced TEFRA (Robert Wood Johnson Foundation, 1994). By 1991 health care costs continued to rise in spite of numerous efforts to contain them. In 1992 the Resource-Based Relative Value Scale (RBRVS) was enacted (Robert Wood Johnson Foundation, 1994). Through this, Medicare reimbursed physicians using three components: (1) a relative value for each procedure, (2) a geographic adjustment factor, and (3) a dollar conversion factor.

The 1990 Health Objectives Planning Act was the result of several years of effort by both the private and public sectors. Title XVII of the Public Health Service Act directed the secretary of DHHS to establish national preventive health goals. The Public Health Service (PHS) in 1979 identified goals to reduce premature mortality and morbidity for all age groups. The first report published was "Healthy People, The Surgeon General's Report on Health Promotion and Disease Prevention" (1979).

In 1980, a second report that included specific objectives for the year 1990 was called "Promoting Health, Preventing Disease, Objectives for the Nation." According to Scott, Tierney and Waters (1991), the Year 2000 health objectives reflect the "second installment of a continuing Federal initiative to adopt 'management by objectives' techniques for health status improvement in the nation."

The Year 2000 objectives were developed with considerable input from a wide range of national, state, and local health organizations. The Association of State and Territorial Health Officials (ASTHO) worked to structure a relationship between the national health objectives and state and local public health efforts. ASTHO was also concerned with the functions of public health as presented in the Institute of Medicine (IOM) 1988 report. All 57 state and territorial health departments were invited to participate in the development of the Year 2000 objectives. Public hearings were conducted in Birmingham, Los Angeles, Houston, Seattle, Denver, Detroit, and New York. These efforts resulted in the IOM re-port "Healthy People 2000" (1990). The efforts of ASTHO, as represented in this document, resulted in the introduction to Congress of the Health Objectives Act 2000 in October 1990. The final document, Public Law 101-582, was passed by the 101st Congress on November 15, 1990. Initial funding authorization ($10 million) was not as much as hoped for, it but did set the direction for health promotion and disease prevention as priorities in health care. A complementary document, "Healthy Communities 2000: Model Standards," published by the American Public Health Association (1991), assists the individual community in setting achievable targets for the future. For a report of how well the United States is achieving the health status objectives, see the appendix Healthy People 2000: Midcourse Review and 1995 Revision (U.S. Public Health Service, 1995).

Redefining Health: A Basis for Health Care

An effective health care system evolves from an understanding of health. The definition of health is dynamic and evolved over time; each definition represents the values and beliefs of a given culture at a particular time. Past definitions served as the basis for the next definition. The classic definition of health is that of C. E. A. Winslow. In recent times the definition most widely used is that of the World Health Organization (WHO). (Both definitions are presented in Chapter 1.)

With the changing nature of health problems of individuals (increasing number of persons with chronic disease and increasing number of older adults) and health issues in the environment (pollution) affecting the population, the WHO definition is not adequate. A definition that better reflects the current needs and could be operationalized into a health care system is as follows:

Health is a state characterized by anatomic integrity, ability to perform personally valued family, work, and community roles; ability to deal with physical, biologic and social stress, a feeling of well-being; and freedom from the risk of disease and untimely death.

(STOKES 1982, P. 34)

With use of this definition, the focus of services changes from unlimited illness care to promoting a safe environment, protecting individuals and communities through immunizations, promoting healthier lifestyles, improving nutrition, and providing health services with known efficacy. Measurable outcomes of a health care system based on this definition include life span, disease, discomfort, participation in health care, health behavior, social behavior, and satisfaction (Blum, 1981). This would be the upstream approach described by Butterfield in Chapter 4 of this text.

For information about the World Health Organization, the United Nations Children's Fund, and other international organizations, see Chapter 29 on World Health.

DETERMINANTS OF HEALTH

The outcomes identified in the definition just given are influenced by a number of factors. For example, Blum

(1981) postulated four major inputs that determine health. The four inputs, in increasing magnitude of impact, are heredity, health care services, behavior, and environment. If this is true and evidence supports this notion, then interventions directed toward education to change lifestyle behaviors and making the environment safer are essential if health is to be achieved (Blum, 1981; Haggerty, 1990; McKeown, 1990).

Blum (1981) suggested the following as the appropriate goals of the health care system:

- Promotion of high-level "wellness" or self-fulfillment
- Promotion of high-level satisfaction with the environment
- Minimization of departures from physiologic or functional norms for optimal health
- Prolongation of life through prevention of premature death
- Extension of resistance to ill health and creation of reserve capacity
- Minimization of discomfort (illness)
- Minimization of disability (incapacity)
- Increasing capacity for the underprivileged to participate in health matters (Blum, 1981, pp. 96–100)

Health care services in the model proposed by Blum have less influence on health than do individual personal behavior and habits and the environment (physical characteristics such as climate, topography, and inadequate housing) (Blum, 1981; Haggerty, 1990; McKeown, 1990). The health care system has been slow in changing to incorporate more recent definitions of health, and the lack of achievement of many of the measurable outcomes is evident in the health of populations. The health care system remains relatively static and continues to focus on illness and disease with less attention to health promotion and disease prevention. This is the downstream approach described by Butterfield.

PREVENTION OF DISEASE AND PROMOTION OF HEALTH

The recognition that social and behavioral factors are vital in the health of the nation has prompted the development of new approaches. Control and eradication of communicable diseases, based on the biomedical model, have dominated the health care system since the late 1800s; now, because there is control or eradication of most of the early killers, there is a change in focus toward promotion of health. A new set of health problems exists today. Green and Raeburn (1990, p. 35) referred to a growing international awareness of an ecologic model of health promotion that identifies health as the "product of the individual's continuous interaction and interdependence with his or her ecosphere—that is, the family, the community, the culture, the societal structure, and the physical environment." The health promotional approach focuses on lifestyle of persons, interacting with the ecostructure, rather than heavy reliance on the biomedical model.

The ecological model also fits more precisely with an international and world view of health (see World Health, Chapter 29; also World Health Organization, 1944). Two documents that support such a perspective are the Alma Ata Charter of 1978 (Alma Ata, World Health Organization, and Children's Fund, 1978) and the Ottawa Charter for Health Promotion (1986). Both documents emphasize living standards as critical to health. The Ottawa Charter states clearly that the fundamental conditions and resources for health are peace, shelter, education, food, income, a stable ecosystem, sustainable resources, social justice, and equity. The document further notes that improvement in health requires a secure foundation in these basic prerequisites. The fundamental differences in definition of health promotion between Canada and the United States is reflected in the efforts of the two countries. Since the Ottawa Charter, the Canadian system (which already has health care available to all) has as its focus the general well-being of populations. For example, major efforts are aimed toward incorporating cultural concepts in all aspects of the health care system. The United States, alternatively, has had

a continued focus on lifestyle change (e.g., smoking cessation, safe sexual practices, and exercise). The ideals set forth in the Ottawa Charter and toward which health of the future is directed will take the industrial countries as well as the third world decades to achieve (Confusion Worse Confounded, Prevention, 1990). Nevertheless, the mandate is clear and will increase in importance during the decade of the 1990s.

According to Terris (1990), health promotion in the United States began with a more limited focus. "Healthy People, The Surgeon General's Report" (U.S. Public Health Service, 1979) defined health promotion as a modification of lifestyle to prevent disease, with little attention given to improvement of living standards. Although modification of lifestyle is important, inattention to improvement of living standards is detrimental to health as defined in the broader ecological model.

COMPONENTS OF THE HEALTH CARE SYSTEM

The current health care system consists of a private health care subsystem and a public health care subsystem (Fig. 3–1). The private health care subsystem includes a variety of personal care services from a variety of sources and also numerous voluntary agencies. The public health subsystem has prevention of disease and illness as a major focus. These subsystems are not always mutually exclusive, and their functions sometimes overlap. With the rapid growth of technology and increased demands on both the private and public health care subsystems, the costs have become prohibitive. A major effort of the latter half of the 1990s is cost containment (Robert Wood Johnson Foundation, 1994).

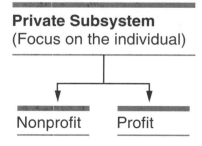

Private Subsystem
(Focus on the individual)

Nonprofit   Profit

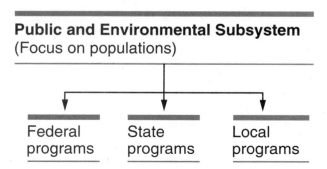

Public and Environmental Subsystem
(Focus on populations)

Federal programs   State programs   Local programs

Figure 3–1
U.S. health care system.

Private Health Care Subsystem

In this subsystem personal health care is provided to individuals. Services in this subsystem include health promotion, prevention and early detection of disease, diagnosis and treatment of disease with a focus on cure, rehabilitative-restorative care, and custodial care. These services are provided on an outpatient basis in clinics, physicians' offices, hospital ambulatory centers, and homes; the services are provided on an inpatient basis in hospitals and skilled care facilities. The majority of personal health care services is provided in the private sector. Increasingly, these private sector services come through HMOs. For persons who do not have access to the private sector, the public health subsystem provides personal care services in clinics, the community, home, or school.

Managed care is the dominant paradigm in health care of the 1990s (Caper, 1995). Basically managed care involves capitation payments for care rather than fee for service. Health care providers, including physicians, hospitals, community clinics, and home care providers, are integrated in a system such as an HMO. Caper (1995) cited the On Lok program in San Francisco as very successful. For the past 20 years On Lok demonstrated the power of capitated payments. They were able to use Medicare and Medicaid dollars in creative ways and coordinated transportation, health services, home care services, and other services needed by the elderly in an effective way.

Health care services in the United States began with a very simple model. Physicians provided care in their offices and made home visits. Patients were admitted to hospitals for general care if they experienced serious complications during the course of their illness. Today, a variety of highly skilled health care professionals provide comprehensive, preventive, restorative, rehabilitative, and palliative care. A broad array of services, general to highly specialized with multidelivery configurations, is available.

Personal care provided by physicians is delivered under five basic models:

- The solo practice of a physician in an office continues to be present in some communities.
- The single specialty group model consists of physicians in the same specialty who pool expenses, income, and offices.
- Multispecialty group practice provides for interaction across specialty areas.

- The integrated health maintenance model that has prepaid multispecialty physicians.
- Community health center—developed through federal monies in the 1960s—addresses broader inputs into health such as education and housing.

The fourth model is the dominant model of the 1990s, including primary care and specialty physicians and, more and more frequently, other nonphysician specialists. Personal health services in the private sector are also provided by a variety of persons other than physicians. Nurse practitioners work in clinics, outpatient departments, and other primary care facilities. The allied health professional group, including physical therapists, occupational therapists, respiratory therapists, and numerous other groups, is one of the fastest growing segments of the health care profession that provides personal health services. A study by the DHHS estimated growth between 1970 and 1990 at 144% (Pew Health Professions Commission, 1995). In addition, there are other kinds of persons who provide many personal health services. Ethnic healers such as curanderos, community folk healers, and acupuncturists are examples of a wide array of folk healers (see Chapter 2).

Voluntary Agencies

Voluntary or nonofficial agencies are a part of the private health care system and developed at the same time that the government was assuming responsibility for public health in the United States. During the first century in the United States, voluntary efforts were virtually nonexistent because early settlers from western Europe were not accustomed to participating in organized charity. Immigration expanded to include slaves from Africa and persons from eastern Europe, and their well-being received little attention. Toward the end of the 19th century, new immigrants brought with them a heritage of social protest and reform. Wealthy business people such as the Rockefellers, Carnegies, and Mellons responded to the needs and set up foundations that provided health and welfare money for charitable endeavors. District nurses such as Lillian Wald established nursing practices in the large cities for the poor and destitute.

Voluntary agencies according to Hanlon and Pickett (1984) fall into several categories. They are those concerned with (1) specific diseases, such as the American Diabetes Association, American Cancer Society, and Multiple Sclerosis Society; (2) organ or body structures, such as National Kidney Foundation

EXAMPLES OF VOLUNTARY AGENCIES

American Cancer Society	National Kidney Foundation
American Heart Association	National Council on Aging
National Safety Council	Planned Parenthood
American Red Cross	Rockefeller Foundation
American Nurses Association	Visiting Nurse Associations
National League for Nursing	United Fund
American Public Health Association	

and American Heart Association; (3) health and welfare of special groups such as National Council on Aging; and (4) particular phases of health such as Planned Parenthood Federation of America. There are also major philanthropic groups that support research and programs. There are, in addition, many professional organizations such as American Medical Association and American Nurses Association. Voluntary organizations provide major sources of help in prevention of disease, promotion of health, treatment of illness, and research. For example, private and voluntary organizations support acquired immunodeficiency syndrome (AIDS) patients today. In many cities, the Chicken Soup Brigade provides meals for AIDS patients who are unable to cook for themselves. AIDS support groups exist in most larger communities. There is frequent overlap of services among the numerous private, voluntary, and public agencies. The private and public agencies provide a wide array of services but because of overlap are sometimes not cost effective. Without both voluntary and official agencies the array of services would be less than what is currently available. The past as prologue to the future is somewhat uncertain for voluntary agencies today, because major changes are occurring in health care. According to the Pew Commission, the emerging health care system will be an amalgam of different public and private forces that will work together to provide integrated, resource-conscious, population-based services (Pew Health Professions Commission, 1995). The system will also be more innovative and diverse in how it provides for health and more concerned with disease prevention and promotion of health.

Public Health Subsystem and Preventive Health Services

To obtain practice in the role of public health nurse or community health nurse and effectively meet responsibilities, one needs to understand the mission, organization, and role of the public health subsystem and the context within which it functions. The public health care subsystem needs to assume a leadership role to identify what is needed to provide a safe environment conducive to health. An organizational framework in which private and voluntary organizations and the government work collectively to prevent disease and promote health is essential. Public health and community health nurses are in a unique position to provide leadership and to facilitate change in the health care system. The public health subsystem, organization, and scope of activities are addressed.

The public health subsystem is mandated by law to address the health of populations. Activities are covered by legal provisions at both state and national levels of government. At the federal level, Congress enacts laws, and rules and regulations are written. The various departments of the executive branch implement and administer them. The U.S. Constitution mandates that the federal government "promote the general welfare of its citizens." Interpretations of and amendments to the Constitution and Supreme Court decisions over time have changed and increased the role of the federal government for health activities. National policies and practices have had an increasing influence on state and local governments in meeting health and social problems. During the past five decades, many laws have been enacted to respond to changing health needs. Two examples of these laws are the Medicare and Medicaid legislation (1965) and the Occupational Safety and Health Act (1970). The former legislation provides for health services for older adults and the poor. The latter law addresses working conditions.

Public health with its focus on populations can be described by the following: Public health is the effort organized by society to protect, promote, and restore the people's health. The program, services, and institutions involved emphasize the prevention of disease and the health needs of the population as a whole. Public health activities change with changing technology and social values, but the goals remain the same: to reduce the amount of disease, premature death, and disease-produced discomfort and disability.

(SHEPS, 1976, P. 3)

The activities of the public health subsystem are directed toward the protection of individuals from hazards in their environment. Thus, the focus of public health is threefold: to search for causes of disease, to develop ways to protect the public against disease, and to establish programs to address community health priorities. The definition of public health has changed over time to reflect the changing health care needs of society. The values of society, principles that guide actions, current knowledge, and social policy determine the public health activities at any given time. For example, as the population has grown and more people live in proximity to each other, it has become necessary for collective action to institute measures to respond to the effects of urbanization (Ellencweig & Yoshpe, 1984).

Public health services are predicated on the principle of social justice. The goal of social justice is to decrease preventable death and disability. The social justice model assumes that everyone is entitled equally to valued ends (e.g., status, income, happiness, and health protection). Therefore, the programs and services target groups who lack the resources and ability to obtain needed health care. However, the market justice model is the one that is most prominent in our country. This model states that persons are entitled to what they can acquire by their own efforts. This belief in individual responsibility affects the health policy of the governmental health agencies. The efforts remain focused on subsidizing the private sector when significant deficiencies are acknowledged (Beauchamp, 1984). The monies awarded in the form of grants and contracts for education (nurse training) and research, monies for construction of health facilities (Hill-Burton), and legislation of Medicare and Medicaid are examples of these efforts. If the social justice model was implemented, health services would be planned and organized with collective action by the private sector in collaboration with governmental agencies. Beauchamp (1984) suggested the following principles that need to be in practice for true social justice to occur:

Controlling hazards of the world to prevent death and disability through organized collective action shared equally by all except where unequal burdens result in increased protection of everyone's health.

(BEAUCHAMP, 1984, P. 309)

ROLE OF GOVERNMENT IN PUBLIC HEALTH

The following discussion describes the organizational structure and the scope of services of the three governmental levels (federal, state, and local). The public health subsystem is organized in multiple levels—federal, state, and local—to more effectively provide services to those who are unable to obtain it without assistance and to establish laws, rules, and regulations to protect the public. The organization of the public health subsystem reflects the values and belief of this country in the separation of powers between the federal government and the states. States have the responsibility for the promulgation of laws to protect the public and for provision of needed public health services. Each level of government has a distinctive role. The public health subsystem is concerned with the health of the population and a healthy environment. The scope of public health is broad in nature and encompasses activities that promote good health. As societal values change and new health and social problems are recognized and we have the knowledge and ability to solve perceived problems, the programs and services of public health will change.

Federal Level

Organization

Most health-related activities are implemented and administered in the DHHS (Fig. 3–2). This department is directed by a secretary, numerous under secretaries, and assistant secretaries. The surgeon general is the principal deputy to the assistant secretary of DHHS. The DHHS has five major agencies: Office of Human Development Services, Public Health Service, Health Care Financing Administration, Social Security Administration, and Family Support Administration.

The Office of Human Development Services is an umbrella agency responsible for programs for special needs of populations such as congregate meals for the elderly. The Health Care Financing Administration administers Medicare and Medicaid programs and carries out activities related to assurance of quality care. The Social Security Administration coordinates all activities related to implementing the Social Security law, including Supplemental Security Income for the Aged, Blind, and Disabled (SSI). The Family Support Administration carries out functions to strengthen the family unit.

The U.S. Public Health Service has six units. The

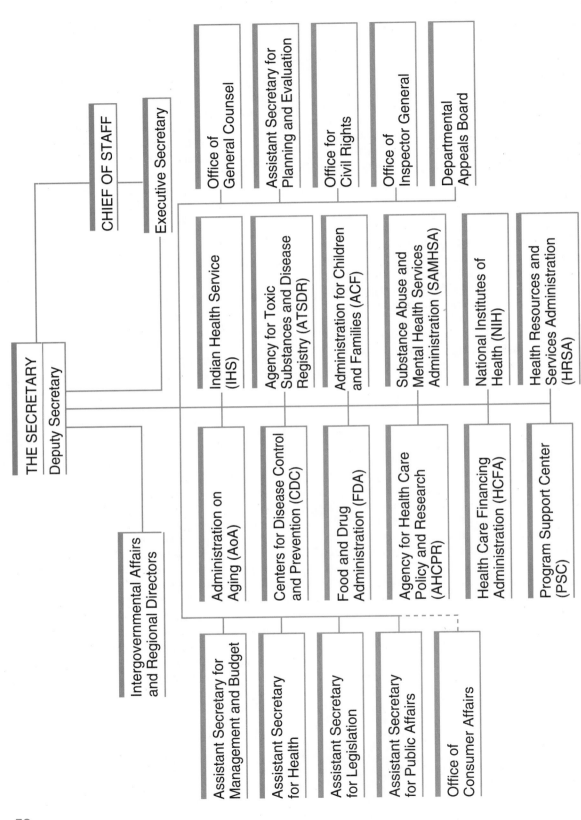

THE SECRETARY
Deputy Secretary

CHIEF OF STAFF
Executive Secretary

Intergovernmental Affairs and Regional Directors

Office of General Counsel

Assistant Secretary for Planning and Evaluation

Office for Civil Rights

Office of Inspector General

Departmental Appeals Board

Indian Health Service (IHS)

Agency for Toxic Substances and Disease Registry (ATSDR)

Administration for Children and Families (ACF)

Substance Abuse and Mental Health Services Administration (SAMHSA)

National Institutes of Health (NIH)

Health Resources and Services Administration (HRSA)

Assistant Secretary for Management and Budget

Assistant Secretary for Health

Assistant Secretary for Legislation

Assistant Secretary for Public Affairs

Office of Consumer Affairs

Administration on Aging (AoA)

Centers for Disease Control and Prevention (CDC)

Food and Drug Administration (FDA)

Agency for Health Care Policy and Research (AHCPR)

Health Care Financing Administration (HCFA)

Program Support Center (PSC)

Figure 3–2
Agencies that compose the U.S. Department of Health and Human Services.

Centers for Disease Control and Prevention conduct and support programs directed to prevent and control infectious diseases; they assist states during epidemics. In addition, they provide services related to health promotion and education and professional development and training. The Food and Drug Administration provides surveillance over the safety and efficacy of foods, pharmaceuticals, and other consumer goods. Health Resources and Service Administration is concerned with the development of health services programs and facilities. The Division of Nursing is in this unit. A major focus of this agency is funding grants related to education and training. The Indian Health Service is also in this unit; it provides health services for Native Americans and Alaskan Natives. The National Institutes of Health carry out and support research programs. The focus of their efforts is to develop and extend the scientific knowledge base related to their respective areas. The National Institute for Nursing Research is in this agency. The Alcohol, Drug Abuse, and Mental Health Administration awards grants related to problems on substance abuse and mental health. A major activity of these units is the administration of grants and contracts.

Other federal agencies perform activities related to health. For example, the Department of Education is involved with health education and school health; the Department of Agriculture is involved with inspection of meat and milk; in addition, it provides funds for the supplemental nutrition program for women, infants, and children (WIC); for the food stamp program; and for the school-based nutrition program. The Department of Interior is concerned with mining safety and stream pollution.

To facilitate coordination and provide more direct assistance to the states, there are 10 regional offices of the U.S. PHS (see Fig. 3–3). The regional offices carry out selected health programs, activities, and initiatives under the direction of the assistant secretary for health (Last, 1987b; Pickett and Hanlon, 1990; Wilner et al., 1978; Wilson and Neuhauser, 1985).

Scope

The federal government targets three major areas: the general population, special populations, and international health. Activities included in the general population category relate to the protection against hazards, maintaining vital and health statistics, advancing scientific knowledge through research, and providing disaster relief.

In recent years, public health efforts were directed toward changing behaviors by fostering the eating of healthy foods, exercising, and stopping or preventing the use of tobacco, drugs, and alcohol. Other programs have provided nutritional food and food stamps to individuals and families to provide adequate food intake, which reduces the risk of illness resulting from lowered resistance caused by malnutrition.

Services for special populations include protection of workers against hazardous occupations and work conditions and health care for veterans, American Indians, Alaskan natives, federal prisoners, and members of the armed services. In addition, they provide special services for children, older adults, mentally ill, and the vocationally handicapped.

In the international arena, the federal government, a member of WHO, works with other countries and international health organizations to promote various health programs throughout the world (Hanlon and Pickett, 1984; Last, 1987a; Wilner et al., 1978; Wilson and Neuhauser, 1985).

> In sum, with the increasing complexity of health problems, the federal government has a more active role in promoting the health of the citizens of this country. Activities that occur at the federal level include (1) financing Medicare for older adults and Medicaid for persons without means to pay for needed health and support services and (2) regulating health services through establishment of standards and accreditation of health care institutions and professional schools. A major activity at the federal level is the conducting of research and financial support to the scientific community to determine causes of disease, to develop effective measures to prevent and control disease, and to provide effective treatments. Other research efforts are directed to determine more efficient and effective ways to deliver care. Many activities are directed to protect the public through surveillance of communicable diseases and quarantine of imported diseases.

State Level

Organization

States are responsible for the health of their citizens. They are the central authorities in the public health care system. There is wide variation in the organization of public health among the states; and activities vary greatly among the states. In a recent survey in

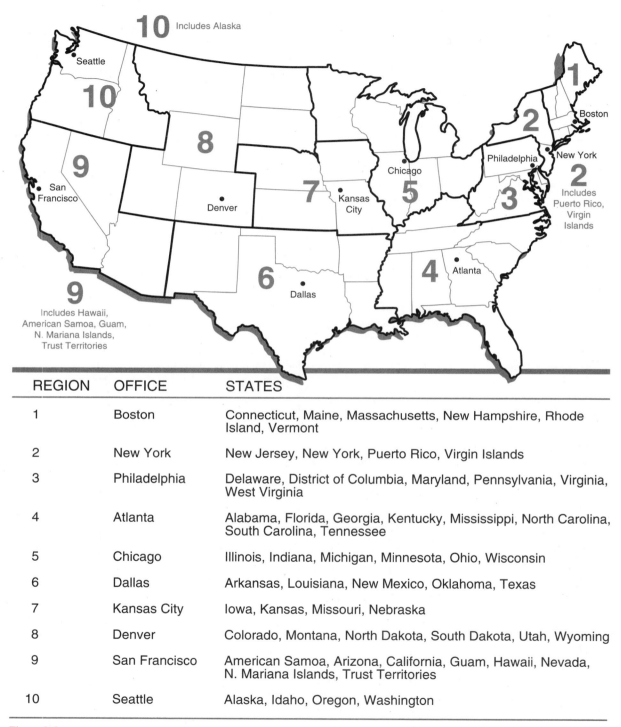

REGION	OFFICE	STATES
1	Boston	Connecticut, Maine, Massachusetts, New Hampshire, Rhode Island, Vermont
2	New York	New Jersey, New York, Puerto Rico, Virgin Islands
3	Philadelphia	Delaware, District of Columbia, Maryland, Pennsylvania, Virginia, West Virginia
4	Atlanta	Alabama, Florida, Georgia, Kentucky, Mississippi, North Carolina, South Carolina, Tennessee
5	Chicago	Illinois, Indiana, Michigan, Minnesota, Ohio, Wisconsin
6	Dallas	Arkansas, Louisiana, New Mexico, Oklahoma, Texas
7	Kansas City	Iowa, Kansas, Missouri, Nebraska
8	Denver	Colorado, Montana, North Dakota, South Dakota, Utah, Wyoming
9	San Francisco	American Samoa, Arizona, California, Guam, Hawaii, Nevada, N. Mariana Islands, Trust Territories
10	Seattle	Alaska, Idaho, Oregon, Washington

Figure 3–3
U.S. Public Health Service regional offices.

which 46 states responded to the question of organizational type, 25 (50%) indicated that they are independent, cabinet-level public health agencies; 13 (26%) were in a department with other services such as social services; and 6 (12%) were in integrated human services departments (Scott et al., 1990).

Most state agencies are directed by a health commissioner or secretary of health. The commissioner/secretary of health is appointed by the state governor. Each state also has a health officer, usually a physician with a degree and experience in public health. In some states, the health officer directs the health department. Twenty-four states have Boards of Health, which determine policies and priorities for allocation of funds. Staffing of the state agency varies among states. Health programs have the largest staff. Nurses represent the largest group of professionals providing health services (Hanlon and Pickett, 1984; Last, 1987b; Wilner et al., 1978; Wilson and Neuhauser, 1985).

Scope

Because each state is responsible for its own public health laws, there is wide variation in state policy among the 50 states. Factors that affect the level of state services include per capita income, political factors related to division of power between state and local health departments, and competition among officials, providers, and the business community. Three major functions that categorize state activities are assessment, policy development, and assurance (IOM, 1988). Assessment activities include collection of data pertaining to vital statistics, health facilities, and human resources; epidemiologic activities such as communicable disease control, health screening, and laboratory analyses; and participation in research projects (IOM, 1988). In the area of policy development, states formulate goals, develop health plans, and set standards for local health agencies. Assurance activities involve inspection in a variety of areas, licensing, health education, environmental safety, personal health services, and resource development.

The IOM in 1988 recommended 13 specific duties of state health departments. A survey of state health officers (n = 50) showed that, although they agreed that the duties were appropriate (>84%), there was a wide variation (26–86%) in the actual implementation of these duties. Two activities less frequently done by states were the integration of mental health services and the establishment of standards for minimum services provided by the state. The two duties most frequently implemented by states were the provision of subsidies and direct assistance to local health departments and the assessment of state health needs. States currently not implementing the duties indicated that they would in the future assess state needs and provide assistance to local health departments (85–100%); fewer states (65%) planned to establish standards; and only 38% planned to integrate mental health services (Centers for Disease Control, 1990a; U.S. Public Health Service, 1990a).

Local Health Departments

Organization

The day-to-day responsibility for protecting the health of citizens resides in the local health departments (LHDs). They are responsible for the direct delivery of public health services. The authority to conduct these activities is delegated by the state and local governments (city, county). Four states—Delaware, Hawaii, Rhode Island, and Vermont—do not have LHDs. The other 46 states have a total of 2262 LHDs. Within the 50 states, there are 3041 counties, 82,290 units of government, and 14,851 school districts that also provide some health-related services (Brecher, 1990, p. 298). The 2262 LHDs were located in the following jurisdictional units: county, 49%; town-township, 13%; city, 10%; 20% were combined departments city-county; and 7% were multiple county (National Association of County Health Officials, 1989, p. 19).

Local health departments are directed by a health officer or administrator appointed by local government. Twenty-one states require the health officer of a local health department to have a medical degree. A multidisciplinary team carries out the activities of the department. Public health nurses and health inspectors represent the two largest groups of professional staff. Other professional staff include dentists, social workers, epidemiologists, nutritionists, and health educators.

The organizational structure of LHDs varies within and among states. Some LHDs function as district offices of the state health department, others are responsible to local government and the state, and still others are autonomous (large cities). Local health departments may be a separate agency or a division within an agency such as health and human services. The population they serve ranges from a few hundred to hundreds of thousands. The relationship between LHDs and state public health agencies varies in the cooperation and sharing of responsibility for programs (Hanlon and Pickett, 1984; Last, 1987b; Wilner et al., 1978; Wilson and Neuhauser, 1985).

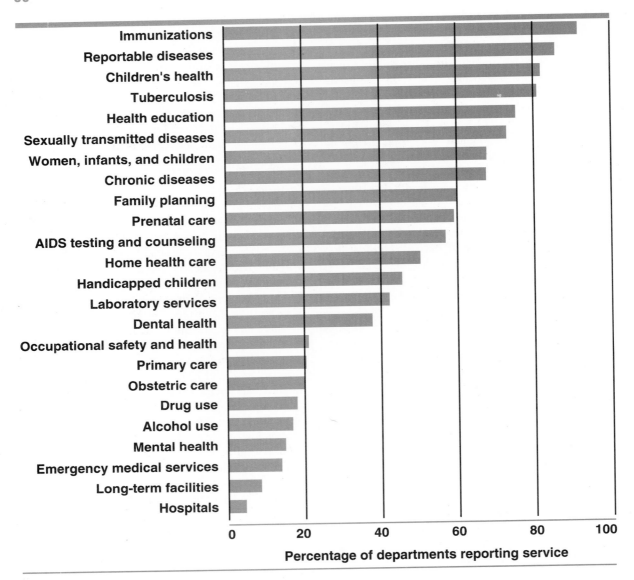

Figure 3–4
Services reported by local health departments. Services are provided very unevenly in the 2262 local health departments reporting. (Redrawn from Centers for Disease Control: Health objectives for the Nation: Selected Characteristics of Local Health Departments—United States, 1989. MMWR (Morb Mortal Wkly Rep) 39:609, 1990a; U.S. Public Health Service, 1990b.)

Scope

The local health departments are responsible for determining the health status and needs of their constituents, identifying unmet needs, and taking action to see that the unmet needs are adequately met. Most services to groups and individuals are provided at the local level. These activities fall into four major categories: community health services, environmental health services, mental health services, and personal health services. Community health services include control of communicable disease (surveillance and immunizations), maternal-child health programs, nutrition, and education. Specific activities include health promotion teaching directed toward changing behavior by eating healthy foods, increasing exercise, and decreasing the use of tobacco, drugs, and alcohol. Other programs provide nutritional food and food stamps to individuals and families to provide adequate food intake, which reduces the risk of illness resulting from nutritional deficit. Preventive screening for potential problems throughout the life span is a major activity of LHDs. Screening leads to early detection of diseases such as genetic disorders, developmental delay, behavior disorders, hypertension, diabetes, and cancer. Environmental health services range from food hygiene (inspection of food producing and processing and restaurant inspection); protection from hazardous substances to control of waste, air, noise, and water pollution; and occupational health. The objective of these activities is to provide a safe environment.

The personal health services provide care to individuals and families in clinics, schools, prisons, and clients' homes. Other activities include disaster planning, programmatic planning within departments and with other agencies, and coordinating programs between the public and private sectors. The scope of services varies among LHDs (Fig. 3–4). These functions and services range from the control of communicable disease, environmental health, food hygiene,

health education, clinic services, screening programs, and home care to disaster planning and coordination of voluntary service agencies.

The data in Table 3–1 indicate that Regions 9 and 10 (West Coast) have been actively involved in providing services related to AIDS testing and counseling, sexually transmitted diseases, immunizations, and tuberculosis; Region 1 has been less active in these functions. To interpret the appropriateness and completeness of the services provided, an understanding of the demographic characteristics and needs of the region is required.

In the preceding description of the three governmental levels that provide public health services, distinctive and overlapping roles have been discussed. The federal government has been assuming a larger role in the protection of the population through regulation and funding. The federal government finances specific programs such as Medicare and categorical programs for mothers and infants and provides direct care to special populations (veterans).

Table 3–1
Percentage of Local Health Departments That Reported Being Active in Selected Functions and Services by Region

Functions and Services	Public Health Service Region									
	1	2	3	4	5	6	7	8	9	10
Reportable disease data collection	75%	92%	97%	94%	87%	88%	80%	77%	96%	96%
Health planning	39%	80%	62%	55%	64%	49%	51%	58%	74%	78%
Food and milk control	83%	82%	94%	81%	66%	73%	42%	49%	73%	70%
Health education	47%	90%	84%	79%	77%	75%	74%	71%	83%	81%
Hazardous waste management	60%	70%	40%	36%	42%	47%	23%	42%	70%	66%
Individual water supply safety	66%	79%	93%	89%	76%	80%	62%	60%	73%	80%
Vector and animal control	57%	85%	81%	77%	77%	70%	41%	57%	77%	72%
AIDS testing and counseling	12%	41%	86%	94%	41%	62%	45%	56%	93%	99%
Child health	35%	96%	92%	99%	86%	94%	89%	83%	91%	93%
Family planning	6%	29%	92%	98%	44%	82%	58%	55%	86%	74%
Immunizations	61%	98%	100%	100%	96%	98%	96%	85%	97%	100%
Prenatal care	10%	50%	76%	93%	53%	77%	43%	59%	52%	82%
Sexually transmitted diseases	20%	77%	97%	99%	68%	92%	55%	63%	99%	95%
Tuberculosis	40%	83%	98%	99%	78%	96%	74%	60%	97%	100%
No. of departments	327	158	124	478	486	239	206	108	69	74

AIDS, acquired immunodeficiency syndrome.

Based on National Association of County Health Officials. NACHO's response to the IOM report: The future of public health. J Public Health Policy 10:95–98, 1989.

States establish health codes, regulate the insurance industry, and license health care facilities and personnel. States also provide funds for services offered through Medicaid. Direct care activities funded by state health departments may include care in mental hospitals, state medical schools, and associated hospitals. Local health departments are the primary agencies that provide the majority of direct services to community, families, and individuals. Local health departments establish local health codes, fund public hospitals (city-county), and provide services to both populations and individuals at risk. Programs and services for both the state and local health departments vary across jurisdictions. The services provided reflect the values of the residents and officials, the available resources, and the perceived needs of their respective populations within their state and local area.

Although the goals of the public health subsystem do not change, the programs and services provided change to meet the changing needs of the public. The leading causes of death illustrate the changing focus of public health. The incidence of pneumonia, diarrhea, and diseases of the heart has decreased in the population. Priorities at this time include activities related to violent and abusive behavior; vitality; independence of older persons; human immunodeficiency virus infection prevention; and health education.

As the role of the government at all three levels evolved, four broad areas of concern emerge: lifestyle behavior, human biology, the environment, and the organization of the system and its programs. The IOM (1988) report stated that the mission of the public health system is to see that vital elements are in place to ensure the conditions in which people can be healthy and provide basic health services to persons who are unable to access the private sector.

Two potential influences on the future of the public health subsystem include the IOM's "The Future of Public Health" (1988) and the Health Objectives 2000 Act (1990), proposed by the Association of State and Territorial Health Officials. These two documents are expected to have a profound influence on the future and can provide the framework for how public health will be structured and how it could function as we move boldly into the 21st century.

The 1988 report from the IOM entitled "The Future of Public Health" remains a very influential document. From a historic perspective, the report stimulated a very productive and extended discussion within the public health community regarding its findings that public health was in disarray nationally and had lost its constituency. Some public health leaders disagree with several premises of the report (Sommer, 1995). With the strong emergence of managed care, many clients previously served by state and local health departments are receiving care from HMOs. Sommer (1995) proposed that the population perspective held by public health places it in a pivotal position to play a dominant role in all health care for the future. He viewed the future public health as developing a data system that truly measures and tracks the health of everyone more effectively. He also saw public health as integrating both curative and preventive services at the levels of the individual and society (Sommer, 1995, p. 661).

The IOM report was also very influential in its articulation of the core functions of public health agencies within the public health system. These were *assessment* (the gathering and analysis of epidemiologic and other community health status information), *policy development* (the blending of the science of public health with community values and politics to formulate strategies to address identified problems), and *assurance* (the process of improving access to health services for individuals and of improving the health status of the community as well as using assessment information in the implementation of policy). These important functions would be at the core of public health reform at the national and state levels throughout the next decade.

The U.S. Conference of Local Health Officers viewed "The Future of Public Health" (1988) as a valuable planning document, useful at all levels. They stated that the IOM report offers a variety of "recommendations that are of value to the future of public health in general and to local public health in particular" (p. 90). Each recommendation contains specific details for implementation. An overarching concept is the importance of partnership among federal, state, and local levels of government and the building of close networks between public and private agencies. Public agencies working with HMOs and other forms of managed care is one strategy.

"Promoting Health/Preventing Disease Objectives for the Nation 1980" (U.S. Public Health Service, 1980) is viewed in concert with the IOM report (Health Objectives 2000 Act, 1990) because together they provide substantive goals for which the organization and structure of the public health subsystem are directed.

GOALS FOR THE NATION

The Year 2000 Health Objectives identify 298 specific health objectives in 22 priority areas. The objectives aim to reduce infant mortality, increase life expectancy, reduce disability caused by chronic conditions, increasing years of healthy life, and decreasing the disparity in life expectancy between white and minority populations.

Various health professionals and organizations use the Year 2000 Health Objectives in setting priorities. "Healthy People 2000, 1994" (National Center for Health Statistics, 1995) reported progress made thus far. Eight percent of the goals have been met; progress is made in 41%. For 16% of the goals, there was movement away rather than toward the goal. An example given was obesity. Overweight among adults and children has increased rather than decreased. However, smoking in adults has decreased, death from automobile accidents has decreased, mammography in women has increased, and deaths from heart disease and stroke are reduced for the population as a whole and for blacks as well. The decrease for blacks declined more slowly than for whites, so the disparity between blacks and whites increased.

FUTURE OF THE HEALTH CARE SYSTEM

There has been a significant shift in thinking about the future of the health care system since the beginning of the 1990s. Congressional elections that focused on the issue of health reform and the emphasis on reform by a newly elected president seemed to signify the emergence of health care reform as a national priority. The defeat of the ambitious national agenda in combination with emergence of a strong antigovernment sentiment called into question the nation's ability to address this issue at all. At the same time, the emergence of public health as a developing—if not full—partner in these discussions seemed to hold promise for community-based services in the future.

The predictions of futurists in the late 1980s and early 1990s were tempered by these events. The innovations carried out at the state level during this period increasingly provided the "testing ground" for reform efforts. The increasing emphasis on public health during this period at the state and national levels offered some hope for a broader definition of health, including substantial emphasis on health promotion and disease prevention, in the future.

Those predicting the future of the health system have their challenges set for them in such changing times. Those authors writing in the late 1980s (Arthur Andersen, 1987; Ebert & Ginzberg, 1988; Kovner, 1990) placed the debate within a national reform context. Those authors writing in the mid-1990s (Butler, 1995; Devers et al., 1994) described a future far more reliant on the marketplace and local initiatives.

Health Care Financing

ACCESS

The current health care system is pluralistic and competitive. By definition, the system provides fragmented and uncoordinated care. Private care agencies-institutions are in competition with each other for clients, health professionals, and resources. Even with recent market reforms, two hospitals in the same geographic area may be competing for the same patients. Hospital home care programs are in direct competition with private home care agencies. Hospitals, as they diversify services to become economically viable, compete with HMOs for the ambulatory market. Public health services can be viewed as indirectly competing for resources (Rice, 1990; Schulz & Johnson, 1990).

The health care agencies functioning in isolation from each other provide fragmented services. Although multiple services are available for the wellness–serious illness continuum, coordination is lacking. Services range from office-clinic, home care, adult day care, acute care institutions, and specialized institutions to skilled nursing facilities. The services provided by one agency or one provider do not help the individual to transit (move) across boundary lines and receive services offered by others. In addition, the services tend to be geographically separated, and each agency has different criteria for access. The focus of services has not kept pace with the changing needs of individuals and populations, and many millions of Americans lack access to health care services and are unable to use available health services because of inadequate financial resources.

Currently, about 40 million Americans do not have health insurance, and an additional 33.4 million cannot afford private coverage and are enrolled in Medicaid (Robert Wood Johnson Foundation, 1994). There are also approximately 4 million illegal immigrants in the

United States who perform domestic work, agricultural work, and services that are not insured. These large numbers of persons have limited, if any, access to a health care system that has become increasingly expensive. By 1993 the national health expenditures reached $884.2 billion dollars, or $3299 per person (Robert Wood Johnson Foundation, 1994). Out-of-pocket health care costs have decreased from 49.8% of health care costs in 1965 to 19.8% in 1991 (Robert Wood Johnson Foundation, 1994), with the change primarily resulting from a shift to payment through health insurance. Today insurance companies are reducing what and how much they will pay in response to employer pressure and market forces. Employers are reducing benefits, and many are requiring employees to pay for a portion of their insurance. These latter trends will influence how much out-of-pocket costs become in the future. Much of what will occur will be dependent on efforts toward cost containment, which are described later.

Although costs continue to increase, and treatments are not too successful in treating chronic diseases and emerging health problems such as AIDS, smoking-related illnesses, and substance abuse, the majority of health care dollars go toward diagnosis and treatment of these conditions rather than prevention. This support is fostered in part by personal attitudes in which individuals tend to seek care only when it is urgently needed (i.e., interference with ability to function) and by reimbursement policies geared to acute illness. In addition, if recovery does occur, it is most frequently attributed to health services received, although evidence supports Scrimshaw's (1974, p. 794) conclusion that "no matter what is done patients get well most of the time."

Over the past decade, privatization of health care has occurred. The public sector, following the enactment of Medicare-Medicaid, channeled governmental dollars into the nonprofit sector to provide needed services. The exception was fee for service to physicians. During the 1980s, the social policy changed from improving access to containing costs. The Omnibus Budget Reconciliation Acts (1981, 1987, 1989, 1990) stimulated competition and deregulation. These acts resulted in increasing amounts of public monies paid to the for-profit sector. Not only did the shift to for-profit providers occur, but at the same time health care dollars did not encourage growth, and the monies for social services was reduced by 20% (Bergthold et al., 1990). The shift toward for-profit providers is based on market principles: ability to pay determines

services attainable. It is a conscious move away from the equity principle: access for all who are in need of the services.

In 1990, the IOM established their Access Monitoring project partly in response to the fact that more than 35 million Americans, most of whom are employed or dependents of someone employed, lacked basic health insurance coverage (Institute of Medicine, 1993). This committee developed a set of indicators to monitor access to health care. Although the committee attempted to be consistent with the Year 2000 Health Objectives, the major focus was use of personal health services, including curative medical services. The committee studied access based on the principles of justice and equity. Fifteen access monitoring indicators were derived and were categorized into a set of national objectives for personal health care, which are as follows:

1. Promoting successful birth outcomes
2. Reducing the incidence of vaccine-preventable childhood diseases
3. Early detection and diagnosis of treatable diseases
4. Reducing the effects of chronic disease and prolonging life
5. Reducing morbidity and pain through timely and appropriate treatment (pp. 5–14)

The debate continues into the mid- and late 1990s regarding what services should be provided, who should have access to them, and how they should be delivered. Changes in the health care system are necessary to meet the changing needs of populations. The personal care subsystem needs to set limits on the care provided, setting criteria for use of technology and, determining which conditions will be treated, which interventions are effective, and who should receive the care (Banta, 1990). The legal and moral issues involved in setting criteria are just beginning to be addressed.

The health care system in the United States is complex, with social policies that favor pluralism, free choice, and free enterprise. The private sector personal care subsystem provides the majority of care to individuals. The private sector includes nonprofit and for profit agencies as well as voluntary organizations. The public health subsystem provides limited personal care services for socially marginal populations but for the most part subsidizes the private sector through Medicare/Medicaid reimbursement to provide these services.

COST CONTAINMENT

The private health care subsystem has up to now been characterized by individual autonomy of both providers and consumers. In the mid- to late 1990s, there is an unprecedented sense of urgency for hospitals, nursing homes, insurance companies, and the various forms of health care providers to join networks of care (Grehan et al., 1995). This movement was originally motivated by prospects of national health care reform but continues as a high priority in an effort to reduce health care costs and maintain quality. The report of the Pew Health Professions Commission (1995) noted that the cost of sustaining the health care system as it currently exists is no longer tenable.

The influx of federal dollars, available through Medicare-Medicaid reimbursement, increased the number of persons who had access to and obtained personal care services from the private sector. These dollars enable the private sector of the health care system to provide highly technical and personal care services (Robert Wood Johnson Foundation, 1994). In the past, the services provided with these federal dollars were based on the biomedical model and focused more on treatment than prevention. Diagnostic practice and treatments continue to depend on the most up-to-date and sophisticated technology. Reliance on expensive laboratory tests and the use of technology for both diagnosis and treatment has increased the cost of care annually. In 1993, more than $782 billion (88.5% of total health expenditures) was spent for personal health services (National Center for Health Statistics, 1995). Chronic conditions such as heart disease and cancer now replace infectious disease as a major health problem. During the 1970s, chronic diseases placed great demands on the personal care system, with treatments providing "relatively marginal benefits" (Banta, 1990; Rice, 1990; Verbrugge, 1990).

Schmitt (1983) concluded that consumers' dissatisfaction with the rising costs of service and health benefits not meeting their expectations caused them to question the right of all individuals to unlimited health care services. There are differing opinions concerning how satisfied or dissatisfied Americans are with the current health care system (Blendon, 1989; Ginzberg, 1990). However, Kovner (1990) did not believe there would be a fundamental break with the current health care system because of the limited power of the uninsured. Change in societal values resulted in policy changes that limited access to health care through the use of caps and rate regulation. Cost-containment policies were implemented in the 1980s. Managed care aims at cost containment in a more aggressive manner than the earlier policies. States see managed care as a solution to rising Medicaid costs and are swiftly converting their fee-for-service Medicaid plans into managed care. Forty-five states and the District of Columbia have Medicaid managed care plans (Robert Wood Johnson Foundation, 1994).

The greatest share of resources is channeled into the personal care subsystem (focus on individuals); this personal care subsystem continues to provide services based on the biomedical model, using high technology for diagnosis and treatment of disease. The public health subsystem provides limited services for socially marginal populations but continues to subsidize the private sector.

The social justice foundation of public health is yet to be realized because many inequities in access to health care still exist. There are more than 34 million (Robert Wood Johnson Foundation, 1994; Thomas et al., 1994) uninsured individuals in the United States at any point in time. Characteristics of uninsured persons reflect a wide range of incomes, races, and occupations. In addition, many individuals underuse the health care system; for example, the following groups do not receive any care: 17% of those with chronic illness; 15% of women in the first trimester of pregnancy; 20% of those with hypertension; and 38% of those who need dental care (Freeman et al., 1990, p. 317).

Health care expenditures in 1993 were $882 billion, 13.9% of the gross domestic product. For 1989 public health expenditures by states was $9669 million. Of this 36.7% was federal grants and contracts (Levit et al., 1994, p. 247). One fifth of public health expenditures was for supplemental food programs for women, infants, and children (WIC). Personal health expenditures accounted for 41% (Thomas et al., 1994). However, the increasing outlay of dollars has not significantly improved the health status of large segments of our society. For example, in 1992, 62.1% of Native American mothers and 63.9% of black mothers received care in the first trimester of pregnancy, whereas 80.8% of white mothers received care (National Center for Health Statistics, 1995). From 1980 to 1992, infant mortality declined by 37% for white infants but declined only 24% for black infants (National Center for Health Statistics, 1995).

Managed care, as indicated earlier in this chapter, is a fast-growing movement of the mid-1990s. Managed care may be a tightly run HMO such as Kaiser-Permanente or an affiliation of physicians and hospitals linked by marketing and formulas. This latter type of managed care is often coordinated by a large for-profit insurance company. According to the Robert Wood Johnson Foundation 1994 annual report, "Cost Containment," for-profit HMOs are the fastest growing types of managed care.

For additional information about primary care and care management, integral components of managed care and of other models of care delivery, which describe nursing's role, see appendix for "Models of Nursing Care Delivery and Case Management: Clarification of Terms" and "Population Management in an HMO: New Roles for Nursing."

An additional concept that extends the notion of networks is that of collaboration (Himmelman, 1995). Implied in a collaborative relationship is the development of partnerships among health care providers and health care consumers with a major focus on health rather than treatment of illness and disease. According to Porter-O'Grady (1995), the focus on health will challenge health care institutions to keep its subscribers from getting ill. "Healthy communities mean the organization partnering with other social institutions and services to address other issues of health, poverty, violence, family issues, children's health and environmental concerns" (p. 11).

State Initiatives in Health Care Reform

States have been in the forefront of reform, usually focusing on services to publicly sponsored residents. The state of Arizona, for example, has had a managed care program for Medicaid clients in place since 1982. Since the mid-1980s, states have increasingly been taking the lead in reform efforts. Accompanying the dramatic changes in the private sector in the late 1980s and early 1990s, states continue to accelerate movement of publicly sponsored patients into managed care. By 1994, seven states had requested or received full waivers from the federal Medicaid program to implement managed care programs (Holahan et al., 1995). These states included Florida, Hawaii, Kentucky, Minnesota, Oregon, Rhode Island, and Tennessee. States such as Minnesota, California, and Washington also began significant efforts to move Medicaid populations into managed care and to make other efforts to control public expenditures. The Robert Wood Johnson Foundation reported that, in 1994, 45

states and the District of Columbia had Medicaid managed care plans, involving 23% of the Medicaid population nationally (p. 14). Many providers previously reluctant to care for the Medicaid population now compete fiercely for the managed care contracts.

Implicit in the move to managed care was greater attention to health promotion and disease prevention. In states such as Oregon, attention was paid to health promotion and disease prevention as aspects of managed care and cost containment. An additional emphasis is on the financial consequences of supporting the medical care system. In Washington State, public health and the benefits of community-based prevention programs were placed at the center of reform efforts.

The Oregon experience remains a very interesting example. The Oregon legislature has legislated and outlined strategies to set priorities for state-funded services. The list of services was generated through public forums and reflects both public values and knowledge related to the efficacy of specific interventions. The budgeting process incorporates the prioritized list of services. If budgets need to be reduced, priorities on the lower end of the list would not be reimbursed. For example, in a rank of 13 community values (Capuzzi and Garland, 1990), prevention ranks first and mental health and chemical dependency rank eighth. With severe budget constraints, Oregon would continue to fund prevention but might have to eliminate or set stringent limits on mental health and chemical dependency. The Oregon form of rationing of health care is closely watched by other states as they continue their efforts at reform.

The Clinton Health Reform Initiative

The country appeared to be ready for health care reform when the Clinton administration took office (Skocpol, 1994). By 1990, support for reform had reached a 40-year high in the polls, and the election of Bill Clinton in 1992 brought health care debate onto the national agenda. Believing reform of the health care system to be part of his election mandate, the new president assembled an ambitious process to produce legislation for national reform of the health care system. The process was initially supported by diverse sectors of the system. As the shape of the Clinton proposals began to emerge, some participants began to distance themselves and ultimately opposed the reform approach. This was true in the case of all the major power constituents: business, physicians, and insurance companies. The insurance sector was probably the most vocal by making its objections known the earliest.

The approach used by the administration was very inclusive, with strong support for public health. The bill eventually proposed in congress included a version of the core functions outlined in the 1988 IOM study "The Future of Public Health." Public health's inclusion in the reform agenda fostered a renewed interest in prevention and health promotion. The focus was to improve health status and also contain costs. On the defeat of reform bills in 1994 and before the influential elections that fall, the consensus emerged that, despite the American public's recognition of the need for reform, there was little recognition that such reform would have specific consequences for individual Americans in terms of cost and choice (Starr, 1993).

A Return to Reform at the State Level

Subsequent to the failure of the Clinton health care initiative, a strong sentiment supporting limitations in the role of government resulted from the 1994 midterm elections. The Clinton reform proposal became a symbol of "big government." Thus, the proposed health care reforms subsequent to this election tended to focus on ways to reduce the role of the federal government.

The re-emergence of the concept of combining categorical funds into block grants and moving them to the states symbolized this movement by the mid-1990s. The concept of combining related federal categorical public health funds to states in block grants first emerged in the mid-1970s with President Nixon's concept of New Federalism. During this era, programs such as the Community Development Block Grant Program were implemented to move more authority to states. In the early 1980s President Reagan reintroduced this concept of block grants, turning a number of categorically funded federal programs into block grants. In addition to the state leadership concept, Reagan also saw the approach as a mechanism for making budget reductions.

Two key health block grants were created during this period—the Maternal and Child Health block grant and the Preventive Health and Health Services block grant, both of which are still in effect today. In the post-1994 emphasis on reducing the role of the national government, the concept was reintroduced for the first time since the early 1980s accompanying proposals to also block grant the Medicaid program and limit growth of Medicare. Significant in this latest emergence of the concept of sending federal health and medical programs to the states as block grants was the level of support for this effort from the states, despite the experience of the early 1980s, which resulted both in reductions in funding levels for such block grants and in continuing federal strings.

The block grant focus in the mid-1990s directly affected funding of community-based public health programs as virtually all of the programs of the federal Center for Disease Control and Prevention were to be combined into one or more block grants. The programs are the main federal funding of public health in most local jurisdictions.

Future of Public Health and the Health Care System

From the vantage point of the late 1990s—with the tremendous change the decade has seen—it is difficult to speculate on the role of community health in the next century. It does seem clear that the community health focus on health promotion and disease prevention and the population-based approach to community assessment are finding a new audience among the leadership of emerging health care systems intent on keeping their enrollees healthy. The concept of upstream thinking is also once again coming to the fore with new listeners. Local and national political leaders must begin to grapple with the health of the population and the need to reduce the levels of health care expenditures in a voluntary environment.

Public health must remain a full partner in these discussions. This has, of course, historically not been the case. Most futurists rarely identify the public health subsystem as a component of the health care system. Perhaps the historic involvement of the public health subsystem with the poor and disenfranchised is a major influence in inattention to their problems. The assumptions underlying the ecological model demand that attention be paid to the poor and underserved, but the political aspects of health care frequently demand a focus in another direction. Terris (1990) stated that international and domestic political and economic factors play a major role in public health policy now and in the future. A major change in policy will require fundamental changes in United States ideology and political stance.

Health promotion, disease prevention, and medical care must all remain priorities for programs proposed for the future. Whether future efforts in reform will be conceived within the framework of the ecological model and incorporate attention to living standards remains uncertain. Focus on environmental influences on population is critical for the future health of any nation.

As we have emphasized in this chapter, the goals for health care reflect the values of society. Last (1987a) pointed out that predicting future trends in human values is more difficult than predicting scientific discoveries or the patterns of disease. Thus, predicting the future is very difficult. However, Koop (1989) stated that the ultimate test of the public health subsystem is whether it effectively serves the people by *their* measurements, not those of the public health profession.

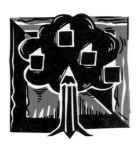

Learning Activities

1. Describe the organization of your state and local health departments.

2. Visit your local health department and learn what services are provided. Compare your health department's services with those listed in Figure 3–4 and identify possible gaps in local services.

3. Identify the regional and state services where you live and compare them with those described in the chapter (see Table 3–1).

4. Visit one voluntary agency; determine the services they offer and how the agency collaborates with the local public health agency.

5. Determine how your state health department has operationalized health goals for the year 2000.

6. Interview a public health nurse regarding perceptions of the Institute of Medicine report on nursing practice.

REFERENCES

Alma Ata World Health Organization and Children's Fund: Primary Health Care: A Joint Report. Geneva: World Health Organization, 1978.

American Public Health Association: Healthy Communities 2000: Model Standards, 3rd ed. Washington, DC, 1991.

Andersen Arthur & Co: The Future of Health Care: Changes and Choices. Chicago: American College of Health Care Executives, 1987.

Banta HD: What is health care? In Kovner AR (ed). Health Care Delivery in the United States, 4th ed. New York, Springer, 1990, pp. 8–30.

Beauchamp DE: Public health as social justice. In Lee PR, Estes CL, Ramsay NB (eds). The Nation's Health, 2nd ed. San Francisco, Boyd and Fraser, 1984, pp. 306–313.

Bergthold LA, Estes CL, Villanueve A: Public light and private dark: The privatization of home health services for the elderly in the U.S. Home Health Care Services Q 11:7–33, 1990.

Blendon RJ: Three systems: A comparative survey. Health Management Q 2:185–192, 1989.

Blum HL: Health and the Systems Approach, 2nd ed. New York, Human Sciences Press, 1981.

Brecher C: The government's role in health care. In Kovner, AR (ed): Health Care Delivery in the United States, 4th ed. New York: Springer, 1990, pp. 297–323.

Butler RN: What to do now on health care system reform. JAMA 273:253–254, 1995.

Caper P: The next shift: Managed care. Public Health Rep 110:682–693, 1995.

Capuzzi C, Garland M: The Oregon plan: Increasing access to health care. Nursing Outlook 38:260–263, 1990.

Centers for Disease Control: Health objectives for the nation. MMWR Morb Mortal Wkly Rep 39:607–610, 1990a.

Centers for Disease Control: Strengthening public health practice: Survey of state health officers. MMWR Morb Mortal Wkly Rep 39:773–776, 1990b.

Cohen SS: The politics of Medicaid: 1980–89. Nursing Outlook 36:229–233, 1990.

Confusion worse confounded: Health promotion and prevention (editorial). J Public Health Pol 11:144–145, 1990.

Devers KJ, Shortell SM, Gillies RP, et al.: Implementing organized delivery systems: An integration scorecard. Health Care Management Rev 19:7–20, 1994.

Ebert RH, Ginzberg E: The reform of medical education. Health Affairs Suppl 7:5–38, 1988.

Ellencweig AY, Yoshpe RB: Definition of public health. Public Health Rev 12:65–78, 1984.

Freeman HE, et al.: Americans report on their access to health care. *In* Lee PR, Estes CL, eds.: The Nation's Health, 3rd ed. Boston, Jones and Bartlett, 1990, pp. 309–319.

Ginzberg E: A non-conforming view. Health Management Q 12:20–22, 1990.

Green LW, Raeburn J: Contemporary developments in health promotion: Definitions and challenges. *In* Bracht N, ed. Health Promotion at the Community Level. Newbury Park, CA, Sage, 1990, pp. 29–42.

Grehan ML, Mannheim LM, Hughes SL: Predicting agency participation in interorganizational networks providing community care. Medical Care 33:441–451, 1995.

Haggerty RJ: The boundaries of health care. *In* Lee PR, Estes CL, (eds). The Nation's Health, 3rd ed. Boston, Jones and Bartlett, 1990, pp. 112–117.

Hanlon G, Pickett J: Public health administration and practice, 8th ed. St. Louis, Times Mirror/Mosby, 1984, pp. 143–156.

Health Care Financing Administration: Health Care Financing Program Statistics: Medicare and Medicaid Data Book (publication no. 03270). Washington, DC, Health Care Financing Administration, 1988, pp. 59–123.

Health Objectives 2000 Act, S2056. Washington, DC, U.S. Government Printing Office. February, 1, 1990.

The health objectives 2000 act. Our first and foremost legislative goal (editorial). J Public Health Policy 2:141–143, 1990.

Himmelman, AT: On the theory and practice of transformational collaboration: Collaboration as a bridge from social service to social justice. Unpublished manuscript, March, 1995.

Holahan J, Coughlin T, Ku L, et al.: Insuring the poor through Section 1115 Medical waivers. Health Affairs 14 (1): 199–216, 1995.

Institute of Medicine: The National Academy of Science: The Future of Public Health. Washington, DC, National Academy Press, 1988.

Institute of Medicine: Access to Health Care in America. Washington, DC, National Academy Press, 1993.

Koop CE: An agenda for public health. J Public Health Policy 10:7–18, 1989.

Kovner AR (ed): Health Care Delivery in the United States, 4th ed. New York, Springer, 1990.

Last JM: Organization of public health services. *In* Public Health and Human Ecology. East Norwalk, CT, Appleton and Lange, 1987a, pp. 1–26.

Last JM: Public Health and Human Ecology. East Norwalk, CT, Appleton and Lange, 1987b.

Levit KR, Sensenig AL, Cowan CA, et al.: Health Care Financing Rev 16:247–294, 1994.

McKeown T: Determinants of health. *In* Lee PR, Estes, CL (eds). The Nation's Health, 3rd ed. Boston, Jones and Bartlett, 1990, pp. 6–13.

National Association of County Health Officials: NACHO's response to the IOM report: The future of public health. J Public Health Policy 10:95–98, 1989.

National Center for Health Statistics, Health United States, 1994. Washington, DC, U.S. Government Printing Office, 1995.

Ottawa Charter for Health Promotion 1986. Ottawa, Canadian Public Health Association, 1986.

Pew Health Professions Commission: Critical challenges: Revitalizing the health professions for the twenty-first century. San Francisco: UCSF Center for the Health Professions, 1995.

Pickett G, Hanlon JJ: Public Health Administration and Practice, 9th ed. St. Louis, Times Mirror/Mosby, 1990, pp. 97–133.

Porter-O'Grady TC: Managing along the continuum: A new paradigm for the clinical manager. Nurs Admin Q 19:1–12, 1995.

Rice DP: The medical care system: Past trends and future projections. *In* Lee PR, Estes CL (eds). The Nation's Health, 3rd ed. Boston, Jones and Bartlett, 1990, pp. 72–93.

Robert Wood Johnson Foundation: Annual Report: Cost Containment. Princeton, NJ.

Schmitt GH: How we deliver care. Issues Health Care 4:8–11, 1983.

Schulz R, Johnson AC: Management of Hospitals and Health Services, 3rd ed. St. Louis, CV Mosby, 1990.

Scott HD, Tierney JT, Waters WJ: The future of public health: A survey of the states. J Public Health Policy 11:296–304, 1990.

Scott HD, Tierney JT, Waters WJ: The year 2,000 national health objectives. J Public Health Policy 12:145–147, 1991.

Scrimshaw N: Myths and realities in international health planning. Am J Public Health 64:792–797, 1974.

Sheps CG: Higher education for public health: A Report of the Milbank Memorial Fund Commission. New York, Prodist, 1976.

Skocpol T: From social security to health security? J Health Politics, Policy and Law 19:239–242, 1994.

Sommer A: Whither public health? Public Health Rep 110:657–661, 1995.

Starr P: The framework of health care reform. N Engl J Med 329:1666–1672, 1993.

Stokes J III, Noren JJ, Shindell S: Definitions of terms and concepts applicable to clinical preventive medicine. J Community Health 8:33–41, 1982.

Terris M: Public health policy for the 1990's. J Public Health Policy 11:281–295, 1990.

Thomas RK, Pol LG, Sennert WF: Health Care Book of Lists. Winter Park, FL, PMD Publishers Group, 1994.

U.S. Public Health Service: Healthy People—The Surgeon General's Report on Health Promotion and Disease Prevention. Washington, DC, U.S. Government Printing Office, 1979.

U.S. Public Health Service: Promoting Health, Preventing Disease, Objectives for the Nation, 1980. Washington, DC, U.S. Government Printing Offices, 1980.

U.S. Public Health Service: Healthy People 2000, National Health Promotion and Disease Prevention Objectives. Washington, DC, U.S. Government Printing Offices, 1990a.

U.S. Public Health Service: Healthy People 2000: Midcourse Review and 1995 Revisions. Washington, DC, U.S. Government Printing Offices, 1995.

U.S. Public Health Service: United States Health and Prevention Profile, 1989 (Publication no. PHS 90-1232). Washington, DC, U.S. Government Printing Office, 1990b, pp. 1–5.

Verbrugge LM: Longer life but worsening health? Trends in health and mortality of middle-aged and older persons. *In* Lee PR, Estes CL (eds). The Nation's Health, 3rd ed. Boston, Jones and Bartlett, 1990, pp. 14–34.

Wilner M, Walkley RP, O'Neill EJ: Introduction to Public Health, 7th ed. New York, Macmillan, 1978, pp. 25–68.

Wilson FA, Neuhauser D: Health Services in the United States, 2nd ed. Cambridge: Ballinger, 1985, pp. 131–236.

World Health Organization: The Constitution of the World Health Organization. WHO Chronicle I:29, 1944.

Zimmerman MA: Citizen participation in rural health: A promising resource. J Public Health Policy 11:323–340, 1990.

The Art and Science of Community Health Nursing

Thinking Upstream: Conceptualizing Health from a Population Perspective

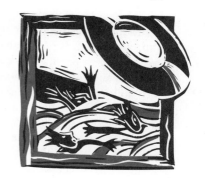

Upon completion of the chapter, the reader will be able to:

1. Describe the concept of theoretical scope as it applies to the protection and promotion of health in community health nursing.

2. Differentiate between upstream interventions, which are designed to alter the precursors of poor health, and downstream interventions, which are characterized by efforts to modify individuals' perceptions of their health.

3. Critique a theory in regard to its relevance to facilitating an understanding of population health dynamics.

4. Recognize theory-based practice as the means of achieving community health nursing's goals to protect and promote health in populations.

Patricia G. Butterfield

A thorough understanding of factors contributing to population health is critical to the practice of community health nursing; this fundamental principle differentiates our practice from other nursing specialties. For many of us, the emphasis on population health requires a change in perspective from our original orientation to nursing practice. As novice nurses we are frequently acculturated to nursing in a hospital or skilled nursing facility; these settings are designed, for the most part, for intervention on behalf of individuals. The structure of such organizations, albeit the important role they play in the health care system, is not conducive to developing an understanding of population health.

The chapter begins with a brief overview of nursing theory followed by a discussion of the scope of community health nursing in addressing population health concerns. Later, several theoretical approaches are compared and contrasted for the purpose of demonstrating how different conceptualizations can lead to different conclusions about the range of interventions available to the nurse. Throughout the text, the analogy of upstream versus downstream thinking is used as a literary tool to differentiate between strategies that are population directed versus those that are directed toward the individual.

THINKING UPSTREAM: LOOKING BEYOND THE INDIVIDUAL

In his description of the frustrations of medical practice, McKinlay (1979) used the image of a swiftly flowing river to represent illness. In this analogy physicians are so caught up rescuing victims from the river that they have no time to look upstream and see who is pushing their patients into the perilous waters. The author used this story to demonstrate the ultimate futility of "downstream endeavors," which are characterized by short-term, individual-based interventions, and he challenged health care providers to focus more of their energies "upstream, where the real problems lie" (McKinlay, 1979, p. 9). Upstream endeavors focus on modifying economic, political, and environmental factors that have been shown to be the precursors of poor health throughout the world.

Although the story cites medical practice, it is equally fitting to the dilemmas of nursing practice. In addition, even though nursing has a rich historical record of providing preventive and population-based care, it has been well substantiated that our current health system, which emphasizes episodic- and individual-based care, has done little to stem the tide of chronic illness, to which 70% of the American population succumbs.

At several points in this chapter I return to this analogy to analyze different theories from an upstream, or **macroscopic,** perspective versus a downstream perspective. Although these categories are not mutually exclusive, the use of the term *upstream* can provide a point of reference to evaluate a theory's potential for understanding population health.

HISTORICAL PERSPECTIVES ON NURSING THEORY

Florence Nightingale is widely regarded as the first member of the nursing profession to formulate a conceptual foundation for nursing practice. However, in the years after her leadership, nursing practice became largely atheoretical and based primarily on reacting to the immediacy of patient situations and medical staff. Thus, nursing's perspective on health and scope of practice was defined primarily by hospital administrative and medical personnel. Nursing leaders, seeing their profession defined by others, began to take proactive action to consolidate their ideas and advance the scientific foundation of nursing practice.

One of the means to move nursing forward was to propose theoretical formulations to guide nursing practice. Several of the early nursing theories were extremely myopic and depicted situations in which persons other than a single nurse and patient (e.g., family members, other health professionals) were noticeably absent from the context of care. This type of characterization may have been a historically appropriate response to the constraints of nursing practice and the need to emphasize the activities of the nursing profession that were independent of medicine.

Although not without some value, theories that address health from a microscopic rather than macroscopic perspective are of limited use in the current context of community-based nursing; they were simply not designed to incorporate the social and environmental variables on which community health is predicated. **More recent advances in nursing theory development take into account the dynamic**

Portions of text have been adapted from Butterfield PG: Thinking upstream: Nurturing a conceptual foundation of the societal context of health care. Adv Nurs Sci 12(2):1–8, 1990, with permission of Aspen Publishers, Inc., © 1990.

nature of health-sustaining and/or damaging environments and address the nature of a collective versus an individual client.

ISSUES OF FIT

Sometimes students are not acquainted with a sufficient range of theoretical approaches and select an individual-oriented theory to give them insight into a population-based health problem. **A related problem occurs when students like a particular theoretical perspective and attempt to use it in all situations regardless of its fit with the clinical scenario; this is analogous to putting the cart before the horse. Because nursing is a practice profession, it is important to recognize that the organizing framework for nursing should be selected to fit the care situation rather than the antithesis.** The results of a *forced fit* do a disservice to both the theory, which was not designed for such application, and the student. It

is easy to understand why students become perplexed and often frustrated when they begin to practice in the community and learn that their cadre of theoretical approaches is of limited help in understanding or guiding their practice. Like other professional disciplines, nursing has many theoretical tools of the trade, and it is important to know when to pick a hammer when a hammer is required versus when to pick a wrench when a wrench is required. A primary goal of this chapter is to enable readers to select, among alternate conceptualizations, theoretical approaches that are compatible with a population perspective of health.

DEFINITIONS OF THEORY

Like other abstract concepts, different nursing authors have defined and interpreted theory in different ways. Figure 4–1 provides a list of definitions of theory as proposed by several authors. The lack of uniformity

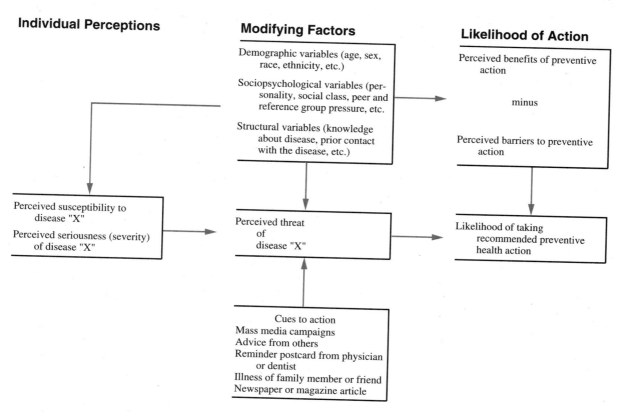

Figure 4–1
Variables and relationships in the health belief model. (Redrawn from Rosenstock IM: Historical origins of the health belief model. *In* Becker MH (ed): The Health Belief Model and Personal Health Behavior. Thorofare, NJ, Charles B. Slack, 1974, pp. 1–8.)

among these definitions, although often frustrating for students, reflects the evolution of the profession's thinking as well as individual differences in the conceptualization of the relationships among theory, practice, and research. The definitions also reflect the difficulty in describing something as complex and diverse as theory within the constraints of one definition. Reading several definitions can foster an appreciation of the richness of theory as well as help the reader identify one or two definitions that are particularly meaningful. Within our profession, definitions of theory typically refer to a set of concepts, relational statements, and the goal or purpose of theory. The theoretical perspectives presented in this chapter are congruent with a fairly broad definition of theory, one that is in step with the definitions proposed by Dickoff and James (1968), Torres (1986), and Barnum (1990).

DEFINITIONS OF THEORY AS PROPOSED BY NURSING THEORISTS

- "A systematic vision of reality; a set of inter-related concepts that is useful for prediction and control." (Woods and Catanzaro, 1988, p. 568.)
- "A conceptual system or framework invented for some purpose; and as the purpose varies so too must the structure and complexity of the system." (Dickoff and James, 1968, p. 198.)
- "A set of concepts, definitions, and propositions that projects a systematic view of phenomena by designating specific interrelationships among concepts for purposes of describing, explaining, and predicting." (Chinn and Jacobs, 1987, pp. 207–208.)
- "A statement that purports to account or characterize some phenomenon. A nursing theory, therefore, attempts to describe or explain the phenomenon called nursing." (Barnum, 1990, p. 1.)
- "Theory organizes the relationships between the complex events that occur in a nursing situation so that we can assist human beings. Simply stated, theory provides a way of thinking about and looking at the world around us." (Torres, 1986, p. 19.)

THEORY TO WHAT END?

The goal of theory is to improve the practice of nursing. Chinn and Jacobs (1987) stated that this goal is best achieved by using theories or parts of theoretical frameworks to guide practice. Students often perceive theory as intellectually burdensome and cannot see how something so seemingly obtuse can help improve their care. However, because theory-based practice guides the process of data collection and interpretation in a clear and organized manner, it is easier for the nurse to make appropriate diagnoses of problems and then to devise means by which to address those problems. In this way, through the process of integrating theory and practice, you can focus on those factors that are critical in understanding the situation at hand. As Barnum (1990) stated, "A theory is like a map of a territory as opposed to an aerial photograph. The map does not give the full terrain (i.e., the full picture); instead it picks out those parts that are important for its given purpose" (p. 1). Using a theoretical perspective to plan nursing care not only guides you in the assessment of a nursing situation, but it also "allows you to plan and not get lost in the details or sidetracked in the alleys" (J. M. Swanson, personal communication, May, 1992).

MICROSCOPIC VERSUS MACROSCOPIC APPROACHES TO THE CONCEPTUALIZATION OF COMMUNITY HEALTH PROBLEMS

In many ways an understanding of population health requires each of us to make a transformation—a new way of seeing and interpreting the complexity of forces that shape the health of a society. This transformation can best be achieved through the integration of population-based practice and theoretical perspectives that conceptualize health from a macroscopic versus microscopic perspective. Table 4–1 differentiates between these two approaches to the conceptualization of nursing problems.

It is helpful to use the analogy of a target to understand the concept of microscopic versus macroscopic. Think of individuals, with the health problem of interest (e.g., pediatric exposure to lead compounds) as the bull's eye. In this context, a microscopic approach to assessment would focus exclusively on individual children who have been diagnosed with lead poisoning; nursing interventions would focus the identification and removal of sources of lead in the home. It is easy to recognize the importance of these nursing activities; it is imperative that all children with elevated serum lead levels be removed from all suspect

Table 4–1	
Microscopic Versus Macroscopic Approaches to the Delineation of Community Health Nursing Problems	
Microscopic Approach	**Macroscopic Approach**
Examines individual (and sometimes family) responses to health and illness	Examines interfamily and intercommunity themes in health and illness
	Delineates factors in the population that perpetuate the development of illness or foster the development of health
Often emphasizes behavioral responses to illness or lifestyle patterns in an individual	Emphasizes social, economic, and environmental precursors of illness
Nursing interventions often aimed at modifying individual's behavior through changing his or her perceptions of belief system	Nursing interventions may include modifying social or environmental variables (i.e., working to remove barriers to care, improving sanitation or living conditions)
	May involve social or political action

sources of exposure as quickly as possible. However, there are broader ways in which to view this problem; one can address the issues relating to health threats to individuals and also examine interperson and intercommunity factors in the development and perpetuation of lead poisoning as a national health problem. Think of this approach as including the bull's eye as well as concentric circles that extend out from the center of the target. A macroscopic approach to the problem of lead exposure may include activities such as examining trends in the prevalence of lead poisoning over time, gathering estimates of the percentage of older homes (which may contain lead pipes or lead-based paint surfaces) in a neighborhood, as well as locating industrial sources of lead **emissions.** Such efforts are not usually addressed by one nurse alone but most frequently involve the cooperative efforts of nurses from school, occupational, and other community settings.

How does a theoretical focus on the individual preclude understanding of a larger perspective? Dreher (1982) used the term *conservative scope of practice* in describing frameworks that focus their energies ex-

clusively on intrapatient and nurse-patient factors. She stated that such frameworks often adopt psychological explanations of patient behavior. In this mode of thinking, low compliance, missed appointments, and reluctance to participate in care are all attributed to motivation or attitude problems on the part of the patient. Nurses are charged with the responsibility of altering patient attitudes toward health rather than altering the system itself "even though such negative attitudes may well be a realistic appraisal of health care" (Dreher, 1982, p. 505). The nurse who views the world from such a perspective does not entertain the possibility of working to alter the system itself or empowering patients to do so.

ASSESSING A THEORY'S SCOPE IN RELATION TO COMMUNITY HEALTH NURSING

The issue of theoretical scope is especially salient to community health nursing because of the many levels of practice within this specialty area. For example, a home health nurse who is caring for ill persons after hospitalization has a very different scope of practice than a nurse epidemiologist or health planner. Although it is certainly important that all nurses practice with an understanding of population health, it is most critical for those nurses whose practice is founded on inter- rather than intrapopulation dynamics. Unless a given theory is broad enough in scope to address health and determinants of health from a population perspective, it will be of limited utility to community health nurses. Although there have been many advancements in the development of nursing theory within the past 25 years, there continues to be some lack of clarity about the theoretical foundation of community health nursing (Batra, 1991). The application of the terms *microscopic* and *macroscopic* to health situations may help to fill this void and stimulate theory development in community health nursing.

How does the concept of "macroscopic" relate to the upstream analogy presented earlier? Although these concepts are similar, the term *macroscopic* refers to that of a broad scope, which incorporates many variables to aid in the understanding of a health problem. Upstream thinking would fall within this domain; this orientation to viewing a problem emphasizes variables that precede or play a role in the development of health problems. Think of macroscopic as the broad umbrella concept and upstream as a more specific concept under the umbrella. Both of these related concepts and the meanings they portray can help nurses develop a critical eye in evaluating a theory's relevance to population health.

FORMAT FOR REVIEW OF THEORIES

Several theoretical approaches are contrasted to demonstrate how they may lead the nurse to draw very different conclusions not only about the reasons for client behavior but also about the range of interventions available to the nurse. Two theories, one that originated within nursing and one that is based in social psychology, will be used to exemplify individual microscopic approaches to community health nursing problems. Likewise, two other theories, one from nursing and another with its roots in phenomenology, have been selected to demonstrate the examination of nursing problems from a macroscopic perspective. The format for this review is as follows:

1. The individual as locus of change
   a. Orem's self-care deficit theory of nursing
   b. The health belief model
2. Thinking upstream: society as the locus of change
   a. Milio's framework for prevention
   b. Critical social theory

The Individual as Locus of Change

OREM'S SELF-CARE DEFICIT THEORY OF NURSING

The theoretical foundations of the self-care deficit theory of nursing were based on Dorothea Orem's initial experiences as a staff and private duty nurse and her later work as faculty at Catholic University of America. In 1958, Orem began to formalize her insights about why individuals required nursing care and the purpose of nursing activities (Eben et al., 1986). The theory is prefaced on the assumption that self-care needs and activities are the primary focus of nursing practice. Orem outlined her general theory of nursing and stated that this general theory is actually a composite of three related constructs: (1) the theory of self-care deficits, which provides criteria for identifying those who need nursing, (2) the theory of self-care, which explains self-care and why it is necessary, and (3) the theory of nursing systems, which specifies the role of nursing in the delivery of care and how persons can be helped through nursing.

The major concepts from Orem's Self-care Deficit Theory (Orem, 1985, p. 31) include the following:

- *Self-care:* "The production of actions directed to self or to the environment in order to regulate one's functioning in the interest of one's life, integrated functioning, and well-being."
- *Therapeutic self-care demand:* "The measures of care required at moments in time in order to meet existent requisites for regulatory action to maintain life and to maintain or promote health, development, and general well-being."
- *Self-care agency:* "The complex capability for action that is activated in the performance of the actions or operations of self-care."
- *Self-care deficit:* "A relationship between self-care agency and therapeutic self-care demand in which self-care agency is not adequate to meet the known therapeutic self-care demand."
- *Nursing agency:* "The complex capability for action that is activated by nurses in their determination of needs for, design of, and production of nursing for persons with a range of types of self-care deficits."
- *Nursing system:* "A continuing series of actions produced when nurses link one way or a number of ways of helping to meet their own actions or the actions of persons under care that are directed to meet these persons' therapeutic self-care demands or to regulate their self-care agency."

The basic concepts of this theory evolved almost exclusively from observing the chronology of illness in hospitalized patients. The theory is based on the premise that nursing is a response to one's incapacity to care for self because of one's health. Nursing assumes the role of providing some or all self-care activities on behalf of the patient (Orem, 1985). Because of this focus, the content and scope of the theory have better utility to nurses practicing within an institutionalized setting than within the community. Although Orem briefly specified the role of nursing for populations in the third edition of her book *Nursing: Concepts of Practice* (1985), the concepts of self-care, self-care deficit, and self-care agency are so embedded in an individual orientation to disease that the application of these concepts to a population can become awkward and trying. In this theory, the process of assessing a patient's abilities **supersedes** upstream concepts (environmental, social, economic) that may explain the development and perpetuation of health problems in the community.

Application of Self-Care Deficit Theory

In a discussion of theory-based initiatives, a British nurse lamented the mandate by nursing supervisors that Orem's self-care deficit theory be adopted as the primary theory for her specialty area of occupational health nursing. Her frustration was evident as she argued that many of the model's assumptions seemed incongruous with the realities of her daily practice. Kennedy (1989) maintained that the self-care deficit theory assumes that persons are able to exert purposeful control over their environments in the pursuit of health; however, in the work place, persons may have little control over the physical or social aspects of the work environment. On the basis of this thesis, she concluded that the self-care model is incompatible with the practice domain of occupational health nursing.

Kennedy exemplified the dissonance that nurses feel when they are forced to put the conceptual cart before the horse. Although it is easy to recognize the salience of Orem's concepts to many arenas of nursing practice, it is also apparent that this gestalt has limited utility for understanding antecedents of population health. Kennedy clearly articulated this position when she stated that "the many facets of the occupational health nurse's role may 'fit in comfortably with Orem's self-care model.' But will Orem's model fit into the many facets of the occupational health nurse's role? That is the key question we should be asking" (p. 354).

THE HEALTH BELIEF MODEL

The second theory that focuses on the individual as locus of change is the *health belief model*. The model evolved from the premise that it is the world of the perceiver that determines what one will do. The model had its inceptions during the late 1950s, when America was breathing a collective sigh of relief after the development of the polio vaccine. Although a life-saving vaccine had finally been found, health professionals were stymied when some people chose not to bring themselves or their children into clinics to be immunized. The health belief model resulted from the efforts of social psychologists and other public health workers who recognized the need to develop a more complete understanding of the factors that influence preventive health behaviors.

The model's core dimensions were derived primarily from the work of Kurt Lewin, who proposed that behavior is primarily based on the current dynamics confronting an individual rather than prior experiences (Maiman and Becker, 1974). Within this framework, diseases are regarded as regions of negative valence, which act to repel the individual. An assumption of the model is that the major determinant of preventive health behavior is the avoidance of disease. Major concepts include perceived susceptibility to disease x, perceived seriousness of disease x, modifying factors, cues to action, perceived benefits minus barriers of preventive health action, perceived threat of disease x, and the likelihood of taking a recommended health action; arrows are used to specify the direction between concepts. The model was not designed to be generalized across disorders; disease x represents a particular disorder that an individual believes may be prevented by a health action. This means that actions that relate to preventive health behaviors for breast cancer will be different from those relating to measles; in the former a cue to action may involve a public service advertisement encouraging women to make an appointment for a mammogram; for the latter, the same concept may be operationalized in the form of hearing of a measles outbreak in a neighboring town. Figure 4–1 outlines the variables and relationships in the health belief model.

Application of the Health Belief Model

Over the years, a number of authors have proposed modifications to the health belief model both to broaden its scope to address health promotion and illness behaviors (Kirscht, 1974; Pender, 1987) and to merge its concepts with other theories that describe health behavior (Cummings et al., 1980). This conceptualization of health and health behaviors represented my first encounter with the power of theory-based practice, and I would like to share a brief personal chronology of my perceptions of the strengths and limitations of the model.

My first class in nursing theory followed a format much like that of many other courses throughout the country. Each week we were introduced to a new theoretical perspective; we covered the background of the theorist, the assumptions of the theory, and the theory's concepts and relational statements and discussed the application of the theory to nursing practice. Like many other students, I was experiencing some mixed feelings about the class. I found most of the content intellectually interesting but had difficulty relating it to the patients whom I saw each week in the neighborhood clinics and during home visits. Several weeks into the class, we covered the health belief model. My interest was immediately piqued; the model soon captured my thoughts in a way that no other framework had. After the seminar, I went to the library and checked out *The Health Belief Model and Personal Health Behavior* by Marshall Becker (1974) and quickly became absorbed in the book.

The model's focus on compliance was something I could relate to in my own clinical practice. The health belief model offered me, for the first time, some insight into my patients' behaviors and helped me organize my thoughts about why persons choose to disregard the instructions of well-intended nurses and doctors. I was most intrigued by the way the model interpreted behaviors from the patient's, rather than nurse's, perspective. Concepts such as "perceived seriousness," "perceived susceptibility," and "cue to action" afforded me new insights into the dynamics of health decision making. All in all, the health belief model provided me with answers to problems that I encountered in my practice every day.

I soon began using my interpretation of the model to guide my work with some families; I recall one family in particular who had an 18-month-old son who had never been immunized. The father owned a health food store and was strongly immersed in a culture in which natural foods and medicines were emphasized and the use of anything deemed "unnatural" was shunned. Childhood immunizations for polio, tetanus, measles, and such certainly belonged, in that family's eyes, in the "unnatural" group. I assessed that the failure to immunize the child resulted from the parents' low perceived susceptibility to and perceived seriousness of childhood illnesses coupled with modifying factors, such as a reference group that disdained most traditional medical practices, which favored inaction over action. During the next few weeks I mapped out my strategy; I would work toward raising the parents' perceived susceptibility to childhood illnesses by providing them with information about communicable diseases. I took time during the next two or three visits to inundate the family with literature and pictures that graphically demonstrated the sequelae of diphtheria, polio, and pertussis. Eventually my efforts culminated in the parents taking their son to an immunization clinic for his first shot, much to my delight.

Fifteen years later I still have mixed feelings when I recall this family and the means I used to drive their compliance to the accepted standard of pediatric health care.

> I believe that their actions were based, for the most part, on their desire to please me and "get me off their backs" rather than any true insight into the risks and benefits of childhood immunization. As a community health nurse, I have a very real understanding of the risks of the failure to protect children against communicable diseases. However, I also understand that, for infectious disease prevention to be effective at the population level, the decision to immunize needs to originate within a collective notion of families within the community. Nurses can be most effective by working within schools, industries, and civic organizations to provide education and a supportive milieu for a healthy choice to occur.

In the years since this experience, I have become more skilled in the assessment and labeling of patient problems and have gained a better appreciation of the strengths and limitations that any theoretical framework imposes on a situation.

Limitations of the Health Belief Model

The health belief model places the burden of action exclusively on the client and assumes that only those clients who have distorted or negative perceptions of the specified disease or recommended health action will fail to act. In practice, the result of using this model as the foundation for practice is to focus the nurse's energies on interventions designed to modify the client's distorted perceptions; this is certainly the approach that I took in attempting to change the behavior of those patients with whom I was working.

True to its historical roots, the model offers an explanation of health behaviors that, in many ways, is similar to a mechanical system. From the health belief model, one easily concludes that compliance can be induced by using model variables as catalysts to stimulate action. For example, an intervention study based on health belief model precepts sought to increase follow-up in hypertensive clients by increasing their perceived susceptibility and seriousness to the dangers of hypertension (Jones et al., 1987). In addition, patients received education over the telephone or in the emergency department, which was designed to increase their perception of the benefits of follow-up. According to the authors, the interventions resulted in a dramatic increase in compliance. However, they noted several patient groups that failed to respond to the intervention, most notably a small group of patients who had no available child care. Although this study demonstrates the predictive power of health belief model concepts, it also exemplifies the limitations of the model. The health belief model may be effective in promoting behavior change through the alteration of patients' perspectives, but it does not acknowledge responsibility for the health professional to reduce or ameliorate barriers to health care.

The health belief model is but a prototype for the type of theoretical perspective that has dominated nursing education and thus nursing practice. It is precisely a strength of the model—its narrow scope—that is its limitation: one is not drawn outside it to those forces that shape the characteristics that the model describes.

The Upstream View: Society as the Locus of Change

MILIO'S FRAMEWORK FOR PREVENTION

Milio's framework for prevention (1976) provides a thought-provoking complement to the health belief model and a mechanism for directing attention upstream and examining opportunities for nursing intervention at the population level. Milio outlined six propositions that relate the ability of an individual to improve healthful behavior to a society's ability to provide options for healthy choices that are both accessible and socially affirming. Through these statements, Milio moved the focus of attention upstream by pointing out that it is the range of available health choices rather than the choices made at any one time that is critical in shaping the overall health status of a society. In addition, she maintained that the range of choices widely available to individuals is shaped, to a large degree, by policy decisions in both governmental and private organizations. Rather than concentrate efforts on imparting information to change patterns of individual behavior, she viewed national-level policymaking as the most effective means by which to favorably impact the health of most Americans.

Milio (1976) proposed that health deficits often result from an imbalance between a population's health needs and its health-sustaining resources, with affluent societies afflicted by the diseases associated with excess (obesity, alcoholism) and the poor afflicted by diseases that result from inadequate or unsafe food, shelter, and water. Viewing the situation

SET OF PROPOSITIONS PROPOSED BY MILIO

1. "The health status of populations is the result of deprivation and/or excess of critical health-sustaining resources."
2. "Behavior patterns of populations are a result of habitual selection from limited choices, and these habits of choice are related to: (a) actual and perceived options available; (b) beliefs and expectations developed and refined over time by socialization, formal learning, and immediate experience."
3. "Organizational behavior (decisions or policy-choices made by governmental/nongovernmental, national/non-national; not-profit/for-profit, formal/non-formal organizations) sets the range of options available to individuals for their personal choice-making."
4. "The choice-making of individuals at a given point in time concerning potentially health-promoting or health-damaging selections is affected by their effort to maximize valued resources."
5. "Social change may be thought of as changes in patterns of behavior resulting from shifts in the choice-making of significant numbers of people within a population."
6. "Health education, as the process of teaching and learning health-supporting information, can have little significantly extensive impact on behavior patterns, that is, on personal choice-making of groups of people, without the easy availability of new, or newly-perceived alternative health-promoting options for investing personal resources."

From Milio N. (1976). A framework for prevention: changing health-damaging to health-generating life patterns. Am J Public Health 66:436–437.

within this context, the poor in affluent societies may experience the least desirable combination of factors. Milio cited the socioeconomic realities that deprive many Americans of a health-sustaining environment despite the fact that "cigarettes, sucrose, pollutants, and tensions are readily available to the poor" (1976, p. 436).

The range of health-promoting or health-damaging choices available to individuals is affected by their personal resources and their societal resources. Personal resources include one's awareness, knowledge, and beliefs and those of one's family and friends as well as money, time, and the urgency of other priorities. Societal resources are strongly influenced by community and national locale and include the availability and cost of health services, environmental protection, safe shelter, and the penalties or rewards given for failure to select the given options.

Milio challenged the commonly held assumption in health education that knowing health-generating behaviors implies acting in accordance with that knowledge, and she cited the lifestyles of health professionals in support of her argument. She proposed that "most human beings, professional or nonprofessional, provider or consumer, make the easiest choices available to them most of the time" (1976, p. 435). Therefore, health-promoting choices must be more readily available and less costly than health-damaging options if individuals are to be healthy and a society is to improve its health status. Milio's framework can enable a nurse to reframe this view by understanding the historic play of social forces that have limited the choices truly available to the involved parties.

Comparison of Health Belief Model and Milio's Conceptualizations of Health

One cannot help but note the similarities between Milio's health resources and the concepts in the health belief model. The purpose of the health belief model is to provide the nurse with an understanding of the dynamics of personal health behaviors; broader contextual variables, such as the constraints of the health care system, are specified only as they influence the decision-making processes of the individual. In contrast, Milio's framework is prefaced on an assessment of community resources and their availability to individuals. This differs from the health belief model, which may assume that each of us has been dealt a full deck of health resources and free will. By assessing such factors up front, the nurse is able to gain a more thorough understanding of the resources, or "cards," that persons actually hold. Milio offered a different set of insights into the health behavior arena by proposing that many low-income individuals are acting within the constraints of their limited resources. Furthermore, she delved beyond the downstream focus and the health of populations by examining choices made by significant numbers of people within a population.

Because Milio's framework provides for the inclusion of economic, political, and environmental health determinants, compared to the health belief model, the nurse is given broader range in the diagnosis and interpretation of health problems. Whereas the health belief model allows for only a dichotomous outcome ("acts" or "fails to act according to recommended health action"), Milio's framework encourages the nurse to understand health behaviors in the context of the societal milieu in which they reside.

Implications of Milio's Framework to the Current Health Delivery Systems

Through its broader scope, Milio's model allows for nursing interventions at many levels: assessing the personal and societal resources of individual patients as well as analyzing social and economic factors that may inhibit healthy choices in populations. Population-based interventions may include such diverse activities as mobilizing comprehensive smoking cessation programs in schools and work places and political activity encouraging an end to federal subsidization of health-damaging industry.

Our health care system's current emphasis on efficient care has favored the employment of nurse practitioners and advanced practice nurses in settings previously dominated by physician practice. Such settings include, but are not limited to, managed care and health maintenance organizations. Overall, this change is favorable because of the level of independence and autonomy this type of practice allows. However, the goal of efficient care in the short term may preclude broader-based interventions that require significant amounts of nursing time (i.e., individualized patient education, anticipatory guidance). Because such care is poorly quantified in billing taxonomies and may not yield immediate results, it may not be viewed as cost effective and may be discouraged at the system level. Indeed, Barnes and colleagues (1995) cautioned that the provision of primary care from a narrow perspective of health determinants leads to nursing's perpetuation of institutionally driven and controlled medical care rather than providing broad-based health care grounded in essential human needs. The authors emphasize those facets of nursing care that address the provision of education and care services through the most direct, simple, and inexpensive means possible. This type of practice requires a conceptual and operational appreciation of "the larger sociopolitical context within which the health care is delivered and in which health evolves, that is, to the inextricable relationships between health status and levels of poverty, employment, education, quality of life, and general community development" (Barnes et al., 1995, p. 10).

Overall, current health care delivery systems are at their best when responding to persons with diagnostic-intensive and acute illnesses. Those persons experiencing chronic debilitation or with less intriguing diagnoses generally fare worse in our system despite efforts by community- and home-based care to "fill the gaps" as best they can. Nurses in both hospital and community-based systems often feel constrained by profound financial and service restrictions imposed by third-party payers. Nursing care is often ordered to be terminated after resolution of the latest immediate health crisis; opportunities for a continuing dialogue promoting long-term health improvements are not compensable and, therefore, not allowed. Because many health systems use nursing standards and reimbursement mechanisms that originate from a narrow, compartmentalized view of health, it is imperative to practice nursing from a broader understanding of health, illness, and suffering.

Issues of health care access are often discussed in both nursing and health services literature; this topic is of particular interest because of the tremendous disparities in access between insured and uninsured persons in this country. Access to care, because of its strong association with economic, social, and political factors, can be a primary determinant of health status and survival, depending on the needs of the individuals and populations of interest. Recently, structural variables, which encompass concepts such as race-ethnicity, educational status, gender, and income, have received attention as being highly predictive of health status. These types of factors, which are also strongly grounded in the sociopolitical and economic milieu, are another way of identifying risk factors for poor health and opportunities for community-based interventions. Bird and Bauman (1995) used a unique combination of structural variables (e.g., percentage of persons who are high school graduates, median earnings ratio between men and women, number of times Republican presidential candidates carried each state in the past 20 years) to explain 65% of the variation in infant mortality rates by state. This type of provocative research, because of its broad conceptualization of health determinants, succeeded in reestablishing direct associations among demographic, social, and economic variables and infant death rates. Such projects close the gap between the precursors of mortality and their effects on individuals and the collective health of our society.

The opportunities for a society to make healthy choices have been a central theme throughout Milio's work. In a related article (1981) she elaborated on this theme.

> *Personal behavior patterns are not simply "free" choices about "lifestyle," isolated from their personal and economic context. Lifestyles are, rather, patterns of choices made from the alternatives that are available to people according to their socioeconomic circumstances and the ease with which they are able to choose certain ones over others.*
>
> (Milio, 1981, p. 76.)

CRITICAL SOCIAL THEORY

Just as Milio used societal awareness as an aid to understanding health behaviors, critical social theory uses similar means to expose social inequalities that limit people from reaching their full potential. This theoretical approach is based on the belief that life is structured by social meanings that are determined, rather one-sidedly, through social domination. Proponents of this theoretical approach maintain that social exchanges that are not distorted from power imbalances will stimulate the evolution of a more just society (Allen et al., 1986). Critical theory assumes that standards of truth are socially determined and that no form of scientific inquiry is value free. As Allen and colleagues (1986, p. 34) stated, "One cannot separate theory and value, as the empiricist claims. Every theory is penetrated by value interests."

Application of Critical Social Theory

Application of the theory uses one's processes of inductive reasoning; rather than superimposing concepts onto a situation, relevant concepts are revealed to the nurse through an ongoing process of data collection and analysis. Interviews with critical informants, news articles, and transcripts of governmental proceedings may all serve as sources of data. For example, suppose the domain of interest involves child care options for employees of a large microcomputer manufacturer. Data sources may initially include the age and gender distribution of the workers, review of work site policies on parental leave, and interviews with both workers and administrative officials. Further into the analysis, the nurse may choose to incorporate additional sources of data; such data may include interviews with shift workers' addressing the difficulties with accessing evening and nighttime child care or statistics on job turnover among child care workers.

The methodological approaches adopted in critical social theory may also differ from those suggested by other nursing theories. No specific method of analysis is mandated; rather, methods are chosen because they are congruent with the focus of study. The dialectic is often used as a methodological tool; this refers to a process in which the investigator seeks understanding by examining contradictions within the phenomena of interest. Continuing with the previous example, the nurse may apply critical social theory to an examination of child care by contrasting an organization's policies with interviews from those workers who have found the organization to be an impediment to achieving quality care for their children. Data analysis may also include an examination of the interests of both workers and administration in promoting social change versus maintaining the status quo.

Wild (1993) used critical social theory to analyze social, political, and economic conditions associated with the cost of prescription analgesics and the commensurate financial burden faced by clients who require these medications. Trends in pharmaceutical pricing were compared to inflation rates of other commodities. Pharmaceutical sales techniques, primarily through marketing directly to physicians, were depicted as an example of distancing the needs of ill clients from the industry whose products are intended to relieve those needs. A critique of this issue from a client perspective revealed limited access to information addressing the extreme variations in cost among different analgesics (e.g., greater than a 10-fold difference in cost among similar drug formulations). Through this analysis, Wild (1993) specified nursing actions, such as challenging pricing policies on behalf of client groups, that would not be considered by a downstream analysis of this prevalent health problem.

Challenging Assumptions About Preventive Health Through Critical Social Theory

The health belief model and Milio's model for prevention both focus on personal health behaviors, either from a disease avoidance or preventive health perspective; this phenomenon may also be analyzed using critical social theory. I now return to the analogy about the health workers who were so busy fishing persons out of the river of illness that they had no time to look upstream to see who was pushing them in. Later in the same article McKinlay used his upstream analogy to ask the rhetorical question, "How preventive is prevention?" (1979, p. 22). He used this tactic to critically examine different intervention strategies aimed at enhancing preventive behavior. Figure 4–2 shows McKinlay's model contrasting different modes of prevention. He related both curative and lifestyle modification interventions by health professionals to a downstream conceptualization of health; the majority of so-called preventive actions fail to alter the process of illness at its origin. Political-economic interventions

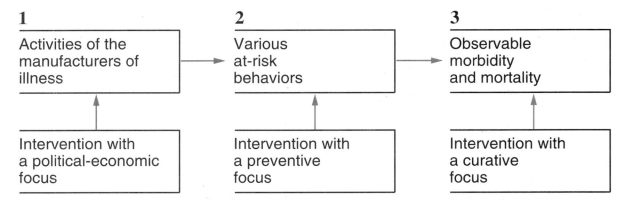

Figure 4–2
Continuum of health behaviors and corresponding intervention foci. (From McKinlay JB: A case for refocusing upstream: the political economy of illness. *In* Proceedings of an American Heart Association Conference: Applying Behavioral Science to Cardiovascular Risk. Seattle, Washington, June 17–19, 1974, pp. 7–17. Reproduced with permission. Copyright © American Heart Association.)

remain the most effective way to address population determinants of health and ameliorate illness at its source.

McKinlay further delineated the activities of the "manufacturers of illness—those individuals, interest groups, and organizations which, in addition to producing material goods and services, also produce, as an inevitable byproduct, widespread morbidity and mortality" (1979, pp. 9–10). Through embedding desired behaviors in the dominant cultural norm, the manufacturers of illness foster the habituation of high-risk behavior in the population. Unhealthy consumption patterns become integrated into everyday lives; one needs only to visit the holiday dinner tables of Americans to see stellar examples of "the binding of at-riskness to culture" (1979, p. 12). However, the existing health care system misguidedly devotes its efforts in an attempt to change the products of the manufacturers of illness rather than the processes that create the products.

Waitzkin (1983) continued with this theme by asserting that the health care system's emphasis on lifestyle diverts attention from important sources of illness in the capitalist industrial environment; "it also puts the burden of health squarely on the individual rather than seeking collective solutions to health problems" (p. 664). Salmon (1987) supported this position by noting that the basic tenets of Western medicine promote an understanding of individual factors of health and illness while obscuring the exploration of their social and economic roots. He stated that critical social theory "can aid in uncovering larger dimensions impacting health that are usually unseen or misrepresented by ideological biases. Thus, the social reality of health conditions can be both understood and changed" (1987, p. 75).

SUMMARY

Community health nurses have been instrumental in making many of the life-saving advances in sanitation, communicable disease, and environmental conditions that are now taken for granted. The practice of community health aids in developing a broad context of nursing practice because community environments are inherently less restrictive than that of hospital settings. Clarke and colleagues elaborated on environmental characteristics between community and hospital-based settings and proposed that community settings, because of their dynamic nature, are the most appropriate settings on which to ground the education of professional nurses (Clarke and Cody, 1994).

It may seem disheartening that the daily activities of nurses seeking to provide the broadest context of health-sustaining care on behalf of individuals and communities are restricted, to a large degree, by many delivery systems. However, nursing practice, because it is determined by the needs of those served, is particularly resilient and adaptable to a wide variety of contextual variables.

As nursing has advanced as a profession, so too has the need to formalize the scientific base of nursing practice through the development and dissemination of nursing theories. The richness of community health nursing comes from the challenge of conceptualizing and implementing strategies that will enhance the health of not just one but many. Likewise, nurses in this area of practice need to be provided with theoretical perspectives that address the social, political, and environmental determinants of population health. Through the integration of population-based theory and practice, nurses are given the means by which to impact favorably the health of our global community.

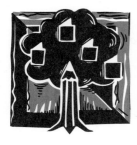

Learning Activities

1. Select a theory or conceptual model with which you are familiar. Evaluate its potential for understanding health in (1) individuals, (2) families, (3) a population of 400 children in an elementary school, (4) 2000 workers within a corporate setting, and (5) a community of 50,000 residents.

2. Identify one health problem (i.e., substance abuse, domestic violence, cardiovascular disease) that is prevalent in the community or city in which you live. Analyze the problem using two different theories or conceptual models: one that emphasizes individual determinants of health and another that emphasizes population determinants of health. What are some of the differences in the ways that these two different perspectives inform nursing practice?

3. Review the American Nurses Association definition of community health nursing practice and the American Public Health Association definition of public health nursing practice (listed in Chapter 1). What do these definitions indicate about the theoretical basis of community health nursing? How is the theoretical basis of community health nursing practice different from that within other specialty areas in nursing?

REFERENCES

Allen DG: Nursing research and social control: Alternate modes of science that emphasize understanding and emancipation. Image J Nurs Sch, 17:58–64, 1985.

Allen DG, Diekelmann N, Benner P: Three paradigms for nursing research: methodologic implications. *In* Chinn P (ed): Nursing Research Methodology: Issues and Implementation. Rockville, MD, Aspen Publishers, 1986, pp. 23–28.

Barnes D, Eribes C, Juarbe T, et al: Primary health care and primary care: A confusion of philosophies. Nurs Outlook 43:7–16, 1995.

Barnum BJS: Nursing Theory: Analysis, Application, Evaluation. Glenview, IL, Scott, Foresman/Little, Brown Higher Education, 1990.

Batra C: Professional issues: The future of community health nursing. *In* Cookfair JM (ed): Nursing Process and Practice in the Community. St Louis, Mosby-Year Book, pp. 613–635, 1991.

Becker MH (ed): The Health Belief Model and Personal Health Behavior. Thorofare, NJ, Charles B. Slack, 1974, pp. 1–8.

Bird ST, Bauman KE: The relationship between structural and health service variables and state-level infant mortality in the United States. Am J Public Health, 85:26–29, 1995.

Chinn PL, Jacobs MK: Theory and Nursing: A Systematic Approach, 2nd ed. St. Louis, CV Mosby, 1987.

Clarke PN, Cody WK: Nursing theory-based practice in the home and community: The crux of professional nursing education. Adv Nurs Sci 17:41–53, 1994.

Cummings KM, Becker MH, Malie MC: Bringing the models together: An empirical approach to combining variables to explain health actions. J Behav Med, 3:123–145, 1980.

Dickoff J, James P: A theory of theories: A position paper. Nurs Res, 17:197–203, 1968.

Dreher MC: The conflict of conservatism in public health nursing education. Nurs Outlook, 30:504–509, 1982.

Eben JD, Nation MJ, Marriner A, Nordmeyer SB: Self-care deficit theory of nursing. *In* Marriner A (ed): Nursing Theorists and Their Work. St. Louis, CV Mosby, 1986, pp. 117–130.

Jones PK, Jones SL, Katz J: Improving follow-up among hypertensive patients using a health belief model intervention. Arch Intern Med 147:1557–1560, 1987.

Kennedy A: How relevant are nursing models? Occup Health, 41:352–535, 1989.

Kirscht JP: The health belief model and illness behavior. *In* Becker MH (ed): The Health Belief Model and Personal Health Behavior. Thorofare, NJ, Charles B. Slack, 1974, pp. 9–26.

Maiman LA, Becker MH: The health belief model: Origins and correlates in psychological theory. *In* Becker MH (ed): The Health Belief Model and Personal Health Behavior. Thorofare, NJ, Charles B. Slack, 1974, pp. 9–26.

McKinlay JB: A case for refocusing upstream: The political economy of illness. *In* Jaco EG (ed): Patients, Physicians, and Illness, 3rd ed. New York, Free Press, 1979, pp. 9–25.

Milio N: A framework for prevention: Changing health-damaging to health-generating life patterns. Am J Public Health, 66:435–439, 1976.

Milio N: Promoting Health Through Public Policy. Philadelphia, FA Davis, 1981.

Orem DE: Nursing: Concepts of Practice, 3rd ed. New York, McGraw-Hill, 1985.

Pender NJ: Health Promotion in Nursing Practice, 2nd ed. Norwalk, CT, Appleton-Century-Crofts, 1987.

Salmon JW: Dilemmas in studying social change versus individual change: Considerations from political economy. *In* Duffy M, Pender NJ (eds): Conceptual Issues in Health Promotion—A Report of Proceedings of a Wingspread Conference. Indianapolis, IN: Sigma Theta Tau, 1987, pp. 70–81.

Torres G: Theoretical Foundations of Nursing. Norwalk, CT, Appleton-Century-Crofts, 1986.

Waitzkin H: A Marxist view of health and health care. *In* Mechanic D (ed): Handbook of Health, Health Care, and the Health Professions. New York, Free Press, 1983, pp. 657–682.

Wild LR: Caveat emptor: A critical analysis of the costs of drugs used for pain management. Adv Nurs Sci, 16:52–61, 1993.

Woods NF, Catanzaro M: Nursing Research: Theory and Practice. St. Louis, CV Mosby, 1988.

Community Assessment and Epidemiology

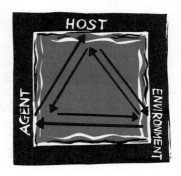

Upon completion of this chapter, the reader will be able to:

1. Discuss the major dimensions of a community.

2. Identify the major sources of information about a community's health.

3. Use epidemiologic methods to describe the state of health of a community or aggregate.

4. Identify epidemiologic study designs for researching health problems.

5. Formulate aggregate diagnoses.

Holly Cassells

The primary concern of community health nurses is to improve the health of the community. Community health nurses use all of the principles and skills of nursing practice as well as those of public health practice to aid the community.

However, what is a community? Towns and cities come to mind immediately. How can a nurse provide services to such a large and nontraditional "client"? A major aspect of the public health philosophy involves applying approaches and solutions to health problems so that the greatest number of people receive the maximum benefit. In this way, time and resources are used efficiently. Despite the desire to provide services to each individual in a community, the community health nurse recognizes the impracticability of this task. An alternative approach is to consider the community itself as the unit of service (i.e., to use the steps of the nursing process in working with the community as an entity).

Another central goal of public health practitioners is primary prevention, or keeping the public healthy and preventing disease from developing. As discussed in previous chapters, these "upstream efforts" are intended to reduce the pain and suffering and the huge expenditures that occur when significant segments of the population essentially "fall into the river" and require downstream resources to be directed at their health problems. In a society that is becoming increasingly intolerant of high health care costs, the need to prevent health problems also becomes dire. In addition to reducing the occurrence of disease in individuals, community health nurses must examine the larger aggregate—its structures, environment, and shared health risks—as a first step in developing improved upstream prevention programs.

This chapter addresses the first steps in adopting a community- or population-oriented practice. Before applying the nursing process, a community must be defined and its characteristics described. Then, the assessment and diagnosis phase of the nursing process can proceed at the aggregate level. Specialized epidemiologic approaches that yield information about a community's health risks are described. Comprehensive assessment data are essential to any effective primary prevention effort in a community.

THE NATURE OF COMMUNITY

Many dimensions are useful in describing the nature of community. The three dimensions addressed are the community as an aggregate of people, the community as a location in space and time, and the community as a social system.

Aggregate of People

Probably the most essential attribute of a community is that it is composed of people, in particular those who share one or more common characteristics. For example, members of a community may share common features, such as citizenship in the same city or membership in the same religious organization, and similar demographic characteristics or traits, such as belonging to a specific age group or having a common ethnic background. Elderly members of a senior citizens group frequently are of similar ages, are retired from the work force, and experience similar economic pressures. It is likely that this group also shares common life experiences, interests, and concerns. Having lived through the many societal changes of the past 50 years, they may also possess similar perspectives on current issues and trends. Many elderly persons share a concern for the maintenance of good health, pursuit of an active lifestyle, and securing of needed services to support a quality life. These shared interests can be translated into common goals and activities, which are defining attributes of a community.

Many human factors help to delineate a community. One such set of "people factors" of particular importance to the community health nurse comprises health-related traits, or *risk factors*. Persons sharing a predisposition to disease or impaired health may identify themselves as a community and join together in a group to learn from and support each other. Parents of disabled infants, persons with acquired immunodeficiency syndrome (AIDS), or those at risk for a second myocardial infarction may consider themselves to be a community. Even when these individuals are not organized, the nurse may recognize that they constitute a form of community or aggregate because of their unique needs.

When individuals come together because of a common problem, a "community of solution" may be said to have formed. These persons may have little else in common with each other but become united by a desire to redress such problems as a shared hazard from an environmental contamination, a shared health problem arising from a soaring rate of teenage suicide, or a shared political concern about an upcoming city council election. The community of solution often disbands after problem resolution but may subsequently identify other common issues to influence.

Each of these shared features may exist among persons who are geographically dispersed or in close proximity to each other. However, in many situations, proximity facilitates the recognition of commonalities and the development of cohesion among members. This active sharing of features in turn fosters a sense of community among individuals.

Location in Space and Time

Regardless of the extent to which features are shared, communities of people may be defined on the basis of geographic or physical location. The dimension of location is best exemplified by the traditional view of community as an entity delineated by geopolitical boundaries. These boundaries demarcate the periphery of cities, counties, states, and nations and are easily identified on maps. Citizens are also members of communities with perimeters that are indicated by less visible boundary lines, such as voting precincts, school districts, water districts, and fire and police protection precincts. Residents may claim membership in each of these entities simultaneously.

Census tracts, which also delineate subsets of larger communities, are used expressly for data collection and population assessment by the U.S. Bureau of the Census. Census tracts facilitate the organization of information about those residing in specific geographic locales in a community. In densely populated urban areas, residents of a tract are frequently part of a neighborhood described by data for one or more census tracts. Therefore, census tract data may be useful in defining and describing neighborhood communities, even though the residents may be unaware of the boundaries or their membership in a census tract (see Census Data).

Finally, the geographic dimension encompasses less formalized types of community or areas that can be identified as communities yet lack official geopolitical boundaries. Neighborhoods may be defined by a geographic landmark (e.g., the East Lake section of the town or the north shore area). Community neighborhoods may also be identified by a style of building construction or by a common time of development (e.g., Co-op City in New York, a housing subdivision on the edge of a city, or a section of historic homes in a central area of a town). Similarly, a dormitory, communal home, or summer camp may also be considered a community. Each shares a close geographic proximity in addition to other characteristics.

Communities are defined not only by location but also by the dimension of time. Their existence and defining characteristics change over time. Although some communities are considered very stable, most tend to change with the demographics and health status of the members, development or decline of the larger community, and various effects of many other factors.

MAJOR FEATURES OF A COMMUNITY

- Aggregate of people

  The "who": personal characteristics and risks

- Location in space and time

  The "where" and "when": physical location frequently delineated by boundaries and influenced by the passage of time

- Social system

  The "why" and "how": interrelationships of the aggregate as they fulfill community functions

Social System

The third major feature of a community relates to the linkages that community members form with each other. By interacting in groups within a community, the essential functions of community are fulfilled. These functions provide members with socialization, role fulfillment, goal achievement, and support. Therefore, a community may be considered a social system, with its interacting members making up various subsystems within the community. These subsystems are both interrelated and interdependent (i.e., they are affected by each other as well as by various internal and external stimuli). These stimuli consist of a broad range of events, values, conditions, and needs.

Health care systems are an example of complex systems that are made up of smaller, interrelated subsystems. Because health care systems interact and depend on other larger systems, such as the city government, they can also be subsystems. Changes in the larger system may not only directly affect that large system but also cause repercussions in many subsystems. For example, when local economic pressures in a community cause a health system to scale back its operations, many subsystems are affected. When programs are eliminated or reduced, service to other health care providers is limited, groups that normally use the system may have reduced access, and families who themselves constitute subsystems in society may be denied needed care. Almost every subsystem in the community may be required to react and readjust to such a financial constraint.

Communities that are very complex systems receive varied stimuli. The ability of a community to respond effectively to changing dynamics is an indicator of productive functioning. Examination of the functioning of the community and its subsystems provides clues to existing and potential health problems.

EXAMPLE OF SYSTEMS INTERRELATIONSHIPS

Health problems can have a severe impact on multiple systems. For example, the AIDS epidemic has required significant funds for direct services to AIDS clients as well as for public AIDS education and prevention. Simultaneously, it has made unrelenting demands on many communities already strapped for funds to meet basic health needs of its citizens. In San Francisco, the allocation of funds for AIDS programs has reduced funding for other programs such as immunizations, family planning, and well-child care.

ASSESSING THE COMMUNITY: SOURCES OF DATA

The essential feature of a community is its members. By traveling through a community and using each of the human senses, the community health nurse becomes familiar with the community and begins to understand its nature. It is through this down-to-earth approach to assessment, which has been called "shoe leather epidemiology," that the nurse begins to establish certain hunches or hypotheses about the community's health, its strengths as well as its potential health problems. For the community health nurse, these initial assessments will have to be better substantiated before a community diagnosis and plan can be formulated.

The use of certain public health tools becomes essential to a nursing practice that is aggregate focused. Demography and the analysis of statistical data provide descriptive information about the population. Epidemiology involves the analysis of data to discover the patterns of health and illness distribution in populations. Epidemiology also involves conducting research to explain the nature of health problems and identify aggregates at increased risk for these problems. The next section addresses these tools and describes ways in which community health nurses can apply them to the assessment of the aggregate.

Census Data

Every 10 years, the U.S. Bureau of the Census undertakes a massive survey of all U.S. families. In addition to this decennial census, intermediate surveys collect specific categories of information. These collections of statistical data describe the characteristics of the nation's population as a whole as well as of progressively smaller geopolitical entities (e.g., states, counties, and census tracts). The census also describes large metropolitan areas that extend beyond formal city boundaries. These are called metropolitan statistical areas, and they consist of a central city with more than 50,000 people and the associated suburban or adjacent counties, for a total metropolitan area of greater than 100,000. Cities with a population of 1 million or more and their associated counties constitute consolidated statistical areas. A census tract, which is one of the smallest reporting units, usually is made up of 3000 to 6000 persons, most of whom share some similar characteristics such as ethnicity, socioeconomic status, or type of housing.

The census combines a broad range of information that is extremely helpful to community health nurses familiarizing themselves with a new community. Among the many demographic variables tabulated in the census are population size; distribution of age, sex, race, and ethnicity; socioeconomic status; and housing characteristics. Variables that describe the health of the community per se are not a part of census data. However, community size numbers can be useful as denominators for morbidity and mortality rates (see Calculation of Rates). Census data are generally found in public and university libraries. Since the 1990 census, data are available on CD-ROM, which allows one to view several variables in combination (e.g., age and ethnicity) and to construct a profile of a community more easily.

The comparison of data with those of other communities and of previous time periods is an essential part of analyzing the data and interpreting their meaning. By comparing data for one census unit, such as a census tract or a city, with those of another community or the nation as a whole, the nurse can identify the attributes that make each community unique. These attributes provide clues to the potential vulnerabilities or health risks of a community. For example, a community health nurse may discover from census reports that a district has many elderly persons. This directs the nurse toward further assessment of the social resources (housing, transportation, and community centers), health resources (hospitals and clinics capable of providing geriatric services), and health problems common to aging persons. By identifying the trends in the population over time, the community health nurse can then modify public health programs to meet the changing needs of that community more effectively.

CENSUS DATA CAN REVEAL "HIDDEN POCKETS" OF NEED

Census data not only are helpful in revealing dominant community features but also suggest the existence of small "hidden pockets" of persons who may have special needs. One nurse who initially assessed her community as an upper-middle-class community was surprised to find 20 families living below the poverty level, 3 of which did not possess running water in their homes. Did these families have particular needs that could be addressed by a community health nurse? Deviations from the central trend, therefore, can be very revealing and important in determining a community health nurse's practice priorities.

Vital Statistics

The official registration records of births, deaths, marriages, divorces, and adoptions form the basis of data included in vital statistics. These events are aggregated and reported annually for the preceding year by city, county, and state health departments. When compared with those of previous years, vital statistics provide indicators of growth or shrinkage in the population size. In addition to supplying information about the number of births and deaths, registration certificates record the cause of death, which is useful in determining morbidity and mortality trends. Similarly, birth certificates document the type of birth (e.g., cesarean) and the occurrence of any congenital malformations. This information is also important in assessing the health status of the community.

Other Sources of Health Data

The U.S. Bureau of the Census conducts numerous other surveys on subjects of interest to the government, such as crime, housing, and labor. Results of these surveys as well as the census and vital statistics reports are usually available in public libraries. The National Center for Health Statistics compiles annual National Health Survey data, which describe health trends in a national sample. Reports are published on the prevalence of disability, illness, and other health-related variables.

In addition to these important sources of information, community health nurses frequently can access a broad range of state and community government reports that contribute to the comprehensive assessment of a population. Local agencies, chambers of commerce, and health and hospital districts collect invaluable information on the health of the communities they serve. Local health systems agencies (discussed in Chapter 7) and other planning organizations also compile and analyze statistical data as part of the planning process. All of these formal and informal resources can be used by the community health nurse in learning about a community or aggregate (Table 5–1).

A community health nurse, however, may require data on certain community aspects for which no formalized collection has been undertaken. Therefore, it may be necessary for the nurse to perform the data collection, compilation, and analysis. For example, school nurses regularly aggregate data from student records to learn about the demographic composition of their population. Their ongoing surveys of classroom attendance and causes of illness are essential to an effective school health program. Thus, the school nurse is not only a consumer of existent data but also a researcher collecting original data for the assessment of the school community.

Calculation of Rates

Collection and compilation of large amounts of descriptive information about the aggregate have been discussed. So far, it has been assumed that data were in the form of counts or simple frequencies of events (e.g., the number of persons with a specific health condition). Community health practitioners interpret these raw counts by transforming them into rates. Rates are arithmetic expressions that allow one to consider a count of an event relative to the size of the

Table 5–1
Community Assessment Parameters

Parameter	Importance to CHN	Sources of Information

Geography
  Topography
  Climate
	Influences nature of health problems and access to health care	Almanac
		Chamber of Commerce

Population
  Size
  Demographic character
  Trends
  Migration
  Density
	Describes population served; suggests their health risks and needs
	
	Suggests growth or decline
		Census documents
		Chamber of Commerce
		Local documents

Environment
  Water
  Sewage and waste disposal
  Air quality
  Food quality and access
  Housing
  Animal control
	Impacts quality of life and nature of environmental health problems
	
	Reflects community resources
	
	Suggests socioeconomic issues
		Local and state health departments
		Newspapers
		
		Local environmental action group
		
		Census documents

Industry
  Employment levels
  Manufacturing
  White vs. blue collar
  Income levels
	Affects social class, access to health care, and resources
	Influences nature of health problems
		Chamber of Commerce
		Almanac
		Employment commission
		
		Census documents

Education
  Schools
  Types of education
  Literacy rates
  Special education
  Health services
  School lunch programs
  Access to higher education
	Influences socioeconomic status, access to health care, ability to understand health recommendations	Census documents
		School districts and nurse

Recreation
  Parks and playgrounds
  Libraries
  Public and private recreation
  Special facilities
	Reflects quality of life, resources available to community, concern for young and disadvantaged	Parks and recreation departments
		Newspapers

Religion
  Churches, synagogues
  Denominations
  Community programs
  Health-related programs
  Community organizing
	Influences values in community, organizing around common interests and concerns
	Reflects involvement of members, community skills, and resources for community needs
		Chamber of Commerce
		Newspapers
		Community center newsletters

Communication
  Newspapers
  Neighborhood news
  Radio and television
  Telephone
  Hotline
  Medical media
  Public service announcements
	Reflects concerns and needs of community
	Networks and resources available for health-related use
		Local libraries
		Newspapers
		
		Local health department
		Medical and nursing society

Table 5–1
Community Assessment Parameters (Continued)

Parameter	Importance to CHN	Sources of Information

Transportation
  Intercity and intracity
  Handicapped
  Emergency transport
	Affects access to services, food, and other resources
	Reflects resources available to community
		Local bus and train service
		Local hospital emergency service

Public services
  Fire protection
  Police protection
  Rape treatment centers
  Utilities
	Affects security of community
	Reflects resources available
		Local police department

Political organization
  Structure
  Methods for filling positions
  Responsibilities of positions
  Sources of revenue
  Voter registration
	Reflects level of citizen activism and involvement, values, and concerns of citizenry
	Mechanism for nurse activism and lobbying
		Newspapers
		Local political party organization
		Local board of elections
		Local representatives

Community development or planning
  Activities
  Major issues
	Reflects needs and concerns of community
	Affects level of involvement of professionals in issues
		Newspapers
		Local and state planning board
		Local community organizations

Disaster programs
  American Red Cross
  Disaster plans
  Potential sources of disaster
	Level of preparedness, coordination, and resources available
	Influences resources and plans
		Local American Red Cross office
		Local emergency coordinating council
		Local fire department

Health statistics
  Mortality
  Morbidity
  Leading causes of death
  Births
	Reflects health problems, trends, and state of community health
	Affects resources needed and CHN services provided
		Local and state health department
		Health facilities and programs
		National vital statistics reports
		National Center for Health Statistics reports
		Morbidity and Mortality Weekly Report

Social problems
  Mental health
  Alcoholism and drug abuse
  Suicide
  Crime
  School dropout
  Unemployment
  Gangs
	Affects health problems and types and amounts of services required
	Influences CHN program priorities
		Local and state department of social services
		Local mental health centers
		Local hotlines
		Libraries

Health manpower	Influences health resources available and nature of CHN practice	Local and state health planning agency Health professional organizations Telephone directory Community service directory
Health professional organizations	Provides support for CHN practice	

Community services
  Institutional care
  Ambulatory care
  Preventive health services
  Nursing services
	Reflects resources available	Local United Way organization
		Local voluntary service directory
		County hospital
		Local health department

CHN = community health nursing.

population from which it is extracted (i.e., the population at risk). Rates are population proportions or fractions in which the numerator is the number of events occurring in a specified period of time. Events described by the numerator are necessarily included as part of the denominator. The denominator consists of all those in the same population at the same specified time period (i.e., per day, per week, or per year). This proportion is multiplied by a constant *(k)* that always is a multiple of 10, such as 1000, 10,000, or 100,000. By using a constant, the resultant number is usually converted to a whole number, which is larger and easier to interpret. A rate can be reported as the number of cases of a disease occurring for every 1000 or 100,000 persons in the population.

$$\text{Rate} = \frac{\text{Numerator}}{\text{Denominator}} = \frac{\text{Number of health events in a specified period}}{\text{Population in same area in same specified period}} \times k$$

When raw counts are converted to rates, the community health nurse can make meaningful comparisons

USING RATES IN EVERYDAY COMMUNITY HEALTH NURSING PRACTICE

The value of rates is exemplified in the following school situation:

On completing tuberculosis screening in the Southside School, the community health nurse identified 15 students with newly positive tuberculin tests among the 500 students at risk for tuberculosis (those tested). The proportion of Southside School students affected was 15/500, or .03 (3%), or a rate of 30/1000 students at risk for tuberculosis. Concurrently, the nurse conducted screening in the Northside School and again identified 15 positive tuberculin tests. This school, however, was much larger than the Southside School and had many more potentially at-risk students (900). To place the number of affected students in perspective relative to the size of the Northside School, the rate was calculated as 15/900, or 0.017 (1.7%), or a rate of 17/1000 students at risk.

On the basis of this comparison, the nurse concluded that, even though both schools had *equal numbers* of tuberculin conversions, Southside School had the *greater rate* of tuberculin test conversions. The nurse then could proceed to explore reasons for the difference in these rates.

with rates from other districts or states, the nation as a whole, and previous time periods. These analyses assist the nurse in determining the magnitude of a public health problem relative to the experience of others and allow more reliable tracking of trends in the community over time.

Sometimes a ratio is used to express a relationship between two variables. A ratio is obtained by dividing one quantity by another, and the numerator is not necessarily part of the denominator. For example, the number of male births could be contrasted to that of female births by using a ratio. Proportions are also commonly used to describe characteristics of a population. A proportion represents the numerator as a part of the denominator and is often expressed as a percentage.

Morbidity: Incidence and Prevalence Rates

The two principal types of morbidity rates (rates of illness) used in public health are incidence rates and prevalence rates. *Incidence rates* describe the occurrence of new disease cases in a community over a period of time relative to the size of the population at risk for that disease during that same period. Because the denominator consists of only those at risk for disease, known cases or those immunized against a disease are subtracted from the total population.

$$\text{Incidence rate} = \frac{\text{Number of new cases or events occurring in the population in a specified period}}{\text{Population at risk during same specified period}} \times k$$

Sometimes the incidence rate is considered the most sensitive indicator of the changing health of a community because it captures the fluctuations of disease in a population. Although incidence rates are valuable for monitoring trends in chronic disease, they are particularly useful for detecting short-term acute disease changes, such as those that occur with infectious hepatitis or measles, when the duration of the disease is typically short.

If a population is exposed to an infectious disease at a given time and place, a specialized form of the incidence rate, the *attack rate,* is used. Attack rates document the number of new cases of a disease in those exposed to the disease. A common example of the application of the attack rate is food poisoning; the denominator used to derive a rate is the number of persons exposed to a suspect food. Therefore, attack rates of illness among those exposed to specific foods can be calculated and compared to identify the critical food sources or exposure variables.

A *prevalence rate* is the number of all cases of a specific disease in a population at a given point in time relative to the population at the same point in time.

$$\text{Prevalence rate} = \frac{\begin{array}{l}\text{Number of existing cases}\\\text{in population at a}\\\text{specified point in time}\end{array}}{\begin{array}{l}\text{Population at same specified}\\\text{point in time}\end{array}} \times k$$

When prevalence rates describe the number of persons with the disease at a specific point in time, they are sometimes called *point prevalences*. For this reason, they are frequently used in cross-sectional studies. Period prevalences represent the number of existing cases during a specified period or interval of time and include old cases as well as new cases that develop in the period of time.

Prevalence rates are influenced by two factors: the number of people who experience a particular condition (incidence) and the duration of the condition. A prevalence rate can be derived by multiplying incidence by duration. An increase in the incidence rate or the duration of a disease increases the prevalence rate of a disease. With the advent of life-prolonging therapies (e.g., insulin for treatment of type I diabetes mellitus), the prevalence of a disease may increase without a change in the incidence rate. As can be seen, those who survive a chronic disease but who are not cured remain in the "prevalence pot" (see Fig. 5–1). For conditions such as cataracts, recent advances in surgical removal permit many persons to recover and thereby move out of the prevalence pot. Although the incidence has not necessarily changed, the reduced duration of the disease lowers the prevalence rate of cataracts in the population.

Morbidity rates are not available for many conditions because surveillance of many chronic diseases is not widely conducted. When available, morbidity rates may be subject to underreporting. Routinely collected rates of births and deaths (mortality rates), which are presented next, are more widely available.

Other Rates

Numerous other rates are useful in characterizing the population. *Crude rates* summarize, for example, the

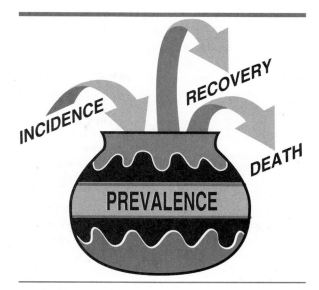

Figure 5–1
Prevalence pot: the relationship between incidence and prevalence. (Redrawn from Morton RF, Hebel JR, McCarter RJ: A Study Guide to Epidemiology and Biostatistics, 3rd ed. Gaithersburg, MD: Aspen Publishers, 1990, p. 30. Copyright © 1990 by Aspen Publishers, Inc.)

occurrence of births (crude birth rate), deaths (crude death rates), or diseases (crude disease rates) in the general population. The numerator is the number of events, and the denominator is the average population size or the population size at midyear (usually July 1) multiplied by a constant.

Because the denominators of crude rates represent the total population and not the population at risk for a given event, these rates are subject to certain biases in interpretation. Crude death rates are sensitive to the number of persons at the highest risk for dying, in particular, the elderly. A relatively older population probably will produce a higher crude death rate than a population in whom the age range is more evenly distributed. Conversely, a young population will have a somewhat lower crude death rate. Similar biases can occur for crude birth rates (e.g., higher birth rates in young populations). This distortion occurs because the denominator reflects the entire population, not only the population truly at risk for giving birth. Age is one of the most common confounding factors that can mask the true distribution of variables. However, many variables such as race and socioeconomic status can also bias the interpretation of biostatistical data. Therefore, several approaches for removing the confounding effect of these variables on rates are reviewed here.

Age-specific rates characterize a particular age group in the population, usually with regard to deaths and births. By determining the rate for specific subgroups of a population and using a denominator that reflects only that subgroup, the bias resulting from age is removed.

$$\text{Age-specific rate} = \frac{\begin{array}{l}\text{Number of cases in a}\\ \text{specific age category in}\\ \text{population at a specified time}\end{array}}{\begin{array}{l}\text{Population in the same age}\\ \text{category at the}\\ \text{same specified time}\end{array}} \times k$$

To characterize a total population using age-specific rates, rates for each category must be computed because a single summary rate (such as a mean) is not being used. Specific rates for other variables may be determined in a similar fashion (e.g., race-specific or gender-specific rates).

Age-adjustment or *standardization* of rates is another method of reducing bias when there are differences in the age distributions of two populations being compared. Two approaches can be used. In the *direct* method, a standard population is chosen, often the population distribution of the United States. Age-specific rates for age categories of the two populations are essentially converted to those of the standard population, and a summary age-adjusted rate for each of the two populations of interest is calculated. This enables one to compare the two rates as if both had the same age structure as the standard population (i.e., without the prior problem of age distortion). See Tables 5–2, 5–3, and 5–4 for examples of the computations involved.

The second method, *indirect standardization,* allows one to compare two populations as though they had similar age distributions (i.e., it removes the effect of age). This is helpful especially when their age-specific rates are unknown or, as in direct adjustment, when there are many strata to be compared. Indirect adjustment involves the calculation of a *standardized mortality ratio* (SMR), which is a single age-adjusted death ratio that compares the observed deaths with those that would be expected if the population of interest had the mortality experience of the standard population.

$$\text{SMR} = \frac{\text{Total observed deaths}}{\text{Total expected deaths}}$$

Table 5–2
Direct Standardization of Mortality Rates by Age for "South Community" and "North Community"

Age (yr)	Size of Population (A)	Percent of Population	Number of Deaths (B)	Age-Specific Death Rate per 1000 (B/A)
South Community*				
<15	5400	30.4	10	1.85/1000
15–44	7300	41.1	16	2.19/1000
45–64	3400	19.2	38	11.18/1000
>65	1650	9.3	84	50.91/1000
Totals	17,750	100	148	
North Community†				
<15	1030	34.2	2	1.94/1000
15–44	1500	49.8	4	2.67/1000
45–64	407	13.5	4	9.83/1000
>65	75	2.5	4	53.33/1000
Totals	3012	100	14	

Step 1: Determine age-specific death rates. Divide the number of deaths by the population size for each age category.
*Crude death rate = 148/17,750 = 8.34/1000.
†Crude death rate = 14/3012 = 4.64/1000.

Table 5–3
Direct Standardization of Mortality Rates

	United States 1990			South Community†		North Community‡	
Age (yr)	Size of Population	Percent of Population (A)*	Age-Specific Death Rate per 1000 (B_1)	Expected No. of Deaths per 1000 ($A \times B_1$)		Age-Specific Death Rate per 1000 (B_2)	Expected No. of Deaths per 1000 ($A \times B_2$)
<15	55,961,000	21.9	1.85	0.405		1.94	0.425
15–44	118,490,000	46.5	2.19	1.018		2.67	1.242
45–64	48,345,000	19.0	11.18	2.124		9.83	1.868
>65	32,283,000	12.7	50.91	6.466		53.33	6.773
Totals	255,079,000	100		10.013			10.308

Step 2: Compute expected number of deaths by multiplying proportion of U.S. population by age-specific death rates. Sum expected deaths to produce age-adjusted death rate.

*Convert to decimal before computing product A × B.

†Age-adjusted mortality rate = 10.013/1000 (sum of $A \times B_1$).

‡Age-adjusted mortality rate = 10.308/1000 (sum of $A \times B_2$).

A ratio of 1 indicates that observed deaths were the same as expected deaths. A ratio greater than 1 indicates that more deaths were observed in the population of interest than would be expected on the basis of rates in the standard population. A ratio of less than 1 indicates the opposite. Standardized ratios as well as rates adjusted by the direct method can be produced for other rates (e.g., birth or morbidity rates) and for other variables (e.g., income or birth weight).

To calculate an SMR, the procedure is in essence the reverse of that used in direct standardization (Tables 5–5 and 5–6). First, age-specific rates from a standard population are applied to each age category of the two populations of interest to produce expected deaths for each stratum. The standard population here may be the U.S. population, as in direct adjustment, or may be the larger or more stable of the two populations being compared. Next, the actual number of observed deaths is divided by the sum of expected deaths for each population to produce an SMR for each population. Note that age-adjusted rates are actually not "real" death rates; rather they are representations of the experience of populations as though their age distributions were like that of the standard population; therefore, they allow comparisons to be made more easily.

The *proportionate mortality ratio* (PMR) is another method used to describe mortality. It represents the percentage of deaths resulting from a specific cause relative to deaths from all causes. As such, it is often helpful in identifying areas in which public health programs might make significant contributions in reducing deaths. In some situations, a high PMR may reflect a low overall mortality or reduced number of deaths resulting from other causes. The PMR thus needs to be considered in the context of the mortality experience of the population.

$$PMR = \frac{\text{Number of deaths resulting from a specific cause in a specific time period}}{\text{Total number of deaths in time period}}$$

Table 5–7 summarizes the advantages and disadvantages of crude, specific, and adjusted rates. Numerous other rates are used in assessing particular

Table 5–4
Summary of Tables 5–2 and 5–3*

Area	Crude Mortality Rate	Age-Adjusted Mortality Rate
South Community	8.34 per 1000	10.013 per 1000
North Community	4.64 per 1000	10.308 per 1000

*When the confounding effect of different age distributions is removed through age adjustment, mortality rates for the two communities are similar.

Table 5–5
Indirect Standardization of Mortality Rates

| Age (yr) | Age-Specific U.S. Death Rates (A)* | Population Size (B) | | Expected Deaths $\frac{(A \times B)}{100,000}$ | |
		South Community	North Community	South Community	North Community
<15	95.18	5400	1030	5.14	0.98
15–44	155.40	7300	1500	11.34	2.33
45–64	788.76	3400	407	26.82	3.21
>65	4922.32	1650	75	81.22	3.69

U.S. age-specific mortality rates are multiplied by population of each community to produce expected deaths, which are summed. Standard mortality ratios are then calculated. Death rates are per 100,000 population.

*1991 data from U.S. Bureau of the Census. (1994). Statistical Abstract of the United States 1994, 114th ed. Washington, DC. Author.

segments of the population. Table 5–8 provides a summary; consult a standard epidemiology textbook, such as *Mausner and Bahn Epidemiology—An Introductory Text* (Mausner and Kramer, 1985) for more detailed background information.

Concept of Risk

The concept of risk and risk factors is familiar to community health nurses whose practices focus on the prevention of disease. *Risk* refers to the probability of an adverse event (i.e., the likelihood that healthy persons exposed to a specific factor will acquire a specific disease). *Risk factor* refers to the specific exposure factor, which frequently is external to the individual, such as exposure to cigarette smoking, excessive stress, high noise levels, or chemicals in the environment. Risk factors may also be fixed charac-

teristics of people, such as age, sex, or genetic make-up. Although these intrinsic factors are not alterable, certain lifestyle changes may reduce their impact as risk factors. For example, positive dietary practices and exercise regimens may modify the effects of aging as a risk factor for certain health conditions.

Epidemiologists describe the pattern of disease in the aggregate and quantify the effect of exposure to particular factors on the rate of disease. To identify specific risk factors, rates of disease for those exposed are compared with those of the nonexposed. One method for comparing two rates is to subtract the rate of nonexposed individuals from that of the exposed. This measure of risk is called the *attributable risk*. It is the estimate of the burden of disease in a population. For example, if the rate of non–insulin-dependent diabetes were 5000 per 100,000 persons in the obese population (those weighing more than 120% of ideal body weight) and 1000 per 100,000 persons in the nonobese population, the attributable risk of non–insulin-dependent diabetes resulting from obesity would be 4000 per 100,000 persons (5000/100,000 minus 1000/100,000). This means that 4000 cases per 100,000 persons can be attributed to obesity. Thus, a prevention program designed to reduce obesity could theoretically eliminate 4000 cases per 100,000 persons in the population. Therefore, attributable risks are particularly important in describing the potential impact of a public health intervention in a community.

A second measure of the excess risk caused by a factor is the *relative risk ratio*. To calculate a relative risk, the incidence rate of disease in the exposed population is divided by the incidence rate of disease in the nonexposed population. In the prior example, a relative risk of 5 was obtained by dividing 5000/100,000 by 1000/100,000. This risk ratio suggests that

Table 5–6
Standardized Mortality Ratio Based on Data from Tables 5–5 and 5–2

Variable	South Community	North Community
Total expected deaths	124.52	10.21
Total observed deaths (from Table 5–2)	148	14
Standardized mortality ratio of deaths (observed to expected)	1.19	1.37

Standardized mortality ratios (SMR) of greater than 1 indicate that more deaths were observed in both communities than would be expected based on the mortality experience of the overall U.S. population. When mortality data for the two communities are standardized to a third or standard population, the SMRs indicate a similar mortality experience.

Table 5–7

Advantages and Disadvantages of Crude, Specific, and Adjusted Rates

Rate	Advantages	Disadvantages
Crude	Actual summary rates Readily calculable for international comparisons (widely used despite limitations)	Because populations vary in composition (e.g., age), differences in crude rates difficult to interpret
Specific	Homogeneous subgroups Detailed rates useful for epidemiologic and public health purposes	Cumbersome to compare many subgroups of two or more populations
Adjusted	Summary statements Differences in composition of groups "removed," permitting unbiased comparison	Fictional rates Absolute magnitude dependent on standard population chosen Opposing trends in subgroups masked

Modified from Mausner JS, Kramer S. (1985). Mausner and Bahn Epidemiology: An Introductory Text, 2nd ed. Philadelphia, WB Saunders, p. 57.

an obese individual has a fivefold greater risk of diabetes than does a nonobese individual.

The relative risk ratio forms the statistical basis for the concept of risk factor. Relative risks are valuable indicators of the excess risk incurred by exposure to certain factors. They have been used extensively in identifying the major causal factors of many common diseases and so direct public health practitioners' efforts to reduce health risks.

Community health nurses may apply the concept of relative risk to suspected exposure variables to isolate risk factors associated with health problems in the community. For example, a community health nurse might investigate an outbreak of probable food-borne illness. The incidence rate among those exposed to potato salad in a school cafeteria can be compared with the incidence rate among those not exposed. The relative risk calculated from the ratio of these two incidence rates indicates the amount of excess risk of disease that was incurred by eating potato salad. A relative risk might also be determined for other suspected foods and then compared with that for potato salad. Incidence rates for specific foods involved in food-borne illnesses are frequently called *attack rates*. A food with a markedly higher relative risk than other foods might be the causal agent in a food-borne epidemic; the identification of the causal agent (a specific food) is critical to the implementation of an effective prevention program, such as teaching proper food-handling techniques.

EPIDEMIOLOGY

Epidemiology is defined as the study of the distribution and determinants of health and disease in the community. It may be described as the principle science of community health practice, and as such it entails specialized methods and approaches to scientific research. Community health nurses working to improve the health of the aggregate use epidemiologic approaches in community assessment and diagnosis and in planning and evaluating effective community interventions. The uses of epidemiology and its specialized methodologies are discussed.

Use of Epidemiology in Disease Control and Prevention

Although the origins of epidemiology may be traced to ancient times, formal epidemiologic techniques were developed in the 19th century. Early applications were focused on identifying factors associated with infectious disease and its epidemic spread in the community. By identifying factors critical to the development of disease, public health practitioners hoped to improve preventive strategies. Specifically, investigators attempted to identify differences among those who were stricken with a disease such as cholera or plague compared with those who remained healthy. These differences might include a broad range of personal factors such as age, socioeconomic status, and health status. Investigators also questioned whether there were differences in location or environment of ill persons compared with healthy individuals and whether these factors influenced the development of disease. Researchers also examined whether factors of time, such as when persons acquired disease, contributed to the cause of the disease. Use of this person-place-time model organized epidemiologists' investigations of the pattern of disease in the commu-

Table 5-8
Major Public Health Rates

Rate Denominator	Rates	Usual Factor	Rate for United States, 1992
Total population	Crude birth rate = $\dfrac{\text{Number of live births during the year}}{\text{Average (midyear) population}}$	Per 1000 population	15.9
	Crude death rate = $\dfrac{\text{Number of deaths during the year}}{\text{Average (midyear) population}}$	Per 1000 population	8.5
	Age-specific death rate = $\dfrac{\text{Number of deaths among persons of a given age group in 1 year}}{\text{Average (midyear) population in specified age group}}$	Per 1000 population	0.22 (5–14 yr) 7.57 (45–64 yr) 25.90 (65–74 yr)
	Cause-specific death rate = $\dfrac{\text{Number of deaths from a stated cause in 1 year}}{\text{Average (midyear) population}}$	Per 100,000 population	285.50 (diseases of the heart) 203.80 (malignant neoplasms)
Women aged 15–44 yr	Fertility rate = $\dfrac{\text{Number of live births during 1 year}}{\text{Number of women aged 15–44 in same year}}$	Per 1000 women aged 15–44 yr	68.90
Live births	Infant mortality rate = $\dfrac{\text{Number of deaths in 1 year of children younger than 1 yr}}{\text{Number of live births in same year}}$	Per 1000 live births	8.50
	Neonatal mortality rate = $\dfrac{\text{Number of deaths in 1 year of children younger than 28 days}}{\text{Number of live births in same year}}$	Per 1000 live births	5.40
	Maternal mortality rate (puerperal) = $\dfrac{\text{Number of deaths from puerperal causes in 1 year}}{\text{Number of live births in same year}}$	Per 100,000 live births	7.80
Rates whose denominators are live births and fetal deaths	Fetal death rate = $\dfrac{\text{Number of fetal deaths in 1 year}}{\text{Number of live births and fetal deaths during same year}}$	Per 1000 live births and fetal deaths	7.40
	Perinatal mortality rate = $\dfrac{\text{Number of fetal deaths} \geq 28 \text{ weeks plus infant deaths} <7 \text{ days}}{\text{Number of live births and fetal deaths} \geq 28 \text{ weeks during the same year}}$	Per 1000 live births and fetal deaths	8.50

Rates from National Center for Health Statistics. (1995). Health, United States, 1994. (Publication No. (PHS) 95-1232). Hyattsville, MD, Department of Health and Human Services, U.S. Public Health Service. Table adapted from Mausner JS, Kramer S. (1985). Mausner and Bahn Epidemiology: An Introductory Text, 2nd ed. Philadelphia, WB Saunders, pp. 92–93.

nity. The study of the amount and distribution of disease constitutes descriptive epidemiology.

In addition to investigating person, place, and time factors related to disease, epidemiologists examined complex relationships among the many determinants of disease. This investigation of the causes, or etiology, of disease is called analytic epidemiology. Even before bacterial agents were identified, public health practitioners recognized that single factors alone were insufficient to cause disease. In exploring the cholera epidemics, for instance, Snow in 1855 collected data about social and physical environmental conditions that might favor disease development, in particular, contamination of local water systems and the pumps where people obtained water. He also gathered information about people who became ill, including their patterns of living, especially related to water use, their socioeconomic characteristics, and their health status. A comprehensive data base assisted Snow in developing a theory about the possible cause of the epidemic. As mentioned, Snow suspected that a single biological agent probably was responsible for the cholera infection, even though the organism, *Vibrio cholerae,* had not been discovered at that time. The comparison of death rates among individuals using one source of water with those among people using a different water pump suggested an association between cholera and water quality.

By examining the interrelationships of host and environmental characteristics, the epidemiologist uses an organized method of inquiry to derive an explanation of disease. This model of investigation has been called the epidemiological triangle because of the three elements that must be analyzed: agent, host, and environment (Fig. 5–2). The development of disease is dependent on the extent of exposure to an agent, the strength or virulence of the agent, the host's susceptibility (either genetic or immunologic), and the environmental conditions (including the biological, social, and physical environment) existing at the time of exposure to the agent (Table 5–9). The model implies that when the balance among these three factors is altered, the rate of disease will change.

The epidemiologic triangle is most applicable to conditions that can be linked to clearly identifiable agents such as bacteria, chemicals, toxins, and other exposure factors. With increased understanding of diseases that do not have single causal agents, other models have been developed that stress the multiplicity of environment and host interactions. An example of such a model is the "wheel model" (Fig. 5–3). The wheel consists of a hub that represents the host with all of its human characteristics such as genetic make-up, personality, and immunity. The surrounding wheel represents the environment and comprises biological, social, and physical dimensions. The relative size of each component in the wheel depends on the health problem being analyzed. Diseases dependent on heredity are represented by a relatively large genetic core. Origins of other health conditions may be more dependent on environmental factors (Mausner and Kramer, 1985). Because the model allows for a multiple-causation rather than a single-causation theory of disease, it is more useful for analyzing complex chronic conditions and identifying factors that are amenable to their intervention.

AN EXAMPLE OF THE EPIDEMIOLOGIC APPROACH

An early example of the use of the epidemiologic approach is John Snow's investigation of an epidemic of cholera in the 1850s. He analyzed the distribution of person, place, and time factors by comparing the rates of death among people living in different geographic sectors of London. Snow noted that those using a particular water pump had significantly higher mortality rates resulting from cholera than those using other sources in the city. Although the cholera organism had not yet been identified, the clustering of disease cases around one neighborhood pump suggested new prevention strategies to public health officials (i.e., that cholera might be reduced in a community by controlling the contamination of drinking water sources) (Snow, 1936).

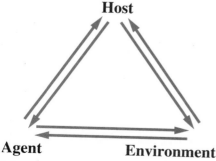

Figure 5–2
Epidemiological triangle.

Table 5–9
A Classification of Agent, Host, and Environmental Factors That Determine the Occurrence of Diseases in Human Populations

Agents of Disease—Etiologic Factors

	Examples
A. Nutritive elements	
Excesses	Cholesterol
Deficiencies	Vitamins, proteins
B. Chemical agents	
Poisons	Carbon monoxide, carbon tetrachloride, drugs
Allergens	Ragweed, poison ivy, medications
C. Physical agents	Ionizing radiation, mechanical
D. Infectious agents	
Metazoa	Hookworm, schistosomiasis, onchocerciasis
Protozoa	Amoebae, malaria
Bacteria	Rheumatic fever, lobar pneumonia, typhoid, tuberculosis, syphilis
Fungi	Histoplasmosis, athlete's foot
Rickettsia	Rocky mountain spotted fever, typhus, Lyme disease
Viruses	Measles, mumps, chickenpox, smallpox, poliomyelitis, rabies, yellow fever, HIV

Host Factors (Intrinsic Factors)—Influence Exposure, Susceptibility, or Response to Agents

	Examples
A. Genetic	Sickle cell disease
B. Age	Alzheimer's disease
C. Sex	Rheumatoid arthritis
D. Ethnic group	—
E. Physiologic state	Fatigue, pregnancy, puberty, stress, nutritional state
F. Prior immunologic experience	Hypersensitivity, protection
Active	Prior infection, immunization
Passive	Maternal antibodies, gamma globulin prophylaxis
G. Intercurrent or preexisting disease	
H. Human behavior	Personal hygiene, food handling, diet, interpersonal contact, occupation, recreation, utilization of health resources, tobacco use

Environmental Factors (Extrinsic Factors)—Influence Existence of the Agent, Exposure, or Susceptibility to Agent

	Examples
A. Physical environment	Geology, climate
B. Biological environment	
Human populations	Density
Flora	Sources of food, influence on vertebrates and arthropods, as a source of agents
Fauna	Food sources, vertebrate hosts, arthropod vectors
C. Socioeconomic environment	
Occupation	Exposure to chemical agents
Urbanization and economic development	Urban crowding, tensions and pressures, cooperative efforts in health and education
Disruption	Wars, floods

HIV = human immunodeficiency virus.
Modified from Lilienfeld DE, Lilienfeld D. (1994). Foundations of Epidemiology. New York, Oxford University Press, pp. 37–38.

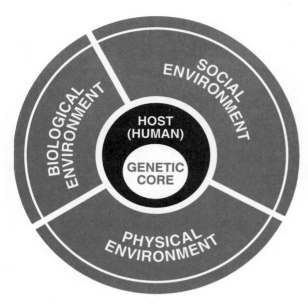

Figure 5–3
Wheel model of human–environment interaction. (Redrawn from Mausner JS, Kramer S: Mausner and Bahn Epidemiology: An Introductory Text, 2nd ed. Philadelphia: WB Saunders, 1985, p. 36.)

As the causative agents of many infectious diseases were discovered, subsequent public health interventions led to a decline in mortality caused by widespread epidemics, particularly in the developed countries. As a result, the focus of public health efforts during the past few decades has shifted to the control of chronic diseases such as cancer, coronary heart disease, and diabetes. These chronic diseases tend to have multiple interrelated factors associated with their origins rather than a single causative agent. Epidemiologists, however, apply approaches to chronic diseases that are similar to those used in infectious disease investigation, thereby developing complex theories about chronic disease control. Of particular importance to chronic disease reduction is the identification of risk factors. As previously discussed, risk factors suggest specific prevention and intervention approaches that may effectively and efficiently reduce morbidity and mortality from chronic disease. For example, the identification of cardiovascular disease risk factors has suggested a number of lifestyle modifications that could reduce the morbidity risk before disease onset. Primary prevention strategies such as reduction of dietary saturated fats, smoking cessation, and hypertension control were developed as a response to previous epidemiologic studies that identified them as risk factors. The web of causation is

a model that can be used to illustrate the complexity of relationships among causal variables identified for heart disease (Fig. 5–4).

Use of Epidemiology in Secondary and Tertiary Prevention Approaches

ESTABLISHING CAUSALITY

As discussed earlier, a principal goal of classic epidemiology is to identify etiologic factors of diseases so that the most effective primary prevention activities might be encouraged and treatment modalities developed. In the last few decades, we have come to understand that many diseases have not one but rather multiple causes. Epidemiologists who examine disease rates and who conduct population-focused research often find multiple factors associated with health problems. For example, cardiovascular disease rates may vary by place, ethnicity, and smoking status. Determining the extent to which these correlates represent associative or causal relationships is important for public health practitioners, who seek to prevent, diagnose, and treat disease.

Six criteria have come to be accepted in establishing the existence of a cause and effect relationship.

- **Strength of association.** Rates of morbidity or mortality must be higher in the exposed group than in the nonexposed group. Relative risk ratios or odds ratios, as well as correlation coefficients, are an indicator of the likelihood that a relation between the exposure variable and the outcome is causal. For example, epidemiologic studies have demonstrated an elevated relative risk for heart disease among smokers compared with nonsmokers (Doll and Hill, 1956).
- **Dose-response relationship.** As exposure to the risk factor increases, there is a concomitant increase in disease rate. The risk of heart disease mortality is higher for those with a history of heavy smoking compared with light smoking (Mattson et al., 1987).
- **Temporally correct relationship.** Exposure to the causal factor must occur before the effect, that is, before the disease. For heart disease, smoking history must precede the development of disease.
- **Biological plausibility.** The data must make biological sense and represent a coherent explanation for the relationship.
- **Consistency with other studies.** Similar associations must be observed in varying types of studies

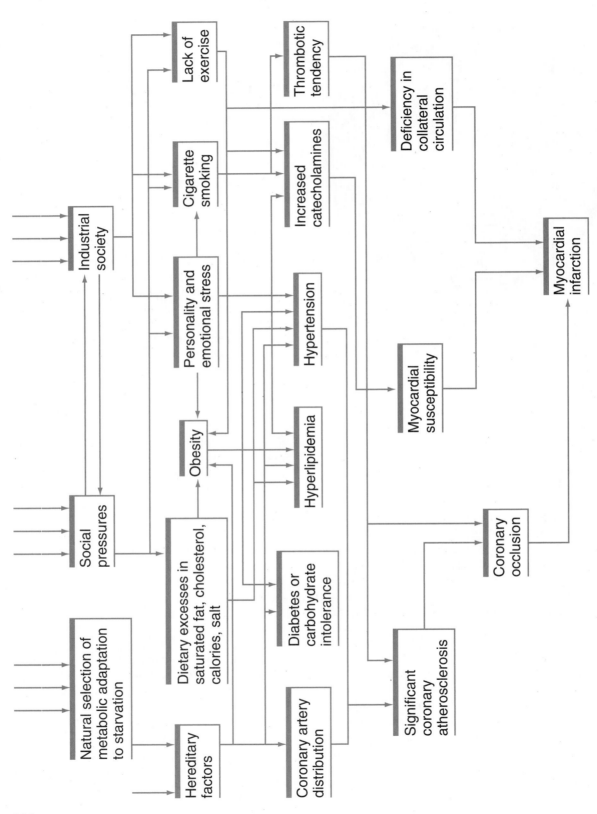

Figure 5–4
The web of causation for myocardial infarction: a current view. (From Friedman GD: Primer of Epidemiology, 4th ed. New York: McGraw-Hill, 1994, p. 4.)

and in other populations. Several studies of different designs must support the relationship between smoking and heart disease.

- **Specificity.** The exposure variable must be necessary and sufficient to cause disease; that is, there is only one causal factor. Although specificity may be strong causal evidence, generally this criterion is considered less important today because diseases do not have single causes; rather they have multifactorial origins.

  In the case of heart disease, the exposure variable, smoking, is one of several risk factors for heart disease. In addition, few factors are associated with only one condition. Smoking is not specific to heart disease alone; rather it is a causal factor for other diseases, notably lung and oral cancers. Further, smoking is not considered "necessary and sufficient" to the development of heart disease, because there are nonsmokers who also experience coronary heart disease. Because of these limitations, specificity as a causal criteria has been more commonly applied to infectious diseases.

Although these criteria are useful in evaluating epidemiologic evidence, it should be noted that causality can never be proven but is always a matter of judgment. In reality, absolute causality is only rarely established. Rather epidemiologists more commonly refer to suggested causal and associated factors. It is difficult to ascertain true relationships between the exposure and outcome variables partly because of the effect of confounding variables. Confounding variables are related independently to *both* the dependent variable and the independent variable and, therefore, may mask the true relationship between these two variables. For example, Buring and Lee (1995) discussed the need to control for dietary fat when examining the relation between physical activity and coronary heart disease. This is necessary because in some populations dietary fat has been shown to be independently related to both physical exercise (Simoes et al., 1995) and heart disease (Willett, 1990). The apparent association between physical activity and heart disease may be attributed to the difference in fat intake between those with and those without heart disease. Those with heart disease may tend to have a higher fat intake and be more sedentary than those without heart disease. The outcome cannot be solely attributed to exercise. On the other hand, Buring and Lee (1995) provided an example in which dietary fat does not act as a confounding variable despite its relation to physical activity. Dietary fat is not a confounder of the relationship of physical exercise and osteoporosis because dietary fat is not a risk factor for osteoporosis, the dependent variable.

By measuring the confounding variable, it is possible to statistically account for its effect in the analysis (e.g., by use of multiple logistic regression analysis or stratification) (see a biostatistics text for discussion of these methods). Alternatively, by matching subjects in treatment and control groups with respect to the confounding variable, the effects of the confounder can be minimized. As discussed earlier, standardization for variables such as age is another method for managing spurious associations, so that true relationships become more apparent. When such relationships are understood, interpretation and application of findings by practitioners are facilitated.

SCREENING

A central aim of epidemiology is to describe the course of disease according to person and time. Observations of the disease process may suggest factors that aggravate or ameliorate its progress. This information also assists in determining usual treatment or rehabilitation patterns (i.e., secondary or tertiary prevention approaches).

Identifying risk factors and diseases in their earliest stages is the purpose of screening programs. Screening is usually classified as a secondary prevention activity because disease is discovered after a pathologic change has occurred, ideally early in the disease process (see Chapter 1, Levels of Prevention). As with all forms of secondary and tertiary prevention, the identification of illness prompts the question, What might have been done upstream to prevent the development of disease?

Screening programs are common activities of community health nurses. A large component of public health nurses' work activities may be consumed by performing physical examinations, promoting client self-examination, or conducting screening programs in schools, clinics, or community settings. Although these secondary prevention activities are important services and provide vital information on the status of a community's health, they are aimed at detecting disease already in process and should be contrasted with primary prevention and anticipatory guidance, which most consider the hallmark of community health nursing practice.

Several guidelines for screening programs have come to be accepted. First, adequate and appropriate follow-up treatment for those with disease must be planned for and carried out as part of the program. The lack of consistent follow-up has been a major criticism of health fairs, a large component of which is screening activity. It should be clear to the nurse in the planning phase that early diagnosis of a particular disease constitutes a real benefit to clients, whether in terms of increased life expectancy or quality of life. Further, some believe that a critical prerequisite to screening is the existence of acceptable and medically sound follow-up and treatment. In the past decade, public health providers have debated the ethical and practical arguments for implementing human immunodeficiency virus (HIV) screening. Concern exists regarding the potential for stigma and discrimination against those who screen positively for a test. Therefore, procedures for ensuring confidentiality have been implemented. These, in conjunction with the development of azidothymidine (AZT) and other antiviral treatments, have encouraged earlier identification of HIV-positive individuals.

Another criterion of a screening program is that procedures must be acceptable to clients and be cost effective. Although sigmoidoscopy is an effective screening procedure for colon cancer, it is not a simple and inexpensive test, nor is it one that many clients readily undergo. Consequently, it has been primarily used for those who demonstrate a high risk for colon cancer. Finally, the cost of the screening program and procedures, the cost of the follow-up of clients who test positively, and the cost of the resultant medical care, each of which can be significant, have bearing on the decision to screen a population.

Issues specific to the validity of the screening test also must be evaluated in developing a screening program. The purpose of screening is to detect those with disease, and the ability of a test to do this correctly is termed *sensitivity*. *Specificity,* on the other hand, is the extent to which a test can correctly identify those who do not have disease. To obtain estimates of these two dimensions, screening results must be compared with those of some definitive diagnostic procedure (Mausner & Kramer, 1985). For a given test, the sensitivity and specificity tend to be inversely related to each other. When a test is highly sensitive, individuals without disease may be labeled as positive. These false-positive tests may cause stress and worry for clients and require further diagnostic testing to confirm a diagnosis. With a highly sensitive test, specificity may be lower, and some with disease may not be detected. These false-negative test results mean that some individuals may be given false reassurance that they do not have the disease and consequently receive no follow-up care. Optimally, a screening test should be maximally sensitive *and* specific. This is dependent to a large extent on the stringency of the cut-off point established for determining a positive case of disease. See Table 5–10 for the formula for calculating sensitivity and specificity.

Sensitivity and specificity reflect the yield of a screening test, which is the amount of disease detected. One measure of yield is the *positive predictive value* of a test, which is the proportion of true positive results relative to all positive test results. On the basis of Table 5–10, the formula is a/a + b. It is dependent on the prevalence of undetected disease in a population. Screening for a rare disease like phenylketonuria will yield a lower predictive value and more false-positive results. In phenylketonuria, a low predictive value is considered acceptable because of the serious consequences of a false-negative result. The predictive value is also affected by the nature of the population being screened. The screening of only individuals at high risk for a disease will produce a higher predictive value and can be considered a more efficient way to identify

Table 5–10		
Sensitivity and Specificity of a Screening Test		
Screening Test	**Those With Disease**	**Those Without Disease**
Positive	True positives (a)	False positives (b)
Negative	False negatives (c)	True negatives (d)

$$\text{Sensitivity} = \frac{\text{True positives} \quad (a)}{\text{All with disease} \; (a+c)}$$

$$\text{Specificity} = \frac{\text{True negatives} \quad (d)}{\text{All without disease} \; (b+d)}$$

those with health problems than the screening of an entire population. For example, screening for diabetes in a Mexican-American or African-American adult population is expected to produce a higher predictive value than screening the general adult population.

SURVEILLANCE

In addition to screening, surveillance is a mechanism for the ongoing collection of health information in a community. Monitoring for changes in disease frequency is essential to effective and responsive public health programs. Identification of trends in the incidence of disease or of risk factor status by location and by population subgroup over time allows the community health nurse to evaluate the effectiveness of programs that are already in place and to implement interventions specifically targeted to high-risk groups. As discussed earlier, identifying new cases for the calculation of incidence rates is particularly useful in evaluating trends in morbidity. Yet this form of surveillance data is among the more difficult to collect and consequently tends to be readily available to public health practitioners for only selected diseases. Prevalence rates, mortality data, and data about risk factors and hospital and health service utilization can also be useful in suggesting program success or areas needing attention.

The U.S. Public Health Service coordinates a system of data collection among federal, state, and local agencies through which numerous sets of data are compiled. Some of these data sets are on the entire population (e.g., vital statistics data), and other collections are based on subsamples of the population (e.g., the National Health Interview Survey). The completeness of data reporting is variable because not all diseases are reportable. For example, only four sexually transmittable diseases (AIDS, syphilis, gonorrhea, and chlamydia) are notifiable to all local and state health departments. Furthermore, not all practitioners report cases on a regular basis, and not all persons with the disease actually seek care. Similar problems of underreporting childhood communicable diseases have been observed. The Centers for Disease Control and Prevention conducts studies to estimate the magnitude of this problem (National Center for Health Statistics, 1995).

Practitioners have a continuing need for comprehensive and systematically collected surveillance data describing the health status of national and local subgroups, such as age and ethnic groups, to evaluate the impact of programs on specific groups in a community. For example, the effectiveness of Healthy People 2000, the national goal-setting process, is dependent on the availability of reliable baseline and ongoing data with which to characterize health problems and evaluate goal achievement. Healthy People 2000 (Public Health Service, U.S. Department of Health and Human Services, 1990) cited the ongoing need to extend the comprehensiveness of such surveillance systems. For example, simply documenting children's mortality rates resulting from injury is insufficient for the development of specific methods of injury prevention. Data on the number of injured children and the nature of injury across the nation would increase the usefulness of surveillance information. At a local level, community health nurses also require regularly reported data about sexually transmitted disease rates, maternal and infant health indicators, and chronic disease morbidity rates, to name a few. To intervene effectively on behalf of communities, nurses need to be able to describe trends by locale and by demographic and risk factor status in a community. They must be able to compare the data for their locale with those of a relevant neighboring area, such as a census tract, city, county, or state or nation, to gain perspective on the magnitude of a local

---

CORONARY HEART DISEASE RISK FACTORS SUPPORTED BY EPIDEMIOLOGIC DATA

- Age: Male, 45 years
  Female, 55 years or premature menopause without estrogen replacement therapy
- Family history of premature coronary heart disease (definite myocardial infarction or sudden death before 55 years of age in father or other first-degree male relative or before 65 years of age in mother or other first-degree female relative)
- Current cigarette smoking
- Hypertension (blood pressure of 140/90 mm Hg or prescribed antihypertensive medication)
- Low high-density lipoprotein cholesterol (35 mg/dL)
- Diabetes mellitus

Data from Summary of the National Cholesterol Education Program (NCEP) Expert Panel on Detection, Evaluation, and Treatment of High Blood Cholesterol in Adults (Adult Treatment Panel II). (1993). JAMA 269:3015–3023.

problem. Ideally, such surveillance data would be available at several different levels and over a period of time. In some instances, community health nurses find it necessary to construct their own surveillance systems that are tailored to specific health conditions or programs in a community. These smaller data collection systems are useful to nurses for program evaluation when the data are readily accessible and compatible with those of large city or statewide surveillance systems.

As discussed, epidemiologists describe the course of disease over time (i.e., they document *secular* trends in disease). Secular trends are changes that occur over a long period of time (years or decades), such as the declining incidence of cancer of the uterus and the increase in cancer of the breast. Frequently, the associated patterns of treatment and intervention are also documented. In many instances, this information is derived from studies conducted by clinical epidemiologists. Cancer registries not only are a form of surveillance of the prevalence and incidence of cancer in a community, but they also document its course, treatment, and associated survival rates. National cancer data are drawn from the registries of 11 U.S. and Puerto Rican cities compiled by the Surveillance, Epidemiology, and End Results Program of the National Cancer Institutes (National Center for Health Statistics, 1995). Denominators of these cancer rates are obtained from the U.S. Census Bureau.

Other community surveys of other segments of a population may need to be conducted to plan adequately for their health. For example, a survey of the disabled population undertaken to assess prevalence may also be used to evaluate the adequacy of present services and to project future needs.

Use of Epidemiology in Health Services

Epidemiology has been discussed regarding the determinants of disease in populations. However, epidemiologic principles are also useful in studying the delivery of health care to populations and, in particular, in describing and evaluating the use of health services by the community. For example, determining the relative number of health care providers in relation to the population size may assist in assessing the system's adequacy in providing care. Also of interest are the reasons that clients initially seek care, methods by which clients pay for their care, and clients' satisfaction with services. Regardless of whether these data are collected by community health nurses or health services researchers, they are essential for those who strive to improve clients' access to quality health care.

HEALTH SERVICES EPIDEMIOLOGY

Health services–focused epidemiology is exemplified by a 1980 study that showed that the poor tend to have higher hospitalization rates than the nonpoor (National Center for Health Statistics, 1981). Although this may imply greater access to health care, a 1981 study found that low socioeconomic status individuals tend to have more chronic disease, which may explain their higher hospitalization rates (Aday and Anderson, 1981).

Epidemiologic studies can be used to evaluate quality of care. An example of this approach is a comparative study of a special geriatric inpatient evaluation ward that used an interdisciplinary program of elderly care (Rubenstein et al., 1984). The outcomes of interdisciplinary care were compared with those of the care usually received by elderly clients on the hospital ward. Patients in the special unit were found to have lower mortality rates, lower morbidity rates, and higher levels of satisfaction. One of the most important findings of this study was the lower costs incurred by clients on the special unit compared with those on other units. This finding suggests another aspect of health services epidemiology: the evaluation of the cost effectiveness of health care and of specific interventions or modes of delivery.

Ultimately, epidemiologic findings must be applied in the practice arena. It is essential that study results be incorporated into prevention programs for communities and at-risk populations. Further, the philosophy of public health and its subspecialty of epidemiology dictates that application be extended to and translated into major health policy decisions. The aim of health policy planning is to achieve positive health goals and outcomes for the good of the majority of society. As a process designed to bring about desirable social changes, policy development is influenced not only by epidemiologic factors but also by history, politics, economics, culture, and technology. The complex interaction of these factors may explain the slow pace of application of epidemiologic knowledge. An example of incomplete progress in implementing effective health policy is lung disease in the United States. The major risk factor, cigarette smoking, was identified and conclusively linked to the continued high rates of lung cancer and heart disease as early as the 1950s (Doll and Hill, 1952). Implemented public policies designed to protect the community include taxation of cigarettes, warning labels on cigarette packages, and, most recently, restriction of smoking in public areas. Nevertheless, other aspects of health policy remain unmodified, in essence, promoting cigarette smoking. One example is the proliferation of billboard and media advertisements targeted to vulnerable segments of the population (i.e., adolescents and black and Hispanic males). This has been vigorously protested and debated in community forums. Recently, the U.S. government endorsed the opening of markets in third world countries for the export of tobacco products; former U.S. Surgeon General Koop called it the export of "disease, death, and disability" (Chen and Winder, 1990, p. 659; see also Barry, 1991).

In 1976, Milio suggested other areas in which public policy had not kept pace with epidemiologic research findings. She asserted that public policy that provides consumers with healthier options such as improved safeguards in the work place, enforcement of higher environmental standards, access to more nutritious food, and incentives to reduce alcohol consumption would significantly benefit the health of consumers. Today, these continue to be among the primary concerns of public health professionals.

In summary, there are innumerable areas in which public health practitioners and epidemiologists have not yet effectively modified public policy in the interest of improved health. Exercising "societal responsibility" in the application of epidemiologic findings is within the province of community health nurses but will necessitate the active involvement of the citizen-consumer. Community health nurses collaborating with community members can most effectively combine epidemiologic knowledge and aggregate-level strategies to effect change on the broadest scale.

EPIDEMIOLOGIC METHODS
Descriptive Epidemiology

Descriptive epidemiology focuses on the amount and distribution of health and health problems within a population. Its purpose is to describe the characteristics of persons who are protected from disease and those who have a disease. Factors of particular interest include age, sex, ethnicity or race, socioeconomic status, occupation, family status, and many other variables. Epidemiologists use morbidity and mortality rates to describe the extent of disease and to determine risk factors that make certain groups prone to acquiring the disease.

In addition to "person" characteristics (or the "who"), the frequency of disease is described by the place of occurrence (or the "where"). For example, certain parasitic diseases such as malaria and schistosomiasis are known to occur in tropical areas. Other diseases may occur frequently in certain geopolitical entities; for example, gastroenteritis outbreaks often occur in communities with lax standards for water pollution. A third parameter that assists in defining disease patterns is time (or the "when"). Incidence rates may be tracked over a period of days or weeks (e.g., epidemics of infectious disease) or over an extended period of years (e.g., trends in the cancer death rate).

These person, place, and time factors can be used to form a framework for the analysis of a disease and may suggest variables that are associated with high versus low rates of disease. Hypotheses about the cause of disease can then be generated from descriptive epidemiology and tested by analytic methods.

Analytic Epidemiology

Analytic epidemiology investigates the causes of disease by determining why a disease rate is lower in one population group than in another. Hypotheses generated from descriptive data are tested and either accepted or rejected on the basis of results of analytic research. The epidemiologist seeks to establish a cause and effect relationship between a preexisting condition or event and the disease (see previous section on causality). To determine this relationship, two major types of research studies may be undertaken: *observational* studies and *experimental* studies.

Although observational studies are frequently used for descriptive purposes, they also are used in discovering the etiologic factors of disease. By observing disease rates in groups of people who are differentiated on the basis of an experience or exposure, the investigator can begin to understand the factors that contribute to disease. To illustrate, differences in the rates of disease may occur in the obese compared with the nonobese, in smokers compared with nonsmokers, and in those with high levels of life stress compared with those with low levels. Variables that define characteristics, obesity, smoking, and stress are called *exposure* variables.

However, unlike experimental studies, observational studies do not allow the investigator to manipulate the specific exposure or experience or, often, to control or limit the effects of other extraneous factors that may influence the development of disease. For example, life stress is known to be related to depression. Those of low socioeconomic status also have high depression rates. Because persons of low socioeconomic status frequently experience greater life stresses, the relationship between stress and depression is difficult to assess. Therefore, the confounding factor of socioeconomic status makes it more difficult to demonstrate the effect of stress on depression.

The three major study designs used in conducting observational research are cross-sectional (Fig. 5–5), retrospective (Fig. 5–6), and prospective (Fig. 5–7).

OBSERVATIONAL STUDIES

Cross-Sectional Studies

Cross-sectional studies, sometimes called *prevalence* or *correlational* studies, examine relationships between potential causal factors and disease at one point in time. Surveys in which information about the risk factors and the disease are collected at the same time exemplify this design. Both the National Health and Nutrition Examination Survey (NHANES) and the subsequent Hispanic Health and Nutrition Examination Survey collected cross-sectional data on persons ranging in age from 1 to 72 years regarding their current dietary practices and physical status (Delgado et al., 1990). The purpose of the two surveys was to detect nutritional deficiencies in the population. Although associations among disease and specific factors can be identified in a cross-sectional study, it is not possible to make causal inferences because the

Time Dimension:

PRESENT

Sample: Subjects sampled from population-at-large at one point in time

Advantages	Disadvantages
Quick to plan and conduct	Cannot calculate relative risk with prevalence data
Relatively inexpensive	
May provide preliminary indication of whether an association between a risk factor and disease exists	Temporal sequence of factor and outcome unknown
Provides prevalence data needed for planning health services	
Hypothesis generating	

Figure 5–5
Cross-sectional, or prevalence, study.

Time Dimension:

PAST

Sample: Subjects sampled with regard to disease and condition

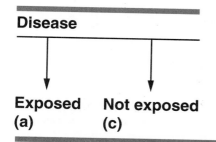

Disease

Exposed (a) **Not exposed (c)**

History of exposure (factors) from the past

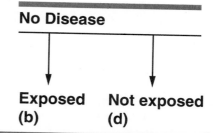

No Disease

Exposed (b) **Not exposed (d)**

Advantages

Can calculate odds ratio (OR), which is an estimate of relative risk:

$$OR = \frac{a}{a + c} \div \frac{b}{b + d} \ast = \frac{ad}{bc}$$

(*If disease is rare.)

Requires fewer subjects than prospective designs do

Possible to study multiple risk factors presumed to be related to a disease

Less expensive and difficult to conduct than a prospective study

Disadvantages

Incidence of disease cannot be calculated

Selection of control group is difficult

Relies on recall or records for exposure information that is subject to bias

Exposure ascertained after disease occurs (temporal relationship)

Figure 5–6
Retrospective, or case-control, study.

temporal sequence of events cannot be established (i.e., the cause preceded the effect). In the NHANES, for example, it is not possible to determine whether high salt intake preceded hypertension and thus is the causal factor or whether the reverse is true. Therefore, cross-sectional studies have limitations with regard to discovering etiologic factors of disease. However, they are useful in identifying preliminary relationships that

may be further explored by other analytic designs and, therefore, may be thought of as hypothesis-generating studies.

Retrospective Studies

Retrospective studies compare individuals known to have a particular condition or disease with those who do not have the disease. The purpose of these studies

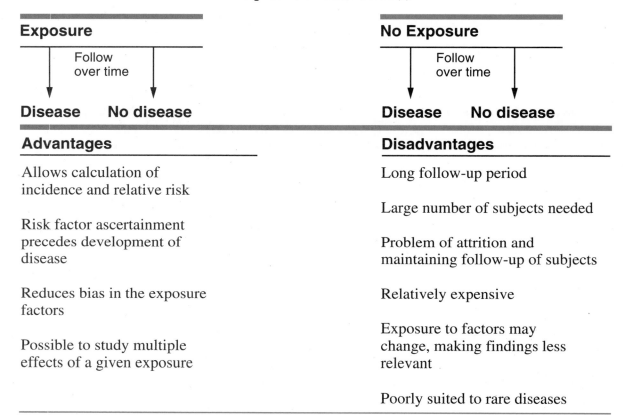

Time Dimension:

FUTURE

Sample: Healthy subjects sampled with regard to exposure or risk factor(s)

Exposure

Follow over time

Disease   No disease

No Exposure

Follow over time

Disease   No disease

Advantages	Disadvantages
Allows calculation of incidence and relative risk	Long follow-up period
	Large number of subjects needed
Risk factor ascertainment precedes development of disease	Problem of attrition and maintaining follow-up of subjects
Reduces bias in the exposure factors	Relatively expensive
Possible to study multiple effects of a given exposure	Exposure to factors may change, making findings less relevant
	Poorly suited to rare diseases

Figure 5–7
Prospective, or cohort, study.

is to determine whether cases (diseased group) differ in their exposure to a specific factor or characteristic relative to controls (nondiseased group). To make unambiguous comparisons, the cases are selected according to explicitly defined criteria regarding the type of case and the stage of disease. Controls are selected from among the general population and should have had the same opportunity of exposure as the cases (i.e., they are similar to the cases in as many ways as possible). Frequently, persons hospitalized for diseases other than the disease under study are selected as controls if they do not share the exposure or risk factor under study. For example, patients with heart disease may be selected as controls in a study of patients with lung cancer; however, this could introduce serious confounding because these patients often share the risk factor of smoking. To prevent the further introduction of bias into the study, the methods of data collection must be the same for both groups. For this reason, it is desirable for interviewers to remain unaware of whether subjects are cases or controls.

In retrospective studies, data collection extends back in time to determine previous exposure or risk factors. Study data are analyzed by comparing the proportion of subjects with disease (cases) who possess the exposure or risk factors with the corresponding proportion in the control group. A greater proportion of exposed cases than controls suggests an association of the disease with the risk factor.

Retrospective study designs are often used because they are better able than cross-sectional studies to address the question of causality. They also require fewer resources and less time in data collection than prospective studies (discussed next). There are many examples of *retrospective*, or *case-control*, studies in the literature. One classic example is Doll and Hill's (1952) investigation of risk factors for lung cancer. They compared exposure rates for those diagnosed with lung cancer (cases) with those of individuals diagnosed with cancer of sites other than the chest and oral cavity (controls). Detailed smoking histories were taken on all subjects. Of the cases, a significantly higher proportion of those with lung cancer smoked compared with controls. From this study, a hypothesis was developed that smoking might be etiologically related to lung cancer.

Prospective Studies

In prospective studies, a group of individuals who are considered free of a disease are monitored forward in time to determine whether and when disease occurs. These individuals, the *cohort,* share a common experience within a defined time period. For example, a birth cohort consists of all persons born within a given period of time. The cohort is assessed with respect to an exposure factor suspected of being associated with the disease and is classified accordingly at the beginning of the study. The cohort then is monitored for the development of disease. The disease rates for those with a known exposure are compared with rates for those who remain unexposed. Because subjects are observed prospectively, data collected over time can be summarized by incidence rates of new cases. As indicated earlier, comparison of two incidence rates produces a measure of relative risk:

$$\text{Relative risk} = \frac{\textbf{Incidence rate among exposed}}{\textbf{Incidence rate among unexposed}}$$

The relative risk indicates the extent of excess risk incurred by exposure to a factor relative to nonexposure. A relative risk of 1 suggests no excess risk resulting from exposure, whereas a relative risk of 2 suggests twice the risk of experiencing disease if there is exposure to the particular factor versus no exposure.

Prospective studies, or *longitudinal, cohort,* or *incidence* studies, are advantageous in that more reliable information about the cause of disease is

obtained than in other study methodologies. The temporal relationship between the presumed causal factors and the effect can be more strongly established than in retrospective and cross-sectional studies. Calculations of incidence rates and relative risks provide a valuable indicator of the magnitude of risk created by exposure to a particular factor.

However, certain disadvantages are inherent in the prospective design. Monitoring a cohort for periods of time is costly in terms of resources and staff and results in subject attrition. These logistic problems may be compounded by problems arising from the nature of chronic diseases. Frequently, chronic diseases have long latency periods between exposure and manifestation of the disease. Furthermore, the onset of chronic conditions may be sufficiently insidious as to make it extremely difficult to document the incidence of disease. In addition, as mentioned previously, many diseases do not have a unifactorial cause but rather are influenced by many interacting factors. These problems do not negate the benefits of prospectively designed epidemiologic studies; rather they suggest a need for careful planning and tailoring of the study to the disease as well as to the study's purpose.

Numerous prospective studies can be found in the literature. In many cases, they have been instrumental in substantiating causal links between specific risk factors and disease. A classic example is an early cohort study of deaths resulting from lung cancer (Doll and Hill, 1956). Questionnaires were originally completed on a cohort of physicians in Great Britain. These subjects were then classified according to several variables but most importantly according to the number of cigarettes smoked. A 4.5-year follow-up of death certificate data revealed an increased mortality rate as a result of lung cancer (as well as coronary thrombosis) among physicians who smoked relative to those who did not smoke. The death rate for heavy smokers was 166/100,000 versus 7/100,000 for nonsmokers. Combining these two incidence rates in a measure of excess risk indicated that heavy smokers were 23.7 times more likely to develop lung cancer than nonsmokers (relative risk: 166/100,000 divided by 7/100,000, or 23.7). These findings in a prospective study provided strong epidemiologic support for smoking as a risk factor for lung cancer.

Another well-known prospective study is the Framingham Study. Findings suggested that serum cholesterol level was associated with the future development of coronary heart disease (Kannel et al., 1971). This and other cohort studies formed the basis for later experimental studies aimed at reducing serum cholesterol through diet modification or drug therapy to ultimately lower the incidence rate of coronary heart disease.

Comparison of Time Factors in Retrospective and Prospective Study Designs

Cohort Study:

Girls with
bacteriuria $\rightarrow$ Women with
renal disease

Girls with
sterile urine $\rightarrow$ Women without
renal disease

Case-Control Study:

Girls with
bacteriuria $\leftarrow$ Women with
renal disease

Girls with
sterile urine $\leftarrow$ Women without
renal disease

PAST---------------PRESENT---------------FUTURE
(BEGINNING)

Comparison of time factors in prospective design (cohort) and retrospective design (case-control) approaches to studying the possible effect of childhood bacteriuria on renal disease in adult women.

EXPERIMENTAL STUDIES

Another type of analytic study is the experimental design (Fig. 5–8). In these epidemiologic investigations, experimental methods are applied to questions regarding the effectiveness of interventions designed to modify the effects of risk factors (i.e., testing of treatment and prevention strategies). The investigator randomly assigns to an experimental or a control group subjects who are determined to be at risk for a particular disease. Only the experimental group is subject to the intervention, but both groups are observed over time for the occurrence of disease. Although theoretically it is possible to introduce an exposure or risk factor as the experimental factor, ethical considerations usually prohibit the use of human subjects for these purposes. Therefore, epidemiologic studies of an experimental nature usually have been restricted to clinical trials of prophylactic and therapeutic measures. For example, experimental testing of vaccines for safety and efficacy is a common application of experimental studies.

The experimental design is also useful in investigating chronic disease. The Multiple Risk Factor Intervention Trial (MRFIT) tested a number of interventions thought to be effective in preventing heart disease: smoking cessation, reduction of dietary cholesterol, and treatment of hypertension (MRFIT Research Group, 1982). The control group was made up of similar high-risk men who were referred to their private physicians for routine medical care. This trial may be considered a public health trial because it tested a set of preventive actions within a community setting.

In contrast, the Coronary Primary Prevention Trial compared the effects of a cholesterol-lowering drug with those of a placebo in a clinical sample (Lipid Research Clinics Program, 1984). The cholesterol-lowering drug reduced the incidence of coronary heart disease by 19% after a 7-year follow-up. Thus, experimental studies are important in determining which of many possible preventive programs should be implemented. Although these studies are of a medical nature, experimental designs may be useful in evaluating community health nursing interventions, such as determining the value of particular prenatal interventions in reducing the incidence of low-birth-weight infants, the effectiveness of a sex education program in preventing high rates of teenage pregnancy, or the feasibility of an AIDS prevention program among intravenous drug users. It is only through the conduct of research that optimal community interventions are identified.

APPLICATION OF THE NURSING PROCESS

The synthesis of assessment data into diagnostic statements about the health of the community is the second step of the nursing process. These statements specify the nature and cause of the actual or potential community health problem. They necessarily direct the plans developed by community health nurses to resolve the problem. A formulation that assists in the writing of a community diagnosis was developed by Muecke (1984). The diagnosis consists of four components: identification of the health problem or risk, aggregate or community affected, etiologic or causal statement, and evidence or support for the diagnosis (Fig. 5–9).

Time Dimension:

FUTURE

Sample: Participants randomized

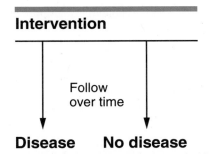

Intervention

Follow over time

Disease   No disease

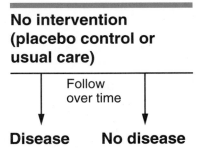

No intervention (placebo control or usual care)

Follow over time

Disease   No disease

Advantages

With randomization, gives confidence that outcome is due to treatment or intervention and not to other unknown factors

Provides strongest evidence that a factor is causal when an effect is seen

Disadvantages

Often impractical to conduct in human populations

Requires relatively long time to conduct, and factors and/or disease may change unrelated to clinical trial

Figure 5–8
Experimental, or clinical trial, study.

Assessment and Diagnosis

The process of collecting data, analyzing it, and deriving community diagnoses is demonstrated in the following example. The identification of a client health problem on a home visit provided the initial impetus for an aggregate health education program. Data collection extended from the individual client level to a broad range of literature and data about the nature of the problem in populations. Formulating a community-level diagnosis then provided direction for the ensuing plan.

THE REFERRAL

The school nurse in a local school district is frequently the person with the knowledge and resources to follow up student health problems with the family at home. In the West San Antonio School District, the school nurse sets aside several hours each week for home visiting. Home visits are initiated by a variety of mechanisms, but in this situation a teacher expressed concern for a student whose brother was dying from cancer. The student, John, was a junior in high school and in a health class had expressed his personal fears about cancer. He generated much interest on the part of his classmates regarding their own risk of cancer and the ways they might reduce that risk.

FAMILY ASSESSMENT

The school nurse visited John's family and learned that the oldest son, age 25 years, was diagnosed 1 year earlier with testicular cancer. Since then, he had

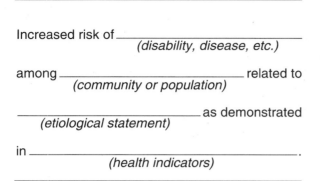

Increased risk of _____
                        (disability, disease, etc.)

among _____ related to
        (community or population)

_____ as demonstrated
    (etiological statement)

in _____ .
        (health indicators)

Figure 5–9
Format for community health diagnosis. (Redrawn from Muecke MA: Community health diagnosis in nursing. Pub Health Nurs *1;*23, 1984. Used with permission of Blackwell Scientific Publications.)

undergone a range of therapies that had been palliative but not curative, perhaps because the cancer was advanced at the time of diagnosis. The nurse spent time with the family discussing care for their son, answering questions, and exploring support available to them and their other children.

The next week at the school nurse staff meeting, the nurse inquired about her colleagues' experiences with other young clients with this type of cancer. Only one nurse remembered a young man in whom testicular cancer had developed. None were familiar with its prevalence, incidence, risk factors, or prevention and early detection approaches. The nurse recognized the high probability that high school students would have similar questions and could benefit from reliable information.

COMMUNITY ASSESSMENT

The school nurse embarked on a community assessment, searching for answers to these questions. The first step was to collect information about testicular cancer. The nurse reviewed the nursing and medical literature for key articles discussing care of clients with this cancer and its diagnosis and treatment. Epidemiologic studies provided additional data regarding its distribution pattern in the population and associated risk factors. She learned that young men aged 20 to 35 years were at greatest risk. No other major risk factors were identified; however, young men who tend to be healthy do not routinely seek regular health care, including testicular cancer screening. They also may be subject to the apprehensions frequently associated with conditions affecting sexual

function. These factors contribute to a delay in prompt detection and treatment. Although only 6100 new cases of testicular cancer were estimated to be diagnosed in 1991 in the United States, it was one of the most common tumors in young men and is amenable to treatment if discovered early (National Cancer Society, 1991).

On the basis of these facts, the nurse reasoned that high school students were a potentially important target for a prevention program. Of importance to a comprehensive assessment, however, was clarifying what students did know, how comfortable they were discussing health problems of a sexual nature, and how interested they were in learning more. Therefore, the nurse's next step was to approach the junior and senior high school students and administer a questionnaire designed to elicit this information. The nurse also queried the health teacher regarding the amount of pertinent information about cancer and sexual development that the students received in the classroom. The nurse considered the latter an important prerequisite to dealing with a sensitive subject such as genital health. The health teacher reported that students did receive instruction about physical development and psychosexual issues. Students expressed a strong 1desire for more classroom time devoted to these subjects, including cancer prevention. They did not, however, have much knowledge of beneficial health practices related to cancer prevention.

COMMUNITY DIAGNOSIS

After collecting a broad range of assessment data, the nurse was able to document that a potential health need existed in the community of high school students. The next step of analyzing and synthesizing data culminated in a community diagnosis. For this aggregate, the community diagnosis was as follows:

There is an increased risk of undetected testicular cancer among young men related to insufficient knowledge about the disease and the methods for preventing and detecting it at an early stage, as demonstrated by high rates of late initiation of treatment.

Planning

Clarifying the problem and its cause provided direction for the nurse as she initiated the planning phase of the nursing process. Planning encompassed several activities, including the discovery of recommended health care practices regarding testicular cancer. The nurse also sought to determine the most effective and

RETRIEVAL OF DATA

Current data on the health of the population of the United States are found in many places. Finding the latest statistics available in an area of interest at the local, state, or national level can be a challenging experience for a student, community health nurse, graduate student, and even a nurse researcher. Statistics are necessary, however, for comparison purposes in identifying the health status of an aggregate or population in a community. The following guidelines are suggested places to begin a search. As experience in gaining access to statistics in an area of interest increases, more resources will become known.

- Reference librarian. The best place to start is in a school or community library or health sciences library if a large campus is available. Cultivate a relationship with the reference librarian and learn from the librarian how to obtain access to the literature of interest to you (e.g., government documents) or how to carry out computer-guided literature searches.
- Government documents. Local libraries have a listing of government depository libraries; these are libraries that have government documents available for use by the public. If the government document needed is not available at a local library, ask the reference librarian at the local library to contact a regional library or state library where an interlibrary loan of the document can be obtained. The Library of Congress in Washington, DC, has a Directory of United States Government Depository Libraries. The number of the national reference service at the Library of Congress is (202) 707-5522, or call for operator in Washington, DC.
- *Health, United States, 1995.* This is an annual publication (*Health, United States, 1996,* and so on) of the National Center for Health Statistics, which reports the latest health statistics for the United States. It presents statistics in areas such as the following: prenatal care; low birth weight; infant mortality; life expectancy; death rates; cancer incidence and survival; trends in AIDS; diabetes; obesity; hypertension; high serum cholesterol; substance use; air pollution; exposure to noise; health status and utilization; national health expenditures; health insurance; Medicaid; Medicare; health maintenance organizations; hospital care; nursing home care; physician contacts; dental visits; diagnostic, surgical, and nonsurgical procedures; mental health services; and enrollment and graduates of health professions schools,

including minorities and women. Graphs and tables are easy to read and interpret with accompanying texts. Many statistics are presented over a selected number of years so that trends may be seen. Also some statistics are presented using comparisons with other countries and for U.S. minority populations.

If this publication is not available locally, it may be ordered from the U.S. Government Printing Office, Superintendent of Documents, 732 N. Capitol Street, NW, Washington, DC 20402. The telephone number is (202) 783-3238, or call for operator assistance in Washington, DC. A new edition of this publication is produced each spring and is available in paperback.
- *Morbidity and Mortality Weekly Report.* This publication, known as *MMWR,* is prepared by the Centers for Disease Control and Prevention in Atlanta, Georgia. It provides weekly reports compiled by state health departments on the numbers of cases of selected notifiable diseases such as AIDS, aseptic meningitis, encephalitis, gonorrhea, hepatitis, legionellosis, Lyme disease, malaria, measles (rubeola), meningococcal infections, mumps, pertussis, rubella, syphilis, toxic shock syndrome, tuberculosis, tularemia, typhoid fever, typhus fever, and rabies, and deaths in 121 U.S. cities by age categories. It also reports accounts of interesting cases, environmental hazards, outbreaks, or other public health problems of interest. An annual index is helpful for locating articles and the latest statistics on areas of interest. It is published weekly by the Massachusetts Medical Society, 1440 Main Street, Waltham, MA 02154. It is found in local and state health departments and many local and health sciences libraries. A subscription is available from the Massachusetts Medical Society.
- Centers for Disease Control and Prevention. Commonly called the CDC, the Centers for Disease Control and Prevention compiles information on the following topics: tobacco, violent and abusive behavior, educational and community-based programs, unintentional injuries, occupational safety and health, environmental health, oral health, diabetes and chronic disabling conditions, sexually transmitted diseases, immunization and infectious diseases, clinical preventive services, and surveillance and data systems. The Centers for Disease Control and Prevention is located at 1600 Clifton Rd NE, Atlanta, Georgia 30333.

appropriate approaches for male and female high school students. Identifying helpful community agencies was an essential part of the process. The local chapter of the American Cancer Society offered consultative services and invaluable information and materials. The media center of a nearby nursing school and the faculty of this school were also very supportive of the program development.

After formalizing objectives, the nurse presented her plan to the teaching coordinator and principal of the high school. Their approval was necessary before any further investment could be made in the project. After eliciting their enthusiastic support, the nurse proceeded with more detailed plans. Classroom instruction methods and activities were selected and developed that would maximize involvement of high school students in their learning. A film and physical models for demonstrating and practicing testicular self-examination were also ordered. Group process exercises designed to relax students and assist them in being comfortable with sensitive subject matter were prepared. The nurse scheduled two 40-minute sessions dealing with testicular cancer as part of the junior-level health class. As a final step of the planning phase, evaluation tools were designed that assessed knowledge levels after each class session as well as the extent to which health practices were integrated into students' lifestyles at the end of the junior and senior years.

The nurse was now ready to proceed with implementation of a testicular cancer prevention and screening program. She had initiated the assessment phase by identifying an individual client and family with a health need, and she extended the assessment to the high school aggregate. Collection of data at the aggregate level (for both the general population and the local high school population) assisted in formulation of a community diagnosis. The diagnosis directed the development of a community-specific health intervention program and its subsequent implementation and evaluation.

Intervention

Each of the two sessions was conducted as part of a health education class. Students participated in group exercises at the beginning of the class period and then were asked about their current knowledge about testicular cancer. A film was shown in the classroom; then the nurse guided a discussion about cancer screening. In the second session, the use of testicular models was introduced, and the self-examination procedure was demonstrated. Students were supervised as they practiced the examination procedure on the models. Male students were advised about the frequency of self-examination. Females discussed the need for young men to be aware of their increased risk, and a parallel was drawn with breast self-examination.

Evaluation

After completing the class sessions, the nurse administered the instruments that assessed the students' knowledge. It was gratifying that knowledge levels were very high immediately after the classes. In addition, students were pleased that the subject of testicular cancer was frankly discussed and that they had the opportunity to ask questions and receive clear responses about such a sensitive subject. Feedback from teachers also was very positive. The nurse reported that her image as a knowledgeable health resource in the high school was enhanced.

Intermediate-term evaluation occurred at the end of the students' junior and senior years. A 15-minute evaluation was arranged during other classes. The integration of positive health practices and, in particular, testicular self-examinations into students' lifestyles was evaluated. As expected, the prevalence of regular self-assessment was significantly lower than knowledge levels at the end of the school year. However, 30% of male students reported regularly practicing self-examinations at the end of 1 year, and 70% reported they had performed a self-examination at least once during the past year.

For long-term evaluation, the compilation of incidence data is ideal and documents the reduction of a health problem in a community. Because testicular cancer is very rare, incidence data are not reliable and may not be feasible to collect. However, for other more prevalent conditions, the collection of objective statistics is helpful in revealing decreases and increases in disease trends, which in turn may be related to the strengths and deficiencies of health programs.

It is evident that epidemiologic data and methods are essential to each phase of the nursing process. The community health nurse compiles a range of assessment data that support the nursing diagnosis. Epidemiologic studies help in planning a program by establishing the effectiveness of certain interventions and the specificity of each for different aggregates. This information supports the nurse's implementation

COMPREHENSIVE PERINATAL PROGRAM IMPROVES BIRTH OUTCOMES IN TEENAGE MEDICAID CLIENTS

A collaborative project among a graduate nursing student, a graduate public health student, and a private, nonprofit, community-based medical center, using an epidemiologic design (retrospective, cross-sectional), was carried out to evaluate the effect of enrollment in two special perinatal programs—the Comprehensive Perinatal Services Program (CPSP) and the school-based Comprehensive Teenage Pregnancy and Parenting Program (CTAPPP)—on the occurrence of adverse perinatal outcomes in teenage Medicaid clients who delivered at the medical center. The project was in response to staff nurses' observations of a recurring clinical problem: questionable perinatal outcomes among teenage girls giving birth at the medical center, a clinical problem with implications for the health of the community.

The CPSP program is a comprehensive program that provides perinatal services including medical, nursing, nutritional, psychosocial, childbirth, and parenting educational interventions that must be provided by a physician or a certified nurse midwife, a certified nutritionist, a social worker with a master's degree, and a certified nurse educator,

respectively. The CTAPPP offers academic, health, nutrition, perinatal, and parenting education support and case management services to pregnant and parenting teenagers.

Adverse perinatal outcomes were defined as one of the following: (1) low birth weight (<2500 g; (2) gestational age less than 37 weeks; or (3) admission to a neonatal intensive care unit not related to congenital syphilis.

Using historic data, pregnancy outcomes were compiled on 312 Medicaid, largely African-American (75.9%) clients, 12 to 18 years of age, who delivered at the medical center between June 1991 and June 1992. Adverse perinatal outcomes were found in 10.9% of the study sample; 35% received substandard prenatal care. Enrollment in CPSP was associated with reduced adverse perinatal outcomes; however, enrollment in CTAPPP was not. A more comprehensive prenatal program, such as CPSP, may improve birth outcomes in high-risk teenage populations. The project presents a model for linking data on birth outcomes to data on program participation among Medicaid clients to assess the efficacy of existing programs.

(Perkocha, Novotny, Bradley, Swanson, 1995.)

of tailored intervention strategies. Finally, epidemiologic data are important for the community health nurse's documentation of program effectiveness, especially in the long term.

SUMMARY

Communities are formed for a variety of reasons and can be homogeneous or heterogeneous in their composition. To help assess the nature of a given community, community health nurses study and interpret data from sources such as the census, morbidity and mortality reports, vital statistics, and information from local government agencies. Through the use of epidemiologic studies, they can glean valuable information about the causes and prevalence of health and disease in a community. On the basis of this information, the community health nurse is able to apply the nursing process, expanding assessment, diagnosis, planning, intervention, and evaluation from the individual client level to that of a targeted aggregate in the community.

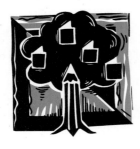

Learning Activities

1. Walk through your community neighborhood, and compile a list of variables that are important to describe with demographic and epidemiologic data. Write down your hunches or preconceived notions about the nature of the population in this community for later comparison with the statistical data you collect.

2. Walk through your neighborhood and describe the information you gain through your senses (i.e., smells, sounds, and sights observed in this area). How do each relate to the community's health?

3. Compile a range of relevant demographic and epidemiologic data for your community by examining census reports, vital statistics reports, city records, and other sources available in libraries and agencies.

4. Using the data you have collected, identify three health problems of this community and formulate three community health diagnoses.

REFERENCES

Aday LA, Anderson RM: Equity of access to medical care: A conceptual and empirical overview. Med Care 19(suppl 12): 4–27, 1981.

Barry M: The influence of the U.S. tobacco industry on the health, economy, and environment of developing countries. N Engl J Med 324:917–920, 1991.

Buring JE, Lee I-M: Annotation: Confounding in epidemiologic research. Am J Public Health 85:164–165, 1995.

Chen TT, Winder AE: The opium wars revisited as US forces tobacco exports in Asia. Am J Public Health 80:659–662, 1990.

Delgado JL, Johnson CL, Roy I, Trevino FM: Hispanic Health and Nutrition Examination Survey: Methodological considerations. Am J Public Health 80 (suppl):6–10, 1990.

Doll R, Hill AB: Study of the aetiology of carcinoma of the lung. BMJ 2:1271–1285, 1952.

Doll R, Hill AB: Lung cancer and other causes of death in relation to smoking. BMJ 2:1071–1081, 1956.

Friedman GD: Primer of Epidemiology, 4th ed. New York, McGraw-Hill, 1994.

Kannel WB, Castelli WP, Gordon T, McNamara PM: Serum cholesterol, lipoproteins and the risk of coronary heart disease: The Framingham Study. Ann Intern Med 74:1–12, 1971.

Lilienfeld DE, Stoley PD: Foundations of Epidemiology. New York, Oxford University Press, 1994.

Lipid Research Clinics Program: The Lipid Research Clinics Coronary Primary Prevention Trial results: Parts 1 and 2. JAMA 251:351–374, 1984.

Mattson ME, Pollack ES, Cullen JW: What are the odds that smoking will kill you? Am J Public Health 77:425–431, 1987.

Mausner JS, Kramer S: Mausner and Bahn Epidemiology: An Introductory Text, 2nd ed. Philadelphia, WB Saunders, 1985.

Milio N: A framework for prevention: Changing health-damaging to health-generating life patterns. Am J Public Health 66:435–439, 1976.

Morton RF, Hebel JR, McCarter RJ: A Study Guide to Epidemiology and Biostatistics, 3rd ed. Gaithersburg, MD. Aspen Publishers, 1990.

Muecke MA: Community health diagnosis in nursing. Public Health Nurs 1:23–35, 1984.

Multiple Risk Factor Intervention Trial Research Group: Multiple Risk Factor Intervention Trial. JAMA 248:1465–1477, 1982.

National Cancer Society: Career Facts and Figures—1991. Atlanta, GA, American Cancer Society, 1991.

National Center for Health Statistics: NHANES—Dietary Intake Findings, United States, 1971–1974 (Vital Health Statistics: Series 11, National Health Examination Survey No. 202, Publication No. [HRA] 77-1647). Hyattsville, MD, Department of Health, Education, and Welfare, National Center for Health Statistics. 1977.

National Center for Health Statistics: Health, United States, 1980. Hyattsville, MD, Department of Health and Human Services, U.S. Public Health Service, 1981.

National Center for Health Statistics: Health, United States, 1994. Hyattsville, MD, Department of Health and Human Services, U.S. Public Health Service, 1995.

Perkocha VA, Novotny TE, Bradley JC, Swanson JM: The efficacy of two comprehensive perinatal programs on reducing adverse perinatal outcomes. Am J Prevent Med 11 (suppl 1):21–29, 1995.

Public Health Service, U.S. Department of Health and Human Services. Healthy People National Health Promotion and Disease Prevention Objectives DHHS Publication No. (PHS) 91-50212). Washington, DC, U.S. Government Printing Office, 1990.

Rubenstein L, Josephson KR, Wieflan GD et al.: Effectiveness of a geriatric evaluation unit. N Engl J Med 311:1664–1670, 1984.

Simoes EJ, Byers T, Coates R, et al.: The association between leisure-time physical activity and dietary fat in American adults. Am J Public Health 85:240–244, 1995.

Snow J: On the Mode of Communication of Cholera, 2nd ed. London, Churchill, reproduced in Snow on Cholera. New York, Commonwealth Fund, 1936.

Summary of the National Cholesterol Education Program (NCEP) Expert Panel on Detection, Evaluation, and Treatment of High Blood Cholesterol in Adults (Adult Treatment Panel II). JAMA 269:3015–3023, 1993.

U.S. Bureau of the Census. Statistical Abstract of the United States: 1994, 114th ed. Washington, DC, 1994.

Willett W: Diet and coronary heart disease. In Willett, W (ed). Nutritional Epidemiology. New York, Oxford University Press, pp. 341–379, 1990.

Community Health Planning and Evaluation

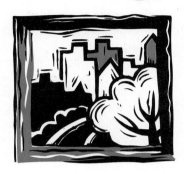

Upon completion of this chapter, the reader will be able to:

1. Define what is meant by "aggregate as client."

2. Apply the nursing process within a systems framework to the larger aggregate.

3. Describe the steps in the health planning model.

4. Identify the level of prevention and the system level appropriate for nursing interventions with aggregates.

5. Compare and contrast goals and outcomes of health planning legislation from the Hill-Burton Act to the National Health Planning and Resources Development Act.

6. Identify the advantages of comprehensive health planning and evaluation.

7. Describe the community health nurse's role in health planning and evaluation.

Deborah Godfrey Brown
Patricia M. Burbank
Barbara S. Morgan

Health planning for and with the community is viewed as an essential component of community health nursing practice. What does the term *health planning* actually mean? At first glance, the terminology appears simple enough, but the underlying concept is more complex. Like many other components of community health nursing, it tends to vary somewhat when applied to different aggregate levels. Health planning with an individual or a family may focus on direct care needs or self-care responsibilities; at the group level, the primary goal may be health education; and at the community level, health planning may involve prevention of diseases within a population or control of environmental hazards.

An example may help to demonstrate the interaction of community health nursing roles with health planning for a variety of aggregate levels. Nancy Jones is the high school nurse in a small suburban community. She notes an increasing incidence of school dropouts as a result of pregnancy. The nurse at the junior high school confirms a corresponding increase among the younger teenagers. Current articles in nursing and other professional journals as well as in the general media indicate what appears to be a national epidemic of unwed pregnant teenagers.

Why is this happening in an era of increased knowledge and more readily available and more effective contraceptive techniques? Nancy's assessment of the problem at the local level includes several findings. The teenagers who are sexually active often do not use contraception on a regular basis because they want their actions to seem "spontaneous" rather than "planned." They also do not perceive themselves as vulnerable to pregnancy because of a variety of misconceptions regarding the reproductive process, for example, "I will not become pregnant if I do not have regular periods or if my boyfriend does not ejaculate inside me." Teenagers also find many contraceptive methods difficult or embarrassing to obtain. In addition, there is no family planning clinic in the area, and local physicians admit to reluctance to counsel or prescribe for teenagers without parental permission. The nurse also discovers that an attempt several years ago to institute a sex education class in the school system was stopped by a group of parents who believed this responsibility belonged in the home.

Nancy's plan of action takes all of these factors into consideration. Meetings with teachers and school officials indicated a willingness to deal with this sensitive issue within the school system if parents could be convinced of its validity. Parents revealed in meetings with her that they were not entirely comfortable with the topic and did need assistance with their teenaged children. They were concerned, however, about the possibility of the mechanics of reproduction being taught without any attention to the obligations involved in relationships and in making moral decisions. Their willingness to support such a program would be facilitated by participation in the planning of the curriculum and by the chance to meet the teachers before the program began. This was a compromise from a previous plan to have parents sign a consent form for each teenager's participation. The students themselves believed this was stigmatizing and said they would attend only if it was required. The family planning agency in a nearby metropolitan area was asked to consider opening a part-time clinic in this suburb. A home tutoring program was proposed to maintain pregnant teenagers' education and encourage their return to school.

Implementation of such a comprehensive plan is time consuming and requires resources and involvement with many people in the community. The nurse enlists the aid of school officials and other professionals in the community for this ambitious project. Time will be needed to evaluate the long-term effectiveness in reducing the incidence of teen pregnancies.

This example shows how nurses can and should become involved in health planning. Nancy identified an important need: Teen pregnancy is a significant health risk for the individual and often predicts lower education and socioeconomic status, resulting in further health problems. Her assessment and planned interventions included individual teenagers, their parents and families, the school system, and the resources of the community.

In this chapter, we provide an overview of health planning and evaluation from a nursing perspective, a model for student involvement in health planning projects, and a review of significant health planning legislation.

OVERVIEW OF HEALTH PLANNING

One of the major criticisms of current community health nursing practice involves the shift away from the community and larger aggregate focus to primary involvement with family caseload management or agency responsibilities. While focusing on the individual or family as the client, nurses must remember that these clients are members of a larger population group or community and are influenced by factors within this environment. By carrying out an assessment of the aggregate or community as a whole, important factors influencing the health of individuals and families can be identified, and interventions can be planned to meet these health needs (Fig. 6–1).

Historically, the community as client is not a new concept. The focus on the community as client is exemplified by Lillian Wald's work in New York City at the Henry Street settlement in 1893–1895. She and others worked with the extremely poor immigrants in the area, caring for the ill in their homes while also working for social reform on a larger scale.

The "case" element in these early reports of hers [Wald] got less and less emphasis; she instinctively went behind the symptoms to appraise the whole individual, saw that one could not understand the individual without understanding the family, saw that the family was in the grip of larger social and economic forces, which it could not control."

(DUFFUS, 1938)

It is clear that the early beginnings of public health nursing itself incorporated not only the nurses' visits

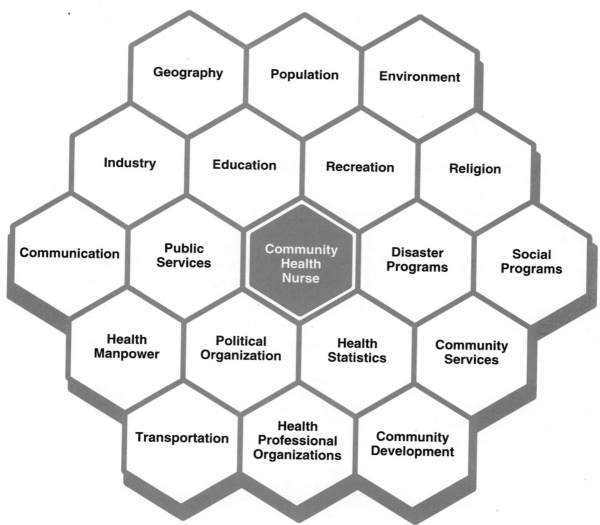

Figure 6–1
The community as client. Assessment parameters from Chapter 5 (Table 5–1) help identify the client.

to people in their homes but also application of the nursing process to larger aggregates and communities to improve the health of a greater number of people. Silverstein (1985) identified Wald's goals and those of public health nursing as health promotion and disease prevention for all people. To accomplish this, health planning at the aggregate or community level is necessary.

A trend beginning in the mid-1960s through the present has been a shift from public health nursing with an emphasis on the community as the focus of care to community health nursing, which encompasses all nursing activities performed outside the hospital setting. The focus of public health nursing, from the time of Wald through the 1950s, was on mobilizing communities to solve their own problems, treating primarily only the poor, and working to improve environmental conditions that fostered disease. Social changes that began in the 1950s have altered the role of the nurse, including increases in family mobility, suburbanization, and government expenditures for a variety of health programs. Currently, as health care reform is being debated, trends are emerging. Primary

health care that uses more nurses as primary care providers is growing in importance (American Nurses Association, 1993). Home health care services are the fastest growing industry in the United States. As the shift into the community continues, community health nurses must become more visible and vocal as leaders in health care reform (Shalala, 1992).

With this increased focus on the community setting, the larger aggregate is emphasized as the client or unit of care in an effort to reestablish the role of the nurse in improving the health care of groups. By becoming involved again in health care at the larger aggregate level, the community health nurse should not lose sight of nursing care at the individual and family levels but rather use information about communities and insight gained to understand the health problems of these individuals and families and ultimately work toward improving their health status (Table 6–1).

Before nurses can be expected to participate in health care planning, however, they must be knowledgeable about the process and comfortable with the concept of community as client or focus of care. It is essential that the "how to" be an integral part of the

---

Table 6–1
Levels of Community Health Nursing Practice

Client	Example	Characteristics	Health Assessment	Nursing Involvement
Individual	Lisa McDonald	An individual with a variety of needs	Individual strengths, problems, needs	Client-nurse interaction
Family	Moniz family (five members)	A family system with individual and group needs	Individual and family strengths, problems, needs	Interactions with individuals and with family as a group
Group	Boy Scout troop; Alzheimer's support group	Common interests, problems, and/or needs; interdependency	Group dynamics, fulfillment of goals	Group member and/or leader
Population group	AIDS patients in a given state; pregnant adolescents in a school district	Large, unorganized group with common interests, problems, and/or needs	Assessment of common problems, needs, and vital statistics	Application of nursing process to identified needs
Organization	A work place; a school	Organized group in a common location with shared governance and goals	Relationship of goals, structure, communications to strengths, problems, and needs	Consultant and/or employee; application of nursing process to identified needs
Community	Italian neighborhood; Anytown, USA	An aggregate of people in a common location with organized social systems	Analysis of systems, strengths, characteristics, problems, and needs	Community leader, participant, health care provider

AIDS = acquired immunodeficiency syndrome.

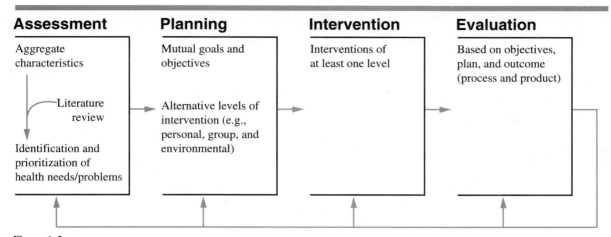

Assessment

Aggregate characteristics

Literature review

Identification and prioritization of health needs/problems

Planning

Mutual goals and objectives

Alternative levels of intervention (e.g., personal, group, and environmental)

Intervention

Interventions of at least one level

Evaluation

Based on objectives, plan, and outcome (process and product)

Figure 6–2
Health planning model.

undergraduate and graduate curricula. If health planning is included in basic and advanced nursing education, the student becomes aware of not only the process but also the opportunities for professional involvement at many levels.

Recognizing the need to provide learning experiences for students in the investigation of community health problems, Hegge (1973), in early efforts, described the use of learning packets for independent study, and Ruybal et al. (1975) provided opportunities for students to apply epidemiologic concepts in community program planning and evaluation. Neither of these approaches, however, presented a complete model that used the nursing process as a framework for health planning. Several other authors such as Hamilton (1985) and Mahon (1991) and their colleagues described and gave examples of the community health planning process. None of these models, however, follows the entire process through use of practical examples for actual student implementation.

HEALTH PLANNING MODEL

In response to this need for a population focus, a model was developed that applies the nursing process within a systems framework to the larger aggregate, with the objective of improving the health of this aggregate (Fig. 6–2). Incorporated into a health planning project, it can be used to assist students in viewing larger aggregates as the client and gaining knowledge and experience in the health planning process. The specific

objectives are based on a model for group intervention by Hogue (1985). Use of the model requires careful consideration of each step in the process (Table 6–2).

Several considerations affect the choice of a specific aggregate for study. The community in which the nurse works may have extensive or limited opportunities appropriate for involvement; each community offers different possibilities for health intervention. An urban area, for example, might have a broader variety of industrial and business settings that need assistance, whereas a suburban community may offer a wider choice of family-oriented organizations such as boys and girls clubs, parent-teacher associations, and so on.

When selecting an aggregate for intervention, a nurse should also consider personal interests and strengths. Are you more interested in teaching health promotion and preventive health or in planning for organizational change? Are your communication skills better suited to large or small groups? Do you prefer working with the elderly or with children? Thoughtful consideration of these and other variables in interaction with the choices available in your community will facilitate beginning an assessment of an appropriate aggregate.

Assessment

Gaining entry is not only a necessary first step but also an important one when establishing a professional relationship with the chosen aggregate. The nurse's communication skills are essential to establish contact and make a positive first impression. An appointment

Table 6–2
Health Planning Project Objectives

I.   Assessment
  A. Specify level of aggregate selected for study (e.g., group, population group, or organization). Identify and provide a general orientation to the aggregate (e.g., characteristics of aggregate system, its suprasystem, and its subsystems). Include why this aggregate was selected and the method used for gaining entry.
  B. Describe specific characteristics of the aggregate including
    1. Sociodemographic characteristics—age, sex, race or ethnic group, religion, educational background and/or level, occupation, income, marital status, and so on.
    2. Health status—work or school attendance, disease categories, mortality, health care use, and measurements of population growth and population pressure (e.g., rates of birth and death, divorce, unemployment, drug and alcohol abuse). Select indicators appropriate for chosen aggregate.
    3. Suprasystem influences—existing health services available to improve health of aggregate and existing or potential impact (positive and negative) of other community-level social system variables on aggregate. Identify methods of data collection used.
  C. Provide relevant information gained from literature review, especially in terms of characteristics, problems, or needs that one would anticipate finding with this type of aggregate. Include comparison of health status of chosen aggregate with other similar aggregates, the community, the state, and/or the nation.
  D. Identify health problems and/or needs of specific aggregate based on comparative analysis and interpretation of data collection and literature review. Include input from clients regarding their perceptions of needs. Give priorities to health problems and/or needs and indicate how these priorities are determined.

II. Planning
  A. Select one health problem and/or need for intervention and identify ultimate goal of intervention. Identify specific, measurable objectives as mutually agreed on by student and aggregate.
  B. Describe alternative interventions necessary to accomplish objectives. Include consideration of interventions at each systems level where appropriate (e.g., aggregate system, suprasystem, and subsystems). Select and validate intervention(s) with highest probability of success. (Note: Intervention may include using existing resources and/or developing new resources.)

III. Intervention
  A. Implement at least one level of planned intervention when possible. If intervention was not implemented, provide rationale.

IV. Evaluation
  A. Evaluate objectives, plan, and outcomes of intervention(s). Include aggregate's evaluation of project as well. Evaluation should include consideration of both process and product and of both appropriateness and effectiveness.
  B. Make recommendations for further action based on evaluation and communicate these to appropriate individuals or systems levels. Discuss implications for community health nursing.

should be made for the first meeting to facilitate a welcome.

The nurse must initially clarify his or her position and organizational affiliation, knowledge, and skills; mutual expectations regarding what can be accomplished; and available time. Once entry has been established, negotiation continues in terms of maintaining a mutually beneficial relationship.

Meeting with the aggregate on a regular basis will allow for an in-depth assessment. Determination of sociodemographic characteristics (e.g., distribution of age, sex, race) may help to determine both health needs and appropriate methods of intervention. For example,

adolescents need information regarding drug and alcohol use and abuse, nutrition, and the development of other-gender relationships. They usually do not enjoy being lectured to in a classroom-like atmosphere, but it requires much skill to get them involved and participating on a small-group level. The average educational level of an adult group will affect not only their knowledge base but also their comfort with formal versus informal learning settings. If the focus is an organization or a population, the aggregate members may be more diverse, and it may be more difficult to coordinate time and energy commitments. Information regarding sociodemographic characteristics may be gathered from a variety of sources, including the nurse's own observations, consultation with others who work with the aggregate (e.g., the nurse in a factory or school, a Headstart teacher, the resident manager in a high-rise apartment building for senior citizens), records or charts if available, and members of the aggregate (verbally or via a short questionnaire).

In assessing the health status of the aggregate, it is important to consider both positive and negative factors. The presence of disease or unemployment may suggest specific health problems, but low rates of absenteeism at work or school may indicate that preventive interventions are more appropriate. The specific aggregate will determine which measures of health status are relevant. Immunization levels are an important index for children and are usually ignored for adults; however, with the elderly, one may want to consider the need for influenza injections. Similarly, one would expect less incidence of chronic diseases with the young, whereas the elderly obviously have higher morbidity and mortality rates.

The suprasystem in which the aggregate is located may facilitate or impede health status. Differing organizations and communities provide various resources and services to their members. Some are obviously health related, such as the presence or absence of hospitals, clinics, private practitioners, emergency facilities, health centers, visiting nursing associations, and health departments. Support services and facilities are also important. For example, does the area provide group meal sites or Meals on Wheels to the elderly? Are there recreational facilities and programs for children, adolescents, and adults? The use of services is further determined by the availability of transportation, reimbursement mechanisms or sliding-scale fees, community-based volunteer groups, and so on. Assessment regarding these factors requires exploration of public records (e.g., from town halls, telephone directories, and community services directories) and talking with health professionals, volunteers, and key informants in the community. The nurse's role is to augment existing resources or possibly even create a new service; merely duplicating what is already available to the aggregate is not the goal.

A literature review is an important means of comparing the aggregate with the "norm." During the winter, children in a Headstart setting, day care center, or elementary school may appear to exhibit a high rate of upper respiratory tract infections. According to the pediatric literature, what is a normal incidence for children of this age range in group environments? Is a factory's experience with on-the-job injuries within an average range for that type of manufacturing? If the aggregate appears especially healthy, what does available information offer about the potential problems one might expect (e.g., developmental stage stresses for adolescents or work or family organization stresses for adults)? Comparison of the foregoing assessment with currently available research reports, statistics, and health information will help to determine and prioritize health problems and needs for the aggregate.

The last phase of the initial assessment is identification and prioritization of the health problems and needs of the specific aggregate. This should be directly related to both the assessment and the review of the literature and should include a comparative analysis of the two. It is also very important that this step reflect the incorporation of the aggregate members' perceptions of the needs. Depending on the aggregate, this may come directly from aggregate members or from consultation with others who work with them (e.g., a Headstart teacher). Interventions are seldom successful if input from the clients has been omitted or ignored at this level. Last, the identified problems and needs must be prioritized to plan effectively.

The following factors should be considered when determining priorities:

- Aggregate's preferences
- Number of individuals in the aggregate who are or could be affected by this health problem
- Severity of the health need or problem
- Availability of potential solutions to the problem
- Practical considerations such as individual skills, time limitations, and available resources

In addition, priorities may be further refined by the application of a framework such as Maslow's (1968) hierarchy of needs (e.g., lower level needs have priority over higher level needs) or Leavell and Clark's (1965) levels of prevention (e.g., primary prevention may take priority for children, whereas tertiary prevention might be of higher priority for the elderly) (see Chapter 1, Table 1–1).

Assessment is ongoing throughout the nurse's relationship with the aggregate; however, once an initial assessment is complete, the nurse should proceed to the planning stage. It is particularly important at this step in the process to link it with the other stages; that is, planning should stem directly and logically from the assessment and be realistic in terms of implementation.

Planning

Selection of the problem or need for intervention should be determined by the prioritization as described previously. Then the ultimate goal for intervention must be identified. For example, are you interested in increasing the aggregate's level of knowledge on a particular topic, or do you expect health behaviors to change as a result of your plan? It is important to be specific with the goals and objectives and make them measurable. This will facilitate not only the nursing interventions but also the evaluation.

Planning the intervention is actually a multistep process. First, determine the levels (e.g., subsystem, aggregate system, or suprasystem) at which you plan to intervene. Second, plan interventions for each appropriate system level that will accomplish your objectives. Interventions may be focused on any of the three levels of prevention: primary, secondary, or tertiary. These levels apply to aggregates and communities as well as to individuals. Primary prevention consists of health promotion and activities directed at providing specific protection from illnesses or dysfunctions. Secondary prevention includes early diagnosis and prompt treatment to reduce the duration and severity of disease or dysfunction. Tertiary prevention is carried out when irreversible disability or damage has occurred. Rehabilitation and restoration of an optimal level of functioning are the goals of tertiary prevention. Plans should include goals and activities that reflect the level of prevention appropriate for the identified problem. Third, validate the practicality of the planned interventions according to available personal, aggregate, and suprasystem resources. Although teaching is often a major component of community health nursing, consider other potential forms of intervention (e.g., personal counseling, group process, game therapy, role modeling, or creation of a community service). Last, plan the scheduling of the interventions with the aggregate to maximize participation (Table 6–3).

Intervention

The intervention stage may be the most enjoyable stage for both the nurse and the clients. Careful assessment and planning before this step should help ensure the receptivity of the aggregate. Generally, implementation of plans should proceed as previously

Table 6–3
Systems Framework Premises

I.   Each system is a goal-directed collection of interacting, interdependent parts (subsystems)

II. System as a whole continually interacting with and adapting to environment (suprasystem)

III. Hierarchical (suprasystem → system → subsystems)

IV. Each system characterized by
  A. Structure—arrangement and organization of parts (subsystems)
    1. Organization/configuration—e.g., traditional versus nontraditional; greater variability (no right or wrong; no proper vs. improper form)
    2. Boundaries—open versus closed; regulate input and output
    3. Territory (spatial and behavioral)
    4. Role allocation
  B. Functions—goals and purpose of system—and activities necessary to ensure survival, continuity, and growth of system
    1. General
      a. Physical—food, clothing, shelter, protection from danger, provision for health and illness care
      b. Affectional—meeting emotional needs of affection and security
      c. Social—identity, affiliation, socialization, controls
    2. Specific—each family also has own individual agenda regarding values, aspirations, cultural obligations, and so on
  C. Process and dynamics
    1. Adaptation—attempt to establish and maintain equilibrium; balance between stability and differentiation and growth; self-regulation and adaptation → equilibrium and homeostasis
      a. Within family—between family members
      b. External—family interaction with suprasystem
    2. Integration—unity, ability to communication
    3. Decision making—power distribution; consensus, accommodation, authoritarian

set forth, but the nurse should also be prepared to be flexible in dealing with unexpected contingencies (e.g., bad weather, transportation problems, a smaller or larger group than anticipated, a competing event; see examples of unsuccessful student projects in the next section). If for some reason intervention becomes impossible, carefully consider the various potential causes of this.

Evaluation

Evaluation is an important component of understanding the success or lack of success of the project. It may include feedback from the participants (verbally or in writing) as well as the nurse's in-depth analysis. Evaluation of the process includes reflecting on each previous stage to determine strengths and weaknesses. Were plans appropriate but based on an incomplete assessment? Was adequate input from the clients allowed for? Were the interventions realistic or unrealistic in terms of available resources? Were all levels of prevention considered? Evaluation also includes consideration of the product, or outcomes. Were the stated goals and objectives accomplished? Were the participants satisfied with the interventions? Are you comfortable with what was accomplished? Do you believe that the outcomes reflect growth by the aggregate and the nurse? It is important to be able to evaluate honestly and comprehensively both positive and negative aspects of each experience.

After the project is completed, the final step is often short changed. Without communicating recommendations for follow-up to the aggregate and other appropriate persons, the impact of the intervention may be limited. Although not every experience lends itself to continuing activity, most at least indicate the need for additional interventions. These may be generated from within the aggregate or from community agencies and resources.

A comprehensive, fulfilling health planning project involves both careful consideration of each step in the process and a close working relationship with the aggregate.

HEALTH PLANNING PROJECTS

The following are examples of student projects using this health planning model with different types of aggregates: group, organization, population group, and community. The interventions with these aggregates occur at the three systems levels: subsystem, aggregate system, and suprasystem (Table 6–4).

Successful Projects

OBESE CHILDREN

While working in a Headstart setting, a student and the nurse identified two obese boys from the same family. After contacting the boys' mother, the student made a home visit and learned that the parents were separated and the children spent time in each parent's home as well as with the grandparents. Obesity appeared to be a family problem; both parents were obese. The student worked with the boys individually and together, carried out teaching with the mother and grandparents, and met once with the boys' father. Both the boys' mother and grandparents were included in the planning. A variety of interventions were carried out, including a food diary with the adults, teaching regarding low-calorie snacks and menu planning, a food collage, and a "Food Land" game made up by the student for the boys. Positive changes were noted in dietary patterns for the mother and boys by the end of the semester. The Headstart nurse also was kept informed of the family's progress so that continued reinforcement could take place after the student left the situation.

TEXTILE INDUSTRY

A student selected for study a textile plant with approximately 470 employees and no occupational health nurse. For data collection, she used Serafini's (1976) assessment guide for nursing in industry. Three major problems or needs were identified through collaboration with management and union representatives. First, the most common, costly, and chronic employee accident-related injury in the plant was lower back injury. Second, there was a generalized concern among employees about the possibility of

Table 6–4
Interventions by Type of Aggregate and System Level

Project	Type of Aggregate	System Level for Intervention
Obese children	Group	Subsystem and aggregate system
Rehabilitation group	Group	Subsystem and aggregate system
Textile industry	Organization	Aggregate system and suprasystem
Housing for elderly	Population group	Aggregate system
Bilingual students (case study)	Group, organization, population group	Aggregate system and suprasystem
Crime watch	Community	Aggregate system and suprasystem

undetected hypertension. Third, the first aid facilities were disorganized and involved no accurate inventory system. Interventions were then planned and implemented for all three identified areas.

On the suprasystem level, plans were formulated by the student with the company's physicians and communicated to management for enactment of an employee training program on proper lifting techniques. Concise and specific job descriptions and requirements were proposed to facilitate medical assessment of the health status of potential employees. In addition, the first aid supplies were organized and clearly labeled, and an inventory system was developed. On the aggregate system level, a hypertension screening program was planned and conducted. Approximately 85% of the employees were screened, and 10 persons were identified with elevated blood pressure readings, conditions that were later diagnosed as hypertension.

As a result of the project, management representatives recognized that workers' health could be improved or maintained at optimal levels through a variety of nursing interventions. Consequently, the student was hired as an occupational health nurse on graduation to facilitate this goal.

HOUSING FOR THE ELDERLY

Another project involved the residents of a housing complex for the elderly. The student met with 20 interested women and assessed their needs through a short questionnaire. Findings revealed that exercise was the highest priority need. Investigation of existing resources revealed that the community's YWCA offered a senior exercise class that met three times a week at a cost of $1 per session. This information was shared with the population group, but use of the program was not considered feasible by members. The alternative plan on which they agreed was to have weekly sessions led by the student at the housing complex (aggregate system level intervention) using exercises described by Frenkel and Richard (1977).

In evaluating outcomes, subjective comments from the participants indicated they felt better about themselves as a result of exercising and maintaining their range of motion. It also was a positive experience for the student; not only did she learn more about the elderly in general, but she also gained skill in applying the nursing process to a larger aggregate within a community.

CRIME WATCH

One student was concerned with the rising incidence of crime in a community and organized a crime watch program. This involved periodic meetings with local residents (aggregate system) as well as with the police. Interventions included posting signs in the neighborhood and more frequent police patrols (suprasystem level). The program increased the residents' awareness of potential problems as well as the need to be more concerned with neighborhood safety.

REHABILITATION GROUP

After working at a senior citizens' center for a few weeks, a student began a careful assessment of the clients served by the center. In addition to interviewing clients already active in the center, he made home visits to speak with homebound clients served by the center's social workers and Meals on Wheels program. A need for socialization and rehabilitation was identified by several of the homebound clients. A significant factor in considering plans to meet this need was the center's recent purchase of a van equipped to transport handicapped people in wheelchairs. After the student further assessed the clients' health and functional status and determined mutual goals, four of these homebound clients expressed a desire to attend a rehabilitation program at the center, if one were available. A weekly program was initiated on the basis of these clients' needs and included van transportation, a coffee hour, an exercise class, a noontime meal, and a craft class. After some initial reluctance to participate and the withdrawal of one man from the group, the group functioned very well. Progress was made toward meeting the goals of increased socialization and rehabilitation.

Unsuccessful Projects

When a project is not completed successfully, its failure can usually be related to problems with one or more stages of the nursing process. This is often not discovered until the evaluation phase. The following examples of unsuccessful projects illustrate failures at different steps of the nursing process (Table 6–5).

HEADSTART PROGRAM

One problem that occurs periodically is the lack of time to follow through with implementation. Among the reasons for this may be the initial

Table 6–5
Unsuccessful Projects

Project	Problematic Step of Nursing Process
Headstart program	Assessment (gaining entry)
Prenatal clinic	Assessment of aggregate system
Group home for mentally retarded adults	Assessment (mutual identification of health problems and needs)
Safe Rides program	Planning (mutual identification of goals and objectives) Evaluation (recommendations for follow-up)
Manufacturing plant	Implementation

problem of *gaining entry*. For example, a student who was aware that one community had a large number of low-income families decided to investigate the feasibility of beginning a Headstart program for the children in the area (a population group). After many frustrating weeks of telephone calls to leaders in the community (which often were not returned), she was finally able to locate the person in charge. By this time, the semester was almost completed. Needless to say, she was disappointed at the end result.

This example illustrates the importance of identifying a *key informant* early (i.e., someone who is familiar with the community), particularly if you are new to the area. Unfortunately, such persons are not always obvious because they may not be considered community leaders. For example, although the key informant in one community may be the director of a neighborhood health center, in another community it may be the person in charge of a local thrift shop in an underserved area.

PRENATAL CLINIC

After working for a few weeks in a prenatal clinic serving a primarily lower income population, the student identified several needs among the clients. Realizing that she needed to gather information regarding what the clients perceived as their needs, she developed a questionnaire that listed several possible topics for discussion and left space for the clients to write in what they would like to learn more about. Also included were spaces for clients to fill

in times when they would be able to attend a health education workshop and whether they had transportation available. After the student collected and tallied the questionnaires from 25 clients, she determined that infant feeding, whether breast or bottle, was the topic most frequently mentioned by the clients and that Tuesday evening was the best time. Transportation was not listed as a problem. With this information, the student set a date for her teaching project, made posters for the clinic, mailed notices describing the program to the clients, and planned her teaching. The evening of the program arrived, and the student was extremely disappointed to find that no clients attended.

What happened? There are many possible reasons for such occurrences. One explanation offered by the student was that returning to the clinic in the evening was too much of an inconvenience, even though this was the time when most clients said they could attend. Possibly health education may not have been a priority for this group of clients; the questionnaire assumed that it was important and merely asked about interests. Also the neighborhood surrounding the clinic may not have been perceived as safe during the evening hours.

This example illustrates the importance of careful assessment and the possible results if assessment is incomplete. The student recommended communicating health education information to clients during clinic hours and using more individual counseling, posters, and other media within the clinic setting.

GROUP HOME FOR MENTALLY RETARDED ADULTS

Another example of an unsuccessful project involved a student who identified as her aggregate six women living in a group home for mentally retarded citizens in the community. From her observations, she noted that they were all overweight, and she decided that she would institute a weekly weight reduction program for them. She then proceeded to meet with the women weekly, at which time she weighed them, discussed diets, and talked about food choices. At the end of an 8-week period, her evaluation revealed that not only had the women not lost weight but that a few of them had gained weight! The student had failed to consider the women's perceptions of their needs and priorities. The women did not consider their weight a problem. Furthermore, their boyfriends provided positive reinforcement regarding their appearance.

SAFE RIDES PROGRAM

One student assessed a university student community through a questionnaire and identified the problem of drinking and driving.

Seventy-seven percent of those she surveyed stated that they had driven while under the influence of alcohol, and 16.5% had been involved in an alcohol-related car accident. After identifying the problem, the student worked with the campus alcohol and drug resource center to plan and implement a Safe Rides program. In this program, which was modeled after one implemented elsewhere, student volunteers manned a hot line and drivers were on call to pick up students who had driven themselves or had ridden with another who was now unsafe to drive. Student interest in the program was also determined. Many unforeseen complications were resolved, such as the need for liability coverage for all individuals participating in the program and funds to cover expenses such as gas reimbursement. The student formulated a 12-hour, 3-week training program to prepare student volunteers for their involvement in Safe Rides. By the end of the semester, the Safe Rides program was ready to begin. However, by this time, the student—the prime motivating force—had graduated. Although others were committed and involved, apparently no provision had been made for another person to coordinate and follow through with the program after the student had left. Because the Safe Rides program required ongoing efforts for coordination, the program was never fully implemented in the student's absence.

MANUFACTURING PLANT

Even careful planning does not always eliminate all potential obstacles.

One student chose to work in an occupational setting involving heavy industry. Her entry into the organization was approved by both the occupational health nurse and the nurse's supervisor in personnel.

After reviewing the literature, working for several weeks with the nurse, and assessing the organization and the employees, the student identified the potential for back injury as a primary problem. Her plan was to decrease the risk factors involved in back injuries by distributing information about proper body mechanics to the workers in a teaching session. This plan was resisted, however, by the personnel manager. Despite his recognition of the need for such instruction, he initially resisted implementation because of an unwillingness to allow the employees to attend the session on company time. A compromise was reached by allowing attendance during coffee breaks, which would be extended by 5 minutes. Before the program could be implemented, however, it was canceled by the personnel manager because negotiations for a new union contract were under way and there was a high probability of a strike. Consequently, management was unwilling to allow any changes in the usual routine.

The student had proceeded appropriately and even received clearance from the proper officials, but the union problems could not have been anticipated or circumvented. The student could only share her information and concern with the nurse and the personnel manager and encourage them to implement her plan when contract negotiations were completed.

Discussion

Each of these projects addressed or was designed to address a particular level of prevention. Most of these examples focused on primary prevention and health promotion because they were conducted by students and were time limited (Table 6–6). However, for the community health nurse working on a regular basis with an aggregate (e.g., in the occupational health setting), interventions would be targeted for all three levels of prevention and at a variety of system levels. It is useful to view nursing interventions with aggregates within a matrix structure to ensure that all opportunities for intervention are being addressed. The matrix gives examples of how the occupational health nurse may intervene at all systems levels and all levels of prevention (Table 6–7). In practice, most interventions occur at the individual level and include all levels of prevention. Interventions at the aggregate level usually are less frequent. For many occupational health nurses, time does not allow for intervention at the suprasystem level. However, industries are integral parts of the community system. Factors that affect the health of communities also affect the health of employees and vice versa. Some industries take their reciprocal relationship with the surrounding community quite seriously. For nurses in these industries, interventions at the suprasystem level may become a reality, thus improving the health of both the community and the workers. This is a good example of refocusing upstream, addressing the "real" sources of problems. Although occupational health nursing has been used as an example here, a similar matrix can be constructed for interventions carried out by any nurse working with aggregate systems.

The projects just discussed illustrate the variety of opportunities available for health planning with ag-

Table 6–6
Level of Prevention for Each Project

Primary Prevention	Secondary Prevention	Tertiary Prevention
Textile industry (first aid and back injury prevention)	Obese children	Rehabilitation group
Housing for elderly	Textile industry (blood pressure screening and counseling)	
Crime watch	Group home for mentally retarded adults	
Headstart program		
Prenatal clinic		
Safe Rides program		
Manufacturing plant		

gregates. In addition, they exemplify the application of the nursing process within various types of aggregates at different systems levels and at each level of prevention. A review of these examples demonstrates the vital importance of each step of the nursing process. Assessments of aggregates must be thorough, as exemplified by the textile industry project. Assessment included answers to key questions about the aggregate's health and demographic profile as well as a comparison of this information with the picture of similar aggregates presented in the literature. Careful planning is a necessity, and mutual goals acceptable to both the nurse and the aggregate must be agreed on. The housing for the elderly and rehabilitation group projects illustrate such mutual planning. Interventions also need to include aggregate participation and must be designed to meet the mutual goals, as exemplified by the Crime Watch project. Last, evaluation must include both process and product evaluation and be conducted with aggregate input.

HEALTH PLANNING FEDERAL LEGISLATION

Health planning at the national level is another example of planning for aggregates. The national level can be considered a broader extension of the suprasystem level and as such impacts on each of the other levels described. Again, this is where upstream change

Table 6–7
Occupational Health: Levels of Prevention for System Levels

System Level	Primary Prevention	Secondary Prevention	Tertiary Prevention
Subsystem (individual)	Yearly physical examination for each employee	Regular blood pressure monitoring and diet counseling for each employee with elevated blood pressure	Referral for job retraining for employee with a back injury
Aggregate and group system	Incentive program to encourage departments to use safety devices	Weight reduction group for overweight employees	Support group for employees who are recovering from problems with alcohol or drug use
Suprasystem (community)	Health fair open to the community as well as employees	Counseling and referral of members of community with elevated blood pressure or cholesterol on the basis of health fair findings	Media advertising to encourage people with substance abuse problems to seek help, including community resources where assistance is available

occurs. National health planning has been minimally influenced by nurses but has a tremendous effect on nurses and nursing practice. Because of the necessity for understanding planning on a national level, a discussion of present health planning legislation follows.

Early History

Although health planning activities existed in the United States before the 1940s, these were usually directed toward specific health problems (e.g., services for maternal and child health, provision of health care activities). Furthermore, these activities were usually initiated by private, nongovernment agencies such as the American Public Health Association or the American Cancer Society, with limited involvement by the federal government. For example, in the 1930s, Blue Cross and the United Fund in New York City were responsible for starting local health planning, but it was mostly provider oriented. The Health and Planning Council of New York was formed to implement local health planning.

The federal government's involvement in health planning changed, however, at the end of World War II, when the government turned its attention to issues raised by the private sector. At this point, there was a general shortage of hospital beds and a lack of coordination among hospitals. Rural areas were especially needy in terms of hospital beds as well as medical personnel (Braverman, 1978).

Hill-Burton Act

To address the need for better access to hospitals, Congress passed the Hospital Survey and Construction Act (Hill-Burton Act, PL 79-725) in 1946, which provided federal aid to states for hospital facilities. This is generally considered to be the first major effort by the federal government to promote health planning.

To be eligible for funds under the Hill-Burton Act for hospital construction and modernization, a state had to submit a plan documenting resources available and estimates of need. As a result, vast sums of money were spent; the outcome was an increase in the number of beds, with the majority in general hospitals.

Although the act and its amendments are often criticized for focusing too narrowly on construction, the act improved the quality of care in rural areas and introduced systematic statewide planning (Stebbins and Williams, 1972).

Regional Medical Programs

The Hill-Burton Act provided for planning related to construction, but the Heart Disease, Cancer, and Stroke Amendment of 1965 (PL 89-239) was more comprehensive and established regional medical programs. These programs were intended to make available to community health care providers the latest technology from existing medical centers for the treatment of the leading causes of death.

To achieve this, 56 health regions across the country were established and charged with evaluating the health needs within each region. Priorities, objectives, and regional programmatic approaches were then developed. As a result, not only was local participation in planning mandated, but also funds were provided for both planning and operating (Hyman, 1982).

Although regional medical programs have been credited with the regionalization of certain services and the introduction of innovative approaches to the organization and delivery of care, some observers believed that the reforms were not comprehensive enough. Also because the regional medical programs were not incorporated into existing federal and state programs, there were both gaps and duplication in delivery of services, personnel training, and research (Stebbins and Williams, 1972).

Comprehensive Health Planning

To broaden the categorical approach to health planning that had characterized previous legislation, Congress signed into law the Public Health Service Act Amendments of 1966 (PL 89-749) relating to comprehensive health planning. Combined with PL 90-174, which was passed in 1967, these amendments created the Partnership for Health Program. The objectives of the program were directed toward promoting and ensuring the highest level of health attainable for every person while at the same time not interfering with the existing patterns of private practice.

A two-level planning system was formulated to meet these objectives. The "A" agencies, with input from an advisory council in which health care consumers were in the majority, were to play a statewide coordinating role. Meanwhile, plans to meet designated local community needs were formulated by the "B" agencies.

Although the comprehensive health plans were the first of the programs previously described to mandate consumer involvement, many believed that they failed in their basic intent. Various reasons have been cited for the perceived failure, including inadequate funding, conflict avoidance in policy formulation and goal establishment, lack of political influence, and, most important, provider opposition (e.g., American Medical Association, American Hospital Association, and major medical centers). The mission appeared to be a discussion of what was wrong with health care delivery rather than the provision of mechanisms for action (DeBella et al., 1986; Roseman, 1972).

Certificate of Need

As a response to increases in capital investments and budgetary pressures, state governments developed the idea of obtaining prior government approval for certain projects through the use of a certificate of need. The first state certificate-of-need law was passed in New York State in 1964, requiring government approval of major capital investments by hospitals and nursing homes. This certificate-of-need requirement ultimately became a component of the health legislation to follow (PL 93-641) and thus was required of all states. At the end of the 1980s, certificate-of-need reviews were still required in 33 states and the District of Columbia; by the fall of 1994, 40 states required certificates of need for selected expenditures.

National Health Planning and Resources Development Act

Given the perceived failure of the comprehensive health planning program, the federal government focused on a new approach to health planning. Of great concern was the cost of health care, which had escalated since the end of World War II; the uneven distribution of services; the general lack of knowledge of personal health practices; and the emphasis on more costly modalities of care. The National Health Planning and Resources Development Act of 1974 (PL 93-641) combined the strengths of the Hill-Burton Act, regional medical programs, and the comprehensive health planning program to forge a new system of single-state and areawide health planning agencies.

The goals and purposes of the new law were increased accessibility, acceptability, continuity, and quality of health services; restraint of the rising costs of health care services; and prevention of unnecessary duplication of health resources. Of particular interest were the needs of the underserved and the concern for providing quality health care. Not only would the provider and consumer be involved in the planning and improvement of health services, but also the system of private practice would be placed under scrutiny.

At the center of the program was a network of local health planning agencies that composed the health system agency, which developed a health systems plan for its geographic service area. These plans were then submitted to a state health planning and development agency, which integrated the plans into a preliminary state plan. This preliminary plan was then submitted to a statewide health coordinating council for approval. The law mandated that the council be composed of at least 16 members appointed by the governor, with 50% of its members representatives of health system agencies and at least 50% consumers. One major function of this council was to prepare a state health plan that reflected the goals and purposes of the act. Once formulated, the tentative plan was presented at public hearings throughout the state for discussion and possible revisions.

Despite careful deliberations by health planners with input from consumers, the health system agency was not always blandly accepted at the grassroots level. For example, Rhode Island's state health plan was commended by federal officials as a considerable achievement and given high praise. However, when the plan was first presented at seven public hearings throughout the state in 1980, approximately 10,000 persons attended, many essentially to protest two of the recommendations.

One recommendation was to move in the direction of a smaller number of larger hospitals, and the second was to reduce the number of hospital beds. In Newport, persons argued vehemently that if the maternity unit of the local hospital was closed and women were forced to deliver in other communities, there would be no more "native Newporters." The same recommendations precipitated a candlelight march in Westerly, a suburban community, with the slogan, "Save Our Hospital."

What happened? Why did a plan aimed at "promoting quality of care while constraining costs" meet with such resistance? In retrospect, planners agreed that although much time was spent introspectively developing the plan, the public was not prepared for the recommendations, which were very ambitious. Furthermore, there was a perception in the state that the council had more power than it actually had; finally, members of the hospital community went out of their way to discredit the plan. The second state health plan was presented in 1983 with the two recommendations substantially modified, and it was met with little or no opposition from the public. By this time, the functions of the council were better known, and the recommendations were more conservative.

Changing Focus of Health Planning

Under the Reagan administration, competition within the health care system was encouraged, and emphasis was placed on cost shifting and cost reduction. This approach, combined with a cutback in funding, dealt a death blow to federal health planning, which ended in 1986 because the expectation that health care costs would be contained was not met (Mueller, 1993).

As a result of the cutbacks, the role of health system agencies was redefined, and the federal government recommended their elimination. Because of a reduction in federal funding and the influence of medical lobbies, some health system agencies did close. Those that remained experienced a decrease in staff, which resulted in a decrease in overall board functioning and a reordering of priorities. In an effort to compensate for the decrease in federal funding, some health system agencies sought nonfederal funding or tried to build coalitions to provide the power base necessary for change.

As previously stated, by the end of the 1980s, certificate-of-need reviews were still required in 33 states and the District of Columbia. Within these programs, requirements for approval were more liberal, expedited reviews were conducted, and certain projects were exempted from review (American Public Health Association, 1989). With the 1990s, reviews were extended to include nursing homes, psychiatric facilities, and expensive equipment.

Under the Clinton administration's plan for health care reform, planning would have been revitalized at the national level. The failure of the legislation to pass left planning efforts again with state and local agencies. As of the fall of 1994, 30 states had statewide health plans in place, with 40 requiring certificates of need for selected expenditures. An example of health planning on the state level is New York State's 1993 legislation, New York Prospective Hospital Reimbursement Methodology—Fifth Version (NYPHRM V), which provided for comprehensive hospital reimbursement reform and expanded the responsibilities of the state's eight health systems agencies while ensuring their continued funding (Health Systems Agency of New York City, Inc., 1994). Other examples include Kentucky, which created the Health Policy Board to collect cost, charges, quality, and outcome data for all providers; Florida, which passed the Health Care and Insurance Reform Act; and Arizona, where the state was divided into 102 primary care areas, developing 88 profiles for each (American Health Planning Association, 1995).

The implementation of managed care by health care providers and health insurers represents one of the more recent attempts at cost management and planning for the health of population groups. This model of organized service delivery links health care financing to care delivery in an effort to maximize the quality of care while minimizing costs (American Nurses Association, 1993). Although reformers envision managed care as an opportunity to provide universal access to consumers, insurers and providers have focused on decreasing costs via group enrollments, limiting standard packages of services, decreasing hospital stays, and downsizing staffing. Consequently, it is anticipated that the restructuring concomitant with the advent of managed care may actually decrease access for consumers and increase the competition for nursing positions (Henneberger, 1994; Weil and Stack, 1993).

Although managed care focuses on health planning and evaluation at the aggregate level, it has the potential for negatively impacting the health of communities. Nurses must remain vocal and committed to the managed care model, which restructures service delivery to the benefit of consumers.

Case Study

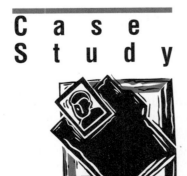

José Mendez, a bilingual community health nursing student, was assigned to a community with a large Portuguese subsystem. He chose as his aggregate the students who were enrolled in the town's bilingual program within the school system. His contacts included the school nurse and the teachers in this program.

Assessment

Included in José's assessment of aggregate characteristics were the specific group of students, members of the organizational level of the school system, and the population group of Portuguese-speaking residents in the town. One problem identified through observation of the children, interviews with teachers and community residents, and a literature review was the lack of primary disease prevention for this subsystem. Further assessment and prioritization revealed the problem to be related to a lack of knowledge rather than to a lack of concern.

Diagnosis

Individual Inadequate preparation at home regarding basic hygiene, dental care, nutrition, and healthy lifestyles

Family Inadequate knowledge base regarding basic hygiene, dental care, nutrition, and healthy lifestyles

Community Inadequate resources for communicating basics of hygiene, dental care, nutrition, and healthy lifestyles to the Portuguese community

Planning

Contracting and goal setting were facilitated by the teachers and staff of the bilingual program, reinforcing the need for mutuality at this step of the process. A variety of alternative interventions would be needed to accomplish the following goals:

Individual

Long-Term Goal: Students will regularly practice good hygiene, preventive dental care, good nutrition, and exercise and adequate sleep habits.

Short-Term goal: Students will learn the basics of good hygiene, preventive dental care, a healthy diet, regular exercise, and adequate sleep habits.

Family

Long-Term Goal: Families will regularly practice and teach their children good hygiene, good nutrition, exercise, and adequate sleep habits.

Short-Term Goal: Families will learn the basics of good hygiene, preventive dental care, a healthy diet, regular exercise, and adequate sleep habits.

Community

Long-Term Goal: Systematic programs will be established to provide families and their children with education and information regarding the basics of good hygiene, preventive dental care, a healthy diet, regular exercise, and adequate sleep habits.

Short-Term Goal: Information will be translated to Portuguese and disseminated to families regarding the basics of good hygiene, preventive dental care, a healthy diet, regular exercise, and adequate sleep habits.

Intervention

Student projects sometimes are more limited than the "ideal" identified in the planning stage; here interventions were limited to one grade level.

Individual Within the aggregate system, the children were taught many basics of healthy lifestyles, including nutrition, hygiene, and dental care. Information was presented in class in both Portuguese and English languages.

Family The content taught to the children was summarized in each language as well as in pictures and then was sent home to all parents.

Community When the local teachers communicated to their state-level coordinators what the student had been doing, the materials developed by the student were incorporated into the bilingual program throughout the state.

Evaluation

This community health planning project not only had an impact on the individuals in the specific aggregate but also had broader implications for the family systems and the community suprasystem. The outcomes, or product, were a huge success! The process, developed from the mutually identified goals and objectives, incorporated input from a variety of sources. Resources were adequate both from the student's perspective and from the support received from the bilingual program. Although only primary prevention was addressed, the continuing nature of the project will allow teachers, the school nurse, and the families to assess for problems related to the content taught. Thus, future implementation might also address secondary and tertiary prevention.

NURSING IMPLICATIONS

One method of strengthening local and national health planning is through increased nursing involvement. Nurses' use of this health planning model facilitates a systematic approach to improving health care at the aggregate level. Through application of this model, aggregates from small groups through population groups can be assessed; their health needs can be identified; and planning, intervention, and evaluations can be carried out. If nurses were to reemphasize the larger aggregate as client, the health of individuals and families as well as of groups would improve.

SUMMARY

Community health nurses have a responsibility to incorporate health planning into their practice. The unique talents and skills of nurses, augmented by the comprehensive application of the nursing process, can facilitate improvement of the health of populations at various aggregate levels. Health planning policy and process constitute a part of the knowledge base of the baccalaureate-prepared nurse. Systems theory provides one framework for application of the nursing process in the community. Interventions are possible at subsystem (individual), system (aggregate or group), and suprasystem (population or community) levels using all three levels of prevention.

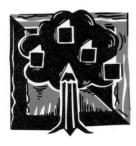

L e a r n i n g
A c t i v i t i e s

1. Assess a neighborhood or local community using exploratory techniques: drive through the area and identify types of houses, schools, churches, health related-agencies, and businesses; look for potential environmental and safety hazards; interview a clerk at the town hall, a senior citizen at a meal site or day care center, a newspaper reporter, a visiting nurse, a police officer, a social worker, or a school nurse regarding the community; call the local, county, or state health department for morbidity and mortality statistics; or attend a town council or school committee meeting. Compare and contrast your findings with those of your classmates.

2. Construct a matrix similar to that of Table 6–7 using interventions from the school nurse setting.

3. As a class project, identify 10 to 15 questions that will elicit important health information from young adults. Have each student in your class write answers to these questions. Tally the students' responses and, as a group, draw conclusions from this assessment. Identify problems or potential problem areas, and construct a plan to solve or prevent these problems.

4. Attend a health system agency meeting or a meeting about health planning at the local level. Observe the number of health care providers and consumers present. Compare the issues being discussed with the goals of improving quality of care and reducing health care costs.

5. Interview a health planner at the state or local level to determine the status of health planning and certificate-of-need review in your community or state.

REFERENCES

American Health Planning Association: National Directory of Health Planning, Policy, and Regulatory Agencies, 6th ed. Washington, DC, American Health Planning Association, 1995.

American Nurses Association: Nursing's Agenda for Health Care Reform. Washington, DC, American Nurses Association, 1993.

American Public Health Association. Most states continue health planning program. Nation's Health 19:24, 1989.

Braverman J: Crisis in Health Care. Washington, DC, Acropolis Books, Ltd., 1978.

DeBella S, Martin L, Siddall S: Nurses' Role in Health Care Planning. Norwalk, CT, Appleton-Century-Crofts, 1986.

Duffus RL: Lillian Wald: Neighbor and Crusader. New York, Macmillan, 1938.

Frenkel LJ, Richard BB: Exercises to help the elderly live longer and stay healthier, and be happier. Nursing 77:58–63, 1977.

Hamilton PA, Barbato HL, Hawley LJ, et al.: Decision Making in Community Health Nursing. Boston, Little, Brown, 1985.

Health Systems Agency of New York City, Inc.: Perspectives 18: (1), 1994.

Hegge ML: Independent study in community health nursing. Nurs Outlook 21:652–654, 1973.

Henneberger M: For nurses, new uncertainties. New York Times, August 21, 1994, pp. 45, 48.

Hogue C: An epidemiologic approach to distributive nursing practice. *In* Hall JE, Weaver BR (eds). Distributive Nursing Practice: A Systems Approach to Community Health, 2nd ed. Philadelphia, JB Lippincott, 1985, pp. 288–303.

Hyman H: Health Planning: A Systematic Approach. Rockville, MD, Aspen Systems Corp., 1982.

Leavell HR, Clark EG: Preventive Medicine for the Doctor in His Community. New York, McGraw-Hill, 1965.

Mahon J, McFarlane J, Golden K: De Madres a Madres: A community partnership for health. Public Health Nurs 8:15–19, 1991.

Maslow AH: Toward a Psychology of Being. New York, Van Nostrand Reinhold, 1968.

Mueller K: Health Care Policy in the United States. Lincoln, NE, University of Nebraska Press, 1993.

Roseman C: Problems and prospects for comprehensive health planning. Am J Public Health 62:16–19, 1972.

Ruybal SE, Bauwens E, Fasla MJ.: Community assessment: An epidemiological approach. Nurs Outlook 23:365–368, 1975.

Serafini P: Nursing assessment in industry. Am J Public Health 66:755–760, 1976.

Shalala D: Nursing and society—The unfinished agenda for the 21st century. *In* National League for Nursing, Perspectives in Nursing 1991–1993. New York, National League for Nursing Press, 1992, pp. 3–8.

Silverstein NG: Lillian Wald at Henry Street, 1893–1895. Adv Nurs Sci 7:1–12, 1985.

Stebbins EL, Williams KN: History and background of health planning in the United States. *In* Reinke WA, (ed). Health Planning: Qualitative Aspects and Quantitative Techniques. Baltimore, MD, Waverly Press, 1972, pp. 1–19.

Weil TP, Stack MC: Health reform—Its potential impact on hospital nursing service. Nurs Economics 11:200–207, 1993.

Community Organization: Building Partnerships for Health

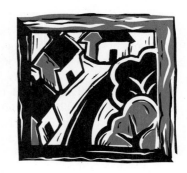

Upon completion of this chapter, the reader will be able to:

1. Define community organization, community development, social planning, and social action.

2. Explain major concepts, models, theoretical frameworks, and strategies of community organization.

3. Discuss the relationships among community health development, social justice, and nursing care of aggregates.

4. Describe strategies for building community partnerships for health promotion and disease and injury prevention.

5. Explain appropriate use of community organization models and conceptual frameworks in nursing care of aggregates.

6. Apply knowledge of community organization to primary, secondary, and tertiary prevention of priority community health problems.

Peggy Hickman

A universal goal of nursing is assurance of access to basic health care for all people (American Nurses Association [ANA], 1985; International Council of Nurses, 1981; World Health Organization [WHO], 1974). In 1978, the United States joined 138 other nations in the WHO in affirming that access to basic health care is a right of all people. Basic health care was defined as provision of the full range of resources essential to human health. The year 2000 was set as the target date for achieving the international goal of health for all.

Because community health nurses encounter many situations in which human rights and freedoms may be in jeopardy, the ANA (1986) stated that major responsibilities of community health nurses are to advocate for individuals and families, identify and rectify gaps in health care, and influence health and social policies that are inconsistent with the rights of humans. Of particular concern to nurses are the barriers that limit access to basic health care for individuals, families, aggregates, and entire communities. A variety of factors, such as socioeconomic status, environment, health care infrastructure, and public policy, work together to form these barriers (Table 7–1). An upstream view requires nurses to address health promotion and disease and injury pre-

vention in a community-wide context. The WHO (1978) stated that health is an integral part of the overall social and economic development of the community and that community members have the "right and duty to participate individually and collectively in the planning and implementation of their health care." Achieving improvements in health and access to basic health care requires cooperative action by all sectors of the community.

BASIC HEALTH CARE (WHO, 1978)

- Education about prevailing health problems, including methods of prevention and control
- Promotion of adequate food supply and proper nutrition
- Provision of safe water and basic sanitation
- Maternal and child health care, including family planning
- Immunization against the major infectious diseases
- Prevention and control of locally endemic diseases
- Appropriate treatment of common diseases and injuries
- Provision of essential drugs

Table 7–1
Examples of Factors Limiting Access to Basic Health Care

Factor	Individual Family Examples	Community Examples
Socioeconomic conditions	Lack money for adequate food, housing, and health care	Lack funds for adequate social, educational, and public health services
Lack of knowledge or skills	Do not know how to prevent or cure common health problems; lack knowledge about available resources	Unable to attract and retain economic and health resources; providers cannot speak language of consumers
Geography-environment	Distance or terrain limits access to centralized services; wood- and coal-burning stoves pollute air	Water and soil pollution caused by improper sewage-refuse disposal
Beliefs, values, and norms	Health promotion not valued; lack of health-promoting and disease-preventing behaviors	Health promotion not valued; lack of preventive services
Situational appropriateness	Health care services not available during nonworking hours	Health care and social services not culturally appropriate
Lack of comprehensive planning	Health care utilization is episodic and illness oriented	Fragmentation or duplication of services; cure-solution not linked to determinants of problem
Public policy	Healthy choices and basic services not available	Lack or maldistribution of resources, including money, personnel, and infrastructure

Much of the success of community health nursing practice is directly related to the nurse's skill in enabling individuals, aggregates, and communities to promote, protect, and restore their health through organized community efforts. The ANA (1986) stated that community health nursing practice entails the understanding and application of

- Concepts of community and public health
- Skills of community organization and community development
- Nursing care of selected individuals, families, and groups for health promotion, health maintenance, health education, and coordination of care

In this chapter, the major concepts, models, processes, and strategies of community organization are discussed and applied to community health nursing practice focused on promotion, protection, and restoration of the health of aggregates.

CONCEPTUAL BASIS OF COMMUNITY ORGANIZATION

Community organization and community health nursing share common roots in theories and concepts of social change and social interaction. The concepts of social systems, social change, and community participation are discussed to provide a basis for understanding selected community organization models and their application to community health nursing practice.

Social Systems Theories

Social scientists view communities as systems that have wholeness, boundaries, organization, openness, and feedback. Each community consists of interrelated subsystems, including aggregates and sectors. Aggregates are groups within the community that share common characteristics, such as age, gender, race, socioeconomic status, culture, occupation, and location of work or dwelling. Sectors are functional divisions of the community such as health, welfare, education, economics, energy, agriculture, religion, transportation, communications, business and industry, recreation, safety, and government and politics. Within systems theory, all sectors and aggregates of the community are interrelated. A change in one subsystem will affect all other subsystems as well as the community as a whole. Similarly, communities are parts of larger systems called suprasystems. Changes

in the suprasystem will also affect a community system and its subsystem aggregates and sectors (Anderson and Carter, 1990).

When promoting the health of aggregates, the community health nurse may intervene at varied levels of the community system. The term *focal system* denotes the system level that is the primary focus of community care. However, within the community systems framework, the nurse must consider the focal system, its subsystems, and the suprasystem as a single entity when planning nursing care. Therefore, when planning health intervention in one aggregate or sector of the community, it is necessary to analyze the effects of the proposed change on all other components of the community. Furthermore, health promotion in the community cannot be achieved by the health care subsystem alone. Community health is brought about by the cooperative effort of all sectors of the community. Recognizing the multiple determinants of human health, the WHO (1978) recommended that health promotion be a collaborative effort of scientific health services, traditional health services, agriculture, animal husbandry, food, industry, education, housing, public works, communication, and all other sectors of community development.

A general nursing model fitting social systems theory is Betty Neuman's health care systems model. Neuman (1995) defines health as the condition in which all parts and subparts are in harmony with the whole. At the aggregate level, Neuman's model indicates that community health nurses must assess all of the aggregates and sectors making up the community, not just the traditional health sectors, as a part of the nursing process. Anderson and McFarlane's (1988, 1995) community-as-client/partner model incorporates the concept of a multisectoral basis for health into Betty Neuman's model in a systems-oriented framework for comprehensive community health nursing practice.

Social Change

The social scientist most frequently associated with *change theory* is Kurt Lewin. Lewin (1951) identified a three-stage process of social change that included

- Unfreezing: the breakdown of existing mores, values, and traditions
- Changing: the identification and internalization of new values and behavior patterns
- Refreezing: the integration of the new values into the community mores and traditions

Lewin also proposed the concept of force field analysis. Community systems (fields) are affected by forces that promote or inhibit change. Driving forces promote or support change. Restraining forces inhibit or oppose change. When the driving and restraining forces are of equal strength, the social system is at equilibrium. Change occurs when the combined strength of one set of forces is greater than the combined strength of the opposing set of forces. To plan effective health promotion programs, community health professionals must analyze the nature and strength of each set of forces (force field analysis) and determine how to increase the strength of forces supporting the health of aggregates and decrease the strength or change the direction of forces opposing health promotion (Hickman & Hustedde, 1995). Although Lewin's concepts have much useful application to community health nursing practice, one must examine carefully the ethics of changing community

values, mores, and traditions unless the community members freely initiated and directed the process.

Community Participation

Community participation has been identified as one of the variables associated with healthy communities and is incorporated into some definitions of community health (Lackey et al., 1987; Woelk, 1992). Research has been conducted on the relationship between community participation and the change process. In a 1953 study of group communication patterns, Bavelas found that groups develop greater problem-solving skills when a participatory, rather than a directive, pattern of communication is used. The exception was in emergency situations, when directive communication was needed for immediate resolution of the problem. Building on Bavelas' research, Hersey and Blanchard (1982) developed a model that identified

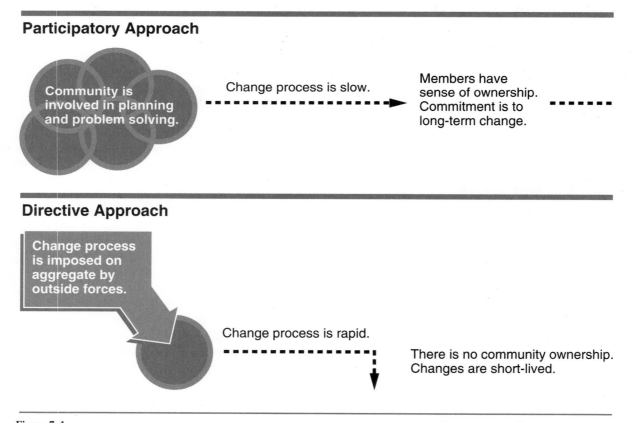

Figure 7–1
Two approaches to change in a community. (Data from Hersey P, Blanchard K: Management of Organizational Behavior: Utilizing Human Resources. Englewood Cliffs, NJ, Prentice-Hall, 1982.)

two approaches to change: participatory and directive. In participatory change, members of the aggregate affected are involved in planning and problem solving at all levels of the change process (Fig. 7–1). Hersey and Blanchard's research has found the participatory approach to be most effective when working with mature, competent communities that can take ownership of the change process. Although the participatory change process is slow, change effected is long lasting because community members develop a sense of ownership and commitment to the change. In contrast, directive change imposed on the community by outside forces has the advantage of bringing about change more rapidly, but without community ownership of the process changes tend to be short lived.

In recent years, community participation has frequently taken the form of coalitions or partnerships among agencies, organizations, and individuals for the purpose of achieving mutual health-related goals. A coalition is defined as a **group of diverse agencies, organizations, and individuals that work together to address a common interest or concern.** Research has found that successful coalitions tend to be issue oriented, structured, action oriented, focused on specific goals external to the organization, and committed to recruiting members with diverse talents and resources (Butterfoss et al., 1993; Francisco et al., 1993; Gottlieb, et al., 1993). Nurses and other health professional are organizing coalitions within their practice and research as a means of increasing community participation focused on prevention of major community health problems, such as agricultural injuries, human immunodeficiency virus, smoking, heart disease, and cancer (Couto et al., 1995; Herman et al., 1993; Lexau et al., 1993; McKinney et al., 1992; Ockene et al., 1991; Rogers et al., 1993; Russell, 1992; Thompson et al., 1993). In addition, nurses and other health professionals are active in coalitions as member-representatives of their employing agencies.

Within community health, community empowerment is the most active level of community participation. **Empowerment is a process whereby individuals, organizations, and communities gain mastery over their lives.** Citizens actively participate in democratic community processes and have full ownership of community decision making about issues that affect their lives, including health promotion and disease and injury prevention (Labonte, 1994; Minkler, 1992; Rappaport, 1987; Skelton, 1994; Wallerstein, 1992, 1993; Wallerstein & Bernstein, 1994). Inherent within

community empowerment are the concepts of community capacity, community self-efficacy, and community self-care agency.

Although community organization research reinforces Hersey and Blanchard's findings that community participation in all aspects of the planning process increases the strength and longevity of the change, recent community health research suggests that the most effective level of participation brings community members, agencies, organizations, and mediating structures together with health professionals in partnerships that address health collaboratively (Daly and Angulo, 1990; Flynn et al., 1991, 1994; Hickman, 1990; Jones and Harris, 1987; Kumpfer et al., 1993). In applying community participation research to clinical practice, community health nurses should consider the situation, the nature of the aggregate, and the relative merits of speed versus longevity when planning community change strategies.

DEFINITION OF COMMUNITY ORGANIZATION

Community organization may be defined as a process, a social structure, and a goal. The process of community organization, sometimes called community organizing, refers to the series of activities related to developing competent community action systems and to the technical tasks associated with these activities. Bracht (1990) identified a five-stage community organization process that parallels the steps of the nursing process (Table 7–2). Both processes begin with a definition and in-depth analysis (assessment) of the focal system (i.e., the aggregate or community).

Table 7–2
Comparison of Community Organization and Community Health Nursing Processes

Stages of Community Organization Process	Stages of Nursing Process
Community analysis	Community health assessment Community diagnosis
Design, initiation	Community health planning
Implementation	Implementation
Maintenance, consolidation	
Dissemination, reassessment	Evaluation

Bracht recommended that the analysis include an assessment of the aggregate's needs, resources, structures, capacities, and priorities. The resulting data (including the community diagnosis) form a basis for subsequent decision making and collaborative health planning.

Community organization also describes the social structure of subsystems within a community. Subsystems includes agencies, organizations, and mediating structures as well as the aggregates and sectors within the community. The term *community organization,* when defined as a social structure, includes not only the subsystems themselves but the relationships among the subsystems. Nursing interventions at the aggregate level may include coalition development, where community subsystems are organized into working partnerships focused on health promotion or disease and injury prevention.

In addition, community organization is defined as a goal of community health nursing practice. In this context, community organization refers to the ability of a community to develop a means of grouping and arranging its parts into a whole working system (Anderson and Carter, 1990). Community organization may include outcome goals that specify the desired structure, change, or action being pursued and process goals that define adjunct outcomes desired as a result of the methods used to bring about a change (Table 7–3). Cottrell (1976) used the term ''community competence'' to describe the ability of community subsystems to collaborate effectively in identifying needs, establishing priorities, setting goals, planning, implementing, and evaluating solutions. Subsequent research by Goeppinger (1982), a community health nurse, linked community competence to aggregate health. Cottrell and Goeppinger described competent (healthy) community systems as having commitment, active participation, articulateness, effective communication, self-other awareness, clarity of situational definitions, conflict containment and accommodation,

and management of relations with larger society (Goeppinger and Shuster, 1992).

Within the remainder of this chapter, community organization is defined as **the process whereby community change agents empower individuals and aggregates to solve community problems and achieve community goals.** Within the context of community health nursing, the definition is operationalized as the process whereby the nurse empowers individuals, aggregates, and communities to solve priority community health problems and to achieve community health-related goals. The process implies upstream thinking as community problems or goals, such as universal access to basic health care, are addressed in a sustainable manner that addresses underlying social, economic, political, and environmental factors.

COMMUNITY ORGANIZATION MODELS

A variety of community organization models have evolved over the years. Many of the current models developed during the social and political activism of the 1960s and 1970s, including several typologies of community organization practice. The typologies are based on a consideration of a variety of elements, including the character of the community action system, setting or locality, substance of the problem being addressed, character of the issues being generated, kind of aggregate most directly affected, organizational structures being developed, sponsor of the community organizing project, and role of the professional worker, in this case, the community health nurse (Kramer and Specht, 1975). As community health professionals have become more aware of the need to involve aggregate and community members in planning and decision making, new community organization models specific to health have evolved.

Table 7–3
Comparison of Process Goals Versus Outcome Goals in Child Health Promotion

Client Focus	Process Goal	Outcome Goal
Individual or family	Development of problem-solving skills	Healthy children
Aggregate	Development of collaborative planning skills by nurses and aggregate members	Establishment of a well-child clinic in a low-income neighborhood
Community	Community competence	Community health

Rothman's Community Organization Typology

A typology of community organization practice frequently used by community health professionals is that of Rothman. Rothman (1972) synthesized the various definitions and approaches to community organization practice into three models: social planning, social action, and locality development.

In the social planning model, community decisions are based on fact gathering and rational decision making. Emphasis is placed on the task rather than on the process. Because rapid problem solution is a primary goal of social planning, the directive approach to social change that emphasizes "expert" planning is used. Roles of the community health nurse using a social planning approach would be as facilitator, fact gatherer, expert analyst, and program implementer.

In the social action model, community change is accomplished by polarization of the community around selected issues followed by confrontation or conflict between persons with opposing viewpoints. Whether the concentration is on process or goals, the major focus of social action is the transfer of power to the aggregate level (Alinsky, 1971). Social action organizers may be revolutionary or evolutionary (Archer et al., 1984). Revolutionary social activists focus on the transformation of society, whereas evolutionary social activists work within the existing social system. Within the social action model, the roles of the community health nurse would be as community activist, agitator, and negotiator.

Locality development, more commonly known as community development, is a model that places emphasis on community involvement, self-direction, and self-help in determining and solving problems (Rothman, 1972). The Community Development Society (CDS), an international organization of community development professionals (including nurses), published the *Principles of Good Practice*, which reflect a shared belief in the importance of grassroots community involvement in planning and decision making (CDS, 1985).

Within the community development model, the empowerment that occurs as individual and aggregate skills are developed during the problem-solving process is an important element of the solution to the problem. Therefore, the roles of the community health nurse would be as an empowerer, a process facilitator, and a teacher of problem-solving skills (Hickman,

COMMUNITY DEVELOPMENT SOCIETY (CDS) PRINCIPLES OF GOOD PRACTICE (ADOPTED BY THE CDS MEMBERSHIP IN JULY 1985)

1. Promote active and representative citizen participation in decision making so that community members can meaningfully influence decisions that affect their lives.
2. Engage community members in problem diagnosis so that those affected may adequately understand the causes of their situation.
3. Help community leaders understand the economic, social, political, environmental, and psychological impact associated with alternative solutions to the problem.
4. Assist community members in designing and implementing a plan to solve agreed upon problems by emphasizing shared leadership and active citizen participation in that process.
5. Disengage from any effort that is likely to adversely affect the disadvantaged segments of a community.
6. Actively work to increase leadership capacity (skills, confidence, and aspirations) in the community development process.

1990; Lassiter, 1992). Paterson and Zderad's humanistic model of nursing (1976) and Orem's self-care nursing model (1980) tend to support the concept of empowerment as a major role of nursing. Corcega (1991) characterized community development as caring at the community level. As nurses and community members work together, entire communities are empowered with the skills, knowledge, and confidence to prevent the root causes of disease, discomfort, and disability.

Rothman's three models of community organization are not intended to be mutually exclusive. Collectively, Rothman's models represent a spectrum of approaches that take into account a wide range of variables affecting community organization practice. As such, the three models present community health nurses with alternative approaches to community organization based on the desired nursing role (Table 7–4). The preferable community organization approach varies with the aggregate's social and cultural context, the nature of the issue or health problem being addressed, and the cultural and ethical values of the nurse serving as community organizer. Community organization strategies should be selected after careful

Table 7–4

Nurses' Roles in Three Community Organization Models

Model	Major Concepts	Nurses' Roles
Social planning	Data collection Rational decision making	Fact gatherer Expert analyst Program implementer Facilitator
Social action	Polarization Confrontation-conflict	Community activist Agitator Negotiator
Community development	Community involvement Self-direction Self-help	Enabler Teacher-educator

consideration of the situation, the nature of the problem or issue being addressed, the social and political context, and the values and beliefs of both the aggregate and the community health nurse. The caveats related to the use of the social planning and social action models are similar to those discussed earlier in relation to social change and community participation theories.

Community Health Development

Community health development describes the approach to community organization that combines concepts, goals, and processes of community health and community development. In the community health development approach, health-related needs are identified, and health goals are established, met, and evaluated through community-professional partnerships (ANA, 1986; American Public Health Association, 1981; Christenson and Robinson, 1989; Green and Kreuter, 1991; Hayes, 1986; Hickman, 1990; Lackey et al., 1987; Nugroho, 1993; WHO, 1978, 1991).

The community health development model (Fig. 7–2) is a paradigm that shows the relationship among key concepts, goals, and processes that must be addressed within community organization practice focused on health promotion (Hickman, 1995). Core concepts of the model include partnership, health, attitudes-values, participation, capacity, and leadership. The mutual partnership between communities

and health professionals, represented by the outer circle, reflects the understanding that the combined expertise of both is needed to develop health promotion strategies that are scientifically sound and situationally relevant.

The attributes of healthy communities, represented by the triangle, include participation, capacity, and leadership. Participation refers to active involvement of all community subsystems, including individuals, families, aggregates, sectors, and agencies-organizations, in comprehensive planning and health promotion. Capacity means that community members are collectively empowered with the knowledge, skills, and techniques requisite to carrying out the tasks and functions of community health promotion. Leadership indicates the development of a broad base of leadership needed for healthy community functioning. Communities need leaders of varied ages, ethnic backgrounds, race, gender, and abilities who can organize and sustain task performance and mobilize widespread community involvement in the task (Garkovich, 1989). The lines connecting the points of the triangle represent attitudes and values conducive to health promotion.

The focal point of the model is the community as a whole. The arrows pointing inward to "Healthy Community" represent the interaction of all the elements of the model to achieve the mutually shared goal of community health. Within community health development, the term *community health* is used to denote both the achievement of a designated qualitative level of well-being and the possession of a set of attributes essential to the achievement of that goal.

The primary role of nurses in the community health development model is that of partner. Other roles will evolve out of that partnership. For example, nurses engaged in leadership development and capacity building may be teachers, empowerers, and facilitators, but the teaching, learning, and empowerment are mutual. Health promotion activities may require the nurse to step into the role of expert, but information should be shared in such a way that community members learn how to obtain, interpret, and use health data in subsequent activities. Nurses attempting to increase community participation in health promotion may assume leadership roles to facilitate coalition development, but leadership should be shared with community members and other professionals.

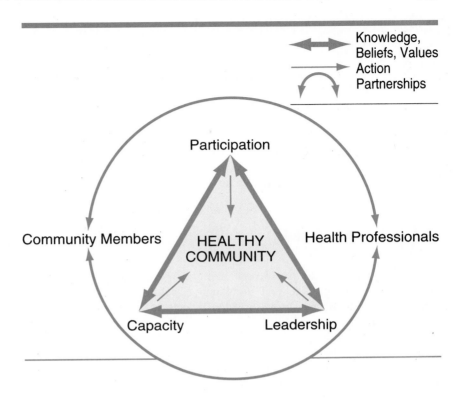

Knowledge, Beliefs, Values
Action
Partnerships

Participation

Community Members

HEALTHY COMMUNITY

Health Professionals

Capacity

Leadership

Figure 7–2
Community health development model.

Primary Health Care

A widely used international framework that synthesizes community organization and community health practice is primary health care. Primary health care refers to community-based provision of essential health care that is accessible to all members of the community (WHO, 1978). Essential health care includes the basic health care services described earlier. Primary health care is based on scientifically sound methods and technologies that are practical, affordable, and socially and culturally acceptable. Community health services are based on prevailing community needs and social, political, economic, cultural, and religious characteristics. Within the context of primary health care, basic community health services should be made universally accessible to individuals and aggregates in the community through their full participation and "at a cost that the community and country can afford to maintain at every stage of development in the spirit of community self-reliance and self-determination" (WHO, 1978). Furthermore, primary health care "forms an integral part both of the country's health care system, of which it is the central function and main focus, and of the overall social and economic development of the community" (WHO, 1978).

The role of nursing in community-based primary health care has been well defined by international health organizations. The WHO (1974) described nursing as a system of care consisting of community health nurses, midwives and other clinical specialists, paraprofessionals, teachers, researchers, administrators, and community members. The WHO (1974, 1985) and the Pan American Health Organization (1977) identified the role of the community health nurse, in partnership with the community, as that of assessing the health status of individuals, families, and communities; prioritizing health needs; identifying resources and groups at risk; planning ways to meet priority health needs; implementing health promotion, disease prevention, case finding, and curative services in the community; promoting development of individual, family, and community competence to identify and meet their health needs; and evaluating community health services and outcomes. Primary health care is endorsed by the ANA (1986) as the preferred approach to community health nursing practice.

Primary health care sets the framework for community organization practice by nurses in several respects. First, it specifies the approach to community organization as one of partnership with individuals, aggregates, and all sectors of the community. Second, it indicates outcome goals of equitable distribution, appropriate technology, and focus on prevention and a process goal of community participation. Third, it defines the primary health care system as the preferred community organization structure. These three components—process, outcome, and structure—set the parameters for the choice of community organization models selected by nurses to guide their practice.

Public Health Models and Frameworks

The field of public health has incorporated principles from primary health care and community health development into several health-oriented models of community organization. Public health models such as the planned approach to community health (PATCH), model standards, the assessment protocol for excellence in public health (APEXPH), and the healthy cities model attempt to provide long-term solutions to population-wide health problems by organizing community members into multidisciplinary partnerships that address local health problems and their precursors.

The PATCH model is promoted by the Centers for Disease Control and Prevention. Within PATCH, community members identify, prioritize, and act on their aggregate health needs through a process of community organization and local decision making (Kreuter, 1992). Emphasis is placed on building long-term solutions to health problems by addressing the social, economic, environmental, and political precursors in collaborative partnerships between health and other sectors of the community.

Two models—model standards and APEXPH—use community organization strategies to involve local communities in planning viable ways to meet Healthy People 2000, the national health objectives. Within the first, model standards, nurses and other health professionals develop community coalitions to establish specific local health objectives for reducing preventable morbidity and mortality and to specify the services needed to achieve these objectives (American Public Health Association, 1991). The second, APEXPH, emphasizes building working partnerships between health departments and the communities they serve in a collaborative approach to addressing federal, state, and local health objectives and priorities (National

Association of Community Health Officers, 1991). Both models were developed jointly by national organizations such as the American Public Health Association, Association of State and Territorial Health Officials, and National Association of Community Health Officers, and federal public health agencies such as Centers for Disease Control and Prevention.

The healthy cities model (sometime known outside of the United States as the health communities model) is an international model developed under the auspices of the WHO. This model uses action research to empower communities to take action for health. Community organization processes are used to place health on the community's political agenda and to build constituencies for healthy public policy (Flynn et al., 1994; Hancock, 1988).

Community health nurses are involved in a variety of ways in the public health models of community organization. Within local agencies, community health nurses may serve as fact gatherers, community activists, facilitators, and program implementers, according to the stage of partnership development and the nurse's position and role in the agency.

FROM THEORY TO PRACTICE: COMMUNITY ORGANIZATION FOR NURSING CARE OF AGGREGATES

Community organization is practiced by professionals from a variety of disciplines, including nursing, and by volunteers in civic associations and social action groups. Interventions are oriented toward changing community institutions and solving community problems. Central to community organization practice is the concept of social justice, with resources being allocated in an equitable manner and priority given to individuals, families, and aggregates at the greatest risk or with the greatest need. Models of community organization that best contribute to social justice are those empowering communities to promote and achieve health for all by addressing the precursors to poor health.

Nursing, Community Organization, and Upstream Thinking: A Historic Overview

The incorporation of community organization as a part of community health nursing practice is not new. Nursing history is rich with examples of civic-minded, community-oriented persons who have alleviated community health problems and social injustices by mobilizing effective community action systems. Florence Nightingale recognized the need for aggregate-level intervention to bring about changes in health. As Nightingale focused on the promotion and restoration of health through improvement of the environment, she analyzed the power structure and intervened at the appropriate level to bring about change. In *Notes on Nursing,* Nightingale (1859) observed that the creation of a healthy environment is not the sole responsibility of the nurse and is better accomplished by involving other persons in the health-promoting activities.

The theme of community organization as a component of nursing practice was carried into 20th-century community health nursing practice by organizations such as the National Organization for Public Health Nursing (NOPHN). In a nursing textbook published in 1935, upstream thinkers in the NOPHN identified general objectives for community health nursing practice, including education of individuals, aggregates, and communities "to protect their own health," to "adjust" social conditions affecting health, to "correlate" health and social programs for the welfare of the family and community, and to develop "adequate public health facilities."

Community organization is both implicit and explicit in current descriptions and standards of community health nursing practice. The ANA (1986, 1996) and the WHO (1974, 1978, 1985a, 1985b) identified community organization as a basic community health nursing skill, with the preferred approach to community organization being community development. The term *partnership* is used repeatedly by the ANA (1986) in the process criteria to describe the relationship between the community health nurse and the individual, aggregate, or community. In a review of major U.S. nursing theories, Meleis (1985) identified the roles of nurses associated with each theory. On the basis of Meleis' analysis of role definitions, it appears that social planning is the practice model most universally supported by nursing theories. This finding should give the nursing profession food for thought because community development is the community organization model considered by social science researchers to be most congruent with U.S. traditions, values, and beliefs (Christenson and Robinson, 1989) and is recommended by international health and nursing organizations as most appropriate for nursing practice.

Community Organization Strategies for Nurses

The selection of a community organization approach or strategy is dependent on the aggregate's social and cultural context, the nature of the issue or health problem being addressed, and the cultural and ethical values of the nurse serving as community organizer.

In 1969, Warren identified three major groups of community organization strategies for achieving social change: collaborative strategies, campaign strategies, and contest strategies. The strategies correspond to Rothman's models of community organization practice.

Collaborative strategies are those that fit with the community development typology of community organization practice. Collaborative strategies are used in situations in which there is basic agreement or likelihood of basic agreement that an issue or problem should be resolved. Within collaborative strategies, the role of the nurse as change agent is as an empowerer or a facilitator. During the assessment phase, the nurse and community members jointly identify community health needs and resources. Depending on the time frame and community context, the nurse gathers data from community members through surveys, town meetings, and interviews and presents the findings to community members for validation, prioritization, and decision making or teaches community members to conduct their own needs assessment. During the planning phase, the nurse fosters community decision making by facilitating community-controlled decision making and teaching problem solving and planning skills as necessary. When implementing the plan, the community health nurse may teach self-care to individuals, families, and aggregates; train community workers to prevent, detect, and treat selected health problems; or provide community-based nursing care when indicated. Collaborative approaches to evaluation of community health and nursing interventions can be fostered by involving community members in the design of evaluation mechanisms that are easy to implement and interpret.

Campaign strategies are linked with the social planning approach to community organization. Campaign strategies are appropriate in situations in which there are different opinions about the substance of an issue or the proposed solution of the issue but the possibility of consensus. Within the campaign model, the role of the nurse as change agent is as persuader and expert witness. As a community health expert, the nurse uses epidemiologic methods to gather data and identify major problems and groups at risk. On the basis of the epidemiologic diagnosis, the nurse recommends solutions and plans appropriate nursing interventions. A major part of the implementation process may be marketing the program to the community. Campaign methods include mass media campaigns, one-on-one persuasion, letters, endorsement by well-known people, public presentations, activation of support groups, and other persuasive techniques.

Contest strategies are most closely linked to social action approaches. Contest strategies, including social action, nonviolence, and civil disobedience, are appropriate when there is refusal of the power structures to recognize a problem or strong opposition to a proposed solution. The predominant role of the change agent is that of advocate, agitator, or contestant. Within the social action model, the nurse addresses inequities in health and health care by working within the system to bring about change or by assisting the client to confront the system and force change. Although nurses may attempt to improve community health through confrontation tactics such as strikes or civil disobedience, more popular contest strategies in contemporary U.S. community health practice are political mobilization and legislation.

No single community organization strategy is universally appropriate. Situational models of leadership suggest that a more directive approach may be appropriate in the early stages of organizational development, whereas a participatory approach should be used as task maturity increases (Hersey and Blanchard, 1982). In actual practice, community organization strategies should be selected after careful consideration of the situation, the nature of the problem or issue being addressed, the social and political context, and the values, beliefs, and capacities of both the aggregate and the community health nurse.

Application of the Nursing Process Through Community Organization

Nurses engaged in promoting, protecting, and restoring community health may select from several community organization models to guide their practice (see Table 7–4). The role of the nurse in relation to community health assessment, diagnosis, planning, intervention, and evaluation varies according to the model selected to guide each phase of practice. The application of social planning, social action, and community development is discussed briefly in relation to the nursing process in the care of aggregates.

The nurse who has selected social planning is a gatherer and analyzer of facts during community assessment.

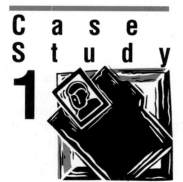

C a s e
S t u d y
1

Social Planning for Tertiary Prevention of Substance Abuse

Assessment Epidemiologic analysis conducted by a large urban health department indicated that substance abuse had reached epidemic proportions. In one of the health districts, nurses were involved in a program of prevention and early intervention for potential teenage drug abusers. The program had been initiated at the local community's request and was financially supported by churches, businesses, and various civic organizations. Because of the success in primary and secondary prevention of drug abuse, community health planners proposed a program of tertiary prevention in the same district. Citing the same epidemiologic data that had triggered the teen program, the county health department unilaterally planned a federally funded methadone maintenance program to rehabilitate hard-core heroin abusers.

Diagnosis Alteration existed in community aggregate function as a result of heroin abuse.

Planning and Goal Long-term heroin abusers will become productive members of the community.

Intervention A methadone program was begun in the clinic that had sponsored the teen drug use prevention program. Community health nurses were called on to implement the new program in the community. Using a variety of campaign strategies, the nurses were able to convince the community to start a methadone program.

Outcomes Two years later, the drug programs were evaluated. County health planners judged the methadone program to be effective because a large number of addicts were enrolled in the program and were experiencing varying degrees of success in heroin withdrawal. However, the teen drug prevention program had disappeared. The methadone program had been linked by community residents to an increase in theft in the area of the clinic. Because of the presence of hard-core drug users in the clinic, parents, schools, and law enforcement agencies no longer referred teenagers to the prevention and early treatment program that was in the same building. All community funds for the teen program were withdrawn. Community mistrust of the health department, including the nursing staff, was high, and staff morale and satisfaction were low.

Evaluation A few adults in the methadone maintenance program ceased heroin use, maintained steady jobs, and were judged to be productive members of the community. Therefore, the goal of tertiary prevention was partially met in an aggregate of adults. However, the unintended outcome—the loss of primary and secondary prevention programs—resulted in an overall increase in heroin use in the community, primarily among teenagers and young adults.

The community diagnosis is based on empirical data and recommendations presented by the nurse. Planning is a process of rational decision making by the nurse and other expert planners. The selected nursing interventions are implemented and evaluated by the nurse. The relationship of the nurse to the community and its aggregates is that of provider to consumer. In the late 20th century, the social planning model has been the model of community organization most frequently used by U.S. nurses in traditional community health agencies and organizations. The advantages of this approach are speed and control of the planning process. A major drawback is a lack of community or aggregate ownership of the goal or solution, often resulting in underuse or nonuse of community health nursing services.

Within the social action model, the focus of nursing assessment is on crystallization of issues.

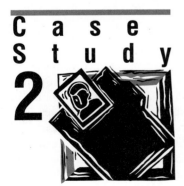

C a s e
S t u d y
2

Social Action in Primary Prevention for Older Adults

Assessment In recent years, state and federal budget crises have affected services for many aggregates. In one state, budget cuts threatened services for the elderly. Comprehensive health promotion was targeted for reduction or termination. In both urban and rural areas, elderly persons faced the potential loss of community-based programs of primary prevention.

Diagnosis Primary prevention was impaired, as evidenced by termination of community health promotion programs for the elderly. Planning and goals for the community will promote, protect, and restore the health of all residents.

Interventions A social action approach using contest strategies was chosen. The State Nurses Association in conjunction with senior citizens' coalitions and the State Public Health Association organized a mass write-in and direct-contact campaign to inform legislators of potential health and political ramifications of the budget cut.

Outcome The campaign resulted in funds being returned to community health programs for the elderly.

Evaluation The community's capacity to provide primary prevention for aggregates of elderly citizens was restored.

Prioritization of issues and selection of intervention strategies initially may be the nurse's prerogative. Later, community or aggregate members may be actively involved in selection and prioritization of issues and action to be taken. Interventions include polarization around issues to shift the balance of power within the community system and its supra-systems and subsystems. Evaluation is conducted jointly by the nurse and aggregate members, possibly during "debriefing" sessions. The relationship of the nurse to the aggregate might be that of advocate, agitator, activist, power broker, or negotiator on behalf of the aggregate. The social action model is often selected by nurses desiring political action or policy changes by governments and corporations. An advantage of this approach is the ability to effect change for aggregates with scarce resources. A disadvantage is that polarization around issues is difficult to reverse and interferes with mutual problem solving should that option be desired in the future.

Within the community development model, community health assessment encompasses multiple sectors of the community system and focuses on community or aggregate identification of perceived needs and potential resources.

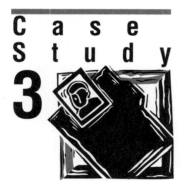

C a s e S t u d y 3

Community Development for Primary and Secondary Prevention of Rural Health Problems

Assessment A nursing student was assigned to conduct a comprehensive community health nursing assessment of a rural midwestern community. One of the important social structures within the community was an active Protestant church. The student chose a community development approach to the assignment and taught church members how to conduct and interpret a neighborhood survey. The survey indicated that a major community need was promotion of individual, family, and aggregate physical and mental health. In addition to identifying community health nursing needs, the student observed that the survey initiated linkages between church members and non–church member community residents.

Diagnosis Optimal community health with potential for achievement was evidenced by community participation in needs assessment.

Planning and Goal The community will engage in self-care by planning and implementing programs of primary prevention for all aggregates.

Interventions As a graduate, the former student returned to the community as a parish nurse. Church members, in partnership with the parish nurse, planned a series of programs to meet neighborhood health promotion needs. The nurse facilitated church leadership in the planning process and provided technical assistance regarding health promotion strategies.

Outcomes Church members, in consultation with community residents, began a weekly diet, exercise, and Bible study group for women; an after-school recreation program for grade school–aged children and teenagers; and a family counseling center. The program was implemented by the church primarily using church and neighborhood personnel and resources. The nurse was called on at times to provide selected community health nursing services such as health teaching. However, ownership of the program belonged to those who had conducted the survey and planned and implemented appropriate solutions.

Evaluation Simple evaluation methods such as group attendance and perceived success in meeting personal health promotion goals indicated successful outcomes for the program. Furthermore, not only had selected neighborhood health needs been met by using collaboration strategies to carry out the nursing process, but the competence of the community had been improved as it became able to identify and solve its own health problems.

Diagnosis is based on the community's priorities. Nursing interventions are focused on community self-help and capacity building, mobilization of resources, and integration of health care services. Direct care of individuals and aggregates may be provided when such services are related to promotion of health of the entire community. Evaluation is a joint procedure involving process, outcome, and context components. As a community developer, the nurse approaches community health practice with two goals. First, individuals and aggregates in the community will become active partners in carrying out each step of the nursing process. Second, as a result of the manner in which the nurse implements the nursing process, individuals and aggregates will acquire the skills and knowledge needed to promote, protect, and restore their community's health in the future. Nursing roles include those of collaborator, enabler, empowerer, and partner. Advantages of this approach include broad-based solutions to complex community health problems and community ownership of health. A disadvantage is the length of time needed to effect change.

As noted earlier, the nurse is not confined to a single community organization model in the practice of community health nursing. All three models are useful. In a similar vein, the nurse may mix models used as situational variables change during the stages of the nursing process. The knowledge of community organization concepts, models, and strategies is part of the science of nursing. The skill with which the nurse uses these concepts, models, and strategies in community health practice is an art.

SUMMARY

Community organization is, as a skill, basic to effective community health nursing practice. The theoreti-

cal basis of community organization has been discussed. Community health development and primary health care have been presented as frameworks for understanding the pertinence of community organization to community health nursing practice. Guidelines for selection of community organization models and strategies appropriate to community health nursing have been suggested. Three models of community organization practice—social planning, social action, and community development—have been presented. Application of the three models to community health nursing practice has been discussed. Although all three models have use in nursing care of aggregates, the model preferred by community health and nursing organizations is community development. Community development emphasizes community participation and multisector collaboration in planning affordable, acceptable solutions to priority health problems. Because of the emphasis on developing interventions that target long-term prevention of the precursors of poor health for aggregates and populations, community development also is the model of community organization that most closely fits with upstream thinking in nursing practice.

Community organization is a powerful tool when used appropriately and skillfully by community health nurses. Communities empowered to mobilize effective community action systems for the promotion, protection, and restoration of health become full partners in achieving the goals of equal access to basic health care services and promotion of health for all people. As many nurses have discovered, the most important reason for incorporating community organization into community health nursing practice is very practical: it truly works!

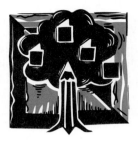

Learning Activities

1. Identify and interview social planners, social activists, and community developers in your community. Compare the similarities and differences in their approaches to community organization.

2. Play a simulation game, such as "The World Game," that demonstrates the interrelatedness of multiple community sectors.

3. Draw a model depicting your understanding of nursing and primary health care.

4. Conduct a mock community health planning forum in which various members of the groups are assigned different community organization roles. Discuss your observations and reactions after the exercise.

5. Write community health nurse job descriptions for each of the three models of community organization.

6. Write a "concept paper" discussing your views of the art and science of community organization in community health nursing practice.

REFERENCES

Alinsky SD: Relief for Radicals: A Pragmatic Primer for Realistic Radicals. New York, Random House, 1971.

American Nurses Association: Code for Nurses with Interpretive Statements. Kansas City, MO, ANA, 1985.

American Nurses Association: Standards of Community Health Nursing Practice. Kansas City, MO, ANA, 1986.

American Nurses Association: Standards of Community Health and Population-Focused Nursing Practice. Kansas City, MO, ANA, 1996 (draft).

American Public Health Association: Definition and Role of Public Health Nursing in the Delivery of Health Care. Washington, DC, APHA, 1981.

American Public Health Association: Healthy Communities 2000: Model Standards. Washington, DC., APHA, 1991.

Anderson ET, McFarlane JM: Community as Client. Philadelphia, JB Lippincott, 1988.

Anderson ET, McFarlane JM: Partner. Philadelphia, Davis, 1995.

Anderson RE, Carter I: Human Behavior in the Social Environment. New York, Aldine de Gruyter, 1990.

Archer SE, Kelly CD, Bisch SA: Implementing Change in Community: A Collaborative Process. St Louis, CV Mosby, 1984.

Bavelas A: Communication patterns in task oriented groups. In Cartwright D, Zander A (eds): Group Dynamics: Research and Theory. Evanston, IL, Roe, Peterson & Co., 1953, pp. 669–682.

Bracht N: Health Promotion at the Community Level. Newbury Park, CA, Sage, 1990.

Butterfoss FD, Goodman RM, Wandersman A: Community coalitions for prevention and health promotion. Health Educ Res, 8:315–330, 1993.

Christenson JA, Robinson JW Jr (eds): Community Development in America. Ames, IA, Iowa State University Press, 1989.

Community Development Society: Principles of good practice. Presented at the 1985 Annual Meeting of the Community Development Society, Milwaukee, WI.

Corcega TF: Caring through community development. Paper published as the 1991 Felicitas de la Cruz-Millman Professional Chair for Nursing, Azusa Pacific University, Azusa, CA.

Cottrell LS: The competent community. In Kaplan BH, Wilson RN, Leighton AH (eds). Further Explorations in Social Psychiatry. New York, Basic Books, 1976, pp. 195–209.

Couto RA, Simpson NK, Harris G: Sowing seeds in the mountains: Community-based coalitions for cancer prevention and control. Washington, DC, National Cancer Institute, 1995.

Daly IM, Angulo J: People-centered community planning. J Comm Dev Soc 21:88–103, 1990.

Flynn B, Rider M, Ray D: Healthy cities: Indiana model of community development in public health. Health Educ Q 18:331–347, 1991.

Flynn B, Rider M, Ray D: Empowering communities: Action research through healthy cities. Health Educ Q 21:395–405, 1994.

Francisco VT, Paine AL, Fawcett SB: A methodology for monitoring and evaluating community health coalitions. Health Educ Res 8:403–416, 1993.

Garkovich L: Local organizations and leadership in community development. In Christenson JA, Robinson JW Jr (eds). Community Development in America. Ames, IA, Iowa State University Press, 1989, pp. 196–218.

Goeppinger J, Lassiter PG, Wilcox B: Community health is community competence. Nurs Outlook 30:464–467, 1982.

Goeppinger J, Shuster G: Community as client. In Stanhope M, Lancaster J (eds). Community Health Nursing, 3rd ed. St. Louis, CV Mosby, 1992, pp. 244–276.

Gottlieb NH, Brink SG, Gingiss PL: Correlates of coalition effectiveness. Health Educ Res 8:375–384, 1993.

Green L, Kreuter M: Health Promotion Planning. Mountain View, CA, Mayfield, 1991.

Hancock T. The future of public health in Canada: Building healthy communities. Can J Pub Health 79:416–419, 1988.

Hayes SE: Toward the Development and Validation of a Conceptual Model for Community Health Nursing. Unpublished doctoral dissertation. International University, San Diego, 1986.

Herman KA, Wolfson M, Forster JL: The evolution, operation, and future of Minnesota SAFPLAN: A coalition for family planning. Health Educ Res 8:331–344, 1993.

Hersey P, Blanchard K: Management of Organizational Behavior: Utilizing Human Resources. Englewood Cliffs, NJ, Prentice-Hall, 1982.

Hickman P: Community health and development. Soc Prac 8:125–132. 1990.

Hickman P: Community health development. *In* Hickman P (ed): Healthy Homeplace Program: Central Highlands Appalachian Leadership Initiative on Cancer. Lexington, KY, University of Kentucky, 1995.

Hickman P, Hustedde R: Force field analysis. *In* Hickman P (ed). Healthy Homeplace Program: Central Highlands Appalachian Leadership Initiative on Cancer. Lexington, KY, University of Kentucky, 1995.

International Council of Nurses: Health Care for All: Challenge for Nursing. Geneva, ICN, 1981.

Jones ER, Harris WM: Conceptual scheme for analysis of the social planning process. J Comm Dev Soc 18:18–41, 1987.

Kramer RM, Specht H: Readings in Community Organization Practice. Englewood Cliffs, NJ, Prentice-Hall, 1975.

Kreuter M: PATCH: Its origin, basic concepts, and links to contemporary public health policy. J Health Ed 23:135–141, 1992.

Kumpfer KL, Turner C, Hopkins R, Librett J: Leadership and team effectiveness in community coalitions for the prevention of alcohol and other drug abuse. Health Educ Res 8:359–374, 1993.

Labonte R: Health promotion and empowerment: reflections on professional practice. Health Educ Q 21:253–268, 1994.

Lackey AS, Burke R, Peterson M: Healthy communities: The goal of community development. J Comm Dev Soc 18:1–17, 1987.

Lassiter PG: A community development perspective for rural nursing. Fam Community Health 14:29–39, 1992.

Lewin K: Field Theory in Social Sciences. New York, Harper & Row, 1951.

Lexau C, Kingsbury L, Lenz B, et al.: Building coalitions: A community-wide approach for promoting farming health and safety. AAOHN J 41:440–449, 1993.

McKinney MM, Barnsley JM, Kaluzny AD: Organizing for cancer. Int J Technology Assess Health Care 8:268–288, 1992.

Meleis AI: Theoretical Nursing Development and Progress. Philadelphia, JB Lippincott, 1985.

Minkler M: Community organizing among the elderly poor in the United States: A case study. Int J Health Serv 22:303–316, 1992.

National Association of Community Health Officers: APEXPH. Washington, DC, NACHO, 1991.

National Organization for Public Health Nursing: Manual of Public Health Nursing. New York, Macmillan, 1935.

Neuman B: The Neuman Systems Model. Norwalk, CT, Appleton & Lange, 1995.

Nightingale F: Notes on Nursing. Philadelphia, JB Lippincott, 1992 (commemorative issue), p. 247. (Originally published in 1859.)

Nugroho G: Partnership for community health development. World Health Forum 14:168–171, 1993.

Ockene JK, Lindsay E, Berger L, Hymowitz N: Health care providers as key change agents in the community intervention trial for smoking cessation (COMMIT). Intl J Community Health Educ 11:223–237, 1991.

Orem DE: Nursing Concepts of Practice. New York, McGraw-Hill, 1980.

Pan American Health Organization: The Role of the Nurse in Primary Health Care. Washington, DC, PAHO, 1977.

Paterson JG, Zderad LT: Humanistic Nursing. New York, Wiley, 1976.

Rappaport J: Terms of empowerment/exemplars of prevention: Toward a theory for community psychology. A J Community Psych 15:121–145, 1987.

Rogers T, Howard-Pitney B, Feighery EC, et al.: Characteristics and participant perceptions of tobacco control coalitions in California. Health Educ Res 8:345–357, 1993.

Rothman J: Three models of community organization practice. *In* Zaltman G, Kotler P, Kaufman I (eds). Creating Social Change. New York, Holt, Rinehart & Winston, 1972, pp. 477–478.

Russell K: Strengthening black and minority community coalitions for health policy action. J Natl Black Nurses Assoc 6:42–47, 1992.

Skelton R: Nursing and empowerment: Concepts and strategies. J Adv Nurs 19:415–423, 1994.

Thompson B, Corbett K, Bracht N, Pechacek T: Community mobilization for smoking cessation: Lessons learned from COMMIT. Health Promotion J 8:69–83, 1993.

Wallerstein N: Powerlessness, empowerment, and health: Implications for health promotion programs. A J Health Prom 6:197–205, 1992.

Wallerstein N: Empowerment and health: The theory and practice of community change. Community Dev J 28:218–227, 1993.

Wallerstein N, Bernstein E: Introduction to community empowerment, participatory education, and health. Health Educ Q 21:141–148, 1994.

Woelk GB: Cultural and structural influences in the creation of and participation in community health programmes. Soc Sci Med 35:419–424, 1992.

World Health Organization: Community Health Nursing. Geneva, WHO, 1974.

World Health Organization: Primary Health Care. Geneva, WHO, 1978.

World Health Organization: A Guide to Curriculum Review for Basic Nursing Education. Geneva, WHO, 1985a.

World Health Organization: Primary Health Care in Industrialized Countries. Geneva, WHO, 1985b.

World Health Organization: Community Involvement in Health Development: Challenging Health Services. Geneva, WHO, 1991.

Community Health Education

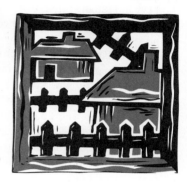

Upon completion of this chapter, the reader will be able to:

1. Describe the aims of health education within the community.

2. Discuss the role of the nurse as educator within a political and social context.

3. Select a learning theory and describe its application to an individual, family, or aggregate.

4. Select teaching and learning strategies that exemplify client-centered health education for individual, family, or aggregates.

5. Compare and contrast Freire's approach to health education with an individualistic health education model.

6. Outline a systematic process for developing health education messages and programs.

7. Identify resources of health education materials and describe their application for a given individual, family, or community as client.

8. Describe factors that enhance relevancy of health materials for an intended target group.

9. Prepare a teaching plan and evaluation criteria for individual, family, and aggregate.

Cathy D. Meade

Health education "is any combination of learning experiences designed to facilitate voluntary actions conducive to health that people can take on their own, individually or collectively, as citizens looking after their own health or as decision makers looking after the health of others and the common good of the community"

(GREEN AND KREUTER, 1991, PP. 14, 17).

Nurses may be tempted to ask such questions as: Why doesn't she stop smoking? Why doesn't he take his medications? Why don't mothers and fathers bring their children in on schedule for their immunizations? Why don't more people attend the free cancer screenings at the clinic? Why does this community have such an alarming rate of teenage pregnancy? Such questions point to the desire for nurses to better understand the link between health behaviors and health education, yet they do little to empower patients and find answers to these complex questions. In fact, such questions are not helpful in addressing the real issues at the root of health problems and, in fact, may be considered "blaming the victim" in nature (Israel et al., 1994).

In reframing the previous questions to empower individuals, families, and groups, the nurse might ask: What other life situations or stressors are my patients coping with while trying to quit smoking? What are the learning needs of the target audience members and how can they be addressed? What types of barriers might be preventing families from bringing their children in for their immunizations; what system strategies and changes can decrease the barriers? What creative and innovative teaching methods can be activated to reach more groups in the community for free cancer screenings? What social, physical, cultural, or structural factors contribute to the high teenage pregnancy rate and should be considered when planning programs aimed at reducing pregnancies?

Consider the following story:

Mr. Podboy often visits the neighborhood senior center to play cards and have lunch. Once a month he takes part in the blood pressure clinic offered by the health department. The health department has established a variety of clinics at senior centers as part of their outreach services and are particularly pleased with the increase in numbers of individuals who use the clinic. Since Mr. Podboy has limited resources, this opportunity provides him with valuable access to health information. On his second visit, his blood pressure is 188/94 (the reading was 184/92 on his first visit). He states that he has

been treated for high blood pressure for more than 5 years at the "county hospital" and was put on medication about 6 months ago.

Assessment by the nurse reveals that Mr. Podboy takes his medication but only when he doesn't "feel good." Why doesn't Mr. Podboy take his medication? He states that he was told by the doctor to take his medicine regularly (which he believes he does faithfully when he doesn't feel quite right). He also states that he remembers getting some papers about his medications but found them too confusing so he threw them out. The nurse's educational assessment reveals that Mr. Podboy has an eighth-grade education, does not read much, enjoys television over print, and likes to learn from pictures. His low reading skills have impacted on his ability to act upon health instructions given to him: many messages are taken literally (e.g., take regularly was interpreted to mean take consistently only when "I don't feel right" vs. taking the pills on an ongoing regular schedule).

What strategies will best communicate health information to Mr. Podboy? To better facilitate learning, the nurse, with input from Mr. Podboy, establishes a teaching plan. This plan involves the communication of health instructions in more relevant ways (e.g., use of pictures, drawings, mnemonics, or videotapes). The nurse also establishes a plan of follow-up.

HEALTH EDUCATION IN THE COMMUNITY

Health education is viewed as an important and integral aspect of the professional nurse's role in the community in the promotion of health and the prevention of disease. Teaching has been viewed as a significant responsibility of nurses since the early work of Florence Nightingale (1859). In 1936, Gardner, in the third edition of *Public Health Nursing*, emphasized that one of the most fundamental principles of the nurse is health teaching and that "a nurse, in even the most obscure position must be a teacher of no mean order" (p. 101). The nurse's involvement in health education is further supported by Nurse Practice Acts, by professional statements of the American Nurses Association (ANA) (1975), by the American Hospital Association's (AHA) (1972) Patient's Bill of Rights, and by the Joint Commission on Accreditation of Healthcare Organizations (JCAHO) (1995).

More health activities and services are occurring outside hospital walls within a variety of settings such as churches, WIC (Women, Infants, and Children) sites, grocery stores, homeless shelters, community-based organizations, health maintenance organization settings, schools, senior centers, and mobile health units. The community is a vital link to health care and provides the nurse with many windows of opportunity for health education within neighborhoods. The goal of health education is both to understand health behavior and to translate knowledge into relevant interventions and strategies for health enhancement, disease prevention, and management of chronic illness (Glanz et al., 1990; Stanton, 1990). In general, health education aims to enhance wellness and decrease disability and attempts to actualize the health potential of individuals, families, communities, and society. Health education is not just information giving, but it encompasses activities designed to guide persons through a decision-making process about their health (Duryea, 1983). Steuart and Kark (1962), stated that "health education must achieve its ends through means that leave inviolate the rights of self-determination of the individuals and their community." A major challenge for community health nurse educators is to ensure that the contributions of individuals are valued while conditions that promote powerlessness are addressed (Wallerstein and Bernstein, 1994). Milio (1981) reminded nurses that health choices are often made on the basis of the ease with which individuals can choose certain options depending on their socioeconomic situation. Health is not necessarily a state or an achievement but rather the response of people to their environments.

As cogently pointed out by Butterfield (1990) and discussed in an earlier chapter in this text, most health literature focuses on the individual relationships that shape a patient's health behaviors. She purported that this downstream thinking seriously restricts nurses' abilities to consider the multitude of external factors that can influence behavior (e.g., environment, culture, social roles, economics). Upstream endeavors or a macroscopic perspective can help nurses gain insight into a more global perspective of behavior and help to address better the complexity of the larger, more powerful systems that can influence behaviors. When viewing human responses to health and illness within the sociopolitical-economic structure, nurses are better able to identify and understand any power imbalances within the community that can prohibit groups from achieving their full potential. She suggested that the use of social critical theory can help nurses create innovative ways to explore societal forces that shape and limit choices of individuals.

The community-as-client approach views the target as the total community aggregate, which includes individuals, families, and groups and is focused on primary, secondary, and tertiary levels of preventions (Anderson et al., 1986). Health education within the community is based on practical, relevant, and scientifically sound methods and technology made accessible to members of the community. In viewing the community health care system, Kleinman (1978) described it as one that is both social and cultural and consists of relating external factors (e.g., economical, political, epidemiologic) to internal factors (e.g., behavioral, communicative). This view of the health care system as a sociocultural system grounds health education activities within the sociopolitical structures, especially within local environmental settings (Jezewski, 1993).

Nurses cannot singularly set the priorities for the individual, family, or community. The lasting effect of cognitive and behavioral changes relies greatly on the active versus passive participation of the learners. In

HEALTH EDUCATION ROLES AND ACTIVITIES OF THE NURSE IN THE COMMUNITY

- Advocate
- Caregiver
- Case manager
- Consultant
- Culture broker
- Educator
    Recognizes dimensions of health choices
    Promotes self-care
    Knows about resources
    Facilitates health-promoting behaviors
- Information broker
- Innovator
- Mediator
- Negotiator
- Policy analyst, change agent
- Promotor of collaborative partnerships
- Role model
- Sensitizer
- Social activist

(Based on data from Clark, 1992; Jezewski, 1993; Rankin and Stallings, 1990; Spellbring, 1991.)

order for change to occur, learners must be included in the determination of health needs and health practices (Green and Kreuter, 1991). Community health nurses are well positioned to impact the health behaviors and practices of community members through a variety of nursing activities and roles; however, continual refinement of skills and knowledge in community-focused practice is needed (Armstrong 1989; Kuehnert, 1995). The role of nurses as health educators is congruent with national priorities as put forth by the year 2000 health objectives for the nation (U.S. Department of Health and Human Services, 1991).

LEARNING THEORIES, PRINCIPLES, AND HEALTH EDUCATION MODELS

Learning Theories

Theories of learning are helpful in understanding and sorting out how individuals, families, and groups learn. They have developed from the field of psychology and provide a picture about how stimuli from the environment result in specific responses. Theories aid in recognizing the mechanisms whereby knowledge, attitudes, and behaviors are potentially modified. Bigge (1982) described learning as an enduring change that may involve a modification of insights, behaviors, perceptions, or motivations or a combination of these. Although many learning theories are described in great detail in psychology textbooks, several broad categories are briefly reviewed for the nurse's application in a community setting: stimulus-response conditioning (behavioristic), cognitive, humanistic, and social learning (Table 8–1).

The nurse should keep in mind that no theory is wholly right or wholly wrong. Different theories work well in different situations. Knowles (1989) related that the purpose of behaviorists is to program individuals through stimulus-response mechanisms to behave in a certain fashion. The purpose of humanistic theories is to facilitate the development of individuals toward their unique potential in a self-directing and holistic manner. Cognitive theorists recognize the potential of the brain to think, feel, learn, and problem solve, and the purpose of education is to train the brain to maximize those functions. Although social learning theory is largely a cognitive theory, it also combines threads of behaviorism (Bandura, 1977b). Its premise is based on explaining behavior and enhancing learning through the use of the concepts of efficacy, outcome expectations, and incentives.

LINKING THEORY TO PRACTICE: AN EXAMPLE OF AIDS EDUCATION

"Why should we as black women be concerned with AIDS?" was the beginning question of an acquired immunodeficiency syndrome (AIDS) prevention intervention designed to increase self-efficacy regarding the ability to implement condom use. On the basis of the theoretical tenets of perceived efficacy, the conviction that one can successfully execute a behavior to achieve the desired outcomes and outcome expectancies, defined as a person's estimate that a behavior will lead to specific consequences, this project was developed for African-American adolescents. The three-session intervention combined a variety of methods, including lecture, discussion, brainstorming, role playing, and skill building, and incorporated media such as videos, games, and exercises intended to influence the variables theoretically important to behavior change. A practice session was held to reinforce the correct application and removal of a condom using a banana, and the use of spermicide with nonoxynol: 9 (Jemmott and Jemmott, 1992).

The authors found in their study of 109 sexually active African-American females that a culturally sensitive social-cognitive AIDS risk reduction intervention was significantly related to increased self-efficacy and more favorable expectancies about the use of condoms on sexual enjoyment and sexual partners' support for condoms use than was knowledge about AIDS. Simply put, knowing the risk of AIDS was not sufficient to change intent of risky behaviors. In summary, the study supported the notion that a culturally sensitive social-cognitive AIDS risk reduction intervention was related to stronger intentions to use condoms after the educational program than before the program. Although continued research is needed to further validate and refine strategies that reduce human immunodeficiency virus risk-associated behaviors, it is recommended that nurses incorporate theoretical variables in the planning, design, and testing of their health education interventions (Jemmott and Jemmott, 1992).

Knowles' Assumptions About Adult Learners

Several assumptions about adult learners have been outlined by Knowles (1980, 1989), who contended

Table 8–1
Learning Theories and Their Relationship to Health Education

Learning Theory	Characteristics	Application to Health Education	Example
Cognitive or Gestalt learning: Lewin, Piaget, Wertheimer (aids in developing high-quality insights)	Depicts learners as active processors of information. Behaviors are determined by the way they are perceived, the manner in which the perception is represented, and the relationship of the perception to the past. Learners are influenced by their past experiences. A search for underlying meanings, feelings, beliefs, and past influences should be considered. Thinking is reflective. Learners interact with their environment on an ongoing basis. Learners make choices based on their own interpretations. Learners may perceive health messages differently in different environments. The environment may not correspond to reality. The whole is more important than individual pieces.	Recognize that new insights can reorganize perceptions and thoughts. Consider earlier learning experiences. Recognize that the nurses' perceptions may differ vastly from those of the individuals, families, or groups and community. Organize learning to match the group's developmental stage or earlier experiences. Organize pieces of information in meaningful ways. Recognize that the environment and individuals and groups are interacting constantly and thus perceptions may change.	Student nurse Bill Driver works with individuals (survivors) whose family members were victims of murder. He designs a support group based on their previous experiences, keeping in mind their developmental stages and their social-family roles. The nurse is aware that such devastating experiences are likely to change the families' perceptions of themselves as well as how they relate to others in their family and community. The nurse, through the support group, leads the discussion to help group members gain insight and understanding about the changes and feelings they are experiencing.
Humanistic: Maslow, Rogers (focuses on feelings)	Emphasis is placed on feelings, beliefs, and emotions as well as on observations of behaviors. Emphasizes what is learned by the process of learning. Affective learning and self-expression are valued. Learners are more self-directed when the teacher is warm, accepting, and empathic to the learner's feelings and thoughts. Inner nature is shaped by unconscious thoughts and experiences.	Consider hierarchy of needs: for individuals, families, or groups. Recognize that lower order needs should be met first. Assist patients, families, and groups in their learning. Administer warm, compassionate nursing care.	Nursing student Kate Winer was assigned to conduct a health assessment with a woman seeking care at a homeless shelter. During planning, the student attempts to have the patient sign up to return to have her cholesterol checked at the free screening that the other students are offering. Although well intentioned, the nursing student soon realizes that her priorities are not consistent with those of the woman. The patient tells the student, "I know you want to help me, but I am more

Table continued on following page

Table 8-1
Learning Theories and Their Relationship to Health Education (*Continued*)

Learning Theory	Characteristics	Application to Health Education	Example
	The uniqueness of the individual is valued: learner-centered education. Individuals and groups do what is congruent with their needs: lower needs must be met before higher needs are realized (from low to high: physiologic, safety-security, love, affection, belongingness, esteem, and self-actualization).		worried about my two sick children and getting them food and a warm bed than trying to get here for your screening!" The nursing student's priorities shift to planning nursing care directed at meeting the lower needs of Maslow's hierarchy.
Behavioral (stimulus-response [S-R]): Pavlov, Thorndike, Skinner (promotes acquisition of S-R responses)	Patients learn in a structured systematic way. Learning is based on conditioning or reinforcement. Observable data are most relevant for patients. Connectionism aids in joining S-R: connections are strengthened when used often and weakened when used infrequently. Actions that are rewarded are more likely to be repeated.	Create ways to provide immediate feedback to patients and groups. Involve patients in perceptual features of learning (seeing and hearing). Help individuals, families, and groups make connections between ideas. Change or eliminate antecedent events.	Within a community-based nursing center, an interactive video module on nutrition assists mothers in learning about the selection and identification of healthy foods and offers tips on economical food preparations. The computerized program provides an organized method of presenting information while providing immediate feedback about the nutritive value of the selections made by the users.
Social learning: Bandura (1977b) (aims to explain behavior and facilitate learning)	Learning is influenced by four main sources: 1. Personal mastery 2. Vicarious experiences 3. Persuasion 4. Physiologic feedback Learner centered. Enhancement of self-confidence and self-efficacy can lead to desired behaviors and outcome.	Provide links for individual, families, and groups to others with similar health education needs. Offer educational materials and media that convey subject information or enhance self-confidence (brochures, audiocassettes). Involve patients in planning. Coach patients in skill building and in progress made. Provide a network for role models. Create interventions that enhance self-confidence.	Based on a needs assessment, a fitness program for senior men is implemented at a church by the group of parish nurses. The educational program consists of general information about fitness through discussion by the nurses, brochures, and video (persuasion) to gain mastery of topic; a light snack and conversation period for them to share information about experiences; and a walking program to allow for 30 minutes of physiologic feedback as they gain fitness (less stiffness, pulse change, overall feeling of vitality).

Based on data from Bandura, 1977b; Bigge, 1982; Lewin, 1938; Maslow, 1970; Pavlov, 1957; Piaget, 1980; Rogers, 1989; Skinner, 1984; Thorndike, 1969; Wertheimer, 1959.

that adults learn better when the environment is more facilitative rather than restrictive and structured as with children. Familiarity with these assumptions can help nurses develop teaching strategies that are motivating for and interesting to individuals, families, and groups and that encourage their active participa- tion in the learning process. Nurses can help create a learning environment that is self-directing and self-empowering. Consider these characteristics and how they impact on learning: need to know, self-concept, experience, readiness to learn, orientation to learning, and motivation (Table 8–2).

Table 8–2
Characteristics of Adult Learners

Characteristics	Application to Health Education
Need to know: Adults need to know why they need to learn.	The nurse gets in touch with the reasons why individuals, families, and groups want to learn. The nurse assists individuals in recognizing the need to learn, similar to Freire's 1973 consciousness raising (discussed later).
Self-Concept: Adults have a self-concept that has developed from dependence to independence. It moves from others' direction to self-direction. Adults want to be treated as capable of self-direction.	The nurse acknowledges that individuals, families, and groups are able to make choices and decisions. The nurse creates an environment in which feelings can be expressed. The nurse recognizes that individuals, families, and groups can learn from their selected actions and can take self-direction and responsibility for such behaviors.
Experience: Adults have many life experiences from which to draw. Such experiences serve as powerful resources for learning and are enriching.	The nurse assesses individuals, families, and groups for life experiences related to health issues. The nurse helps facilitate connections between previous and present experiences. The nurse allows individuals, families, and groups to share experiences with others in a supportive manner. The use of experiential methods, problem solving, case method, and discussion can help uncover experiences of the learner. The nurse aids in clarifying previous and present experiences: this is especially helpful if experiences have been negative or biased.
Readiness to learn: Developmental tasks and social roles impact on readiness to learn. Timing learning experiences with developmental tasks is important.	The nurse assesses and identifies individual, family, and group roles, key developmental tasks (e.g., caregivers, single parents). The nurse seeks understanding about the impact of such roles and tasks on learning. The nurse organizes learning around life application categories. The nurse creates role-modeling experiences.
Orientation to learning: Learning is present oriented and "now" based. Learning is directed to the immediate need and is problem centered.	The nurse assesses the learning needs of individuals, families, and groups on the basis of their priority. The nurse recognizes the everyday stresses and hassles and addresses them within their learning context. The nurse provides health information, gives responses to their immediate needs, and offers problem-solving skills.
Motivation: Internal drives and factors are powerful motivators (e.g., self-esteem, life goals, quality of life, responsibility).	The nurse determines individual, family, and group motivators. The nurse assesses for barriers that block motivation (e.g., poor self-esteem, lack of resources) and provides appropriate education, counseling, and referrals.

Content adapted from Knowles MS: The Making of an Educator. San Francisco, Jossey-Bass, 1989, Chapter 4; and Knowles MS: The Modern Practice of Adult Education: From Pedagogy to Andragogy. Upper Saddle River, NJ, Globe Fearon, 1980.

APPLICATION OF CHARACTERISTICS OF ADULT LEARNERS TO THE DEVELOPMENT OF A COMMUNITY SUPPORT GROUP

In 1984, I and a colleague began a community support group for individuals with amyotrophic lateral sclerosis (ALS) and their family members and friends. (ALS is a degenerative neuromuscular disease that affects the function of nerves and muscles and the ability of the brain to control muscle movement. There is no known cure.) The group began based on feedback obtained from community target members who identified the need for education and support. At that time, no support group in Southeast Wisconsin existed. This initial dialogue provided the organizing framework for the start-up of the support group, which is now in its 11th year of existence. On the basis of my observations and interactions at the monthly meetings, an illustration of Knowles' assumptions follows:

Need to know. At the support group, topics are introduced by the facilitator-nurse describing the reason for the discussion and rationale for the selected subject (e.g., identified by patients, common concerns expressed by family members). As group members introduce themselves, they are asked by the nurse to comment on what they would hope to learn from the presentation to set the stage for the discussion. In some cases, members are not sure of their reasons for gaining more information on a given topic but indicate that they are here to listen. Because progression of the disease is variable, the need to know is facilitated by the nurse as well as other patients who have already noted the importance of specific learning tasks (e.g., need for an assistive walking device, need for financial planning).

Self-concept. A comfortable, informal environment allows patients to express their feelings and frustrations about this disease. Members are told that it is okay to say what is on their minds: mutual respect and trust among participants are cultivated. Members can see and hear that others are in a similar situation, and they share their concerns. Hugs are common. Opportunities are given to group members to voice their desire about ways to manage their own disease (e.g. life support decisions). Acceptance of those feelings is recognized without value judgments being imposed, even if the choices are not congruent with their own. Patients and family members receive acknowledgment from the facilitators and from each other about their feelings. The facilitators and group members are equal partners in the learning process.

Experiences. Some patients and family members have gone through other difficult life experiences (e.g. other illnesses, deaths in the family). Strengths gained from such experiences are often shared with other members and are assistive in helping others cope with the management of ALS. Additionally, individuals and family members who are going through varying stages of the disease process are able to share their experiences (e.g., obtaining home care, selecting a computer, managing feeding and breathing difficulties). Tips and time-saving strategies are shared with each other. Newly diagnosed families learn from those diagnosed before them.

Readiness to learn. Family members often assume many roles when someone is ill, especially with a chronic illness such as ALS. The redefinition of roles creates opportunities for learning, but this may also hinder learning if it is too overwhelming. For example, the well spouse may assume additional roles as caregiver, parent, and financial supporter. Identification of resources to help the family cope with roles is helpful (e.g., respite care).

Orientation to learning. Learning a variety of psychomotor skills is necessary in caring for the ALS patient (e.g., suctioning, positioning, using a feeding tube, toileting). The time frame for learning such skills is variable depending on the course of the illness. Presenting information about such skills too early in the course of the disease may be frightening and anxiety producing. Families often are not responsive to learning such tasks until the need is readily apparent. In some cases, this may be evidenced at a crisis point (e.g., a fall, choking incident, severe respiratory distress). However, such topics are introduced slowly (planting seeds of information) via the support group, newsletter, printed brochures, and one-on-one discussions.

Motivation. Individuals and families experience a shift in life goals when faced with ALS. Such shifts may create opportunities for learning that are aimed at enhancing their quality of life and maintaining self-esteem. For example, one individual with ALS (college professor) strived to keep his link to the university. He was highly motivated to continue his research work and to supervise his graduate students. Learning how to manage his breathing (use of a ventilator), arranging for transportation to the university, obtaining nursing care, and creating methods for communication (computer) were important and necessary for his academic work to continue.

Health Education Models

In addition to learning theories, the application of health education theories and principles to situations involving individuals, families, and groups helps to show how ideas fit together, offers explanations for health behaviors or actions, and aids in planning community nursing interventions. Such theoretical elements form the basis of understanding health behavior, and I refer to them as the "nuts and bolts." Glanz and colleagues (1990) related that theories give educators the power to assess the strength and impact of interventions and are intended to be enriching, informative, and complementary to practice. Theoretical frameworks offer nurses a blueprint for interventions that promote learning and provide them with an organized approach to explaining relationships of concepts (Padilla and Bulcavage, 1991). "What the health practitioner needs is not a single theory that would explain all that he or she hears, but rather a framework with meaningful hooks and rubrics on which to hang the new variables and insights offered by different theories. With this customized meta-theory or framework, the practitioner can triage new ideas into categories that have personal utility in his or her practice" (Green, 1990, p. 2).

Models of Individual Behavior

Two models that are frequently used to explain determinants of preventive behavior include the health belief model (HBM) (Table 8–3) (Becker et al, 1977; Hochbaum, 1958; Kegeles et al., 1965; Rosenstock, 1966) and the health promotion model (HPM) (Pender, 1987). Both models are similar in that they are multifactorial, are based on the idea of value expectancy, and address individual perceptions, modifying factors, and likelihood of action. The HBM is based on social psychology and has undergone much empirical testing, mostly attempting to predict compliance on singular preventive measures. It was first developed to help understand why people did not participate in health education programs to prevent or detect disease, specifically participation in tuberculosis screening programs (Hochbaum, 1958). Subsequent studies have addressed other preventive actions and factors related to adherence to medical regimens.

Primarily, the HBM addresses factors that promote health-enhancing behavior rather than the inhibiting factors. It is disease specific and focuses on an avoidance-orientation. Dimensions considered by the

Table 8–3
Health Belief Model

Components	Example and Explanation
Perceived susceptibility	Belief that disease state is present or likely to occur
Perceived severity	Perception that disease state or condition is harmful and has serious consequences
Perceived benefits	Belief that health action is of value
Perceived barriers	Belief that health action would be associated with hindrances (e.g., cost)
Self-efficacy	Belief that actions can be performed to achieve the desired outcome
Demographics	Age, sex, ethnicity
Cues to action	Influencing factors (e.g., billboards, newspapers)

For a more detailed description of the health belief model, the reader is directed to Becker (1974).

HBM include perceived susceptibility, perceived severity, perceived benefits, perceived barriers, and other sociopsychological and structural variables. The variable of self-efficacy (the notion that an individual can act successfully on a given behavior to produce the desired outcome) (Bandura, 1977A, 1977B) was added to the HBM (Rosenstock et al., 1988; Strecher et al., 1986). In a review of 46 studies using the HBM, the most powerful predictive element within the model was identified as perceived benefits, whereas perceived severity had the lowest associative value (Janz and Becker, 1984).

Glanz and coworkers (1990) provided an analysis of HBM, and raised several criticisms. In general, the HBM purports that if individuals perceive themselves as susceptible to an illness or condition, if they perceive serious consequences from a given course of action, if they perceive benefits from a course of action, and if the benefits outweigh the barriers, they will seek preventive action. The model, however, is focused on individual determinants of behavior and is less focused on socioenvironmental factors. They related that this view may promote blaming the victims for their health problems. Additionally, the model is focused greatly on the influence of individuals' beliefs and values on health. From a practical perspective, how changeable are these? Although the HBM is recognized for bringing to light an array of variables important in explaining individual health, such variables should also be viewed within a larger societal perspective.

Pender's HPM (1987) offers modifications of the HBM and is more focused on predicting behaviors directed toward health promotion (Table 8–4). It is meant to provide an organizing framework to help explain why individuals engage in health actions. Two individual factors were added: perceived control and perceived importance of health. Within modifying factors, Pender added the variable of interpersonal influence (interactions with family members, health professionals, expectations of others).

In a review of 23 studies conducted from 1983 to 1992, Gillis (1993) reported that the theoretical framework most commonly used in health promotion studies was Pender's HPM. Gillis identified that the strongest determinant of participation in a health-promoting lifestyle was self-efficacy followed by social support, perceived benefits, perceived barriers, and one's definition of health education. The least important determinant was identified as locus of control (although this has been studied the most).

The HBM and HPM are two tools that can assist community health nurses in examining factors relating to an individual's health choices and decisions. The models offer nurses a cluster of variables that provide important insight into explaining health behavior. The usefulness of such models relies not on trying to fit an individual into all the categories, which is an overwhelming task for nurses, but rather trying to view the determinants as helpful cues to consider when interacting and planning health education interventions. Simply put, models are helpful aids to guide nurses in their patient assessment and in developing, selecting, and implementing relevant educational interventions.

In applying the models, think for a moment about your own health behavior related to exercise. Consider the following questions:

- Do you feel that you or others in your family are susceptible to heart disease or stroke?
- Do you consider yourself continually striving for improved health?
- Do work, school, or family responsibilities get in the way of your exercise plans?
- Does a family history of cardiovascular disease spur you and others on to exercise?

- Has any family member, friend, or health professional recently reminded you of the benefits of exercise and encouraged you to start exercising?
- Do you feel that you have the ability to initiate and incorporate an exercise program into your lifestyle, or do you need external reinforcement and cues?

Table 8–4
Health Promotion Model Components

Cognitive-Perceptual Factors	Example and Explanation
Importance of health	Perceived value of health to functioning and life
Perceived control of health	Perceived ability to control health: external, internal, chance
Perceived self-efficacy	Perceived ability to perform the necessary behaviors to achieve an outcome
Definition of health	Views of what health means for self: may vary from absence of illness to self-actualization
Perceived health status	Perception of how individual views health: may range from wellness to illness
Perceived benefits of health-promoting behaviors	Perception of positive outcomes that can occur from health-promoting behavior (e.g., look good, smell good)
Perceived barriers to health-promoting behaviors	Perception of things that obstruct health-promoting behaviors (e.g., money, transportation

Modifying Factors	Example and Explanation
Demographics	Age, sex, race
Biological	Body fat and weight
Interpersonal influences	Interactions with family, nurses
Situational factors	Environmental determinants that make health-promoting options available
Behavioral	Previous knowledge or skills
Cues to action	Influencing factors: internal cues (e.g., feeling good about self); external cues (mass media)

The reader is directed to Pender (1987) for a more comprehensive description and explanation of the health promotion model.

- Do money or safety issues pose any barriers to your planning an exercise program?
- In viewing your health, how important are exercise behaviors when weighed against other health behaviors you may wish to modify (e.g., cutting down on fat intake, getting relief from work and school stresses)?

Analyze the answers to these questions to assist in developing an action plan that is tailored to *your own* needs and capabilities.

Model of Health Education Empowerment

The models previously described (HBM and HPM) focus on individual strategies for achieving optimal health and well-being. Although such approaches may be appropriate to changing individual behaviors, they do not take into account fully the complex relationships among social, structural, and physical factors in the environment such as unemployment, lack of social support systems, inaccessible health services, and racism (Israel et al., 1994). Kendall (1992) suggested that nurses must move away from being focused on adaptation and coping and rather develop leadership strategies to help emancipate patients from the oppressive forces that they live under. This means taking race, gender, and class seriously and recognizing the structural and foundational changes needed to effect changes for the socially, politically, and economically disadvantaged oppressed groups. This type of thinking may help nurses to assist individuals in moving from simply coping with their oppressed situations to fighting back.

Features of a new health promotion and health education movement embrace a broader definition of health that does address the social, political, and economic aspects of health (Labonte, 1994). Reconceptualizing health beyond the individual to the collective group has been viewed as moving the health education field beyond a narrow lifestyle focus to one that is based on empowerment and community participation (Robertson and Minkler, 1994). Such a theoretical perspective is congruent with community education because it supports learner participation and learner involvement. Three principles supportive of empowering health education and social justice are the neighborhood as base, development of comprehensive education strategies and programming, and community empowerment, which is a combination of process and outcome of organized community members gain-ing control over their lives (Eisen, 1994). Citizen participation is key for effective and successful health promotion and disease prevention programs (Braithwaite et al., 1994).

Empowerment education evolved out of the work of Paulo Freire's successful work in literacy in Brazil in the 1950s. His work was based on a problem-solving approach to education, which is in contrast to what he referred to as *banking education,* which places the learner in a passive role or as a receptacle of the teacher's information. By allowing for active participation and ongoing dialogue, problem-solving education encourages learners to be critical thinkers and reflective about health issues. He suggested that powerlessness exists when individuals assume the role of objects, letting the environment control them, rather than as subjects who can exert influence on environmental factors that affect their lives and their community. Community members (subjects) are viewed as the best resources to make change a reality (Freire, 1970, 1973).

Freire's approach to health education means that knowledge about health issues is gained through a participatory group process. This process seeks to explore the nature of the problems and address the deeper issues behind the problems. The nurse (facilitator-educator) is a resource person and relates as an equal partner to the other group members. This first phase, listening, is important to gain an understanding about the issues. The exchange of ideas and concerns leads to a problem-posing dialogue and the identification of problems or generative themes. The root causes of the problems are further discussed and explored. Last, group members create relevant action plans that are congruent with their own reality (Freire, 1973).

At the core of the empowerment process is information, communication, and health education (World Health Organization, 1994). Involving individuals, families, and groups in their learning validates the important role of learners and helps to ensure the relevancy of interventions (Rudd and Comings 1994; Wallerstein 1992).

Nurses can use empowerment strategies to aid people in developing skills in problem solving, networking, negotiating, lobbying, and information seeking to enhance health. The Freirian approach may appear similar to health education's emphasis on helping people take responsibility for their health by providing them with information, skills, reinforcement, and support. However, Freire purported that knowledge that is imparted by the collective group is significantly more powerful than information provided by health educators. This approach attempts to uncover the social and political aspects of problems and encourages group members to define and develop strategies for action. Because changes in health are complex and do not usually have immediate solutions, the term *problem posing,* instead of *problem solving,* has been suggested to better describe this empowerment process (Bernstein et al., 1994; Wallerstein and Bernstein, 1988).

EXAMPLES OF EMPOWERMENT EDUCATION

1. **The use of photonovella (picture stories) as an empowerment strategy was described by Wang and Burri (1994).** This participatory process integrated empowerment education, feminist theory, and documentary photography to bring about changes in consciousness. In this project, 62 rural Chinese women were trained in the technique and process of photonovella. Issues related to social, economic, cultural, and biomedical factors affecting women's health were explored through the village women's documentation of their own everyday lives. The images created by the women were used as educational tools to increase their individual and collective knowledge about their health status, to empower them to mobilize for social change, and to communicate their reality to policymakers. Facilitated group discussions validated their concerns about family, self, and community; aided in problem identification; and challenged them to create strategies for action. The photographs were used in presentations to county-level officials to convey the significance of the identified problems and to pose solutions to them. Empowerment resulted in access to knowledge, resources, networks, and decisions for the women.

2. **Wallerstein and Bernstein (1988) described a collaborative Alcohol and Substance Abuse Prevention (ASAP) program developed in 1982 as a school-based prevention project in New Mexico.** The aim was to empower teenagers by engaging them in critical thinking about drugs and alcohol. On four occasions, students visited local hospital emergency rooms and detention centers and interacted with patients and jail residents. Along with facilitators and other students, they attempted to explore the root causes of drug and alcohol abuse in their community. Students examined the reasons for such problems, explored their own role in solving them, and discussed creative ways to address the problems. The students and health professionals were co-learners in attempting to understand social knowledge about substance abuse and identify ways to address this complex health issue in their community. The ASAP program emphasized empathy, feelings, group connectiveness, and individual emotional growth as a motivator for social responsibility.

3. **The empowerment model was used in the design and development of the de Madres a Madres program in Houston's inner-city Hispanic community described by McFarland and Fehir (1994).** The program was developed to increase access to prenatal care and to decrease barriers. Unique to this program was the belief that information is power and that women, if provided with culturally relevant social support in combination with community resource information, would use the information even before they entered the traditional health care system. Key elements of this program were respect and reverence for individual and cultural differences, volunteerism, empowerment of indigenous women through unity, validation of women as key health promoters, and the belief that community members could identify and address their own health needs. Community members were active decision makers at every level of the program, further enhancing their leadership skill development and investment in the outcomes. The group shared responsibility for decisions and actions in the community. Information was provided to any pregnant resident through channels such as local businesses, schools, churches, media, health clinics, elected officials, or social services agencies. At the end of the 5-year community empowerment process, outcome data revealed that the women's own personal strengths were enhanced and their ability to work within the system for improved community health had increased.

Robertson and Minkler (1994) pointed out that even though the adoption of empowerment education, community participation, and a broader socialized definition of health fit the new definition of health promotion, this definition may potentially undervalue individual empowerment. Although this approach provides a socialized conceptualization of health and separates individuals from their health status, it also minimizes the very real associations between people and their everyday difficulties in managing their health and illnesses. This strong push to embrace collective empowerment may negate the value of professionally based direct health services. Rather, they suggested an empowerment continuum that acknowledges the value and interdependence of individual and political action strategies aimed at the collective. This thinking is supported by Labonte (1994), who identified the community as the engine of health promotion and a vehicle for empowerment. He described five spheres of an empowerment model that focus on different levels of social organization: interpersonal (personal empowerment), intragroup (small group development), intergroup (community), interorganizational (coalition building), and political action. Therefore, it seems that both micro- and macro-viewpoints of health education are needed to provide nurses with multiple opportunities for intervention across a broad continuum.

Community Empowerment

Effecting change at the community level requires the nurse to be knowledgeable about key concepts central to community organization (Table 8–5). As a methodologic tool, this approach enables nurses to be partners with the community to identify common goals to develop strategies and to mobilize resources to increase community empowerment and community competence. Key concepts inherent in community health education programming are empowerment, community competence, principle of relevance, principle of participation, issue selection, and creation of critical consciousness (see Table 8–5) (Minkler, 1990).

Keck (1994) indicated that successful community health relies on learning how to empower citizens to assume responsibility for decision making about their own health and the health of the community. Empowering the citizenry means that power shifts away from the health providers toward community members to set and tackle health priorities. The basic tenets of community empowerment are not new. However, what is new is the belief that this framework is of value and important. Collaboration and cooperation among community members, academicians, clinicians, health agencies, and businesses can help ensure that science, community needs, sociopolitical needs, and environmental needs are brought together in a humanistic manner. In Milwaukee, the Silver Spring Neighborhood Community Nursing

---

EXAMPLE OF COMMUNITY EMPOWERMENT–COLLABORATION–PARTICIPATION: SILVER SPRING NEIGHBORHOOD COMMUNITY NURSING CENTER (SSCNC) MILWAUKEE, WI

In 1987, SSCNC, an innovative academic nursing center program, opened its doors, providing easy access to primary care, health promotion, and intervention services to residents of the largest subsidized housing development in Wisconsin. Located in and developed in partnership with the Silver Spring Neighborhood Center, a large multi-program social service agency, this community nursing center (CNC) developed a comprehensive coordinated model for primary health care with a strong emphasis on primary prevention through health education. Mechanisms for ongoing input and dialogue with community members were viewed as an essential component for developing relevant programs and health interventions. Supported by multiple private and public funders, the CNC is staffed by a team of advanced practice nurse clinicians, community health nurses, and outreach workers. Approximately 50% of all services offered at the SSCNC are group education and support programs focusing on such topics as parenting, stress management, lifestyle modification, domestic violence, self-protective behaviors, and management of chronic illness.

The success of these programs with a population that is often considered "noncompliant" in follow-through on health-focused activities has been in large measure based on the willingness of the advanced practice nurses in the setting to develop educational programs and take the programs "to where the people are." Classes are conducted in various settings, including patients' homes, as well as integrated into aspects of the neighborhood center programs, including the day care program, alternative school classrooms, cultural arts center, an elderly congregate meal site, a family resource center, day camp, food pantry, and job skills program. The other 50% of interventions provided at the SSCNC each year are associated with individual or family visits through the nursing clinic at the SSCNC. The nursing center staff provides approximately 8000 direct encounters annually. In 1994, a total of 17,289 individual interventions were coded by nurses at the SSCNC using the Omaha Classification System, with health teaching guidance and counseling being the most widely used nursing intervention strategy.

Data from S. Lundeen, personal communication, 1995; Lundeen and Friedbacher (1993).

Table 8–5
Community Organization Practice

Key Concepts	Application to Health Education (Nursing Actions)
Empowerment: Helping individuals, families, and groups through problem solving and dialogue to gain insight and mastery over life situations	The nurse works with community members in identifying and defining issues and creates mechanisms for (1) discussion and problem solving and (2) identification of other factors impacting on everyday lives.
Community competence: Helping the community through collaboration to achieve desired goals	The nurse identifies key leaders and members to work collaboratively on identification and setting of goals and priorities. The nurse gets in touch with social and political leaders and networks.
Principle of relevancy: Begin where the people are	The nurse allows the community members to define their own issues while assisting them to focus on objectives. Hold town hall meetings to let members share concerns and issues of importance. Allowing community to define issues enhances their ownership of issue.
Principle of participation: learn by doing	The nurse facilitates community members to make decisions about health programs and messages. The nurse encourages group feelings of support. The nurse recognizes that active vs. passive participation results in greater likelihood of attitudinal and behavioral changes.
Issue selection: identification of community problems that are felt by the community as specific, meaningful, and able to be won	The nurse uses problem-solving techniques to help group members identify issues of relevance vs. troubling problems (e.g., use of door-to-door surveys, group process activities).
Creation of critical consciousness: highlights a relationship of equality and mutual respect among group members and educators to identify problems behind problems and generate appropriate action plans.	The nurse uses problem-posing dialogue (Freire, 1973) to understand root issues and devises creative and innovative methods to transform situations.

Content adapted from Minkler M. (1990). Improving health through community organization. *In* Glanz, Lewis, Rimer (eds). Health Behavior and Education. San Francisco, Jossey-Bass, pp. 266–274. Used with permission.

Center is an illustration of how the basic philosophic tenets of community organization resulted in a nursing center model bringing together members of the university, businesses, health agencies, and, most importantly, the community.

THE NURSE'S ROLE IN HEALTH EDUCATION: THE CEMENT

Although learning theories and health education models provide a useful framework when planning health interventions (the nuts and the bolts), key to their application is the nurse's ability to facilitate the education process and become a partner with individuals and communities. At the core of health education is a therapeutic relationship that develops between the nurse and individuals, families, and the community. Nurses are the cement of the process and serve as catalysts for change by delivering humanistic care. Nurses can move ideas into action, offer appropriate interventions, identify resources, and facilitate group empowerment. Rankin and Stallings (1990) described four key characteristics of nurses in facilitating the teacher-learner process: confidence, competence, caring, and communication. It is beyond the scope of this chapter to detail communication techniques, but a brief reminder about the value of inclusion and trust before the delivery of content is offered to the reader.

Enhancing Communication

Inclusion → Trust → Content

The critical step of inclusion sets the foundation for possible health action to occur. It is the cement that solidifies the relationship. Examples of ways to enhance inclusion may be greeting individuals, families, and groups in a timely and warm fashion, introducing one's self, asking participants about their day, providing for comfort needs (comfortable setting, taking coats, identifying bathroom areas), and attending to their immediate concerns or stress. Educating does not begin with the first instructional word but rather starts with establishing an atmosphere conducive to learning. By attending to inclusion, individuals, families, and groups will begin to trust the nurse and then the health message. This trust will be evident by active participation and a commitment to the education process. The content or the health message has a greater chance of being received and acted on if a positive, proactive, and personalized relationship has been established.

Community empowerment is reflective of participatory decision making and planning from the bottom up and is culturally sensitive (Bernstein et al., 1994). As minority populations in the United States continue to grow, nurses are key in creating and delivering culturally competent health messages and programs. Sociopolitical and environmental forces must be addressed within cultural expressions. The reader is directed to Chapter 17 for a detailed perspective on cultural diversity and community health nursing. Davis and colleagues (1992) outlined several principles to help nurses be sensitive to cultural diversity and to global health care needs:

- Confront one's own racism and ethnocentrism.
- Be sensitive to intergroup and intragroup cultural diversity and commonalities in ethnic minority populations.
- Seek knowledge about the dynamics in biculturalism (e.g., how a particular ethnic group may be a synthesis of several cultures).
- Seek understanding of how social and structural factors influence and shape behaviors.
- Avoid a "blame the victim" ideology.

Ask yourself the following questions and respond by noting frequency ("very often," "often," "not often," "rarely").

Do you interact with people of color on an ongoing basis? Do you feel comfortable when teaching a diverse group of learners? How often do you ask people of color for new ideas on solving problems? Can you deal with cultural differences without taking them negatively? Do you feel comfortable when you are alone in an elevator with a person of color? Do you have high expectations of people of color? Are you aware of and confront stereotypic expectations about attitudes, values, communication patterns, or health behaviors based on skin color? Do you alter your teaching based on situations and on individuals, families, or groups?

For questions to which you responded "not often" or "rarely," reexamine assumptions that may obstruct effective and relevant health teaching. Consider ways to modify your thinking to include cultural considerations into nursing care. Examine ways to overcome barriers to effective communication (American Management Association, 1993).

Cultural assessment and cultural negotiation are two processes that can enhance health teaching. In using these processes, nurses use information gathered from their assessment (e.g., issues related to religion, patterns of decision making, preferred communication styles to plan relevant care). Cultural brokering is then used to translate instructions and messages to match the individuals, families, or groups. Centralizing the cultural experiences of the group enhances cultural sensitivity (Airhihenbuwa, 1994; Tripp-Reimer and Afifa, 1989). For example, Hall (1988) described the development of a diabetes control program for Mexican-Americans in California. Of importance was the development of culture-specific communications, culturally sensitive instructors who respected cultural differences in beliefs, and the development of culturally appropriate print materials. Health messages incorporated the use of folk medicines (use of herbal teas) along with the recommended diabetes regimen for diet planning. Additionally, cooking instructions provided were consistent with their current practices (e.g., pictures showing the palm of the hand for measuring vs. traditional measuring spoons). Menus were modified to reflect regional and individual food habits. The diabetes program was tailored to the intended target members based on ongoing feedback and dialogue from the group.

Effective health education in the community can be realized through the expert knowledge and skills of nurses. Nurses are key in making community education happen. Shalala (1993), in her keynote address to the 20th Biennial Convention of the National League for Nursing, commented,

But who will slay the dragon of disadvantage? Who will step in with the wand, the ruby slippers, the handful of magic beans? It will not be one individual, not one profession, not one tower of vision. It must be a consortium of professionals, a combined vision of many different parts and different life stories: corporate leaders politicians, teachers, leaders of nursing professionals. Yes, very importantly, nurses, whose profession is not just a career, but a lifework. Nurses who have one foot high on the crystal, tower of knowledge and theory and one foot in the dust and grit of human need. . . . (p. 291)

PUTTING MODELS AND THEORIES INTO ACTION

Within the community, the nurse's target audience may be an individual, a family, a group, or many segments of the community. Using a systematic approach to the development and delivery of health messages provides the nurse with an organized yet user-friendly approach to deliver health messages.

Although nurses can draw from a variety of educational models, theoretical frameworks, and teaching and learning principles as described earlier in the chapter, the National Cancer Institute suggested the "Framework for Developing Health Communications" when creating a variety of health education messages and programs (U.S.DHHS, 1992) (Fig. 8–1). The six stages depict a circular loop that mirrors that of the nursing process (assessment, planning, implementation, and evaluation) and provide a sequential path for continuous assessment, feedback, and improvement. This model is based on principles of social marketing, health education, and mass communication theories. An appealing feature of this framework is that it relies heavily on target audience assessment to guide the process. It is also congruent with Freire's model of empowerment education, which encourages ongoing dialogue with the potential consumers of health services. Although this model focuses on communication strategies aimed at a programmatic level, the basic elements are applicable to individual, family, and group systems.

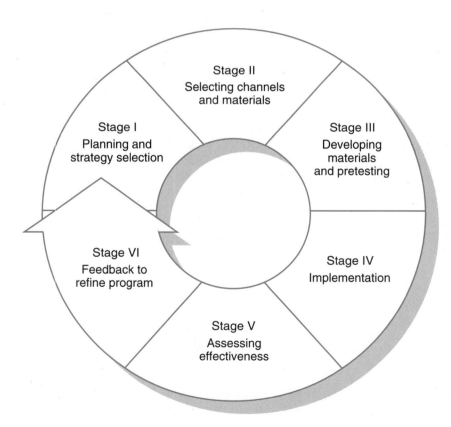

Figure 8–1
Framework for developing health communications. The National Cancer Institute suggests using this model to develop health education messages. (Data from U.S. Department of Health and Human Services, 1992.)

The ideas contained in this model are intended to be a practical scheme for planning and implementing health education communications programs. Nurses are encouraged to use the model as a guideline in planning health education messages and programs: use all or portions of the steps as necessary. It is more important to use an organized and systematic approach rather than to try and fit your health education plan into all the steps. Each of the six stages is discussed, key points are highlighted, methods to accomplish each stage are described, and examples are identified. To illustrate the process, consider the following scenario:

Launching of a Mobile Mammography Van

In 1989, a community volunteer-leader felt a lump in her breast, obtained a mammogram, and shortly thereafter obtained a biopsy. The whole experience, she described, was very stressful and gave her pause to wonder about her fellow community members who might not have access to the type of care that she had. Current statistics revealed that the incidence of breast cancer had been steadily increasing and that the mortality from breast cancer for minority women was alarmingly high. The volunteer had served her community for a number of years and had cultivated significant relationships with community and governmental members. She met with the mayor to convey the extreme need for action to make health screening accessible. This initial meeting resulted in the mayor calling together a task force of representatives from state and public health agencies, business, health care professionals, and private citizen volunteers to devise new stategies to combat fear of breast cancer and mammography among target clients. To first identify the root issues behind the problem and select the relevant issues to address, focus groups (meetings with community members) were held. Information was also gathered from a variety of community and health sources. The outcomes of the focus groups provided a description of the intended target audience (underserved, uninsured, and underinsured women) and the identified need: culturally relevant education, accessible mammography service, and follow-up care within the community. A year of planning and fund raising resulted in a mobile mammography van hitting the streets in October 1990. During the first 5 years of service, more than 21,000 women received educational materials, and 9800 received mammograms. What made this initiative successful?

Stage I: Planning and Strategy Selection

The planning stage provides the foundation for the entire communication process. Of key importance in putting health education into action is an understanding of the learning needs of the target audience and targeting the program or message to the audience. This step reinforces the philosophical tenets put forth by Freire in which the needs of the target audience are ascertained and an open dialogue is created.

QUESTIONS TO ASK

- Who is the target audience?
- What is already known about the audience and from what sources?
- What are the objectives and goals?
- What evaluation strategies will I use?
- What is the health issue of interest?

COLLABORATIVE ACTIONS TO TAKE

- Review available data from health statistics, local sources, libraries, newspapers, and local or community leaders.
- Obtain new data: interviews, focus groups (problem-posing dialogues).
- Determine the target group's needs and perceptions of health problems: identify audiences.
  - Physical (sex, age, health history)
  - Behavioral (lifestyle characteristics, health-related activities)
  - Demographic (income, years of schooling, cultural characteristics)
  - Psychographics (beliefs, values, attitudes)
- Identify issues behind the issues.
- Identify existing gaps of health knowledge.
- Write goals and objectives that are specific, attainable, prioritized, and time specific.
- Assess your resources (money, staff, materials).

Illustration: Description of Health Issue and Target Audience

Health statistics revealed that the incidence of breast cancer had increased and the death rates among minority women were alarmingly high. A gap in health service was identified: the lack of mammography screening and education for high-risk economically disadvantaged women residing in the city of Milwaukee. The target population was under-served, uninsured, or underinsured women who had limited access to the services. In considering this service, women identified that they wanted and needed health information about breast health but were dealing with many everyday survival issues and struggles. A root issue to be addressed was to create a health service within the neighborhoods delivered by culturally sensitive providers. Women 40 years of age and older, as well as those 30 years and older with a family history of breast cancer, were eligible, Breast cancer is higher among women aged 50 years and older, and particular emphasis was placed on this group. The intended target audience included women from diverse ethnic backgrounds, including Caucasian, African-American, Hispanic, Hmong, Laotian, and Vietnamese.

Goal. To prevent premature death and disability from breast cancer

Objectives. To increase the number of high-risk economically disadvantaged women residing in Milwaukee each year who obtain education, mammograms, clinical breast examinations, and follow-up.

Stage II: Selecting Channels and Materials

Decisions made in Stage I can help guide the nurse in selecting appropriate communication channels and produce effective and relevant materials. The nurse needs to consider how to reach the target audience. The community nurse needs to consider how best to reach the audience and what methods should be used. *Channel* refers to how the nurse will reach target churches, schools, clinics, libraries, nurses, or community-based organizations. *Format* refers to how the health message will be communicated (e.g., one-on-one, group discussion) (Table 8–6). *Materials/Media* are defined as the tools of a program, not the program itself (Table 8–7). Remember that education is a human activity and should not focus on the use of audiovisuals only.

QUESTIONS TO ASK

- What channels are best?
- What formats should be used?
- Are there existing resources?

COLLABORATIVE ACTIONS TO TAKE

- Identify messages and materials to be used.
- Decide whether to use existing materials or to produce new ones.
- Select the channels and formats.

Illustration

A combination of channels were selected to communicate health information about the prevention of breast cancer, screenings, and detection methods (e.g., community-based clinics, home visits, churches, or senior centers). Nurses used one-on-one interactions at the mobile site and during follow-up home visits. Group discussions about breast health were offered at many of the community sites. Extensive collaboration with community agencies and hospitals ensured that sites for the screening were in place and follow-up care would be provided.

A variety of health materials were collected on the topic of breast cancer from national, state, and local sources, and it was determined that many of the printed materials were not culturally or educationally relevant (written at difficult-to-read levels). Because appropriate materials were not available, the task force created their own written materials and pretested them with the intended target audience.

Stage III: Developing Materials and Pretesting

Several different types of communication concepts may be developed in the first stages and can be tested with the audience for feedback.

QUESTIONS TO ASK

- In what ways can the message be presented?
- How will the target audience react to the message?
- Will the audience understand, accept, and use the message?
- What changes might improve the message?

COLLABORATIVE ACTIONS TO TAKE

- Develop relevant materials with the target audience.
- Pretest materials and message and obtain feedback from the audience (interviews, questionnaires, focus groups, readability testing). Pretesting helps to ensure comprehension, acceptability, and personal relevance.

Table 8-6
Teaching-Learning Formats

Teaching Format	Application to Health Education
Brainstorming session	Allows participants the freedom to generate ideas and discuss them in a group setting. Creativity is cultivated. Fosters empowerment to let members identify the issue and come up with solutions.
Community-wide programs	Can reach large numbers of community members through a systematic plan. May include individual or group approaches with defined target audience.
Demonstration	Effective in learning perceptual motor skills. Aids in visual identification
Group discussion	Members can learn from each other and receive support. Teaching content can be tailored to group needs. Ideal for groups combining patients and families. Groups can be led by nurses, other health professionals, or lay members. Facilitator needs to be comfortable with group method and familiar with characteristics of group.
Lecture	Formal oral presentations can be used with varying group sizes. Expertise and experiences of group members are shared. Presenter must be comfortable and possess speaking ability. Requires organizational skills and ability to highlight key points in interesting and creative ways. Lecture can be combined with media to enhance learning. Audience participation is linked to presenter's speaking style and ability. Audience feedback is limited.
One-on-one discussion	Allows for individual assessment and identification of literacy, cultural barriers, physical impairments, learning needs, and anxiety. Promotes tailoring of health education plans. Ideal to capture the "teachable moments." Does not allow for sharing and support from others. High cost of staff time
Role playing	Effective in influencing attitudes and opinions. Encourages problem-solving and critical thinking skills. Enhances learner participation: some members may be hesitant to become involved.
Task force-committee	Brings together individuals with diverse backgrounds and expertise to achieve a goal. Many interests can be represented.

Based on data from Babcock and Miller, 1994; Lancaster, 1992; Rankin and Stallings, 1990; Redman, 1994.

Illustration

Local newspaper ads publicized the mammography screening service. Printed schedules were distributed to area community agencies, churches, and senior centers. Printed materials about breast self-examination were developed by the task force members with input from target members. Breast self-examination literature was printed in five languages. Efforts were made to have translators on the van. At present, the task force group is exploring creative ways to obtain funding for a more culturally relevant videotape. Ongoing dialogue with community members and health agencies aided in refining the screening process and the education component of the service to ensure effectiveness, efficiency, and appropriateness.

Stage IV: Implementation

At this point, the health education message and programs are introduced to the target audience, and necessary components are reviewed and revised.

Table 8–7
Materials and Media

Media	Considerations in Health Education Settings
Audiotapes	Requires no reading; portable and small Can be used at home in a comfortable setting: can be replayed and used at individual's own pace Economical Helpful for individuals with visual difficulties and for those with low reading skills.
Bulletin boards	Inexpensive and easy to develop Directs attention to a specific message; uses few words
Exhibits/displays	Graphics offer appeal Placement in high-traffic areas (e.g., waiting rooms, exam rooms can reach wide audiences)
Flip charts, chalkboards	Excellent format to enlarge teaching concepts or to cue reader to salient points; graphics/diagrams can be added Chalkboards can be reused; flip charts have replacement pads. Inexpensive
Games/simulations	Involves patients in a fun manner; effective in involving the entire family Highly effective with children
Graphics	
Drawings/visuals	Can convey important points in a salient and visual fashion Can aid understanding for low-literacy audiences Humorous messages may attract the attention of target members Visual messages should be pretested to ensure acceptability, understandability
Interactive videotapes	A variety of computer programs, interactive videodisks, and computer-assisted instructions are available and are being tested; algorithms and branching decisions aid patients in decision making, problem solving, and fact acquisition (Alterman & Baughman, 1991; Campbell et al., 1994) Interactive patient education is becoming more common via kiosks in waiting rooms Computer comfort level should be assessed Software development may be time intensive and costly
Models/real objects	Brings the teaching concept to the patient in a familiar way
Demonstrations	Helpful when conveying psychomotor skills; encourages patient involvement and tactile learning (e.g., colostomy bag, penis model for condom placement) No reading needed Helpful in individual and group instruction Models and real objects can be incorporated into displays or fairs
Overhead slides	Can be used in small and large group settings Can be used to highlight key points and help patient focus ideas Use of color and advance organizers, large type, and key points are recommended; avoid busy and cluttered overheads Can be prepared in advance Inexpensive
Photographs/picture books/ album slide series	Helps to promote understanding by showing realistic images and real situations; aids patients in making connections to their life; can be used alone or in combination with other photographs, slides; can be placed in an album Helpful for patients with limited literacy skills; offers visual presentation of concepts Effective with individual and small groups: self-study/reflection Can be updated easily

Table 8–7
Materials and Media (*Continued*)

Media	Considerations in Health Education Settings
Printed materials (brochures, leaflets, booklets)	Portable, widely available, economical Useful in reinforcing health concepts and interactions Patients can set and adjust the pace and refer back to information later Can be effective with individuals, families, groups, or community-wide dissemination Materials written at simple levels can be effective and acceptable for both low-level and high-level readers (Meade et al., 1989) Materials that are personalized are highly effective (Skinner et al., 1994) Issues of readability, design, layout, cultural relevance, and appropriateness of content should be assessed
Programmed materials, self-help guides, slide/tape programs	May involve printed materials combined with visuals to allow for self-pacing Helpful to learn facts Nurse should assess individual or group to determine whether independent learning style is preferred
Teaching cards	Portable, uses few words, offers visual interpretations
Flashcards	Can be created economically by the nurse and easily updated. Effective with individual, small group, or family instruction
Radio/newspapers	Reaches large audiences within the community Effective in conveying general health information in a user-friendly manner Nurses can play an active role in disseminating health information (Meade, 1992)
Television, cable television	Reaches large audiences within the community Can help to enhance general health and well-being of community members Effective in influencing attitudes and behaviors Offers a familiar medium for viewers to learn about health topics Nurses can play key roles in reaching community (Meade, 1992)
Videotapes	Combines audio and visual medium to convey realistic images Videotapes that incorporate role modeling concept are recommended (Gagliano, 1988) Expensive to produce and update; access to audiovisual equipment needed and sites for viewing required Videotapes may be costly to produce, purchase, and update. Tailoring of content to target audience enhances effectiveness
On-line resources (Internet, simple dial-up services)	Electronic information sources can link individuals, families, and groups to health information, data bases, bulletin board services, and so on Common Internet providers are America On-Line and Prodigy World-Wide-Web is a widely used software system that facilitates the creation and sharing of multimedia across Internet New technologies can help consumers find health information, advice, and support

Media are tools of a health education program and encounter. They can be used to inform, reinforce, and convey health messages. Education is a human activity and should not be reduced to the use of only audiovisuals. Media should be selected keeping in mind the target audience. If developing new media, field test the media with members of the target group to ensure relevancy.

Based on data from Babcock and Miller, 1994; Breckon et al., 1994; Lancaster, 1992; Rankin and Stallings, 1990.

QUESTIONS TO ASK

- Is the message and program getting to the target audience?
- Do any channels need to be altered?
- What are the strengths of the health program?
- What changes would enhance effectiveness?

COLLABORATIVE ACTIONS TO TAKE

- Work with community organizations, businesses, and other health agencies to enhance effectiveness.
- Monitor and track progress.
- Establish process evaluation measures (e.g., follow-up with users of services, number of women who used services, expenditures).

Illustration

The mass media were used to introduce the service at a press conference. Several spokespersons helped facilitate this event and kick it off. Lists publicizing the identified sites for the mobile unit stops were distributed in the community. At each screening site, women were greeted by mobile unit staff inside the clinic or center where the unit was stationed for the morning. Information about the woman's history and current health situation was obtained. Questions about the procedure and follow-up were also answered. Additionally, child care was provided if needed. Women were escorted to the mobile unit and then viewed a videotape on breast self-examination. Staff consisted of a registered nurse, a radiological technologist, driver, program coordinator, and outreach worker. Funding for the service was supplied by the governor and mayor with private donations from local foundations, businesses, and individuals.

Stage V: Assessing Effectiveness

The program and health message are analyzed for effectiveness. The mechanisms identified in Stage I should be tracked. Both process and summative evaluations can be helpful. Process evaluation examines the procedures and tasks involved in the program or message such as monitoring of media, identifying interim reactions from target audience, and addressing internal functioning (e.g., work schedules, expenditures). Outcome evaluation looks at short-term or long-term results such as the number of sites covered, inquiries made about the program or service, change of audience awareness, knowledge, attitude and behaviors, number of women reached, and change in mortality and morbidity figures.

QUESTIONS TO ASK

- Were objectives met? What was the impact (change in morbidity or mortality)?
- How well did each step work (process evaluation)?
- Were the changes realized as a result of the program or other factors (outcome evaluation)?

COLLABORATIVE ACTIONS TO TAKE

- Conduct process and outcome evaluations.

Illustration

Process Evaluation. A number of newspaper, television, and radio advertisements publicized the free mammography service and highlighted breast health. Eight hospitals provided follow-up service. The number of staff since 1990 has increased by two and now includes a program coordinator, nurses, site coordinator, technologist, driver, receptionist, and outreach worker. Continual improvements in the on-site logistics of the service were made. Public health nurses also were added to support the program by providing follow-up. Women responded well to the service based on their formal and informal feedback. Women have responded well to the educational materials; however, a need continued for a culturally relevant videotape on breast self-examination. The mobile van was frequently out of service because of its age (the mobile van was previously used for tuberculosis screenings) and caused multiple interruptions to the delivery of the service. This inefficiency was serious, and ways to rectify this problem were addressed.

Outcome Evaluation. The number of community sites that participated in the service has increased from 16 to more than 300. The number of women reached (screened) has steadily increased and during its first 5 years resulted in 9800 women being screened. More than 40 cases of breast cancers were discovered, and these patients were referred for follow-up care; others were being further evaluated. The number of calls from community sites requesting the service has increased as has the number of calls from women requesting health information.

Stage VI: Feedback to Refine Program

The information gained from the audience, the channels of communication, and the program's intended effect can now be used to prepare for a new cycle of development. This phase helps to continually refine the health message and make it responsive to the needs of the target audience. Information gained from this stage aids in validating the strengths of the programs and allows for necessary modifications. Feedback is necessary to continually refine the message.

QUESTIONS TO ASK

- What was learned?
- What can be improved on?
- What worked well and what did not work so well?
- Are the goals and objectives relevant?
- Has anything changed about the target audience?
- Was the assessment complete?
- Did the audience perceive the problem?
- Are the methods and formats tailored to the target audience?
- Were some barriers overlooked?
- Overall, what lessons were learned, and what modifications could be made to strengthen the health education activity?

COLLABORATIVE ACTIONS TO TAKE

- Reassess goals and objectives. Revise them as needed.
- Modify strategies or activities that did not succeed.
- Generate continual support from businesses, health care agencies, and other community groups for ongoing collaboration and partnerships.
- Summarize the health education program or message in an evaluation report.
- Provide justification for continuing the program or for ending one.

Illustration

Reports describing process and outcome evaluation and analysis of the service have continually been documented by the health department outlining and describing the program. Such reports serve to apply what has been learned and to outline ways to enhance and improve the efficiency and effectiveness of the service. The mobile mammography van continues to provide service to Milwaukee women. As a result of successful fund raising, a new van was purchased in January 1994. The number of women receiving the service has continued to increase each year. The program continues under the auspices of the city's health department, and sources of funding are being addressed. Recent monies were obtained from the Centers for Disease Control and Prevention. New partnerships with area community organizations, businesses, and agencies are ongoing.

The reader is encouraged to consider how other health messages or programs can be planned using this model, which mirrors that of the nursing process. Complete the exercise in Figure 8–2 to organize your ideas systematically.

HEALTH EDUCATION RESOURCES

A variety of health education materials and resources are available from local, state, and national organizations and agencies. Such associations can provide helpful information about their services, educational materials, and linkages to support groups or self-help groups. Often materials (both printed and electronic) are available free or at a nominal cost. Nurses can help individuals, families, and groups access needed materials, services, or equipment loan programs. By being knowledgeable about available resources, nurses can support community education programs and messages. Additionally, identification of gaps in services or resources can provide nurses with data to create the needed service or material. For example, in Milwaukee, no breast cancer support group existed that was targeted to African-American women. Even though many support groups were established by cancer-related organizations, they were perceived as not meeting the needs of women of color and were not located in convenient locations within the community's central city neighborhood. Several community members and nurses who had experienced breast cancer or who were at high risk took the lead to initiate a support group called Women Supporting Women. This support group meets monthly and is open to all breast cancer survivors and their friends and significant others, but it is specifically targeted to African-American women. It continues to thrive after 4 years and meets at a well-known community site (M. Leigh-Gold, and J. McCord, personal communication, July 1995).

A summary of major organizations and resources follows. This general guide provides the reader with categories of health resources. One source for a comprehensive listing of resources is Rankin and Stallings' (1990) *Patient Education: Issues, Principles, Practices* (Chapter 8, Appendix B).

Planning Your Health Education Message

Instructions: Think about a target group that you are currently working with and for which you are planning to deliver/create a health education program or message. Complete the exercise by asking yourself the following questions:

Questions to Ask	Action Plan
• What is the overall intended message/goal? What are my reasons for planning this message? How do I know that it is needed or wanted by the target audience?	
• Who is the intended audience? (Write a brief statement describing the characteristics of the target group.)	
• What will be the benefits of this message to the target group?	
• What channels will I use to deliver the message? Provide a rationale.	
• Will I need to create materials? Are there available materials that are appropriate for my target group?	
• How will I know if my message gets across to the target audience? Did the target audience respond? How many people were reached? Who responded?	
• Was there change? What are the reasons the message was or was not effective? What can be modified to strengthen the message?	

Figure 8–2
Planning your health education message.

The nurse can contact the following sources for health education information.

- Local and regional hospitals, clinics, libraries, health education centers, businesses.
- Local and state governmental sources: health departments, social service agencies (check the yellow pages for listings).
- Community-based organizations (consider those that advertise and those that do not but are known through community leaders).
- Universities and colleges, academic nursing centers
- Professional organizations (e.g., AHA, American Public Health Association, ANA, National Black Nurses Association.
- Commercial organizations: pharmaceutical, medical supply companies; patient and health education companies (both written and audiovisual sources: catalogues are often available).
- Federal government sources: This is one of the largest and most comprehensive sources and in-

cludes such health-related sources as the National Institutes of Health (e.g., National Cancer Institute, National Heart, Lung, Blood Institute), Public Health Service, Centers for Disease Control and Prevention, National AIDS Clearinghouse, Office of Minority Health, Office on Smoking and Health).

- Voluntary agencies and their local affiliates such as the American Heart Association, Amyotrophic Lateral Sclerosis Association, American Council for Drug Disorders, American Dairy Council, American Lung Association, and so on.
- DIRLINE (Directory of Information Resources onLINE) (database available on the National Library of Medicine's software package called Grateful MED). This database offers a directory of organizations providing information services. For application, call 1-800-638-8480.
- Internet searches.

Assessing the Relevancy of Health Materials

It is critical that materials used in health education initiatives are appropriate for the intended target audience. Ask the following questions:

- Is there a good fit between material and target audience?
- Are the materials appealing?
- Is the message contained in the materials clear and understandable?
- Will the target audience identify and relate to the content, the visuals, and the written style?

Literacy and Health

In her 1944 text *The Public Health Nurse in the Community,* Rue stated that the illiteracy level of the people of the community is an important factor in planning health programs. This factor continues to be a significant issue in the planning of health education programs and materials. Millions of Americans are unable to process and use information often vital to their own survival. This means that approximately one of every five Americans is faced with the challenges of illiteracy. A survey from the U.S. Department of Education indicated that more than half of the population 16 years of age and older have very basic reading skills and have difficulty with critical thinking skills (Educational Testing Service, 1993). Have you

ever been left wondering, Will the parents know what to do if their infant gets a fever? Do they know how to read a thermometer? Does she or he know how to take those four different types of medications? Will this family understand how to get through the health care system? Are food labels understandable, and do they make sense to community members? Are printed immunization schedules clear? Can the warning messages be heeded if they are written in complex technical language? Unfortunately, research shows that there is a serious disparity between the reading levels of materials and the reading skills of most Americans (Ledbetter et al., 1990; Meade and Byrd, 1989; Meade et al., 1992; Swanson et al., 1990; Meade et al., 1994; Wells et al., 1994).

Weiss and colleagues (1992) reported significant links between health status and literacy even while adjusting for sociodemographic variables. The relational mechanisms between literacy and health are not clearly defined; however, individuals with very low literacy skills are at an increased risk for poor health. The Doaks, who are recognized for bringing the literacy issue to the forefront in public health, indicated that

The health community is a written culture. Unfortunately, many written instructions are over the heads of patients. There is often a serious mismatch between the readability levels of their instructions and the reading skills of patients. Health care providers have control over the literacy levels of their instructions, and have a responsibility to reduce the mismatch. Techniques to accomplish this are available and easily applied. (L. Doak and C. Doak, personal communication, September 1995)

The reader is referred to their excellent book, *Teaching Patients with Low Literacy Skills* (1995), in which practical suggestions and tips are offered for preparing and testing materials.

Nurses can assume important roles in the creation and dissemination of relevant health materials and media. Within Stage I of the previously described model, the nurse should use assessment skills to determine the reading level of the intended target audience. For example, ask your patients a series of simple questions to provide a better indication of their reading skills. Ask them whether they read, whether they enjoy reading, what they like to read, and how often they read. Skilled readers like to read and enjoy a variety of materials. Determine how they like to get their health information; is it from written sources? Ask your patients to read aloud a paragraph from a health material. Skilled readers like to read, read with fluency, are able to grasp the content, look up unfamiliar words, and are able to interpret the meaning of words. Limited readers read slowly and miss the intended meaning, take words literally, tire quickly from reading, and skip over uncommon words. Also, ask them a few questions about the information that they have just read. Can they answer questions about the content (Doak et al., 1995)? Remember that reading skills are not necessarily equated with years of schooling. In fact, a three- to four-grade-level difference has often been noted (Meade and Byrd 1989; Meade et al., 1994; Streiff, 1986).

Such informal assessment techniques can be coupled with more formal but easy to administer assessment methods to create a reading profile for your patients. Helpful tools include the use of the Wide-Range Achievement Test, Level III (Jastak and Wilkinson, 1993), or a newer tool entitled Rapid Estimate of Adult Literacy in Medicine (REALM) by Davis and colleagues (1993) (Fig. 8–3). When developing health programs and materials for groups within the community, the nurse should apply informal or formal assessment techniques with a sample of potential target members to ensure a match between health communications and readers.

HELPFUL TIPS FOR EFFECTIVE TEACHING*

- Assess the reading skills of target members using informal and formal methods.
- Determine what the target members know and want to know.
- Stick with the essentials. Limit the number of items. The focus may need to be on critical survival skills.
- Set realistic goals and objectives. Take your cues from your patients about what they want to learn and how you can help them learn.
- Use clear and concise language. Avoid technical terms if possible. For example, substitute the word *problem* for *complication.* Use the term *stick to* instead of the word *compliant,* or use the word *chance* instead of *possibility.* However, do not needlessly simplify if the intended meaning is taken away. Even though the words *infection* and *chemotherapy* may be polysyllabic words, cancer patients are usually familiar with them. See Example 1.
- Consider developing a glossary or vocabulary list

---

*These data are from Doak et al., 1995, 1996; Lange, 1989; Michielutte et al., 1992; Plimpton & Root, 1994; Wells et al., 1994.

for common words on the health topic. For example, in teaching a family about dental health, create a list of common words about that topic for them: toothbrush, flossing, cavity, decay, check-ups, x-rays.
- Space your teaching. Incorporate health education activities into other activities. For example, ask patients about their smoking habits at every prenatal visit. Relate teaching to their everyday life concerns.
- Personalize health messages. Use the active voice. For example, instead of saying, "It is important for patients who want to cut down on their fat intake to read labels, say "Learn to read food labels. This can help you to cut down on the amount of your fat intake." See Example 2.
- Build in methods of illustration and demonstration and real life examples. Connect the health message to everyday events.
- Give and get. Plan on review. Ask the patient questions before, during, and after teaching.
- Summarize often. Provide the patient with feedback. Obtain feedback from your target audience.
- Be creative. Use your imagination in conveying difficult concepts (e.g., use of picture cards, drawings, real objects).
- Use appropriate resources and materials to enhance teaching and convey ideas, e.g., videotapes, flip charts, bulletin boards).
- Try to put your patients at ease. Focus on inclusion and trust before delivering content.
- Praise your patients but do not overdo to the point of patronizing them.
- Be encouraging throughout the educational steps.
- Allow time for patients to think and ask questions.
- Remember that understanding takes time and practice. Ongoing feedback is needed to help in refocusing the teaching encounter. Conduct learner verification to ensure understanding of message.

Assessing Materials: Become a Wise Consumer and User

Within community sites, materials are collected, stored, and disseminated as needed. In many instances, pamphlets are distributed but not read or are superficially reviewed with little impact on the reader. "People of this country have had so much pamphlet materials passed out to them free that some have lost respect for free literature. Health educators may have contributed to this delinquency by passing out health literature carelessly and indiscriminately. The nurse who expects the pamphlet to take the place of the

RAPID ESTIMATE OF ADULT LITERACY IN MEDICINE (REALM)©
Terry Davis, PhD • Michael Crouch, MD • Sandy Long, PhD

Reading
Level _____

Grade
Completed_____

Patient's name/
Subject #_____   Date of Birth_____

Date_____ Clinic_____ Examiner_____

List 1		List 2		List 3	
fat	_____	fatigue	_____	allergic	_____
flu	_____	pelvic	_____	menstrual	_____
pill	_____	jaundice	_____	testicle	_____
dose	_____	infection	_____	colitis	_____
eye	_____	exercise	_____	emergency	_____
stress	_____	behavior	_____	medication	_____
smear	_____	prescription	_____	occupation	_____
nerves	_____	notify	_____	sexually	_____
germs	_____	gallbladder	_____	alcoholism	_____
meals	_____	calories	_____	irritation	_____
disease	_____	depression	_____	constipation	_____
cancer	_____	miscarriage	_____	gonorrhea	_____
caffeine	_____	pregnancy	_____	inflammatory	_____
attack	_____	arthritis	_____	diabetes	_____
kidney	_____	nutrition	_____	hepatitis	_____
hormones	_____	menopause	_____	antibiotics	_____
herpes	_____	appendix	_____	diagnosis	_____
seizure	_____	abnormal	_____	potassium	_____
bowel	_____	syphilis	_____	anemia	_____
asthma	_____	hemorrhoids	_____	obesity	_____
rectal	_____	nausea	_____	osteoporosis	_____
incest	_____	directed	_____	impetigo	_____

SCORE
List 1_____
List 2_____
List 3_____
Raw
Score_____

Figure 8–3
The Rapid Estimate of Adult Literacy in Medicine (REALM) is a screening instrument to assess an adult patient's ability to read common medical words and lay terms for body parts and illnesses. It is designed to assist medical professionals in estimating a patient's literacy level so that the appropriate level of patient education materials or oral instructions may be used. The test takes 2 to 3 minutes to administer and score. (Reprinted with permission of Dr. Terry Davis, Louisiana State University.)

Figure continued on following page

DIRECTIONS:
1. Give the patient a laminated copy of the REALM and score answers on an unlaminated copy that is attached to a clipboard. Hold the clipboard at an angle so that the patient is not distracted by your scoring procedure. Say:
   "I want to hear you read as many words as you can from this list. Begin with the first word on List 1 and read aloud. When you come to a word you cannot read, do the best you can or say "blank" and go on to the next word."
2. If the patient takes more than 5 seconds on a word, say "blank" and point to the next word, if necessary, to move the patient along. If the patient begins to miss every word, have him/her pronounce only known words.
3. Count as an error any word not attempted or mispronounced. Score by marking a plus (+) after each correct word, a check (√) after each mispronounced word, and a minus (−) after words not attempted. Count as correct any self-corrected words.
4. Count the number of correct words for each list and record the numbers in the "SCORE" box. Total the numbers and match the total score with its grade equivalent in the table below.

Raw Score	GRADE EQUIVALENT Grade Range
0–18	**3rd Grade and Below** Will not be able to read most low literacy materials; will need repeated oral instructions, materials composed primarily of illustrations, or audiotapes or videotapes.
19–44	**4th to 6th Grade** Will need low literacy materials; may not be able to read prescription labels.
45–60	**7th to 8th Grade** Will struggle with most patient education materials; will not be offended by low literacy materials.
61–66	**High School** Will be able to read most patient education materials.

Figure 8–3 *Continued*
See legend on page 181.

health teacher is employing weak measures in the health education program" (Rue, 1944, p. 215). It is important today as in the past for nurses to evaluate health materials before they are disseminated to individuals, families, or the general public. Health materials are intended to strengthen the teaching already done and are meant to be used as an adjunct to health instruction.

An assessment guide for reviewing health materials is shown in Figure 8–4 and can be used when critiquing printed materials; however, nurses can make slight modifications to it when assessing other types of

EXAMPLE 1: PROSTATE CANCER AND TREATMENT OPTIONS

Original text (harder to grasp)
Your doctor has recently communicated to you that you have localized prostate cancer, commonly labeled as Stage I. In addition to managing the anxieties associated with a life-threatening illness, patients must carefully consider the available treatment modalities while taking into account the potential effect each one may have on quality of life. Patients must seriously evaluate the benefits and side effects of each treatment modality and determine the most efficacious one for their lifestyle.

Revised text (easier to grasp)
You have recently been told by your doctor that you have early-stage prostate cancer. Deciding on a treatment is important but hard. Besides dealing with fears that go along with having cancer, you must look at your treatment options.

- Get to know the benefits and the side effects of each treatment.
- Think about how each treatment will affect your life.
- Ask questions.
- Choose the treatment best for you.

EXAMPLE 2: TESTICULAR SELF-EXAMINATION

Version A (Use of passive voice; more complex words; more difficult to grasp)	Version B (Use of active voice, simpler words; easier to grasp)
Performing testicular self-examination can increase the likelihood that any abnormal growths can be located early. Current recommendations state that men should perform this procedure regularly every month after a warm bath or shower. This procedure is not difficult to perform and involves several minutes.	You can increase your chances of finding any growths or lumps early by doing a simple exam called testicular self-exam (TSE). Do TSE once a month after a warm bath or shower. It is easy to do and takes only a few minutes.

health resources (e.g., videotapes, interactive modules). This tool provides a systematic method for reviewing health materials for their appropriateness for the intended target audience. The assessment of materials should focus on the following criteria: format-layout, type, verbal content, visual content, and aesthetic quality.

- **Format-layout**
  - Is the information organized clearly?
  - Are headers or advance organizers used to cue the reader?
  - Is there a 50%-50% allocation of white and black space?
  - Does the information appear easy to read or cluttered?
- **Type**
  - Is the type or font a readable size? (Consider the age of your target group and whether visual difficulties are likely to be present.)
- **Verbal content**
  - Is the information current, accurate, and relevant to the target group?
  - Are difficult terms explained?
  - What is the reading level?
- **Visual content**
  - Are the graphics accurate, current, and relevant to the target group?
  - Is there cuing to aid the reader in connecting the printed words to the pictures?
  - Are the intended meanings of the pictures understood?
  - Do the pictures on the outside of the material reflect the material on the inside?
  - Do the pictures reflect the diversity of the target audience?
- **Aesthetic quality-appeal**
  - Is the material appealing?

- Are there any special features that are helpful (e.g., a glossary, space for notes, and useful telephone numbers)?

Assessment of Reading Level. Part of the assessment of written materials is reading level. A number of formulas are available for estimating the readability grade level of the printed text, including the SMOG readability formula (see Fig. 8–5). Although readability formulas are objective quantitative tools that measure sentence and word variables, they do not take into account factors related to understanding such as motivation, need to know, or experience (Meade and Smith, 1991). They do, however, provide an overall estimate of reading ease and guidelines for assessing and rewriting health information.

Learner Verification. By far, the best way to identify the suitability of materials is to take them directly to the target audience to obtain feedback about how acceptable, understandable, and useful the materials are. The ongoing process of learner verification engages target members in dialogue and helps to uncover unsuitable aspects of the material, whether in content, visuals, or format. Materials should be evaluated by members of the targeted audience during a preproduction phase (Doak, Doak, and Root, 1995).

When the nurse determines that a need exists for the creation of new educational materials, the incorporation of Freirian principles can be helpful in producing empowering products. The Freire approach supports learner participation in the development process, includes the learner as the active subject of the educational experience, and allows learners to define the content and outcomes (Rudd and Comings, 1994; Wallerstein, 1992). Freire's approach focuses on drawing on the people's experiences and ideas and creating themes to address them.

Directions:
Assess your printed material using the following tool. Use the rating scale of 1–4 for each item in a major category: *1=poor, 2=fair, 3=good, 4=very good, N/A = not applicable.* For each category, give it an overall category rating of *(+) effective, (–) not effective, or (X) unsure.*

Name of brochure:_____.

Author:_____.

Intended target audience:_____.

Cost/availability/producer: _____.

Category/criteria	Rating 1 to 4	Overall rating (+) (–) (x)	Comments
Format/layout			
Organizational style	_____		_____
White/black space	_____		_____
Margins	_____		_____
Grouping of elements	_____		_____
Use of headers/advance organizers	_____	_____	_____
Type			
Size	_____		_____
Style	_____		_____
Spacing	_____	_____	_____
Verbal content			
Clarity	_____		_____
Difficulty	_____		_____
Quantity	_____		_____
Relevancy to target group (i.e., age, gender, ethnicity)	_____		_____
Use of active voice	_____		_____
Readability level	_____	grade level _____	_____
Accuracy	_____		_____
Currency	_____	_____	_____

Figure 8–4
Assessment guide for reviewing health materials. (Adapted from Effective Patient Education Materials Workshop, University of Kentucky, 1980.)

Category/criteria	Rating 1 to 4	Overall rating (+) (−) (x)	Comments

Visual content

Tone/mood
Clarity
Cueing
Relevancy to target group
    (i.e., age, gender, ethnicity)
Currency
Accuracy
Detail

Aesthetic quality/appeal

Attractiveness
Color
Quality of production
    space for notes, glossary,
    personalized instructions

Comments:

_____

_____

_____

Overall, based on your scoring of 1 to 4 and an evaluation of its effectiveness with the target audience, how would you rate this educational tool? Circle one.

1 = poor: probably won't work with my target group. I would probably never use it.

2 = fair: has a low likelihood of success with my target group. I would use it rarely and only in combination with other sources.

3 = good: has a good likelihood of being suitable and relevant for about half of my target group. I would use it sometimes.

4 = very good: has a high likelihood of being suitable and relevant for most of my target group. I would most definitely use it!

Figure 8–4 *Continued*
Legend appears on page 184.

SMOG Readability Formula

Directions

- Count off 10 consecutive sentences near the beginning, in the middle, and near the end of the text (total of 30 sentences).

- Circle all polysyllabic words (those containing 3 or more syllables). This includes repetitions of words. Total the number of polysyllabic words.

- Estimate the square root of the total number of polysyllabic words counted. This is done by finding the nearest perfect square and taking its square root.

- Add a constant of 3 to the square root. This number gives the SMOG number, grade, or the reading grade level that a person must have reached to understand the text being evaluated.

Tips:

Count hyphenated words as one word.

Count a sentence as a string of words with a period (.), an exclamation point (!), or a question mark (?).

Count proper nouns.

Count numbers that are written out or, if in numeric form, pronounce them to assess whether they are polysyllabic.

Figure 8–5
SMOG formula for estimating readability grade level of printed text. (Adapted from McLaughlin GH: SMOG grading: a new readability formula. J Reading 12:639–646, 1969, used with permission.) For more detailed information about the application of SMOG formulas, refer to U.S. Department of Health and Human Services publication (1992); for information on other readability formulas, refer to Redman (1994) (see references).

Even though the strategies described here are especially helpful when working with individuals with low literacy, it should be emphasized that people at all literacy levels tend to prefer and understand simply written and concise materials and find materials more motivating when they are relevant to their own perceived learning needs.

SUMMARY

Teaching is a significant component of community health nursing and impacts on virtually every activity in which nurses are involved. The goal of health education is to facilitate a process that allows individuals, families, and groups to make well-informed decisions about their health practices. Inherent in community health education is an understanding of the nature of learning and theoretical frameworks that can help explain behaviors and health actions. No one theory has been shown to explain human behavior; multiple theories and approaches are required.

The success of health education strategies rests largely on nurses being knowledgeable about the social, cultural, political, and environmental forces affecting the health of its community members. Health education, which is relevant for a target group, is based on the consideration of both individual variables as well as social, structural, political, cultural, and economic factors within the larger context of community. The development of relevant teaching interventions is based on a thorough assessment of the target audience members and their characteristics and the use of an organized and systematic approach in the delivery of health messages and programs. The use of social action strategies such as advocating health-promoting lifestyles, creating an environment for problem-posing dialogues with community members, and providing linkages to health resources supports the philosophy of critical consciousness. Nurses can facilitate the principle of social justice by being experts in the delivery of health information while being committed to the creation of empowerment strategies that equip individuals, families, and communities with the knowledge and skills for healthy lifestyles and environments.

Nurses can select from and use a variety of methods, materials, and media to support their health education activities. Such resources should be reviewed and evaluated for their appropriateness for the intended target group. Key to meeting the needs of individuals, families, and communities is embracing the notion that health education is an ongoing interactive process influenced by many internal and external factors. With knowledge, spirit, and a commitment to empowering strategies, nurses can make important contributions to the prevention of disease and promotion of personal and community health.

APPLICATION OF THE NURSING PROCESS

The following case study and teaching plan provide an example of the use of selected teaching approaches for the individual, family, and community and their respective learning needs.

Case Study

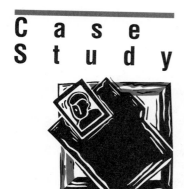

Emma Jackson is a 29-year-old woman who obtains her ongoing health care at a community-based clinic in her neighborhood. She has just seen the nurse practitioner, who confirmed that she is 2 months pregnant. She is married and has a 4-year-old child. Mrs. Jackson tells the nurse that she is a smoker, would like to try to quit, but was unsuccessful in quitting during her last pregnancy. She tells the nurse "I smoke when I get stressed, I have so many things on my mind." Her husband is also a smoker. The nurse refers Mrs. Jackson to the community nursing student (Irene Green) for counseling, education, and follow-up.

Assessment

Irene recognizes that smoking during pregnancy has detrimental effects on the unborn infant and has unhealthy effects directly on Mrs. Jackson and her other child (second-hand smoke) (DiFranza and Lew, 1995; MacLeod and MacLain, 1992). The nurse also knows that smokers often go through stages of readiness in their attempts to quit smoking and that relapse is often part of the process (Prochaska and DiClemente, 1983). She notes that family and community support systems are also important.

The nurse on an individual level assesses Mrs. Jackson's

- Smoking history, pattern, previous quit attempts
- Support systems: family, friends, peers
- Perceived barriers to quitting
- Perceived benefits to quitting
- Perceived priority in addressing this health issue versus other everyday stresses
- Perceived effect of smoking behavior on family communication patterns
- Feelings of confidence in being able to quit

Assessment of other groups includes family, neighborhood, churches, community organizations, and environmental messages that promote smoking cessation.

Diagnosis

Individual

- Ineffective individual coping related to inadequate resources and supportive networks as evidenced by unsuccessful management with stressors
- Decisional conflict (feelings of lack of confidence in ability to quit smoking) related to previous unsuccessful attempts
- Altered health maintenance (tobacco use) in response to personal stressors, lack of knowledge of available resources, and insufficient family and personal support systems
- Health seeking behaviors (wanting to quit smoking) for self and her family

Family

- Potential for altered family processes related to lack of agreement about household smoking patterns

Community

- Inadequate organized smoking cessation programs and initiatives for populations at risk related to lack of economic resources and community-building coalitions

Planning, Goals, and Interventions

Individual
Short-Term Goals

- Mrs. Jackson will recognize that continued smoking is unhealthy for both her and her unborn infant.
- Mrs. Jackson will become aware of ways to enhance her confidence while stopping smoking.
- Mrs. Jackson will identify situations and stressors that influence her smoking patterns.
- Mrs. Jackson will state two strategies to cope with stressful situations.
- Mrs. Jackson will decrease the number of cigarettes smoked.

Long-Term Goal

- Mrs. Jackson will quit smoking.

Planning and interventions involve encouraging the expression of feelings, offering positive reinforcement, helping the patient use adaptive mechanisms to cope, providing culturally and educationally relevant materials and media, and offering appropriate smoking cessation strategies. The nurse can apply the National Cancer Institute's "4 A's" approach to smoking cessation counseling (Ask, Advise, Assist, and Arrange). The nurse offers empowering strategies to help Mrs. Jackson cope not only with smoking cessation attempts but also with identified everyday hassles and stressors. Tailored smoking cessation messages are given along with culturally and educationally appropriate materials. A follow-up plan is initiated and mutually agreed on.

Family
Short-Term Goals

- The Jacksons will acknowledge the benefits of being a smoke-free family.
- Mr. Jackson will recognize the need to quit smoking.
- The Jacksons will recognize the need to support each other in their smoking cessation endeavors.

- Specific supportive actions will be mutually identified and discussed by the Jacksons during the smoking cessation phases.
- The Jacksons will identify another person or network system to enhance support.

Long-Term Goal
- The Jacksons will quit smoking and be a smoke-free family.

Planning and interventions involve the awareness of the need for strong support systems within the home and family. The nurse provides education and counseling aimed at promoting family self-care and recognizes that the husband's support or lack of support needs to be addressed and incorporated into the plan of care. Linkages to community resources are made (e.g., health classes, support groups, networking with other women and men who have quit or are trying to quit) to build Mrs. Jackson's self-confidence and support systems.

Community
Short-Term Goals
- A coalition of community members will be formed to develop and implement policies to support a smoke-free environment.
- A consortium of health care agencies and community-based organizations will recognize the need to develop partnerships with each other in creating smoking cessation strategies to affect the community system.

Long-Term Goals
- The community will support and endorse a smoke-free environment and publicize such efforts through billboards and other media.
- Community agencies and organizations will integrate smoking cessation programs and messages into their other health-related activities.
- Cigarette advertising will be eliminated.

Planning and interventions are carried out on an aggregate level to identify key community leaders, agencies, legislators, and lay members who are committed to tackling smoking cessation initiatives at a sociopolitical level (e.g., producing counter-billboard advertising, creating smoking cessation initiatives at various channels within the community). The development of program initiatives are based on assisting community members to define the issues and the solutions to the effects of smoking on individual, family, and community groups. The development of coalitions and partnerships among community-based organizations, health care groups, governmental agencies, and target audience members is key through dialogue and consciousness raising.

Evaluation

Evaluation is a systematic and continuous process focused on the individual as well as the family and community.

Individual
- An evaluation of Mrs. Jackson's smoking habits is made at points of contact within the health system and within the community (e.g., clinics, WIC). Both process (number of cigarettes cut down to) and outcome (quit or not quit) endpoints are addressed.

- Increases in Mrs. Jackson's coping skills and support systems are evident when evaluating her personalized care plan.
- Smoking cessation messages have been tailored to Mrs. Jackson.
- Follow-up (telephone, letter, in-person visit) with Mrs. Jackson is carried out.

Family

- Development of family or significant other patterns of support for smoking cessation initiatives were included in plans of care.
- Family health patterns were assessed. Screenings for at-risk behaviors were offered to families.
- Family communication patterns and support have been identified and are addressed in care plan.

Community

- Smoking cessation programs and smoking prevention initiatives have been introduced to at least two channels (e.g., churches, schools, work sites, community-based organizations).
- Smoking cessation messages are infused throughout the community and evidenced on radio, television, and billboards.
- Community task forces and coalitions are present that demonstrate a collaborative partnership among lay members, community leaders, organizers, and legislators to address smoking-related health issues.

Learning Activities

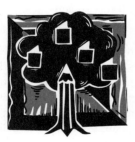

1. In groups of two to four students, describe the utility of theoretical frameworks in helping to explain health behaviors. Identify strengths and limitations of using models that are focused on individual determinants of health versus models that encompass sociopolitical factors.

2. Identify a specific target group with which you are working in the community. Describe their characteristics and identify the methods used for obtaining these data.

3. Select an aggregate (e.g., students, pregnant women, preschoolers, homeless). Describe how you would apply Freire's model of empowerment education to address health issues (identify with community members, develop generative themes, and prioritize their view of the problems).

4. Select a health education brochure, and apply the assessment criteria for evaluating its relevancy for a selected target audience. Evaluate the relative strengths of the printed material and potential areas for improvement.

5. Review the electronic or printed media in your community (television, radio, or newspaper) for the identification of health issues of concern (closing of hospital or clinic, smoking bans in restaurants). Discuss sociopolitical issues that impact this health issue. Outline specific activities and roles in which the nurse in the community can engage to educate people regarding the health issue.

REFERENCES

Airhihenbuwa CO: Health promotion and the discourse on culture: Implications for empowerment. Health Educ Q 21:345–353, 1994.

Alterman AI, Baughman TG: Videotape versus computer interactive education in alcoholic and non alcoholic controls. Alcoholism Clin Exp Res 15:39–44, 1991.

American Hospital Association: A patient's bill of rights. Chicago, AHA, 1972.

American Management Association: Fifth annual multicultural forum: Gaining the competitive edge. New York: American Management Association, 1993.

American Nurses Association: The professional nurse and health education. Kansas City, MO, ANA, 1975.

Anderson E, McFarlane J, Helton A: Community-as-client: A model for practice. Nurs Outlook 34:220–224, 1986.

Armstrong ML: Orchestrating the process of patient education: Methods and approaches. Nurs Clin North Am 224:597–604, 1989.

Babcock DE, Miller MA: Client education: Theory and practice. St. Louis, CV Mosby, 1994.

Bandura A: Self-efficacy: Toward a unifying theory of behavioral change. Psych Rev 84:191–215, 1977a.

Bandura A: Social Learning Theory. Englewood Cliffs, NJ, Prentice-Hall, 1977b.

Becker MH (ed): The Health Belief Model and Personal Health Behavior. Thorofare, NJ, Charles B. Slack, 1974.

Becker MH, Maiman LA, Kirscht JP, et al.: The health belief model and prediction of dietary compliance: A field experiment. J Health Social Behav 18:348–366, 1977.

Bernstein E, Wallerstein N, Braithwaite R, et al.: Empowerment forum: A dialogue between guest editorial board members. Health Educ Q 21:281–294, 1994.

Bigge ML: Learning Theories for Teachers, 4th ed. New York, Harper & Row, 1982.

Breckon DJ, Harvey JR, Lancaster RB: Community Health Education: Settings, Roles, and Skills for the 21st Century, 3rd ed. Gaithersburg, MD, Aspen 1994.

Braithwaite RL, Bianchi C, Taylor SE: Ethnographic approach to community organization and health empowerment. Health Educ Q 21:407–416, 1994.

Butterfield PG: Thinking upstream: Nurturing a conceptual understanding of the societal context of health behavior. In Saucier KA (ed). Perspectives in Family and Community Health. St. Louis: CV Mosby, 1990, pp. 66–71.

Campbell MK, DeVelis BM, Stretcher VJ, et al.: Improving dietary behavior: The effectiveness of tailored messages in primary care settings. Am J Public Health 84:783–787, 1994.

Clark MJ: The health education process. In Clark MJ (ed). Nursing in the Community. East Norwalk, CT, Appleton & Lange, 1992, pp. 126–141.

Davis L, Dumas R, Ferketich S, et al.: AAN Expert Panel report on culturally competent health care. Nurs Outlook 40:277–283, 1992.

Davis TC, Long SW, Jackson RH, et al.: Rapid estimate of adult literacy in medicine: A shortened screening instrument. Fam Med 25:56–57, 1993.

DiFranza JR, Lew RA: Effect of maternal cigarette smoking on pregnancy complications and sudden infant death syndrome. J Fam Pract 40:385–394, 1995.

Doak LG, Doak CC, Meade CD: Strategies to develop effective cancer education materials. Oncol Nurs Forum 23:1305–1312, 1995.

Doak CC, Doak LG, Root JH: Teaching Patients with Low Literacy Skills. Philadelphia, JB Lippincott, 1995.

Duryea EJ. Decision making and health education. J School Health 53:29, 1983.

Educational Testing Service: Adult Literacy in America: A First Look at the Results of the National Adult Literacy Survey Washington, DC, Office of Educational Research and Improvement, US Department of Education, 1993.

Eisen A: Survey of neighborhood-based, comprehensive community empowerment initiatives. Health Educ Q 21:235–252, 1994.

Freire P: Pedagogy of the oppressed. New York, Herder and Herder, 1970. Translated from original manuscript, 1968.

Freire P: Education for Critical Consciousness. New York, Seabury Press, 1973.

Gagliano ME: A literature review on the efficacy of video in patient education. J Med Educ 63:785–792, 1988.

Gardner MS: Public Health Nursing, 3rd ed. New York, MacMillan, 1936, p. 3.

Gillis AJ: Determinants of a health-promoting lifestyle: An integrative review. J Adv Nurs 18:345–353, 1993.

Glanz K, Lewis FM, Rimer BK (eds): Health Behavior and Health Education. San Francisco, Jossey-Bass, 1990.

Green L: Introduction to behavior change and maintenance: Theory and measurement. In Shumacker S, Schon E, Ockene J (eds). The Handbook of Health Behavior Change. New York: Springer, 1990, pp. 1–3.

Green LW, Kreuter MW: Health Promotion Planning: An Educational and Environmental Approach, 2nd ed. Mountain View, CA, Mayfield, 1991.

Hall TL: Designing culturally relevant educational materials for Mexican American clients. Diabetes Educ 13:281–285, 1988.

Hochbaum GM: Public participation in medical screening programs: A sociopsychological study (Public Health Service Publication No. 572). Washington, DC, Government Printing Office, 1958.

Israel BA, Checkoway B, Schulz A, Zimmerman M: Health education and community empowerment: Conceptualizing and measuring perceptions of individual, organizational, and community control. Health Educ Q 32:149–170, 1994.

Janz NK, Becker MH: The health belief model: A decade later. Health Educ Q 11:1–47, 1984.

Jastak S, Wilkinson GS: The Wide-Range Achievement Test III: Revised Administration Manual. Wilmington, DE, Jastak Associates, 1993.

Jemmott LS, Jemmott JB: Increasing condom-use intentions among sexually active Black adolescent women. Nurs Res 41:273–279, 1992.

Jezewski MA: Culture brokering as a model for advocacy. Nurs Health Care 14:78–85, 1993.

Joint Commission on Accreditation of Healthcare Organizations: 1996 Accreditation Manual for Hospitals. Vol. 1. Oak Brook, IL, JCAHO, 1995.

Keck CW: Community health: Our common challenge. Fam Commun Health 172:1–9, 1994.

Kendall J: Fighting back: Promoting emancipatory nursing actions. Adv Nurs Sci 15:1–15, 1992.

Kegeles SS, Kirscht JP, Haefner DP, Rosenstock IM: Survey of beliefs about cancer detection and papanicolaou tests. Public Health Rep 80:815–823, 1965.

Kleinman A: Concepts and a model for the comparison of medical systems as cultural systems. Social Sci Med 12:85–93, 1978.

Kuehnert PL: The interactive and organizational model of community as client: A model for public health nursing practice. Public Health Nurs 12:9–17, 1995.

Knowles MS: The Making of an Adult Educator: An Autobiographical Journey. San Francisco, Jossey-Bass, 1989.

Knowles MS: The Modern Practice of Adult Education: From Pedagogy to Andragogy. Chicago, Association Press/Follett, 1980.

Labonte R: Health promotion and empowerment: Reflections on professional practice. Health Educ Q 21:253–268, 1994.

Lancaster J: Education models and principles applied to community health nursing. In Stanhope M, Lancaster J (eds). Community

Health Nursing Process and Practice for Promoting Health, 3rd ed. St. Louis, CV, Mosby, 1992, pp. 180–199.

Ledbetter C, Hall S, Swanson J, Forrest K: Readability of commercial versus generic health instructions for condoms. Health Care Women Int 11:295–304, 1990.

Lewin K: The conceptual representation and the measurement of psychological forces. Durham, NC, Duke University Press, 1938.

Lundeen S, Friedbacher B: Healthy families/healthy children initiative: A report to the Helen Bader Foundation. Milwaukee, WI, University of Wisconsin—Milwaukee School of Nursing, 1993.

MacLeod C, MacLain K: The effects of smoking in pregnancy: A review of effects of approaches to behavioral change. Midwifery 8:19–30, 1992.

Maslow AH: Motivation and Personality, 2nd ed. New York, Harper & Row, 1970.

McFarland J, Fehir J: De madres a madres: A community, primary health care program based on empowerment. Health Educ Q 21:381–394, 1994.

Meade CD: Approaching the media with confidence. Public Health Nurs 9:209–214, 1992.

Meade CD, Byrd JC: Patient literacy and the readability of smoking education literature. Am J Public Health 79:204–206, 1989.

Meade CD, Byrd JC, Lee M: Improving patient comprehension of literature on smoking. Am J Public Health 79:1411–1412, 1989.

Meade CD, McKinney WP, Barnas G: Educating patients with limited literacy skills: The effectiveness of printed and video-taped materials about colon cancer. Am J Public Health 84:119–121, 1994.

Meade CD, Diekmann J, Thornhill D: Readability of American Cancer Society patient education literature. Onc Nurs Forum 19:51–55, 1992.

Meade CD, Smith CF: Readability formulas: Cautions and criteria. Patient Educ Counseling 17:153–158, 1991.

Michielutte R, Bahnson J, Dignan MB, Schroeder EM: The use of illustrations and narrative text style to improve readability of a health education brochure. J Cancer Educ 7:251–260, 1992.

Milio N: Promoting Health Through Public Policy. Philadelphia, FA Davis, 1981.

Minkler M: Improving health through community organization. In Glanz K, Lewis K, and Rimer BK (eds). Health Behavior and Education. San Francisco, Jossey-Bass, 1990, pp. 257–287.

Nightingale F: Notes on Nursing. New York, Appleton-Century Crofts, 1859.

Padilla GV, Bulcavage LM: Theories used in patient/health education. Semin Oncol Nurs 7:87–96, 1991.

Pavlov IP: Experimental Psychology, and Other Essays. New York, Philosophical Library, 1957.

Pender NJ: Health Promotion in Nursing Practice, 2nd ed. Los Altos, CA, Appleton & Lange, 1987.

Piaget J: Adaptation and Intelligence: Organic Selection and Phenocopy. Chicago, University of Chicago, 1980.

Plimpton S, Root J: Materials and strategies that work in low literacy health communication. Public Health Rep 109:86–92, 1994.

Prochaska JO, DiClemente CC: Stages and processes of self-change of smoking: Toward an integrative model of change. J Consult Clin Psychol 51:390–395, 1983.

Rankin SH, Stallings KD: Patient Education: Issues, Principles, Practices, 2nd ed. Philadelphia, JB Lippincott, 1990.

Redman BK: The Process of Patient Education, 7th ed. St. Louis, CV Mosby, 1994.

Robertson A, Minkler M: New health promotion movement: A critical examination. Health Educ Q 21:295–312, 1994.

Rogers CR: A Carl Rogers Reader. Boston, Houghton Mifflin, 1989.

Rosenstock I: Why people use health services. Milbank Memorial Fund Q 44:94–127, 1966.

Rosenstock IM, Strecher VJ, Becker MH: Social learning theory and the health belief model. Health Educ Q 15:175–183, 1988.

Rudd RE, Comings JP: Learner developed materials: An empowering product. Health Ed Q 21:313–327, 1994.

Rue CB: The Public Health Nurse in the Community. Philadelphia, WB Saunders, 1944.

Shalala DE: Nursing and society: The unfinished agenda for the 21st century. Nurs Health Care 14:289–291, 1993.

Skinner BF: About Behaviorism. New York, Knopf, 1974.

Skinner CS, Strecher VJ, Hospers H: Physician's recommendations for mammography: Do tailored messages make a difference? Am J Public Health 84:43–49, 1994.

Spellbring AM: Nursing's role in health promotion. Nurs Clin North Am 26:805–813, 1991.

Stanton M: Health education. In Bullough B, Bullough V (eds). Nursing in the Community. St. Louis, CV Mosby, 1990, pp. 104–125.

Steuart GW, Kark SO: A practice of social medicine: A South African Team's Experiences in Different African Communities. Edinburgh, Livingstone, 1962.

Strecher VJ, DeVellis BM, Becker MH, et al.: The role of self-efficacy in achieving health behavior change. Health Educ Q 13:73–92, 1986.

Streiff L: Can clients understand our instruction? Image: J Nurs Scholar 18:24–52, 1986.

Swanson JM, Forest K, Ledbetter C, et al.: Readability of commercial and generic contraceptive instructions. Image: J Nurs Scholar 22:96–100, 1990.

Thorndike EL: Educational Psychology. New York: Arno Press, 1969.

Tripp-Reimer T, Afifa LA: Cross-cultural perspectives on patient teaching. Nurs Clin North Am 24:613–619, 1989.

U.S. Department of Health and Human Services, Public Health Services. Healthy people 2000: National health promotion and disease prevention objectives 1991 (Publication No. PHS 91-50212). Washington, DC, U.S. Government Printing Office, 1991.

U.S. Department of Health Human Services: Making health communication programs work (NIH publication No. 92-1493). Bethesda, MD, Office of Cancer Communications, National Cancer Institute, 1992.

Wallerstein N: Health and safety education for workers with low-literacy or limited English skills. Am J Industrial Med 22:751–765, 1992.

Wallerstein N, Bernstein E: Introduction to community empowerment, participatory education, and health. Health Educ Q 21:141–148, 1994.

Wallerstein N, Bernstein E: Empowerment education: Freire's ideas adapted to health education. Health Educ Q 15:379–394, 1988.

Wang C, Burris MA: Empowerment through photo novella: Portraits of participation. Health Educ Q 21:171–186, 1994.

Weiss BD, Hart G, McGee DL, D'Estelle S: Health status of illiterate adults: Relationship between literacy and health status among persons with low literacy skills. J Am Board Fam Practice 5:257–264, 1992.

Wells JA, Ruscavage D, Parker B, McArthur L: Literacy of women attending family planning clinics in Virginia and reading levels of brochures on HIV prevention Fam Plan Perspect 26:113–131, 1994.

Wertheimer M: Productive Thinking. New York, Harper, 1959.

World Health Organization: Health Promotion and Community Action in Developing Countries. Geneva, UHO, 1994.

Policy, Politics, Legislation, and Public Health Nursing

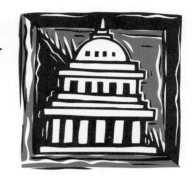

Upon completion of this chapter, the reader will be able to:

1. **Describe the role nurses have played in influencing the public's health through policy development.**

2. **Analyze public policy as the critical basis for protecting the public's health.**

3. **Identify the legislative process involved in establishing state or federal health policy.**

4. **Identify the political processes that influence health policy development.**

5. **Discuss political activities through which nurses can affect the health policies of their community and country.**

Ruth F. Stewart

Acknowledgment is given to Madalon O'Rawe Amenta for contributions to this Chapter.

Policy, politics, and legislation are the forces that determine the direction of public health programs at every level of government. These programs are critical to the health and well-being of the nation and of every individual. Public health, however, lacks the drama of highly technical medical "cures" and thus requires continual and dedicated efforts to ensure population-focused health protection and promotion.

POLITICS: THE SCIENCE OF GOVERNMENT

Dictionary definitions of politics refer to it as the science of government: the policies and aims of a nation, state, or other institution. The common elements in all of the definitions are power, capacity to influence, and authority in interpersonal or intergroup relationships. We also commonly recognize the allocation of always-scarce resources as a function of politics.

Because resources are finite, the process of deciding who gets what, when, where, and how is critical to all groups, whether personal, professional, or societal. In a family with teenagers, a decision has to be made about who will get the car for the evening. In a community health nursing agency, decisions about continuing education opportunities, student preceptoring, salary increases, and promotion possibilities have to be made. In any work setting, there is continuous allocation of time, money, human resources, equipment, and supplies, and conflict inevitably arises among those competing to control them. Politics, influenced by the balance of power, determines the outcomes. According to Donna Diers, "politics is the use of power for change" (Diers, 1985).

Politics and legislation are processes through which sound public health policies can be instituted. In this chapter I describe the interrelationships of these and the importance of nurses' efforts in these processes.

NURSES WHO MADE A DIFFERENCE

Two stories of political action by nurses are related in this chapter. One story is famous, that of Florence Nightingale and her care of British foot soldiers in the Crimea in the mid-1800s. The other concerns a contemporary nurse who worked with Hispanic fami-lies living along Luckey Road in Monaco, Texas, more than 100 years later. In each case, a nurse effectively used the political process to improve health conditions for clients. Nightingale's well-known sanitary reforms at Scutari saved thousands of lives. Carrie Long, a nursing student in Texas, acted to depollute the water supply and sewage disposal along Luckey Road, thus potentially reducing the risk of enteric infection.

Florence Nightingale

The appointment of a woman to the position of superintendent of the nursing staff by the secretary of the British Army, Sir Sidney Herbert, was a radical move in the 1850s. He made the appointment in response to reports in *The London Times* that "the soldiers in Crimea die without the slightest effort to save them . . . [and the] sick appear to be tended by the sick, and the dying by the dying" (Kalisch and Kalisch, 1978). In contrast, French troops fighting alongside their British allies were being admirably nursed by the Sisters of Charity.

Sir Sidney realized the need for drastic action and thought immediately and only of Nightingale, whose ability and commitment to nursing were widely recognized.

Although he knew Parliament would oppose sending women into the war zone, he took the risk and invited Nightingale to organize and supervise a nursing service for the wounded and ill soldiers. She readily accepted.

Nightingale recruited a group of 38 nurses and immediately went to Turkey. The situation they found at Scutari was, if anything, worse than that described. The Barrack Hospital was filthy, vermin ridden, and overcrowded, with 3000 to 4000 men occupying a space suitable for half that number. It was not surprising, therefore, that three fourths of the wounded soldiers contracted cholera, dysentery, and typhoid fever as a result of being hospitalized, not as a result of battlefield conditions.

Although the soldiers worshipped Nightingale, military and government officials blocked her efforts at every turn. The medical officers not only resisted the intrusion of the nurses but on a deeper level also resented the implication of incompetence that was inherent in Nightingale's proposed reforms. Although few of them cooperated with her, she persisted. Because she was from a wealthy and politically active family, she used her personal resources and influence in London to obtain food, dressings, and other necessary supplies. When the "Nightingale Nurses" arrived, 60% of the patients were dying. At the end of the war, the mortality rate was reduced to slightly greater than 1% (Kalisch and Kalisch, 1978).

This dramatic change was wrought not by a miracle but rather by Nightingale, and her nurses, counteracting neglect and outright sabotage through the canny use of power. She wielded great power through her wealthy family and politically powerful friends. After the war, she achieved power in her own right as a result of the extraordinary recognition accorded her by the British public for her humanitarian work at Scutari.

Carrie Long

Luckey Road in Monaco, Texas, had not been lucky for the people who shared the development built there by a contractor with an eye on a quick cash return. The boxlike wooden houses on small plots of land appealed to people seeking reasonably priced housing for their families. The contracts of sale required no down payment and offered several poor Hispanic families a means to realize their dream of owning a home.

These families were pleased to have electricity, running water, and indoor flush toilets. At first, they did not worry that their sewage drained into an open pit behind each house into which children or animals might fall. Nor did they realize that the hazards of this pit included the danger of acute and protracted infections and, perhaps, death.

These hazards were recognized, however, by Carrie Long, a student in a university community health nursing course who was working with the Saenz family. While doing the family assessment, she asked Mrs. Saenz about the household sewage disposal. She thought she had misunderstood when told it drained into "a hole in the back" but knew that she had heard correctly when she visited the yard. Outside she found a 3 × 4-foot pit filled to the brim with raw sewage. Mrs. Saenz explained that it was not always so full; recent rains had raised the level.

Further data collected from neighbors confirmed that not only was this sewage situation common but that there also were other problems. One family was transporting household water from 10 miles away because they could not get it piped into their house from the rural water supply. None of the families knew who was responsible for repairs and upkeep in the development. All they were sure of was where to mail the monthly payments: a lumber company's post office box. Only one family held a deed to their property.

Knowing that the problem was potentially explosive, Carrie began carefully collecting more data. She confirmed that Texas state law requires approved septic tanks for households in such rural areas and that the county health department has enforcement authority. Her companion concern, however, was that the families might be evicted and their plight made even worse if action were taken against the owners.

Carrie and two classmates had scheduled earlier, as part of their student project, a meeting with the county (administrative) judge to discuss health services and needs from the viewpoint of an elected official. During this meeting, she brought up the Luckey Road problems and showed the judge pictures of the open-pit sewage. The pictures were "worth a thousand words." On seeing it, the judge expressed rage that such conditions existed within the county.

In discussing the situation, Carrie stressed her concern that the families not be evicted or harassed by the owners. They agreed that this would be a prime consideration in any corrective action. The judge asked for Carrie's cooperation and, after a conference with her instructor, she agreed to help.

Once Carrie began working with the officials by providing the necessary names and addresses, the judge's office swung into action. They contacted the county health and the public works departments. The judge called on the media to raise public interest and support. A television miniseries exposé was planned, with Carrie acting as liaison to the Luckey Road families. Because she suspected that her position as an "outsider" would hamper efforts to convince the families of her sincerity, she approached Don Martinez, a local leader who was well known for his strong religious convictions and commitment to helping others. Once aware of the situation, Mr. Martinez, better known as "Deacon," agreed to help.

In an effort to gather more information, the pair made house-to-house visits. Not only did they gain the cooperation of many neighborhood families, but some families agreed to describe their plight for the television production and to allow filming in and around their houses.

It was on this round of visits that Carrie met the Culebra family. Mr. Culebra's reaction to inquiries about sewage disposal was explosive, leaving no question about his anger and frustration. This family had to transport all water for household use 10 miles. Their water pipes, intact and laid to the road where the water main passed in front of the house, had been disconnected before they purchased the home. All efforts to get them reconnected, whether through assistance from the developer or the rural water board, had come to a dead end.

Mr. Culebra was especially upset because his wife had just returned from the hospital after having surgery, and she had to irrigate her drainage tubes twice daily. He was so angry that he reverted to Spanish during the conversation. Mr. Culebra agreed to tell his story on television.

Unfortunately, instead of arousing public concern, the television exposé failed miserably. Because the original investigative reporter had been subpoenaed in a court case at the same time that filming was scheduled, a substitute was assigned. The new reporter was not interested in the situation, let alone in portraying it sympathetically. He had the camera-person film a few shots of the Culebra's yard and open pit but refused to go inside. Mr. Culebra was offended, later telling Carrie that the reporter thought "he was too good to go into a Hispanic's house."

The story that appeared on the evening news was a brief clip of the Culebra yard and pit, with Carrie describing the health implications. Public response was negligible. The program did, however, attract the attention of two affluent community members, who told Carrie to "lay off" because sewage improvements would generate higher taxes.

To counter this argument, Carrie went to the county hospital for information. She learned that the amount of tax money spent for a 3-day hospital stay of one infant with severe diarrhea or one adult with surgical wound infection could be as high, if not higher, than the cost of installation of a septic tank. She learned that preventive health measures are a sound financial as well as human investment for society.

The judge's efforts with the health and the public works departments met with somewhat more success, a result of his legitimate power in county administration. Engineers, sanitarians, and others evaluated the situation and verified official records relating to the housing development. On one visit to the neighborhood, Carrie by chance met several of the public health inspectors. They were not eager to be involved and told her emphatically that any attempt to change conditions would be futile. She believed that they resented the meddling of nurses in their domain.

The inspectors' report nevertheless objectively and comprehensively documented the problems. Bureaucratic response outlining corrective action was slow, but there has been progress. The interest and support of Carrie and her nursing colleagues sustain hope for the Luckey Road residents that improvements will occur.

POWER: THE KEY TO CHANGE

Despite the common notion that power is inherently evil, it is, in reality, neutral. It attains value only in context. Power is the ability to change the behavior of others in desired ways, the ability to influence what others do, or, conversely, the ability to cause others to stop doing something. Parent power socializes worthy citizens; gang power promotes delinquent behavior. The term *power of the press* denotes the media's strong impact on thinking and, hence, behavior. The source of empowerment for any person or agency is its position or potential as perceived by others.

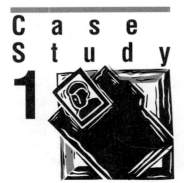

Case Study 1

Assessment

Carrie Long observed that open cesspools rather than adequate waste disposal existed in backyards of homes. She interviewed family and community members, who lacked awareness of the potential danger and hazards to health and affirmed that no action had been taken by individuals, families, or the greater community to remedy the situation. The cesspools were located where people could fall into them. The nurse confirmed that state law required approved septic tanks in rural areas and that enforcement authority was the county health department. She verified that preventive measures are more cost effective than a hospital stay for gastrointestinal disease or a wound infection.

Diagnosis

Individual
- Potential for injury related to open sewage pits
- Potential for infection related to open pits containing human waste

Family
- Impaired home maintenance management related to accumulated wastes
- Ineffective family coping related to stress resulting from care of injured or ill family members

Community
- Decreased ability to communicate because of imbalances in power between home buyers and contractor; at risk for community dysfunction resulting from inadequate systematic channels for linking families in potential crises to community resources
- At risk of environmental hazards because of inadequate inspection of new housing units by county authorities

Planning

Individual
- Children and adults need to avoid pits

Family
- Education, mutual goal setting, and collaboration will result in the family identifying hazards and using collective activity and support to eliminate hazards

Community
- Dissemination to individuals, families, informal and formal leaders, and public officials in the community about the existence of the environmental hazards
- Dissemination of information that standard public health polices exist to protect the public at large from the consequences of these hazards
- Coordination of efforts to bring pressure onto perpetrators of hazardous conditions and public officials responsible for taking action to eliminate hazards

Intervention

- Education and lobbying of individuals, families, and community members, including informal and formal leaders, politicians, health officials, and citizens, through the media regarding threat to health from environmental hazards in housing
- Follow-through with community members until corrective action is initiated

Evaluation

- Feedback from individuals, families, and community, including informal and formal leaders, politicians, health officials, and citizens, regarding knowledge and understanding of potential for injury and illness from environmental hazards

- Degree of coordination of efforts to bring pressure onto perpetrators of hazards to correct situation
- Outcomes of efforts taken for corrective action

LEVELS OF PREVENTION

Primary

- Assessment, teaching, and referral related to prevention of accidents and infection related to environmental hazard

Secondary

- Screening for signs of infection and risk factors related to accident-prone behavior and environment
- Pressuring health officials to inspect all new housing developments adequately

Tertiary

- Coordinate processes that lead to correction of environmental hazard

NURSES: AGENTS OF CHANGE

Although historically nurses have been recognized as a necessary resource during wars and other emergencies, since the 1950s all levels of government have begun to consider nurses indispensable in ordinary times (Aiken, 1982). The public now also recognizes nurses as necessary and valued national resources. In

---

Table 9–1
Sources for Legislative Information

Government Level	Information Available	Location
Federal	Background of members of Congress, committee assignments, terms of service	*Congressional Directory,* Government, Documents section of selected public or university libraries
	Congressional news, vote tabulations	*Congressional Quarterly Weekly Report,* Government Documents section of selected public or university libraries
	Bills in process or legislated (bill number needed)	U.S. Congressperson U.S. Senator (may have local office)
	Health and nursing issues in U.S. Congress; American Nurses Association political action committee *(The American Nurse)*	American Nurses Association 600 Maryland Ave, SW Suite 100 Washington, DC 20024 (202) 554-4444
	Public health issues in U.S. Congress *(The Nation's Health)*	American Public Health Association 1015 15th St. NW Washington, DC 20005 (202) 789-5600
State	Bills in process or legislated (bill number needed)	State representative State senator (may have local office)
	Health and nursing issues in state legislature; state political action committees for nursing	State nurses association; for location, see *American Journal of Nursing* April directory issue

Table 9–2
Sources for Electoral Information

Government Level	Information Available	Location
State	State government operations Political subdivisions Legislative information telephone number State election laws and procedures Campaign finance reports	Secretary of state, state capitol Alaska and Hawaii, office of lieutenant governor, state capitol
County, municipal	Similar to above as appropriate to local government Political jurisdictions for each household address	County clerk, county court house, city clerk, city hall
General	Government information Political jurisdictions for each household address Names of current office holders in local jurisdictions	League of Women Voters 1730 M Street, NW Washington, DC 20036 (202) 429-1965 Telephone directory (major cities)

their advocacy role, nurses are seen as professionals whose knowledge, skill, and concern are used to promote society's well-being through a disciplined change process.

Because of their unique status in the lives of patients, because they are interpreters of the health care system to the public, and because their most basic professional activities are profoundly influenced by government-funded programs, public health nurses must know how to participate in the political process. To do this effectively, they need a sound knowledge of community, state, and national government organization and function and a clear understanding of how they interact as a system. They must know how to influence the creation of health care legislation and how to contribute to the election and appointment of key officials. In addition, because policy is fundamental to governance, they need to know about the formulation of public policy and the acts of government and its agencies (Tables 9–1 and 9–2).

PUBLIC POLICY: BLUEPRINT FOR GOVERNANCE

Policy deals with values. It treats the "shoulds" of a situation (Diers, 1985). Policy articulates the guiding principles of collective endeavors, establishes direction, and sets goals. It influences and, in turn, is influenced by politics. Through the political process, policy directives may become realized or obstructed at any step along the way.

Policy Formulation: The Ideal

In ideal circumstances, health care policy would be created by duly authorized bodies that would rationally—on the basis of valid evidence or data—determine what should be done. These groups would decide what is right and then develop the political strategies to effect the desired outcomes (Diers, 1985). The question of whether a particular policy is advocated or adopted would depend on the degree that a group or the society as a whole might benefit without harm or detriment to subgroups (Spradley, 1985). Of all the seemingly limitless factors that might influence policy formation, group need and group demand should be the strongest determinants. The premises supporting the goals of health policy should be equitable distribution of services and the assurance that the appropriate care is given to the right people, at the right time, and at a reasonable cost.

Policy Formulation: In the Real World

Real world policy for health care, alternatively, exemplifies both conflict and social change theories. It is the product of a continuous interactive process in which "interested" professionals, citizens, institutions, and other groups compete with each other for the attention of various branches of government (Aiken, 1982). The most obvious and prominent among these is the legislative branch, although policy is also made through executive orders, regulatory mechanisms, and court decisions. It may also issue from the recommendations of fact-finding commissions established by the legislative or executive branch. Occasionally, policy derives from formal planning. Sometimes, policy is created in the private sector. This occurs when private foundations mount demonstration projects in obvious areas of need (e.g., the homeless, high-risk adolescents) and, on the basis of the findings, official bodies act (Diers, 1985).

EXAMPLE OF HEALTH POLICY FORMULATION IN THE UNITED STATES

The National Health Planning and Resource Development Act of 1974 (PL 93-641) was a major step in the direction of the statement of a coherent health policy for the United States. After almost 50 years of advocacy on the part of various health care, business, and citizen groups, health planning finally was placed on the agenda. The law created a national network of local, regional, and state health planning organizations called health systems agencies and incorporated the certificate-of-need process (Diers, 1985). This policy initiative was short lived, however, because during the 1980s the Reagan administration encouraged competition within the health care system. The emphasis on cost shifting and reductions, as well as cuts in federal funding "dealt a death blow" to federal health planning (Morgan, Burbank and Godfrey, 1993). This notable beginning was not only the first but also remains the last such example of comprehensive health planning for this country.

Health policy is rarely created through discrete, momentous determinations in relation to single problems or issues (Aiken, 1982). Most often, it evolves slowly and incrementally as an accumulation of many small decisions. It also changes slowly because changes in the social beliefs and values that underlie established policy develop within the context of actual service delivery. Most often, once a direct health care service is offered, especially an official, tax-funded

service, it is difficult to discontinue it. Existing programs create tradition by establishing vested interest or a sense of entitlement on the part of the public or the recipients of the service as well as on the part of a bureaucracy that invests itself not only in the delivery of the service but also in its own jobs, status, and income. This "tradition" also, in a natural effort at self-preservation, exerts political influence (Spradley, 1985).

Steps in Policy Formulation

The tangible formulation of public policy begins with the most critical step: defining the problem and then "getting it on the agenda" (Aiken, 1982; Diers, 1985). The next step is the commitment of resources, most often, as indicated previously, through the passage of legislation. Then, a regulatory schedule for the implementation of the law into program is formulated; finally, an evaluation process is designed that satisfies both regulatory and legislative remedies should they be needed (Aiken, 1982).

Policy Analysis

Unlike advocacy, which is subjective, analysis of health policy is an objective process that identifies both the sources and consequences of decisions in the context of the factors that influence them (Spradley, 1985). Health policy analysis identifies those who benefit and those who experience a loss as the result of a policy (Fig. 9–1). These considerations are critical to ensure health policies that are fair to all those affected.

President Clinton's attempt to reform health care reflects ethical and practical considerations for a national health policy. The fundamental principle was access to health care for all Americans. Those benefiting would be the American public, both as consumers of health care as well as payors for health care through tax-supported and insurance programs. On the other side were those envisioning major financial losses from the proposed changes. Among these, the insurance industry was a dominant antagonist, with some provider groups joining the opposition forces.

The public, the targeted beneficiaries, were confused by the complexity of the issues and thus wary of change. This effort to make an overdue change in health care policy was doomed to failure.

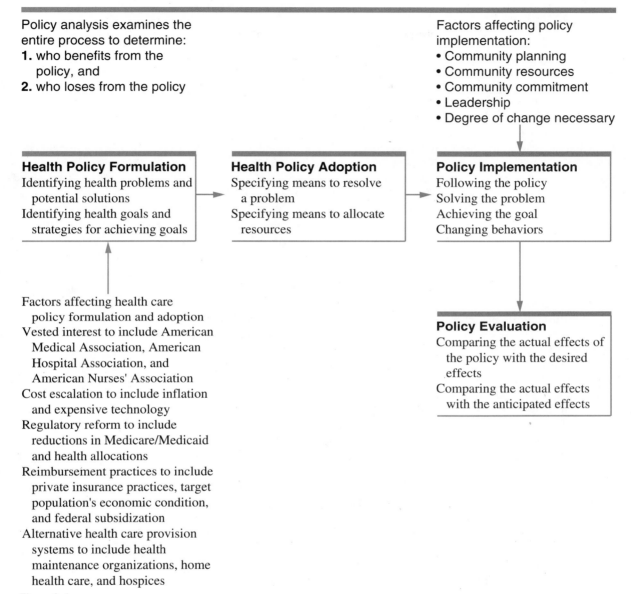

Policy analysis examines the entire process to determine:
1. who benefits from the policy, and
2. who loses from the policy

Factors affecting policy implementation:
• Community planning
• Community resources
• Community commitment
• Leadership
• Degree of change necessary

Health Policy Formulation
Identifying health problems and potential solutions
Identifying health goals and strategies for achieving goals

Health Policy Adoption
Specifying means to resolve a problem
Specifying means to allocate resources

Policy Implementation
Following the policy
Solving the problem
Achieving the goal
Changing behaviors

Factors affecting health care policy formulation and adoption
Vested interest to include American Medical Association, American Hospital Association, and American Nurses' Association
Cost escalation to include inflation and expensive technology
Regulatory reform to include reductions in Medicare/Medicaid and health allocations
Reimbursement practices to include private insurance practices, target population's economic condition, and federal subsidization
Alternative health care provision systems to include health maintenance organizations, home health care, and hospices

Policy Evaluation
Comparing the actual effects of the policy with the desired effects
Comparing the actual effects with the anticipated effects

Figure 9–1
Policy analysis model. (Redrawn from Spradley B: Community Health Nursing, 2nd ed. Boston, Little, Brown, 1985, p 589.)

HEALTH CARE REFORM AND THE NURSING AGENDA

Few nurses will argue that the health-illness system in this country needs revamping. In virtually every practice arena, nurses see all too clearly the inequities and inadequacies that diminish the nation's level of wellness. Identifying problems is an important initial step, but developing direction for their correction is essential follow-up. Recognizing this, *Nursing's Agenda for Health Care Reform* was developed through collaborative efforts of the American Nurses Association (ANA) and the National League for Nursing. Once completed, more than 75 nursing associations added their endorsements (de Vries and Vanderbilt, 1994).

The agenda was distributed to thousands of nurses and was also used to explain nursing's values to other groups. Each member of Congress received a copy, with staff briefed on the primary issues. Keen interest was reflected by both Republican and Democratic members, with heightened awareness of nursing as a valuable national resource.

The agenda was a powerful tool to promote understanding of nursing and its special contributions to health care. Candidates for office in the 1992 election cycle were among those targeted with this information. Bill Clinton, Democratic candidate for president, was especially enthusiastic. Reform of health care was a major issue of his campaign, and *Nursing's Agenda for Health Care Reform* supported many of his own beliefs. He spoke often, both to television audiences and in private discussions, about nursing and its position on health care reform. He frequently commented about nurses' political activism in achieving needed change. Undoubtedly his response was influenced by a childhood sensitization to nursing, because his mother was a registered nurse anesthetist. Because of his positions on nursing and health care, Bill Clinton was endorsed for president by the bipartisan ANA Political Action Committee [PAC] Board of Directors in a unanimous vote in July 1992 (ANA-PAC, personal communication, July 13, 1992). Clinton's election the following November brought visions of improved health care systems, with an influential role for nurses in the process.

Nurses were active participants in the Clinton health-related endeavors during the ensuing months. Myra C. Snyder, PhD, RN, an activist in California health politics, joined the president-elect's transition team to assist in advising a health policy (ANA, 1992). President Clinton moved forward quickly, appointing a health care reform task force in early January, soon after his inauguration. The seriousness of his intent was underscored by his appointing first lady Hillary Rodham Clinton to head the initiative (ANA, 1993g).

The task force and its multitude of consultants, including nurses, forged ahead to design a universal and usable plan. ANA President Virginia Trotter Betts, JD, MSN, RN, and other nursing association representatives were involved in many discussions. Of particular concern were two issues critical to nursing: reducing barriers to practice for advanced nurse practitioners and redesigning personnel systems for nurse utilization in a reformed system (ANA, 1993a).

President Clinton delivered his Health Security Act to Congress in September 1993. He proclaimed that it "literally holds the key to a new era for our economy," providing coverage for all Americans in a way that reduces costs and maintains quality while still preserving choice of plans and providers (ANA, 1993c). The campaign began! Congressional committees, provider groups, the press, and the public began heated debates on the proposed plan. Nurses, along with their association representatives, began grassroots lobby efforts in support of reform. They were credible interpreters of the health care issues and of the changes needed.

As the debate progressed, nurse representatives were invited to participate in White House briefings. ANA articulated its continued support for health care reform and cost containment but maintained that quality of care for consumers and preparation and placement of nurses must be ensured (ANA, 1994f).

Nurses' significance to President Clinton's reform endeavors was highlighted by Hillary Rodham Clinton in the keynote address to the ANA convention on June 11, 1994. The first lady affirmed the special contributions of nurses and pleaded for them to "redouble and retriple your efforts and to bring allies in the entire health care field with you." Her focus on "the moral imperative" basic to the vision for America was a germane opening for the convention theme "Nurses: Charting the Course for a Healthy Nation" (ANA, 1994a).

The unprecedented effort to redesign the health care system to benefit the American public continued, but with massive opposition by the insurance industry and some provider groups. The complexity of the plan as well as the issues involved confused the public. Despite general acknowledgment of the problems with the health care system, many were wary of the changes proposed. The momentum engendered by an enthusiastic beginning faltered. By fall of 1994, Capitol Hill efforts to push through the president's plan were discontinued. For the time being, the inequities and inadequacies in health care would continue. However, nurses will continue "charting the course for a healthy nation."

GOVERNMENT: THE HALLMARK OF CIVILIZATION

Government is broadly defined as the exercise of political authority, direction, and restraint over the actions of inhabitants of communities, societies, or states.

Government is crucial to human interdependence and the concomitant necessity for cooperative action.

Among its purposes are the regulation of conditions beyond individual control, providing the individual protection through population-wide focus. Sewage treatment is one example of this.

The delineation of the government's responsibility for health in the United States has evolved from statements of policy that express the values of the founders of the country. These statements have been issued in a series of historic documents. The earliest was the Mayflower Compact (1620) through which the Pilgrims committed themselves to making "just and equal laws" for the general good (Beard and Beard, 1944). The Declaration of Independence (1776) later established the doctrine of "inalienable rights . . . life, liberty and the pursuit of happiness" (Beard and Beard, 1944). The U.S. Constitution (1788), the bedrock of U.S. democracy as well as the supreme law of the land, established the responsibilities of the federal government, including the responsibility to "promote the general welfare." The following year, the first 10 amendments of the constitution, the Bill of Rights, ensured the sovereignty of the states in all areas not constitutionally reserved for the federal government. The Bill of Rights also emphasized specific individual freedoms (Hanlon and Pickett, 1984).

Intermediary policies have developed as needed to provide more specific guidance to government in its day-to-day operations. Some of these policies have been explicitly declared, and some have been implied through programs or other activities. An implicit policy basic to public health programming is that the right to health of the majority must be preserved over individual freedoms. For example, a corporation may not dump hazardous wastes into a river that is a source of drinking water for a community. The welfare of the people must prevail over short-term corporate profits.

GOVERNMENT AUTHORITY FOR THE PROTECTION OF THE PUBLIC'S HEALTH

The authority for the protection of the public's health is largely vested with the states, and most state constitutions specifically delineate this responsibility. Municipal subdivisions of states, such as counties, cities, or towns, usually have the power of local control of these services conferred by the state legislature (Fig. 9–2).

The responsibility of local, state, and federal governments for health services under varying conditions sometimes complicates attempts to determine the locus of political decision making. Because the supremacy of the state prevails in most situations, the state is a critical arena for political action. An example is the state's authority to license health professionals such as nurses and physicians as well as health care institutions such as hospitals, nursing homes, and day care centers.

Each state establishes policies or standards for goods or services that impact the health of its citizens. As noted, however, that authority may be affected by a number of factors. For example, the standards for pasteurization of milk sold within a state are determined by that state, but if the milk is to be sold in another state, it comes under the interstate commerce jurisdiction of the federal government. This could mean that a higher standard must be met, which in effect negates the state standard. Alternatively, when public health authority is delegated to political subdivisions within the state, they too may impose a standard that is higher (never lower) than that of the state (Hanlon and Pickett, 1984).

The federal government also has a strong influence on health services. Constitutionally, this authority is derived from the federal role in regulation of interstate commerce (e.g., meat inspection) and through broad interpretation of the general welfare clause (e.g., Medicare). Because states vary considerably in resources needed to provide health programs, significant de facto authority derives from the promise of revenues. Many of the programs discussed in this and other chapters are funded fully or partially through federal funds.

Conformance by states to federal program standards is voluntary, but the advantage of the revenue, which is withheld from the states if they do not comply, is seldom ignored. Programs such as control of sexually transmitted diseases and the statistical reporting system are standardized across the country because of the indirect but marked effect of federal funding.

BALANCE OF POWERS: SAFEGUARD OF GOVERNMENT

Decisions affecting the public's health are made not only at every level of government but also, as mentioned, in each branch. The separation of powers is a principle as important to the health as it is to the economic or military status of the country.

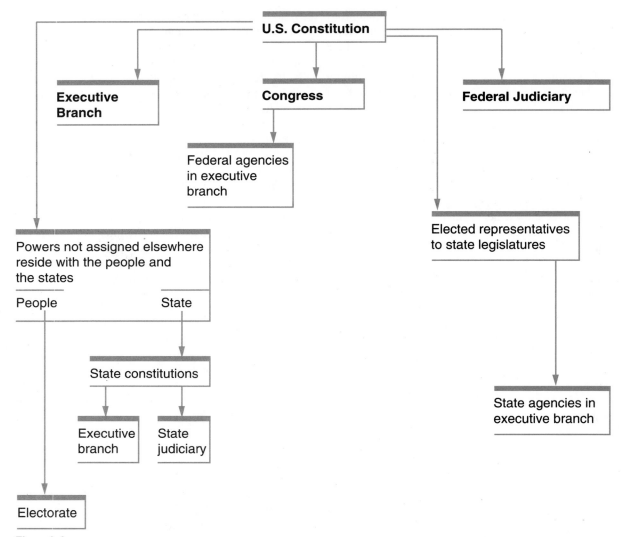

Figure 9–2
Mandate of powers. (Redrawn from Bagwell M, Clements S: A Political Handbook for Health Professionals. Boston, Little, Brown, 1985, p. 23.)

CHECKS AND BALANCES ON IMMUNIZATION REQUIREMENTS

Immunization requirements for school attendance are an example of the checks and balances among the three branches of government. To protect the public welfare, most state legislatures have passed laws mandating that all primary school children be immunized against certain communicable diseases. The appropriate executive agency, usually the state health department, develops the regulations through which the law is implemented and enforced. The legislative branch has no further power over the administration of the law except to change it when necessary through amendment or repeal. The few parents who object to their children being immunized have recourse through the judicial system to have the law waived in their case.

The legislative branch (Congress at the federal level and the legislature, general assembly, or general court at the state level) enacts the statutory laws that are the basis for governance. The laws, which are broad in scope, are administered and enforced by the executive branch through regulatory agencies. These agencies, in turn, define more specifically implementation of the statutes through rules and regulations known as regulatory or administrative law. The judiciary body, the third branch of government, provides protection against oppressive governance and against professional malpractice, fraud, and abuse. Its function, through the courts, is to determine the constitutionality of laws, to interpret them, and to decide on their legitimacy when they are challenged (Beard and Beard, 1944). The courts also have jurisdiction over specific infractions of laws and regulations.

THE LEGISLATIVE PROCESS: POLITICS IN ACTION

The saying, "If you love the law and you love sausage, you shouldn't try to find out how either one is made," reflects a common cynicism about the decision-making process of public governance. For professional and business groups, it apparently does not pay to be too fastidious because most of them are knowledgeable about the process and adept at finding the points most sensitive to outside pressure. Medical and hospital associations are widely recognized for their shrewdness in this area. Until very recently, their success in influencing health care legislation has been remarkable. Many of the decisions that these associations have successfully influenced, however, have benefited their institutional interests, not consumers of health care or nurses as providers of that care.

How a Bill Becomes a Law

The procedure through which legislation must pass to eventually become law is similar for all U.S. legislative bodies. Once a concept has been drafted into legislative language, it becomes a bill, is given a number, and moves through a series of steps. The bill's passage is sometimes smooth, but more often than not the bill may be extensively altered through amendments or even "killed" at various stages.

In the Congress and the 49 states that have a bicameral legislature, a bill must succeed through two legislative bodies, the House and the Senate. A bill that has moved successfully through the legislative process has one final hurdle: the chief executive's approval. The approval may be a clear endorsement, in which case the governor or president signs it. If the executive neither signs nor vetoes it, the bill may become law by default. An explicit veto conclusively kills the bill, which then can be revived only by a substantial vote of the legislature to override the veto. This is another example of the checks and balances of the government process (Archer and Goehner, 1982).

Issues that find their way into the legislative arena are commonly controversial, and proponents and opponents quickly align themselves. Because defeating a bill is much easier than getting one passed, the opposition always has the advantage. Health legislation, which usually requires preventive action (e.g., toxic waste management) or creates a new service (e.g., nursing center organizations for Medicare recipients), is at a disadvantage from several other standpoints as well.

Few elected officials are knowledgeable about the health care field. Although health is readily recognized as a national resource, it is not easily quantified into the economic terms that make the essence of an issue easy to grasp. Other disadvantages are the backgrounds, biases, and ambitions of each legislator. Frequently, the decision to run for public office is made in keeping with personal goals that are likely to differ considerably from health values or the public good.

Despite these obstacles, good health laws can be passed when concerned nurses and other health care workers understand the legislative process and use it effectively. For nurses, this is yet another mode of intervention on behalf of clients. It is as crucial to have legislation passed to reduce abuse of all children as it is to care physically and emotionally for the individual abused child.

THE NURSE AS LOBBYIST: PERSUASIVE POLITICS

To lobby is to try to influence legislators. A lobbyist is, by definition, a person who represents special interests (Kalisch and Kalisch, 1982).

Influencing lawmakers to pass effective health legislation requires the participation of individual nurses as well as their organizations. The initial step in this process involves a telephone call to make an appointment with an elected official. Although there are exceptions, most officials are interested in meeting only with their own constituents (i.e., those registered to vote in their political jurisdiction). The power of generating votes is the primary determinant of political influence!

The goal of the first contact with the official is to establish oneself as a concerned constituent as well as a credible source of information on health issues. The

NEW HAMPSHIRE NURSES LEARN TO LOBBY

New Hampshire nurses faced political reality when their licensing board was abolished. The Sunset Law, a good-government means of making boards and agencies accountable, requires periodic legislative reenactment of boards, or they literally fade into the sunset. This occurred in New Hampshire during the 1981 legislative session.

Some New Hampshire legislators wanted to consolidate selected licensure under an umbrella board, and nurses became their initial target. Nurses believe they were selected because they were expected to be "clean, quiet, and cooperative and to leave by the servants' exit."

Nurses knew about the Sunset Law review but expected the nursing board to be reauthorized with no problem. They assumed the legislators would appreciate the role of nurse licensure in protecting the public. However, the legislative session ended in June 1981 with no legislation for a nursing board.

A coalition of nurses rallied under the leadership of the New Hampshire Nurses Association, calling itself the Coalition for Action in Nursing, and prepared for an upcoming special legislative session. They learned quickly how to lobby!

A friend in the state legislature, Representative Peter C. Hildreth (D), explained that "the swift passage of the bill to recreate the board of nursing was a direct result of the political clout of nurses. When they flexed their muscles, the politicians listened." New Hampshire nurses are ensuring that politicians continue to listen (ANA, 1982)!

image of nurses as caring and helping people is a definite advantage here. In communities where nurses have already established strong political credentials, their colleagues will be more readily accepted. A person who establishes a reputation as a reliable and accurate resource as a lobbyist, has substantially greater influence. This is simply an expression of the exchange principle, or quid pro quo, which is a firm political reality.

Legislators rely heavily on lobbyists for education on issues, and they usually want to hear from opposing sides before taking a position. Because of this dependence, the official must trust lobbyists to give accurate, though predictably biased, informa-

INSTITUTE OF NURSING RESEARCH

The National Center for Nursing Research became a reality in November 1985 through broad-based bipartisan support in the U.S. Congress. The lop-sided vote to override President Reagan's veto of the center reflected the awareness of Congress of the contribution to health care made by the nursing profession. The center, within the National Institutes of Health (NIH), was a negotiated compromise from an earlier attempt to establish a separate Institute of Nursing Research.

During the floor debates preceding the successful override vote, numerous friends of nursing spoke passionately about the importance of nursing research. Senator Orrin Hatch (R-UT) objected to the veto argument that the funding for such a center was a major obstacle. He retorted:

A proposal for nursing research to have one-one thousandth of the NIH budget is too much? My fellow Senators, don't you believe it. It is high time that nursing research took its rightful place in those NIH halls of ivy (ANA, 1985a).

Senator Bill Bradley (D-NJ) was another articulate supporter of the veto override, explaining:

The president claims that such research will not help with disease-oriented research. I disagree. The care of patients is of the utmost importance in curing them of disease. Nurses play an extremely important role in helping patients learn how to participate in patient care. They also help to prevent illness and determine how to provide patient care in nonacute care settings (ANA, 1985a).

Nursing research, focused in National Center for Nursing Research, was established as an important component of NIH. In June 1993 the center was redesignated as the National Institute of Nursing Research, making it a full partner in NIH. In celebrating this significant event in nursing history, nurse researchers recognized the notable efforts of (former) Representative Carl Purcell (R-MI), Senator Daniel Inouye (D-HI), and Senator Tom Harkin (D-IA) (ANA, 1993e).

tion. If a lobbyist does not have information requested, it should be obtained and given to the official quickly.

Each official represents a constituency with varied needs and interests, and each vote must be weighed within this context. It is important to realize that the positions taken by legislators will not always be to one's liking, and evaluation of their performance should be based on their overall voting patterns, not on their votes on isolated issues. Jesse Unruh, a political sage and former speaker of the house of the California legislature, explained, "Had I slain all my political enemies, I would have no friends today" (ANA, 1986). The ANA and the American Public Health Association (APHA) regularly tally and publish the records of each federal legislator on all issues related to the organization's priorities. This information can be very helpful in evaluating elected officials.

THE POLITICAL PROCESS: CAMPAIGNING, A MEANS TO AN END

Helping someone win an election is a sure way of gaining influence. All candidates are grateful for campaign assistance and usually remember those who have helped. Although campaign contributions are commonly thought of as being financial, they can also take the form of campaign activities.

Because nurses are frequently unable to contribute much money, they can provide these invaluable services. For the novice, there are always veteran campaigners who are eager to help them "learn the ropes." Initially, one can address or stuff envelopes for mailings. One can also invite friends and neighbors for a social gathering to meet the candidate, thereby providing an opportunity to discuss issues of concern with constituents.

Telephone banks help a candidate identify supporters, opponents, and the critical "undecided" voter. These latter voters, who can make the definitive difference on election day, are courted by all candidates. The telephone interviews are highly structured and easily handled by inexperienced campaign workers. Direct contact with potential voters may occur later in the form of house-to-house "block walks" or election day poll work. The confidence this requires comes with experience and a strong commitment to the candidate and the cause.

Hosting a social function to allow nurse colleagues to meet the candidate is a welcome contribution to the campaign. Because nurses are substantial in number and their voting record is humanistic, they are valued as a political force. ANA-PAC promotes awareness of this through its buttons and bumper stickers that proclaim there are "5000 nurses in every congressional district."

Policies about political activity may restrict political activism by government employees. Nurses employed at any level of government need to know whether such prohibitions affect them. The military services have specified policies for their personnel (Archer & Goehner, 1982). The Hatch Act was amended in 1993 to permit most federal civil service employees to participate in partisan political activities on their off-duty time. For more than 50 years, this act prevented federal workers from participating in the political processes that determined so much of their lives. The restriction was considered by many to be an unconstitutional abridgment of free speech and was finally modified by Congress (ANA, 1993d). The Office of Personnel Management (OPM) later issued interim regulations to clarify the congressional action (ANA, 1994b). Nurses who are employed by a federal agency should contact its human resources or legal staff for interpretation (OPM, personal communication, March 2, 1995).

POWER OF NUMBERS

Nurses' interest in affecting health policies and legislation has burgeoned in recent years as they realize the impact on their practice and profession. As a body of more than 2 million (ANA, personal communication, March 3, 1995), they can wield enormous power.

This power of numbers is never more apparent than in the legislative process. A legislator carefully weighs the number of constituents supporting or opposing a bill before deciding how to vote. A sizable block of constituents on one side of an issue can significantly affect that vote. "Representing the district" is important to a legislator for ethical reasons as well as for political pragmatism (Fig. 9–3).

To maximize the nursing influence during the debate on health care reform, ANA initiated the Nurses Strategic Action Team in 1993. Members of state nurses associations responded eagerly to the call for grassroots activists to assist ANA and state nurses associations in responding to various health issues (ANA, 1993b).

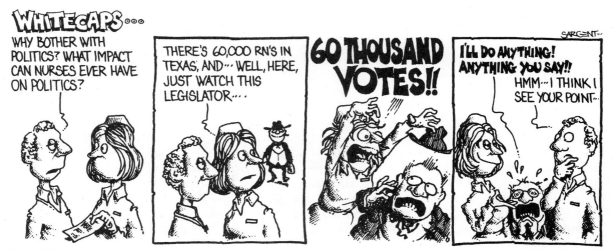

Figure 9–3
The power of numbers. (With permission from Texas Nursing, September 1976. Copyright Texas Nurses Association, 1976.)

Professional Associations and Lobbying

Collective action by nursing and health care organizations such as ANA and APHA is critical to their goals. These associations monitor legislative activity related to health issues and link the process to their membership. This continual surveillance of the legislative environment is critical: even seemingly minor amendments can have profound effects on health services.

Thorough monitoring requires the participation of people who are knowledgeable about not only nursing and health care but also the political intricacies of the legislative process. The ANA and the APHA have full-time staff lobbyists who work with Congress. Many of their state constituent associations also work with state legislatures. However, regardless of the effectiveness of association lobbyists in promoting the interests of nurses and society, they always need grassroots cooperation to deliver the real punch. In the final analysis, it is sufficiently high numbers of communications—letters and telephone calls—from individual constituents that have the greatest influence.

PACs

Since the 1970s, other important sources of collective influence have been PACs. These nonpartisan entities promote the election of candidates believed to be sympathetic to their interests. PACs are established by professional associations and business and labor groups under federal and state laws that stipulate how they may contribute financially to campaigns. The advantage of a PAC is that small donations from many members, when added together, make an impressive addition to a campaign fund in the name of an organization. This gains the attention of the candidate and earns good will for the group.

Cogent arguments are advanced—primarily by Common Cause, the self-styled citizens' lobby—against PACs. There is valid concern about the correlation of major PAC contributions and the legislator's votes on special interest legislation. As long as PACs are a reality of political life, however, nurses need to recognize their power and support those that are committed to electing candidates sympathetic to health care issues.

Most national associations of health care providers have PACs. Among the strongest are those representing hospitals, nursing homes, home health agencies, pharmaceutical interests, and insurance companies. A PAC that makes major political contributions is the AMPAC, sponsored by the American Medical Association. State medical associations also have strong PACs. This means that organized medicine has a powerful influence on national and state elections and thus on health care legislation.

The ANA-PAC has developed considerable influence in Washington as nurses throughout the country respond to the reality of political impact on nursing practice. In 1994, ANA-PAC endorsed more than 200 candidates for federal office, and an impressive 70% of these candidates won their races (ANA-PAC, personal communication, February 9, 1995). The endorsed candidates, Republicans and Democrats, have demonstrated commitment to the beliefs and values basic to the nursing profession. Their influence will be invaluable to the decision-making processes that result in health policy.

Nurses contributed more than $1 million to ANA-PAC to promote the election of these favored candidates. The costs of political campaigns are enormous, and financial support can make a considerable difference in the election day outcomes. Apart from the dollar assistance from ANA-PAC, endorsed candidates were also aided by the many nurses who contributed time, energy, and skill to the grassroots campaign essential to a winning campaign (ANA, 1994d, 1994e).

Coalitions

When two or more groups join to maximize resources, thus increasing their impact and improving their chances of success in achieving a common goal, it is called a *coalition*. Coalitions of health care providers often work together on issues such as family violence and fluoridation of water supplies. An outstanding example of such cooperative action has been the establishment of rehabilitation programs for health professionals whose practice has been impaired by substance abuse or mental health problems.

Nursing and consumer groups often form coalitions to advance their shared interests in health promotion. The Grey Panthers is one consumer group that is a frequent and valued ally of nursing because of its concern for quality of life and health care for the aging. Groups like the National Women's Political Caucus and the National Organization for Women share an interest in promoting the rights of women and are natural collaborators with nurses, for whom equity is an issue.

POLITICAL ACTION: ONE PUBLIC HEALTH NURSE'S STORY

Joan Diamond, RN, a public health nurse in rural Texas, has been a long-time activist both professionally and politically. She was acutely aware of the inequities that were causing higher-than-average communicable disease and infant mortality rates in her region. The affluence of most Texans stood in sore contrast to the poverty experienced by the people in her case load. However, she knew that her nursing care interventions, however skilled, could never improve individual client health without changes in the area's economic, environmental, and educational conditions.

These changes could never be realized unless the system designed to support the status quo was changed. Her frequent contacts with local appointed and elected officials were gaining her nothing except a reputation as "the nagging nurse." Rumblings of discontent from others in the area, however, were being heard by the district delegation to Austin, the state capital. Out of this activist ferment emerged a young businessman who stood as a "reform" candidate for the state legislature.

NURSES RALLY AGAINST REGISTERED CARE TECHNOLOGISTS

The "innovative solution to the shortage of bedside personnel" proposed by the American Medical Association (AMA) in 1988 enraged nurses and brought them together as had nothing else in history. The position of registered care technologist (RCT) was designed to "help" nurses and the nursing shortage through the training of individuals to "continuously monitor and implement physicians' orders at the bedside" and report to the physician. Although the AMA assured nurses that it had their practice needs in mind, nursing was not consulted about this. The legal and ethical implications to licensed nurses were not addressed.

The reaction by nurses and all major nursing organizations was instantaneous, universal, and volatile! Nurses unified to protect their patients and their role. Coalitions of nurses (licensed vocational, licensed practical, and registered) developed strategies to refute the AMA proposal and articulate the methods under way to increase the ranks of nurses.

Nurses were not alone in their concern for the quality of patient care by the RCTs, and many physician groups stood in opposition. Consumer groups, such as the American Association of Retired Persons, expressed opposition, and numerous major newspapers editorialized against the AMA.

Although the AMA continues to support its RCT plan, as of 1990, it had not begun any of the four proposed demonstration projects. Nurses realized their power possible through unity (Stewart, 1988).

Joan found Carl Findley's philosophy of government bracingly different from that of the incumbent and compatible with her own. All Findley knew about health care, however, was that he was "for it." He was nevertheless eager to learn, and he asked Joan to serve on his campaign advisory committee. He also asked her to develop a position paper describing the health problems in the district presenting goals for intervention through his legislative representation.

Joan consulted with clients and colleagues while writing the position paper and involved them in presenting it to the candidate for his approval and education. Findley was pleased to have the information, especially the statistics that so convincingly documented the problems.

Meanwhile, Joan began actively recruiting colleagues to work in the campaign. The political activity for most of these nurses had been limited to voting. They found the idea of political involvement both tantalizing and terrifying, but Joan was persuasive. She argued that if they really cared about promoting health, they should be helping to send a sympathetic and knowledgeable legislator to Austin. A macroscopic approach to health policy could do far more to improve health conditions for their clients than all their concerned interventions at the local level. Perhaps he could initiate legislation requiring use of child safety seats in moving vehicles, which would get parents' attention far faster than the public health nurses' persuasion.

Under Joan's tutelage, the nurses, several of whom brought their children and friends to help, manned the campaign office for two nights a week. They prepared mailings, handled the telephone work, and dispatched yard sign crews. In addition, they organized neighborhood coffee klatches and campaign rallies. They distributed and displayed bumper stickers advocating Findley's election. Several walked house to house in key neighborhoods handing out campaign leaflets and presenting themselves as nurses supporting Findley to obtain better health care for the district. They almost always had animated discussions with the residents.

Although the campaign was long and arduous, election day brought sweet reward; Findley won. In his victory address, he gave glowing praise to Joan and the other nurses for their contribution to his success.

Once in office, the Honorable Carl Findley's record showed he had learned that to be in favor of health meant working for better health legislation. He consulted regularly with Joan about health-related or nursing-related legislation—a significant 200 to 250 bills of the approximately 2000 bills filed in each legislative session. He also helped the Texas Nurses Association staff in lobbying his colleagues on health issues.

Findley is recognized by his constituents as representing the district well, and they reelected him six more times. As for the basic health issues of the people on her caseload that got Joan involved in politics in the first place, progress, albeit slow, has been made.

A major health initiative that received a great deal of attention in the Texas legislature in 1985 was passed only because of Joan's influence with Findley. The Indigent Health Care Legislation was a bare-bones effort to provide programs, especially perinatal and preventive services, for the poor. The need for state action had been well documented by a select committee of legislators, professionals (including one registered nurse), and business people. Coalitions, pro and con, were formed. The Texas Nurses Association aligned itself with public hospitals, community health centers, and numerous consumer groups to promote the program. When the final vote was imminent, the Texas Nurses Association staff were astounded to learn that Findley was going to vote against it. They wasted no time in tracking down Joan in a North Texas well-infant clinic, and they told her the problem. She immediately called Findley, and her call was transferred to him on the floor of the House (an example of her power with him). At the very last minute, she was able to convince Findley that he should support the bill for the good of his district.

One vote is always important, but Findley's vote had special significance: it created a tie. This required the speaker of the house to break the tie, which he did with a dramatic "aye." Without Findley's support, this bill would have been defeated by one vote. Because of Joan's professional concern and political activism, the poor of Texas received better health care.

NURSING AND THE HEALTH OF THE NATION: A SOCIAL CONTRACT

A profession derives its status from a contract with society to provide essential services under conditions of altruism and trust. Nurses are demonstrating this professionalism by serving the healthy and the sick and by serving future generations through their influence in promoting wellness as public policy. Nurses are a powerful political force.

If every public official had at least one nurse consultant to help put health issues in perspective, health policies would be improved. Although some nurses contribute to health policy development, more are needed. Both nurses and the public should be constantly attuned to opportunities to promote the appointment or election of nurses to policymaking positions.

The first nurse to serve in the U.S. Congress is Eddie Bernice Johnson (D-TX), reelected to a second term in 1994. Representative Johnson is recognized for her promotion of health and human service programs. Although other nurses have run for Congress, strongly supported by ANA-PAC, no others have won as yet.

More and more nurses are serving in state legislatures across the country. According to the ANA, in 1995 about 48 were serving the public (personal communication, July 19, 1995). These nurse-legislators play a crucial role in interpreting health issues and influencing appropriate legislation. Important, also, are the nurses serving in county and city government as well as on special governing bodies such as school boards.

Nurses are also key to sound health policy through politically appointed positions. These appointments are based on individual qualifications for the position but also involve political connections. President Bill Clinton has appointed several nurses to important federal positions. Among these is Shirley Chater, PhD, RN, a former educator and university president, who heads the Social Security Administration. As commissioner of this agency, she manages programs that provide benefits to 44 million people each month (ANA, 1993f).

One of President Clinton's early appointments was Kristine Gebbie, MPH, RN, as coordinator for the nation's AIDS policy. Sound, long-term acquired immunodeficiency syndrome [AIDS] policies were initiated during her tenure, but she was caught in the cross-fire between AIDS advocates and the administration. She resigned after 1 year in office (Lee 1995).

Mary Lou Keener, JD, RN, a nurse and an attorney, won appointments as general counsel of the Department of Veterans' Affairs, thus heading that massive department's legal operations. She is the first woman to hold this position (ANA, 1993h).

Nurses now head 2 of the 10 regional offices of the U.S. Department of Health and Human Services (DHHS). Pat Montoya, MA, RN, is director for Region VI, covering five states, headquartered in Dallas (ANA, 1994c). Pat Ford-Roegner, MS, RN, is responsible for the eight states in Region IV, with her office in Atlanta (P. Montoya, personal communication, March 6, 1995). The regional directors serve as U.S. DHHS Secretary Shalala's representative in coordinating policies within the regions they serve as well as the liaison with other governmental and public interest groups.

The governors of Michigan and Texas have appointed nurses to major public health positions. Bernice David Anthony, MPH, RN, was appointed by Governor John Engle (1990) as director, of the Michigan Department of Health. In this important position, she is responsible for the overall management of all state public health functions (personal communication, April 14, 1995).

In Texas in 1993, Governor Ann Richards appointed Ruth Stewart, MS, RN, as chair of the Texas Board of Health, an important public health policy position. She was not only the first nurse but the first woman to head the board (Texas Nurses Association, 1993).

SUMMARY

Historically, nurses have been able to make significant differences in the quality of life experienced by the members of the communities they serve. The case study of Carrie Long presented in this chapter is an example of how one nurse gathered data and worked with residents, bureaucrats, and the media to effect change in a situation that was negatively affecting public health. By understanding how government works, how bills become law, and how legislators make decisions, nurses can influence policy decisions through individual efforts such as letter writing, participation in political campaigns, and selection of candidates who support policies conducive to improving the health and welfare of all citizens. When organized in lobbying groups, coalitions, and PACs, nurses can be a powerful force that brings about change in the delivery and quality of the health care of aggregates.

**L e a r n i n g
A c t i v i t i e s**

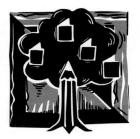

1. Develop an "Insight" bulletin board, with each class member contributing cartoons, anecdotes, and clippings about issues affecting public health or nursing.

2. Develop expertise on a current public health or nursing issue, including an understanding of the causes, effect on the public, and possible solutions. Influence its resolution through any of the following activities:
   - Write a succinct letter to the editor of a local newspaper.
   - Write a position paper and submit it to the "Opinion Page" of a local newspaper.
   - Write to elected or appointed officials whose jurisdiction could be influential on the issue.
   - Meet with an elected or appointed official to discuss the issue. (This can be done in groups of two or three.)
   - Call in to a radio talk show about the issue.
   - Volunteer to speak on the issue to appropriate consumer or professional groups.

3. With a group of two or three, meet with an elected official for a 15-minute appointment to ask about the official's concerns and priorities. If the official is not familiar with health issues, do not preach; instead, begin an educational process.

4. Invite an elected official who is sympathetic to nurses to speak to the local chapter of the National Nursing Students Association to discuss the political process and health policy.

5. Invite an elected official to spend a day with a public health nurse or nursing student in appropriate activities. (Take black-and-white pictures for press use.)

6. Invite a medical reporter from the press, radio, or television to observe public health nursing activities that would appeal to the public.

7. Participate in a group organized around a public health issue (e.g., disposable diapers, toxic waste, fluoride).

8. Serve as a volunteer in a campaign for a candidate who is supportive or potentially supportive of public health or nursing issues.

9. Serve as a volunteer for a political party of choice.

REFERENCES

Aiken L: Nursing in the 1980s. Philadelphia, JB Lippincott. 1982.

American Nurses Association: New Hampshire nurses learn politics the hard way. Polit Nurse 2:1, 1982.

American Nurses Association: NIH veto overridden by wide margin. Capital Update 3:10 (November-December):1, 1985a.

American Nurses Association: Building bridges over troubled waters. Polit Nurse 6:6, 1986.

American Nurses Association: Nurse selected for Clinton transition team. Capital Update 10:14 (December 23):1, 1992.

American Nurses Association: ANA advises on health care reform. Capital Update 11:8 (April 23):1, 1993a.

American Nurses Association: ANA leads grassroots revolution. Capital Update 11:17 (September 24):6, 1993b.

American Nurses Association: Clinton delivers health plan to Congress. Capital Update 11:20 (November 5):1–2, 1993c.

American Nurses Association: Hatch Act reform passes Senate. Capital Update 11:14 (July 23):2, 1993d.

American Nurses Association: "Nightingala" celebrates the National Institute for Nursing Research. Capital Update, 11:22 (December 3):7, 1993e.

American Nurses Association: Nurse appointed to head Social Security Administration. Capital Update, 11:15 (August 6):5, 1993f.

American Nurses Association: President holds bipartisan health care meeting. Capital Update 11:2 (January 29):2, 1993g.

American Nurses Association: Senate confirms Mary Lou Keener, RN. Capital Update, 11:12 (June 25):3, 1993h.

American Nurses Association: Hillary Clinton asks RNs to look to "tomorrow." Convention News June 13:1, 1994a.

American Nurses Association: OPM issues regulations on amended Hatch Act. Capital Update 12:19 (October 14):7, 1994b.

American Nurses Association: Pat Montoya, RN appointed as DHHS regional director. Capital Update 12:18 (September 30):6, 1994c.

American Nurses Association: Political nurse. Am Nurse 26:8 (September):30, 1994d.

American Nurses Association: Political nurse. Am Nurse 26:9 (October):6, 1994e.

American Nurses Association: White House briefs nurses on health care reform. Capital Update 12:8 (April 29):1, 1994f.

Archer S, Goehner P: Nurses: A Political Force. Monterey, CA, Wadsworth, Health Sciences Division, 1982.

Beard CA, Beard MR: A Basic History of the United States. Philadelphia, Blakiston, 1944.

De Vries C, Vanderbilt M: Nurses gain ground during reform debate. Am Nurse 26:10 (November-December):2–3, 1994.

Diers D: Policy and politics. *In* Mason D, Talbott S (eds). Political Action Handbook for Nurses. Menlo Park, CA, Addison-Wesley, 1985, pp. 53–59.

Hanlon JJ, Pickett GE: Public Health: Administration and Practice. St. Louis, Times Mirror/Mosby, 1984.

Kalisch BJ, Kalisch PA: Politics of Nursing. Philadelphia, JB Lippincott, 1982.

Kalisch PA, Kalisch BJ: The Advance of American Nursing. Boston, Little, Brown, 1978.

Lee M: Kristine Gebbie. Am J Nurs 95:34–37, 1995.

Morgan BS, Burbank PM, Godfrey DA: Health planning. *In* Swanson, JM, Albrecht, M (eds). Community Health Nursing: Promoting the Health of Aggregates. Philadelphia, WB Saunders, 1993, p. 125.

Osgood GA, Eliott JE: Federal government. *In* Mason D, Talbott S (eds). Political Action Handbook for Nurses. Menlo Park, CA, Addison-Wesley, 1985.

Spradley B: Community Health Nursing, 2nd ed. Boston, Little, Brown, 1985.

Stewart RF: RCTs: A quick-fix boondogle. Heartbeat 1:3–4, 1988.

Texas Nurses Association: Ruth Stewart to head public health board. Tex Nurs 67:4–6, 1993.

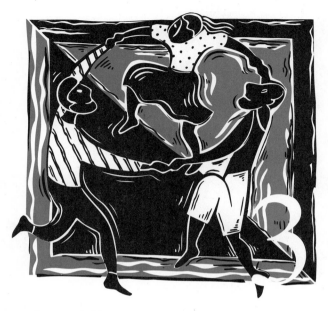

Aggregates in the Community

Child and Adolescent Health

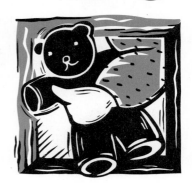

Upon completion of this chapter, the reader will be able to:

1. Identify major indicators of child and adolescent health status.

2. Describe how socioeconomic circumstances influence child and adolescent health.

3. Discuss the individual and societal costs of poor child health status.

4. Discuss public programs targeted to children's health.

5. Apply knowledge of child and adolescent health needs in planning appropriate, comprehensive care at the individual, family, and community levels.

Mary Brecht Carpenter
Susan Rumsey Givens

It is said that a nation's destiny lies with the health, education, and well-being of its children. Although most of this nation's children are healthy and succeed in school, a growing percentage are not in optimal health, are failing academically, and may not reach their full potential as contributing members of society. The mortality and morbidity rates for children in all age groups are unacceptably high. Every year, nearly 35,000 infants die before reaching their first birthday. An additional 300,000 are born with low birth weights, and many suffer long-term debilitating respiratory, vision, or mental conditions. Nearly 1000 children die each year from physical abuse and neglect. More than 1 million teenage girls become pregnant every year. Forty-six percent of youth aged 12 to 17 years will use alcohol, and 20% will use an illegal drug other than alcohol. One in 13 juveniles will be a victim of violent crime, often committed by another juvenile.

The health of a child has long-term implications; it plays a pivotal role in the physical and emotional development of that child and the well-being of the entire family. Children who go to school sick or hungry, who cannot see the chalkboard or hear the teacher, who abuse drugs or miss school frequently, or who are troubled by abusive parents or disruptive living circumstances often do not do as well as healthy children.

In this chapter, we focus on the health status of children and adolescents; medical, socioeconomic, and other factors that must be addressed to improve their health; and the implications for community health nursing. The indicators of child and adolescent health status are discussed, as are the costs to the individual and society of poor child health, public programs targeted to children's health, and strategies to improve child and adolescent health at the individual, family, and community levels.

INDICATORS OF CHILD AND ADOLESCENT HEALTH STATUS

Pregnancy and Infancy

Early child health status is strongly influenced by genetic endowment, maternal health, and intrauterine and neonatal environments. Children who suffer from intrauterine effects of maternal smoking, alcohol use, and illicit drug use; children exposed to maternal conditions such as hypertension, poor nutrition, anemia, and infectious disease; and those who are exposed to unsafe environmental conditions, including lack of preventive health care, are more likely to suffer from chronic conditions that can affect their health and well-being throughout the childhood years and beyond. Because the first year of life is the most hazardous until the age of 65 years, it is particularly important for pregnant women to receive prenatal care and for infants to receive primary health care so that serious and long-lasting health problems can be prevented or at least minimized.

INFANT MORTALITY

Infant mortality is an important gauge of overall children's health status. It is often seen as a marker of the health and welfare of an entire community or society. With a 1992 infant death rate of 8.5 deaths per 1000 live births (Kochanek et al., 1995), the United States ranks poorly among industrialized nations. Its 1990 rate was an abysmal 24th behind other nations, including Japan, Sweden, Canada, and France (Table 10–1).

After two decades of steady improvement in infant mortality in the United States, progress has slowed (Fig. 10–1). African-American infants are more than twice as likely to die in their first year of life as white infants. This disparity is largely accounted for by higher rates of low-birth-weight infants among African-American women. African-American infants are most likely to die from disorders related to short gestation and unspecified low birth weight, whereas white infants are most likely to die from congenital anomalies.

Although declines in infant mortality for African-Americans have been steady, they have not kept pace with improvements in white infant mortality (see Fig. 10–1). Other minority groups, including Hispanics, Asians, and Native Americans, experience infant mortality rates much closer to those of whites, although some minority subgroups (e.g., Puerto Ricans) experience much higher infant mortality rates (Kochanek et al., 1995).

LOW BIRTH WEIGHT

Overall, the leading predictor of infant mortality is low birth weight (infants born weighing less than 5.5 pounds). Every year in the United States, nearly 300,000 infants are born at low birth weight. Despite the development of advanced technologies for keeping small infants alive, the percentage of infants born at low birth weight (7.1%) has risen over the past decade.

Table 10-1 Infant Mortality Rates: Ranking of the Developed Countries, 1990		
Rank	**Country**	**Infant Mortality Rate***
1	Japan	4.60
2	Finland	5.64
3	Sweden	5.96
4	Hong Kong	6.13
5	Singapore	6.67
6	Canada	6.82
7	Switzerland	6.83
8	Federal Republic of Germany	6.98
9	Norway	7.02
10	Netherlands	7.06
11	France	7.33
12	German Democratic Republic	7.33
13	Denmark	7.39
14	Northern Ireland	7.47
15	Scotland	7.73
16	Austria	7.84
17	England and Wales	7.88
18	Belgium	7.94
19	Spain†	8.07
20	Australia	8.17
21	Ireland	8.20
22	New Zealand	8.31
23	Italy	8.53
24	United States	9.22
25	Greece	9.32
26	Israel	9.84
27	Cuba	10.74
28	Portugal	10.99
29	Czechoslovakia	11.25
30	Bulgaria	14.77

*Number of infant deaths per 1000 live births.
†Rate from Spain is from 1988.

From National Center for Health Statistics (1994). Health, United States, 1993. Hyattsville, MD, U.S. Public Health Service.

African-American infants are more than twice as likely as white infants to be born at low birth weight (Ventura et al., 1994).

Although low birth weight affects 7% of infants, these infants account for nearly 60% of all the infant deaths (U.S. Congress, Office of Technology Assessment, 1988). Low-birth-weight infants are almost 40 times as likely to die within the first 4 weeks of life; if raised in disadvantaged households, they have two to three times the risk of physical and mental disabilities such as blindness, deafness, learning disabilities, and mental retardation (Institute of Medicine [IOM], 1985).

Risk factors associated with low birth weight include African-American race, lack of prenatal care, and low socioeconomic status. Unhealthy habits such as poor nutrition, alcohol and drug use, and cigarette smoking also increase the likelihood of low birth weight. The National Center for Health Statistics estimates that 40,000 fewer infants would be born at low birth weights each year if their mothers did not smoke during pregnancy (Ventura et al., 1994).

LACK OF PRENATAL CARE

Inadequate prenatal care is associated with the high infant death rate and low-birth-weight rate in the United States. Nearly one in four pregnant women in the United States fails to receive early, regular prenatal care (Ventura et al., 1994). Infants born to women who receive no prenatal care are three times as likely to be born at a low birth weight as infants of mothers who receive first-trimester care (Ventura et al., 1994).

Through prenatal care, specific causes of infant morbidity and mortality such as maternal anemia, diabetes, hypertension, urinary tract infections, sexually transmitted diseases (STDs), and poor nutrition can be identified and treated. Health education and counseling provide women with the information they need to make lifestyle changes that will help ensure a healthy pregnancy (Kogan et al., 1994). Comprehensive prenatal care is particularly important for low-income women because it helps them obtain needed social services such as the Special Supplemental Food Program for Women, Infants, and Children (WIC), food stamps, housing, child care, job training, treatment for substance abuse, and counseling for domestic violence.

Women who are poor, young, unmarried, or African-American, Hispanic, or Native American; who live in isolated rural areas or medically underserved urban areas; and who have completed fewer than 12 years of education are less likely to obtain adequate prenatal care than are those who are older, married, white or Asian, and better educated.

Financial barriers often block women from receiving the preventive health care they need. An estimated 26% of women of childbearing age lack maternity health insurance coverage even though a large proportion of these women are employed (Snider, 1993). Even with health insurance, it is difficult for many to

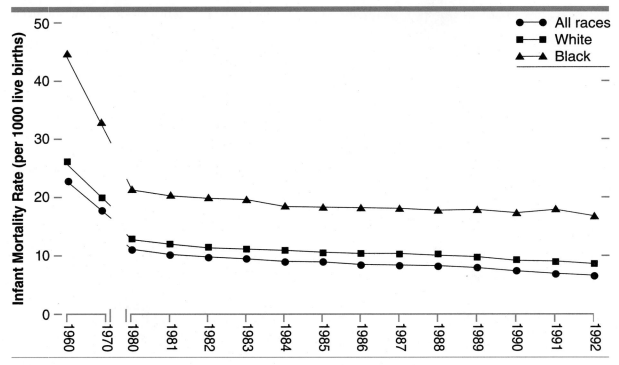

Figure 10–1
U.S. infant mortality rate by race (1972–1992). Based on data from Kochanek and Hudson (1995).

meet costly deductibles and copayments. Other barriers that block access to prenatal care include (IOM, 1985)

- Inadequate supply of health care providers and services, particularly for Medicaid-eligible women
- Bureaucratic red tape; lack of coordinated, user-friendly services; and inhospitable and culturally insensitive conditions at clinics or offices
- Lack of knowledge and personal attitudes and lifestyle conditions that inhibit women from seeking prenatal care

PRENATAL SUBSTANCE USE

Cigarette, alcohol, and illicit drug use are social factors that affect health; their use during pregnancy has profound effects on fetal neurologic and physical development. With the use of any combination of these substances, outcomes are worsened. In 1992, 16.9% of infants were born to mothers who smoked cigarettes during pregnancy, and 2.6% were born to mothers who reported drinking alcohol during pregnancy (Ventura et al., 1994).

Illegal Drug Use. According to the National Pregnancy Health Survey, 5% of women who delivered in 1992 used illegal drugs while pregnant. Illegal drug use was higher among unmarried women, those who had no jobs, and those with less than a college education (Leshner, 1994).

One of the most serious potential consequences of pregnant women's drug abuse is the prenatal transmission of STDs, especially the human immunodeficiency virus (HIV). Women at highest risk of contracting HIV are those whose sex partners have high-risk behaviors (e.g., use of injectable drugs and nonuse of condoms), adolescents, those with multiple sex partners, and those with other STDs. Heterosexual transmission of HIV is the most rapidly increasing route of HIV transmission for women. The second most common means of transmission is through women's use of injectable drugs.

Smoking. By far, smoking is more common than alcohol and illicit drug use during pregnancy, and the elimination of tobacco use among pregnant women would result in significant declines in the percentage of low–birth-weight infants. Maternal cigarette smoking and childhood exposure to secondhand smoke are also linked closely to sudden infant death syndrome (SIDS) (Schoendorf and Kiely, 1992) and childhood asthma (Cunningham et al., 1994).

Alcohol Use. Although the effect of low alcohol consumption during pregnancy is uncertain, high consumption by pregnant women is associated with spontaneous abortion, mental retardation of the child, low birth weight, and a cluster of congenital defects, including the nervous system dysfunction called fetal alcohol syndrome (FAS). FAS has surpassed Down syndrome as the leading cause of mental retardation in the United States (Streissguth et al., 1991).

Childhood

At all ages, medical care plays an important role in children's health status, but other factors, including parental lifestyles and community safety, also exert strong influences over children's well-being. The causes of death among children change with age. The major cause of adolescent death is accidental injury. Parents and the community have important responsibilities in ensuring access to medical care, promoting healthy lifestyles, and creating safe environments by taking steps to protect children from accidental injury and exposure to environmental toxins, abuse, and violence.

ACCIDENTAL INJURIES

After the first year of life, accidental injury (including motor vehicle injury, drowning, burning, and suffocation) is the leading cause of death. Nearly 20,000 children and young adults (younger than 24 years) die each year from accidents (Kochanek, 1995). Low socioeconomic status is linked to injury fatalities (Durkin, 1994).

Motor vehicle accidents account for the greatest danger to children's life and health. Most deaths are due to children not being secured in car seats. Approximately one third of those killed are pedestrians. Head injury from cycling is also a leading cause of death. Although helmets have been shown to reduce the risk of head injuries in biking accidents by 85%, less than 5% of children who ride bicycles wear helmets (American Academy of Pediatrics, 1995). Many of the children who survive serious motor vehicle and bicycle accidents suffer severe permanent neurologic damage.

LEAD POISONING

In the United States, one in every six children younger than 6 years has a dangerously high blood lead level, making lead poisoning the most prevalent disease of environmental origin among U.S. children (National Education Association, 1990). Lead poisoning is a preventable cause of death, mental retardation, cognitive and behavioral problems, and sensory and other disabilities in children. High levels of lead are also associated with lower class standing in high school, increased absenteeism, lower vocabulary and grammatical reading scores, poorer hand-eye coordination, and longer reaction times (Needleman et al., 1990).

Lead is an invisible threat. Sources of lead contamination include lead-based paint, water, food, soil, dust generated during restorations of older homes, and raising and lowering of windows painted with lead-based paint. The United States has gone a long way toward reducing the threat of toxic lead exposure through the elimination of lead from gasoline and the removal of lead from the manufacture of paint. Before 1950, the use of lead-based paint was quite common, but the 1972 Lead Paint Poisoning Prevention Act severely limited the manufacture of lead-based paint. The problem has not been eliminated, however. An estimated 42 million housing units, most but certainly not all of which are located in poor inner city neighborhoods in the United States, still contain lead-based paint.

The neurotoxic properties of lead have been recognized for at least a century, but the nature and extent of subtle long-term effects are just being realized. Unlike the obvious signs of measles or polio, low-level lead poisoning is difficult to recognize in children. To reduce the menace of lead poisoning, the Centers for Disease Control and Prevention have recommended blood lead screening for most infants and toddlers (Centers for Disease Control and Prevention, 1991).

CHILD ABUSE AND NEGLECT

Rates of child abuse and neglect are other indicators of child physical and emotional health status. In 1994, child protection agencies across the country received reports that 3.1 million children were abused and neglected, a 4.5% increase from 1993. Approximately

1000 U.S. children die each year from abuse and neglect (Wiese and Dara, 1995).

Most reported cases involve children younger than 5 years, and the two dominant characteristics of their parents are a history of substance abuse and having been abused themselves as children. A very disturbing trend is the growing population of young children being raised by drug-abusing parents who are ill equipped to cope with the physical and psychological demands of caring for young children. There is a critical need for involvement by community organizations in preventing child abuse and in creating a climate that supports families and provides alternatives to abusive behavior. Tragically, in most communities, such services are in short supply.

Adolescence

In the struggle to gain independence, all too often adolescents engage in risk-taking behaviors that threaten their health, including alcohol and drug abuse, early and unprotected sexual activity, unsafe driving, and participation in delinquent and violent activities. The leading cause of death for those aged 15 to 24 years is accidental injury, but the second and third leading causes of death for older children and young adults are homicide and suicide, respectively (Kochanek, 1995). Injury and violence are by far the leading threats to the health and lives of adolescents.

VIOLENCE

Violence has emerged as a way of life, a way of coping with challenging and difficult situations, and a significant public health problem for too many of our nation's youth (Koop and Lundberg, 1992). Although violence is most predominant in inner cities, adolescents in suburbs and rural areas are increasingly faced with violence and its direct and indirect impact on the entire community.

Homicide is the second leading cause of death for 15- to 24-year-olds in the United States; African-American youths are at greatest risk. Since 1978, homicide has been the leading cause of death among African-American males aged 15 to 24 years (Kochanek, 1995). Handguns are readily accessible to America's youth. One survey revealed that handguns are available to 47% of urban high school boys and 22% of girls (Callahan and Rivara, 1992).

Violence among youth is a multifaceted problem. It disproportionately affects minorities, but this excess is strongly influenced by social factors such as unemployment and poverty (Durant et al., 1994). Factors such as gang exposure; witnessing violence in the home, in the media, and in the community; gun ownership; and being a victim of child abuse, violence, or severe corporal punishment may serve to socialize youth to viewing violence as an expected and unavoidable part of life.

TEEN PREGNANCY

Annually, almost 1 million girls and women younger than 20 years become pregnant. The great majority of pregnancies (between the ages of 15 and 19 years) are unintended, and more than half end in abortions (Alan Guttmacher Institute, 1994). Approximately 13% of births in the United States (518,000) occur to women younger than 20 years (Ventura et al., 1994).

Teen childbearing poses significant health risks to the infant, including death, prematurity, low birth weight, abuse, and neglect. Research studies disagree on the causes of poor outcomes of pregnancy among teenagers. Most point to socioeconomic factors that are associated with young age, such as low income, lack of education, and inadequate prenatal care (Goldenberg and Klerman, 1995). Fifty-nine percent of teenage mothers fail to receive first-trimester prenatal care compared with 24% of all women (Ventura et al., 1994). Early prenatal care is clearly associated with improved prenatal outcomes.

More recent but fewer studies have identified young maternal age as the most powerful influence on outcomes rather than the socioeconomic conditions present in the young woman's life (Goldenberg and Klerman, 1995). Sorting out these conflicting findings are important so that appropriate interventions can be taken to help improve the chances for infants of adolescent mothers.

The problems of teen parenting do not end in infancy. Children of teen parents are more likely to have problems in school, score low on intelligence quotient tests, have emotional problems (Lewit, 1992), and become teen parents themselves. Teen pregnancy has long-lasting social and economic impacts on the young parents as well. Compared with those who begin parenting in their 20s, adolescent parents are less likely to finish high school and less likely to be employed. They are more likely to have low incomes, to face marital disruptions, and to be dependent on welfare.

Since 1990, the proportion of adolescents who

reported being sexually experienced remained stable, whereas an increasing percentage reported using condoms, thus reducing their risk for unintended pregnancy and STDs, including HIV infection. Still, far too many teenagers remain at risk for unintended pregnancy and STDs.

SEXUALLY TRANSMITTED DISEASES

Sexually active teenagers have the highest rates of STDs among heterosexuals of all age groups. In general, STDs are a problem of the young. An estimated 12 million persons in the United States are infected with STDs each year. Eighty-six percent of these cases occur among 15- to 29-year-olds (Morris et al., 1993).

Young men infected with STDs do not suffer the same health consequences as women largely because their symptoms typically appear earlier than they do in women; thus, treatment can begin earlier. Not only is a woman's health affected, especially if the infections go untreated, but infants born to women with STDs are at risk for being infected themselves and can suffer long-term consequences. One of the most tragic of these is the perinatal transmission of HIV. Approximately 7000 infants are born to HIV-infected women in the United States each year. Acquired immunodeficiency syndrome will develop in 15 to 30% of these infants (Centers for Disease Control and Prevention, 1995). Chlamydia and gonorrhea are common STDs among adolescent girls. Untreated, they can progress to pelvic inflammatory disease (PID). Rates of PID are highest among adolescent girls; about 16 to 20% of all cases occur in this group (Morris et al., 1993).

SUBSTANCE ABUSE

Alcohol is the drug most often used and abused by adolescents. A recent survey found that approximately 88% of American high school seniors have tried alcohol at least once (Johnston et al., 1993). Alcohol use among teenagers is strongly associated with a number of health risks, including early and unprotected sex, tobacco use, violence, and traffic fatalities.

Likewise, tobacco use is a prevalent and dangerous problem among adolescents. Despite three decades of health warnings, more than 3 million adolescents in the United States smoke cigarettes or use smokeless tobacco (Johnston et al., 1992). Nearly all initial uses of tobacco occur before high school graduation (Elders et al., 1994). In a report to the nation, then Surgeon General Joycelyn Elders concluded the following (Elders et al., 1994):

- Most adolescent smokers are addicted to nicotine and report that they want to quit but are unable to do so.
- Adolescents with lower levels of school achievement, with fewer skills to resist pervasive influences to use tobacco, with friends who use tobacco, and with lower self-images are more likely than their peers to use tobacco.
- Cigarette advertising appears to increase young people's risk of smoking by affecting their perceptions of the pervasiveness, image, and function of smoking.

As well, illegal drug use is all too common among high school students. In 1991, 15% of students reported current marijuana use, and 2% were current cocaine users (6% reported ever having used cocaine) (Kann et al., 1993).

SOCIAL FACTORS AFFECTING CHILDREN'S HEALTH

As is true for all age groups, children's health is largely determined by social nonmedical factors. Because children, especially the young, are dependent on their families or others for their health and well-being, factors such as parents' or caretakers' education, income, and stability and the security and safety of the home environment significantly impact children's physical and mental health and overall well-being.

Just as family and community can offer important protection to support a child's health, serious risk factors such as poverty may act as threats to good health. Being poor alone does not always mean a child is at risk, but other socioeconomic risks can compound the risks of poverty. For example, many poor children also live in unsafe neighborhoods filled with the danger and influence of crime and drugs. Being in single-parent families, having poor nutrition, and lacking positive and nurturing adult role models also increase health risks. A combination of these factors can contribute to a child's chances of being in poor physical or mental health.

To meet successfully the health needs all children, but especially those with known risk factors, the community health nurse must be cognizant of family and other social influences in a child's life and be prepared to address the child's health needs in that context.

Poverty

Twenty-three percent, or nearly one in four, of the nation's children live below the poverty threshold ($14,763 for a four-person family in 1993), and this percentage is growing. Children are far more likely than adults to live in poverty (Fig. 10–2). Even though children account for a little more than one fourth of the population, they represent 40% of the poor (Baugher and Denavas, 1993). The poverty rate is rising fastest for children younger than 6 years.

Children in poverty experience more health problems than do their peers in higher income families (Klerman, 1991). Deaths from unintended injuries, child abuse, homicide, SIDS, and infectious diseases, including AIDS, are more common. Poor children also suffer more from low birth weight, asthma, dental decay, lead poisoning, and learning disabilities. The extreme living conditions of poor children who are also homeless, migrants, or in foster care usually compound their health problems. These social and economic burdens can create a sense of despair and hopelessness among parents and children that greatly hinders healthy behaviors.

Single-Parent Households

Contributing to the increasing numbers of children born into poverty is a rising proportion of nonmarital births. By far, children in households headed by single women are more likely to be in poverty. In 1993, of children younger than 6 years living with a single mother, 63.7% were poor compared with 13.4% of such children in married-couple families (Baugher and Denavas, 1993).

Children living in single-parent households tend to score lower on many health indicators than those living in two-parent homes. They are more likely to be exposed to drugs and alcohol before birth and not to have a regular source of health care (Klerman, 1991). Young women who become mothers before age 18 years are less likely to graduate from high school and are more likely to be single parents. Their incomes are often quite low, and this, plus a lack of social supports, influences their children's health to be less than optimal.

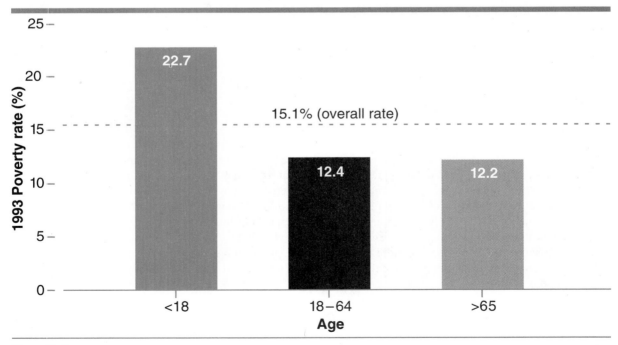

Figure 10–2
Poverty rates by age group (1993). Based on data from Baugher and Denavas (1993).

COMMUNITY HEALTH VISIT

- *Story by Leonard Kaku, RN, MSN*
- *Photography by George Draper*

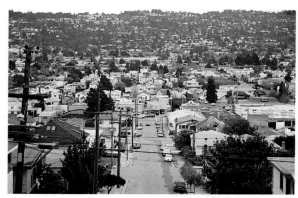

What is community health nursing? The American Nurses Association's definition says it is *a synthesis of nursing practice applied to promoting and preserving the health of populations.* It is, therefore, general, comprehensive, and continuous. The focus of care is directed to individuals, families, or groups (aggregates). Many community health nurses (CHNs) provide care to families in clinic settings.

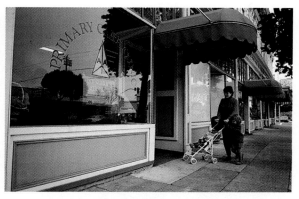

This clinic provides services through the Early Periodic Screening Diagnostic Treatment (EPSDT) Program, which was developed to provide health care for children in low-income families.

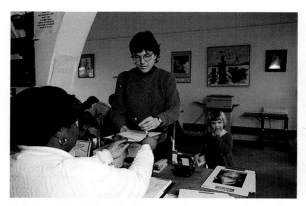

Unfortunately, clinic schedules are often crowded and clients may not be able to get appointments for several weeks.

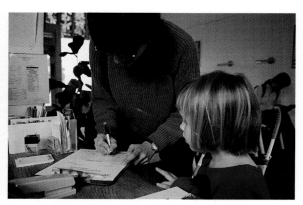

The nurse has an opportunity to observe the client and the family as they register and wait for their appointment. The parent registers the 5-year-old daughter for a school entry health physical. Medicaid insurance is verified for the physical exam.

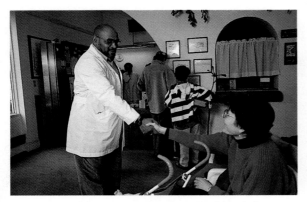

Introduction of the nurse to the client should include your name and role with the agency. It is important to address clients by their proper names and titles—Mr., Mrs., Ms.

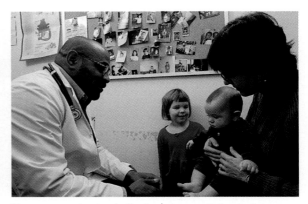

The nurse understands the importance of developing a comfortable atmosphere by beginning with social talk and general questions about the client and family.

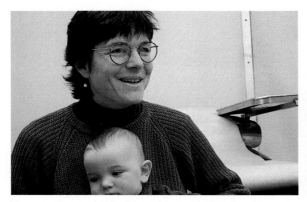

Trust can be established in a short period of time. The nurse can begin by explaining the steps in the clinic process so that the client knows what is expected. Always listen to the client attentively, and allow enough time for the client to reflect and respond to questions.

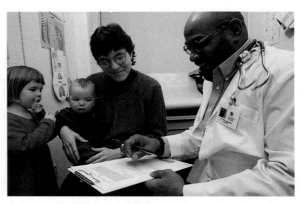

Asking an introductory question, such as "What brought you here today?", provides an open range of responses from the client. The parent's signature is required on a consent form in order for a physical examination and laboratory tests to be performed. The nurse explains the consent form to the parent.

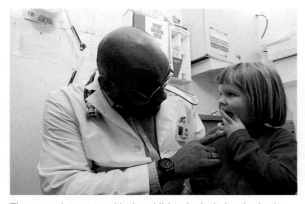

The nurse interacts with the child to include her in the interview process. This provides an opportunity for the nurse to develop a clearer picture of the relationship between the child and parent. It will promote a smoother transition through the examination process.

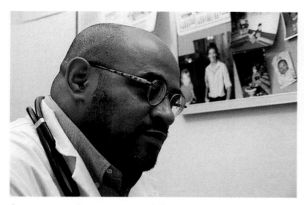

As you move from one part of the history to another, it is helpful to orient the client with brief transitional phrases such as, "Now I would like to ask you some questions about. . . "

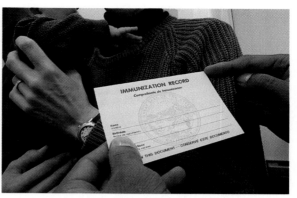

Reviewing immunization records is an important primary prevention role for the community health nurse. This is a teachable opportunity for the nurse to stress the importance of maintaining immunizations for the child. In California parents are provided with a yellow state immunization record for the child, which they should use for recording all immunizations and showing proof of immunizations when needed.

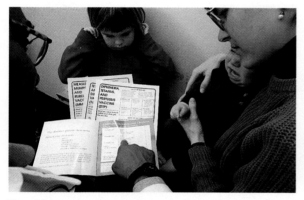

The child requires booster immunizations. The immunization consent forms are given to the parent for a signature. The nurse goes over the consent form with the parent and obtains a signature.

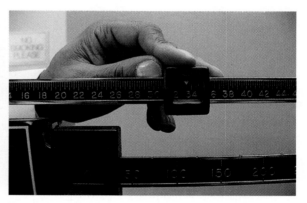

The clinic staff often take vital signs on clients, which include height and weight.

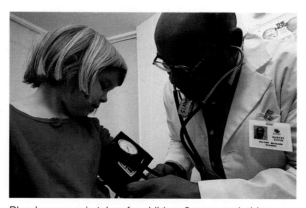

Blood pressure is taken for children 3 years and older.

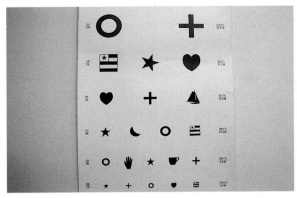

A vision screen is first attempted on a 4-year-old child. If the child is younger, a verbal report is taken from the parent.

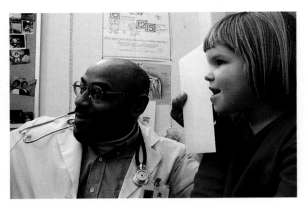

The results of the vision test are: OS: 20/40; OD: 20/50; and OU: 20/50.

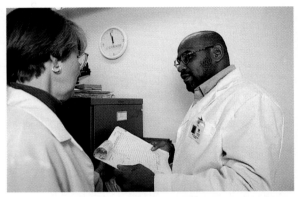

The nurse discusses any concerns about the client with the practitioner prior to the examination. The nurse reports the vision test results to the practitioner as well as any other concerns the nurse may have about the family.

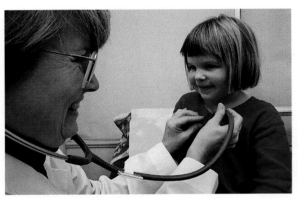

The practitioner performs the physical examination on the child with the help of the parent. The practitioner discusses the result of the vision test with the parent and the need for a follow-up appointment with an ophthalmologist. The child has not had a lead level done and requires booster immunizations. The practitioner orders laboratory tests, immunizations, and a referral to an ophthalmologist.

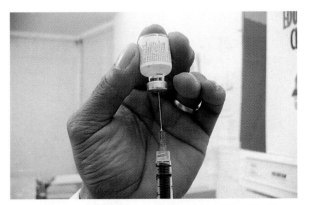

The clinic staff perform the laboratory work: Hct, UA, Pb level. The immunization consent forms have been signed by the parent. The nurse administers the immunizations and takes this opportunity to reinforce the importance of immunizations for both children.

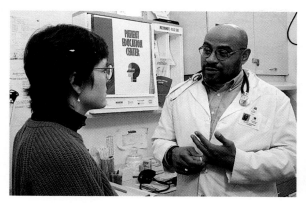

The nurse also offers suggestions to relieve the common side effects of immunizations.

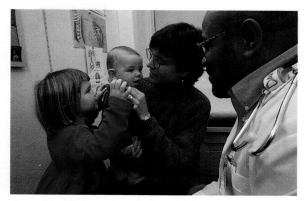

The exit interview provides an opportunity for the nurse to review any issues the parent has raised about the child. The nurse may ask, "Is there anything else I can assist you with?"

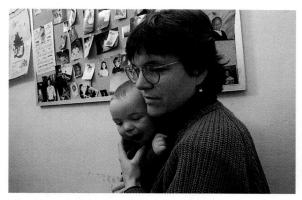

The parent asks about an ophthalmologist who takes Medicaid and about day care facilities in the area for the younger child. The parent also asks about family planning services in the community.

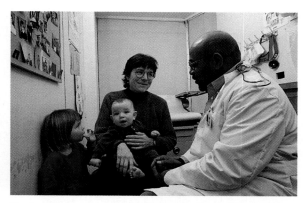

The family agrees to maintain immunizations on the children and to follow-up with appointments with an ophthalmologist and a family planning clinic. The nurse returns the immunization record to the parent documenting today's immunization as well as when the next immunizations are due. The nurse will call with a referral for an ophthalmologist, a family planning clinic, and a day care facility.

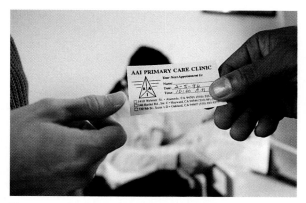

The nurse gives the parent a business card with the nurse's name and agency's address and phone number. The CHN advises the parent to call the nurse if there is anything else that the family may need.

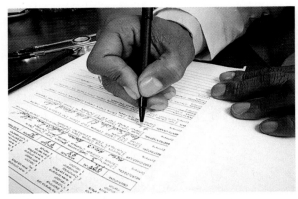

The nurse charts accurately, clearly, and concisely after the clinic visit.

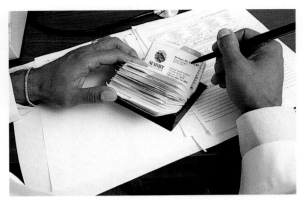

The nurse searches for resources for an ophthalmologist and a family planning clinic that accept Medicaid and a resource for day care providers. The nurse obtains phone numbers for a couple of ophthalmologists, a family planning clinic, and a day care consortium service.

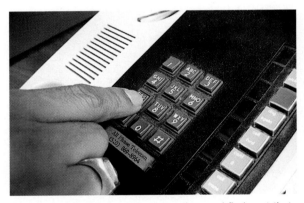

The nurse calls the day care consortium and finds out that there is a list of day care providers available.

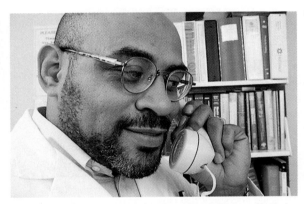

The nurse calls the family with the referrals for an ophthalmologist and a phone number to obtain a list of day care providers.

Adolescence

Adolescence is a period of growing independence and experimentation with risk-taking behaviors. These changes affect the willingness of adolescents to discuss certain matters with parents and other authority figures, including health care providers. During adolescence, the responsibility for health begins to shift from the parent to the child; the community health nurse must be aware of this and directly involve the adolescent in developing and implementing the care plan.

Whether an adolescent obtains needed health and other services is influenced by several factors such as attitudinal or behavioral obstacles presented by adolescents themselves, ability and willingness of health care providers to identify and treat their often complicated needs, and the broad array of social concerns that impact adolescent health. Confidentiality of services has been identified as important to an adolescent's willingness to obtain care, especially for sensitive matters such as sexual behavior, mental health, and substance abuse.

In response to the inadequacies of traditional medicine to meet the complex health needs of the adolescent population, specialized service centers, such as school-based clinics and adolescent health clinics in hospital outpatient departments, have been created. These clinics serve largely low-income clients with multiple health and social needs, and their significance in meeting adolescent health needs is growing.

COSTS TO SOCIETY OF POOR HEALTH AMONG CHILDREN

The best way to ensure the success and well-being of future generations is for each child to start life healthy and to have that health status maintained throughout childhood. Too many children grow up in adverse home conditions with physical and emotional health problems that will impair their ability to reach their full potential. Any health problem—whether hunger, poor vision or hearing, increased blood levels of lead, asthma, anemia, dental caries, illicit drug use, or teen pregnancy—can interfere with school attendance and success and a child's ability to grow and develop normally, to learn, and ultimately to succeed in life.

For no other age group is the prevention of health problems more significant or more cost effective than for children. Each dollar spent on the prevention of physical and emotional problems in children is a sound investment. Primary health care and early intervention for children and families can help prevent costly problems, suffering, and lost human potential.

Prenatal Care

Prenatal care, which costs as little as $1000 per pregnancy, can save hundreds of thousands of dollars by preventing conditions such as low birth weight that can require many expensive medical treatments after an infant has been born. The cost to our nation of low birth weight is astronomic. Hospital costs for each low-birth-weight infant are close to $4500. For each very-low-birth-weight infant (less than 3.3 pounds), the cost rises to $33,000 (U.S. General Accounting Office [GAO], 1992). Among the many additional costs of low birth weight are outpatient care, rehospitalization, special education, and special supplemental income for disabled children. The IOM has calculated that every $1.00 spent on prenatal care for high-risk women can save more than $3.00 on the cost of providing direct medical care during the first year of an infant's life (IOM, 1985).

Lead Poisoning

Removing the sources of lead in our environment is expensive but not nearly as expensive as the long-term consequences of lead poisoning. The Centers for Disease Control and Prevention estimate that preventing a child's blood lead level from reaching dangerous levels saves $3331 per child in avoided special education costs (Needleman, 1991).

Once discovered, lead can never be entirely removed from a child's body, nor can the neurologic damage that has already been done be reversed. Clearly, the most cost-effective treatment is prevention.

Adolescent Pregnancy and Parenting

Preventing pregnancy among school-aged mothers can reduce the dropout rate, welfare dependency, low birth weight, and infant mortality. It has been estimated that the public costs incurred in 1 year for all families that were started when parents were adolescents total $16.65 billion (costs of Aid to Families with Dependent Children program, Medicaid, and food stamps) (Burt and Levy, 1987).

PUBLIC HEALTH PROGRAMS TARGETED TO CHILDREN

A number of public programs have been established to address the health needs of children specifically or in conjunction with a targeted population of the medically underserved or poor. In addition, local and state public health and social service agencies aim to protect the health of an entire community or state through programs such as water fluoridation, sanitation, and the control of infectious diseases. Furthermore, broad-based strategies, such as the elimination of lead-based paint, use of lead-free gasoline, mandatory use of child safety seats in automobiles, bicycle helmet laws, comprehensive school health clinics, and drug and violence prevention programs serve to improve the health of children through community-wide approaches.

Medicaid

Poor children's ability to obtain health care services has improved since the introduction of Medicaid and its Early and Periodic Screening, Diagnosis, and Treatment (EPSDT) program. Medicaid is financed by state and federal governments and pays for health care services delivered to eligible individuals. Between 1985 and 1990, Congress and states passed legislation that expanded Medicaid eligibility for pregnant women, infants, and children in an effort to improve the nation's infant mortality rate and children's health status. Medicaid pays for approximately one third of all U.S. births (U.S. GAO, 1994).

Through EPSDT, children covered by Medicaid can receive a range of health and health-related services that far exceeds those usually covered by private insurance. Services include health, developmental, and nutritional screening; physical examinations; immunizations; vision and hearing screening; certain laboratory tests; and dental services. Unfortunately and contrary to popular belief, not all poor children are eligible for Medicaid, and not all those eligible are enrolled. In 1991, Medicaid assisted only 59% of children living in poverty (National Commission on Children [NCC], 1991). Barriers standing in the way of reaching all eligible children include

- Lengthy application forms and eligibility determination processes
- Stigma of welfare that is associated with Medicaid
- Increasing numbers of physicians unwilling to take Medicaid patients
- Unfriendly, overcrowded, and uncomfortable waiting rooms and public clinics

Medicaid does not provide access to health care for all those without private health insurance coverage. More than 34 million Americans, 8.3 million of whom are younger than age 18 years, are without any type of insurance. This represents approximately 13% of all children (NCC, 1991). Children without Medicaid or private health insurance use fewer medical services than those who are insured, and they are less likely to receive their immunizations (NCC, 1991).

Direct Health Care Delivery Programs

Although Medicaid pays for the health care used by its recipients, several other public programs directly deliver health care services to underserved populations. Although some of these underserved populations are eligible for Medicaid, many have neither Medicaid nor private health insurance. Most live in inner cities or rural areas with few health care providers and facilities.

MATERNAL AND CHILD HEALTH BLOCK GRANT

This program has its roots in a number of smaller, categorical grant programs that were consolidated in 1981. Through the block grant, federal funds are allocated to the states, which in turn add their own funds. These resources are combined with local funding to help ensure the delivery of basic health care to pregnant women and children and additional services to children with special health care needs.

COMMUNITY AND MIGRANT HEALTH CENTERS PROGRAMS

The Community and Migrant Health Centers Programs began in 1965 as two of the early programs of the U.S. Office of Economic Opportunity. Through a network of approximately 550 centers that operate more than 2000 clinics, these health centers provide comprehensive primary health care to more than 6 million low-income people, 2.1 million of whom are children younger than 15 years. Health centers also often obtain funds from local governments, foundations, corporations, clients, and other sources.

NATIONAL HEALTH SERVICE CORPS

The National Health Service Corps (NHSC) is another federal program through which children receive primary health care services. The NHSC sends physicians, nurses, and other health care providers to underserved areas of the country. Through scholarships and loan repayment plans, the program assists students with medical, nursing, and other training in return for a certain number of years of service in a rural or urban underserved area.

Although the NHSC funds were substantially reduced in the 1980s, Congress increased its funding in the early 1990s in response to the continued lack of health care providers, especially obstetric providers, in certain parts of the country.

SPECIAL SUPPLEMENTAL FOOD PROGRAM FOR WOMEN, INFANTS, AND CHILDREN

Although not exclusively a health program, WIC provides highly nutritious foods and nutrition education to more than 2 million low-income pregnant and breast-feeding mothers and their infants and to more than 2 million children younger than 5 years (U.S. GAO, 1994). Women and children who are on Medicaid are automatically eligible for WIC. Women participating in the program are encouraged to obtain prenatal care if they are pregnant. They also are encouraged to obtain preventive health care for themselves and their children, including childhood immunizations, and to maintain healthy diets.

Established in 1972, WIC has been one of the most successful, popular, and cost-effective public health programs. Women participating in WIC have less chance of delivering a low-birth-weight baby than similarly situated women not in the WIC program. The U.S. GAO has concluded that prenatal WIC benefits reduce the rate of low-birth-weight births by 25%. The GAO further estimates that the federal government saves $3.50 for every federal dollar spent on the WIC program (U.S. GAO, 1992).

Despite its successes, WIC has never been funded at a level that allows all eligible women and children to be served. In fact, an estimated 25% of income-eligible women (income up to 185% of the federal poverty level) are not served by the WIC program (U.S. GAO, 1992). Although Congress has steadily increased WIC funding, the current congressional efforts to convert WIC and other nutrition programs into block grants for the states would also reduce funding levels.

HEAD START

Head Start is a federally funded comprehensive early childhood program for low-income children aged 3 to

5 years. Head Start provides not only educational opportunities for children but also medical, dental, mental health, nutritional, and social services. It strongly emphasizes parental involvement on a voluntary or paid-staff basis. Head Start is widely viewed as a successful program, although it does not reach all eligible children. Congress has been steadily increasing the funding level in recent years in an attempt to reach the goal of full enrollment. Considerable ground will have to be covered to reach this goal, however. In 1993, only 36% of eligible children were enrolled in the Head Start program (Children's Defense Fund, 1994).

STRATEGIES TO IMPROVE CHILDREN'S HEALTH

As pointed out earlier, most children in the United States are born healthy and remain so throughout childhood. However, this is not the case for all children. The protective factors operating in the lives of healthy children and the interventions they receive should be available to all children, but they are not. Although the federal and state governments have attempted to provide a "safety net" for children without medical services, the system that has developed over the past three decades fails to address the multiple and interrelated health and social needs of our nation's growing population of poor and at risk. For example, the system may provide emergency care to a 9-year-old injured by gunfire in a drive-by shooting, but it leaves unaddressed the community conditions that perpetuate violence.

Because child health is affected not only by medical factors but also by social and family concerns, responsibility for improving children's health rests with the entire community, including health care professionals, parents, employers, and government. Only as a child gets older can that individual be held responsible for practicing healthy behaviors and obtaining proper health care.

In an effort to involve nationwide activity and support for improving the health of children and of all Americans, the U.S. Public Health Service has established Health Goals for the Year 2000. The numerous goals and objectives that have been set for children provide opportunities to help an individual community health nurse, other health care providers, or a community, state, or the nation focus on efforts to achieve optimal health for all children. To realize these goals, actions are needed by individuals, within families and communities, and at all levels of government.

Parents' Role

Even before conception, a mother's responsibility begins to ensure the health of her fetus. Before and during pregnancy, she must develop healthy behaviors, including proper nutrition and avoidance of smoking, alcohol, drugs, and other behaviors that could harm her fetus. This is particularly important in the early stages of gestation, when fetal organ systems are developing. It is also important for the mother to receive prenatal care early in pregnancy.

Starting with breast-feeding, parents must give their children nutritious food and ensure that they are immunized, receive needed health care services, and acquire healthful lifestyles. One of a parents most important jobs is to model healthy behaviors for their children.

Another important task for parents is doing all they can to ensure that their children have a safe environment at home, in the neighborhood, and at school. They must protect their children from injury, violence, and abuse and neglect. Parents must learn how to nurture, guide, and protect their children effectively through the developmental stages of childhood.

Community's Role

Families need support from their community and society to fulfill their roles and responsibilities. This is particularly true for families living in poverty and for parents who are isolated and disenfranchised. Ensuring access to health care is an important community role, but the responsibilities of communities in promoting complete well-being go far beyond the provision of traditional medical care.

Communities should work to create safe neighborhoods and support the development of community-based, comprehensive health, education, and social service programs. As well, communities can promote community health education campaigns concerning prenatal care, smoking, nutrition, teenage pregnancy, drug and violence prevention, and other health topics. At individual and community levels, they can also sponsor health fairs, immunization drives, bicycle safety helmet campaigns, crime prevention and reduction programs, and other projects that help families develop healthy lifestyles and gain access to needed health services.

Communities are well situated to facilitate integration of health, education, and social services, to eliminate fragmentation and duplication of services, and to better organize more comprehensive and streamlined systems of care. Despite the number of health and social service programs that exist, they are usually poorly coordinated with each other, and there is little collaboration among the professional disciplines (National Commission to Prevent Infant Mortality, 1991). Communitywide initiatives to better organize services and reach out to families through public awareness campaigns and home visits can alert parents to the importance of immunizations, a safer environment, prenatal care, and other services and can provide information on how to obtain these services.

As part of the community at large, the media should be involved with promoting child health. The media significantly influence children's lives and their perceptions of the world and themselves. From developing information campaigns about prenatal care and immunizations to discouraging violence and explicit sex in popular television programs, the media can have a profound effect on improving children's health and well-being.

Employer's Role

Business and industry have an enormous stake in the health of our nation's children. A strong, productive work force is ensured only when the health, social, and educational needs of the next generation of workers are met. Furthermore, health risks cost employers in lost productivity and increased health care costs.

The private sector can play a role in improving the health of individual children or of the community in general. An employer can make health care more accessible to families with children by offering affordable health insurance that covers the employee and dependents. The provision of insurance plans that offer full pregnancy and well-child health care benefits is essential to employee health promotion.

Maintaining a work place that allows flexible leave for prenatal and pediatric health care as well as time off to care for newborn and sick children can also contribute to child health improvements. In 1993, the Family and Medical Leave Act mandated that employers with 50 or more employees must allow a total of 12 workweeks of unpaid leave during any 12-month period for the birth or adoption of a child or for the care of a sick family member.

Employers can sponsor opportunities for employees to learn about healthy diets, healthy pregnancies, how to fight substance abuse, and ways to decrease stress.

Businesses also can offer on-site child care and work with community leaders and public officials to initiate community-wide health promotion projects targeted to children. Employers can also serve as catalysts for linking health, education, and social services for children.

Government's Role

The role of government in the United States in promoting or ensuring the health of children is more limited than it is in other countries. Most other countries have defined policies on children's health; the United States does not. Not only do such policies indicate that children are a priority of the citizenry, but they also help shape the operation of programs and their funding.

In this country, state and federal governments have several public health programs, as discussed earlier, that provide assistance to children, especially to those at risk owing to poverty or other disadvantages. Despite the number of programs and the significant funds committed to each, many children with health problems do not receive the services they need; also the various programs are not well coordinated, making access to those needed more difficult. Although these programs are not a substitute for a family's or caretaker's care and concern, they are important in protecting and promoting health and delivering services to those who would otherwise go without. Increasing access to health care, particularly for poor families, can help to prevent disease and suffering and will lower costs to society of remediating neglected conditions.

To ensure the health of children and other aggregates, particularly as the federal government devolves more responsibilities to lower levels of government and tightens funding, state and local public health agencies must provide leadership in planning for expanded access to services, monitoring program quality, and evaluating the quality of health and social services. Effective programs for underserved populations should be expanded, and the managers and front-line workers such as community health nurses, social workers, physicians, and caseworkers should be encouraged to cross their program lines and professional orientations to collaborate and thereby assist children with problems that adversely impact their health. "One-stop shopping" (i.e., user-friendly, accessible services for children and families) is an important concept for public programs to embrace so that children can receive the services they need, especially preventive health and social services, before a problem becomes a crisis. Outreach efforts through programs such as home visiting should be an integral part of health initiatives to find children in need and link them to the services they require.

Community Health Nurse's Role

From the earliest days of visiting nurses, public health nurses have played pivotal roles in improving the health status of pregnant women and children. Of all of the members of the community, the community health nurse is often the one most aware of children's health status, any barriers that stand between them and the care they need, and other factors that may be adversely affecting their health. Armed with this information and knowledge of the health and other resources available, it is the community health nurse's responsibility to advocate for improved individual and community responses to the needs of children, to participate in publicly funded programs, to promote social interventions that will enhance the living situations of high-risk families, and to network with other professionals to improve collaboration and coordination of services.

One important role of the community health nurse is to help link local health and social services with the school system. Children must be healthy to learn, but often children arrive at the school door with vision, hearing, and other health problems that could have been prevented or alleviated with appropriate education, screening, and treatment. As children move out of the preschool years, sometimes their only connection with the health care system is through the school health nurse. School health nurses can be an important source of primary health care and health information for students and their families.

Community health nurses can act as catalysts to alert the health professional community, business leaders, religious groups, and voluntary organizations to the needs of children and the strategies that can improve their ability to obtain the services they need. Community health nurses, as individuals and groups, can also influence the planning and implementation of necessary changes in the health care system so that children's health is improved and the national health goals for the year 2000 are achieved. As well, they can promote commitment within their own institutions for comprehensive, user-friendly health services.

APPLICATION OF THE NURSING PROCESS

By applying the principles of the nursing process to the individual, family, and community, the community health nurse can provide child health services more systematically and effectively. Most communities offer a range of preventive and other important services needed by children. The community health nurse must thoroughly understand the needs of the individual child and family and be aware of available community resources to act as a catalyst for meeting child health needs.

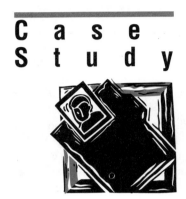

C a s e
S t u d y

Maria Martinez, a community health nurse working for the county health department, received a telephone call from the high school nurse informing her that Tara Parkhurst, a 16-year-old high school student from a low-income family, would be coming in that afternoon for a pregnancy test. Tara had already missed three menstrual periods and was afraid to talk about this with her family, although she and the school nurse had a long discussion. She was going to ask her boyfriend to take her to the health department clinic for the pregnancy test after school.

Assessment

Tara's pregnancy test was positive, and she was estimated to be 3½ months pregnant. She was upset and did not want to talk with Maria at the health department. Maria arranged to make a home visit the next afternoon.

Maria learned from the school nurse that Tara wanted to keep her baby. Knowing that a number of issues needed to be addressed at the first home visit, Maria prepared by developing a list of possible areas of assessment that covered individual, family, and community concerns. Her list included the following:

Individual
- Medical risk factors
- Emotional well-being
- Understanding and acceptance of pregnancy
- Health-promoting and risk-taking behaviors
- Understanding of importance of obtaining preventive care services
- Health insurance status
- Access to transportation

Family
- Adequacy of housing structure
- Safety of neighborhood
- Ability of family members to provide emotional support
- Ability of family to provide financial support

Community
- Prenatal and pediatric care
- Health and social services coordination
- Availability of culturally sensitive health care
- Emotional guidance and counseling
- Educational opportunities for pregnant and parenting teenagers
- Job training
- Nutrition services such as WIC and food stamps
- Pregnancy and parenting education
- Child care availability

Assessment Data

Individual

- The client is already in the early second trimester of pregnancy, with no prenatal care. She engages in risk-taking behaviors (smoking, alcohol use, and poor eating habits).
- During the interview, Tara seemed quiet and reserved. She said that she was excited to have a baby but she feared labor and delivery. Her boyfriend wants her to keep the baby.
- She says that she has not thought much about prenatal care but will probably see a doctor sometime before her delivery. She cannot afford to go to a physician right now.
- She desires to keep the baby and remain in school, yet she does not have a realistic understanding of the responsibilities of parenthood.

Family

- Tara's parents experienced disappointment with news of their only daughter's pregnancy, but her mother expressed a willingness to provide emotional support. Her father, who is emotionally distant, expressed anger.
- Both parents expressed concern about how the family would manage financially.

Community

- Maria determined that prenatal services were available but only during school hours. The only community provider taking Medicaid patients served a predominately middle-class clientele.
- Given her family income, Medicaid coverage and WIC services were probably available but would require lengthy and complex applications at the welfare office.
- Although Medicaid would pay for some prenatal classes, those available were geared to older, married couples.
- Tara's school would encourage her to remain in regular classes until her delivery date and would then provide home study for a limited time.
- No parenting classes were available.
- No child care was available at the high school, making returning to school more difficult.
- Although the community has a lay home visitor program that matches mentors with pregnant and parenting teens to provide health information and encouragement, the project does not serve Tara's neighborhood.

Diagnosis

Individual

- Altered health maintenance related to lack of prenatal care
- Knowledge deficit of effects of nutrition, smoking, and alcohol use on fetal development
- Altered parenting potential related to unrealistic expectations about parenting responsibilities

Family

- Altered family processes related to anger and disappointment over daughter's pregnancy
- Altered financial status because of the addition of another dependent to the family

Community

- Lack of coordinated, culturally sensitive, accessible prenatal and parenting services available to adolescents
- The existing Resource Mother (home visiting) program is a community strength, but the project needs to be expanded to reach all at-risk adolescents.

Planning

To ensure that the action plan is complete, realistic, and successfully implemented, Maria must thoroughly identify the factors affecting Tara's health and well-being. In addition, mutual goal setting among Tara, her family, and Maria must be accomplished.

Individual

Long-Term Goal

- Pregnancy outcome will be healthy.

Short-Term Goals

- Tara will obtain prenatal care.
- Tara will express an understanding of the reasons to change nutrition and substance use habits.
- Tara will plan with the nurse actions to change poor health habits.

Long-Term Goal

- Tara will demonstrate successful parenting behaviors.

Short-Term Goal

- Tara will enroll in parenting class. (If classes are not available in time, reading material, films, videotapes, or visits with experienced parents may be used.)

Long-Term Goal

- Tara will complete high school.

Short-Term Goal

- Tara will remain in school throughout her pregnancy and will use the home study program until she returns to school after the birth of her baby.

Family

Long-Term Goal

- The family's ability to handle crises will improve as evidenced by their ability to discuss problems and engage in mutual problem solving.

Short-Term Goal

- Parents will display supportive behaviors such as accompanying Tara to prenatal care appointments, helping her to engage in healthy behaviors, and assisting her to arrange child care so she can remain in school.

Community

Long-Term Goal

- Accessible, comprehensive, culturally sensitive prenatal and other health care services targeted to adolescents will be established.

Short-Term Goals

- Evening hours at the health department clinic will be extended to accommodate students and working families.
- Home visiting services will be expanded to meet community needs.

- Pregnancy and parenting classes targeted to adolescents will be provided in the community.
- A child care facility will be established in or near the high school.

Intervention

The immediate, mutually agreed-on goals established by the nurse, family, and individual must be addressed to help Tara achieve a healthy birth outcome and begin her role as a successful parent. In addition, the nurse must act as an advocate for community-wide change to ensure that the needs of individuals are being met by the community in which they live. To achieve aggregate-level goals, the community health nurse must communicate the needs of individuals to program managers, community leaders, policymakers, and others in decision-making roles.

For example, the health department director may not be aware that prenatal services are not readily accessed by high-risk groups of women such as adolescents. By bringing this and possible solutions to the director's attention, clinic hours can be expanded to benefit both pregnant teenagers and pregnant working women.

Likewise, it is in the best interest of the pregnant teenager, her child, her family, and the community for her to remain in school and obtain her high school diploma. The community nurse is in an ideal role to stimulate dialogue about the consequences of dropping out of high school and to facilitate action around policies such as child care for parenting teenagers so that they may remain in school.

Evaluation

Evaluation strategies must involve both processes and outcomes on the individual, family, and community levels. For example, evaluating a strategy for an individual might entail considering processes (e.g., the number of prenatal appointments kept by the pregnant woman) or outcomes (e.g., whether the infant was born at full term). Evaluating a strategy at the community level would require assessing whether programs were established (such as an evening prenatal clinic) and whether the establishment of the programs led to improved outcomes such as a reduced rate of preterm births or a reduced rate of dropping out of school by adolescent mothers.

Levels of Prevention

For no other aggregate is prevention more important than for children. In particular, primary prevention strategies, such as early prenatal care, good nutrition, and healthy behaviors among pregnant women, help ensure that a child is born healthy and gets a healthy start in life. The costs to the child, family, and society for not implementing prevention strategies are astronomic.

Primary Primary prevention depends largely on the age of the child. For the youngest children, strategies include preconceptional counseling and the practice of healthy behaviors by mothers before becoming pregnant and by parents and their children. Primary prevention also includes the prevention of unwanted pregnancy; this is especially important for adolescents.

Secondary Once pregnant, the woman must receive early and adequate prenatal care, practice healthy behaviors, obtain any other necessary social and supportive services, and prepare herself for becoming a parent. Although the woman is responsible for many of these practices, it also is incumbent on the community to ensure that adequate preventive health services such as prenatal care, nutrition and dietary counseling, pregnancy and parent education, and social services are available. The community health nurse can alert community leaders to the individual and societal consequences of women not receiving prenatal care or of teenagers not being able to complete high school owing to child care responsibilities. This kind of information can help planners design programs and policies that are in the best interest of the individual and society.

Tertiary Tertiary prevention involves the rehabilitation of individuals and aggregates to maximize their potential functioning. In the case of adolescent pregnancy, the community health nurse is in an ideal position to initiate programs and services that will prevent future unwanted pregnancy among teenagers and will help the parenting teenager provide the best care possible to the child. These programs could include the establishment of parenting classes and support services to help adolescents complete their education; coordination of health and social services for the mother and her child, including family planning services; and well-child care, immunizations, and nutrition services.

SUMMARY

Child and adolescent health status remains an important indicator of the health of the nation. Today's child and adolescent health problems are a reflection of rapidly changing social conditions rather than isolated events. Despite worrisome data that reveal declining child health status, community health nurses can use their experience and "inside knowledge" of barriers to child health to educate others.

Rather than limiting their approach to caring only for the individual and family, community health nurses can maximize their roles to collaborate and forge alliances where needed to solve children's health problems. Nurses are authority figures in places where it may least be expected. Being on the front line of health care is a powerful and very real position to members of Congress, state legislators, mayors, and others. By creatively using this kind of power, community health nurses can contribute greatly to improving the health and well-being of all children.

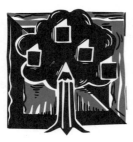

Learning Activities

1. Examine infant mortality statistics in your community and compare the rates with state and national averages. Is infant mortality higher for any particular ethnic groups within your community?

2. Imagine that you are a pregnant teenager without finances or available transportation and determine how you would obtain prenatal care.

3. Accompany a pregnant woman to a local department of social services as she tries to establish Medicaid eligibility for herself and her unborn child.

4. Identify pregnancy and parenting education programs in your community that are available to low-income women.

5. Survey your local medical community to discover the extent to which physicians determine whether children in their care are at risk for high levels of lead in the blood.

6. Survey businesses in your community to find out whether they offer maternity health insurance benefits, paid or unpaid maternity or paternity leave for new parents, and time off for prenatal care appointments. Use this information to develop a strategy to encourage the adoption of family-friendly policies and practices in the business community.

7. If your community has a lay home visitor program, meet with a home visitor and, if possible, accompany her when she makes her home visits.

8. Communicate with those in policy-making positions through writing letters or holding meetings about the needs of children.

9. Develop working relationships with lay and consumer groups to address children's health needs in the community.

REFERENCES

Alan Guttmacher Institute: Sex and America's Teenagers. New York, 1994.

American Academy of Pediatrics, Committee on Injury and Poisoning Prevention: Bicycle helmets. Pediatrics 95:609–610, 1995.

Baugher E, Denavas C: Income, Poverty, and Valuation of Non-Cash Benefits: 1993. Washington, DC, U.S. Department of Commerce, Bureau of the Census, 1993.

Burt MR, Levy F: Estimates of public costs of teenage childbearing: A review of recent studies and estimates on 1985 public costs. *In* Hofferth SJ, Hayes CD(eds). Risking the Future: Adolescent Sexuality, Pregnancy, and Childbearing. Volume II. Washington, DC, National Academy Press, 1987, pp. 15–29.

Callahan CM, Rivara FP: Urban high school youth and handguns: A school-based survey. JAMA 267:3038–3042, 1992.

Centers for Disease Control and Prevention, U.S. Public Health Service: Preventing Lead Poisoning in Young Children. Washington, DC, U.S. Department of Health and Human Services, Centers for Disease Control, 1991.

Centers for Disease Control and Prevention, U.S. Public Health Service: Update: AIDS Among Women—United States, 1994. MMWR Morb Mortal Wkly Rep 44:81–84, 1995.

Children's Defense Fund: The State of America's Children Yearbook, 1994. Washington, DC, 1994.

Cunningham J, Dockery D, Speizer F: Maternal smoking during pregnancy as a predictor of lung function in children. Am J Epidemiol 139:1139–1152, 1994.

Durant RH, Cadenhead C, Pendergrast RA, et al.: Factors associated with the use of violence among urban black adolescents. Am J Public Health 84:612–617, 1994.

Durkin MS, Davidson LL, Kuhn L, et al.: Low income neighborhoods and the risk of severe pediatric injury: A small area analysis in Northern Manhattan. Am J Public Health 84:587–592, 1994.

Elders JM, Perry CL, Eriksen MP, Giovino GA. (1994). The report of the Surgeon General: Preventing tobacco use among young people. Am J Public Health 84:543–547.

Goldenberg RL, Klerman LV. (1995). Adolescent pregnancy—Another look. N Engl J Med 332:1161–1162, 1995.

Institute of Medicine: Preventing Low Birthweight. Washington DC, National Academy Press, 1985.

Institute of Medicine: Prenatal Care: Reaching Mothers, Reaching Infants. Washington, DC, National Academy Press, 1988.

Johnston LD, Bachman JG, O'Malley PM: Monitoring the Future: Questionnaire Responses from the Nation's High School Seniors, 1989. Ann Arbor, MI, University of Michigan, Institute for Social Research, 1992.

Johnston LD, O'Malley PM, Bachman JG: National survey results on drug use from the monitoring the future study, 1975–1992 (NIH Publication No. 93-3597.) Bethesda, MD, U.S. Department of Health and Human Services, National Institutes of Health, 1993.

Kann L, Warren W, Collins J, et al.: Results from the National School-Based 1991 Youth Risk Behavior Survey and Progress Toward Achieving Related Health Objectives for the Nation. Public Health Rep 108(suppl 1): 47–55, 1993.

Klerman LV: Alive and Well? A Research and Policy Review of Health Programs for Poor Young Children. New York, National Center for Children in Poverty, Columbia University, 1991.

Kochanek KD, Hudson BL: Advance Report of Final Mortality Statistics, 1992. Monthly Vital Statistics Report 43(6, suppl). Hyattsville, MD; National Center for Health Statistics, 1995.

Kogan M, Alexander DR, Kotelchuck M: Prenatal care and low birthweight infants. JAMA 271:1340–1345, 1994.

Koop CE, Lundberg GD: Violence in America: A public health emergency. JAMA 267:3075–3076, 1992.

Leshner AI: National Pregnancy and Health Survey. Washington, DC, U.S. Department of Health and Human Services, Public Health Service, National Institutes of Health, National Institute on Drug Abuse, 1994.

Lewit E: Teenage childbearing. *In* The Future of Children: U.S. Health Care for Children. Los Altos, CA: The Center for the Future of Children, The David and Lucile Packard Foundation, 1992.

Morris L, Warren CW, Aral SO: Measuring adolescent sexual behaviors and related health outcomes. Public Health Rep 108(suppl 1):31–36, 1993.

National Commission on Children: Beyond Rhetoric: A New American Agenda for Children and Families. Washington, DC, U.S. Government Printing Office, 1991.

National Commission to Prevent Infant Mortality: One-Stop Shopping: The Road to Healthy Mothers and Children. Washington, DC, U.S. Government Printing Office, 1991.

National Education Association: Testimony presented July 27 before the U.S. Senate Subcommittee on Toxic Substances, Environmental Oversight, Research and Development, 1990.

Needleman HL: Childhood lead poisoning: A disease for the history text. Am J Public Health 18:685–687, 1991.

Needleman HL, Schell A, Bellinger D, et al: The long term effects of exposure to low doses of lead in childhood. N Engl J Med 322:83–88, 1990.

Public Health Service, U.S. Department of Health and Human Services: Healthy People National Health Promotion and Disease Prevention Objectives (DHHS Publication No. [PHS] 91-50213). Washington, DC, U.S. Government Printing Office, 1990.

Schoendorf KC, Kiely JL: Relationship of sudden infant death syndrome to maternal smoking during and after pregnancy. Pediatrics 90:905–908, 1992.

Snider S: Sources of Health Insurance and Characteristics of the Uninsured: Analysis of the March 1992 Current Population Study. Washington, DC, Employee Research Institute, 1993.

Streissguth AP, Aase JM, Sterling K, et al: Fetal alcohol syndrome in adolescents and adults. JAMA 265:1961–1967, 1991.

U.S. Congress, Office of Technology Assessment: Healthy Children: Investing in the Future (Publication No. OTA-H-345). Washington, DC, U.S. Government Printing Office, 1988.

U.S. Department of Health and Human Services: 1989 National High School Senior Drug Abuse Survey. Washington, DC, HHS News, 1990.

U.S. General Accounting Office: Early Intervention: Federal Investments Like WIC Can Produce Savings (Publication No. GAO/HRD-92-18). Washington, DC, U.S. Government Printing Office, 1992.

U.S. General Accounting Office: Medicaid Prenatal Care: States Improve Access and Enhance Services But Face New Challenges. (Publication No. GAO/HEHS-94-152BR). Washington, DC, U.S. Government Printing Office, 1994.

Ventura S, Martin J, Taffel S, et al.: Advance Report of Final Natality Statistics, 1992. Monthly Vital Statistics Report; 43(5 suppl). Hyattsville, MD; National Center for Health Statistics, 1994.

Wiese D, Dara D: Current Trends in Child Abuse Reporting and Fatalities: The Results of the 1994 Annual 50 State Survey. Chicago, National Committee to Prevent Child Abuse, 1995.

Women's Health

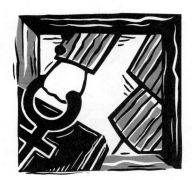

Upon completion of this chapter, the reader will be able to:

1. Discuss the incidence and prevalence of gender-specific health problems.

2. Determine the major indicators of women's health.

3. Relate the impact of poverty on the health of women.

4. Identify barriers to adequate health care for women.

5. Discuss the impact of public policy on the health of women.

6. Apply the nursing process to women's health concerns in the community.

7. Discuss reproductive health in relationship to the work place.

8. Examine prominent health problems among women of all age groups (from adolescence to old age).

9. Discuss primary, secondary, and tertiary prevention stages as they relate to women's health.

10. State the necessity for increased research efforts focused on women's health issues and their needs.

Roma D. Williams
Donna Neal Thomas

To achieve "health for all" by the 21st century, health care services must be affordable and available to all. Women are considered to be the key to realizing this goal; however, a significant number of them and their families face tremendous barriers in gaining access to health care. Additionally, knowledge deficits related to health promotion and disease prevention activities prevent women of all educational and socioeconomic levels from assuming responsibility for their own health and well-being.

The women's movement of the 1970s set high on its agenda a call for the reform of systems affecting the health of women. Women were encouraged to become involved not only as consumers of health services but also as establishers of health policy. More women entered health professions in which they had been previously underrepresented, and those in traditionally female-dominated professions such as nursing and teaching became more assertive in their demands to be recognized for their contributions to society.

Over a decade ago, in her "Preamble to a new Paradigm for Women's Health," Choi (1985) declared that collaboration and an interdisciplinary approach are necessary to meet the health care needs of women. She further stated that "essential to the development of health care for women are the concepts of health promotion, disease and accident prevention, education for self-care and responsibility, health risk identification and coordination for illness care when needed" (Choi, 1985). To realize this paradigm, community health nurses must work with other health care professionals to formulate upstream strategies that modify the factors affecting the health of women.

In this chapter we address the health of women as an aggregate, from adolescence through old age. Major indicators of health, including specific health problems, as well as the socioeconomic, sociocultural, and health policy issues surrounding the health of women are explored. The identification of current and future research aimed at improving the health of women is discussed. An understanding of these points will enable community health nurses to appropriately apply expertise in a community setting to help improve the health of the women among whom they work and live.

MAJOR INDICATORS OF HEALTH

In the United States, data collected on major causes of death are used to indicate the health status of any aggregate, whether gender, age, or ethnicity. Women use health services at a much higher rate than men, and the data can help interpret their levels of health. The primary indicators of health that are covered in this chapter are life expectancy, mortality (causes of death), and morbidity (causes of acute and chronic illness). Many factors that lead to death and illness among women are preventable or avoidable. If certain conditions are detected early and treated, a significant positive impact on both longevity and the quality of life could ensue.

Life Expectancy

Worldwide, women typically experience greater longevity than their male counterparts (except in Bangladesh, Bhutan, and Nepal) (Paolisso and Leslie, 1995). Females born in 1970 in the United States, for example, had an average life expectancy of 74.7 years, or 7.6 years longer than males born in the same year. During the past two decades, this discrepancy has continued: males born in 1992 have a life expectancy of 72.3 years compared with 79.0 years for females (U.S. Bureau of the Census, 1995).

Racial background also influences life span. For instance, although black females born in 1992 gained an additional 6.5 years of life expectancy—up from the projected 69.4 years for those born in 1970—it still falls behind the 79.7 years of life expectancy of white females born in 1992 (Population Today, 1993; U.S. Bureau of the Census, 1988).

Mortality

LEADING CAUSES OF DEATH

Table 11–1 lists the five major causes of death among American women in 1992. The largest percentage of overall deaths is caused by cardiovascular disease (CVD), but it has decreased in the past 40 years, from 424.2 per 100,000 in 1950 to 186.0 per 100,000 in 1991 (American Heart Association [AHA], 1994). Nevertheless, disparities continue related to care of women (Steingart et al., 1991). Annually, all CVDs combined cause more deaths among females (479,359, or 51.8%) than among males (446,702, or 48.2%). Some investigators claim that the problem is not gender bias; rather women do not display typical symptoms that men do, such as a positive exercise test and, therefore, are not treated in the same way as men, such as with cardiac catherization (Mark et al., 1994)

Table 11–1
Five Leading Causes of Death Among Women for All Races and Age Groups in 1992

Age Group (yr)	Cause of Death (in Rank Order)
15–24	Unintentional injury ("accidents") and adverse effects
	Homicide
	Malignant neoplasm
	Suicide
	Heart diseases
25–44	Malignant neoplasm
	Unintentional injury and adverse effects
	Heart disease
	Human immunodeficiency virus
	Homicide
45–64	Malignant neoplasm
	Heart disease
	Cerebrovascular disease
	Chronic obstructive pulmonary disease
	Diabetes mellitus
65–74	Heart disease
	Malignant neoplasm
	Cerebrovascular disease
	Influenza and pneumonia
	Chronic obstructive pulmonary disease

Adapted from U.S. Bureau of the Census. (1994). Statistical Abstract of the United States. Washington, DC, U.S. Government Printing Office.

MATERNAL MORTALITY

Because of their reproductive capabilities, women are uniquely at risk during pregnancy and childbirth, with additional dangers associated with legal and spontaneous abortions. The National Hospital Discharge Survey (National Institutes of Health [NIH], 1993) reported that one in five American women will be hospitalized at least once during pregnancy because of a complication. Some of these women will die.

Since the 1950s, maternal mortality has continued to decline in the United States, a reduction largely attributed to improved prenatal care and education of the woman, early detection of maternal risk factors, blood transfusions, improved anesthesia, and antibiotics (Cunningham et al., 1993). However, in maternal mortality, as in life expectancy, racial discrepancy persists (Table 11–2). Nonwhite women have a threefold greater incidence of death during pregnancy than whites (Cunningham et al., 1993). Major risk

factors include inadequate access to prenatal care, poor nutrition, and substandard living conditions. Despite progress in reducing deaths of nonwhites, their infant death rates remain more than twice that of white women. According to Johnson (1992), this four-decade disparity in mortality between black and white infants provides insight into the social order, one that will respond to actual changes in the well-being of infants and pregnant women.

Pulmonary embolism, according to *Williams' Obstetrics* (Cunningham et al., 1993), is the leading cause of maternal mortality (17%) followed by, in decreasing order of occurrence, hypertension, ectopic pregnancy, hemorrhage, stroke, and anesthesia. Mortality associated with legal surgical abortion is considered rare in the United States. Complications that result in death from abortion relate to the woman's age, type of abortion, and gestational age of the fetus when it is aborted. Recognized or unrecognized health problems, anesthesia, hemorrhage, and infection have also been identified as risk factors in deaths from surgical abortion (Hatcher et al., 1994).

Since 1988 a medical method of abortion using mifepristone, or RU-486, an antiprogestin medication, together with prostaglandins has been used in European countries and China and is reported to be as effective as surgical abortion. However, in the United States, because of public pressure against the use of this method of abortion, only since the Clinton administration has testing, licensing, and manufacturing of RU-486 begun. In mid-1994, RU-486 became available for clinical trials and is expected to be approved for use in the general population within 3 years. Additional research is needed to examine the acceptability of this method among American women, the relationship between medical method abortion and a woman's cultural beliefs, and her decision-making process used to choose between a medical method or

Table 11–2
Maternal Mortality Rate per 100,000 Live Births

Year	Total	Whites	Blacks	Other Nonwhites
1985	7.8	5.2	20.4	18.1
1986	7.2	4.9	18.8	16.0
1987	6.6	5.1	14.2	12.2
1992	7.8	5.0	20.8	18.2

BARRIERS TO USE OF PRENATAL CARE

Women who receive little or no prenatal care are at risk for higher mortality rates for themselves and their infants. Healthy People 2000 (U.S. DHHS, 1991) has set the goal for the nation's maternal mortality rate to be less than 3.3 deaths per 100,000 live births and to reduce the infant mortality rate to no more than 7 deaths per 100,000 births.

Many of the factors associated with maternal deaths have also been related to infant deaths. Because of the wide disparity between deaths in white infants (8.9) and deaths in black infants (17.9), Native American (12.5), and Puerto Rican (12.9) infants, Healthy People 2000 has projected an infant mortality rate of no greater than 11, 8.5, and 8 per 100,000 live births for each group, respectively, by the year 2000.

Several factors make women disinclined to seek prenatal care: (1) perceptions by the woman regarding the usefulness of prenatal care and whether the environment where services are sought is supportive and pleasant, (2) cultural values, and (3) beliefs. Unintended pregnancy or a pregnancy viewed negatively is associated with a delay in seeking prenatal services.

Women receive insufficient prenatal care for several reasons (Institute of Medicine, 1988):

- Financial constraints: absent or inadequate private insurance, lack of public funds for prenatal care, lack of support for public agencies providing maternity care services
- Lack of maternity care providers: inadequate numbers of physicians in some parts of the country, low participation of obstetrician-gynecologists in Medicaid and a decrease in obstetric care because of increasing malpractice premiums; inadequate use of nurse practitioners and certified nurse midwives
- Insufficient prenatal care in agencies in which high-risk groups usually seek services (sites such as community health centers, hospital outpatient departments, and local health departments)
- Environments that shape the context of poor women's lives, where they face violence, death, poverty, unemployment, and despair. Providers report time is spent dealing with basic survival needs (housing and food), and a discussion of prenatal care is often put off repeatedly (J. Maxwell; Better Babies Project, Washington, DC, personal communication, 1988).

surgical abortion. The reader is referred to Donaldson and colleagues' (1995) report for an up-to-date description of the current and potential uses of RU-486; the history, advantages, and disadvantage of medical abortion; and new clinical trials and ethical issues. Abortion is a controversial issue for providers and for the women in their care. An upstream intervention would certainly be the best strategy; however, until that time, nurses must continue to keep abreast of all available pregnancy termination options to provide the best counsel.

Ectopic pregnancy is a sizable mortality threat, accounting for 13% of maternal deaths, 90% of which are due to hemorrhage (NIH, 1993). Primary prevention interventions are critical in reducing a woman's risk for an ectopic pregnancy, because early diagnosis and treatment greatly reduce mortality. Yet in the last two decades, the incidence of ectopic pregnancy has increased fourfold, to 10.7 per 1000 pregnancies among women 15 to 44 years of age (Seltzer and Pearse, 1995). As has been seen before, racial

discrepancy is evident, with a rate of 14.2 per 1000 among nonwhites compared with 9.7 per 1000 in whites. This disparity continues to increase throughout the reproductive years of nonwhite women (Cunningham et al., 1993) possibly because, even though sexually transmitted diseases (STDs) are more frequent among nonwhite women, these patients have less access to health care.

Because the most significant risk for ectopic pregnancy is previous pelvic inflammatory disease or salpingitis, women at risk for acquiring STDs must learn to protect themselves from these diseases. Upstream endeavors targeted to aggregates at risk include school programs that address responsible sexuality. An example of one such successful program is called Postponing Sexual Involvement, a joint effort of Grady Memorial Hospital and Emory University in Atlanta, Georgia (Contraceptive Report, May 1994). Staff discovered that limiting young people to information on human sexuality is not effective in changing sexual behavior, so this innovative educational component was added to the agenda. Based on the social influence theory described as an educational model for reducing negative health behaviors, it maintains that young people are more likely to become sexually involved as a result of social and peer pressures than because of lack of knowledge. The two-part course is taught to 4000 eighth graders in Atlanta. According to Marion Howard, PhD, clinical director of the Teen Services Program, "a unique element of the program [is that] 11th and 12th grade girls and boys . . . are trained by hospital staff to lead the class. These teen leaders are very powerful role models . . . Messages about sexual involvement that come from those close to their own age are particularly powerful influences on young people" (p. 7). This is one of the earliest and best known abstinence intervention programs in the nation. (For more information on the program, contact Dr. Marion Howard, Grady Memorial Hospital, 80 Butler St, SE, Atlanta, GA 30335.)

MALIGNANT NEOPLASMS

Cancer death rates among women increased from 136.0 per 100,000 women in 1960 to 141.9 per 100,000 women in 1990 (American Cancer Society [ACS], 1995). The ACS estimated that 242,277 deaths occurred among women as a result of cancer in 1991. Over the past 30 years, lung cancer has increased 450% in women and 96% in men (Boring et al., 1994). Since 1987, lung cancer surpassed breast cancer as the leading cause of cancer deaths in women. Every year, breast cancer claims the lives of 46,000 women, but an estimated 62,000 women will die from lung cancer in 1995. Colorectal cancer, the third most frequent cause of cancer deaths in women, claims the lives of 28,100 men and 27,200 women annually (ACS, 1995). The good news is that, primarily because of healthy lifestyle changes, in the past 30 years mortality from some cancers has fallen. Colorectal cancer, as an example, is down 29% for women and 7% for men (ACS, 1995).

Five-year survival rates vary according to type of cancer and stage at diagnosis. For instance, the 5-year survival rate for all patients with lung cancer is only 13%. For localized breast cancer it is 94%, but only 18% when diagnosed with distant metastases. Of cancers related to the reproductive tract, ovarian cancer has the lowest survival rate: 42% (ACS, 1995). When diagnosed at an early stage, the 5-year survival rate for women with colon cancer is 93% and for those with rectal cancer, 87%.

Early diagnosis and prompt treatment are major factors in surviving many types of cancer. In addition, certain health choices might reduce an individual's risk of cancer. All women need to replace and avoid health-deteriorating practices by adopting health-promoting behaviors that foster a health-protecting lifestyle. If providers and patients applied everything known about cancer prevention, approximately two thirds of cancer cases would not occur (ACS, 1995). For example, women could reduce their risk for cancer by never smoking or by quitting if they already use tobacco products. Eating a nutritious diet can decrease a woman's risk of heart disease and cancer. Community health nurses play a major role in providing cancer control services, services that should be culturally sensitive and appropriate to the targeted aggregate (Brown and Williams, 1994). Community health nurses must encourage women to maintain healthy weight, and instruct them to use the food guide pyramid as an aid to eating a low-fat, high-fiber diet filled with needed nutrients and calories (Spark, 1994). Limiting alcohol and the consumption of salt-cured, smoked, and nitrite-cured foods should also be recommended (ACS, 1995).

CVD AND DIABETES MELLITUS

Each day more than 2500 Americans die from CVDs. About one in four individuals has one or more forms of CVD, which includes high blood pressure, coronary artery disease, stroke, and rheumatic heart disease. An equal opportunity killer, one in nine women aged 45 to 64 years has some form of CVD, a ratio increasing to one in three after age 65 years. Women of color are more likely than whites to die from CVDs. In 1991, the CVD death rate among white females was 131.2 per 100,000, but it was 68.9% higher for blacks: 221.6 per 100,000 (AHA Heart and Stroke Facts: Statistical Supplement 1994). The coronary heart disease death rates for white females is 66.4 in contrast to 88.3 for black females (33.0% higher). Stroke, although 19% higher for males than for females, is more deadly for women than for men. Black women are more likely to die from stroke than white women: 41.0 and 22.8, respectively (almost 80% higher).

There is currently an increased emphasis on the cardiovascular health of women and studies directed toward women. Health care providers are learning about heart disease in women and learning that women need different interventions than men to protect themselves from this deadly disease (Olson and Labat,

1995). According to Amsterdam and Legato (1993), postmenopausal mortality rates increase, at which time more women than men will die of CVDs. Further declines in CVD rates for women are possible only as individuals become more aware of risk factors and accept increasing responsibility for managing their own health and well-being. This will take concerned and motivated providers to encourage women to practice heart-healthy behaviors.

Diabetes mellitus is another disease with a pronounced gender differential, causing the premature death of many women (Kahn and Weir, 1994). The incidence of non–insulin-dependent diabetes (NIDDM) increases with age and is slightly higher for women than men, except among those 65 to 74 years of age. The highest prevalence of NIDDM is found among the Pima Indians (35%), significantly higher than among Native Americans as a whole (17%). African-Americans have a prevalence rate of 5%, twice that of the general population (2.5%) (Seltzer and Pearse, 1995). Prevalence among blacks is higher than among whites at all ages for both men and women. In the United States, diabetes ranks as the seventh leading cause of death in black women (AHA, 1994; Nesto et al., 1994).

Diabetes is an independent risk factor for the development of coronary artery disease (Nesto et al., 1994). When diabetic patients suffer heart attacks, their overall in-hospital mortality is much higher than for nondiabetic patients. The prognosis for diabetic women after a myocardial infarction (MI) is particularly grave, with an overall in-hospital mortality of 37% compared with 19% for men. A possible explanation for this disparity is that women may have additional diagnoses that men do not have, such as congestive heart failure. Whatever the cause, women with diabetes are at considerable risk of dying when they have an MI. According to Nesto and colleagues (1994), the aggregate at highest risk of mortality seems to be obese, diabetic women. An upstream approach to this downstream problem includes helping women maintain a desirable weight throughout life in an effort to avoid nutrition-related causes of death such as NIDDM and cardiovascular disease (Spark, 1994).

Morbidity

HOSPITALIZATIONS

The 1993 National Hospital Discharge Survey (Graves, 1995) reported that more women than men were hospitalized. Yet the average length of hospital

ization for men (6.4 days) exceeded that for women (6.5 days) until after the age of 65 years. Cerebrovascular disease resulted in the longest average hospital stays (10.9 days), occurring most frequently among women aged 65 years or older. Fractures accounted for an average of 9.4 days, malignant neoplasms for 8.3 days, and diseases of the heart for 7.2 days (Graves, 1995).

After hospitalization for several of these conditions, referrals may be made to community health nurses to provide ongoing nursing care in the home. Because of the prospective payment system for hospitalization, there is an increasing demand for skilled nursing services to be provided in the home. Nurses practicing in home environments must be prepared to deliver high-tech as well as high-touch services.

CHRONIC CONDITIONS AND LIMITATIONS

Women are more likely than men to be limited in activity because of chronic conditions. Arthritis and rheumatism, hypertension, and impairment of back or spine decrease women's activity level more often than they affect their male counterparts. In fact, almost twice as many women (24.6%) as men (12.4%) are limited in activity level because of arthritis and rheumatism. Nevertheless, more men than women have limited activity because of heart conditions (U.S. Bureau of the Census, 1995). Women are more likely than men to have difficulty performing activities such as walking, bathing or showering, preparing meals, and doing housework (U.S. Bureau of the Census, 1995).

Functional limitations require home health care that is supervised and delivered by nurses practicing in community settings. Nursing interventions are planned and implemented based on functional assessments. The care plan facilitates optimal resumption of the individual's independence in personal care activities.

SURGERY

Hysterectomy is the most frequently performed surgery among nonpregnant women 15 years of age or older (Wilcox et al., 1994). The mean age at hysterectomy is reported to be 40.9 years (Ravnikar and Chen, 1994). Although in the United States 562,000 hysterectomies were performed in 1993 compared with 653,000 in 1987, this represents not a decline in the rate of hysterectomy but rather an artifact of the change in design of the National Hospital Discharge Survey (Graves, 1995). Hysterectomy rates for black women are slightly higher than those for white women (61.7 and 56.5 per 10,000 women, respectively), not a significant difference. According to Wilcox and colleagues, uterine fibroids or leiomyoma, the most common reason for hysterectomy, accounts for one third of all such surgeries but considerably more for blacks (61%) than for whites (29%). The most common causes for hysterectomies among white women are endometriosis, uterine prolapse, and cancer.

According to Nora Coffey, founder of Hysterectomy Educational Resources and Services, women need more information about the options to and aftereffects of hysterectomy (personal communication, September 1995). A woman of childbearing age with fibroid tumors, for example, might be counseled to have a hysterectomy instead of an alternative approach to resolving the problem. The surgical approach for hysterectomy seems to depend on the physician's training and diagnosis. The vast majority (75%) of hysterectomies are performed as abdominal surgery. As with any abdominal surgery, there may be an increase in morbidity and a longer hospitalization.

Community health nurses, functioning as advocates for women, could provide health education programs related to indications for hysterectomy and oophorectomy (removal of ovaries) as well as information regarding the type of surgical approach and the purpose of a second opinion. If there is the least doubt as to the necessity for a hysterectomy, women are encouraged to obtain a second opinion. This is, in fact, usually a requirement of insurance plans. Second opinions tend to decrease the rate of hysterectomies, as do higher levels of education (Finkel and Finkel, 1990; Meilahan et al., 1989).

Birth by cesarean delivery, the most prevalent surgical procedure experienced by women in the United States, accounts for one of every four births (Olds et al., 1992). Almost half of these occur among women who have had prior cesareans. Several factors contribute to its increase, including progress in technology that facilitates monitoring of the fetus and physicians' fear of malpractice suits. The practice of vaginal birth after cesarean (VBAC) may decrease America's high cesarean birth rate. As part of the childbirth curriculum, childbirth educators offer information related to the cesarean birth experience. Some hospitals or groups, such as Cesareans/Support, Education and Concern, hold classes in preparation of a repeat cesarean birth or to prepare couples desiring VBAC (Olds et al., 1992).

MENTAL HEALTH

The most frequently occurring interruption in the mental health of women relates to depression. Well-controlled epidemiologic studies consistently demonstrate that young women experience depression at twice the rate of men (Hauenstein, 1991). Symptoms range from depressed mood to apathy, anxiety, irritability, and thoughts of death and suicide (Weissman, 1980; Weissman and Klerman, 1982). Hauenstein found that women were vulnerable to feelings of hopelessness and lowered self-esteem. Those of lower income and educational levels are at greater risk for depression than those of higher educational or economic status. Lacking adequate financial or emotional support, they often express a sense of frustration and futility. Nurses practicing in community health settings should be aware of the signs and symptoms of depression and identify referral sources for professional help within the community.

SIGNS AND SYMPTOMS OF DEPRESSION

The woman experiencing depression may display some of the following signs and symptoms (Smith, 1986):

- Mood disturbance and emotional distress
- Sad, blue, gloomy feelings
- Feelings of helplessness, hopelessness, being inadequate, worthlessness
- Loss of interest in work, friends, family, sex
- Low energy level
- Sleep pattern disturbances
- Loss of appetite or voracious appetite
- Feelings of heaviness in head or chest
- Crying easily and sighing often
- Complaining of headaches, backaches, constipation
- Difficulty in concentrating and making decisions
- Flat to hectic gaiety
- Everything drooping: mouth, eyes, posture (body language)

Other Factors

EDUCATION AND WORK

In the work place, women predominate as librarians, teachers, social workers, and nurses, accounting for

65% of working women in 1990 (Pollard and Tordella, 1993). Yet in the 1980s, more women began to enter professions traditionally held by men (e.g., lawyers, physicians and dentists), so that by 1990 more than half (57%) of the young professionals were women. According to Pollard and Tordella, this is a revolutionary development and the likely trend of the future.

Academically too, statistics are rising. In 1970, 55.4% of all women 25 years of age or older were high school graduates compared with 75.9% in 1988. Of this same age group 17% had completed college in 1988, approximately twice the 1970 rate of 8.2%. In 1987, women earned 51.2% of the master's degrees and 35.2% of all doctorates, about a 10% increase over that in 1970. Increasing numbers of women have been conferred degrees in traditionally male-dominated professions. Table 11–3 reflects recent changes occurring in percentages of women receiving degrees in medicine, dentistry, law, and theology (U.S. Bureau of the Census, 1995).

EMPLOYMENT AND WAGES

In the early 1990s, nearly two of every three women of working age (18–64 years) were employed compared to four of every five men. More than half (57%) of married women with young children (younger than 6 years) are working outside the home. In 1950, only 12% of women were combining these roles (Chadwick and Heaton, 1992). Do these represent true gains and opportunities? According to Riche and Pollard (1994), the American woman of the 1990s resembles the Chinese character for change: more opportunities, but also greater risks.

Table 11–4 depicts median annual income by marital status of women and men. A review of

Table 11–4
Median Annual Earnings by Family Type in Current Dollars for 1970, 1980, 1988, and 1993

Family Type	1970	1980	1988*	1993
Families maintained by a married couple	10,516	23,141	36,389	43,005
Families maintained by women	5093	10,408	15,346	17,443
Families maintained by men	9012	17,519	26,827	29,467

*Based on revised processing procedures: data not directly comparable with prior years. From U.S. Bureau of the Census. (1995). Statistical Abstract of the United States: 1995, 115th ed. Washington, DC, U.S. Government Printing Office, p. 477.

female-dominated versus male-dominated jobs discloses inequities in wage and salary scales; despite the diminishing gap between women's and men's incomes, there is still much room for improvement. Average annual earnings for both black and white women are lower than for their male counterparts. Recent data indicate that women earn only 69.9¢ for every $1.00 earned by men (Tiffany and Johnson-Lütjens, 1993).

Schreiber (1994) discussed nursing as women's work and the gender bias of job evaluation systems. In Illinois, for example, it was demonstrated that charge nurses received as much as $12,540 less annually than did a stationary engineer whose primary duty was to run a boiler system. With the Hay system, a method of allocating points according to education required, responsibility involved, and accountability, charge nurses score 415 points compared with 181 points for the sanitary engineer (ANA, 1984). Some groups have said that the major battle of the last decade of the 20th century will focus on bringing about pay equity between the traditional female- and male-dominated jobs. Valuing nurses' work will help ensure that work of all women is recognized and compensated.

The aggregate fast becoming the poorest in the United States are women and their children, a phenomenon labeled "the feminization of poverty." The nurse working with these families should be aware of social services, child care programs, emergency services, and other resources for families in need (Sidel, 1991). It is often the community health nurse who will act as case manager and advocate

Table 11–3
Percentages of Degrees Received by Women

Degree	1970	1980	1987	1992
Medicine (MD)	8.4	23.4	32.4	35.7
Dentistry (DDS or DMD)	0.9	13.3	24.0	32.3
Law (LLB or JD)	5.4	30.2	40.2	42.7
Theology (BD, MDiv, or MHL)	2.3	13.8	19.3	23.3

From U.S. Bureau of the Census. (1995). Statistical Abstract of the United States: 1995, 115th ed. Washington, DC, U.S. Government Printing Office, p. 192.

for families with social service agencies and other public entities.

WORKING WOMEN AT HOME

Added to inequities outside the home are inequities within the home. A working woman is less likely to have a spouse or partner to help with the home and children. Even when a spouse or partner is present, the burdens of housework and child care usually fall more heavily on women regardless of ethnicity. Mothers spend more time than fathers preparing meals and training and disciplining their children. These multiple-role demands and conflicting expectations contribute to stress (Bonam-Crawford and Orlick, 1994; Haas, 1982).

Changes are occurring, however, as, according to Chadwick and Heaton (1992), younger and older men now report spending more time in family activities compared with middle-aged men. Minority men, blacks, and Hispanics tend to spend a little more time working at family tasks than white men. Today books and articles encourage wives and husbands to make their needs known. As a result, many couples emphasize increased communication between partners. Marriage enrichment programs, often offered through churches and synagogues, teach couples how to communicate more effectively with each other (Chadwick and Heaton, 1992). Such efforts should foster equality between partners.

FAMILY CONFIGURATION AND MARITAL RELATIONSHIP STATUS

Women are members of multiple family configurations (e.g., nuclear families, extended family units, single-parent units, families of group marriages, blended family units, adoptive family units, nonlegal heterosexual unions, lesbian family units, and others). Because of this diversity, women's roles within families are changing. Whether or not they function in a traditional role, most do whatever is necessary to maintain their own integrity and that of their families. Early assessment of the strengths of family units by the community health nurse provides a data base for positive nursing interventions established on upstream strategies to enhance each family's level of health and well-being.

According to Chadwick and Heaton (1992), many women are delaying marriage, and an increasing number are not marrying. It appears that overall marriage rates have remained stable because of the increasing number of remarriages that make up for a declining rate of first marriages. When a relationship does end in divorce or separation, more women than men have the increased responsibility of providing for themselves and their children. According to the U.S. Bureau of the Census (1994), one-parent households now represent 3 of every 10 family groups. Single mothers are most often the head of a single-parent family (6:1). Table 11–5 lists characteristics of black and white female-headed households. Percentages of single-parent households with children include 63% of African-American family groups, 35% of Hispanics, and 25% of whites. However, even in the face of changing lifestyles, divorce, and increased mobility, which leads to long-distance relationships, most Americans report that they remain connected to their extended families through parents, grandparents, siblings, aunts, and uncles (Hugick, 1989). A recent Gallup Poll showed that family ties appear to be intact across America.

One contemporary family configuration involves single women with one or more adopted children. Because there is no legal ban on single-parent adoptions, an increasing number of single women are becoming adoptive parents and express joy in their new role. An often-ignored family structure is one headed by a lesbian parent. Lesbians who become parents are potential clientele and in most respects have needs similar to those of all mothers. Many cities have lesbian-gay parent groups that provide support, anticipatory guidance, and strategies for coping in society (Dickinson, 1990). However, these women often neglect their own health. According to Stevens (1992), this self-neglect may be traced to hostile and rejecting attitudes of health care providers. It is, however, im-

Table 11–5 Characteristics of Black and White Female-Headed Households		
Characteristic	Black	White
Single (never married) (%)	43.00	18.00
Married and spouse absent (%)	20.00	17.00
Widowed (%)	13.00	22.00
Divorced (%)	23.00	43.00
Number of children per	1.28	0.99

Adapted from U.S. Bureau of the Census. (1995). Statistical Abstract of the United States: 1995, 115th ed. Washington, DC, U.S. Government Printing Office, p. 63.

portant to any child's well-being that the parents or guardians remain healthy. A delay in health seeking services could have devastating consequences.

HEALTH BEHAVIOR

Because a woman's ability to carry out her important roles can affect her entire family, it is imperative that women be provided services that promote health and detect disease at an early stage (Northouse, 1991). Early detection and improved treatments for disease allow women to return to work or remain working throughout the course of the disease. Although for many women work is essential to the economic and social well-being of their families, the work place itself provides stress both physically and socially. As more women enter the work force, it is not surprising that their formerly favorable mortality and morbidity rates have been declining.

Milio, professor of health administration at the University of North Carolina, expressed concern for women as well as for the health and welfare of the unborn. What are the long-term effects on the woman's reproductive system in the work place? The task of health care professionals, including occupational health nurses, is to work with management unions and other groups to develop programs in the work place that will increase women's health-promoting options. A few of these options include educational programs, improved nutrition in the area of food service, exercise facilities, stress management clinics, and child care arrangements (Women's health risk, 1981).

Many women seek information that will allow them to be in control of their own health. Since the early 1970s, women have met in self-help groups to develop a better understanding of their own health needs. Some of the health behaviors that women learn in self-help groups are recognition of the early signs of vaginal infections and STDs, awareness of variations in female anatomy and physiology, importance of nutrition, breast self-examination (BSE), pregnancy testing, and contraceptive awareness.

Because of women's desire to become more knowledgeable about their own health, many books written for consumers are available in bookstores, in public libraries, and among the holdings of traditional women groups such as sororities, federated women's clubs, and others. An excellent resource for women is the *FDA Consumer,* the official magazine of the Food and Drug Administration (FDA). The second edition of *Current Issues on Women's Health* reports on FDA studies that cover a variety of women's health issues such as eating disorders, infertility, cosmetic safety, silicone breast implants, osteoporosis, and menopause (U.S. DHHS, 1994b).

Pender's (1987) health promotion model synthesizes the literature on health promotion and wellness. She indicated that "health promoting behaviors are directed toward sustaining or increasing the level of well-being, self-actualization and fulfillment of a given individual or group." This model can be used by the community health nurse in teaching health behaviors that lead to general health promotion among women. However, because many models were developed for the middle class, they may not be useful to community health nurses working with low-income families. Indeed, health promotion for low-income, underserved women might differ from that for their middle-class counterparts. Williams and Lethbridge (1995) studied health promotion in low-income rural women. The ethnographic study of black and white low-income women (N = 49) was aimed at eliciting views and the meaning of health as well as health promotion and maintenance behaviors, barriers, and facilitators. These women identified health as the ability to do for oneself and one's family. Findings revealed that women believed health promotion was the taking of blood pressure medicine and watching what they ate. Many did not think strenuous exercise was good for most women, and their exercise was in the form of walking, gardening, and taking care of children and grandchildren. These women did not distinguish between health promotion and health maintenance, concepts that may be more meaningful to health care providers than to their clientele. It is imperative that rural and other underserved women be self-sufficient and yet have available to them a culturally relevant, accessible, and appropriate health care delivery system that fits within the context of their lives.

Knowledge deficits prevail among women regardless of socioeconomic or educational level when it comes to an awareness of their own bodies. We have found that regardless of whether a group comprises college-educated professional women or women employed as blue collar workers, many of the questions asked are the same: "Will I menstruate after I have a hysterectomy?", "When should I perform a breast self-examination?", "What can I do to prevent recurrent episodes of vaginitis?"

Nurses can play an instrumental role in helping women develop a greater sense of self-awareness. Furthermore, community health nurses can remove the cloak of mystery surrounding the woman's body and give permission to clientele to ask previously unmentionable questions.

HEALTH CARE ACCESS

Approximately 32 million U.S. citizens are unable to receive medical care. This figure, although astronomic, does not include 250,000 to 2 million homeless men, women, and children (U.S. Bureau of the Census, 1989). Owing to the nature of women's employment, they frequently lack health insurance and are not eligible for Medicaid benefits. Young adults, those 16 to 24 years of age, make up approximately 50% of individuals without insurance coverage. A further breakdown of women between the ages of 15 and 44 years by race indicates that 28.5% of Hispanics, 21% of blacks, and 15% of whites are without coverage (Metropolitan Life and Affiliated Companies, 1988). Lacking economic means for meeting the costs of health care, these women are not likely to seek health care delivery until they or a family member is in acute distress. Others may rely on home remedies, over-the-counter drugs, lay midwives, or other folk healers for health care. The elderly, usually covered by Medicare, often delay seeking health care. Elderly women receiving fixed incomes may have difficulty meeting copayments required by Medicare. Many senior citizens have paid hospitalization insurance premiums for policies that fail to meet the gap.

Culture influences one's perception of health. It is essential that nurses become aware of the health practices of the diverse cultural groups that they serve, as demonstrated by the following example. Lynn Saunders, a white junior nursing student, was assigned to make home visits to Joan Peabody, a 15-year-old black girl with a newborn boy. Joan lives with her mother, sibling, and grandmother. On a home visit, Joan informs Lynn that she is going to have to get her 6-week-old baby some asafetida for his "hives," adding that giving a baby asafetida was common in her family. Lynn, unfamiliar with this regimen, sought assistance from her instructor and a local pharmacist. The pharmacist informed the student of the safe dosage range.

Many folk practices surround the mystique of a woman's menstrual cycle. Various herbal teas are given to decrease dysmenorrhea and premenstrual syndrome, to regulate menstrual periods, and to provide greater comfort during menopause. Herbs may also be used in some cultures for vaginal and bladder infections (Rose, 1984). Use of herbs for self-treatment should be approached with caution. Many of the herbal remedies are sold as food products and thus do not have to undergo the rigor of clinical trials. Community health nurses must be aware of some of the more toxic agents used by some groups (McKenry and Salerno, 1992).

Types of Problems

ACUTE ILLNESS

Females report a greater incidence of acute conditions than do males. It is estimated that approximately 5% of primary care visits by women are prompted by symptoms suggestive of bacteriuria (Seltzer and Pearse, 1995). One commonly reported problem is dysuria (painful urination), which most women will experience at some point in life. In fact, 43% of women aged 14 to 61 years report having had a bladder infection, often experiencing their first urinary tract infection during pregnancy or soon after delivery (Clark, 1995). The prevalence of infection directly correlates with age, increasing from about 3.5 to 10% between puberty and 70 years of age (Seltzer and Pearse 1995).

Another common problem—trigonitis, also known as "honeymoon cystitis"—frequently occurs with a change in sexual activity, usually from infrequent or no activity to more vigorous and frequent intercourse. Other acute illnesses specific to the reproductive tract include pelvic inflammatory disease, cervicitis, oophoritis, vulvitis, and toxic shock syndrome (TSS). TSS has declined over the years thanks to media warnings about the use of tampons as well as product changes (Farley, 1994). In 1980, a certain manufacturer removed its high-absorbency tampon from the market and after 1985, tampons that contained polyacrylate rayon were no longer produced. According to Creehan (1995), TSS is still a threat to women's health, and providers must make women aware of this acute illness potential, encourage them to report symptoms early, and exercise caution when using tampons and barrier contraceptive methods. Although TSS occurs most often in women of reproductive age who are menstruating, it has occurred in children and men (Creehan, 1995).

CHRONIC DISEASE

Included among chronic diseases that may affect a woman during her life span are CVD, hypertension, diabetes, arthritis, osteoporosis, and cancer.

Arteriosclerotic heart disease (ASHD) may have its beginnings in the second and third decades of a woman's life, according to clinical evidence. Changing lifestyles are altering these statistics, but some risk factors, such as race or family history of ASHD, are nonmodifiable. Black women are more vulnerable than white women to ASHD and more frequently experience congestive heart failure and angina pectoris after MI (AHA, 1994). Among the modifiable risk factors are

- Elevated serum lipid levels
- A diet high in calories, total fats, cholesterol, refined carbohydrates, and sodium
- Hypertension
- Obesity
- Glucose intolerance
- Cigarette smoking

In comparison, the following modifiable risk factors are considered minor:

- Personality type
- Sedentary lifestyle
- Stress (Phipps et al., 1983)

Hypertension, defined as blood pressure of 140/90 mm Hg or greater, significantly increases the risk of serious morbidity and mortality from coronary heart disease. Essential hypertension is the most common type of chronic hypertensive disorder in women of childbearing age, accounting for 85% of such cases. It is also responsible for approximately one third of all hypertension cases during pregnancy. Hypertension is more common in women than in men and affects more blacks than whites. Additional factors associated with primary hypertension are age (>35 years), family history of hypertension, obesity, cigarette smoking, and diabetes mellitus (AHA, 1994; Neeson and Stockdale, 1981). Because hypertension usually starts with an asymptomatic phase, every woman, beginning in her teenage years, should be screened on an average of every 2 years. Diagnosis is crucial to prevent or modify possible complications of this disease.

According to Kahn and Ware (1994), diabetes in the United States has an overall prevalence of 6.6%, of which only 3.4% is diagnosed. Thus, of the 8 million cases of NIDDM, almost 4 million are undiagnosed. In previous years, community health nurses have worked to educate women to assume responsibility in their management of diabetes mellitus. More recently, community health nurses have been actively involved in educational and screening programs for groups at high risk. Included in these groups are individuals who have a family history of diabetes, who are obese, or who are elderly.

According to Cunningham and coworkers (1993), pregnancy is potentially diabetogenic. The condition may be aggravated by pregnancy, and clinical diabetes may appear in some women only during pregnancy. Consequently, considerable attention has been given to screening for diabetes in pregnancy. There is much controversy regarding the most effective method of screening for diabetes, but regardless of the selected method, the nurse is involved in explaining to the woman the purpose of the screening and how to prepare for the tests. In most public health settings, the nurse is responsible for explaining the results.

Arthritis, which afflicts an estimated 50 million people in the United States, is a major health concern for women. The incidence of osteoarthritis is slightly higher in women than in men, but rheumatoid arthritis afflicts threefold as many women as men (Byyny and Speroff, 1990; Verbrugge, 1995). The cause of arthritis is not known; however, recurring multiple factors in the development of arthritis include diet, environment, and stress. Nursing intervention focuses on aspects of joint deformity prevention and lifestyle modification if necessary.

Osteoporosis, a condition involving diminishing bone density, is a major disorder affecting women. Estimates of its occurrence conflict, ranging from 25 to 50%. Although men may experience osteoporosis, it is more often associated with women and their diminished ovarian function. In fact, of the 24 million Americans who suffer from osteoporosis, 80% of them are women. Every year 1.3 million osteoporosis-related fractures occur (Papazian, 1994). In addition, 300,000 people experience hip fractures, approximately 20% of whom will die within a year because of complications from the injury.

Postmenopausal white women are at highest risk for osteoporosis. In women, loss of bone begins at an earlier age and proceeds twice as rapidly as in men. Because osteoporosis has no cure, prevention is especially important to begin early in life. Strategies involve an awareness of dietary practices such as maintaining a correct balance of calcium, vitamin D, and protein. Exercise is vital for its probable protective effect. Estrogen may be prescribed for both perimenopausal and postmenopausal women to maintain bone.

Nurses in ambulatory health practices should encourage women to become more knowledgeable of the preventive aspects of osteoporosis. The risks and benefits associated with estrogen replacement therapy must be discussed with the woman to facilitate her decision making. For women diagnosed with osteoporosis, nurses may assist in various aspects of management (e.g., education regarding prescribed medication, follow-up care, avoidance of complications, and dietary modifications as needed).

Incidence of breast cancer has been increasing during the past 50 years. Presently, one of every eight women will acquire breast cancer sometime in her life (Marshall, 1993). Risk factors include aging, personal or family history of breast cancer, early age at menarche, late age at menopause, never having had children, or having a first child after age 30 years (ACS, 1995). Female gender and aging are identified as the most significant risk factors for breast cancer.

In the battle against breast cancer, women must understand and practice early detection methods. The practice of monthly BSE should begin in high school. Nurses in any setting where there is an aggregate of women should possess the skills for teaching BSE. (Most chapters of the ACS regularly offer classes.) A breast examination by the woman's health care professional should be performed in addition to her annual pelvic and Papanicolaou (Pap) smear. A baseline mammogram should be done by 40 years of age and every year or 2 for women aged 40 to 49 years. Mammography, which is low-dose radiography, is not usually indicated for women younger than 35 years, but once a woman reaches 50 years, she should have an annual mammogram (ACS, 1995). These recommendations are for asymptomatic women without a personal or family history of breast cancer.

Twenty percent of all malignant diseases in women occur in the genital tract. Carcinoma of the cervix, the most common, accounts for 21% of all new genital tract malignancies (Eisenkop et al., 1988). Because the cervix is accessible to cytologic study, mortality has decreased. Risk factors for cervical cancer include coitus at an early age, multiple sexual partners, history of human papilloma virus and other STDs, or history of exposure to diethylstilbesterol *in utero* (ACS, 1995; Sherwen et al., 1991).

The decline in deaths from cervical cancer is directly related to early detection through an annual pelvic examination that includes a Pap smear. In fact, the incidence of invasive cervical cancer has been estimated to have been decreased 70% through regular Pap tests. A precancerous condition, cervical carcinoma *in situ,* is more frequent than invasive cancer and is detected through early screening. In recent years, there has been debate regarding how often a woman

RESOURCE MATERIALS

American Cancer Society Breast Cancer Resource Materials
Breast Cancer: Nowhere to Hide (pamphlet)
Three Ways to Take Special Care of Your Breasts (card, 5th grade reading level, English on one side and Spanish on the other)*
Breast Health (poster)
BSE—Special Touch (video, instructor's guide, and flip chart)
How to Do Breast Self-Examination (pamphlet)
A Woman's Guide to Mammography (pamphlet)
For copies call 1-(800)-ACS-2345

National Cancer Institute Breast Cancer Resources
A Mammogram Once A Year . . . For a Lifetime (video)
Smart Advice for Women 40 and Over: Have a Mammogram (pamphlet)

Guidelines for Screening Mammography (pamphlet)
A Mammogram Could Save Your Life
Take Care of Your Breasts
For copies call 1-(800)-4-Cancer or NCI at (301) 496-8680

Department of Health and Human Services Health Care Financing Administration
Get a Mammogram: A Picture That Can Save Your Life (pamphlet)
Medicare Covers Mammograms (pamphlet)
For copies and more information call 1-(800)-4-Cancer (1-800-422-6237) (breast cancer/mammograms); 1-(800)-638-6833 (Medicare coverage)

*Specifically designed for low-literacy audiences; some resources in Spanish and English.

should have a Pap smear. However, major authorities now recommend that women who are or have been sexually active or who have reached age 18 years receive an annual Pap test. After three or more annual examinations with normal findings, the test may be performed less frequently at the discretion of the woman and her clinician (U.S. DHHS, 1994c). The test is inexpensive, causes no known harm, and has the capacity for a high degree of sensitivity, yet each year many women die of cervical cancer because they had not been screened by a Pap smear (McKie, 1993).

Carcinoma of the endometrium has increased significantly during the past three decades, commonly in women during their sixth and seventh decades of life: 80% of women with this condition are postmenopausal. Factors believed to be related to its occurrence are obesity, low parity, diabetes mellitus, and conditions in which high circulating estrogen levels are not countered by adequate progesterone levels. The most common sign of endometrial cancer, occurring in 90% of women, is abnormal vaginal bleeding. Postmenopausal women experiencing vaginal bleeding should seek immediate gynecologic evaluation (Gusberg and Runowicz, 1991; Seltzer and Pearse, 1995). A satisfactory screening method permitting early diagnosis would do more to reduce mortality from this disease than would advances in treatment. Until that time, high-risk women should be identified and encouraged to seek ongoing monitoring.

Cancer of the ovary causes more deaths than any other pelvic malignancy. In the United States, its annual incidence usually ranges between 5 and 15 cases per 100,000 women. Approximately 1 in 70 will acquire ovarian cancer, a rate increasing fairly rapidly after age 40 years. Risk factors include increasing age, nulliparity, a history of breast cancer, and a family history of ovarian cancer (ACS, 1995). Because early-stage detection of ovarian cancer is virtually impossible, once discovered it has usually reached an advanced stage. The health professional should be alert to ovarian enlargement with suspicion that ovarian malignancy may be present; this is especially true in postmenopausal women (Seltzer and Pearse, 1995). According to the ACS (1995), the most common sign a woman experiences is abdominal enlargement. She may complain that her skirts and slacks are getting tighter in the waist. Because this is a silent cancer, any woman older than 40 years who experiences vague digestive complaints that persist and are not explained by another cause needs to have a thorough evaluation for ovarian cancer.

The mental health of women is influenced by a variety of circumstances and conditions. Every day women are called on to adapt to a changing environment, and although men live in the same stressful environment, according to Witkin-Lanoil (1984) women have some special stresses of their own. "Women menstruate, become pregnant and go through menopause. They sometimes have to justify their marital status to employers and their sexual behavior to their families. They are expected to be full of energy at the end of a working day and prepared to keep going through the weekend. Women are expected to be sexy, but not sexual; to have a child, but remain childlike; to be assertive, but not aggressive; to hold a job, but not neglect their home" (p. 55).

Women face stressful decisions about career and family, and many express anxiety in these decisions. A woman may say her biological clock is ticking and feel pressured to make decisions regarding childbearing before she has fulfilled career goals. Deciding to focus on a career may mean decreased authority and the suffering of stress in the work place. Women combining motherhood and a career have additional decisions such as working during pregnancy and choice of child care (Houde-Quimby, 1994). More women are occupying middle-management positions, positions known for creating stress-related illness associated with high demands and little or no power. Staats and Staats (1983) compared differences in stress levels between 82 women and 113 men employed in management and professional roles. Women identified higher stress levels involving marital dissatisfaction, interpersonal conflict in the home, incompatibility within the family, marital discord, relationship with parents, criticism by friends, and worries over drug and alcohol problems. They reported more frequent episodes of nervous diarrhea, tension, and migraine headaches. They also indicated problems in the past year for which they should have sought medical or mental health consultation. Staats and Staats recommended stress management programs for women to include assertiveness training, cognitive skills training, and family therapy with role revision plus relaxation training, conflict resolution, and time management activities.

A woman's emotional state has been said to be influenced by ovarian function from the onset of menstruation to the cessation of menstrual periods. Depressive symptoms have been associated with menarche, premenstrual dysphoric disorder or premenstrual syndrome, the postpartum period, and the perimenopause (Gordon and Ledray, 1986; Stotland,

1995). Depression is more prevalent among women than among men; however, some attribute this difference to women's role socialization rather than to biological differences (Radloff, 1980). Others emphasized the interactive biopsychosocial dynamics involved in the phenomenon of depression in women (Jones-Warren, 1995). Community health nurses are in a good position to assess women's mood in diverse aggregates (Woods et al., 1994).

Although some health professionals view the perimenopause as a time of depression and dismay, many women consider this phase of development as a time of fulfillment and creativity. Thomas (1988) found in a study of midlife that, although women experienced a high number of perimenopausal symptoms associated with depression, they also perceived themselves as leaders, as having talents in the visual and performing arts, and as possessing other abilities related to creative expression. It is suggested that nurses planning health promotion activities for an aggregate of midlife women draw on their clients' creative energies and expressions as an intervention to decrease or prevent nonpathologic depression.

REPRODUCTIVE HEALTH

Community health nurses provide a variety of services in the area of women's reproductive health from menarche through the postmenopausal phase. Nurses, in collaboration with other health care professionals, have identified a persisting group of preventable and correctable problems related to maternal-child health. Healthy People 2000 (U.S. DHHS, 1991) lists opportunities for improving maternal and infant health by a reduction of cigarette smoking and alcohol and other drug use, better nutrition, better socioeconomic opportunities, including education, and a decrease in environmental hazards.

One of the most important factors related to a woman's reproductive health focuses on her total life nutritional experience from inception through infancy, childhood, and adolescence. Pregnancy may provide a motivational factor for developing an awareness of proper nutrition. During the nutritional assessment of a prenatal client, the community health nurse can take this opportunity to determine dietary habits and initiate a referral to the Special Supplemental Food Program for Women, Infants, and Children (WIC) program when necessary. WIC provides food vouchers for pregnant or breast-feeding women, infants, and children who are at nutritional risk. Diet must be

developed by taking into consideration factors other than kinds and amounts of foods. Other elements to consider include age, lifestyle, economic status, and culture. When counseling a pregnant adolescent, for example, it may be helpful to include the primary person responsible for meal preparation. However, the adolescent should not be ignored in the planning of her diet but rather should be asked to identify foods she likes from those recommended. The adolescent needs to be made aware of the impact of her nutrition on fetal growth and development, information that must be balanced with the young woman's individual needs.

The community health nurse has many opportunities to provide counseling in the area of family planning. Although the phrase "family planning" has come to imply planned limitation of pregnancies, another important aspect of family planning concerns couples attempting to increase their chances of conception. Infertility occurs in a surprising number of otherwise healthy adults: Approximately 15 to 18% of couples in the United States are unintentionally childless. On the other hand, more than half of all pregnancies occurring in the United States are unintended (Seltzer and Pearse, 1995). In her inaugural address as president of the American College of Obstetricians and Gynecologists, Klein (1984) stated:

A fertile, sexually active woman using no contraception would, on the average, face 14 births or 31 abortions during her reproductive lifetime—a mind-boggling disruption of her life in this period of hoped-for independence and equality for women and in an era of disappearing economic value of children. (p. 287)

Community health nurses are in a strategic position to provide support and guidance for women in the control of their fertility. Numerous factors contribute to the decision of whether to use family planning methods. When counseling women on this matter, a holistic approach is needed. Factors such as age, pattern of sexual activity, cost, and access to health care as well as the woman's and her partner's values and beliefs must be considered. After a discussion with the nurse of benefits and risks, indications and contraindications, and advantages and disadvantages, the client selects a method that she believes to be safe and comfortable. The nurse's insistence on methods that are found to be a messy nuisance or that the woman fears may hurt her may do more harm than good. These and other issues must be considered to ensure the greatest protection from unintended pregnancy.

Health care professionals often neglect to mention natural family planning as a method of family planning. Although many consider this approach to be synonymous with the rhythm method, proponents of natural family planning are describing this method as *natural reproductive technology,* a term that is broader in scope and encompasses the health of a woman's reproductive system. According to certified natural family planning practitioner Rometta Hock, RN, MSN, the fertility awareness method increases women's awareness of their own reproductive processes (Central North Alabama Health Services, personal communication, September 1, 1995). Such knowledge allows for feelings of empowerment and a sense of control of one's fertility. Women experience self-knowledge and thereby gain autonomy in relation to fertility. Family and community health care professionals need to have up-to-date information concerning natural family planning.

Women who have decided that their families are large enough and do not wish to be concerned with temporary methods of fertility control may select voluntary surgical contraceptive (VSC) or contraceptive sterilization by tubal ligation. Vasectomy as a VSC continues to be a simpler, safer, and less expensive procedure than tubal ligation. According to Hatcher and colleagues (1994), VSC is one of the most effective, safest, and cost-effective methods of family planning that is widely used in developed and developing countries. In no other phase of family planning is it more important that the client's decision be based on clear, complete information than it is for sterilization. The reversibility of sterilization procedures is not dependable; if a woman has any doubts about her future childbearing, she should be encouraged to use other methods of fertility control. It is hoped that research in the area of family planning will provide a number of safe options for all women that are designed to meet individual needs.

Promoting responsible family planning is a goal of the International Council of Nurses (ICN). The ICN believes that family planning is basic to the health of the family and to form a strong society and that all couples and individuals have the basic right to decide the number and spacing of their children and to have adequate knowledge to make these critical decisions (ICN, 1993). Major benefits of family planning services and counseling worldwide include prevention of unwanted pregnancies and reduction in the high incidence of abortions. Worldwide, 300 million couples do not want more children but are not using effective methods of family planning. Tragically, more than 50,000 *illegal* abortions every day result in the

deaths of 150,000 women annually (Haller, 1994). Nurses worldwide have a major role to play if the health of women and their families is to improve. Besides being knowledgeable about family planning methods and services, all nurses must work for universally accessible maternal and child health care and seek to protect the rights of couples and individuals to receive good information about family planning. In addition, nurses must be involved in shaping policy that affects every woman's reproductive health.

SEXUALLY TRANSMITTED DISEASES AND HUMAN IMMUNODEFICIENCY VIRUS

In 1992, more than 700,000 cases of gonorrhea were reported, making it the most commonly reported communicable disease in the United States (CDC, 1993). This number is estimated to double when unreported cases are included. Genital chlamydial infections are the most common bacterial STDs in the United States (4 million annually), and case reporting is required in some states (Hatcher et al., 1994). Because a woman may acquire chlamydial infection along with gonorrhea, it is recommended that she be treated presumptively with a regimen effective against both organisms (CDC, 1993). Complications resulting from STDs include tubal occlusion, leading to infertility and ectopic pregnancy, neonatal morbidity and mortality caused by transmission of organism to fetus, genital cancers, and epidemiologic synergy with human immunodeficiency virus (HIV) transmission (Hatcher et al., 1994).

HIV has become a woman's health problem. HIV infection is, in fact, rising more rapidly among American women than any other group. AIDS is the fourth leading cause of death among reproductive-age women. Yet even now, many providers are unfamiliar with the symptoms of HIV disease as it infects women (Clark, et al., 1993). Women at highest risk for becoming HIV seropositive include

- Intravenous drug users who share needles or syringes
- Prostitutes
- Those who have sex with infected partners
- Participants in unprotected sex

An estimated 13 to 39% of infants born to infected mothers acquire HIV infection (U.S. DHHS, 1994a). Community health nurses as well as other health providers, including physicians, nurse practitioners, nurse midwives, physician's assistants, and social workers, must be prepared to provide age-appropriate STD prevention education and counseling. Risk-reduction objectives to decrease the spread of these diseases include the following recommendations (U.S. DHHS, 1991):

- Reduce the proportion of adolescents who have engaged in sexual intercourse to no more than 15% by age 15 years (baseline in 1988: 27% of girls reported in 1988) and not more than 40% by age 17 (baseline in 1988: 50% of girls).
- Increase use of condoms by partners of sexually active young women aged 15 to 19 years to 60% by the year 2000 (baseline in 1988: 25%).

UNINTENTIONAL INJURY (ACCIDENTS)

Older women are at increased risk for accidents such as falls. Falls account for the majority of serious unintentional injuries and lead to 40% of all injury mortality in people older than 75 years. This type of injury is the sixth leading cause of death in individuals 75 years of age and older (U.S. DHHS, 1994b, p. 291). Factors that may be responsible for this major cause of morbidity among the elderly are associated with an unsteady gait, reduced vision, or a hazardous environment. Because older women experience an increasing number of falls, it is important to identify the preventable factors. Nurses, whether working with the elderly in the home or in institutional settings, must be knowledgeable of hazards that may be corrected to decrease the incidence of falls.

Abuse in women is often explained as accidental injury. Approximately 6% of visits made by women to emergency rooms are for injuries that result from physical battering by their husbands, ex-husbands, boyfriends, or lovers. Millions of women from all socioeconomic levels are abused annually; according to the *Clinician's Handbook of Preventive Services* (1994), that all women should be asked directly whether they have been abused or not. Nurses employed in community health settings need to know how to make assessments, provide support, and make referrals to agencies dealing with domestic violence.

DISABILITY

According to Verbrugge (1989), more women than men have disabilities resulting from acute conditions, but women experience fewer disabilities resulting from chronic conditions because they report their symptoms earlier and receive necessary treatment. A disability may reduce the individual's activity; women report proportionately more days of restricted activity than do men. Women average 16.1 days of disability per year compared with 12.7 days for men (U.S. Bureau of the Census, 1990).

A frequently encountered disabling condition is dysmenorrhea, most often associated with ovulatory cycles and one of the most common concerns of women. It affects approximately 50 to 80% of the female population between the ages of 15 and 24 years (Robinson et al., 1992; Sullivan, 1990) but continues to plague women throughout the reproductive years (Seltzer and Pearse, 1995). At least 10 to 20% of women with dysmenorrhea are incapacitated for 1 to 3 days each month (Brown, 1982; Robinson et al., 1992). Dysmenorrhea is the greatest single cause of absenteeism from school and work among young women. It is estimated that dysmenorrhea is the cause of the loss of 140 million working hours annually (Weiss, 1984). The economic impact of this condition is difficult to estimate.

Disabling conditions often limit the physical functional abilities of many women, but the health care delivery system has often overlooked the unique needs of this aggregate. In planning care for disabled women, community health nurses should focus attention on enabling the women to strengthen her capabilities. In addition, nurses should be sensitive to barriers in the clinical setting that affect the access of disabled women to health care services.

MAJOR LEGISLATION AFFECTING WOMEN'S HEALTH SERVICES

Several legislative acts have a direct or indirect impact on the health of women. Many changes have been made in the past decade that have the potential for improving the health and welfare of all women.

Public Health Service Act

The Public Health Service Act, passed in 1982, provides for the following activities:

- Biomedical and health services research
- Information dissemination
- Resource development
- Technical assistance
- Service delivery

During 1984, an inventory was made throughout the U.S. DHHS of government agencies provided for within the Public Health Service Act. The purpose of the inventory was to identify the extent of each agency's involvement in women's health concerns. The scope of activities includes general, reproductive, social, behavioral, and mental health among other female-specific health issues (Women's Health, 1985). Aggregates of women targeted by the CDC, a Public Health Service agency, encompassed those disabled by specific diseases, victims of sexual abuse and domestic violence, recent immigrants, and occupational groups.

In 1981, one agency within the Public Health Service, the Family Planning Assistance Program, assisted more than 4.5 million women in obtaining family planning services. The committee studying the prevention of low-birth-weight infants recommended the following in regard to the continuation of government support for family planning (Institute of Medicine, 1985):

The need for subsidized family planning remains significant and federal funds should be made generously available to meet documented needs. With regard to the particular relationship of family planning and low birth weight, it is important to stress that both young teenage status and poverty are major risk factors for low birth weight . . . As such the program should be regarded as an important part of public effort to prevent low birth weight (p. 128).

The focus of Public Health Service activities regarding women's health issues described most frequently in the inventory was health promotion and disease prevention, with activities directed toward research, evaluation and analysis, and education and training operations. The task force responsible for the inventory recommended the continuation of monitoring and reviewing of activities concerning women's health by the Public Health Service. As advocates and as professionals directly involved with the health care of women, nurses should review the task force's complete report and thus encourage the implementation of goals set by the surgeon general for a complete nation of healthy people, including healthy women.

Civil Rights Act

Title VII of the Civil Rights Act of 1964 prohibits discrimination based on sex, race, color, religion, or national origin in hiring or firing, wages, and fringe benefits. With the amendment of the act in 1978, discrimination was prohibited against pregnant women or conditions involving childbirth or pregnancy. This landmark legislation makes it unlawful for employers to refuse to hire, employ, or promote a woman because she is pregnant. In addition, employee benefit plans that continue health insurance, income maintenance during disability or illness, or any other income support program for disabled workers will have to include disabilities resulting from pregnancy, childbirth, and other related conditions. If employers allow disabled employers to assume lighter or medically restricted assignments, the same considerations must be extended to the pregnant woman (Craven et al., 1993).

The amendment does not require employers to pay health insurance benefits for abortions or abortion-related care unless the mother's life is endangered or she has medical complications after an abortion. Employers are prohibited from firing or refusing to hire a woman because she has had an abortion.

Sexual harassment is a violation of the Civil Rights Act. Sexual harassment is "conduct of a sexual nature . . . unwelcome by the target . . . severe or pervasive enough to create an intimidating work environment" (Women Employed Institute, 1994). Women and men workers may face unwelcome sexual advances or requests for sexual favors or other verbal or physical conduct of a sexual nature. In 1991 a young law professor, Anita Hill, charged that Supreme Court nominee Clarence Thomas had sexually harassed her. This case raised the consciousness of the nation. In fact, since the Thomas hearings, complaints to the U.S. Equal Employment Opportunity Commission have more than doubled in 3 years, from 6883 in 1991 to 14,420 in 1994. According to Suzanna Walters (Knight-Ridder News Service, 1995), a sociology professor at Georgetown University, highly publicized cases like the Hill-Thomas case do have an effect, but it will take more than sensational news stories to eliminate work place harassment. Walters emphasized that men's power in the world is the underlying issue in sexual harassment and to eliminate it will take a reorganization of society.

Social Security Act

The Social Security Act provides monthly retirement and disability benefits to workers and survivor benefits to families of workers covered by the system. Full retirement benefits are available to workers after 10 years of covered employment.

Recent changes in the Social Security Act permit a divorced person to receive benefits based on a former spouse's earning record when that spouse retires, becomes disabled, or dies if the marriage lasted at least 10 years. As of January 1985, a woman who has been divorced for at least 2 years can receive spousal benefits at age 62 if her ex-husband is eligible for benefits regardless of whether he is actually receiving them.

Another benefit covered under Social Security is Medicare. Medicare covers 50% of the medical expenses of the elderly, including payments for physicians, home health care, and other services and supplies after the deductible has been met (Bodenheimer, 1992). Medicaid covers preventive cancer screening for women (such as mammographies and Pap smears), but services vary widely throughout the United States (Moore, 1992).

Occupational Safety and Health Act

The Occupational Safety and Health Act enacted in 1970 ensured safe and healthful working conditions for workers in all businesses affecting commerce throughout the United States. However, in 1995 worker health and safety regulations have been a target of budget cuts by the 104th U.S. Congress (Worthington, 1995). Fortunately, the American Nurses Association was successful in delaying these budget cuts, but other attempts at deregulation are sure to follow. Worthington (1995) stated that "a specific example is the strong opposition by Congress and industry to [Occupational Safety and Health Administration's] Ergonomics Standard, the first formal effort to address work-related musculoskeletal disorders. The government's own data show that over half of all RN occupational injuries requiring time away from work are related to overexertion, primarily affecting the back" (p. 14). Of course, nurses face other hazards that remain uninvestigated and unregulated, such as latex allergy, disinfectants, and diverse air contaminants. The physical and emotional health of nurses is destined to increase with the restructured health care system (fewer staff, increased responsibility, ever-changing shifts, and so on.)

Table 11–6 lists specific positions in which large numbers of women are employed and the potential for health hazards exist.

Although there is an increasing emphasis in the study of the health of women workers, gaps in knowledge exist. Less is known about women who work in cottage industries, in domestic work, as prostitutes, in agriculture, and in the garment industry (Misner et al., 1995). In addition, there are women whose work is classified as "women's work" and includes such things as housework, child care, care-

giver of the sick, and farming (Misner et al., 1995). These women (and certainly some men) experience physical demands and hazards, yet these individuals have not been recognized as workers in government economic reports. However, their contributions to family, community, and society are immeasurable. Investigations of these women workers are needed.

Community health nurses, occupational health nurses, and nurse practitioners need to be cognizant of environmental hazards wherever they find women at work. In taking health histories, data should be collected regarding the client's occupational environment to assess the potential risk to emotional, general, and reproductive health. In addition, nurses individually and as an aggregate must work with their legislatures to maintain strong worker health and safety programs to protect the health of all women.

Family and Medical Leave Act

The Family and Medical Leave Act (FMLA) enacted in 1993 allows an employee a minimum provision of 12 weeks of unpaid leave each year for family and medical reasons such as personal illness; an ill child, parent, or spouse; or the birth or adoption of a child.

Table 11–6
Hazardous Occupations in Which Women are Employed

Occupation	Health Hazard
Clerical workers	Organic solvents in stencil machines, correction fluids, rubber cement; ozone from copying machine
Textile and apparel workers	Cotton dust; skin irritants; chemicals
Hairdressers and beauticians	Hair, nail, and skin beauty preparations
Launderers and dry cleaners	Heat, heavy lifting, chemicals
Electronics workers	Solvents and acids
Hospital and other health care workers	Infectious diseases, heavy lifting, radiation, skin disorders, anesthetic gases
Laboratory workers	Biological agents; flammable explosive, toxic, or carcinogenic substances; exposure to radiation; bites from and allergic reactions to research animals

This act guarantees the employee the same or equivalent job with the same pay and benefits upon the employee's return to work. In addition, health benefits must continue throughout the leave. The FMLA is particularly important to women workers because they are most often the caregivers of the family. According to the Women's Legal Defense Fund, every employee who must be away from work for family and medical reasons loses income; however, the loss is severe for those without job-protected leave. Annual earnings for female workers without job-protected leave were reduced by 29.1% in the first year after giving birth, whereas those with leave lost only 18.2% according to a 1990 Institute for Women's Policy Research study. The FMLA is an important step toward equitable leave policies (Cassetta, 1993).

HEALTH AND SOCIAL SERVICES TO PROMOTE THE HEALTH OF WOMEN

Approximately 5.7 million women of childbearing age are assisted by Medicaid. An additional 1.6 million women aged 45 to 64 years have Medicaid coverage (Current Population Survey, 1992). It is a health insurance program for the poor exclusive of age eligibility, and it is administered by individual states.

Many of the women who are eligible for Medicaid are at high risk for poor pregnancy outcome, including low birth weight. Ideally, women who are at high maternal risk should be seen by a maternity care provider immediately after conception. Often these women seek prenatal care late in the pregnancy or present at the emergency department when delivery is imminent without having received any prenatal care.

Consider the following example. Anita Rogers, a 16-year-old unemployed single woman, comes to the Family Services Health Center seeking initial prenatal care at 36 weeks gestation. She states that for a few days she has noted some brown discharge from her vagina. She tells the nurse practitioner that she knew that she should have begun prenatal care earlier, but when she called several physicians' offices, the receptionist told her that she should bring $50 for her first visit. She said that she did not have that much money, nor did her parents; her father was unemployed, and her mother worked at a cafe as a waitress. She also had difficulty with transportation. Anita was sent to the hospital immediately for an ultrasound examination. The sonogram revealed triplets, but two

of them had died in utero. Anita was hospitalized and soon began to hemorrhage. She delivered a 3-pound infant.

This case is not unusual among those most in need of high-quality prenatal care. However, barriers limit access to prenatal care. The Medicaid program allows for some access to care, but there is a need for greater public awareness of facilities and of maternity care providers who accept Medicaid. However, recent changes in payment plans that allow billing for care at higher rates have increased the numbers of providers that accept patients who were once considered "undesirable." This may not be the best answer to underserved women or to future health care reform. For example, in a small county in California, specialists who until recently would not treat a MediCal obstetric patient (unless referred by the certified nurse midwife) are now accepting these patients. Anecdotal reports indicate that there are additional costs when patients are seen by a specialist, more technology, and an increase in cesarean births (Mills et al., 1994). These changes do not reflect an upstream approach to the reproductive health of women.

Nurse practitioners, certified nurse midwives, and public health nurses may provide ambulatory perinatal care. One large metropolitan city has established a network for perinatal care. Nurses provide prenatal and postpartum care. Family practice residents, obstetric-gynecologic residents, and some private physicians deliver the women and accept referrals of women assessed as being at high risk. The women are assisted with obtaining Medicaid if they are eligible.

Women's Health Services

Since the mid-1970s, women have sought health services other than the conventional mode of care delivery. Many self-help groups have emerged, and new approaches to women's health services have been accepted. Because women have demanded a participatory role and have become more assertive, health care facilities, including physicians' offices, are more responsive to women's perceptions of their health needs. There has been a complete revolution in maternity care with the emergence of freestanding as well as hospital-based birth centers, family- and sibling-attended births, and so on. The health care needs of women go beyond their reproductive status and include their primary health care needs. According to Star and colleagues (1995), the health care needs of women must be addressed more effectively and must include, for example, services for (1) eating disorders, (2) of all forms of abuse, (3) disease prevention, including smoking cessation, and (4) health promotion, focusing on nutrition, exercise, and stress management.

The National Women's Health Network has been a strong advocate for women's concerns and has provided testimony before congressional hearings dealing with women's issues. This organization is concerned with patients' rights, environmental safety, reproductive rights, warnings regarding the effects of alcohol and drugs on the developing fetus, and safety in relation to medical devices. For example, the

network was instrumental in the worldwide recall of the Dalkon Shield intrauterine device. In 1995, approximately 90% of claimants had received compensation for their injuries (International Dalkon Shield Victims Education Association, personal communication, September 11, 1995).

Another concern is that of drug safety, especially concerning drugs that may have teratogenic or carcinogenic effects. For example, the network has attempted to identify women who may have been exposed to diethylstilbestrol in utero. These are just a few of the concerns of the network in regard to improving women's health (Charting a course, 1983).

HEALTH RESOURCES

American Cancer Society
1599 Clifton Rd, NE
Atlanta, GA 30329

American Lupus Society
23751 Madison St
Torrance, CA 90505
(213) 373-1335

National Association of Anorexia Nervosa and Associated Disorders (ANAD)
P.O. Box 7
Highland Park, IL 60035
(708) 831-3438

American Social Health Association
1-(800)-227-8922
STD information

Arthritis Foundation
1314 Spring St, NW
Atlanta, GA 30309
(404) 872-7100
(Check telephone book for local chapters.)

Black Women's Health Project
Martin Luther King Community Center
Suite 157
Atlanta, GA 30120
(405) 659-3854

Boston Self-Help Center
18 Williston Rd
Brookline, MA 02146
(A counseling, consulting, and disability rights organization staffed by and for people with disabilities)

Calcium Hotline
1-(800)-321-2681

Cesareans/Support, Education and Concerns (C/SEC)
22 Forest Rd
Framingham, MA 01701
(508) 877-8266
(Information and support to parents-professionals on cesarean birth, prevention, VBAC)

Coalition for the Medical Rights of Women
2845 24th St
San Francisco, CA 94110
(415) 826-4401
(A health advocacy and information resource; publishes a monthly newsletter *Second Opinion*)

Command Trust Network
Breast Implant Information Service
256 South Linden Dr
Beverly Hills, CA 90212
(213) 556-1738

Gay Nurses' Alliance
44 St. Mark's Pl
New York, NY 10003
(An active group working for both gay rights and health issues; provides educational resources)

Health Research Group
2000 P Street, NW
Washington, DC 20036
(202) 872-0320
(Publishes consumer-oriented books and manuals on drugs, medical devices, occupational and environmental health, health insurance and benefits programs, and related topics)

Box continued on following page

HEALTH RESOURCES *Continued*

Hysterectomy Educational Resources and Services (HERS)
422 Bryn Mawr Ave
Bala Cynwyd, PA 19004
(610) 667-7757
(Provides information and counseling for women who have had hysterectomies and for those to whom hysterectomy has been recommended)

Institutes for the Study of Medical Ethics
P.O. Box 17307
Los Angeles, CA 90017
(213) 413-4997
(An active patients' rights group offering advocacy, documentation, and research; active in monitoring legislation)

National AIDS Network
1012 14th Street, NW
Washington, DC 20005
(202) 347-0309
(Referrals to local groups)

National Council on Child Abuse and Family Violence
1155 Connecticut Ave, NW, Suite 400
Washington, DC 20036
1-(800)-222-2000
(Local referral numbers for assistance and information on detection and treatment of domestic violence)

National Women's Health Network
514 10th St, NW, Suite 400
Washington, DC 20004
(202) 347-1140
(A national consumer-provider membership organization; monitors and works to influence government and industry policies; publishes *Network News*)

National Women's Health Resource Center
514 10th St, NW, Suite 400
Washington, DC 20004
(202) 628-7814

Paul VI Institute
6901 Mercy Rd
Omaha, NE 68106-2604
(402) 390-9168
(Information on the Creighton model of the ovulation method/natural family planning)

Women and AIDS Resource Network
P.O. Box 020525
Brooklyn, NY 11202
(718) 596-6007

National Telephone Hot Lines
American Cancer Society: 1-(800)-ACS-2345
National Cancer Institute: 1-(800)-4-CANCER
National HIV-AIDS Information Line, Public Health Service, U.S. Department of Health and Human Services: 1-(800)-342-AIDS
National Sexually Transmitted Disease Hot Line, American Social Health Association: 1-(800)-227-8922

The National Women's Health Network undertook a special project to encourage health promotion among black women. The Black Women's Health Project's coordinator, Byllye Avery, established self-help groups. The goals of these groups are "to raise the consciousness of women about the severity and pervasiveness of black women's health problems [and] to provide a comfortable, supportive atmosphere for women to explore health issues affecting them and their families."

The nationwide self-help groups have diverse interests. For example, in Monteocho Gordon, Florida, the focus is on reducing high blood pressure; in Chicago, the focus is on learning self-help skills.

Women's health consumers are requesting more emphasis in the area of well-women's health care (i.e., health care aimed at well-being, health promotion, and disease prevention). Several nurses throughout the country have established collaborative practices with other health professionals to meet this demand for nonconventional services.

Other Community Voluntary Services

One of the major movements during the last decade has been that of networking. Networking has been described as a system of interconnected or cooperating individuals. It is the means by which women seek to advance their careers, improve their lifestyles, and increase their income and yet simultaneously help other women to be successful (Flanagan, 1992; Kleiman, 1980).

Business, professional, support, political and labor,

artistic, sports, and health networks have been established throughout the United States. These multiple networks have enabled women to take on new identities and become empowered to achieve mutual goals.

Many private voluntary organizations spend money, time, and energy in attempting to increase health awareness among its members as well as provide direct services to the public. Most urban areas have crisis hot line services in which women volunteer to provide counseling to battered women, battering parents, rape victims, and those considering suicide as well as those with multiple other needs. An example follows.

Helena Rowland arrives by taxi with her 2-year-old child at the Truth Safe House for Women. Her left eye is bloodshot, and her face is bruised and very edematous. It is obvious that she is pregnant (about 20 weeks gestation). She states that "my old man got mad and started beating on me. When he left, I found a friend who gave me some money to come to this place. I just don't know what gets into him, but every time I get pregnant he becomes even more abusive than usual. See my stomach? He kicked me right here" [pointing to the left side of her abdomen]. After the intake worker receives some preliminary information, Ms. Rowland is shown through the shelter and assigned a place for her and her child to sleep. She is greeted by the other six women and their children

(ranging in age from 2 weeks to 12 years). The women are working together to prepare the evening meal. They tell Ms. Rowland to come back to the living room of the house because the nurse who comes to talk and assist them with personal and children's health concerns will be coming shortly.

One of the most effective low-cost, voluntary efforts to assist abused women involves the shelters and safe houses scattered throughout the United States. It is estimated that between 2 and 4 million American women are abused annually and that abuse occurs in approximately 25% of all familial relationships (Clinician's Handbook of Preventive Services, 1994). Many women needing shelter are often turned away from emergency housing. No more than 10% of women and their children will be turned away because of limited space if the nation meets the Healthy People 2000 objectives by the 21st century.

Women's organizations have a long history of voluntary involvement with the community. An increasing number have added to their agenda activities to improve pregnancy outcomes, to prevent teen pregnancy, and to support older women's rights. Organizations such as the Older Women's League, United Methodist Women, other religious denomination women's groups, Urban League, sororities, Junior League, YWCA, National Association of Colored Women's Clubs, and many others have made women's health a major item on their agenda.

APPLICATION OF THE NURSING PROCESS

Case Study

John Lawrence, an educator at the state women's correctional center, contacted Donna Williams, a women's health care nurse practitioner and faculty member at the College of Nursing, and expressed concern for the health of a prisoner, Lela Marvin. According to Mr. Lawrence, Lela, a 19-year-old pregnant primigravida, is seen at the state-supported hospital for antepartal care; however, she is not permitted to attend perinatal education classes. He stated that there were other pregnant women in the facility who could benefit from perinatal education. In fact, approximately 6.1% of female state prison inmates are pregnant when admitted to prison and could benefit from perinatal education (Snell, 1994).

Lawrence's call was followed by a call from Herman Martin, RN, who also expressed concern for the other women's needs for information regarding their personal hygiene. Although a registered nurse, Mr. Martin was not knowledgeable of women's health; his primary clinical focus was emergency and trauma care. He indicated that many of the women were overweight, cared little about themselves, and lacked a general knowledge of how to maintain their health.

Assessment

After gaining clearance by the prison officials, Donna Williams made an assessment of health care information needs and started offering classes. The immediate need was for perinatal education for women in the last weeks of pregnancy. Lela Marvin said she wanted to learn about labor because she had heard only horror stories from other women. Donna noted that there were three other women close to term, and they too seemed eager to learn. Donna knew that students' readiness to learn was key to the courses' success. Success of this course would be crucial to future course offerings.

The traditional perinatal education course is designed to promote healthy birth outcomes and an emotionally satisfying birth experience. These goals are also important to pregnant women in a correctional facility; however, perinatal education must be modified to meet this group's special needs. For example, information on care of the newborn would not be taught because the infant is placed with the mother's family or in foster care.

Assessment of nonpregnant women provided opportunities for other health education classes. The next spring and each spring thereafter, junior nursing students, under the guidance of Ms. Williams, were assigned to develop and carry out a 1-hour weekly health education and awareness session at the correctional facility.

Although each of these students expressed some initial anxiety toward the experience, each evaluated it as being a worthwhile learning experience.

Diagnosis

After assessment the community health nurse proceeds to diagnosing. The nursing diagnosis serves as the pivotal step of the process because the plan of care is based on this (Bobak et al., 1995).

Individual

* Inadequate preparation for childbirth related to lack of resources in prison (Lela Marvin)
* Lack of family support related to separation secondary to incarceration (Lela Marvin)
* Potential for feelings of loss related to separation from infant after birth (Lela Marvin)

Family Because Lela Marvin's family of origin's visits are rare, she has looked for others to provide support during her pregnancy. Lela tells Ms. Williams that her cell mate, Julieanna, has offered, although hesitantly, to be her labor support person.

* Lack of knowledge of her role as a labor support person (Julieanna)

Community

* Knowledge deficit of adequate health-seeking behaviors of women in the correctional facility (pregnant and nonpregnant women)
* Lack of programs to promote health and prevent diseases among women prisoners

Planning

After validating the nursing diagnosis with the individual, family, or community, the plan of care is developed. Examples of long- and short-term goals follow:

Individual
Long-Term Goal
- Individual family members will have a positive birth experience (Lela Marvin).

Short-Term Goal
- Family member or friend will assist Lela to use relaxation techniques to cope with discomforts of labor.

Family
Long-Term Goal
- The family will be strengthened through their newly acquired knowledge and skills.

Short-Term Goal
- The family will demonstrate increased ability to perform role as labor support person.

Community
Long-Term Goal
- The health and well-being of incarcerated women (pregnant and nonpregnant) will improve.

Short-Term Goal
- Health education programs will be instituted to individuals, families, and aggregates in the correctional facility.

Intervention

The community health nurse works with the individual, family, or community to achieve mutually established goals. Intervention is aimed at empowering individuals and groups to take responsibility for self and to form linkages with others to accomplish goals.

Individual Providing a perinatal education program for Lela is Ms. Williams first priority. In addition, counseling related to feelings of loss after birth may be appropriate. Referral to a counselor may be necessary, and Ms. Williams must become familiar with available resources.

Family Teaching the family the roles and responsibilities of a labor support person is an important intervention. In the correctional facility, interventions must be carried out to ensure that Lela Marvin has a labor support person to practice her relaxation techniques and to also be available for the birth. The nurse must negotiate with prison officials to make it possible for Lela to have a labor support person. If a family member is unavailable, then Ms. Williams may call on a childbirth educator in the community to assist during this time.

Community Specific interventions with a group of pregnant women in the correctional facility are carried out based on the specific needs of the group. The community health nurse must then identify prison officials who are supportive of health education programs and request input as to which women should be targeted for such programs. Then the nurse meets with targeted women to assess level of knowledge regarding women's health. For example, survey what they perceive as learning needs (e.g., well-women's care, women's anatomy and physiology, self-care in health promotion, health protection, and disease prevention). Ms. Williams asked each nursing student to select a topic based on the survey and develop a teaching plan for presentation to women prisoners (pregnant and nonpregnant) at least once during spring semester.

Evaluation

The community health nurse compares the actual and predicted outcomes to determine the efficacy of the plan of care and to make revisions.

Individual For example, Lela Marvin learned necessary relaxation techniques that were useful to her in labor and assisted in making the birth experience positive. Follow-up of Lela's psychosocial concerns in postpartum was also important.

Family Evaluation of this nontraditional family would include their level of satisfaction with their role in the birth experience. Evaluation would also include learning how this interaction between family members (Lela and Julieanna) prepared them for other situations.

Community The aggregate evaluation focuses on the community. In the health education programs designed for pregnant and nonpregnant women in the correctional facility, it is important to

- Maintain record of attendance
- Seek feedback from women, referring nurse-educator, and prison officials regarding changes in self-care behavior regarding health
- Obtain student response to learning experience
- Make changes in health education programs based on evaluation

Levels of Prevention

PRIMARY AND SECONDARY

The authors became involved in primary prevention as members of an ACS committee called Stop Cancer Among Minorities (SCAM). The SCAM committee members represented several ethnic groups from the settings of churches, schools, and health care agencies. The committee assessed the needs of a community that revealed a lack of knowledge of health promotion practices necessary to decrease the risk of cancer.

The committee planned a health fair to promote cancer awareness in the community. It was sponsored by the state chapter of the ACS and a local community health center. Nursing students and undergraduate faculty from the local nursing college joined the committee to plan and implement the program.

Nursing students offered nutritious snacks (low in fat, high in fiber and complex carbohydrates) and discussed the relationship of diet to risk reduction for cancer. They also taught BSE and testicular self-examination. Other students shared the risks of starting to smoke and the benefits of quitting. Seven booths located at the fair were associated with the seven danger signals of cancer.

Women's health care nurse practitioners, family nurse practitioners, and midwives from the community and the university baccalaureate nursing program as well as the clinic's medical staff joined together to perform breast and pelvic examinations for each woman. Pap smears were also performed and were sent for cytologic study to the state health department. Follow-up on Pap smear results was carried out by the health center's director of Nursing Services.

SECONDARY

The focus of secondary prevention is on early diagnosis or health maintenance for persons with chronic disorders. Junior-year nursing students from the nursing college involved in a community study identified a population at risk for breast cancer. They gained permission to present a program on BSE to a group of nuns in a local convent. The students prepared themselves by becoming certified by the ACS as instructors in BSE. The ACS provided the students with current knowledge of breast cancer, its treatments, and early detection methods. The ACS also provided helpful films, pamphlets, and models for demonstration. Through the student's assessment, planning, and intervention, a group of women have been provided with skills for early detection of a life-threatening disease.

TERTIARY

Tertiary prevention consists of rehabilitation when sequelae of a condition have occurred. For example, Sandra Smith, a 55-year-old Native American, has had diabetes mellitus for the past 3 years. She attends an urban clinic for monitoring of her diabetes. After the physician examines her, he suggests that she have her annual pelvic examination. She is overdue for this, and she agrees to be seen by the women's health care nurse practitioner. Ms. Smith describes to the nurse symptoms of a yeast infection (e.g., increase in vaginal discharge and itching). Her examination and a wet mount confirmed the diagnosis of *Candida albicans,* a common problem among diabetic women. The woman learns about the nature, predisposing factors, and treatment of the infection.

ROLES OF THE COMMUNITY HEALTH NURSE

Direct Care

The community health nurse provides direct care in a variety of settings. Often this is considered the "hands-on" nursing care given to a client in the home or a clinic. Direct care occurs many times every day in clinics such as those for STDs. The following scene is representative of situations that arise numerous times every day. Jane Beaumont is a 20-year-old white woman who has come to the clinic on the advice of her boyfriend. She appears confused and frightened. She states her boyfriend has "clap" and that he told her to go for treatment. She expresses little anger at this time and states that she knew he had sex with other women.

The nurse sees many opportunities for teaching, but if the client is too anxious she will be unable to integrate new information. The present goal of the nurse is to develop trust so that the young woman will return later for follow-up.

During the interview, the nurse gathers information regarding the behavioral aspects of sexuality, physical symptoms, the client's knowledge of sexual health, and the client's emotional responses to the problem. During the examination, chlamydia and gonorrhea cultures are taken from appropriate sites. After this, the nurse draws blood for serologic diagnosis of syphilis. The patient is diagnosed as having gonorrhea. The client also consents to testing for HIV after the nurse discusses risk factors with her.

After the examination and initiating treatment according to protocol, the nurse answers questions and stresses the importance of follow-up and future protection against STDs. Ms. Beaumont asks why all this is necessary because she "feels okay." The nurse explains that 50 to 80% of all women have no complaints (symptoms) and feel "okay" even though the disease is present. The nurse asks her to return in 1 week for the HIV test results. At this time, the nurse will also evaluate whether the client understands her role in the prevention of STDs, including HIV.

Counselor

The counseling role of the nurse occurs in almost every interaction in the area of women's health. Before beginning counseling in the area of reproductive health, it is essential for effective intervention that the nurse become aware of his or her value system, including how one's biases and beliefs about human sexual behavior affect the counseling role. In a representative scenario, Diana Cook comes to the family planning clinic reporting that she has missed two periods and "feels" pregnant. Ms. Cook is 33 years old and has two children, ages 9 and 12 years. Her pregnancy test is positive, and her pelvic examination is consistent with a 6- to 8-week pregnancy.

Ms. Cook had not planned this pregnancy, and she needs counseling regarding her options. The nurse realizes that this is a crisis in the life of this woman and that she will need support in whatever decision she makes.

RESEARCH IN WOMEN'S HEALTH

Women have long been the major users of the health care (illness care) system; however, there has been less research involving women that provides information enabling prediction, explanation, or description of phenomena affecting health. In the majority of cases, medical treatment for women is based on research in which the subjects were exclusively male. This is true even in conditions that cause more deaths in women, such as CVDs (Amsterdam and Legato, 1993). Fortunately, there has been an increased effort to include women in studies related to cardiovascular health. This emphasis came after federal mandate that research must include women and minorities, or, if women are not included, a rationale must be given for their exclusion.

Community health nursing faculty, interested in the health of women and their children, received funding to offer a comprehensive breast cancer control program. The program is being offered to the female parents or guardians of children enrolled in the Children's Rehabilitation Services (CRS) of Alabama. CRS is a state program that provides family-centered community-based assistance to prevent, correct, or reduce physical disabilities of children. Previous research has documented a decline in the personal health of parents of children with special health care needs. These caregivers, mostly mothers, often disregard personal symptoms of disease and avoid regular health checkups and important cancer detection practices in which delay may be catastrophic. In addition to providing breast health education, clinical breast examinations, and referral for mammography, data are being collected to compile a family profile and assess participants' breast cancer detection practices. This project has allowed the nursing school in cooperation with the CRS staff to assist women in their pursuit of health promotion, provide clinical instruction to nursing students, and conduct needed research in the area of women's health (Williams and Turner-Henson, 1996).

The Office of Research on Women's Health was established in 1990 by the NIH. Through a special task force, NIH recommendations are made for the research agenda for women's health for the next two decades (Healy, 1991). In addition, nurse researchers are encouraged to test interventions and question rituals in nursing (conduct ritual-busting research). Covington and Collins (1994) stated that this will provide the groundwork for change in women's health care. "However, research-driven change endorses the shedding of an antiquated nurse image and practice" (p. 187). Some of the areas for exploration and research among women are as follows:

- Health promotion
- Barriers to care
- Disease prevention
- Health education at various literacy levels
- Wellness across the life cycle
- Differences among women experiencing menopausal symptoms
- Dysmenorrhea
- Contraception, safe and effective
- Promotion of breast-feeding
- Infertility
- Coping with chronic illness such as systemic lupus erythematosus or arthritis
- Discomforts of pregnancy, including morning sickness
- Strengths of single female heads of households
- Adolescent sexuality
- Multiple-role adaptation
- Menstrual cycle variations
- Control of obesity
- Substance abuse and its effect on pregnancy
- HIV infection and pregnancy
- Influence of diet on osteoporosis
- Effect of socialization on role
- Domestic violence

The Women's Health Initiative, a landmark study by the NIH, was launched in 1991. This study includes women of all races and socioeconomic levels and examines major causes of death, disability, and frailty. Specific conditions to be examined include heart disease and stroke, cancer, and osteoporosis (Healy, 1991).

With the increased emphasis on community health, community health nurses can make significant contributions toward the improvement of women's health through scholarly research either as principal investigators or through data gathering. Furthermore, they can become consumers of research and develop nursing interventions based on sound research and recommendations.

SUMMARY

Women's health care has multiple facets. Many areas for community health nursing intervention exist. Nurses are advocates and activists for women's health through their involvement in health policymaking as a profession. Along with other multidisciplinary and consumer groups, professional nurses are in the forefront of making changes in the health care delivery system that will promote an overall quality- and research-based health plan for women. Women are at the center of the health of the nation; therefore, if better models are developed for improving the health of women, the health of the entire nation will benefit.

Learning Activities

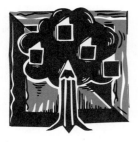

1. Integrate wellness principles and values into your personal and professional life.

2. Model to non-nursing students participatory (the woman as well as the health care provider) care to enhance wellness.

3. Survey examples from everyday life that support or encourage violence against women (e.g., magazines, books, and television advertisements).

4. Survey lay magazine advertisements and determine the percentage of total pages that use a woman's image (including aging, menopause, overweight and obesity, and sexuality) to sell products.

5. Discuss with your female relatives the need for cancer screening based on ACS guidelines.

6. Discuss with your female relatives the need for a heart-healthy nutritional plan based on AHA guidelines.

7. Investigate community resources for sites that offer instruction in BSE, clinical examination, and mammography that is accredited by the American College of Radiology.

8. Identify resources for mammograms and Pap smears for low-income women.

9. Visit with a women's group in your community (e.g., business, church, sorority, Parents Without Partners, and so on) to discuss its members' health care needs and concerns. From these data, develop research questions.

10. Call a family planning clinic and determine the population served (eligibility), services offered, and costs.

11. Use the telephone directory to identify resources providing health care and psychosocial services to men, women, and children with HIV and acquired immunodeficiency syndrome.

12. Query a women's health care nurse practitioner or nurse-midwife regarding the changes made in gynecologic care of women with physical disabilities.

13. Review county or state health department statistics for leading causes of deaths among women of varying ethnic or racial groups.

14. Create a list of upstream strategies that may be used to modify precursors of the causes of death identified in Learning Activity 13.

15. Determine the percentage of women in your county who begin prenatal care during the first trimester.

16. Identify how the health care needs of women are met when they are in the correctional system in your county or state.

REFERENCES

American Cancer Society: Cancer Facts and Figures 1995. Atlanta, GA, ACS, 1995.

American College of Obstetricians and Gynecologists: Periodic Cancer Screening for Women: Statement of Policy. Washington, DC, ACOG, 1980.

American Heart Association: Heart and Stroke Facts: Statistical Supplement, National Center, Dallas, TX, 1994, p. 10.

American Nurses Association: INA file lawsuit, charge unfair wages. Am Nurse 16;11, 1984.

Amsterdam EA, Legato MJ: What's unique about CHD in women? Patient Care 27:21–61, 1993.

Bobak IM, Lowdermilk DL, Jensen MD: Maternity Nursing, 4th ed. St. Louis, CV Mosby, 1995.

Bodenheimer T. Sounding board: Underinsurance in America. N Engl J Med 327(4):274–278, 1992.

Bonam-Crawford D, Orlick M: Helping patients with cancer achieve their work potential. Clin Perspect Oncol Nurs 1:3, 1994.

Boring CC, Squires TS, Tong T, Montgomery S: Cancer statistics, 1994. CA-A Cancer J Clin 44:7–26, 1994.

Brown M: Primary dysmenorrhea. Nurs Clin North Am 17:145–153, 1982.

Brown L, Williams RD: Culturally sensitive breast cancer screening programs for older black women. Nurse Pract 19:21, 25, 26, 31, 35, 1994.

Byyny RL, Speroff L: A Clinical Guide for the Care of Older Women. Baltimore, MD, Williams & Wilkins, 1990.

Cassetta RA, FMLA: A first step toward equitable leave policies. The American Nurse 25(8):21, 1993.

Centers for Disease Control and Prevention: Sexually transmitted disease treatment guidelines. MMWR Morbid Mortal Wkly Rep 42:57, 1993.

Chadwick BA, Heaton TB (eds): Statistical Handbook on the American Family. Phoenix, Oryx Press, 1992.

Charting a course for health and well being. Network News: 8:2, 8, 9, 1983.

Choi M: Preamble to a new paradigm for women's health. Image 17:14–16, 1985.

Clark RA: Infections during the postpartum period. J Obstet Gynecol Neonatal Nurs 24:552–548, 1995.

Clark R, Hankins CA, Hein K, et al: HIV: What's different for women. Patient Care 27(14):119–147, 1993.

Clinician's Handbook of Preventive Services: Injury and violence prevention. Washington, DC, U.S. Government Printing Office, p. 291, 1994.

Contraceptive Report: Postponing sexual involvement. 5:6–9, 1994. Emory University/Grady Memorial Publication.

Covington C, Collins JE: Back to the future of women's health and perinatal nursing in the 21st century. J Obstet Gynecol Neonatal Nurs 23:183–194, 1994.

Craven S, Greenberger MC, Kolker A: Reproductive health: An essential part of health care. A report by the National Women's Law Center, Washington, DC, 1993, p. 14.

Creehan PA: Toxic shock syndrome: An opportunity for nursing intervention. J Obstet Gynecol Neonatal Nurs 24:557–561, 1995.

Cunningham FG, MacDonald PC, Gant NF, et al: Williams' Obstetrics, 19th ed. Norwalk, CT, Appleton & Lange, 1993, p. 4.

Current Population Survey: Employee Benefit Research Institute Analysis, Washington, DC, March 1992, p. 32.

Dickinson C: The postpartum period. In Lichtman R, Papera S (eds). Gynecology: Well-Woman Care. Norwalk, CT, Appleton & Lange, 1990, pp. 394–395.

Donaldson K, Briggs J, McMaster D: RU 486: An alternative to surgical abortion. J Obstet Gynecol Neonatal Nurs 23:555–559, 1995.

Eisenkop SM, Lowitz BB, Casciato DA: Gynecologic cancers. In Casciato D, Lowitz B (eds). Manual of Clinical Oncology, 2nd ed. Boston, Little, Brown, pp. 166–184, 1988.

Farley D: Preventing TSS: Tampon labeling lets women compare absorbencies. FDA Consumer Special Report: Current Issues in Women's Health, 2nd ed. Rockville, MD, DHHS, 1994, pp. 21–24.

Finkel ML, Finkel DJ: The effect of a second opinion program on hysterectomy performance. Medical Care 28:776–783, 1990.

Flanagan L: "What You Need to Know About Today's Workplace: A Survival Guide for Nurses, Washington, DC. American Nurses Publishing. 1992.

Gordon VC, Ledray LE: Growth-support intervention for the treatment of depression in women of middle years. West J Nurs Res 8:263–283, 1986.

Graves, EJ: National Hospital Discharge Survey: Annual Summary, 1993. National Center for Health Statistics. Vital Health Stat 13(121), 1995, pp. 15 and 21.

Gusberg SB, Runowicz CD: Gynecologic cancers. In Holleb AI, Fink DJ, Murphy GP (eds). American Cancer Society Textbook of Clinical Oncology. Atlanta, American Cancer Society, 1991.

Haas M: Women, work and stress: A review and agenda for the future. J Health Soc Behav 23:132–144, 1982.

Haller KB: Family planning for healthy nations (editorial). J Obstet Gynecol Neonatal Nurs 23:547, 1994.

Hatcher RA, Trussell J, Stewart F, et al: Contraceptive technology, 16th ed. New York, Irvington. 1994.

Hauenstein EJ: Young women and depression: Origin, outcome, and nursing care. Nurs Clin North Am 26:601–612, 1991.

Healy B: Women's health, public welfare. JAMA 266:566–568, 1991.

Houde-Quimby C: Women and the family of the future. J Obstet Gynecol Neonatal Nurs 23:113–123, 1994.

Hugick L: Women playing the leading role in keeping modern families close. Gallup Report 286:27–35, 1989.

Institute of Medicine: Prenatal Care: Reaching Mothers, Reaching Infants. Washington, DC, National Academy Press, 1988.

Institute of Medicine: Preventing Low Birthweight. Washington, DC, National Academy Press, 1985.

International Council of Nurses: Healthy families for healthy nations. Geneva: Author. 1993.

Johnson CD: Projecting unmet need for prenatal care. In Kotch JB, Blakely CH, Brown SS, Wong FY (eds). A Pound of Prevention: The Case of Universal Maternity Care in the U.S. Washington, DC, American Public Health Association, 1992, pp. 87–107.

Jones-Warren B: The experience of depression in African American women. In McElmurry BJ, Parker R (eds). Annual Review of

Women's Health, Vol. 11. New York, National League for Nursing, 1995, pp. 267–283.

Kahn CR, Weir GC: Joslin's Diabetes Mellitus, 13th ed. Philadelphia; Lea & Febiger, 1994.

Kleiman C: Women's Networks. New York, Ballantine Books, 1980.

Klein L: Unintended pregnancy and the risks/safety of birth control methods. J Obstet Gynecol 13:287–289, 1984.

Knight-Ridder News Service: Finally, men 'get it' about sexual harassment in workplace. The Huntsville Times, September 1995, pp. 1, 15, 10.

Mark DB, Shaw LK, DeLong ER, et al: Absence of sex bias in the referral of patients for cardiac catheterization. N Engl J Med 330:1101–1106, 1994.

Marshall E: Search for a killer: Focus shifts from fat to hormones. Science 259:618–621, 1993.

McKenry LM, Salerno E.(eds): Psychologic and cultural aspects of drug therapy and self-treatment. In Mosby's Pharmacology in Nursing. St. Louis, CV Mosby, 1992, pp. 117–118.

McKie L: Women's views of the cervical smear test: Implications for nursing practice in women who have not had a smear test. J Adv Nurs 18:972–979, 1993.

Meilahan EN, Matthews KA, Egeland G, Kelsey SF: Characteristics of women with hysterectomy. Maturitas 11:319–329, 1989.

Metropolitan Life and Affiliated Companies: Health insurance of women of childbearing age, United States, in 1985. Statistical Bulletin 69:16–23, 1988.

Mills C, Safriet B, Woodward J, Wysocki S: NP's role: Will it change after health-care reform? Contemp OB/GYN-NP 2(2): 18–25, 1994.

Misner ST, Beauchamp-Hewitt JB, Fox-Levin P: Occupational issues in women's health. In McElmurry BJ, Spreen-Parker R (eds). Annual Review of Women's Health, vol. 11. New York, National League for Nursing, 1995, pp. 107–142.

Moore KG: A survey of state Medicaid policies for coverage of screening mammography and Pap smear services. Women's Health Issues 2:40–49, 1992.

National Institutes of Health: Preventing unintended pregnancy: The role of hormonal contraception. Clinician 11:5, 1993.

Neeson J, Stockdale C: The Practitioner's Handbook of Ambulatory OB/GYN. New York, J Wiley, 1981.

Nesto RW, Zarich SW, Jacoby RM, Kamalesh M: Heart disease in diabetes. In Kahn CR, Weir GC (eds). Joslin's Diabetes Mellitus, 13th ed. Philadelphia: Lea & Febiger, 1994.

Northouse L: Psychologic consequences of breast cancer on partner and family. Semin Oncol Nurs 7:216–223, 1991.

Olds S, London M, Ladewig P: Maternal-newborn nursing, 5th ed. Menlo Park, CA, Addison-Wesley, 1995.

Olson A, Labat J: Women, diet, and heart disease. In McElmurry BJ, Parker RS (eds). Annual Review of Women's Health, vol. 11. New York: National League for Nursing, 1995, pp. 71–92.

Paolisso M, Leslie J: Meeting the changing health needs of women in developing countries. Soc Sci Med 40(1):55–65, 1995.

Papazian R: Osteoporosis treatment advances. In FDA Consumer Special Report: Current Issues in Women's Health, 2nd ed. Rockville, MD, DHHS, 1994, pp. 107–110.

Pender NJ: Health Promotion in Nursing Practice, 2nd ed. Norwalk, CT, Appleton & Lange, 1987.

Phipps W, Long B, Woods N: Medical-Surgical Nursing Concepts and Clinical Practice, 2nd ed. St. Louis, CV Mosby, 1983.

Pollard K, Tordella S: Women making gains among professionals. Population Today 21:1–2, 1993.

Population Today: US reaches its highest ever levels of life expectancy. 21:4, 1993.

Radloff LS: Risk factors for depression: What do we learn from them? In Guttentag M, Salasin S, Belle D (eds). The Mental Health of Women. New York, Academic Press, pp. 93–109, 1980.

Ravnikar VA, Chen E: Hysterectomies: Where are the indications? Obstet Gynecol Clin North Am 21:405–411, 1994.

Riche MF, Pollard KM: PRB census analysis finds U.S. women are anything but "typical." Population Today 22:4–5, May 1994.

Robinson JC, Plichta BA, Weisman CS, et al: Dysmenorrhea and use of oral contraceptives in adolescent women attending a family planning clinic. Am J Obstet Gynecol 166:578–583, 1992.

Rose J: Herbal treatments for women. In Weiss K (ed). Women's Health Care—A Guide to Alternatives. Reston, VA, Reston Publishing, pp. 235–245, 1984.

Schreiber R: Pay Equity for nurses: Comparable worth and gender neutrality. Health Care Women Int 15:577–585, 1994.

Seltzer VL, Pearse WH: Women's Primary Health Care: Office Practice and Procedures. New York, McGraw-Hill, 1995.

Sherwen LN, Scoloveno MA, Weingarten CT: Nursing Care of the Childbearing Family. Norwalk, CT, Appleton & Lange, 1991.

Sidel R: Women and children first: Toward a U.S. family policy. J Health Care Poor Underserved 1:342–350, 1991.

Smith LS: Psychologic concerns. In Griffith-Kenney J (ed). Contemporary Women's Health: A Nursing Advocacy Approach. Menlo Park, CA, Addison-Wesley, pp. 156–175, 1986.

Snell T: Survey of state prison inmates, 1991: women in prison. United States Department of Justice, Bureau of Justice Statistics, Washington, DC, US Government Printing Office, 1994, pp. 1–11.

Spark A: Nutrition counseling. In Edelman CL, Mandle CL (eds). Health Promotion: Throughout the lifespan, 3rd ed. St. Louis, CV Mosby, pp. 265–298, 1994.

Staats MB, Staats TE: Differences in stress levels, stressors, and stress responses between managerial and professional males and females: Vector analysis—research education. Issues Health Care Women 4:165–176, 1983.

Star WL, Lommel LL, Shannon MT: Women's Primary Health Care: Protocols for Practice. Washington, DC, American Nurses Publishing, 1995.

Steingart RM, Packer M, Hamm P, et al: Sex difference in the management of coronary artery disease. N Engl J Med 325:226–230, 1991.

Stevens PE: Lesbian health care research: A review of the literature from 1970-1990. Health Care Women Int 13:91–120, 1992.

Stotland NL: Psychiatric and psychosocial issues in primary care of women. In Seltzer VL, Pearse WH (eds). Women's Primary Health Care: Office Practice and Procedures. New York, McGraw-Hill, pp. 337–376, 1995.

Sullivan N: Dysmenorrhea. In Lichtman R, Papera S (eds). Gynecology: Well-Woman Care. Norwalk, CT, Appleton & Lange, 1990.

Thomas DN: Influences of creativity, depression and psychological well-being on physiological and psychological symptoms in midlife women. Unpublished dissertation, Texas Woman's University, Denton, TX, 1988.

Tiffany C, Johnson-Lütjens LR: Pay inequity: it's still with us. J Prof Nurs 9:50–55, 1993.

U.S. Bureau of the Census, Statistical Abstract of the United States: 1988, 108th ed. Washington, DC, U.S. Government Printing Office, 1988.

U.S. Bureau of the Census, Statistical Abstract of the United States: 1989, 109th ed. Washington, DC, U.S. Government Printing Office, 1989.

U.S. Bureau of the Census, Statistical Abstract of the United States: 1990, 110th ed. Washington, DC, U.S. Government Printing Office, 1990.

U.S. Bureau of the Census, Statistical Abstract of the United States: 1995, 115th ed. Washington, DC, U.S. Government Printing Office, 1995.

U.S. Bureau of the Census: Single parents maintain 3 in 10 family groups involving children. Mother's Day Statistics of the

United States. Washington, DC, U.S. Government Printing Office, 1994.

U.S. Department of Health and Human Services: Healthy People 2000. National Health Promotion and Disease Prevention Objectives—Public Health Service. Washington, DC, U.S. Government Printing Office, 1991.

U.S. Department of Health and Human Services: Clinical practice guideline: Evaluation and management of early HIV infection (AHCPR Publication No. 94-0572). Washington, DC, U.S. Government Printing Office, 1994a.

U.S. Department of Health and Human Services: Current Issues in Women's Health (2nd ed.) (Publication No. FDA 94-1181) Washington, DC, 1994b.

U.S. Department of Health and Human Services. Papanicolaou smear. *In* Put Prevention into Practice. A Clinician's Handbook. Washington, DC, U.S. Government Printing Office, 1994c, pp. 195–196.

Verbrugge LM: The twain meet: Empirical explanations of sex differences in health and mortality. J Health Soc Behav 30:282–304, 1989.

Verbrugge LM: Women, men and osteoarthritis. Arthritis Care Res 8:212–220, 1995.

Weiss K: Women's Health Care—A Guide to Alternatives. Reston, VA, Reston Publishing. 1984.

Weissman MM: Depression. *In* Brodsky AM, Hare-Mustin R (eds). Women and Psychotherapy. New York, Guilford Press, pp. 97–112, 1980.

Weissman MM, Klerman GL: Depression in women: Epidemiology, explanations, and impact on the family. *In* Notman MT, Nadelson CC (eds). The Woman Patient. Vol. 3: Aggression, Adaptations and Psychotherapy. New York, Plenum Press, pp. 189–203, 1982.

Wilcox LS, Koonin LM, Pokras R, et al: Hysterectomy in the United States, 1988–1990. Obstet Gynecol 83:549–555, 1994.

Williams RD, Lethbridge DJ: Health promotion behaviors for women in Third World areas of industrialized countries. Connecting conversations: Nursing scholarship and practice. Book of Abstracts. University of Iceland, Department of Nursing. June 20–23, 1995, p. 176.

Williams RD, Turner-Henson A: Breast health protection of female family caregivers. Sigma Theta Tau International, Eighth International Research Congress, Book of Abstracts. Jamaica, West Indies, May, 1996, p. 126.

Witkin-Lanoil G: The reality of female stress. Health 16:54–60, 1984.

Women Employed Institute: Sexual harassment: The problem that isn't going away. Chicago, Author 1994.

Women's Health—Report of the Public Health Service Task Force on women's health issues. (1985). Public Health Reports 100:73–106, 1985.

Women's Health Risk Expected to Increase. Am Operating Room Nurse J 33:1181, 1981.

Woods NF, Lentz M, Mitchell E, Oakley LD: Depressed mood and self-esteem in young Asian, black, and white women in America. Health Care Women Int 15:243–262, 1994.

Worthington K: Regulatory reform: Will your health and safety be at risk. Am Nurse 27:14. 1995.

Men's Health

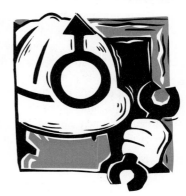

Upon completion of this chapter, the reader will be able to:

1. Identify the major indicators of men's health status.

2. Describe two major explanations for men's health status.

3. Discuss factors that impede men's health.

4. Discuss factors that promote men's health.

5. Describe men's health needs.

6. Apply knowledge of men's health needs in planning gender-appropriate nursing care for men at the individual, family, and community levels.

Janice M. Swanson

It is common knowledge that women live longer than men. Death rates for men are higher than for women for the major causes of death (Kochanek and Hudson, 1995). However, despite increasing interest in health promotion and illness prevention, little attention has been paid to men's health. Although women's health is becoming a specialty area of practice and courses and programs in women's health are available in many colleges of nursing, courses, programs, and a specialty for men's health are not emphasized.

This chapter focuses on the health needs of men and the implications for community health nursing. Specific areas that are discussed include men's health status, theories that attempt to explain men's health, factors that impede men's health, factors that promote men's health, men's health needs, meeting men's health needs, and planning gender-appropriate care for men at the individual, family, and community levels.

MEN'S HEALTH STATUS

Traditional indicators of health include rates of longevity, mortality, and morbidity.

LONGEVITY AND MORTALITY IN MEN

Major differences between the sexes in rates of longevity and mortality show that men are disadvantaged despite marked increases in medical care and access to health services. In contrast, higher morbidity rates are experienced by women, who are more likely to use health services. Sex differentials have been associated with behavioral factors, which place men at greater risk of death. Antecedents of sex-linked behavior in men, however, are compounded by social and environmental factors of major public health concern. These factors, together with men's reluctance to seek preventive and health services, have marked implications for community health nursing.

Longevity

Rates of longevity are increasing for both men and women. We can expect to live more than 20 years longer than our forefathers and foremothers at the turn of the century. Infants born in the United States in 1992 can expect to live 75.8 years, whereas those born in 1900 lived an average of 47.3 years (Kochanek and Hudson, 1995). Although life expectancy has increased, the gender gap—differences between males and females—has also increased. Males born in 1992 will live an average of 72.3 years (Kochanek and Hudson, 1995). Females born in 1992, however, will live an average of 79.1 years. At the turn of the century, women lived an average of only 2 years longer than men. The gender gap increased from 5.5 to 7.8 years between 1950 and 1975, with females gaining over males each year. That trend reversed and men started to catch up, as evidenced by a decline from 7.8 years in 1975 to 6.8 in 1992. Overall, however, differences in longevity rates between males and females suggest that males have become disadvantaged over the course of this century.

STANDARDIZED TERMINOLOGY

In the fields of demography and sociology, the following terms are standardized:
Persons of all ages: males, females
Children (younger than 18 years): boys, girls
Adults (18 years of age or older): men, women
Sex: the distinction, biologically, between males and females
Gender: the attitudes and behavior of men and women that are shaped by socialization and have a potential to be changed
Role: the part one plays in society

Adapted from Skelton R. (1988). Man's role in society and its effect on health. Nursing 26:953–956; Verbrugge LM, Wingard DL. (1987). Sex differentials in health and mortality. Women Health 12:103–145.

The United States has been the only Western industrialized nation that has failed to routinely report many health and vital statistics by socioeconomic status (Navarro, 1989). Educational attainment as reported on the death certificate has been tabulated only since 1989 (Kochanek and Hudson, 1995). Income (family) is more likely to be tabulated in reports of morbidity (rates of illness) than in reports of mortality (see, e.g., reports of mortality and morbidity in *Health, United States, 1993* (National Center for Health Statistics [NCHS], 1994). In England, life expectancy is closely associated with socioeconomic status (Skelton, 1988). Reports of health and vital statistics in the United States by race and sex show that underserved populations in the United States, especially minorities, live significantly fewer years. For example, of those born in 1992, black males will live

Table 12–1
Life Expectancy at Birth According to Sex and Race, United States, 1900–1993

Year	All Races			White			Black		
	Both Sexes	Male	Female	Both Sexes	Male	Female	Both Sexes	Male	Female
1900	47.3	46.3	48.3	47.6	46.6	48.7	33.0	32.5	33.5
1960	69.7	66.6	73.1	70.6	67.4	74.1	63.2	60.7	65.9
1992	75.8	72.3	79.1	76.5	73.2	79.8	69.6	65.0	73.9

Data compiled from National Center for Health Statistics (1995). Health, United States, 1994, Hyattsville, MD, Public Health Service.

65.0 years and white males will live 73.2 years; black females will live 73.9 years and white females will live 79.8 years (Kochanek and Hudson, 1995). Data for Hispanic populations had not been available until recently because they had been traditionally classified as white in the United States and considered an ethnic group. The United States lags behind a number of other countries; in 1991 the rating was 25th in life expectancy for men and 16th in life expectancy for women (Table 12–1) (NCHS, 1995).

Mortality

Males in industrialized countries have higher death rates than do females (Waldron, 1995b). In the United States, males lead females in rate of mortality in each of the leading causes of death (Table 12–2). Men are about seven times as likely as women to die from acquired immunodeficiency syndrome (AIDS). Men are more than four times as likely as women to die from suicide, about four times as likely to die from

Table 12–2
Ratio of Age-Adjusted Death Rates for 12 Leading Causes of Death for the Total Population by Sex and Race: United States, 1992

Rank Order	Cause of Death (Ninth Revision, International Classification of Diseases, 1975)	Ratio	
		Male to Female	Black to White
	All causes	1.72	1.61
1	Diseases of the heart	1.88	1.48
2	Malignant neoplasms	1.45	1.37
3	Cerebrovascular diseases	1.18	1.86
4	Chronic obstructive pulmonary disease and allied conditions	1.70	0.81
5	Accidents and adverse effects	2.63	1.27
—	Motor vehicle accidents	2.35	1.03
—	All other accidents and adverse effects	2.97	1.57
6	Pneumonia and influenza	1.69	1.44
7	Diabetes mellitus	1.14	2.41
8	Human immunodeficiency virus infection	6.97	3.69
9	Suicide	4.28	0.58
10	Homicide and legal intervention	3.98	6.46
11	Chronic liver disease and cirrhosis	2.42	1.48
12	Nephritis, nephrotic syndrome, and nephrosis	1.53	2.76

Data compiled from Kochanek KD, Hudson BL (1995). Advance report of final mortality statistics, 1992. Monthly vital statistics report; 43 (6 suppl.). Hyattsville, MD: National Center for Health Statistics.

homicide or legal intervention, and two to three times as likely to die from accident or chronic liver disease or cirrhosis. They are nearly twice as likely as women to die of diseases of the heart, chronic obstructive pulmonary disease, and pneumonia and influenza and lead in deaths resulting from cancer, kidney disease, cerebrovascular disease, and diabetes (Kochanek and Hudson, 1995). The age-adjusted sex-to-mortality ratio for all ages has increased between 1950 and 1992 from 1.5 to 1.72.

Black men are more than four times as likely to die from human immunodeficiency virus (HIV) infection as are black women, nearly three times as likely to die from vehicle accidents, and more than 1.6 times as likely to die from diseases of the heart or from cancer (NCHS, 1995). The highest sex-to-mortality ratios shared by both white and black men were for HIV infection, homicide, and legal intervention (Kochanek and Hudson, 1995).

Morbidity

In health interviews in which people are asked to report their view of their health status, men have consistently reported their health status higher than have women (Verbrugge and Wingard, 1987). In the National Health Interview Survey of 1993, 9.4% of men stated their health was "fair or poor" compared with 11.5% of women. However, 40.3% of men rated their health as "excellent" compared with 35.0% of women (Benson and Marano, 1994).

SOURCES OF DATA

- National Center for Health Statistics

  Through the National Vital Statistics System, the National Center for Health Statistics collects data from each state, New York City, the District of Columbia, the U.S. Virgin Islands, Guam, and Puerto Rico on births, deaths, marriages, and divorces in the United States.

- National Health Interview Survey

  The National Health Interview Survey is a continuing nationwide sample survey in which data are collected by personal interviews about household members' illnesses, injuries, chronic conditions, disabilities, and use of health services.

Morbidity rates, or rates of illness, are very difficult to obtain and have been available usually only in Western industrialized countries. In the United States, for example, reports of analyses of morbidity by gender lag several years behind analyses of mortality by gender. Gender differences in morbidity reported here reflect the latest available reports. Common indicators of morbidity are:

- Incidence of acute illness
- Prevalence of chronic conditions
- Use of medical care

Although variations exist, in general, women are more likely to be ill, whereas men are at greater risk for death.

ACUTE ILLNESS

The incidence rate is higher for women than for men for acute infective and parasitic disease, digestive system conditions, and respiratory conditions (Benson and Marano, 1994). The only exception is for injuries, which in 1993 were 12% greater for men. The incidence rate for injuries for men is about the same as for women. Acute conditions associated with the childbearing role of women are included. When these female conditions are excluded, however, the incidence rate for women is still 18% greater than that for men.

In the 1993 National Health Interview Survey, men and women differed in their response to acute conditions. Women slowed their activities and rested in bed more often than men. The number of restricted-activity days associated with acute conditions per 100 persons is 33% greater for women than for men; similarly, the number of bed days associated with acute conditions per 100 persons is 38% greater for women than for men (Benson and Marano, 1994). In this survey, an acute condition was considered a type of illness or injury that usually lasted less than 3 months and either resulted in restricted activity (e.g., causing a person to limit daily activities for at least half a day) or caused the patient to receive medical care.

CHRONIC CONDITIONS

A chronic condition was considered a condition that lasted at least 3 months or belonged to a group of conditions that was classified as chronic regardless of time of onset, such as tuberculosis, neoplasm, or arthritis (Benson and Marano, 1994). Women, in general, have higher morbidity rates than do men.

Major sex-to-morbidity ratios are presented in Table 12–3. Women are more likely than men to have a higher prevalence of chronic diseases that cause disability and limitation of activities but do not lead to death. Men, however, have higher morbidity as well as mortality rates for conditions that are the leading causes of death.

USE OF MEDICAL CARE

Medical care may occur as use of ambulatory care, hospital care, preventative care, or other health services. Here, the gender gap again appears.

Use of Ambulatory Care

Men seek ambulatory care less often than do women. According to the 1993 National Health Interview Survey, the physician's office is the primary setting for ambulatory care for both men and women. In this report, a physician contact is defined as consultation with a physician or with another person working under the physician's supervision, in person or via telephone, for the purposes of examination, diagnosis, treatment, or advice (Benson and Marano, 1994). Women had 6.2 physician contacts outside a hospital (physician's office or via telephone) in 1993, whereas men had 4.3 contacts. Men are seen more frequently than women for conditions that correspond with their leading causes of mortality, such as ischemic heart disease. On the other hand, women are seen more frequently than men for the chronic diseases found to be more prevalent among them. Visit rates for boys and girls younger than 18 years old are about the same (4.2 vs. 4.0).

Men were less likely than women to report seeing a physician in the past year (72.8% vs. 84.1%) (Benson and Marano, 1994). Also men were more likely than women to report intervals of last contact with a physician between 1 and 2 years (11.1% vs. 8.3%), 2 and 5 years (11.2% vs. 5.5%), and 5 years or more (4.9% vs. 2.1%).

Use of Hospital Care

The literature indicates that hospitalization rates also vary by sex. For example, in 1993, rates of discharges from short-stay hospitals were lower for males (9.1 per 100 population) than for females (12.3 per 100 population) even when discharges for deliveries are excluded (9.7 per 100 population) (Benson and Marano, 1994). Males, however, had a longer length of stay in the hospital than females (6.1 vs. 5.5 days). Boys up to the age of 15 years are hospitalized more than girls, but females aged 15 to 44 years are hospitalized more often than males in this age group (Verbrugge and Wingard, 1987). Discharge rates increase for both men and women after the age of 45; rates for men, however, increase more rapidly. After age 65, men's discharge rates continue to be higher than women's.

Table 12–3
Morbidity Sex Ratios by Age, United States, 1993

Type of Condition	Male-Female Ratio per 1000 Persons		
	<45 Years	45–64 Years	≥65 Years
Gout, including gouty arthritis	11.00	2.70	2.00
Absence of extremities (excludes tips of fingers or toes only)	5.50	7.10	7.40
Ischemic heart disease	2.27	2.45	1.63
Intervertebral disc disorders	1.50	1.40	.94
Hypertension	1.08	.94	.85
Asthma	1.00	.51	.82
Hay fever or allergic rhinitis without asthma	.88	.87	.79
Ulcer	.79	.62	.84
Arthritis	.76	.65	.74
Enteritis or colitis	.68	.42	.62

Data compiled from Benson V, Marano MA. (1994). Current estimates from the National Health Interview Survey, 1993. National Center for Health Statistics, Vital Health Statistics Series 10, No 190.

Use of Preventive Care

Preventive examinations are necessary for early diagnosis of health problems. National health surveys indicate that women are more likely than men to receive physical examinations (NCHS, 1994). Women's examinations are also more likely to be recent than are men's examinations. Young women to age 35 are more likely to have health insurance than young men; after age 35, there is no difference (Salem, 1995).

Use of Other Health Services

Women are more likely to be admitted for psychiatric services to outpatient psychiatric settings such as community mental health centers that are federally funded and to be admitted for psychiatric services to private mental hospitals and psychiatric care units of nonfederal, general hospitals (NCHS, 1995). Women also are more likely to reside in nursing homes owing to their longer life expectancy (NCHS, 1994). Men are more likely to be admitted for psychiatric services to state and county mental hospitals (NCHS, 1995).

THEORIES THAT EXPLAIN MEN'S HEALTH

It is clear that there is a gender gap in health. The data reviewed raise many questions for community health nurses to explore regarding sex differences in health and illness. Although men have shorter life expectancy and higher rates of mortality for all leading causes of death, women have higher rates of morbidity, including rates of acute illness and chronic disease, and use of medical and preventive care services. What theories exist to explain men's health status? Or, as asked by Verbrugge and Wingard (1987), how is it that "females are sicker, but males die sooner?" (p. 135). Is it simply that we aggregate more mortalities of men and more morbidities of women, or is it more a matter of how males and females respond to health problems? There are several explanations for this paradox.

Traditionally, adult health was viewed within a developmental framework (Erikson, 1963); only later was there a focus specifically on the development of men (Levinson, 1978). Developmental theory has traditionally been used by nurses to explain individual behavior; less has been written about the many factors and combinations of factors that in-

fluence sex differences in the health and illness of populations.

Possible explanations proposed by Waldron (1995a–e) and Verbrugge and Wingard (1987) attempt to account for sex differences in this important area:

- Biological factors including genetics, effects of sex hormones, and physiological differences, which may be influenced by genetics, hormones, and environment
- Socialization
- Orientations toward illness and prevention
- Reporting of health behavior

Biological Factors

Sex differences in mortality and morbidity are influenced by a number of biological factors, including genetics, effects of sex hormones, and physiological differences, which may be influenced by genetics, hormones, and environmental factors (Waldron, 1995a–e). More male births occur than female births in both developed and developing countries (Waldron, 1995c). Sex ratios at birth favoring males range between 104 and 107 in developed countries and 103 and 106 in developing countries (Waldron, 1995c). Sex ratios at birth appear to be lower for births to older fathers, black fathers, higher order births (such as second, third, or fourth births), and births after induced ovulation. It is unknown whether or not sex ratios at birth are influenced by sex ratios at conception or sex differentials in mortality before birth. Current evidence suggests that greater than two of three prenatal deaths occur before clinical recognition of the pregnancy. Sex differences in late fetal mortality, once favoring males in developed countries, have decreased since the early and mid-20th century; currently, no differences exist due to improved medical care and maternal health (Waldron, 1995c). These factors have decreased deaths resulting from difficult labor, injuries at birth, and maternal diseases and accidents. Even though females have had higher rates of late fetal mortality as a result of congenital malformations, one condition that has increased, the male excess in late fetal mortality, has disappeared.

After birth, however, the picture changes. For example, in 1992, the neonatal (less than 28 days) mortality rate for males was higher than for females (5.8 vs. 4.9), as was postneonatal (28 days to 11 months) mortality rate (3.5 vs. 2.7) and infant (less than 1 year) mortality rate (9.4 vs. 7.6) (Kochanek and Hudson, 1995). Males' experience of higher mortality for perinatal conditions is attributed to biological disadvantages such as males' greater risk of premature birth, higher rates of respiratory distress syndrome, and infectious disease mortality in infancy resulting from the influence of male hormones on the developing lungs, brain, and possibly the immune system of the male fetus (Waldron, 1995c). Sex chromosome–linked diseases such as hemophilia and certain types of muscular dystrophy are more common among males than among females (Waldron, 1995c). Biological advantages for females may also exist later in life because of the protective mechanism produced by estrogen against heart disease, although studies must be interpreted cautiously (Waldron, 1995d). Some evidence supports the hypothesis that men's higher testosterone levels contribute to men's lower high-density lipoprotein levels. Body fat distribution also appears to contribute to sex differences in ischemic heart disease risk, specifically the tendency for men in Western countries to accumulate abdominal body fat versus the tendency for women to accumulate fat on the buttocks and thighs (Waldron, 1995d). Men's higher levels of stored iron are also thought to contribute to their risk of ischemic heart disease.

Socialization

A second theory for explaining sex differences in health is socialization. Acquired risks may be different between males and females owing to differences in work, leisure, and lifestyle. These differences may be influenced by sex-role socialization.

More men than women are employed on a full-time basis in work environments outside the home. Usually, men's occupations are more hazardous than are positions held by women. Accidents on the job contribute significantly to higher accident rates and represent a major killer among men (NCHS, 1994; Waldron, 1995b). Men's higher exposure to carcinogens at the work site is associated with high rates of mesothelioma and coal worker's pneumoconiosis (NCHS, 1994). In the United States, men score higher than women on measures of hostility and one's trust of others, which may place them at higher risk of ischemic heart disease (Matthews et al., 1992). Although occupational hazards to women's health are being identified, evidence indicates that, unlike men, employment of U.S. women outside

the home has had a positive effect on their health (Waldron, 1995b).

FOUR DIMENSIONS OF STEREOTYPED MALE SEX-ROLE BEHAVIOR

No Sissy Stuff: The need to be different from women
The Big Wheel: The need to be superior to others
The Sturdy Oak: The need to be independent and self-reliant
Give 'Em Hell: The need to be more powerful than others, through violence if necessary

Adapted from David DS, Brannon R. (1976). The male sex role: Our culture's blueprint of manhood, and what it's done for us lately. In David DS, Brannon R (eds). The Forty-Nine Percent Majority: The Male Sex Role. Reading, MA, Addison-Wesley, p. 12.

Leisure, sports, and play activities also place men at high risk of injury. Greater risk-taking behavior by males is supported by boys' higher rates of accidents caused by riskier play (Rosen and Peterson, 1990), men's faster driving rates and higher rates of traffic violations and motor vehicle fatalities (Waldron, 1995a), and men's greater use of illegal psychoactive substances, higher rates of alcohol consumption, and higher rates of cigarette smoking (NCHS, 1994). Of interest is that Waldron (1995e) cited evidence that supports higher accident mortality in males as due to both biological factors (prenatal hormones) and socialization. For example, male fetuses are more active during the third trimester of pregnancy than female fetuses because of the effects of male prenatal hormones on activity levels (Eaton and Enns, 1986). Boys are encouraged to be active and to be strong both physically and psychologically.

Orientations Toward Illness and Prevention

Illness orientations (i.e., one's ability to note symptoms and take appropriate action) may also differ between the sexes. That boys in our society are socialized to ignore symptoms was noted more than three decades ago by Mechanic (1964). The reporting of symptoms may be more socially acceptable for girls (Waldron, 1995a). Women are more likely to cut down their activities when ill, to seek health care, and to report more details to health care providers (Waldron, 1995a).

MEN'S REPRODUCTIVE HEALTH NEEDS

Reproductive health needs are beginning to be recognized as important to men's health as well as to women's health. Usually the term "reproductive health" is applied to women of childbearing age. Used here, the term "reproductive health" applies to the health of reproductive organs, which develop in utero and with which a person is born, in both males and females, regardless of whether a person has sex or not or reproduces or not, throughout one's lifetime. Males may have reproductive health needs whether child or adult, straight or gay, or virgin or sexually experienced.

Many STDs are at epidemic proportions in the United States and are a major health hazard for many men as well as women. There are sex differences in the incidence of STDs. It is well known that AIDS in the United States is more likely to occur in males. For the 12-month period ending September 30, 1994, males 13 years of age and older accounted for 64.3 cases of AIDS per 100,000 population, whereas females of the same age accounted for only 12.6 cases of AIDS per 100,000 population (NCHS, 1995). Less well known, perhaps, is that many STDs are considered to be intrinsically "sexist," because clinical evidence, more overt in men, is more likely to facilitate a correct diagnosis in men than in women. For example, in 1993, the rate of primary and secondary syphilis was higher for men (11.3/100,000 population) than for women (9.6/100,000 population) (Centers for Disease Control [CDC], 1994). The rate of gonorrhea was higher among men (185.1/100,000 population) than among women (147.2/100,000 population), because men are more likely to be treated for these STDs than are women (CDC, 1994). It is easier to detect these STDs in men because men are more likely to be symptomatic; in addition, laboratory tests are more reliable in men; efficiency of transmission is greater from male to female; and men are more likely to seek care for STDs, which are symptomatic in men (CDC, 1994; Ehrhardt and Wasserheit, 1991; Temmerman, 1994; Wasserheit, 1994).

Testicular cancer is most likely to affect young men, ages 15 to 35 years, and was estimated to account for 7100 new cases in 1995, up from an estimated 6100 in 1991 (American Cancer Society, 1991; Wingo et al., 1995). The incidence of testicular cancer has increased three- to four-fold worldwide since the 1940s (Giwercman et al., 1993).

Cancer of the prostate is a leading cause of death from cancer in men and was estimated to account for 244,000 cases in 1995, up from an estimated 76,000 cases in 1984 (NCHS, 1992, 1995). The increase in the incidence of cancer of the prostate has been attributed to factors such as improved methods of detection and increased exposure to environmental carcinogens.

Incidence rates for all types of cancer increased between 1975 and 1979 and 1987 and 1991, but age-adjusted rates were higher among males (18.6%) than females (12.4%), which was largely due to rising rates of prostate cancer among men (Devesa et al., 1995). On the other hand, mortality rates for all cancers were less, at 3% among men and 6% among women, largely because of rising rates of lung cancer mortality, whereas death rates for the majority of other types of cancer were stable or declining.

Many occupational and environmental agents associated with adverse sexual and reproductive outcomes in men have been identified and include pesticides, anesthetic gases in the operating room and dental office, inorganic lead from smelters, painting, printing, carbon disulfide from vulcanization of rubber, inorganic mercury manufacturing and dental work, and ionizing radiation from x-rays (see Chapters 26 and 27; Cohen, 1986; McDiarmid et al., 1991); Whorton, 1984). Nonchemical agents have also been identified as hazardous in men; for example, hyperthermia experienced by firefighters has been linked to male infertility (Agnew et al., 1991).

Many pharmacological agents, including prescription, over-the-counter, and recreational drugs, have been found to affect the reproductive outcomes or sexual functioning of men (Zilbergeld, 1992). Examples include drugs from the following categories: antihypertensives, antipsychotics, antidepressants, hormones, sedatives, hypnotics, stimulants, chemotherapy agents used in cancer treatment, amphetamines, opiates, and alcohol, marijuana, cocaine, barbiturates, and lysergic acid diethylamide (LSD).

A focus on gay men's health has come about largely through the advent of the AIDS epidemic. For the role of the clinician in assessment, education, counseling, and providing support related to the reproductive health of the gay male client, see Swanson and Forrest (1984).

REPRODUCTIVE HEALTH AND RIGHT TO KNOW RESEARCH

Reproductive health hazard descriptions were analyzed on nearly 700 Material Safety Data Sheets (MSDAs), important sources of information regarding health risks caused by exposure to toxic chemicals (e.g., lead or ethylene glycol ether–containing products). The descriptions were submitted by businesses in central Massachusetts to the Department of Environmental Protection under the provisions of the Massachusetts Right-to-Know Law. More than 60% of the MSDAs failed to mention effects on the reproductive system, and among those that did, developmental risks rather than male reproductive effects were most often addressed. Those from larger firms (100 or more employees) were more likely to mention reproductive effects than those from smaller firms (Paul and Kurtz, 1994).

Prevention orientations (i.e., one's ability to take action to prevent disease or injury) may also vary between the sexes. Women's higher likelihood of seeking preventive examinations includes their need for routine reproductive health screening—the Papanicolaou test and breast examination. This examination includes some general screening, such as check of blood pressure and tests of urine and blood for chronic problems. Men do not have routine reproductive health checkups that include screening, which would also detect other health problems at an early stage. With the advent of managed care, those men who are eligible for coverage will have access to routine health screening. If, indeed, they respond to available health checkups, it is still unknown whether their reproductive health concerns will be addressed by primary care professionals.

MEN'S REPRODUCTIVE HEALTH SERVICES

Men's reproductive health services in family planning settings have existed but have been sorely underutilized by men (Swanson and Forrest, 1987). A national survey of 600 family planning clinics that were publicly funded with Title X money, conducted by The Urban Institute in 1993 (Schulte and Sonenstein, 1995), indicates that the trend continues. For example, of the 388 clinic managers who responded to the survey, only 13% reported that greater than 10% of their clients were men; many services were available for men, including provision of condoms and contraceptive counseling, yet few men used them. Other services available to men in some clinics · included testing, counseling, and treatment for STDs; HIV testing and counseling; vasectomy; infertility testing and counseling; and work and sports physicals.

Actual sex differences in preventive health behavior are variable and must be viewed with caution for two reasons: (1) little research has been carried out, and (2) the efficacy of many of the behaviors is still in question (Waldron, 1995a). In addition, existing research shows decreasing gender differences for some health behaviors and increasing gender differences for others.

In the 1990 National Health Interview Survey of Health Promotion and Disease Prevention, women were more likely than men to report wearing seatbelts, to have had blood pressure checks, to have had their blood cholesterol checked, and to seek help for an emotional or personal problem in the past year (Piani and Schoenborn, 1993). On the other hand, men tended to spend more time in leisure time activities than did women, including the playing of sports regularly. Men were, however, less likely to have exercised by walking in the past 2 weeks. Only a borderline difference was found regarding eating breakfast. Of note is that only 4.9% of men and 5.5% of women knew that exercise periods of 20 minutes per session three times per week are necessary to strengthen the heart and lungs.

OVERTRAINING AFFECTS MEN'S REPRODUCTIVE HEALTH STATUS

Overtraining physically, or strenuous exercise, has been recognized for its effect on the suppression of ovarian functioning in women. A study confirmed that overtraining in men affects their reproductive functioning also. Five endurance-trained men with normal spermatogenesis and hormone profiles engaged in overtraining, which doubled their average weekly mileage. After overtraining, basal testosterone levels decreased, basal cortisol levels increased, and sperm count decreased, the latter by 43%. Three months after overtraining, sperm count decreased by 52%, a

Box continued on following page

significant decrease; the normal length of spermatogenesis is 72 ± 2 days. Although semen changes were also evident, such as the presence of immature sperm, semen reductions were within the normal range. Three months after resumption of normal training, testosterone and cortisol profiles returned to normal (Roberts et al., 1993).

Other studies are also suggestive of sex differences in preventive health behavior. Women are more likely to make dental visits (NCHS, 1994). In addition, women are more likely to be trying to lose weight (Piani and Schoenborn, 1993). Women's consumption of fruit, vegetables, and vitamin pills is greater than men's, contributing fiber and antioxidants such as vitamin C, which are thought to contribute to lower ischemic heart disease risk in women (Waldron, 1995d).

Females' illness and prevention orientations, in particular, their likelihood of seeking routine medical and dental care, contribute to their higher morbidity rates. In addition, women are generally the caretakers of the health of the family; they observe signs of illness, learn about sources of health care, set health care appointments and escort family members, and give direct care to ill family members. Although most women have more flexible schedules, their flexibility in scheduling time to see a physician balances out with men's as a result of the little differences in the time it takes to carry out their respective role obligations; men may work more hours, but women generally have more family demands (Waldron, 1995a).

Reporting of Health Behavior

A number of differences in how health behavior is reported may affect sex differentials (Verbrugge and Wingard, 1987). Most health surveys are conducted face to face or via telephone by women interviewers. Women may be better respondents than men, more likely to remember their health problems and actions, and more likely to talk with someone about aspects of their illness and health. A woman may respond more openly to another woman; a man may be more inhibited. Women are usually called on in health surveys to report the health behavior of men; therefore, women are proxies, and proxies have a tendency to underreport behavior (Montiero, 1976). Under these conditions, women may recall and report more health problems than do men. Men may be less willing to talk, may not recall health problems, and may lack a health vocabulary.

Discussion

INTERPRETING THE DATA

Verbrugge and Wingard (1987) cautioned that all four factors (biology, socialization, illness and prevention orientations, and health-reporting behavior) must be taken into consideration when interpreting data. When only diagnostic data from examinations or laboratory tests are considered (a highly medical perspective), sex differentials are most likely the result of inherited and acquired risks. On the other hand, when data have the potential to be affected by social factors such as sex differences in illness and prevention orientations and health-reporting behavior, these factors should not be ignored. As the authors stated, "a sex differential in emphysema partly reflects risks men and women incur, but also whether they are aware of the condition or feel like reporting it" (Verbrugge and Wingard, 1987, p. 134). Health interview data such as those from the National Health Interview Survey and the National Survey of Health Promotion and Disease Prevention are the most common types available concerning a population's health; Verbrugge and Wingard (1987) cautioned that the social factors of sex differences in illness and prevention orientations and health-reporting behavior are, therefore, critical in interpreting health interview data.

Many issues are raised for community health nurses, who usually are women and usually interact with women clients. Because the data obtained and interpreted by community health nurses may be influenced by one or more of these factors, the following questions must be considered.

- What are the differences in reporting of health histories between male and female clients?
- How do data obtained by male nurses differ from those obtained by female nurses?
- What are the differences in data from health histories given by female "proxies" of absent members of the household or group and those given by the individual?
- What is the caretaking role of women in the family, and how can they be supported in the caretaking role?
- How do these questions apply to men in the caretaking role (e.g., parent, partner, or other caretaker of a person with chronic disease)?

In response to the question of why "females are sicker, but males die sooner," Verbrugge and Wingard

(1987) provided several reasons. First, conditions that affect morbidity (e.g., arthritis and gout) do not significantly impact mortality, and conditions that affect mortality (e.g., heart disease) may not erupt as troublesome on a day-to-day basis. Second, there is a difference in how the sexes respond to their health problems. Although mortality is in large part the outcome of inherited or acquired risks, sex differences in illness and prevention orientations and the reporting of health behaviors suggest that social and psychological factors affect morbidity. Although males have higher prevalence and death rates for "killer" chronic diseases as well as for injuries and accident mortalities, females have higher prevalence rates for a greater number of nonfatal chronic conditions. In addition, adult women report higher rates of morbidity from acute conditions than do adult men. The authors stated that "females' greater willingness and ability to take care of themselves when ill, to seek preventive help, and to talk about health all boost their morbidity rate" (Verbrugge and Wingard, 1987, p. 136).

SEX-LINKED BEHAVIOR

The largest sex differences in mortalities occur for causes of death associated with sex-linked behavior and suggest that sex-linked behavior, which is more prevalent and encouraged in men in our society, correlates with the following major categories of death (Harrison (1984):

- Smoking: lung cancer, bronchitis, emphysema, asthma
- Alcohol consumption: cirrhosis, accidents, homicide
- Poor preventive health habits and stress: heart disease
- Lack of other emotional channels: cirrhosis, suicide, homicide, accidents

Smoking, alcohol consumption, preventive health habits, and use of emotional channels are lifestyle factors that may be compounded by social and environmental conditions. These conditions include major public health concerns, both physical and psychological, such as occupational hazards (e.g., carcinogens, stress), unemployment, and massive advertising campaigns that use sex and sex roles to sell alcohol and tobacco. These lifestyle factors are compounded by men's lack of willingness to seek preventive care such as screening and to seek health care when a symptom arises. These concerns call for a major public health approach to men's health.

IMAGES OF MEN AND THE NEED FOR MARKETING

For years, women have been writing about the harmful, sex-role–stereotyped images of women as passive, unintelligent, dependent sex objects in print as well as in audio and visual media (Bird, 1970; Steinem, 1983). Less has been written about the damaging sex-role–stereotyped images in the media's portrayal of men as aggressive, independent, and powerful, yet aloof (Allen and Whatley, 1986). Community health nurses are in a position to overcome the traditional medical and scientific approach to men's health as the presentation of "facts" only by marketing gender-appropriate health information directly to men. Recognizing the difference between the damaging sex-role–stereotyped images of men and the use of male culture as a way of communicating with men is important in marketing health concepts to men. For example, an early self-care book for men, *Man's Body: An Owner's Manual* (Diagram Group, 1976) uses language with which men can identify in their culture ("an owner's manual"). Another example of using this concept in marketing health information to men is an advertisement for seminars on fatherhood, "Come to Our Fatherhood Seminar . . . Because Babies Don't Come With an Owner's Manual."

Another example of marketing to men occurred within an HMO in Portland, Oregon (Ann Plunkett, Health Educator, Kaiser Permanente, personal communication, October 1995). When traditional advertising of a series of 12 weeks of weight reduction classes, "Freedom From Fat" targeting men, in the HMO's health education catalog failed to bring a response, an article about the class was placed in the business section of the daily newspaper. The response was immediate, and three classes of men signed up to take the series of classes, which were open to both members and nonmembers and required a fee. Many men may not read health education catalogs; more men may read the business section of the newspaper. It is important to use a knowledge of men's culture in efforts to market programs and services to men.

UNEMPLOYMENT AND MEN'S HEALTH

Although unemployment is not viewed as a major cause of mortality or morbidity, it has long been recognized as a health risk (Hibbard and Pope, 1987; Lewis, 1988). Consequences of unemployment include a loss of personal and social identity, a life crisis and major change, loss of income or poverty, and higher rates of illness (e.g., cardiovascular disease, hypertension, myocardial infarction, cerebrovascular accidents, cirrhosis, and psychosis). Other increases noted are smoking, drinking, depression, aggression, and child abuse. For example, a study of employed persons free of major depression reported that, on follow-up interview, those who had become unemployed had more than twice the risk of increased depressive symptoms and clinical depression than those persons who did not become unemployed (Dooley et al., 1994). These authors reported additional findings of initial and follow-up interviews with persons who were initially employed and not violent. Those who were unemployed at reinterview had nearly six times the risk of violent behavior compared with those persons who remained employed (Catalano et al., 1993). Another study reported that the incidence of clinically significant alcohol abuse is greater among persons who have lost their jobs than among persons who have not (Catalano et al., 1993). The current economic situation in a country may have marked implications for men's health. A U.S. study that investigated the relationship between states' public welfare spending and suicide rates from 1960 through 1990 reported that in 1990 states that spent less for public welfare had higher suicide rates (Zimmerman, 1995). The consequences of unemployment are felt not only at the individual level but also by the family and the community. Community health nurses may experience the deprivation associated with a community that experiences high rates of unemployment.

To counter these types of factors, research is needed to determine alternative methods of education and practice aimed at health promotion, illness prevention, and political processes to create safer environments to enhance the well-being of both males and females.

FACTORS THAT IMPEDE MEN'S HEALTH

Many factors have been viewed as barriers to men's health. Men's higher rates of mortality, greater risk taking, less use of the health care system, gaps in preventive health behavior, and differences in illness and health orientations and reporting of health behavior all contribute to a diminished health status for men. A number of other barriers have been proposed, including the patterns of medical care provided in the United States, access to care, and lack of health promotion.

Medical Care Patterns

As DeHoff and Forrest (1984) stated over a decade ago, "the usual pattern of medical care in this country—'the system'—has contributed indirectly to men's health problems" (p. 5). During his lifetime, a man is likely to come into contact, first, with a pediatrician; then, with a school nurse; next, with a college, military, or company physician; and, last, with a family practitioner, internist, or geriatrician by the time he develops chronic disease later in life. Many health professionals provide care for men with complex health needs in a wide variety of settings, yet these authors pointed out that men have had no specialist to whom they could go for care that "feels right" for them. As medical care became increasingly specialized, there has been a noticeable effort to reestablish general health care, particularly with the shift to managed care in the United States. This has been attempted by creating yet another specialty—family practice—and by reincorporating the discrete specialties of internal medicine, pediatrics, obstetrics/gynecology, and geriatrics into "primary care specialties." Men were overlooked as new medical specialties were developed. Urologists, who may see men for genital abnormalities or diseases of the prostate, are not primary care physicians, and they also see women. The medical specialty andrology, which originated in Europe to treat problems of fertility and sterility, is considered too narrow in focus to treat "the whole man." Without a primary care specialty that focuses specifically on men's needs, many needs, such as sexual and reproductive problems and sex-role influences on health and lifestyle, may not be attended to by anyone. In addition, these specialists and generalists have most likely not received training that would enable them to focus on men's health needs specifically as occurs in women's health as a specialty area of practice. In the current era of managed care, men will still be left without a primary care provider with training to focus specifically on their needs.

Access to Care

Mission Orientation. Public interest in men's health has in large part focused on efforts necessary to maintain an effective work force (DeHoff and Forrest, 1984). Mission-oriented health care is a priority for large industries and organized sports. More general health care, however, may be provided through insurance programs such as that provided by health maintenance organizations (HMOs). Perhaps the most complete care is currently offered by the military. However, even in the military, marked deficiencies exist in the lack of a focus on prevention and health promotion at the individual and aggregate levels as well as inattention to policy regarding, for example, environmental hazards.

Financial Considerations. Another barrier to health care for men is financial ability. A man may receive an annual physical examination if he belongs to an HMO or is an executive or an airline pilot, but many private insurance companies will reimburse more fully for a diagnosed condition (e.g., for pathology) and less fully for preventive care. A man is more likely to be insured for acute or chronic illness conditions than for health education, counseling, or other types of preventive health care. Unlike women, who have had annual gynecological examinations that include screening for other conditions and allow a woman to express other physical or psychological needs, men have lacked entrée to the health care system for a physical examination on a routine basis. Now, under managed care, it will be of interest to note whether gender differences in routine physical examinations for preventive reasons continue as they have in the past. Socialization, however, is a marked influence on behavior, and current trends may prevail in spite of current trends in health care delivery.

Time Factors. That men may not have access to the health care system as readily as women because of men's greater participation in the work force, time periods that usually correspond to when clinicians are available, is no longer true (Waldron, 1995b). Dif-

ferences in role obligations balance out because of family demands on women, even though more men are employed. Men may still be reluctant to take time from work for a medical visit, fearing loss of income or the stigmatization of being "weak," "ill," or "less of a man."

Lack of Health Promotion

A concept of health that considers health as merely the absence of disease is limiting. Traditional measures of mortality and morbidity, although reflective of the state of "health" of a population, fall short of desired health outcomes and tend to divorce the biological from the psychosocial (Choi, 1985). For example, the absence of overt pathology, even in the presence of behavioral risk factors such as smoking, alcohol consumption, obesity, and a sedentary lifestyle, is enough to give one a "clean bill of health." Physical recovery after impairment, illness, or injury is considered satisfactory. Although touted as the means to cost containment in managed care, prevention and health promotion are not always within the scope of the current system.

PRECURSORS OF MORTALITIES

Which precursors of today's mortalities are frequently not addressed by the present health care system?

Heart disease and stroke

- Hypercholesterolemia
- Hypertension
- Diabetes mellitus
- Obesity
- Type A personality
- Family history
- Lack of exercise
- Cigarette smoking

Cancer

- Sunlight
- Radiation
- Occupational hazards
- Water pollution
- Air pollution
- Dietary patterns
- Cigarette smoking
- Alcohol
- Heredity
- Certain medical conditions

The disease focus of the present health care system persists and is limited in addressing the precursors of today's mortalities. Many disciplines are needed to prevent today's health problems. Nursing's contribution to practice and research is instrumental in this process.

In a review, McKinlay and colleagues (1989) cited evidence supporting the lack of impact of medical measures on mortality and morbidity in the United States. Coronary heart disease, cancer, and stroke are three conditions that account for two thirds of all mortality and the greatest use of resources. However, these authors contended that medical measures have not made a substantial impact on mortality. An increase in life expectancy has occurred but usually has resulted in an increase in years of disability.

COMMUNITY HEALTH NURSING SERVICES FOR MEN

A male can be seen by a community health nurse in a well-baby clinic, by a school nurse, by an occupational health nurse, and finally by a community health nurse or home health nurse on a home visit for follow-up of a chronic disease. However, men are less likely to be seen by a community health nurse than are women. Not only is a major focus of many health departments maternal and child health, but also neither a medical nor a nursing specialty within a health department routinely exists to specifically address men's health. Preventive reproductive health care (family planning, prenatal care, and cancer screening) and associated general screening are not routinely available for men. The hours of services offered by health departments do not usually provide ready access for men. The community health nurse's commitment to health for all requires an increased awareness of men's health issues in their social and cultural context and individual and group action that will improve men's physical, psychological, and social well-being.

Mortality rates for coronary heart disease, the top killer, declined approximately 40% between 1968 and 1987 (McKinlay et al., 1989). The causes of the decline are not clear and have been associated with changes in risk behaviors. McKinlay and colleagues (1989) cited evidence that the effects of pharmaco-logical intervention, emergency response in the community, coronary care units, and coronary bypass surgery have been negligible with the exception of some benefits from beta-blocking agents in postmyo-cardial infarction patients (Goldman and Cook, 1984).

Age-adjusted mortality rates for all types of cancer, the second top killer, increased slowly between 1950 and 1982 (McKinlay et al., 1989). Despite known environmental and personal risk factors for major cancers, funds and other resources have been allotted disproportionately into treatment and cure rather than into public health measures and primary prevention.

Mortality rates for stroke have been declining since the turn of the century (McKinlay et al., 1989). Although the declines occurred well before antihypertensive therapy was available, McKinlay and associates (1989) cited evidence for the contribution of medical treatment to only about 12 to 25% of the decline since 1970.

SOCIAL DEMOGRAPHY AND SOCIAL EPIDEMIOLOGY

Epidemiology is the method of research used to determine the nature and distribution of a health problem in a community (see Chapter 5). *Social demographers* and *social epidemiologists* study social and psychological factors that affect the distribution of health problems in a community. Factors associated with the occurrence of the problems can be identified, and resources can be focused on prevention. Social epidemiologists have identified men as a population at risk for premature death. What concentrated efforts can be made to improve men's health?

Financial resources have been invested in traditional curative care rather than in public health action. An inordinate amount of funds is poured into the health care system each year, with only a minimum allotted to public health approaches (see Chapter 3). For example, in 1992, total health expenditures accounted for 13.6% of the gross domestic product, an increase from 5.9% in 1965 (NCHS, 1995). Of every $1.00 spent on health care in 1993, approximately $0.46 went to hospital care and physician services, which are in large part curative in focus, and less than $0.03 went to preventive government public health activities.

In view of the facts that finite resources have been allocated to traditional curative care rather than to public health and that the present health care system is limited in addressing the precursors of today's mortalities, the following question may be asked: Is medical care, or even another medical specialty, the answer to men's health needs when social, occupational, environmental, and "lifestyle" factors place men at risk?

Prevention and health promotion, when available, often are not applied at the aggregate and population levels. Milio (1983) asserted that healthy lifestyles are not a matter of free choice but rather result from opportunities that are not always equally available to people. As health policies shape opportunities for both individuals and aggregates, environmental and occupational changes beyond the control of the individual are among those needed to improve the health of the population. Community health nurses can be involved in political activities that develop health policies that will make a difference in men's health as well as in the health of the population. Such activities are congruent with the philosophy of public health as "health for all" (see Chapter 29) and a commitment to a social justice ethic of health care rather than a market justice ethic of health care. Examining men's health affords the community health nurse the opportunity to observe the impact of the market justice ethic of health care not only on the health of men in the United States but ultimately, because of men's traditional roles in the family, also on the health of women, family, and community. The community health nurse can play a vital role in contributing to a social justice ethic of health care, particularly in relation to promoting men's health. What is needed is "upstream thinking," (see Chapter 4), with a focus on health promotion and prevention at the aggregate and population levels rather than "downstream thinking" with a focus on treatment and cure.

FACTORS THAT PROMOTE MEN'S HEALTH

Factors that promote men's health can be found in the community, including interest groups in men and men's health, men's increasing interest in physical fitness and lifestyle, policy related to men's health, and health services for men.

GAINING SKILLS NECESSARY TO ADDRESS MEN'S HEALTH NEEDS

Assessment skills necessary to carry out screening activities with men to detect reproductive health needs may be lacking in nursing education. One community health nurse who worked in a rural health department felt unable to respond to male partners' requests for genital examinations when couples came to seek family planning services. The community health nurse requested to work for specified periods of time with a urologist and in a STD clinic in a large urban area to gain the necessary skills. On return to the rural health department, she felt comfortable with male patients and taught the skills she had learned to nurse colleagues.

Interest Groups in Men and Men's Health

Unlike the consumer movement that occurred on behalf of women's health in the 1960s and early 1970s, there is no consumer movement advocating men's health (Allen and Whatley, 1986). However, a viable men's consumer movement is increasingly being heard. The National Organization for Changing Men is interested in redefining the male role, particularly those aspects of the male role that are confining to the health and growth of men in our society. The American Assembly for Men in Nursing sponsors annual meetings that address issues such as men's health, men's work environments, research on men's health, and networking and support among men who are nurses. During the past two decades, nursing has responded to consumer issues raised by feminists advocating a health care system sensitized to women's health care needs. Researchers are now pushing to define women's health beyond that limited to women's reproductive role (e.g., occupational risks). Researchers are also beginning to define and study men's health beyond that limited to men's occupational role (e.g., reproductive health) (Flaming and Morse, 1991; Smith and Babaian, 1992; Swanson, 1995).

Men's Increasing Interest in Physical Fitness and Lifestyle

Although cardiovascular diseases are a major health hazard for men, research on the validity and usefulness of preventive and treatment modalities is an issue of considerable debate (Waldron, 1995d). Men's interest in altering behavior that places them at risk of cardiovascular and other major diseases is increasing. For example, men's smoking behavior has changed dramatically. Between 1965 and 1993, the age-adjusted percentage of men who smoked decreased from 51% to 27% (NCHS, 1995). As stated previously, more men report being physically active in leisure time sports in the past 2 weeks than do women (36.6% vs. 22.6%) and more men report exercising or playing sports regularly than women (44% vs. 37.7%) (Piani and Schoenborn, 1993).

It is of interest, however, that those health behaviors that have reported the greatest change in a positive direction have been those most influenced by legislative action (e.g., example, seatbelt use, use of smoke detectors, and drunk driving) (Piani and Schoenborn, 1993).

Policy Related to Men's Health

Nurses are working to set policy related to men's health, particularly in the area of family planning. The Task Force on Male Involvement in Family Planning and Reproductive Health of the American Public Health Association (APHA), in which nurses are active members, was instrumental in passing resolutions that called for greater access to family planning for men (1981) and that called for counting and reporting the number of men who seek care from federally funded family planning services (1987) (APHA, 1988). A resolution on men's health submitted to the Governing Council of the APHA by the Medical Care Section in 1985, however, failed to pass.

Health Services for Men

Although Allen and Whatley (1986) argued that medicine "has largely focused on the problems of men" (p. 7), there is a lack of health care clinics tailored to the special needs of men, as have evolved to meet the special needs of women. The "well-man clinic" model has been developed by male public health nurses in Scotland, called "health visitors," to expand the role of the health visitor and the National Health Service in screening and health education of the marginal- and low-income man (Sadler, 1979). For a description of the well-man clinic and its expansion (Brown and Lunt, 1992; Fareed, 1994; Woodland and Hunt, 1994), see "New Concepts of Community Care" p. 286. Gender-specific care may fade in the era

of managed care, as both men and women receive primary care from the same health services. Some health services that have contracts to offer primary care to both men and women have traditionally given care to only one gender, which could be problematic. For example, some Planned Parenthood clinics have expanded their repertoire of services to include primary care for both men and women. Selected Planned Parenthood clinics are providing primary care, under managed care, to men. Whether all men delegated to receive primary care from a Planned Parenthood clinic, which has traditionally served women, will readily attend a "woman's clinic" or not will be of interest to this group of providers of care.

In some instances, Planned Parenthood clinics have used strategies such as combining with a community-based clinic and changing the name of the clinic to reflect the merger. An example is the merger of the Planned Parenthood clinic in Santa Cruz, California, with the Santa Cruz Westside Community Health Clinic, which has changed its name to Westside Health Center, now offering primary care to both men and women (D. Seamster, Clinic Manager, personal communication, October 1995).

MEN'S HEALTH CARE NEEDS

DeHoff and Forrest (1984) delineated men's health care needs that draw from both the biological and the psychosocial causes of men's distinctive health situation. According to these authors, men need the following:

- Permission to have concerns about health and to talk openly to others about them
- Support for the consideration of sex-role and lifestyle influences on their physical and mental health
- Attention from professionals regarding factors that may cause illness or impact a man's expression of illness, including occupational factors, leisure patterns, and interpersonal relationships
- Information about how their bodies function, what is normal, what is abnormal, what action to take, and the contributions of proper nutrition and exercise
- Self-care instruction, including testicular and genital self-examination
- Physical examination and history taking that include sexual and reproductive health and illness across the life span

- Treatment for problems of couples, including interpersonal problems, infertility, family planning, sexual concerns, and sexually transmitted diseases
- Help with fathering (i.e., being included as a parent in the care of children)
- Help with fathering as a single parent, in particular, with a child of the opposite sex, in addressing the child's sexual development and concerns
- Recognition that feelings of confusion and uncertainty in a time of rapid social change are normal and may mark the onset of healthy adaptation to change
- Adjustment of the health care system to men's occupational constraints regarding time and location of source of health care
- Financial ways to obtain these goals

Additional health care needs of men are for primary prevention as well as for secondary and tertiary prevention at the individual, family, and community levels, to address the precursors of mortality that impact males so greatly. Because men are less likely than women to be seen as consumers in the health care system, alternative approaches must be developed that address their health needs. The most significant approaches in the future will be those that reach men in the community, in schools, in the work place, and in public settings. This calls for political processes that set policy, for health marketing techniques, and for advocacy.

MEETING MEN'S HEALTH NEEDS

Meeting the health needs of men requires approaches that extend beyond the traditional health care services and include new concepts of community care. Interdisciplinary efforts are needed to address the many factors that impact the health of men. Major legislation and health and social services that meet the needs of men and women are complex and have been covered extensively in Chapter 3.

Traditional Health Services

Traditional health services for males are available in both government and private arenas. Services have been diagnostic and treatment oriented rather than preventive, although that may be changing with the shift to managed care. Government health services also stem from legislation, such as that reviewed in

DOOR OPENERS: WAYS TO ADDRESS MEN ABOUT HEALTH CONCERNS

Strategies to address men about health concerns include the following:

- Ask a man to talk about the last time he had a physical examination, what was done, why it was done, where, and what were the recommendations.
- Ask a man how he feels about his health insurance coverage, and if he lacks health insurance, ask about the resources that have been used for medical care for him and his family.
- Ask a man about how he spends his leisure time, what he is doing to take care of himself, and what his usual physical activities are.
- Observe a man for signs of stress such as moist palms, nail biting, posture, and nervous movements. If signs of stress are present, ask about how he is coping with an identified health problem, family problem, being unemployed, and so on.
- Observe a man for difficulty clearing airway (smoking) and flushing of the face (alcohol). Inquire as to habits of smoking and drinking and whether these habits have increased since the occurrence of the particular health or social problem.
- Involve men in decision making about health care to instill a sense of control over events.

Chapter 3. Government health insurance programs include Medicare and workers' compensation. Government health assistance programs include Medicaid and maternal-child health services. Payment for health services may also be out of pocket or through private insurance such as Blue Cross, Blue Shield, and HMOs. Health service programs that benefit men in particular are also sponsored by the government for specific population groups such as for veterans, military personnel, merchant marines, and federal employees. All of these programs are being restructured in some way according to congressional mandates (see Chapter 3).

Local and state health departments have also provided services that benefit men as well as women and children, although major changes are taking place as the restructuring of public health occurs across the country (see Chapter 3). State departments of health provide policy and leadership and disburse state and federal funds for programs carried out by local health departments. These programs include the gathering of vital statistics, laboratory services, environmental and occupational health, and control of communicable disease, including sexually transmitted disease (STD). Personal health services are usually operationalized through maternal-child health programs and programs for the disabled and elderly, although individual programs vary somewhat. The public health function and personal health services provided by health departments are changing in many locations across the nation with the shift to managed care.

New Concepts of Community Care

Specific services for men within health departments have been usually lacking in the United States, with the exception of STD clinics and selected family planning service models. An innovative public health nursing program directed at men was started in Glasgow, Scotland, by two male health visitors (British term for public health nurses) from the National Health Service (NHS) (Sadler, 1979). Health visitors Bill Deans and Bob Hoskins set up a nurse-run Well-Man Clinic with the help of the NHS and the Scottish Council for Health Education. On home visits to a caseload of mothers and infants, Deans and Hoskins observed that fathers excused themselves and left for the local pub when they arrived. Noting characteristics of the male population of their community such as overweight, heavy smoking, drinking, and high unemployment, they decided to modify their practice to the needs of their clients. One afternoon per week, the clinic, which is based on a nursing model rather than on a medical model, offers health screening, health education, and primary prevention to men. Marketing is important, and men are referred from general practitioners' and specialists' practices and recruited through newspaper advertisements. Clients with clinical signs and symptoms are referred back to their physicians. Lifestyle counseling and education are offered in areas such as fat and fiber content in diet, smoking, alcohol use, and exercise.

Deans and Hoskins consider the clinic as a way of extending the health visitor's role as well as extending the NHS's efforts in health education with an aim to "nip potential diseases in the bud" (Sadler, 1979, p. 18). Deans and Hoskins are concerned that the NHS does not provide male services and are quite clear that "the unemployed chain-smoking husband needs as much care and health education from the health visitor as do his wife and baby" (Sadler, 1979, p. 18). Today, the Well-Man Clinic as well as the Well-Woman Clinic models can be found in a number of communities throughout Great Britain and have been expanded to serve inmates in prison (Fareed, 1994; Woodland and Hunt, 1994). For a description of the establishment and evaluation of a Well-Man Clinic and discussion of its ability to meet the health needs of men, see Brown and Lunt (1992).

Public health nurses working in the Benton County Health Department in Corvallis, Oregon, responded to the challenge of teen pregnancy in the 1970s by launching a communitywide effort that included developing a men's health clinic and marketing reproductive health services directly to teenage boys and men (Fig. 12–1). An early effort was establishing an advisory committee that included persons from churches, schools, and health care facilities. An extensive education program was launched in the high school by a public health nurse health educator and focused on decision-making processes and services available in the community. Later efforts involved establishing the clinic for men. Teenage boys were members of a consumer advisory committee established by the nurses that recommended the wording and format for advertisements about the clinic that were run in the high school newspaper. The advisory committee also recommended a format for flyers that would be attractive to males. Specifically, they requested a card with information about how to use condoms and about the clinic that would be small enough to discretely fit into their wallets and yet be available to share with peers (Fig. 12–2).

Today, the nurses have expanded their focus to create inclusive service environments in which teenage girls and boys and adult men and women will feel accepted and comfortable. Particular attention is given to the clinic decor and advertising, reading materials, and posters, so that a message that includes offering health care for males as well as females is transmitted. Clinic staff will see males or females at any time, however; a room in which staff see men has decor geared toward men (i.e., no gynecological stirrups on the examining table), pamphlets available for men on topics such as testicular cancer, chewing tobacco, and so on. Integrated services exist in the areas of family planning, STDs, and HIV counseling and testing (Susan Hines, Program Manager, personal communication, July 1995).

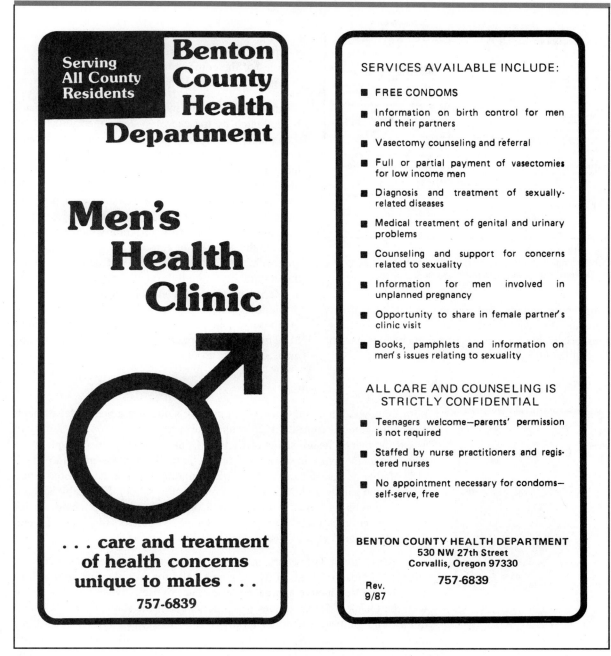

Figure 12–1
Men's Health Clinic brochure, Benton County Health Department, Corvallis, Oregon. Reprinted with permission.

APPLICATION OF THE NURSING PROCESS

Community health nurses are in an ideal position to address the health needs of men at the individual, family, and community levels. The community health nurse may promote self-care in male members of the family, facilitate men's health by addressing changes needed at the family level such as diet, buttress women's roles as caretakers of the family's health, and

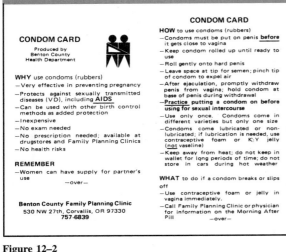

Figure 12–2
Condom card, Benton County Health Department, Corvallis, Oregon. Reprinted with permission.

bring about change that impacts policy that affects men at the community level. Planning gender-appropriate care for males is presented by examples of the following:

- Application of the nursing process at the individual, family, and aggregate levels initiated via a home visit
- Application of the levels of prevention
- Roles of the community health nurse
- Research and men's health

Application of the nursing process to aggregates is facilitated by the use of systems theory, in which the nurse identifies the system and subsystems involved. The nurse may use a deductive or an inductive approach. A deductive approach would involve, first, carrying out a community assessment and identifying an area or areas such as a program needed by the community. Planning, implementation, and evaluation of the program would be carried out at the family or group level. An inductive approach, on the other hand, would involve entering the community system through a person or client via a referral about a problem or concern. Assessment of the individual would be followed by identification of those groups such as family and community to which the client belongs as well as assessment of those groups.

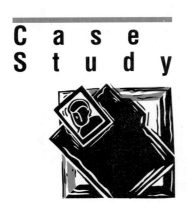

Case Study

Beth Lockwood, a community health nursing student at a health department, received a referral from the high school nurse to visit the Connors family to assess the mental health status of Richard Connors, a 16-year-old sophomore whose academic work in school had declined rapidly after the premature death of his father at age 46 from a myocardial infarction, which he suffered while cleaning the garage with Richard one evening after school. Efforts by Richard and the neighbors failed to revive Mr. Connors, for which Richard carries feelings of guilt. Household members include Mrs. Connors (44 years old) and Richard's sister, Yvonne, who is 12.

Assessment The referral that Beth received to assess the Connors family after the premature death of Mr. Connors calls for an inductive approach to assessment. A deductive approach is used later by Beth, when her experience with the Connors family piques her concern about the status of men's health in the community in which her family resides. Beth must assess Richard, his mother, and his sister as household members of the family. She must not stop with the immediate family, however, but continue to identify the other groups within the community to which each individual family member belongs. Viewing the community as a system and focusing on systems and subsystems will help Beth organize the data she collects during assessment. Knowing that "the whole is greater than the sum of its parts," Beth prepares for her visit by reviewing adolescent theories of development and family theory. Beyond individual assessment, she notes factors related to the development of sex-role–related behavior that may impact on health. Examples of areas of assessment include the following:

- Family configuration, traditional or nontraditional
- Sex-role–related behavior of parents, including work patterns in and out of home, division of household labor, and decision-making patterns
- Patterns of parenting: mothering, fathering, and substitute father figure(s)
- Ability of male children to disclose feelings to family members and others
- Degree of assertiveness in female children
- Ability of family members to give emotional and physical support during crises and noncrises
- Ability of family members to trade off role-related behavior during crises and noncrises
- Risk-taking health behaviors
- Processing of stress and grief
- Communal lifestyle patterns that place individual or family at risk (e.g., lack of exercise, poor diet, smoking, drinking)
- Family history of morbidity and mortality
- Health care–taking patterns of family members
- Preventive health behaviors
- Leisure time activities

Assessment of other groups includes neighborhood and other peer groups, school environment, sports, and church and civic activities.

Diagnosis

Through induction, a nursing diagnosis is made for each individual and each system component, including family and the community. Examples of diagnoses follow.

Individual

- Loss of interest or involvement in activity related to conflicting stages of grief process secondary to premature death of father (Richard)
- Expressed dissatisfaction with parenting role related to feelings of helplessness and hopelessness secondary to premature death of husband (Mrs. Connors)
- Risk of interpersonal conflict resulting from prolonged, unrelieved family stress secondary to premature death of father (Yvonne)

Family

- Decreased ability to communicate related to family stress secondary to premature death of father
- At risk of family crisis related to disequilibrium

Community

- Inadequate systematic programs for linking families in crisis to community resources
- Inadequate systematic programs for populations at risk of premature death related to inadequate planning among community systems

Planning

Planning involves contracting and mutual goal setting and is an outcome of mutually derived assessment and diagnosis. A contract with the family alone is shortsighted and may provide little community benefit over time. Examples of other aggregates with whom a contract may be established include the following:

- The school subsystem that does not provide ongoing counseling but will meet periodically to evaluate pupil progression with family members
- The school subsystem that provides physical education in football, basketball, and baseball (nonaerobic, nonlifetime sports) but offers extramural aerobic, lifetime sports such as swimming and track after school hours
- The American Red Cross, which does not offer cardiovascular pulmonary resuscitation (CPR) courses on evenings or weekends but offers to consider doing so for a defined minimum-size community

Mutual goal setting requires collaboration regarding long- and short-term goals. Again, mutually defined needs and diagnoses are important to this process. Regardless of the diagnosis, each individual in the family and the subsystem must participate in developing a plan of care. Examples of goals follow.

Individual

Long-Term Goal
- Individual family members will be able to trade off role-related behavior.

Short-Term Goal
- Individual family members will express feelings related to abandonment and loss.

Family

Long-Term Goal
- The family will exhibit increased ability to handle crisis as evidenced by ability to discuss roles and interdependencies.

Short-Term Goal
- The family will identify specific ways to recognize and use support services.

Community

Long-Term Goal
- Systematic programs will be established for populations at risk of premature death from coronary heart disease as evidenced by local planning bodies with ongoing evaluation of programs.

Short-Term Goals
- Dissemination is provided to individuals, families, groups, and planning bodies in the community about the incidence of coronary heart disease.
- Existing programs are identified that address coronary heart disease.
- Existing programs are coordinated to bridge gaps and avoid duplication of effort.

Intervention

The nurse, family, and other aggregates each carry out interventions contracted during the planning phase to meet the mutually derived goals. Most importantly, the nurse empowers the family and community to develop the networks and linkages necessary to care for themselves.

Individual   Individual counseling regarding loss and grief may be beneficial to each family member, but options may need to be explored, and referrals may need to be reevaluated for members of the rural family. Education regarding preventive measures to combat risk factors for heart disease include those aimed at individual family members and address such areas as diet, exercise, smoking, alcohol use, and ways of handling stress.

Family   Examples of interventions with the family include counseling, education, and referral aimed at promoting family self-care. For example, Beth's interventions with the Connors family are dependent on the family's ability to solve problems, to investigate community resources, and to create linkages between family and resources. Periodic family conferences at school and more inclusive family therapy may be initiated to enable the family to work through the death of Mr. Connors; this results in the development of new roles and the communication necessary to maintain family equilibrium. Education regarding preventive measures to combat risk factors for heart disease may need discussion at the family level as well as at the individual level (e.g., diet, exercise, smoking, alcohol use, and stress management).

Community   Interventions must also be carried out with other aggregates. These may involve activities such as educating, facilitating program expansion, or tailoring programs to meet community needs. Intervention at the aggregate level calls for group and community work. The nurse carries out interventions at this level in several ways (e.g., by communicating community statistics from a community analysis, relating anecdotes from families served, or linking family experience to program need by acting as an advocate and by bringing family members to board meetings or hearings on community health issues).

Education regarding preventive measures to combat risk factors for heart disease also includes those interventions aimed at the community. A rationale for the development of lifetime aerobic sports is needed not only by Richard but also by school districts. Exploring options with the school nurse and reviewing the school district health education curriculum would be beneficial. A community assessment of heart disease awareness, including determination of the availability of resources such as emergency response and CPR courses, is an aggregate intervention. Taking the outcome of the assessment in the form of statistics and the anonymous anecdotal story of the Connors family to planning bodies in the community also is intervention at the aggregate level. Creative programs used by other communities (e.g., teaching CPR within the school system) should be investigated and proposed.

Evaluation

Evaluation is multidimensional and ongoing. Using a systems approach to evaluation, the nurse evaluates each component of the system, from individual family member to family and community, in terms of goal achievement. Evaluation includes noting degrees of equilibrium established, degree of change, how the system handles change, whether the system is open or closed, and patterns of networking. Ongoing evaluation includes noting referrals and follow-up of the individual, the family, and other aggregates in use of resources.

Individual For example, use of resources such as support groups by the individual family member may be noted. These resources may include a support group for teens, a women's support group, support groups for those experiencing the loss of a spouse or other family member, reentry programs for women at a local junior college or university, and parents without partners.

Family Evaluation of the Connors family would also include follow-up of their use of support services specifically for the family, such as counseling options for the family as a unit. Evaluation would also focus on the family's ability to handle crises in the future.

Community Aggregate evaluation would focus on the community. For example, to what extent do school programs encourage sports options that promote lifetime aerobic activities and prevent premature death from heart disease? Are programs systematically planned in the community for populations that are at risk of premature death from heart disease?

Levels of Prevention

Society's expectations of men and women are in transition. Application of levels of prevention by the community health nurse must take into account men's health status, socialization of men, men's use of health care services, men's primary needs for prevention and health promotion, and the role of women as caretakers of the family's health.

Primary Because men are more likely to engage in risk-taking behavior than women and are less likely to engage in preventive behaviors, primary prevention must be marketed specifically to men. Examples of primary prevention for the Connors family are applied at the individual, family, and community levels:

Individual. Assessment, teaching, and referral related to diet and exercise behaviors

Family. Assessment and teaching related to food selection and preparation at home and fast-food restaurant food selection; teaching and role-modeling gender roles that allow male members of the family to use alternative expressions of emotion

Community. Provision of CPR courses for members of the community; consultation with schools regarding need for aerobic activities in physical education and sports programs

It is important to pull men from the family, work place, or other aggregates into involvement with family planning, education, antepartum and postpartum care, parenting, dental prophylaxis, and accident prevention. In addition, assessing need for immunizations and classes (e.g., retirement preparation) is considered action aimed at primary prevention.

Secondary Because men have higher mortality, morbidity, and health care use rates for many of the leading causes of death but are second to women in overall use of health care services, including preventive physical examinations and screening, early diagnosis and prompt intervention must also be tailored to meet men's needs. Examples of secondary prevention regarding the Connors family include the following:

Individual. Screening for risk factors related to cardiovascular disease in the individual such as how the individual handles stress

Family. Screening for risk factors related to cardiovascular disease in the family such as how stress is processed by the family

Community. Organizing screening programs for the community such as health fairs

It is important to screen individuals and aggregates of men according to lifestyle risk factors, mortality at different age levels, morbidity, and occupational health risks.

Tertiary Activities that rehabilitate individuals and aggregates and restore them to their highest level of functioning are aimed at tertiary prevention. The nurse in the community is ideally situated to locate people in need of rehabilitation services. Evaluation and physical, mental, and social restoration services may be provided. Men in need of rehabilitation may have special needs because their disability impacts not only themselves but also their families and, ultimately, their communities. Financial assistance and vocational counseling, training, and placement may be priorities for the well-being of the family. Because of socialization, men may find it hard to admit they need help. Community health nurses who teach men with chronic disease to rest at specified periods during the day or to continue with medical regimens or speech or occupational therapy are providing tertiary prevention. Working with couples as a unit is also important because caretaking patterns may shift owing to chronic disease and disability. Encouraging men to express their concerns about their health, their families, and their jobs as well as frustration with themselves is important. Examples of tertiary prevention with the Connors family are the following:

Individual. Assist individual family members in dealing with grief from the loss of father/husband.

Family. Assist family in dealing with grief and assuming alternate roles.

Community. Assist community in dealing with loss of fully functioning family by providing grief support services that include males or target males as well as females.

ROLES OF THE COMMUNITY HEALTH NURSE

Alternative approaches to reaching men will depend on creative marketing of multiple options for men. Community health nurses can fill multiple roles that address men's health now and in the future. Some examples follow.

Health Educator

Tailoring messages to the needs of men is imperative. Market surveys of brochures and posters designed for men or to include men may be crucial. For example, the "pregnant man" poster, which was designed to involve men in family planning services, may be accepted by one population yet found to be offensive by another. Health fairs for men are another example of health education efforts. Asking a car dealer to display a new car in which infant car seats are promoted may attract men to the fair. Emergency medical personnel can be asked to volunteer tours of emergency medical vehicles and give information at health fair sites to attract men and boys in particular.

Education can address the need for changing societal attitudes that encourage negative health behaviors, including risk taking among males regarding, for example, attitudes toward drinking, reckless driving, and wearing seat belts. Supporting or possibly working with a legislator to even introduce legislation that mandates positive health behaviors is also important. Teaching the caretaking role to both men and women is important. School programs that teach child care to boys open up new roles as nurturers and caretakers to fathers of the future. If such programs exist for girls in the community, what can be done to enlist support for parallel programs for boys?

Facilitator

The community health nurse may carry out the role of facilitator of change at several levels. Adult role models in the home and in the media may equate concern with health and health problems as "feminine." Facilitating change by promoting healthy lifelong behaviors by parents and other family members is important. The community health nurse may also facilitate change at the aggregate level by assessing the community's needs and resources specifically designed for men (e.g., help for batterers) (see Chapter 21).

Community health nurses working in an agency may review health education literature (e.g., family planning or parenting brochures) for sex-role–related content and messages. Organizations that publish the literature can be contacted, and options can be offered based on feedback gathered by the nurses from the population they serve.

Facilitation of change also reaches the congressional district level; a community assessment may point out highway safety problems or a common occupational health hazard. Community organization efforts also need to be initiated and supported where indicated (see Chapter 7)).

At the professional level, the community health nurse needs to join organizations and create awareness of men's health as an issue. A review of nursing and other professional literature for men's health and

a review of indexes in nursing texts for men's health or men's reproductive health or fathering can be carried out.

RESEARCH AND MEN'S HEALTH

Will we allow men and women more options in the future? As women progress even more into the work place, will their mortality rates be more like those of men? Or will men be allowed to explore more flexible roles and live longer, like women? It is appropriate to ask how community health nurses can buffer the process by allowing more alternative choices for men in lifestyles as well as in health services. Charged with the public's health, community health nurses must ensure a safe work place and environment for both men and women. Community health nurses have traditionally also provided for the disadvantaged, who may not have the economic freedom to choose from a range of options. Research directed toward men's health is an appropriate response to these concerns.

Nursing research is more and more addressing health aspects of men's roles in the family, for example, in family planning (Swanson, 1985, 1988), in childbearing (Chapman, 1992), and in parenting (Ferketich and Mercer, 1995a, 1995b). Further research is needed on fathering and on gender effects on the delivery of health services. Structural components of service delivery such as hours and services for men and for couples are another area of research need. Research is also needed on new models of service delivery in both the public and the private sector, as the nation embraces principles of managed care. A cross-disciplinary approach is needed because approaches to men's health have social and psychological dimensions.

Last, research must include two important approaches: population-based research (Williams, 1992) and qualitative research (Chenitz and Swanson, 1986; Morse, 1994). Defining who in the community has hypertension, where they are, and the best method of reaching them is an example of population-based research (Williams, 1992). The second approach involves using qualitative research methods (e.g., interview and participant observation) to find out from men, couples, families, and groups, in their own words, about their experiences. Through this approach, researchers are better able to target research needs that are grounded in the experience of the people and reflect the complexity of human experience. Community health nurses can improve the health of the community by using knowledge that exists, by identifying problems for research, and by participating in research efforts.

SUMMARY

The gender gap is not new, nor is it confined to political arenas. The gender gap in health presents a serious paradox that has marked implications for community health nursing. Men in industrialized countries have higher death rates and live shorter lives than do women (Waldron, 1995a). Although major advances in medical care and access to care have occurred in the United States during this century, men have suffered a disadvantage. However, the health of females appears to be worse than the health of males. Morbidity rates are higher for women because women are more likely to experience illness that does not cause death, to receive disability days, and to use health services (NCHS, 1995). Evidence suggests that sex differences in health may be related to behavioral and biological determinants, such as men's propensity to engage in risk-taking behaviors related to lifestyle. Antecedents of the largest sex differentials in mortality are associated with sex-linked behavior that is more prevalent in men: smoking, alcohol consumption, poor preventive health habits, stress, and lack of other emotional channels. These factors, however, are compounded by social and environmental conditions of major public health concern: occupational and environmental hazards, both physical and psychological; unemployment; accidents, including motor vehicle and sport; suicide; and homicide. These concerns call for a major public health approach to men's health. These factors, compounded by men's lack of willingness to seek preventive and health care, have marked implications for community health nursing. Factors that impede men's health include medical care patterns based on acute care rather than on prevention. Factors that promote men's health include interest groups in men and men's health, men's increased interest in physical fitness and lifestyle, policy making related to

men's health, and models of health services for men. Men's health care needs are psychosocial as well as medical, and they require prevention and health promotion marketed specifically for men. Current attempts to meet men's health care needs are made through the provision of both traditional and innova-

RESOURCES ON MEN'S HEALTH

The National Organization for Changing Men
P.O. Box 451
Watseka, IL 60970
The American Assembly for Men in Nursing
c/o College of Nursing, Rush University
600 South Paulina, 474-H
Chicago, IL 60612
Coalition of Free Men, Inc.
P.O. Box 129
Manhasset, NY 11030
American Divorce Association of Men, Inc.
1008 West White Oak St
Arlington Heights, IL 60005
Men's Rights, Inc.
P.O. Box 163180
Sacramento, CA 95816
National Gay Task Force
80 Fifth Ave
New York, NY 10011
Gay Men's Health Crisis Employer Consulting Service
129 W. 20th St
New York, NY 10011
Check the WEB sites for current resources

tive services. Community health nurses can plan gender-appropriate care for males by applying the nursing process to individuals, families, and communities using the three levels of prevention. Research related to men's health is in an early stage of development. Community health nurses can improve the health of the community by using knowledge that exists and by participating in research efforts.

ADDITIONAL READING: MEN'S HEALTH

Bozett FW, Forrester DA. (1989). A proposal for a men's health nurse practitioner. Image J Nurs Sch. 21:158–161.
Brabant S, Forsyth C, Melancon C. (1992). Grieving men: Thoughts, feelings, and behaviors following deaths of wives. Hospice J 8:33–47.

Brown I, Lunt F. (1992). Evaluating a "well man" clinic. Health Visitor 65:12–14.
Chalmers K. (1992). Working with men: An analysis of health visiting practice in families with young children. Int J Nurs Stud 29:3–16.

Box continued on following page

DiPasquale JA. (1990). The psychological effects of support groups on individuals infected by the AIDS virus. Cancer Nurs 13:278–285.

Flaming D, Morse J. (1991). Minimizing embarrassment: Boys' experiences of pubertal changes. Issues Comprehensive Pediatric Nurs 14:211–230.

Franciosa D, Shaw S. (1994). Breast cancer and benign breast disease in men. Nurse Pract Forum 5:56–58.

Go K. (1992). Recent advances in the treatment of male infertility. Clin Issues Perinat Women's Health Nurs 3:320–327.

Gregory DM, Peters N, Cameron CF. (1990). Elderly male spouses as caregivers: Toward an understanding of their experience. J Gerontol Nurs 16:20–24.

Hahn W, Brooks J, Hartsouogh D. (1993). Self-disclosure and coping styles in men with cardiovascular reactivity. Res Nurs Health 16:275–282.

Julian T, McKenry P, McKelvey M. (1992). Components of men's well-being at mid-life. Issues Ment Health Nurs 13:285–299.

Lovejoy N, Morgenroth B, Paul S, et al. (1992). Potential predictors of information-seeking behavior by homosexual/bisexual (gay) men with a human immunodeficiency virus seropositive health status. Cancer Nurs 15: 116–124.

MacIntyre R. (1991). Nursing loved ones with AIDS: Knowledge development for ethical practice. J Home Health Care Pract 3:1–10.

Mackey V. (1992). Another look at the circumcision debate: Opinions of nursing-home caregivers. Nurse Pract 17:63–64.

Mellick E, Buckwalter K, Stolley J. (1992). Suicide among elderly white men: Development of a profile. J Psychosocial Nurs Ment Health Serv 30:29–34.

Smith D, Babaian R. (1992). The effects of treatment for cancer on male fertility and sexuality. Cancer Nurs 15:271–275.

Stoller EP. (1990). Males as helpers: The role of sons, relatives and friends. Gerontologist 30:228–235.

Underwood S. (1992). Cancer risk reduction and early detection behaviors among Black men: Focus on learned helplessness. Jo Commun Health Nurs 9:21–31.

Wilson S, Morse JM. (1991). Living with a wife undergoing chemotherapy. Image J Nurs Sch 23:78–84.

Woodland A, Hunt C. (1994). Healthy convictions . . . Well-man clinic for the inmates of Lindholme prison. Nurs Times 90:32–33.

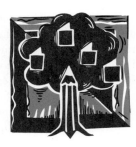

L e a r n i n g
A c t i v i t i e s

1. Examine the vital statistics in your community and compare the sex-specific differences in mortality.

2. During a 1-week period, determine the frequency of newspaper articles in your major newspaper that identify the top 12 causes of mortality for men.

3. Survey the billboards in your community and determine the frequency of those that depict sex-linked behavior of men associated with risk-taking behavior.

4. Survey local businesses and industries in your community to find out what health promotion and prevention programs are available and used by men and women.

5. Select a family from your caseload that has a man in the household who is accessible to you. Select two "door openers" appropriate to initiate discussion of health concerns with this man. Devise a gender-appropriate nursing care plan that includes primary, secondary, and tertiary prevention for this man as an individual, for his family, and for the community in which he resides.

6. Select a family from your caseload that has a man in the household with whom you do not have ready access. Interview the woman caregiver in the household and obtain information by proxy about the man's health. If possible, arrange to meet the man for lunch, at work, or after work, and obtain information about his health. Compare the information obtained by proxy with that obtained from the client.

7. Review major nursing texts (e.g., medical-surgical) you have used as a student; examine the tables of contents and the indexes for content on men's health versus women's health.

REFERENCES

Agnew J, McDiarmid MA, Lees PS, Duffy R: Reproductive hazards of fire fighting: I. Non-chemical hazards. Am J Ind Med 19:433–445, 1991.

Allen DG, Whatley M: Nursing and men's health: Some critical considerations. Nurs Clin North Am 21:3–13, 1986.

American Cancer Society: Cancer Facts and Figures—1991. Atlanta, Georgia, ACS, 1991.

American Public Health Association: Recording of males served by federally funded family planning programs. Policy statements. Am J Public Health 78:204–205, 1988.

Benson V, Marano MA: Current estimates from the National Health Interview Survey, 1993. National Center for Health Statistics. Vital Health Stat Series 10, No. 190, 1994.

Bird C: Born Female: The High Cost of Keeping Women Down. New York, Pocket Books, 1970.

Brannon RC: No "sissy stuff": The stigma of anything vaguely feminine. In David D, Brannon B (eds). The Forty-Nine Percent Majority: The Male Sex Role. Reading, MA, Addison-Wesley, 1976, pp. 49–50.

Brown I, Lunt F: Evaluating a "well man" clinic. Health Visitor 65:12–14, 1992.

Catalano R, Dooley D, Novaco RW, et al.: Using ECA survey data to examine the effect of job layoffs on violent behavior. Hosp Community Psychiatry 44:874–879, 1993.

Catalano R, Dooley D, Wilson G, Hough R: Job loss and alcohol abuse: A test using data from the Epidemiologic Catchment Area project. J Health Soc Behav 34:215–225, 1993.

Centers for Disease Control: Sexually Transmitted Disease Surveillance, 1993. Atlanta, GA, U.S. Department of Health and Human Services, Public Health Service, CDC, 1994.

Chapman L: Expectant fathers' roles during labor and birth. J Obstet Gynecol Neonatal Nurs 21:114–120, 1992.

Chenitz WC, Swanson JM (eds): From Practice to Grounded Theory: Qualitative Research in Nursing. Palo Alto, CA, Addison-Wesley, 1986.

Choi MW: Preamble to a new paradigm for women's health care. Image: J Nurs Scholarship 17:14–16, 1985.

Cohen FL: Paternal contributions to birth defects. Nurs Clin North Am 21:49–63, 1986.

David DS, Brannon R: The male sex role: Our culture's blueprint of manhood, and what it's done for us lately. In David DS, Brannon R (eds). The Forty-Nine Percent Majority: The Male Sex Role. Reading, MA, Addison-Wesley, 1976 pp. 1–45.

Deans W: Well man clinics. Nursing 26:975–978, 1988.

DeHoff JB, Forrest K: Men's health. In Swanson J, Forrest K (eds). Men's Reproductive Health. New York, Springer, pp. 3–10, 1984.

Devesa S, Blot W, Stone B, et al.: Recent cancer trends in the United States. Cancer Inst 87:175–182, 1995.

Diagram Group: Man's Body: An Owner's Manual. New York, Paddington Press Ltd., 1976.

Dooley D, Catalano R, Wilson G: Depression and unemployment: Panel findings from the Epidemiologic Catchment Area study. Am J Community Psychol 22:745–765, 1994.

Eaton WO, Enns LR: Sex differences in human motor activity level. Psychol Bull 100:19–28, 1986.

Ehrhardt AA, Wasserheit JN: Age, gender, and sexual risk behaviors for sexually transmitted diseases in the United States. In Wasserheit JN, Aral SO, Holmes KK (eds.) Research Issues in Human Behavior and Sexually Transmitted Diseases in the AIDS Era. Washington, DC, American Society for Microbiology, 1991.

Erikson E: Childhood and Society. New York, WW Norton, 1963.

Fareed A: Equal rights for men. Nursing Times 90:26–29, 1994.

Ferketich SL, Mercer RT: Paternal-infant attachment of experienced and inexperienced fathers during infancy. Nurs Res 44:31–37, 1995a.

Ferketich SL, Mercer RT: Predictors of role competence for experienced and inexperienced fathers. Nurs Res 44:89–95, 1995b.

Flaming D, Morse JM: Minimizing embarrassment: Boys' experiences of pubertal changes. Issues Comprehensive Pediatric Nurs 14:211–230, 1991.

Francoeur RT: Becoming a Sexual Person. New York, Macmillan, 1991.

Giwercman A, Carlsen E, Keiding N, Skakkebaek NE: Evidence for increasing incidence of abnormalities of the human testis: A review. Environ Health Perspect 101 (suppl 2):65–71, 1993.

Goldman L, Cook EF: The decline in ischemic heart disease mortality rates: An analysis of the comparative effects of medical interventions and changes in lifestyle. Ann Intern Med 101:825–835, 1984.

Harrison JB: Warning: The male sex role may be dangerous to your health. In Swanson J, Forrest K, (eds). Men's Reproductive Health. New York, Springer, 1984, pp. 11–27.

Hibbard JF, Pope CR: Employment characteristics and health status among men and women. Women Health 12:85–102, 1987.

Kochanek MA, Hudson BL: Advance Report of Final Mortality Statistics, 1992. Monthly vital statistics report; vol 43, no 6 (suppl). Hyattsville, MD, National Center for Health Statistics.

Levinson D: The Seasons of a Man's Life. New York, Alfred A. Knopf, 1978.

Lewis T: Unemployment and men's health. Nursing 26:969–974, 1988.

Matthews KA, Woodall KL, Engebretson TO, et al: Influence of age, sex, and family on type A and hostile attitudes and behaviors. Health Psychology 11:317–323.

McDiarmid MA, Lees PS, Agnew J, et al.: Reproductive hazards of fire fighting: II. Chemical hazards. Am J Ind Med 19:447–472, 1991.

McKinlay JB, McKinlay SM, Beaglehole, R: A review of the evidence concerning the impact of medical measures on recent mortality and morbidity in the United States. Int J Health Serv 19:181–208, 1989.

Mechanic D: The influence of mothers on their children's health attitudes and behavior. Pediatrics 33:444–453, 1964.

Milio N: Primary Care and the Public's Health. Lexington, MA: Lexington Books, 1983.

Montiero L: Monitoring Health Status and Medical Care. Cambridge, MA, Ballinger, 1976.

Morse JM (ed): Critical Issues in Qualitative Research Methods. Thousand Oaks, CA, Sage, 1994.

National Center for Health Statistics: Health, United States, 1991. Hyattsville, MD, U.S. Public Health Service, 1992.

National Center for Health Statistics: Health, United States, 1993. Hyattsville, MD, U.S. Public Health Service, 1994.

National Center for Health Statistics: Health, United States, 1994. Hyattsville, MD, U.S. Public Health Service, 1995.

Navarro V: Race or class, or race and class. Int J Health Serv 19:311–314, 1989.

Paul M, Kurtz S: Analysis of reproductive health hazard information on material safety data sheets for lead and the ethylene glycol ethers. Am J Ind Med 25:403–415, 1994.

Piani A, Schoenborn, C: Health promotion and disease prevention, United States, 1990. Vital and Health Statistics, Series 10, No. 185, 1993.

Roberts A, McClure R, Weiner R, et al: Overtraining affects male reproductive status. Fertil Steril 60:686–692, 1993.

Rosen BN, Peterson L: Gender differences in children's outdoor play injuries: A review and an integration. Clin Psychol Rev 10:187–205, 1990.

Sadler C: DIY male maintenance. Nurs Mirror 160:16–18, 1979.

Salem N: Health insurance coverage and receipt of preventive health services—United States, 1993. Morb Mortal Wkly Rep 44:219–224, 1993.

Schulte MM, Sonenstein RL: Men at family planning clinics: The new patients? Fam Plann Perspect 27:212–216, 225, 1995.

Skelton R: Man's role in society and its effect on health. Nursing 26:953–956, 1988.

Smith DB, Babaian RJ: The effects of treatment for cancer on male fertility and sexuality. Cancer Nurs 15:271–275, 1992.

Steinem G: Outrageous Acts and Everyday Rebellions. New York, Signet, 1983.

Swanson J: Men and family planning. *In* Hanson S, Bozett F, (eds). Dimensions of Fatherhood. Beverly Hills, CA, Sage, 1985, pp. 21–48.

Swanson J: The process of finding contraceptive options. West J Nurs Res 10:492–503, 1988.

Swanson J: Overview of men's health. Invited paper presented at the continuing education program, "Including Men in Reproductive and Family Health," at the American Public Health Association's 123rd Annual Meeting, San Diego, CA, October 28, 1995.

Swanson J, Forrest K (eds): Men's Reproductive Health. New York, Springer, 1984.

Swanson J, Forrest K: Men's reproductive health services in family planning settings: A pilot study. Am J Public Health 77:1462–1463, 1987.

Temmerman M: Sexually transmitted diseases and reproductive health. Sex Transm Dis 24 (suppl 2):S55–S58. 1994.

Verbrugge LM, Wingard DL: Sex differentials in health and mortality. Women Health 12:103–145, 1987.

Waldron I: Changing gender roles and gender differences in health behavior. *In* Gochman DS (ed). Handbook of Health Behavior Research. New York, Plenum, 1995a, in press.

Waldron I: Contributions of changing gender differences in behavior and social roles to changing gender differences in mortality. *In* Sabo D, Gordon D (eds). Men's Health and Illness: Gender, Power, and the Body. Thousand Oaks, CA, Sage, 1995b, pp. 22–45.

Waldron I: Factors determining the sex ratio at birth. *In* United Nations (eds). Sex Differentials in Infant and Child Mortality. New York, United Nations, 1995c, in press.

Waldron I: Contributions of biological and behavioral factors in changing sex differences in ischaemic heart disease mortality. *In* Lopez A, Caselli G, Valkonen T (eds). Adult Mortality in Developed Countries: From Description to Explanation. New York, Oxford University Press, 1995d, pp. 161–178.

Waldron I: Sex differences in infant and early child mortality—Major causes of death and possible biological causes. *In* United Nations (eds). Sex Differentials in Infant and Child Mortality. New York; United Nations, 1995e, in press.

Wasserheit JN: Effect of changes in human ecology and behavior on patterns of sexually transmitted diseases, including human immunodeficiency virus infection. Proc Nat Acad Sci U S Am 91:2430–2435, 1994.

Whorton MD: Environmental and occupational reproductive hazards. *In* Swanson J, Forrest K (eds). Men's Reproductive Health. New York, Springer, 1984, pp. 193–203.

Williams C: Community-based population-focused practice: The foundation of specialization in public health nursing. *In* Stanhope M, Lancaster J (eds). Community Health Nursing: Process and Practice for Promoting Health, 3rd ed. St. Louis, CV Mosby, 1992, pp. 244–252.

Wingo PA, Tong T, Bolden S: Cancer statistics, 1995. CA—Cancer J Clin 45:8–30, 1995.

Woodland A, Hunt C: Healthy convictions . . . well-man clinic for the inmates of Lindholme prison. Nursing Times 90:32–33, 1994.

Zilbergold B: Appendix: The effects of drugs on male sexuality. *In* Zilbergold B (ed): The New Male Sexuality. New York, Bantam Books, 1992, pp. 537–546.

Zimmerman SL: Psychache in context: States' spending for public welfare and their suicide rates. J Nerv Ment Dis 183:425–434, 1995.

Addressing the Needs of Families

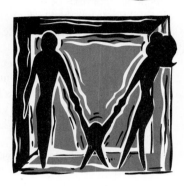

Upon completion of this chapter, the reader will be able to:

1. State a personal definition of "family."

2. Identify characteristics of the changing family that have implications for community health nursing practice.

3. Describe strategies for moving from intervention at the individual level to intervention at the family level.

4. Describe strategies for moving from intervention at the family level to intervention at the aggregate level.

5. Discuss the application of one conceptual framework to studying families.

6. Discuss a model of care for communities of families.

7. Apply the steps of the nursing process to individuals within the family, to the family as a whole, and to an aggregate of which the family is a part.

Janice M. Swanson

Joe Hudson is a 74-year-old alcoholic who is being treated at an outpatient department in a large medical center. He lives in a hotel room in downtown Salt Lake City. He has one living relative of whom he is aware, a 76-year-old brother. Mr. Hudson states, "I had a falling out with my brother some 20 years ago. . . . I never hear from him. I reckon he's still in Boston, if he's alive at all." Mr. Hudson frequently falls out of bed, dislodging the telephone that the desk clerk has placed precariously close to the bed, which signals the desk clerk that something is amiss. The clerk then goes to Mr. Hudson's room and puts him back to bed. Mr. Hudson's source of income is a check sent him the first day of the month by an acquaintance, a minister, who lives in a town 75 miles away. The desk clerk cashes Mr. Hudson's check and assists him in paying his bill from the hotel, which provides congregate dining facilities.

Lai Chan is a Chinese refugee from Vietnam who moved with her family to San Francisco 3 months ago. Mrs. Chan is a single parent; Mr. Chan died in an automobile accident shortly after arriving in the United States. Mrs. Chan has two children: an 11-year-old son and a 5-year-old daughter. The family resides in a one-room efficiency apartment in the Tenderloin district in downtown San Francisco.

Jaime Gutierrez, a 72-year-old Mexican-American man, lives with his 36-year-old son, Roberto; his 34-year-old daughter-in-law, Patricia; and his three grandchildren, who are 14, 13, and 12 years old. Mr. Gutierrez was in good health until he fell from a tree while helping his son make roof repairs on the house in 1985. He suffered a concussion, right hemothorax, and fracture of T-11 and T-12. Confined to bed, he is receiving home health care. He requires intermittent catheterization but feels uncomfortable when the nurse suggests that his daughter-in-law is willing to carry out this procedure for him. Therefore, Roberto quit work to provide this personal care to his father. Consequently, the family of six lives on Mr. Gutierrez's retirement income, which consists of $239 from Social Security and $244 from a pension plan per month. Roberto would like to increase his job skills while at home. He has finished the 4th grade and has failed the Graduate Equivalency Degree exam twice. Patricia would also like to return to school and pursue job training. Although agreeable to Patricia's interests, Roberto is hesitant to support active steps taken by Patricia to initiate her plan.

These three families, which include today's broad contemporary definitions of family, are examples of families carried in caseloads by undergraduate community health nursing students. Assessments made by students during home, office, and hospital visits with these families triggered interventions that linked the families to resources provided by the community and, in turn, triggered questions about health needs of groups of families or larger aggregates living in the same communities.

Families have major health care needs that are not usually addressed by the health care system. Instead, the individual is the unit most frequently addressed by the health care system. This holds true for nursing interventions within the health care system. The majority of nurses work in hospitals where interventions traditionally occur at the individual client level. Nurses, however, are on the forefront of a trend toward intervention at the family level.

NURSING AN INDIVIDUAL CLIENT VERSUS NURSING A FAMILY AS CLIENT

These authors discuss the similarities and differences between nursing an individual as client versus nursing a family as client. Using the Betty Neuman systems model as a guide, they present factors that contribute to the decision to use one approach versus the other. These factors include the following:

- The perception of the client as to the need for nursing
- The nature of the stressors as affecting only one member of the family or other family members
- The risk of instability to the family as a whole posed by the health status of an individual member
- The feasibility of the family-nurse collaboration (i.e., the availability of family members and the availability of nursing time to meet with family members)
- The knowledge and skill of the nurse

Using a case study, the authors then make comparisons between an individual approach and a family approach by applying the nursing process to an individual client and to the family client.

Data from Ross MM, Helmer H: A comparative analysis of Neuman's model using the individual and family as the units of care. Public Health Nurs 5:30–31, 1988.

The family is composed of many subsystems and, in turn, is tied to many formal and informal systems outside the family. The family is imbedded in social systems that have an impact on health (e.g., education, employment, housing, and more). Many disciplines are interested in the study of families; interdisciplinary perspectives and strategies are necessary to understand the impact of the family on health and the impact of the broader social system on the family. Traditionally, nursing, and even community health nursing, has relied heavily if not solely on theoretical frameworks for intervention with families from disciplines of psychology or social psychology, which target individuals (e.g., Duvall, 1977; Erikson, 1963; Maslow, 1970). Dreher (1982) questioned the usefulness of these frameworks for the public health nurse "who is ministering to the health of socially and economically diverse populations. . . . Such psychological themes often draw our attention away from broader social issues that are the essence of public health nursing" (p. 505).

Intended for clinical rather than for public health use, these models do not address why some social and economically advantaged populations are more likely to become self-actualized or why, in the experience of death, some populations experience greater mortality rates than other populations. Improvement, stated Dreher (1982), must come about by addressing the socioeconomic conditions that make some families more dysfunctional than others and to alter the system itself that produces such inequities. Dreher cautioned that socioeconomic causes cannot be interpreted as psychological symptoms. Thus, social and policy changes are necessary to alter the conditions under which families function. How community health nurses work with families within communities to bring about healthy conditions for families at the family, social, and policy levels is addressed in this chapter. This chapter will focus on five areas:

- The changing family
- Approaches to meeting the health needs of families
- Family theory approach to meeting the health needs of families
- Extending family health intervention to larger aggregates and social action
- An example of the nursing process applied to a family

THE CHANGING FAMILY
Definition of the Family

Definitions of the family are many. Essentially, the term "family" as used here is defined as an aggregate made up of a body of units, the individuals that represent the whole sum, or the family. Definitions of the family vary by discipline, by the professional, and by distinct groups of families. For example, psychologists may define the family in terms of personal development and intrapersonal dynamics; the sociologist has used a classic definition of the family in terms of a "social unit interacting with the larger society" (Johnson, 1984, p. 333). Other professionals have classically defined the family in terms of kinship, marriage, and descent (Farber, 1973):

[A family is] a cluster of people, whose relationship is stipulated by law in terms of marriage and descent, and whose precise membership varies according to the circumstances.

(p. 2)

Other professionals have defined the family in terms of household membership, as "a primary group of people living in a household in consistent proximity and intimate relationships" (Helvie, 1981, p. 64). The concept of family, according to Stuart (1991, p. 40), has five critical attributes:
1. The family is a system or unit.
2. Its members may or may not be related and may or may not live together.
3. The unit may or may not contain children.
4. There is commitment and attachment among unit members that include future obligation.
5. The unit caregiving functions consist of protection, nourishment, and socialization of its members.

Wright and Leahey (1994) stated that "the family is who they say they are" (p. 40). Most important, according to McGoldrick (1982), is the definition of "family" given by different family groups within the population:

The dominant American (WASP) definition focuses on the intact nuclear family. Black families focus on a wide network of kin and community. For Italians, there is no such thing as the 'nuclear' family. To them family means a strong, tightly knit three- or four-generational family, which also includes godparents and old friends. The Chinese go beyond this and include in their definition of family all their ancestors and all their descendants.

(p. 10)

The community health nurse interacts with communities made up of many types of families. When faced with the great diversity in the community, the community health nurse must formulate a personal definition of the family and yet be aware of the changing definition of the family held by other disciplines, professionals, and family groups. The community health nurse who interacts with Mr. Hudson, the alcoholic who lives in a hotel, must have a broad conceptualization of the family. The surveillance activity of the hotel manager and the financial support of the minister-friend could both be accounted for in Jordheim's (1982) definition of the family as a "relationship community of two or more persons" (p. 61) whether from the same or different kinship groups.

Characteristics of the Changing Family

The characteristics of the U.S. family are changing. The typical family, the nuclear family, has traditionally been defined as "a small group consisting of parents and their non-adult children living in a single household" (Farber, 1973, p. 2). The stereotypical view of this family as father, mother, and nonadult children is eroding. For example, in 1970, 85% of children younger than age 18 were living with two parents; in 1993, this proportion declined to 70% (Saluter, 1994). Over the past 23 years, the percentage of African-American children living with both parents decreased from 58.5% (in 1970) to 35.6% (in 1993). Seventy-seven percent of white children lived with both parents in 1993, whereas 64.5% of children of Hispanic origin lived with both parents.

Cohabitation, which is defined as "two unrelated adults of the opposite sex (one of whom is the householder) who share a housing unit with or without the presence of children under 15 years old," has also increased over time (Saluter, 1994, p. vii). Cohabiting unmarried persons increased from 523,000 in 1970 to 3.5 million in 1993. In other words, "there are 6 unmarried couples for every 100 married couples in 1993, compared to only 1 for every 100 in 1970" (Saluter, 1994, p. viii). In 1993, about one third of the cohabiting-couple households included children.

Single parenting has also increased over time. Between 1970 and 1993, the proportion of children living with one parent grew from 12 to 26.7% (Saluter, 1994). Between 1983 and 1993,

The proportion of one-parent children who lived with a divorced parent declined form 42.0% to 37.1%, while the proportion who lived with a never-married parent continued to rise, from 24.0% to 35.0%.

(SALUTER, 1994, P. XII)

The proportion of children younger than 18 years who are living with their grandparents (i.e., their grandparents own or rent their home) is also growing. In 1970, only 3% of children lived with their grandparents. By 1993, this figure rose to 5% of all children (3.4 million).

A homosexual family is made up of a cohabiting couple of the same sex who have a sexual relationship. The homosexual family may or may not have children. Estimates of the number of children who live in lesbian or gay-parented families (including children conceived in heterosexual marriages) range from 6 to 14 million (Singer, 1994). There are between 1 and 5 million lesbian mothers in the United States and between 1 and 3 million gay fathers (Patterson, 1992). These numbers are estimates because the U.S. Bureau of the Census does not count the number of lesbians and gay men. However, the 1990 census does report that of 3,187,772 "unmarried partners," 145,130 were counted as same-sex couples (Saluter, 1994). Studies have been conducted by Overlooked Opinions, a Chicago polling organization that has demographic data on gay and lesbian Americans (Singer, 1994).

Divorce is associated with the financial well-being of children. In 1991, 39% of divorced women with children lived in poverty and 55% of those with children younger than 6 years were poor (Teachman and Paasch, 1994). During the same year, the poverty rate for all children was 22%.

APPROACHES TO MEETING THE HEALTH NEEDS OF FAMILIES

Community health nursing has long viewed the family as an important unit of health care, with an awareness that the individual can be best understood within the social context of the family. Observing and inquiring about family interaction enable the nurse in the community to assess the impact and influence of family members on one another. Direct intervention at the family rather than the individual client level, however, is a new frontier for many nursing students, most of whom have experience in acute care settings before the community setting. A family model, largely a community health nursing or psychiatric-mental health intervention model, is now expanding into the areas such as birthing and parent-child, adult day care, chronic illness, and home care. Nursing assessment and intervention must not stop with the immediate social context of the family, however, but must consider the broader social context of the community and society as well. As Dunn (1961) stated, "the family stands in-between individual wellness and social wellness. You can't really have high-level wellness for either individuals or social groups unless you have well families."

Moving From the Individual to the Family

Community health and home care nurses have traditionally focused on the family as the unit of service; with the move to managed care throughout the United States, most of these nurses continue to focus their practice on individuals residing in the home. As a result of the current era of cost containment, constraints on the community health nurse as well as on nurses working within hospitals and in other settings will increase. Reimbursement, for example, which is almost entirely calculated for services rendered to the individual, is a major constraint toward moving toward planning care for families as a unit. A variety of creative approaches to meeting the health needs of families are needed, approaches reflecting interventions appropriate to the needs of the population as a whole.

FAMILY INTERVIEWING

Approaches to the care of families are needed and must be creative, flexible, and transferable from one setting to another. Community health nurses are generalists who bring previous preparation in communication concepts and in interviewing to the family arena. Wright and Leahey (1994) proposed the realm of *family interviewing* rather than family therapy as an appropriate model. In this model, the community health nurse uses general systems and communication concepts to conceptualize health needs of families and a family assessment model to assess families' responses to "normative" events such as birth or retirement or to "paranormative" events such as chronic illness or divorce. Intervention is straightforward, as in asking a family to read a book about sex education of prepubescent teenagers, or dealt with through referral if the level of intervention is beyond the preparation of the nurse. For the purposes of this

text, the model is extended to include intervention at the level of the larger aggregate. For example, the index of suspicion based on the health needs of a particular family for information would prompt the community health nurse to assess the need for similar information and the resources for intervention with other families in the community, in schools, churches, or other institutions. Family interviewing requires thinking "interactionally" not only in terms of the family system but also in terms of larger social systems.

Creative family interviewing calls for interviewing families in many types of settings. The future prediction of decreased hospitalization supplemented by a wide variety of health care settings ranging from acute to ambulatory to community centers calls for flexible, transferable approaches. Clinical settings for family interviewing are reviewed by Wright and Leahey (1994) and include inpatient and outpatient ambulatory care and clinic settings in maternity, pediatrics, medicine, surgery, critical care, and mental health. According to these authors, community health nurses have many opportunities besides the traditional home visit to engage the family in a family interview. Community health nurses are employed in ambulatory care centers, occupational health and school sites, housing complexes, day care programs, residential treatment and substance abuse programs, and other official and nonofficial agencies. In each of these sites, community health nurses meet families and can assess and intervene at the family and community levels.

For example, the community health nurse can implement preventive programs for family units. The family is particularly appropriate because it experiences similar risk factors: physiological, behavioral, and environmental. For example, in a classic study conducted by Manley and Graber (1977) in a community hospital, family members of patients with coronary heart disease were invited to attend preventive screening and educational programs. Family members were evaluated for hypertension, smoking, and triglycerides. Findings were similar to those in large epidemiological studies: 25% had lipid abnormalities, 44% were overweight, 12% smoked, and 15.5% had previously undetected hypertension. Such programs can occur in community health settings and demonstrate the need to go beyond intervention with the individual family to groups of families, thus serving the population as a whole. A community health nurse working with Mexican-American families with diabetes could implement such a program, basing assessment on both needs of the individual families and biostatistics that reflect populations at risk. For example, the risk of diabetes in Mexican-Americans is three times that found in whites, and of all ethnic groups, Mexican-Americans are less likely to see a physician (Council of Scientific Affairs, 1991).

Involving family members in newborn assessments can aid the community health nurse in assessing the family's adjustment to the newborn and parenthood. It can be done in the home, clinic, or other health care center. Family members should be involved during the first contact or visit, and if they do not attend, a telephone call explaining the nurse's interest in them should take place (Wright and Leahey, 1994). More husbands and family members are becoming involved in the pregnancy and delivery phases of childbirth. The community health nurse in the well-baby clinic may often see parents for whom a family interview or home visit may be valuable. A general statement may be used to introduce the commonality of hurdles faced by new parents: "Many new parents face similar problems, which usually last only a short period of time. We find that bringing all of the family members together is important as the entire family is affected when a new baby comes into the home."

HOME VISITS BY NURSES TO POOR, UNMARRIED, TEENAGE WOMEN PROMPT MORE RAPID RETURN TO SCHOOL, INCREASE EMPLOYMENT, AND RESULT IN FEWER SUBSEQUENT PREGNANCIES

A program of home visits by nurses is described that provided comprehensive care to poor, un-married, and white teenagers bearing their first children in a semirural county in upstate New York. The study found that women who re-ceived home visits from the prenatal period through 2 years after the birth of their child were more likely than women who did not receive home visits to return to school more rapidly, to increase the number of months they were em-ployed, to have fewer subsequent pregnancies, and to postpone the birth of their second child.

Data from Olds DL, Henderson CR, Tatelbaum R, Chamberlin R: Improving the life-course development of socially disadvantaged mothers: A randomized trial of nurse home visitation. Am J Public Health 78:1436–1445, 1988.

The community health nurse working with single-parent families may face particular challenges. Mothers in single-parent families report a higher incidence of children's academic and behavioral problems than do mothers in two-parent families. For example, in the National Health Interview Survey, 1988, researchers found that children 3 to 17 years of age living with a formerly married mother were more than three times as likely to have received treatment for emotional or behavioral problems in the preceding 12 months (8.8%) as children living with both biological parents (2.7%) (Dawson, 1991). It is important to remember, however, that children living in a nuclear family who experience severe conflict may have as many problems as children from a disrupted household. Children in these families need a chance to express their concerns; the family interview is important in giving care to these families.

THE SCHOOL NURSE

The school nurse has a unique opportunity to compare the child in the school system—classroom, lunchroom, playground, and so on—with the child in the family system. The school nurse is increasingly becoming involved in planning special programs in the schools. Astute assessment of children's needs within the context of their families in interviews at school or in the home can lead to innovative interventions such as leading support groups for children with chronic illness. Other areas of assessment and intervention that benefit from a family approach include learning or behavioral problems and absenteeism (Wright and Leahey, 1994).

THE OCCUPATIONAL HEALTH NURSE

The nurse in the occupational health setting can also use a family approach to care to improve the health of the worker and contribute to overall productivity. For example, alcohol and chemical abuse account for much absenteeism in the work place. Effective intervention with these families has been demonstrated (Steinglass, 1985). Assessment of occupational haz-ards may involve conducting reproductive histories in an effort to determine the effects of a chemical or agent on the reproductive capacity of the couple (Swanson, 1984). Toxic agents can also be transferred to family members from the work place via clothes and equipment (Whorton, 1984). An awareness and high degree of suspicion of risks of occupational hazards common to industries in the community in which the community health nurse works are necessary. Obtaining an occupational history from all family members who have entered the work place and referral for screening and health education of family members will contribute to unraveling occupational hazards and effects in the future. In addition, the community health nurse should be aware of the many family-related work issues that may trigger stress-related illness, such as promotion or loss of job and shift work.

INTERVENTION IN CASES OF CHRONIC ILLNESS

The community health nurse working with families coping with chronic illness in a child, adult, or elder is aided by the family interview. As Glaser and Strauss (1975) in their classic work on chronic illness state, chronic illness interjects change into various areas of family life:

Sex and intimacy can be affected. Everyday mood and interpersonal relations can be affected. Visiting friends and engaging in other leisure time activities can be affected. Conflicts can be engendered by increased expenses stemming from unemployment and the medical treatment . . . different illnesses may have different kinds of impact on such areas of family life, just as they probably will call for different kinds of helpful agents.

(P. 67)

Changes in family patterns, fears, emotional responses, and expectations of individual family members can be assessed in the family interview. Special needs of the primary caretaker—often, the spouse, daughter, or daughter-in-law—can be assessed. The community health nurse making family visits to the elderly and terminally ill is able to assess intergenerational conflict and stress and to influence positively family interaction (Wright and Leahey, 1994).

Moving From the Family to the Community

Dreher (1982) stated that the practice of public health nursing is distinct from that of other specialties in nursing because of its scope and orientation to the care of the public, not because of its practice setting. Preparation of the public health nurse, according to this author, cannot be limited to "'following a family in the community'—paltry preparation for a career in caring for the health of the public" (p. 509). The care of entire populations is the major focus, as stated by Freeman in her classic work (1963):

The selection of those to be served . . . must rest on the comparative impact on community health rather than solely on the needs of the individual or family being served. . . . The public health nurse cannot elect to care for a small number of

people intensely while ignoring the needs of many others. She must be concerned with the population as a whole, with those in her caseload, with the need of a particular family as compared to the needs of others in the community.

(P. 35)

The challenge to the community health nurse, then, is to provide care to communities and populations and not to focus only on the levels of the individual and family. How does the community health nurse, who traditionally may carry a caseload of families, extend practice in the field with families to include a focus on the community? To do so, an aggregate, community, and population focus must serve as a backdrop to the entire practice.

For example, families must be viewed as components of communities. The community health nurse must know the community. As stated in Chapter 5, a thorough community assessment is necessary to practice in the community. By way of review, it is important to remember that communities must be compared not only in terms of differences in health needs but also in terms of differences in resources to effect intervention that will have an impact on policies and redistribute resources to ensure that the health needs of these communities and the families residing within them are met. As Dreher (1982) stated:

Data gathered about the physical, social, and demographic variables of the population being served are essential to provide an empirical basis for the development and delivery of nursing services. Unless these data, however, are viewed within a larger context—across communities—they will never serve to develop either the more encompassing theories which explain the relationship between society and health or the policies which will be most effective in assuring health and health care.

(P. 508)

SOURCES OF DATA ABOUT THE COMMUNITY'S HEALTH

National data are available from resources such as *Health, 1994* (NCHS, 1995, published annually), *Health Status of Minorities and Low Income Groups* (Department of Health and Human Services, 1991), and the *Morbidity and Mortality Weekly Report* (MMWR). State data are also provided in these publications. More in-depth data at the state level may be obtained from state department of health publications that give mortality and morbidity statistics. Local data are available from the census, city planners, and city or county departments of health (see Chapter 5).

Community health nurses must then compare city data with county data and then county data, state data, and national data. In addition, they may need to compare local census tract data and areas of a city or county with other areas of the city or county.

For example, community health nursing students in San Antonio who were planning home visits to families of pregnant adolescents attending a special high school compared local, state, and national statistics on infant mortality as a part of a community assessment. They found higher rates of infant mortality in San Antonio in census tracts on the south side of the city in which the population was predominantly Mexican-American. They also found the population to be younger, to have a higher rate of functional illiteracy among adults, to be less educated, to be more likely to drop out of high school, to have higher fertility rates, to have higher birth rates among adolescents, and to be more likely to be unemployed. They found that specific health needs varied among census tracts. Common major health needs of this subpopulation were thus identified from the community assessment, which assisted the students in planning care for these families. Their goals, for example, were broadened from carrying out interventions at the individual level to interventions at the family and community levels. In addition to targeting good perinatal outcomes for the individual teenage parent, nursing students planned to include assessments of functional literacy at the individual and family levels, and arranged for group sessions in clinic waiting rooms that informed and referred individuals and family members to alternative resources to enable teenage parents to complete school, take classes in English as a second language, and use resources for family planning and employment at the community level.

In addition to the cross-comparison of communities, the community health nurse also cross-compares the needs of the families within the communities and sets priorities. As the students just mentioned found that specific health needs varied among census tracts, so too the nurse in the community finds that specific health needs vary among families. The nurse must account for time spent with families and choose those families on the basis of their needs compared with the needs of others in the community.

DELEGATION OF SCARCE RESOURCES

Although the community health nurse serves the community or population as a whole, fiscal con-

DOUBLE STANDARD TOLERATED IN PUBLIC HEALTH

A double standard is tolerated in public health. Although the government is responsible for the maintenance of health, a minimal amount of health care is guaranteed each person because of the limitations of public resources. As Smith (1985) stated:

This prohibits discrimination based upon traits of persons that are not matters of free choice: for example, race, sex, and other congenital conditions; and wealth, poverty, or geographic location when these cannot be altered by the individual. (P. 143)

Thus, a minimum is established for all, yet as demonstrated with Medicare and Medicaid (see Chapter 3), unequal care exists as a result of differences in income (Medicare) and geographical location (Medicaid). In a market system, the wealthy can purchase all the health care services they desire; the poor cannot. The few supplemental resources provided by the government to ensure a minimum for all vary among communities, states, administrations, and countries.

straints hold the nurse accountable for the best delegation of scarce resources. Time spent on home visits has traditionally allowed the community health nurse to assess the environmental, social, and biological determinants of health status among the population and the resources available to them. Fiscal accountability, nevertheless, means setting priorities. Anderson and her colleagues in 1985 listed the factors that impact public health nursing practice, especially home visits, as "the need to justify personnel costs in a time of fiscal constraint, the increasing number of medically indigent who turn to local public health services for primary care, and the change in reimbursement mechanisms by the federal government and some states" (p. 146). In the shift to managed care, Anderson's observations still hold a decade later.

In a period of cost containment, the focus of community health nurses on prevention and health maintenance, areas difficult to justify, must carefully legitimate home visiting services by identifying aggregates in need of care. As stated in the definition of public health nursing by the Public Health Nursing Section of the American Public Health Association (1981):

Identifying the subgroups (aggregates) within the population which are at high risk of illness, disability, or premature death and directing resources toward these groups is the most effective approach for accomplishing the goal of public health nursing.   (P. 4)

Prioritizing groups at highest risk and using home visits to them in conjunction with planning for needs of larger aggregates are necessary. Hand-in-hand with this activity goes working for social and policy changes to alter the conditions that place these families at high risk. Little research has been done on the necessity for home visits in conjunction with group instruction or other agency-based care. Anderson and her colleagues (1985) reported a study of the integration of public health nursing and primary care in northern California. They found that "the teaching component of primary care and the continuity of nursing care from hospital to clinic and home for patients served by county medical services was strengthened" (p. 146). Populations at high risk that may benefit from home visiting are being identified (Brooten et al., 1986; Olds et al., 1988). Evidence indicates that costs are cut by home visits for high-risk infants in combination with other support systems such as social and medical services (Brooten et al., 1986).

What are the approaches to meeting the health needs of families? Many schools of thought exist among community health, community mental health, and public health nursing professionals. Dreher (1982) stated that the traditional basis for community health nursing intervention has a focus that has long endorsed psychological and social psychological theories to explain variations in health and patterns of health care, such as those set forth by Erikson (1963), Maslow (1970), and Duvall (1977). She stated that what is needed are "more encompassing theories which explain the relationship between society and health [and] the policies which will be most effective in assuring health and health care" (p. 508). To help bridge this gap, two approaches will be presented: meeting family health needs through the application of family theory, and extending family health intervention to larger aggregates and social action.

THE FAMILY THEORY APPROACH TO MEETING THE HEALTH NEEDS OF FAMILIES

There are many reasons why the community health nurse should work with families. Friedman (1992) listed the following six reasons:

- The belief that within the family unit any "dysfunction" (e.g., separation, disease, or injury) that affects one or more family members probably will affect other family members and the family as a whole.
- The wellness of the family is highly dependent on the role of the family in every aspect of health care, from prevention to rehabilitation.
- The level of wellness of the whole family can be raised through care that reduces lifestyle and environmental risks by emphasizing "health promotion, 'self-care,' health education, and family counseling" (p. 5).
- Commonalities in risk factors and disease shared by family members can lead to case finding within the family.
- A clear understanding of the functioning of the individual can be gained only when the individual is assessed within the larger context of the family.
- The family as a vital support system to the individual member needs to be incorporated into treatment plans.

For example, 10-year-old Jean Wilkie was referred by her teacher to the school nurse. She was withdrawn, had no school friends, and was dropping behind in her schoolwork. The school nurse talked to Jean in her office. Jean said that she had no friends because the other girls stayed overnight with each other "all the time" and that she did not want to bring her friends home because her father "drank all the time." The school nurse decided that Jean's problems needed assessment within the context of the family and arranged to visit the family at home. The father refused to participate in the family interview, but Jean's mother, her 13-year-old brother Peter, and Jean expressed concerns that the father had changed jobs several times in the past year, was frequently absent from work, and had been in two recent car accidents while "drinking." Thus, the school nurse was able to verify the family context as the basis of Jean's "problems" and to continue her family assessment and plan for intervention at the family level. In addition, she was prompted to assess the community's preventive efforts directed toward drinking and the ability to provide ongoing care for families of alcoholics.

Nurses have relied heavily on the social and behavioral sciences for approaches to working with families. These approaches include psychoanalytical, anthropological, systems or cybernetic, structural-functional, developmental, and interactional frameworks (for reviews, see Friedman, 1992; Whall and Fawcett, 1991; Wright and Leahey, 1994).

Three conceptual frameworks (systems, structural-functional, and developmental), often used by nurses in providing health care to families, are described.

Systems Approach

The systems approach has been widely used in diverse areas such as education, computer science, engineering, and communication. General systems theory (von Bertalanffy, 1968, 1972, 1974) has been applied to the study of families. General systems theory (see Chapter 3) is a way to explain how the family as a unit interacts with larger units outside the family and with smaller units inside the family (Friedman, 1992). The family may be affected by any disrupting force acting on a system outside it (suprasystem) or on a system within it (subsystem). Allmond and colleagues (1979) compared the family as a system with a piece of a mobile suspended from the air that is in constant movement with the other pieces of the mobile. At any time, the family, like any piece of the mobile, may be caught by a gust of air and become unbalanced, moving "chaotically" for a while; however, eventually, the stabilizing force of the other parts of the mobile will reestablish balance.

MAJOR DEFINITIONS FROM SYSTEMS THEORY

System: "A goal-directed unit made up of interdependent, interacting parts which endure over a period of time" (Friedman, 1992, p. 115); a family system is not concrete. It is made up of suprasystems and subsystems and must be viewed in a hierarchy of systems. The system under study at any given time is called the focal, or target, system. In this chapter, the family system will be the focal system.

Suprasystem: The suprasystem is the larger system of which the family is a part, such as the larger environment or the community (e.g., churches, schools, clubs, businesses, neighborhood organizations, gangs, and so on).

Subsystem: Subsystems are the smaller units of which the family consists, such as sets of relationships within the family (e.g., spouse, parent-child, sibling, or extended family).

Hierarchy of Systems: The hierarchy comprises the levels of units within the system and its environment that in their totality make up the universe. Higher level units are composed of lower level units (e.g., the biosphere is made up of communities, which are made up of families). Families are made up of family subsystems, and, in turn, family subsystems are made up of individuals, who are made up of organs, which are made of cells, and cells are made of atoms.

Boundaries: A boundary is an imaginary definitive line that forms a circle around each system and delineates the system from its environment. Auger (1976) conceptualized the boundary of a system as a " 'filter' which permits the constant exchange of elements, information, or energy between the system and its environments. . . . The more porous the filter, the greater the degree of interaction possible between the system and its environment" (p. 24). Families with rigid boundaries may lack necessary information and resources pertinent to maintaining family health or wellness.

Open System: An open system interacts with its surrounding environment—it gives outputs and gets inputs necessary to survival. An exchange of energy occurs. All living systems are open systems. However, if a boundary is too permeable, the system may be too open to input new ideas from the outside and may be unable to make decisions on its own (Wright and Leahey, 1994).

Closed System: A closed system theoretically does not interact with the environment. This is a self-sufficient system; no energy exchange occurs. Although no system has been found that exists in a totally closed state, if a family's boundaries are impermeable (i.e., less open as a system), needed input or interaction cannot occur. An example is the refugee family from Vietnam living in San Francisco; they may remain a closed family for some time because of differences in culture and language.

Input: Input is information, matter, or energy that the open system receives from its environment that is necessary to survival.

Output: Output is information, matter, or energy dispensed into the environment as a result of receiving and processing the input.

Flow and Transformation: The system's use of input may occur in two forms: some input may be used in its original state, and some input may have to be transformed before it is used. Both original and transformed input must be processed and flow through the system before being released as output (Friedman, 1992).

Feedback: Feedback is "the process by which a system monitors the internal and environmental responses to its behavior (output) and accommodates or adjusts itself" (Friedman, 1992,

p. 117). The system controls and modifies both inputs and outputs by "receiving and responding to the return of its own output" (Friedman, 1992, p. 117). Internally, the system adjusts by making changes in its subsystems. Externally, the system adjusts by making boundary changes.

Equilibrium: Equilibrium is a state of balance or steady state that results from self-regulation or adaptation. As with the concept of a system as a mobile in the wind, balance is dynamic and, with change, is always reestablishing itself.

Differentiation: Differentiation is the tendency for a system to actively grow and "advance to a higher order of complexity and organization" (Friedman, 1992, p. 117). Energy inputs into the system make this growth possible.

Energy: Energy is needed to meet a system's demands. Open systems will require more input through porous boundaries to meet high energy levels needed to maintain high levels of activity.

CHARACTERISTICS OF HEALTHY FAMILIES

In a classic work, Pratt (1976) characterized healthy families as "energized families" in the following ways:

- Members interact with each other repeatedly in many contexts.
- Members are enhanced and fulfilled by maintaining contacts with a wide range of community groups and organizations.
- Members make efforts to master their lives by becoming members of groups, finding information and options, and making decisions.
- Members engage in flexible role relationships, share power, respond to change, support growth and autonomy of others, and engage in decision making that affects them.

The following conceptual frameworks have been found useful in studying the family. Community health nurses have found them helpful in assessing the characteristics of families and their strengths and weaknesses and in planning interventions.

Structural-Functional Conceptual Framework

With the structural-functional conceptual framework approach to the family, the family is viewed according to its structure or the parts of the system and according to its function, or what the family does.

STRUCTURAL

Wright and Leahey (1994) stated that three aspects of family structure can be examined: internal structure, external structure, and context. *Internal structure* of the family refers to the following five categories:

ROLE RELATIONSHIPS

When Edna Smith, a 64-year-old client with severe arthritis, was diagnosed with diabetes, her longtime friend, Frank Gardens, a widower of several years, moved in with her and assumed a caretaker role. The community health nurse assessed the dietary habits of Mr. Gardens and Mrs. Smith and found that Mr. Gardens did the shopping and the cooking because Mrs. Smith's mobility was severely restricted as a result of her arthritis. Because Mr. Gardens did the cooking, he purchased canned fruits and vegetables rather than fresh or frozen. Cooking, which was a new role for Mr. Gardens, was perceived by him as demanding. After several visits, he disclosed to the nurse that his resistance to preparing fresh or frozen fruits and vegetables came from "the time it takes to clean the darn things, cook 'em, store 'em, and clean up the 'fridge when they go bad on ya." He stated unequivocally that it was stressful caring for Mrs. Smith and that he wanted to do it, but it was "much easier" to just "open a can" and "heat it in a pan" than to take the time and energy that preparation of fresh or frozen foods would require. The shift in roles that is often required of couples when one is diagnosed with a chronic illness can have an impact on the health of the family. For additional reading about how couples manage with chronic illness, see Corbin J, Strauss AL: Unending Work and Care: Management of Chronic Illness at Home. San Francisco, Jossey-Bass, 1988.

- Family composition, or who is in the family and changes in family constellation
- Gender
- Rank order, meaning positions of family members by age and sex

- Subsystem or labeling the subgroups or dyads (e.g., spouse, parental, interest) through which the family carries out its functions
- Boundary, or who participates in the family system and how (e.g., a single parent mother who does not allow her 17-year-old son to let his girlfriend spend the night in their home)

External structure refers to the extended family and larger systems (Wright and Leahey, 1994). It includes the following two categories:

- Extended family, including family of origin and family of procreation
- Larger systems, including work, health, and welfare

Context refers to the background or situation relevant to an event or personality in which the family system is nested (Wright and Leahey, 1994). It includes the following five categories:

- Ethnicity
- Race
- Social class
- Religion
- Environment

FUNCTIONAL

Wright and Leahey (1994) also dichotomized *family functional assessment,* or how family members behave toward each other, into two categories: instrumental functioning and expressive functioning. *Instrumental functioning* refers to activities of daily living (e.g., elimination, sleeping, eating, or giving insulin injections). This area takes on important meaning for the family when one member of the family becomes ill or disabled and is unable to carry out daily functions and must rely on other members of the family for assistance. For example, an elder may need assistance getting into the bathtub or a child may need to have medications measured and administered.

The second type of family functional assessment is *expressive functioning,* or affective or emotional aspects. This aspect has nine categories.

1. *Emotional communication:* Is the family able to express a range of emotions, including happiness, sadness, and anger?
2. *Verbal communication,* which focuses on the meaning of words. Do messages have clear meanings rather than distorted meanings? Wright and Leahey (1994) gave the example of masked criticism when a father states to his child, "Chil-

dren who cry when they get needles are babies" (p. 83).
3. *Nonverbal communication,* which includes, for example, any sounds, gestures, eye contact, touch, or inaction. An example is when a husband remains silent and stares out the window when his wife is talking to him.
4. *Circular communication* is commonly observed between dyads in families. A common example is the blaming, nagging wife and the guilty, withdrawn husband.
5. *Problem solving* refers to how the family solves problems. Who identifies problems? Someone inside or outside the family? What kinds of problems are solved? What patterns are used to solve and evaluate tried solutions?
6. *Roles* refer to "established patterns of behavior for family members" (Wright and Leahey, 1994, p. 88). Roles may be developed, delegated, negotiated, and renegotiated within the family. It takes other family members to keep a person in a particular role. Traditional roles are being challenged and are changing with economic and feminist changes; many women are entering the work force outside the home. Formal roles, with which the larger community agrees, may come into conflict with roles set by family and influenced by religious, cultural, and other belief systems.
7. *Influence* refers to methods used to affect the behavior of another. Instrumental influence refers to the use of reinforcement via objects or privileges (e.g., money, watching television, and so forth). Psychological influence refers to the influence of behavior through the use of communication or feelings. Corporal control refers to use of body contact (e.g., hugging, spanking, and so forth).
8. *Beliefs* refer to assumptions, ideas, and opinions that are held by family members and families as a whole. Beliefs shape the way families react to chronic or life-threatening illness. For example, if a family of a person with colon cancer believes in alternative treatments, then acupuncture may be a viable option for it to pursue.
9. *Alliances and coalitions* are important within the family. What dyads or triads appear to occur repeatedly in the family? Who starts arguments between dyads? Who stops arguments or fighting between dyads? Is there evidence of mother and father against child? When does this change to parent and child against the other parent? The balance and intensity of relationships be-

tween subsystems within the family are important to note. Questions may be asked regarding the permeability of the boundary. Does it cross generations?

SUMMARY OF FAMILY FUNCTIONAL ASSESSMENT

I. Instrumental functioning
   A. Activities of daily living
II. Expressive functioning
   A. Emotional communication
   B. Verbal communication
   C. Nonverbal communication
   D. Circular communication
   E. Problem solving
   F. Roles
   G. Influence
   H. Beliefs
   I. Alliances and coalitions

Data from Wright LM, Leahey M: Nurses and Families: A Guide to Family Assessment and Intervention, 2nd ed. Philadelphia, FA Davis, 1994.

DEVELOPMENTAL

Nurses are familiar with developmental states of individuals from prenatal through adult. Duvall (Duvall and Miller, 1985), a noted sociologist, is the forerunner of a focus on *family* development. In her classic work, she identified eight stages that normal families traverse from marriage to death.

FAMILY LIFE CYCLE

1. Beginning family (marriage)
2. Early childbearing family (eldest child is in infancy through 30 months old)
3. Preschool children (eldest child is 2.5–5 years old)
4. School-aged children (eldest child is 6–12 years old)
5. Teenage children (eldest child is 13–20 years old)
6. Launching family (oldest to youngest child leaves home)
7. Middle-age family (remaining marital dyad to retirement)
8. Aging family (retirement to death of both spouses)

Data from Duvall EM, Miller BC: Marriage and Family Development, 6th ed. New York, Harper & Row, 1985.

The community health nurse must comprehend these phases and the struggles that families go through during them to assess the family. Wright and Leahey (1994) called attention to the need to distinguish between "family development" and "family life cycle." They stated that the former is the *individual, unique* path a family goes through, whereas the latter is the *typical* path many families go through.

The following developmental categories outline the six stages of the middle-class North American family life cycle (Carter and McGoldrick, 1988; Wright and Leahey, 1994) and the tasks necessary for the family's resolution of each stage. The stages may be used by nurses to delineate family strengths and weaknesses.

STAGES AND TASKS OF MIDDLE-CLASS NORTH AMERICAN FAMILY LIFE CYCLE

I. Launching: the single young adult leaves home
   A. Coming to terms with the family of origin
   B. Development of intimate relationships with peers
   C. Establishment of self: career and finances
II. Marriage: The joining of families
   A. Formation of identity as a couple
   B. Including spouse in realignment of relationships with extended families
   C. Parenthood: making decisions
III. Families With Young Children
   A. Integration of children into family unit
   B. Adjusting tasks: childrearing, financial, and household
   C. Accommodation of new parenting and grandparenting roles
IV. Families With Adolescents
   A. Development of increasing autonomy for adolescents
   B. Reexamine midlife marital and career issues
   C. Initial shift toward concern for the older generation
V. Families as Launching Centers
   A. Establishment of independent identities for parents and grown children
   B. Renegotiation of marital relationship
   C. Readjust relationships to include in-laws and grandchildren
   D. Dealing with disabilities and death of older generation
VI. Aging Families
   A. Maintenance of couple and individual functioning while adapting to the aging process
   B. Support role of middle generation
   C. Support yet allow autonomy of older generation

D. Preparation for own death and dealing with the loss of spouse and/or siblings and other peers

Data from Wright LM, Leahey M: Nurses and Families: A Guide to Family Assessment and Intervention, 2nd ed. Philadelphia, FA Davis, 1994.

It is important to note, however, when reviewing these stages and tasks, that the profiles of families living in North America and in many other parts of the world are changing dramatically from what they have been in the recent past, both in structure and in form (Wright and Leahy, 1994). Language used in reference to the family should be inclusive of many kinds of "families," be they dual-career families, single parents, unmarried couples, gay or lesbian couples, including children, or remarried couples, and so on. Thus, terms such as "working mother," "children of divorce," or "fatherless home" should no longer be used when speaking of the family.

ALTERATIONS IN FAMILY DEVELOPMENT: DIVORCE AND REMARRIAGE

Alterations to the life cycle occur, as seen in previously reviewed statistics of separation, divorce, single-parent families, and remarriage. Carter and McGoldrick (1980, 1988) identified phases involved in the processes of divorce, postdivorce, and remarriage (Tables 13–1 and 13–2). The family must engage in emotional work as a result of divorce, a process that may occur suddenly or be long and drawn out. In her classic study, Stern (1982a) interviewed stepfather families in their homes and conceptualized the integration of the blended family once remarriage occurs as integration of two distinct family cultures. In addition, Stern (1982b) identified a set of affiliating strategies that can be taught to families that lead to stepfather–child friendship.

Assessment Tools

Many tools exist for the community health nurse to use in assessing the family (Friedman, 1992; Wright and Leahey, 1994). Reviewed here are the genogram, the ecomap, the family health tree, and a family health assessment.

GENOGRAM

The genogram is a tool that helps the nurse to outline the family's structure. It is a way to diagram the family

PERSONAL GOALS OF RECENTLY DIVORCED WOMEN

From divorce records in three counties, the authors identified recently divorced women with children. Of 528 women contacted by mail and by telephone, 252 completed questionnaires and interviews. The women described eight categories of personal goals. The most frequently cited goals were, in order of frequency, independence, employment, and education. Older women were more likely to choose employment and environmental goals over mental health goals than were younger women.

Data from Duffy ME, Mowbray CA, Hudes M: Personal goals of recently divorced women. Image J Nurs Sch 22:14–17, 1990.constellation, or "family tree." It is possible to fill out

the blank genogram (Fig. 13–1) for three generations of family members with the generally agreed-on symbols (Fig. 13–2) to denote geneology. Children are pictured from left to right, beginning with the oldest child.

The community health nurse may use the genogram during an early family interview, starting with a blank sheet of paper and drawing a circle or a square for the person initially interviewed. The nurse tells the family that several background questions will be asked to gain a general picture of the family. Circles may be drawn around family members living in separate households (Fig. 13–3). The Chan family, a refugee family from Vietnam, is a nuclear family. With the death of Mr. Chan upon the family's arrival in San Francisco 3 months before the first home visit (Fig 13–3), the family became a single-parent family. Although Mr. Chan is no longer physically present in the family, his presence is still felt, because the nurse learns the family has yet to express affectively their loss. Some families may be very cooperative in helping to fill out the genogram, freely relating significant information such as divorces and remarriages. Other families may be sensitive to such information, particularly when it is shown to recur with each generation.

FAMILY HEALTH TREE

The family health tree is another tool that is helpful to the community health nurse (Fig. 13–4). Based on the genogram, the family health tree provides a mechanism for recording the family's medical and health histories (Diekelmann, 1977; Friedman, 1992). Causes

Table 13–1
Dislocations of the Family Life Cycle Requiring Additional Steps to Restabilize and Proceed Developmentally

Phase	Emotional Process of Transition; Prerequisite Attitude	Developmental Issues
Divorce		
1. The decision to divorce	Acceptance of inability to resolve marital tensions sufficiently to continue relationship	Acceptance of one's own part in the failure of the marriage
2. Planning the breakup of the system	Supporting viable arrangements for all parts of the system	a. Working cooperatively on problems of custody, visitation, and finances b. Dealing with extended family about the divorce
3. Separation	a. Willingness to continue cooperative coparental relationship b. Work on resolution of attachment to spouse	a. Mourning loss of intact family b. Restructuring marital and parent-child relationships; adaptation to living apart c. Realignment of relationships with extended family; staying connected with spouse's extended family
4. The divorce	More work on emotional divorce: Overcoming hurt, anger, guilt, and so on	a. Mourning the loss of intact family: giving up fantasies of reunion b. Retrieval of hopes, dreams, and expectations from the marriage c. Staying connected with extended families
Postdivorce family		
1. Single-parent family	Willingness to maintain parental contact with ex-spouse and support contact of children and ex-spouse and ex-spouse's family	a. Making flexible visitation arrangements with ex-spouse and ex-spouse's family b. Rebuilding own social network
2. Single-parent (noncustodial)	Willingness to maintain parental contact with ex-spouse and support custodial parent's relationship with children	a. Finding ways to continue effective parenting relationship with children b. Rebuilding own social network

From Wright LM, Leahey M. Nurses and Families: A Guide to Family Assessment and Intervention. Philadelphia, FA Davis, 1984, p. 52, as adapted from Carter E, McGoldrick M (1980). The family life cycle and family therapy: An overview. *In* Carter E, McGoldrick M: The Family Life Cycle: A Framework for Family Therapy. New York, Gardner Press, 1980, pp. 3–28.

Table 13–2		
Remarried Family Formation: A Developmental Outline		
Steps	**Prerequisite Attitude**	**Developmental Issues**
1. Entering the new relationship	Recovery from loss of first marriage (adequate "emotional divorce")	Recommitment to marriage and to forming a family with readiness to deal with the complexity and ambiguity
2. Conceptualizing and planning new marriage and family	Accepting one's own fears and those of new spouse and children about remarriage and forming a stepfamily Accepting need for time and patience for adjustment to complexity and ambiguity of: a. Multiple new roles b. Boundaries: space, time, membership, and authority c. Affective issues: guilt, loyalty conflicts, desire for mutuality, and unresolvable past hurts	a. Work on openness in the new relationships to avoid pseudomutuality b. Plan for maintenance of cooperative coparental relationships with ex-spouse(s) c. Plan to help children deal with fears, loyalty conflicts, and membership in two systems d. Realignment of relationships with extended family to include new spouse and children e. Plan maintenance of connections for children with extended family of ex-spouse(s)
3. Remarriage and reconstitution of family	Final solution of attachment to previous spouse and ideal of "intact" family: Acceptance of a different model of family with permeable boundaries	a. Restructuring family boundaries to allow for inclusion of new spouse-stepparent b. Realignment of relationships throughout subsystems to permit interweaving of several systems c. Making room for relationships of all children with biological (noncustodial) parents, grandparents, and other extended family d. Sharing memories and histories to enhance stepfamily integration

From Wright LM, Leahey M. Nurses and Families: A Guide to Family Assessment and Intervention. Philadelphia, FA Davis, 1984, p. 53, as adapted from Carter E, McGoldrick M (1980). The family life cycle and family therapy: An overview. *In* Carter E, McGoldrick M: The Family Life Cycle: A Framework for Family Therapy. New York, Gardner Press, 1980, pp. 3–28.

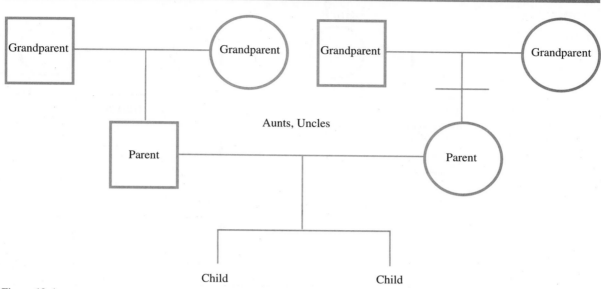

Figure 13–1
Genogram. (Redrawn from Wright LM, Leahey M. Nurses and Families: A Guide to Family Assessment and Intervention, 2nd ed. Philadelphia: FA Davis, 1984.)

of death of deceased family members, when known, are important. Genetically linked diseases, including heart disease, cancer, diabetes, hypertension, sickle cell anemia, allergies, asthma, and mental retardation, can be noted. Environmental and occupational diseases, psychosocial problems such as mental illness and obesity, and infectious diseases should also be noted. From health problems, familial risk factors can be noted. Risk factors can also be noted by inquiring about what family members do to prevent illness, such as having periodic physical examinations, Papanicolaou smears, and immunizations. Lifestyle-related risk factors can be assessed by asking what family members do to "handle stress" and to "keep in shape." The family health tree can be used in planning positive familial influences on risk factors, such as dietary, exercise, coping with stress, or pressure to have a physical examination.

ECOMAP

The ecomap (Fig. 13–5) is another classic tool that is used to depict a family's linkages to their suprasystems (Hartman, 1979; Wright and Leahey, 1994). As originally stated by Hartman (1978):

The eco-map portrays an overview of the family in their situation; it depicts the important nurturant or conflict-laden connections between the family and the world. It demon-

strates the flow of resources, or the lacks and deprivations. This mapping procedure highlights the nature of the interfaces and points to conflicts to be mediated, bridges to be built, and resources to be sought and mobilized.

(P. 467)

As with the genogram, the ecomap may be filled out during an early family interview, noting persons, institutions, and agencies significant to the family. Symbols used in attachment diagrams (see Fig. 13–2) may be used to denote the nature of the ties that exist. For example, in Figure 13–6, the Chan family ecomap suggests that few contacts occur between the family and the suprasystems. The community health nursing student was able to use the ecomap to discuss with the family the types of resources in the community and the types of relationships they wanted to establish with them.

These tools for family assessment can be used with families in every health care setting to increase the nurse's awareness of the family within the community and to help guide the nurse and the family in the assessment and planning phases of care.

FAMILY HEALTH ASSESSMENT

Many agencies in the community have developed guidelines for assessment of the family that help practitioners identify the health status of individual

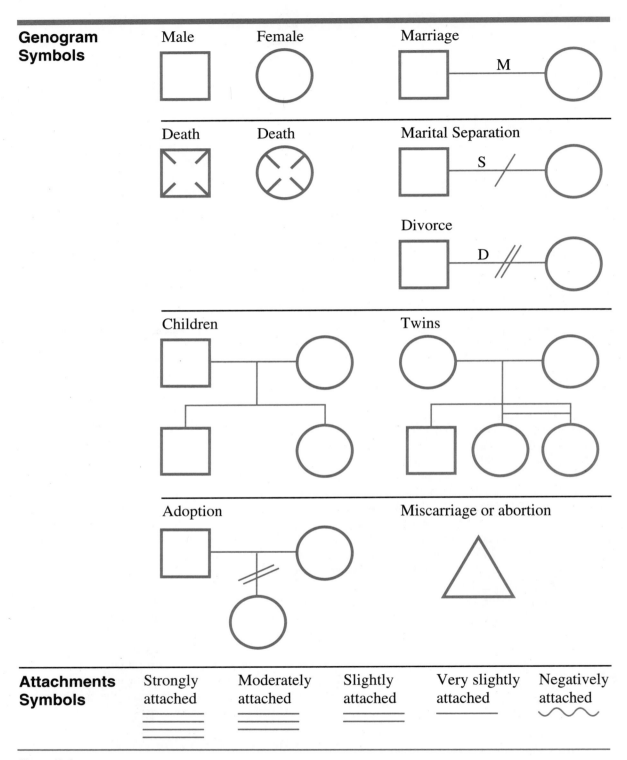

Figure 13–2
Genogram and attachment symbols. (Redrawn from Wright LM, Leahey M. Nurses and Families: A Guide to Family Assessment and Intervention, 2nd ed. Philadelphia: FA Davis, 1984.)

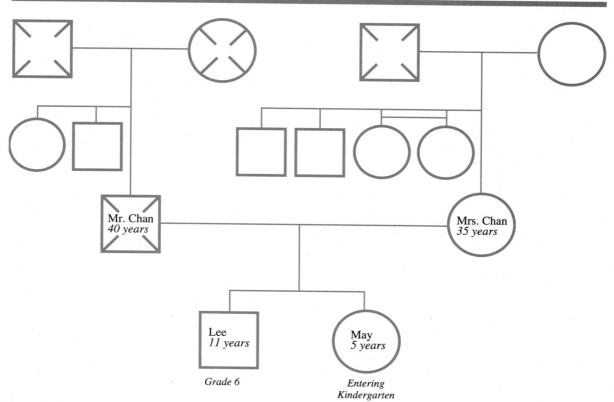

Figure 13–3
Sample genogram of Chan family.

members of the family and aspects of family composition, function, and process. Often included in family health assessment guidelines is information about the environment, or community context, as well as information about the family. The Family Health Assessment (Fig. 13–7) is an example of a guideline that may be used to assist in data collection and organization of the data collected from families over time. Bergman et al. (1993) reviewed four key family characteristics that can impact how persons recover from and function over time following health-related disruptions: *family cohesion,* or emotional bonding of family members and the degree of individual autonomy of each person in the family; *family adaptation,* or the degree of flexibility evidenced by the ability to change roles, relationships, and power structures in response to stress; *family social integration* or the degree of social network with neighbors, friends, other family members, and religious or social organizations; and *the degree of stress experienced by the family,* including com-

binations of stressors that may impact the family. Information for the Family Health Assessment may be obtained by interviews of one or more family members individually, interviews of subsystems within the family, such as dyads of mother-child, parent-parent, sibling-sibling, and so on, or group interviews with more than two members of the family. Information may also be obtained through observation of individual family members, dyads, and the entire family and observation of the environment in which the family lives, including housing, the neighborhood, and the larger community. Family assessment tools have been developed both by nurses and by other professionals such as sociologists, social workers, and psychologists working with families to assess a range of dimensions of the family such as marital satisfaction, parental coping abilities, and family dysfunction (see Hanson and Mischke, 1996, for a review and listing of family assessment tools). An example is the Family Adaptability and Cohesion Evaluation

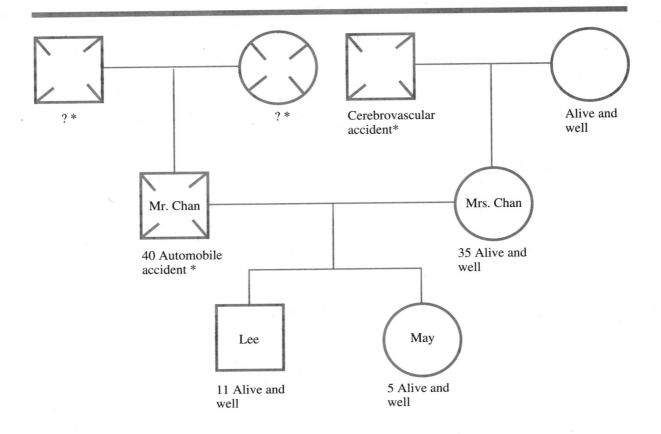

? *   ? *   Cerebrovascular   Alive and
                                    accident*   well

Mr. Chan   Mrs. Chan

40 Automobile   35 Alive and
accident *   well

            Lee   May

            11 Alive and   5 Alive and
            well   well

* Cause of death.

Figure 13–4
Chan family health tree. (Modified from Diekelman N. Primary Health Care of the Well Adult. New York, McGraw-Hill, 1977. Reproduced with permission of McGraw-Hill, Inc.)

Scale (FACES I), which assesses family interactions, cohesion, and adaptability, although completed by each individual in the family (Olson et al., 1979). Observation of communication and behavior of the individual, a dyad, or a family can also provide important information. For example, a mother's self-report about her communication with her husband may be different from observation of interaction between the couple. The "ability to negotiate" is a characteristic that cannot be attributed to one person but may be obvious from observation of the couple. "Conflict avoidance" may be obvious from observation of the entire family. It is important, however, not to attribute a characteristic of the entire family, such as "flexible," to each individual in the family because an individual family member, away from the family, may be quite rigid (Copeland,

1990). The Family Health Assessment addresses family characteristics, including structure and process, and family environment, including residence, neighborhood, and community. Not all dimensions on the Family Health Assessment will be appropriate for every family; content of the assessment guideline should thus be modified and adapted as necessary to fit the individual family. The guidelines should serve as a guide only, as a means to record pertinent information about the family that will assist the nurse in working with the family. Information in the assessment should be gathered spontaneously over several contacts with the family and with various members and dyads within the family. It should also include multiple forays into the community, neighborhood, and home in which the family resides. Thus, several contacts with the family will no doubt be required to complete the Family Health Assessment.

SOCIAL AND STRUCTURAL CONSTRAINTS

In addition to the tools just reviewed, an important aspect of family assessment and planning for intervention is the need to make note of the social and structural constraints that prevent families from achieving a state of health or receiving care, in particular, the health care they need. These constraints explain why some families differ in mortality rates, in ability to achieve "integrity" rather than "despair," or in ability to "self-actualize." Social and structural constraints are usually based in social and economic causes, which affect a wide range of conditions associated with major health indicators (mortality and morbidity), such as literacy, education, and employment. Families most frequently served by the community health nurse are the disadvantaged, those who are unable to buy health care from the private sector. Constraints to obtaining needed health and social services by these families are well documented, however, and may more often be due to characteristics of the health and social services rather than individual limitations of the family. These constraints may be noted on the ecomap, because they influence each

family's ability to interact with a specific agency. For example, in addition to noting the strength of the relationship between family and agency or institution, those constraints that prevent use or full use of the resource should be noted. Constraints include hours of service, distance and transportation, availability of interpreters, and criteria for receiving services such as age, sex, and income barriers. Specific examples include the different guidelines posed by each state for Medicaid and by each community for home-delivered meals to the homebound.

Helping families understand constraints and linking them to accessible resources is necessary, but intervention at the family level is not sufficient. The common basic human needs of families in a community add up, and structural constraints faced repeatedly by families must be tallied by the community health nurse and compared with those of families in other communities. Intervention may then be planned and carried out at the aggregate level. Muecke (1984) reported the process of community health nursing diagnosis carried out by undergraduate community health nursing students among households in Seattle of Mien refugees from Laos. The following section is an overview of how community health nurses can extend intervention at the family level to larger aggregates and social action.

EXTENDING FAMILY HEALTH INTERVENTION TO LARGER AGGREGATES AND SOCIAL ACTION

Institutional Context of Family Therapists

Many theories exist to help bridge the gap between the application of nursing and family theory to the family and broader social action on the behalf of communities of families. Most family theorists view the family as a system that interfaces with outside suprasystems or institutions only when there is a problem to be addressed, such as in the school or a courtroom. Examples of three approaches that go beyond the family as a system to address the interaction between the family and the larger social system are the following:

- The ecological approach
- Network therapy
- The transactional model

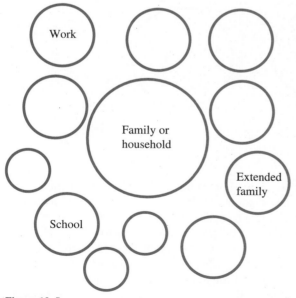

Figure 13–5
Ecomap. (Redrawn from Hartman A. Diagrammatic assessment of family relationships. Soc. Casework 59;469, 1978.)

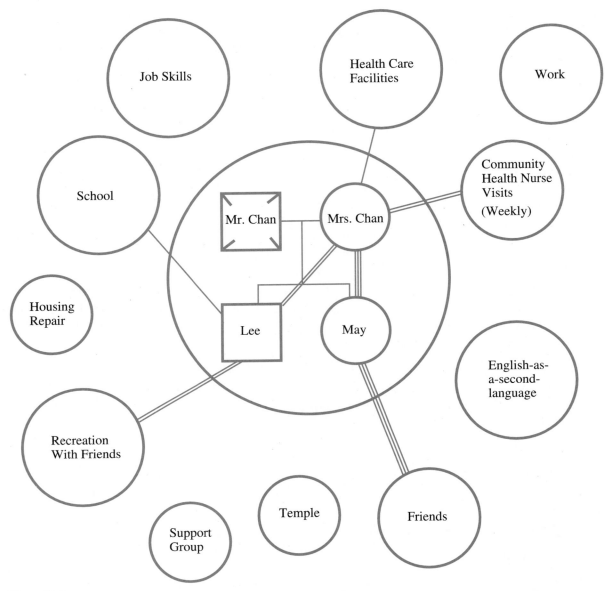

Figure 13–6
Sample ecomap of Chan family.

ECOLOGICAL APPROACH

The ecological approach indicts the specialization and fragmentation seen in the social and health service structure based on Western concepts of time and space. This approach focuses on providing a more complex and flexible structure. Helping families transcend rigid boundaries and intake procedures of agencies that they need to maintain themselves in their environment is essential, as is changing the social and health service

structure. For example, Koepke (1994), in a study investigating health care settings as resources for giving information to parents, found less than a third of 82 physicians' waiting rooms to provide parenting information. A majority of the physicians, however, agreed to display parenting pamphlets for a trial period; all found them helpful to patients and desired additional pamphlets. A simple intervention can aid families in a traditional health care setting. Another example of a study using an ecological approach is one

Text continued on page 326

FAMILY HEALTH ASSESSMENT

Family surname: _____

Household members (name, age, relationship to head of household): _____

_____

_____

_____

_____

Family composition: _____

_____

_____

Genogram:

Family health tree (include health problems of individual members):

Ecomap (for social and health agencies include hours of service, distance and transportation, availability of interpreters, and criteria for receiving services such as age, sex, and income barriers):

Family Characteristics	**Source(s) of Information**	**Date**
Extended family Relatives living outside household		
Location of relatives		
Frequency and duration of contact		

Figure 13–7

Family Characteristics	Source(s) of Information	Date
Means of communication		

Family mobility
Length of time living in residence

Location of previous residence

Frequency of geographic moves

Country/area of origin

Family structure
Educational experiences

Employment history

Financial resources

Leisure time interests

Division of labor

Allocation of roles

Distribution of authority and power

Family cohesion
Emotional bonding of family members

Degree of individual autonomy

Family adaptation
Flexibility in role change

Flexibility in power structures

Figure 13–7 *Continued*

Family Characteristics	**Source(s) of Information**	**Date**

Family processes
How members communicate

_____

How decisions are made

_____

How problems are solved

_____

How conflict is handled

_____

Family social integration
Language(s) and/or dialect(s) spoken; where

_____

Literacy; ability to read or write in language(s)

_____

Degree of racial or cultural identity

_____

Degree of social network with neighbors, friends, other family members

_____

Network with religious organizations

_____

Network with social organizations

_____

Degree of stress experienced by the family
Combinations of stressors:

1. _____

2. _____

3. _____

_____

Family health behavior
Activities of daily living (how family spends typical day)

_____

Health history

_____

Health status (problems, priorities)

_____

Risk behaviors

_____

Figure 13–7 *Continued*

Family Characteristics	Source(s) of Information	Date
Self-care (health promotion, prevention)		

Health care resources
  Professionals, lay healers
  Working with family, agencies		

Family strengths		
Family priorities		
Family–nurse contract(s)		

Family cultural influences
  Values, attitudes, and beliefs about
    Spirituality

    Rituals (holidays, celebrations)

    Customs

    Dietary habits

    Child-rearing practices

    Health

    Folk diseases, folk medicine

    Cultural healers

    Care of ill family member

    Role of spiritual leader in care of ill family member

Family Environment	Source(s) of Information	Date
Family residence Adequacy of size		
Structurally safe		
Sanitation: water, sewage, garbage		
Adequacy of sleeping arrangement		

Figure 13–7 *Continued*

Family Environment	Source(s) of Information	Date
Cooking and refrigeration		
Storage of medicines, cleaning agents		
Loose rugs		
Smoke alarm		
Emergency numbers		

Family neighborhood
　Location (e.g., urban, rural)

　Type (e.g., semicommercial)

　Age composition

　Safety
　　Traffic patterns

　　Lighting

　　Security (police)

　Density (noise, crowding, poverty, crime)

　Modes of transportation

　Resources
　　Grocery shopping

　　Pharmacy

　　Recreational (e.g., parks)

　　Educational

　　Religious

　　Emergency (fire, hospital)

Figure 13–7 *Continued*

Family Environment	Source(s) of Information	Date
Neighborhood interaction		

Family community
Industry, business

Leadership

Government

Migration (in and out of community)

Community memberships/interaction

Social services

Health services
Primary care

Institutions (e.g., hospital, nursing home)

Figure 13–7   *Continued*

that assessed health risk in homeless urban elderly and described various hazards within a single geographical area over a 24-hour period (Reilly, 1994). The spatial-temporal distribution of resources, factors in the natural environment, including temperature and patterns of daylight and dark, and factors in the human-created environment, such as crime and traffic patterns, were identified as hazards within the urban environment. Hazards of importance to homeless elderly also included the social milieu, the effects of aging, homelessness, and behavior such as alcohol abuse. The interactive effect caused by the convergence of hazards and nursing interventions to reduce risk is presented.

NETWORK THERAPY

This involves changing the network of families, be it extended family or friends, who tend to maintain a dysfunctional status quo in the nuclear family. This is done by replacing the network with others from the wider system who would be able to provide more support and therefore enhance the functioning of the family. Examples of network therapy are drawn from community mental health. In a study evaluating the social networks of 24 persons with schizophrenia 1 year after social network therapy, 12 of the 24 persons showed significant improvement in their social network (Gillies et al., 1993). In comparison to the unimproved group, the improved group had an increase in the number of reciprocal relationships, an increase in the number of confidants, and improvement in scales measuring psychotic symptoms, anxiety, and depression. In Britain, a review of the literature about social networks of persons with long-term mental illness showed that larger social networks are associated with a more favorable prognosis than smaller social networks (Brewer et al., 1994). A day care approach to care of persons with long-term mental illness, the Community Group Network model, is presented as advantageous to these persons over other day care approaches. Biegel and colleagues (1994) described a model to aid mental health case managers who desire to increase the natural support systems of their clients through community resource development and building of community ties. Building support systems for vulnerable populations such as the chronically mentally ill remains a challenge in the community, yet may be enhanced through social network therapy.

TRANSACTIONAL MODEL

In this model, the term "transaction" refers to a system in process with a system, where the focus is on process as opposed to a linear approach, which may lead to blaming or labeling. The family as an institution, along with other institutions whether religious, educational, recreational, or governmental, is said to be culturally anchored. That is, each holds a distinct set of beliefs and values about the nature of the world and about human existence. An awareness of culture (e.g., beliefs and values) as it is expressed in each system, in particular, as it is expressed in mainstream U.S. values, versus the value patterns of the family is important. Examples of research using the transactional model are the following. A study of parent influences on the self-esteem of children from economically disadvantaged families used data from both parents and their children and reported the influence of the parents on the child's self-concept and self-esteem, parental support, children's competencies, childrearing practices, and family conflict (Killeen, 1993). A study of common stressors and coping strategies in rural adolescents defined coping as "a cognitive and transactional process between a person and the person's environment" (p. 50) and included events related to school, family, friendship, health, and transportation (Puskar et al., 1993). In working with culturally and ethnically diverse families, in particular, an awareness of the culture of origin, how the family's values are changing according to where they are in the process of acculturation, and the family's interpretation of the mainstream U.S. values is essential to viewing the transaction of systems with each other.

Models of Social Class and Health Services

Social class places major limitations on access to medical care. For example, the poor have long been known to use health services at lower rates than the middle class. For example, in 1991 to 1993, poor or near-poor children received less ambulatory care than nonpoor children (National Center for Health Statistics [NCHS], 1995). The average number of physician contacts per year for poor or near-poor children was 23 to 26% less (4.3–4.4 visits) than for nonpoor children (5.4 visits). In 1993, the age-adjusted percent of persons who did not see a physician in the preceding 2 years was more than 50% greater in persons with low family incomes (less than $14,000) than among persons with high incomes ($50,000 or more) (8% vs. 13%, respectively).

Between 1980 and 1993, the age-adjusted percentage of persons younger than 65 years of age without health care coverage increased from 12.5% to 17.3% (NCHS, 1995). *Those without health care coverage included persons not covered by private insurance, Medicaid, Medicare, or military plans.* In 1993, 35% of those with family incomes of less than $14,000 were without health care coverage compared with 5% of those with family incomes of $50,000 or more.

Among a number of other differences in access to health care in the United States are race and region of the country. For example, in 1993, Hispanic persons were more than twice as likely as white persons to be without health care coverage (34% vs. 16%, respectively) (NCHS, 1995). African-Americans were also less likely to have coverage than white persons (23% vs. 16%, respectively). A greater proportion of persons living in the southern part of the United States were less likely to have any health care coverage (21.9%) than those living in the Midwest (11.9%), in the Northeast (14.3%), and in the West (19.0%).

Another difference in access, affected by income, is the setting in which persons receive health care. In 1992, the location of visits where ambulatory care occurred was different for white and African-American persons. Sixteen percent fewer African-Americans used physicians' offices than did whites (263 and 312 per 100 persons, respectively) (NCHS, 1995). Use of hospital outpatient departments by African-Americans was double that for whites (40 vs. 20 visits per 100 persons). African-Americans were also more likely to receive ambulatory care in hospital emergency rooms than were whites (55 vs. 34 visits per 100 persons).

A classic theoretical perspective used to explain the reasons for these disparities was suggested three decades ago by medical sociologists as a *culture of poverty view* of life that discouraged self-reliance

(Lewis, 1966). Reasons for lack of use of health services included a crisis-orientation, a living-for-the-moment attitude, a low value of health, and a lack of psychological "readiness." Another explanation is the *structural view*, which considers constraints that limit use of medical care, such as material constraints (money to buy services), and characteristics of health care settings for the poor, in contrast to private office practices available for the nonpoor, such as hours available, waiting time, transportation, block appointments, specialty clinics, and disease-oriented rather than preventive care.

Research has looked at use of health care using attitudes and beliefs to test the culture of poverty explanation and using financial and systems barriers to test the structural explanation (Riessman, 1984). Although studies have acknowledged some problems methodologically and with generalizability, evidence supports the findings that unequal use of health care is more a result of the system of care rather than of individual characteristics of persons seeking care. For example, Patrick (1992) compared health status and health care utilization of the insured and uninsured residents of Washington State and found that both health status and health care utilization were influenced by insurance coverage. The uninsured had more sinus problems than insured families after family characteristics were controlled for (income, family size, education, ethnicity). The uninsured also used health services less frequently, as they made fewer ambulatory visits to health care providers and reported fewer hospitalizations. Yet the uninsured reported more often that the emergency room was their usual source of care and even attributed limited access of health care to cost barriers.

With recent cutbacks in services and the increased closing of public hospitals, increasingly more persons are forced to attend overcrowded public clinics where professionals have little control over the nature of their work and little time to establish ongoing relationships with clients. Riessman (1984) stated that increasing clients' access to these kinds of services is not in itself sufficient. Instead, she noted changes called for by a new generation of medical sociologists (i.e., changes in the culture of medicine with its technological approach to human problems that separates the provider from the consumer and the consumer from a network of family and friends in society). Although managed care settings provide access to a primary care provider who will see the patient over time, the amount of time clinicians can spend with patients is usually closely regulated; also, the amount of control over their work has yet to be established, as well as the ability of the provider to link the consumer to a network of family and friends.

Models of Care for Communities of Families

Models exist to guide the community health nurse in providing care to communities of families in special need of services that improve access, equality between consumer and provider, and sensitivity to human need. Riessman (1984) reviewed two classic models; one, initiated by consumer efforts, is an alternative childbirth center, Su Clinica Familiar. This center is located in the Rio Grande Valley in South Texas. It is situated in a "family-oriented rural health clinic" and serves mostly low-income Mexican-American agricultural worker families. Services (93%) were given by nurse-midwives between 1972 and 1979. Prenatal care and professionally assisted deliveries that encouraged family participation were made available to women who previously lacked access to care. Outcomes showed lower rates of prematurity than the state average, favorable birth weights, and positive Apgar scores.

A second model was initiated by a pediatrics department within an urban teaching hospital. This alternative delivery model offered home care for chronically ill children of poor, largely black and Hispanic families in New York City. A team focus that involved home visits by pediatric nurse practitioners was compared with usual in-hospital care. No difference existed between the families receiving home care and standard hospital care at 6 months in impact on the family and functional status of the child. Significant differences did exist at 6 and 12 months, however, for psychological adjustment of the child and the mother's satisfaction with medical care: the home care group was favored.

Riessman (1984) stated that these alternative programs were strategies to change the structural barriers that prevent access to care for low-income families. Professional role functions changed as nurses provided health care rather than physicians. Active self-care was promoted, and health and medical knowledge was shared. Assistance by family and social networks was encouraged. Riessman warned, however, that although both programs addressed aspects of the cultural critique of medicine, the programs did not "address the social determinants of disease." Neither program addresses the health-damaging conditions that poor persons face, such as poor housing, malnutrition, and environmental hazards at the work place and in the community. Although these programs represent steps in the right direction, changes in access to medical and health services is not enough; social changes are also necessary.

Two health care delivery models initiated by community health nurses to promote access to care for families are presented, the Block Nurse Program and the De Madres a Madres program.

BLOCK NURSE PROGRAM

A block nurse program was initiated in St. Paul, Minnesota, by community health nurses (Jamieson, 1990; Jamieson and Martinson, 1983; Martinson et al., 1985). The program links registered nurses who live closest to families that have elders who need care with nursing services, medical supervision, and support services such as social work and volunteers. Based on a community needs assessment, census data showed that the 1-square-mile geographical area of St. Anthony's Park had a population of 6969. Of this population, 12.5% (872) were age 65 or older. Of these elders, more than half lived in family households, 33% lived in nonfamily households, and approximately 17% lived in "group quarters." Annual incomes of households were below the poverty level ($7500) for 26%, which accounted for approximately 5.2% of all elders living in the district.

Eighteen of more than 40 registered nurses who lived in the same district signed up to assist their elderly neighbors by making nursing services available to them to keep them out of hospitals and nursing homes. They were also involved in prevention and case finding. The nurses became roster nurses for the Ramsey County Public Health Nursing Service and completed 60 hours of gerontological nursing courses. Services are covered by Medicare, Medicaid, third-party insurance, and private funds. Private funding was needed because many of the nursing services needed by persons with chronic illness are not covered under current reimbursement guidelines. Careful documentation of services that are not covered will be useful to show the need for health policy and programs to cover services in the home that ultimately cut the cost of more expensive hospitalization and nursing home care.

With the projected increase of the elderly population and the early discharge from hospitals related to managed care and case management to cut costs, the need for nursing services for this aggregate of elders is clear. Keeping persons with chronic illness in the home is a priority for the future.

DE MADRES A MADRES PROGRAM

A partnership for health program was initiated in Houston, Texas, by community health nursing faculty at the College of Nursing, Texas Women's University using the empowerment education model as developed by Freire (Freire, 1983; Mahon et al., 1991; McFarlane and Fehir, 1994). Funded by the Houston March of Dimes and the W. K. Kellogg Foundation, the program originally linked the general public, businesses, volunteer mothers, and a community health nurse with a targeted community of high-risk Hispanic mothers in need of early prenatal care, a major public health and community problem. The peer education program, named by the volunteer mothers, De Madres a Madres (from mothers to mothers), trains volunteer Hispanic women to identify women at risk of late prenatal care in the community, to provide culturally relevant information about resources in the community, and to give social support. Methods of providing information in culturally acceptable milieus was a priority. Examples include group meetings in a food pantry in the community, in the homes of the volunteers, or in the homes of the women at risk. During the first year of the program, 14 volunteer mothers contacted more than 2000 women at risk of delayed prenatal care. The program grew and eventually a home was rented, a volunteer mother was hired to manage the center, and two community health nurses were hired to assist in the development of the community coalition. The center became a hub of community activity and the source of empowerment of women as it responded to community needs such as the inaccessibility of eligibility cards for health care. Men and children came with the women and received information about not only health care, but also about food, shelter, child care, legal aid, and employment. Outreach efforts extended to schools, banks, bakeries, and supermarkets within the community. By the end of the fifth year, the volunteers changed their mission statement from targeting prenatal care for high-risk pregnant women to providing support for families in the Near North Side of Houston. The transfer of power from the professionals occurred as the professionals taught grant development skills, budgets, and networking with funding agencies to the volunteers. A grant from the Hogg Foundation for Mental Health was given to reach high-risk Hispanic families with a "parent-to-parent" support program. The volunteers have purchased the building, secured operating funds from foundations, and now have paid staff. In addition, they have begun a business to create and market handicrafts to fund their outreach efforts. As necessary for true community empowerment, the professionals have left; they now serve as volunteers on the board of directors and the advisory board.

Clearly, these programs initiated by community health nurses also represent steps in the right direction to overcome barriers to medical and health services among the elderly and high-risk women and families. The need to address social determinants of health, such as poor housing, malnutrition, and poverty, call for such efforts and even more proactive social change programs by nurses, the community, and the country. For additional reports of action research by community health nurses at the community level, which address many of the social determinants of health, see Flick and associates' (1994) report of building community for health, and Flynn and colleagues' (1994) report of their Healthy Cities projects.

APPLICATION OF THE NURSING PROCESS

The Home Visit

Home visiting is increasing in popularity in some contexts and coming under increased scrutiny in others. Providing health care in the home to persons with an identified health problem has been shown to be cheaper than hospital care (Berg and Helgeson, 1984; Brooten et al., 1986). The shift in financial structure to proprietary or for-profit corporations in home health care poses difficult questions for community health nursing. Although the home health care client has the same basic human needs now as before the shift to a market system, the shift creates an ethical dilemma: that of belief in market justice versus social justice. Questions about cost effectiveness of home visiting to well families in face of limited public health resources have resulted in home visiting to largely high-risk populations. Setting priorities and visiting groups (families) in the community at high risk of illness, disability, or premature death is becoming ever necessary because of the current focus on cost constraints. Financial and other considerations are made in conjunction with an agency's policy regarding home visits (see Chapter 28).

This section will present the application of the nursing process to a family on a home visit. The example will note the use of the home visit to identify a high index of suspicion of needs of larger aggregates within the community and consequent programs planned to meet those needs, which ultimately will benefit a population of families in the future.

The home visit is a crucial experience for both the student and the family (Warner et al., 1994). Important factors that may impact the home visit include the family's background experience with the health care system, the agency in which the student is working, the family's experience with previous students who have visited the family, and the background of the student. For example, student characteristics may vary; the student brings differing levels of knowledge of medical and nursing practice, of self, and of the community.

The student brings previous learning about families, family-related theory, the growth and development of members of different ages within a family, disease processes, and access to the health care system. Because curricula within schools of nursing vary, some students will also bring preparation in all specialties—medical-surgical, childbearing, parent-child nursing, and psychiatric and mental health nursing—to the experience. Others may be taking basic clinical courses such as pediatrics and psychiatric–mental health nursing concurrently with community health. Thus, the need for review of appropriate theory, health education, and standard assessment tools for individuals and for families will vary.

The student's knowledge of self, previous life experience, and values are also important. Research reveals that conflict related to culture exists in the delivery of health care (see Chapters 17, 18, 19, and 20). For example, in a study of community health nurses' conceptions of low-income black, Mexican-American, and white family lifestyles and health care patterns, Erkel (1985) found that respondents could not identify major health care delivery problems in giving care to different ethnic groups. Yet only half the respondents felt they could work equally well with each group. Students must recognize their strengths and weaknesses in these areas in preparation for entering a new community.

Knowledge of the community and level of comfort with a new environment, in particular, one outside the student's previous experience, are also important. Additional preparation by all students will be necessary before the first home visit is made, depending on the content of the referral.

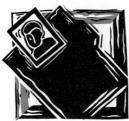

Case Study

The first home visit is usually initiated by a referral. The source of a referral may be, for example, a clinic, a school, a private physician, or an agency responsible for the care of a particular aggregate. Doris Wilson received a referral to visit the Chan family from the Intercultural Agency, a private agency responsible for follow-up of refugees from Southeast Asia. The referral traditionally lists family members, names, and ages; address; telephone number; identifying characteristics of family; reason for referral; and response to referral.

The Chan family consists of Mrs. Chan, 35 years old; Lee, 11 years old; and May, 5 years old. The referral notes that the Chan family is a Chinese refugee family from Vietnam who have been in the United States 3 months. Mrs. Chan was recently widowed after her husband was killed in a hit-and-run automobile accident. Mrs. Chan speaks some English. The referral requests a home visit to assess health needs, immunization status, and knowledge of sources of health care.

Doris reviews previous learning in anticipation of her initial home visit and assessment of the family. She brings many skills such as interviewing, knowledge of pediatrics and adult health, and specific nursing care skills. She reviews what is expected in terms of growth and development parameters for each family member. She also reviews the grieving process, its effect on the widow and the children, and supportive interventions. To provide anticipatory guidance to the family, she will need to research areas in which she is lacking information or skill such as immunization needs, school requirements, and nutritional needs. She researches carefully the cultural health beliefs, values, and practices of the Chinese and Vietnamese. She collaborates with the Chinese community health nurse working in the health center for additional insight and guidance. She also investigates the health care resources and facilities available to refugee clients. She ensures that she has basic emergency telephone numbers to give to the family for ambulance, fire, and police service in their neighborhood. She reviews both agency policy and university or college policy regarding safety (see Chapter 28).

She engages in work on behalf of the family, known as *parafamily work,* to ready herself for the visit. If she has any questions about the family that must be answered (e.g., if the referral did not state the family's ability to speak English), she should contact the agency of referral. If necessary, she would then seek an interpreter through the agency to make the initial appointment and accompany her on home visits. She may also contact agencies with which she is unfamiliar that may provide needed services to the family. She will elicit from them information about criteria, location, available hours, and name of

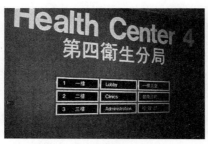

The Public Health Center is one setting in which community health nurses work.

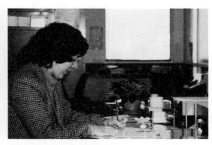

The community health nurse reviews a referral before making a home visit.

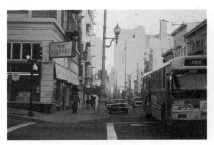

As the nurse enters the neighborhood of her clients, she observes the density of housing, the bus services, and other aspects of the community.

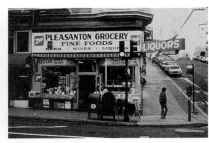

The nurse visits a neighborhood store to assess the types and price of foods available.

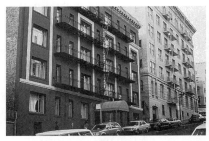

Arriving at the client's apartment building.

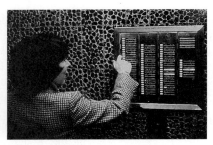

Many nationalities are represented here. If she has difficulty locating the family, the nurse may seek help from the apartment house manager.

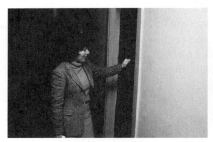

After knocking on the door, it is important for the nurse to announce who she is because some people will not respond to a knock on the door for safety reasons.

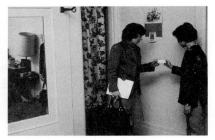

The nurse presents her card from the health department and states the purpose of her visit.

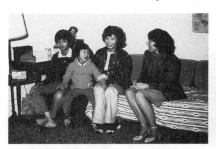

The importance of social talk in establishing a relationship and trust is understood by the nurse and she takes time to chat with the family before beginning any tasks.

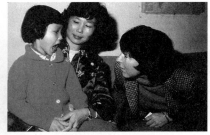

After first establishing a relationship with the adult, the nurse directs a question to a young child, who is far more comfortable on her mother's lap.

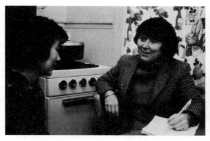

Periods of silence may be necessary while the client reflects on her thoughts and feelings.

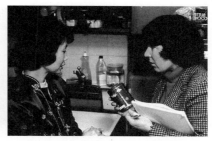

The nurse may observe folk health practices during a home visit, which helps her learn more about the family health beliefs and needs.

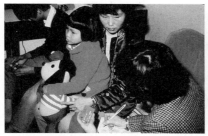

A mutually agreed-upon goal was keeping the daughter healthy.

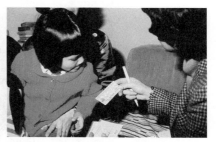

Finding a source of dental care is agreed upon as a first priority, and a referral is made.

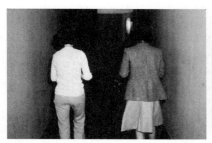

At the end of the home visit, the client accompanies the nurse to the elevator.

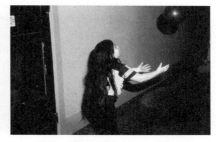

The nurse remains observant as she is leaving the client's apartment and notices children playing in a dark and poorly maintained hallway.

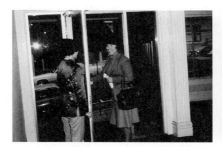

The client accompanies the nurse to the apartment building's front door.

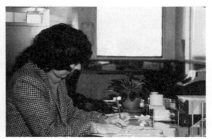

The community health nurse returns to the health center and records the visit. Charting objectively and promptly and according to agency policy is part of the responsibility of making a home visit.

a contact for the family. Examples of such agencies for the Chan family include the local health department for immunizations, the medical center dental clinic for low-cost dental care, and several primary care clinics at public and private hospitals. She will continue to do parafamily work throughout her visiting, as she contacts with the family and shares with them the exploration of resources.

Doris obtains a city map and rapid transit maps for both bus and subway. She familiarizes herself with the neighborhood in which the Chan family lives, where the nearest schools and hospitals are located, and the bus lines between the hospitals, other health care agencies, and where the family lives. She plans her own route and method of transportation to visit the family. She plans to visit during the day, if possible, but after school hours when Lee and May should be home.

She visits the neighborhood, engaging in a "community walk" in which she uses her five senses to observe and experience the community to familiarize herself before she makes her visit (see Chapter 5). She notes the high density of apartment housing, the high number of cars, the bus services, and the ages and numbers of people on the sidewalks. She notes children playing on the street, which is on a very steep hill. She notes that the busy, steep hill is the children's neighborhood, their community, their playground; that is where they spend their time. She also observes groups of older men clustered at street corners and talking. She observes the availability of grocery stores, largely "mom and pop" stores, and the lack of supermarkets. She enters one store near the Chan apartment and notes the availability and price of staples such as fresh produce, meat, rice, and milk; she plans to compare these prices with those of a supermarket in the suburbs. She also notes the location of the nearest pharmacy, private physicians' offices, and clinics. The wide variety of entertainment available ranges from an elite theater to "adult" entertainment; she asks herself if these are types of entertainment her family might choose or could afford to choose.

Initial Contact Because Mrs. Chan has a telephone and speaks English, Doris calls for an appointment, announcing, "My name is Doris Wilson. I am a student community health nurse from the University, working with the San Francisco Health Department. The Intercultural Agency is concerned about how you and the children are doing and if you have found places to get health care. They have asked me to stop by and visit you. I would like to see Lee and May, too. I have time on Tuesday or Thursday at 3:00 PM. It would probably take about an hour. Would 3:00 PM allow me to visit after school is out?"

As mentioned in Chapter 28, if families do not have telephones, the community health nurse may stop by the home and ask for an appointment for a later time that is convenient to the family. The nurse must be prepared for a visit, however, even when "dropping by" with a note, as the family may be very receptive, invite the nurse in, and proceed with a visit. When the family is not home, a card from the agency with a message asking them to call the nurse or setting a tentative time when the nurse will stop by again should be left on the door. Leaving personal cards or other messages in a mailbox is illegal. However, a note with a card may be mailed to the family. If there still is no response within 1 week, the nurse should return to the home and ask the apartment manager and neighbors if the family is still living in the residence. Apartment managers can aid in helping nurses locate families. Wright and

Leahey (1994) reviewed the methods of dealing with family members who are reluctant or never present for a family interview, particularly men and fathers. Letting reluctant family members know they have a unique and important view of the family, one only they can provide, is important. The nurse must also realize that some families will reject visits by not being at home at the arranged time, by simply not answering the door, by closing it once they identify who is there, or by asking the nurse not to return.

Gaining Entrée Coordinating visits with bus schedules or parking meters is important to allow ample time for the student to devote complete attention to gaining entrée and carrying out a successful first home visit. Doris notes that there are many different names representing many different nationalities, including several families named "Chan," on the roster of the large apartment building and is thankful that the apartment number was noted on the referral. When Mrs. Chan answers through the speaker system, Doris announces clearly who she is, that she spoke with Mrs. Chan on the telephone, and that she is now here for the visit they agreed on.

Finding her way to the elevators and through the apartment maze, Doris walks down a darkly lit hallway, yet she notices a large hole in the hallway door with wooden splinters and makes a mental note of this environmental hazard. Doris knocks on the door and states, "This is Doris Wilson, Mrs. Chan, the student community health nurse." It is important to announce who is knocking, because for safety reasons some people will not respond to a knock on the door. Mrs. Chan takes a moment to open the door, and Doris hears the shifting of several latches, a cue that safety may be a concern to the family. Doris realizes she is a guest, says hello, shakes Mrs. Chan's hand, and again states who she is, showing Mrs. Chan her university identification card and a card from the agency. She again states the purpose of her visit and sets the approximate time limit to the visit:

"I'm from the health department, and I'm a community nursing student at the university. The Intercultural Institute asked me to visit with you to talk about your family's immunizations and where you and your family might go to see a physician, nurse, or dentist. Here is my card with my name and office telephone number. I can stay about an hour, if that is all right with you."

She reassures the family that in the United States nurses make visits in the home and that she is not from the Immigration and Naturalization Service.

Assessment

Throughout the visit and on each succeeding visit, Doris assesses and reassesses the family in its home environment within its particular neighborhood in the community. Doris uses the conceptual framework of systems theory to organize her approach to the family. Her view of the community as a suprasystem and the family as a system composed of subsystems will help her not only to organize the data she collects during the assessment phase but also to carry out the other steps of the nursing process at the individual, family, and community levels. In assessing the family as client, Doris is aware that data about the family should be collected from as many members of the family as possible to accurately reflect its situation rather than from one individual only.

Developing rapport and trust between the community health nurse and the family is essential (Wright and Leahey, 1994). There may be a natural reluctance on the part of the student to enter the family's territory and to do so without "props" such as stethoscopes, blood pressure cuffs, and thermometers relied on so heavily in the acute care setting. There may be a tendency to immediately take the client's blood pressure, for example, so the nurse will feel more comfortable with something familiar to do. Wright and Leahey (1994) stated that the first stage of the interview is very important; it is during this phase that an alliance can begin to be established.

The importance of social talk in establishing a relationship and as a means of assessment cannot be overstressed. Kendall (1993) explored the extent to which clients participated in encounters with health visitors (British public health nurses) on home visits. The study found that participation by the client was rarely initiated by the client and also rarely elicited by the health visitor. Morgan and Barden (1985) examined nurses' interactions with perinatal patients during home visits and found that the majority of the nurses' visits (53.8%) were categorized by nurse-observers as "asks for information" or "gives information." Very few visits (7.9%) were reported as "seems friendly." Patients, however, agreed that the nurses were friendly to them and to others present. Nurses appeared to be more critical of visits than were patients. When focused on allowing the family to express itself, the social phase can cut down on information asking and giving by the nurse, promote friendly interaction, and elicit data appropriate to the assessment phase.

In a study by Berg and Helgeson (1984) of students' first home visits, time spent socializing during the first home visit ranged between 5% and 100%; 13 of 15 students reported obtaining important data during the socializing phase of the visit. Important verbal and nonverbal cues can be noted (e.g., smiling, maintaining eye contact, shaking hands, and inviting the student to sit down). Environmental as well as behavioral cues, when noted and mentioned, can serve to elicit a family's history, biographical aspects, and biographical exchange between the nurse and the family. For example, noting photographs of family members, a record collection, types of books and magazines, or plants or pets can serve as cues that elicit much information about the family because such cues are based on the family's world, and their response interprets the meaning of that world as the family sees it. That is not to discount health-related cues such as bottles of Alka-Seltzer or commercial soups in the home of a family member on a low-sodium diet or herbal teas and folk treatments in the home of an immigrant, but the nurse should concentrate on establishing a trusting relationship before discussing health-related topics.

Fostering the relationship involves letting the family express their concerns before bringing up sensitive topics such as source of income. Agency assessment forms need not always be completed on the first visit; they can best be completed after the relationship is established. For example, Doris says hello to May, who is clinging to her mother, and to Lee, who is working on a puzzle, but knowing the respect due elders in Asian cultures, she directs her main conversation first to Mrs. Chan. Comments may be made about everyday topics such as the weather and about the family. "How long have you lived here?" "Where is the rest of your family?" "What are the neighbors like?" The social phase, which should be repeated as an informal phase at the beginning of each visit, sets the stage for the rest of the visit. It is a way to informally check in with the family to find out what is happening in their world, and it prepares the family for the more-focused phase of the visit by giving them a chance to renew their acquaintance with the nurse and to relax.

Having created a social footing on which the nurse and the family establish communication and rudimentary elements of trust, the focused phase of the visit allows the nurse and family to communicate more intensely around areas of concern to each and to determine needs, plans, and actions that need to be taken.

In this phase, the use of focused questions can elicit more details about the family important to assessment, such as the following. "Tell me how you got to San Francisco." (This may elicit a life review.) "Tell me, how do you spend your day?" (This may elicit activities of daily living or social interaction or lack thereof.) This question is repeated at different times with other members of the family.

In addition to gaining the information just discussed, the community health nurse is able to observe family dynamics. This includes the relationships and patterns of communication among family members, roles that are taken, the division of labor or how things get done, and whether the family as a system is open or closed (see "The Family Theory Approach to Meeting the Health Needs of Families"). The nurse uses the five senses in making an ongoing assessment, attending to what is seen, heard, felt, smelled, and, on occasion, even tasted.

Doris directs a question to May: "How old are you, May?" May, sitting on her mother's lap, grins and buries her face in her mother's shoulder, without verbally responding. Mrs. Chan states that May will be starting kindergarten in the fall, and she expresses her concern that May has not been to a dentist and that she would like to take her now so she will be ready for school. In addition, neither Lee nor Mrs. Chan has received dental hygiene. Mrs. Chan does not know whether May needs an immunization. Mrs. Chan invites Doris into the kitchen where she keeps a shoe box full of papers. She shows Doris all their immunization records. Doris, prepared for the visit, assesses that May needs her fifth diphtheria-pertussis-tetanus immunization (second booster) and must have it before school starts.

A corner at the kitchen table in the small apartment gives Doris a chance to talk to Mrs. Chan alone.

"How are *you* doing, Mrs. Chan?" (Mrs. Chan is silent.) Nursing students bring communication and psychiatric skills with them to the community setting. The community health nurse knows to allow periods of silence while the client reflects on her thoughts and feelings.

"My husband is gone . . ." [Mrs. Chan covers her face with her hands.]

"It must be hard to be alone . . . and with the children," Doris reflects. [Mrs. Chan shakes her head.] "I don't want to talk right now," she says. Doris realizes that support at a later date, once rapport is better established, is appropriate. A sensitive issue such as this cannot be pushed, but it must not be overlooked in the long term. Assessment will continue on a following visit, perhaps when the children are in school. She notes mentally that she will need to assess at a later date the children's response to their father's death.

Doris observes several unusual kinds of teas and asks Mrs. Chan if she uses any special medicines. Mrs. Chan shows Doris one of the special teas she uses when May has an upset stomach. She details that each of the different teas has a use for a specific ailment. An important exchange occurs, and Doris has the opportunity to learn of the folk health practices of the family.

Doris observes the kitchen, in particular, the techniques of food storage of new refugees. Many refugee families are unfamiliar with how to prepare foods for storage and are unaware of which foods need refrigeration. Assessment of these seemingly routine food-handling tasks and instruction requires tact and ingenuity.

Doris summarizes in her mind the following areas as appropriate to consider in her assessment of the Chan family:

Individual

- Language ability of individual members
- Sex-role–related behavior of family members
- Lifestyle patterns that place individuals at risk (e.g., poor diet, inadequate exercise, use of alcohol or drugs, and so on)
- Patterns of self-care in health and illness
- How leisure time is spent
- Utilization of preventive health services (physical examinations, dental hygiene, immunizations)

Family

- Family configuration; traditional beliefs and signs of acculturation
- Division of household labor and decision-making patterns
- Pattern of parenting
- Ability of family members to disclose feelings to each other and to others
- Ability of family members to give emotional and physical support to each other during times of crisis and noncrisis
- The manner in which family members process grief
- Family history of morbidity and mortality
- Family interaction with groups in neighborhood and community

Community

- Resources available to the family, particularly Asian refugee families, in the community, such as school, sports, or religious activities
- Physical environment of apartment, building, and neighborhood
- Resources in the community for recreation and leisure
- Neighborhood safety

Diagnosis

Doris mentally makes a nursing diagnosis for each individual in the family and a tentative diagnosis for the family as a whole and poses community diagnoses. Ross and Helmer (1988) stated that nursing diagnoses for the *individual* usually stem from using approaches such as lifestyle, activities of daily living, and symptomatology. These authors state that nursing diagnoses for a *family* often differ from those for the individual and are developed from using approaches such as a systems framework, structural-functional framework, problems in communication or roles, and value conflicts. Wright and Leahey (1994) preferred the generation of a list of strengths and problems of the family rather than diagnoses, noting that the list is limited in that it is the perspective of one observer, not necessarily the "truth" about a family.

Individual

- Alterations in health maintenance related to lack of routine dental hygiene (May, Lee, and Mrs. Chan)
- Alterations in health maintenance related to lack of immunizations for age (Carpenito, 1984) (May)
- Grieving related to loss of husband (Mrs. Chan)
- Knowledge deficit related to language and cultural differences (Mrs. Chan)

Family

- Alterations in health maintenance related to failure to seek health care despite awareness that such health care is needed
- At risk of family crisis resulting from prolonged stress secondary to premature death of father
- Alteration in family processes related to situational cross-cultural relocation
- Potential accidental wound related to faulty maintenance of apartment building environment

Community

- Inadequate systematic programs for linking Asian refugee families to community resources
- Inadequate systematic programs for maintaining environmental safety of apartment dwellers as a result of faulty upkeep of buildings

SOURCES OF NURSING DIAGNOSIS IN THE COMMUNITY

The following resources are available to aid in the formulation of appropriate nursing diagnoses in the community.

Alex WM: Nursing diagnosis with the family and community. *In* Logan BB, Dawkins CE (eds). Family Centered Nursing in the Community. Menlo Park, CA, Addison-Wesley, 1983, pp. 227–246.

Hamilton P: Community nursing diagnosis. Adv Nurs Sci 5:21–36, 1983.

Houldin A, Salstein S, Ganley K: Nursing Diagnoses for Wellness. Philadelphia, JB Lippincott, 1987.

Lee HA, Frenn MD: The use of nursing diagnoses for health promotion in community practice. Nurs Clin North Am 22:981–986, 1987.

Martin KS, Scheet NJ: The Omaha System: A Pocket Guide for Community Health Nursing. Philadelphia, WB Saunders, 1992.

Muecke MA: Community health diagnosis in nursing. Public Health Nurs 1:23–35, 1984.

Neufeld A, Harrison M: The development of nursing diagnoses for aggregates and groups. Public Health Nurs 7:251–255, 1990.

Porter E: Administrative diagnosis—implications for the public's health. Public Health Nurs 4:247–256, 1987.

Porter E: The nursing diagnoses of population groups. *In* McLane A (ed). Classification of Nursing Diagnoses: Proceedings of the Seventh Conference. St. Louis, CV Mosby, 1987, pp. 306–314.

Planning

In Morgan and Barden's (1985) study of nurse–client interactions on home visits, both nurses and clients "were uncertain as to whether or not they had agreed on goals to work toward" (p. 165). The authors conclude that the client should be more involved in the process of goal setting. Planning with the family is essential. Planning involves mutual goal setting between nurse and family; mutual setting of objectives to meet goals; prioritizing, or setting short- and long-term goals with the family; contracting, or establishing the division of labor between nurse and family that will meet the objectives; and evaluation of the process and outcome.

Contracting is defined as "any working agreement, continuously renegotiable, between nurse and clients" (Sloan and Schommer, 1991, p. 306). The purpose of the contract is to delineate jointly the change needed and how it will come about. Contracting carried out jointly will involve the family as an active participant. In a study of contracting by senior community health nursing students, Helgeson and Berg (1985) found that contracts were rated as important to the majority of students and families but were not appropriate to all. For example, written contracts were not appropriate for families who did not read or write. Written and oral contracts were not appropriate for families in crisis situations. In addition, some families did not grasp the idea of a contract and did not agree to its use.

Individual

Short-Term Goals

Doris planned and contracted verbally with Mrs. Chan around a mutually agreed-upon goal: keeping May healthy so she will be ready for school. Receiving dental care for May was a priority for Mrs. Chan, who stated she would seek the immunization after the source of dental care was found. Doris agreed to Mrs. Chan's plan, realizing that the dental care may have a more visible, concrete outcome for the family and thus reinforce the benefits of the family's efforts in seeking this care. Doris offered a known resource to Mrs. Chan, the dental clinic at the medical center. Mrs. Chan felt she could take May by bus to the clinic but asked if Doris would call for an appointment for her "because I'm still afraid to speak on the phone." Doris answers, "I'll be glad to call. It can be difficult until you practice. I'll make this call and then you can try the next call, later, for the immunizations." An informal contract has now been established with the student calling first and giving Mrs. Chan support in her ability to try to make the second call, later, for the immunizations. Mrs. Chan and Doris then set a time frame in which Doris would call and make the appointment and inform Mrs. Chan, and Mrs. Chan agreed to keep the appointment time with May. A brief, reasonable, specific, and realistic contract is more likely to lead to the desired outcome. In addition, contracts must be continually reviewed, evaluated, and negotiated anew (Helgeson and Berg, 1985).

Long-Term Goal

Doris noted mentally the long-term need of teaching the importance of immunizations.

Family

Short-Term Goal

Short-term plans included assisting the family in expressing their feelings of loss in the grieving process.

Long-Term Goal

Long-term plans included fostering the ability of the family to find and use appropriate support services for both physical and mental care.

Community

Short-Term Goal

In addition to planning at the family level, Doris was aware that planning was needed at the community level. For example, she planned to identify existing programs that specifically addressed the physical and mental health needs of Asian refugees and to see whether coordination of such programs included creating awareness of the programs in the referral systems of agencies such as the Intercultural Institute.

Long-Term Goal

Planning at the community level also included an investigation into the process of how to initiate responsibility for obtaining repairs to the inner-city apartment in which the Chan family lives.

Intervention

Doris realized that many interventions would need to be carried out at the individual, family, and community levels.

Individual   An example of an intervention at the individual level is referral for preventive health examinations for each family member.

Family   At the family level, an example of an intervention is referral to a support group for the family's experience of grief.

Wright and Leahey (1994) categorized direct interventions offered by the nurse as those directed at family functioning at the following levels:

- Cognitive
- Affective
- Behavioral

At the cognitive level, new information is provided to the family, usually educational, that promotes problem solving by the family. An example would be giving to Mrs. Chan the location of a dental care resource and information regarding the immunization needed by May. At the affective level, families are encouraged to express intense emotions that may be blocking their efforts at problem solving. An example would be Doris' planned validation of Mrs. Chan's emotions to allow her to work through the grieving process. Finally, at the behavioral level, tasks are negotiated to be carried out either during the family interview or as homework between visits. An example is the dental appointment to which Mrs. Chan will take May between visits. The nurse may also counsel a family to stop doing something it is doing, using changes in the same three areas just mentioned: providing information; encouraging the expression of affect that may be acting as a barrier, such as anger; and jointly assigning tasks to be carried out.

Community   In addition, Doris realizes she has already used the referral process. She must engage in self-preparation and ongoing parafamily work to identify how the community is mobilized to provide physical and mental health care to families of refugees. Does anyone at the dental clinic speak Chinese or Vietnamese? Are there interpreters there and at the health department or at the clinics and the hospitals? If any exist, where are they? Where do most refugee families receive health care and social support? Is there anyone working with widows? Are there any English-as-a-second-language classes for Asians? Are there any job skills courses or programs for women approaching midlife? Questions such as these bring up many areas of assessment Doris will need to make with the Chan family and the community in the future, but her visit is over, and she must plan ongoing evaluation and terminate the visit.

Evaluation

Evaluation includes taking note of progress made during two phases: the ongoing process of carrying out the contract, and the outcome at the termination of the relationship and the home visits (Helgeson and Berg, 1985).

Individual Doris reviews the basic informal contract with Mrs. Chan that will lead to an appointment and dental care for May. Doris will evaluate with Mrs. Chan the progress made during the next home visit.

Family Upon termination of the visit to the family, Doris will evaluate the overall outcomes for the family in terms of changes in risk factors and health status. Using a systems approach, she will evaluate each component of the system, individual family members, dyads within the family, and the family as a whole in terms of goal achievement. For example, she will note whether the family system is open or closed, the degree of equilibrium established, and the degree of change on the part of the family in finding and seeking care in the suprasystem.

Community In addition to evaluating the family system, she will also evaluate the ability of the suprasystem—the community—to provide culturally acceptable health resources and environmental safety needed by the family and will continue to intervene at the community level as needed to ensure that these resources are available to this and other families in the future.

Terminating the Visit

At the end of the home visit, Doris reviewed the needs that were identified and summarized the plan that each would carry out. Doris asked the family whether they had any questions and instructed Mrs. Chan to call her at the number of the agency on the card she had given her upon entry to the home. They jointly agreed on a date and time for the next home visit, planning to meet earlier in the day before Lee was home from school, when May would have a neighbor with whom to play to allow them more privacy. Doris also set realistic expectations to the visits by telling Mrs. Chan that she would be available to visit her over the course of the next 12 weeks.

As she leaves, she notices that May and a friend are now playing in a darkly lit hallway. A large hole in the hallway door with wooden splinters reminds her that nurses in the community need to be aware of the environmental conditions that their families are encountering. With this information, to which most other health professionals do not have access, the nurse can act as an advocate and collaborator in mobilizing the community to take action in addressing housing and environmental health concerns. Mrs. Chan accompanies Doris to the entrance of the apartment building as she leaves.

Postvisit

The community health nurse is not finished with the visit. She must return to the agency and record the visit. Should Mrs. Chan call and need a visit before she returns to the field the following week, the community health nurse who responds to her call will know that a visit was made, what occurred, and what the future plans are. The observations made should be recorded objectively, and the charting carried out according to agency format and policy. A written referral may need to be made to the dental clinic. The referral from the Intercultural Institute must be answered and returned.

As she considers future plans for her visits, Doris feels overwhelmed, that she has only assessed the tip of the iceberg. She feels that there is much more she needs to know about Mrs. Chan, May, and Lee. She also feels she needs to review carefully how to assess the family as a whole. Are they a closed or an open system? How does Mrs. Chan get support? What kinds of friends does Lee have? What roles does he play in the family now that he is without a father? How do culture and the process of acculturation affect family functioning? What are the family's resources, both financial and social?

In addition to questions about the family, Doris had many questions about other families who were faced with similar conditions. Cues from the home visit triggered thinking about the needs of larger aggregates: single-parent refugee families; women in midlife without English-speaking skills, education, or job skills; and preteenagers and teenagers who enter U.S. schools with little English-speaking ability. What supports or group activities are available to meet their special needs?

Levels of Prevention

Society's expectations of the family are in transition. Application of the levels of prevention to families by the community health nurse must take into account the changing family configuration; the financial, emotional, and physical burdens often compounded in the single-parent family; and the lack of resources such as no health insurance or inadequate health insurance experienced by many families today.

Primary

Examples of primary prevention for the Chan family are applied at the individual, family, and community levels.

Individual Assessment, teaching, and referral related to self-care behaviors such as immunization and dental hygiene

Family Teaching, role modeling, and reinforcing roles that allow family members to express feelings

Community Providing health centers in the community where culturally acceptable preventive services are readily available to Southeast Asian refugees

Secondary

Examples of secondary prevention for the Chan family are applied at the individual, family, and community levels.

Individual Screening for dental caries, cervical cancer, and alterations in growth and development

Family Screening for risk factors related to family dysfunction concerning how stress is processed by the family

Community Organizing screening programs in community centers and distributing informative flyers in multiple languages in markets where non–English-speaking persons shop for native foods

Tertiary

Examples of tertiary prevention for the Chan family are applied at the individual, family, and community levels.

Individual Assist family members to express feelings related to grief in the loss of the father or the husband. Assist family members to seek repair of dental caries

Family Assist family to deal with grief, assume flexible roles, and support each other in other ways

Community Assist community to provide support services for widows and families experiencing grief

SUMMARY

This chapter has highlighted the community health nurse's work with families. Families have major health care needs that have been little addressed by the health care system. The nature of the family is changing, challenging traditional definitions and configurations. Approaches to meeting the health needs of families must go beyond that of the traditional health care system, which addresses the individual as the unit of care. Strategies are given for expanding notions of care from the individual to the family and from the family to the community. Common theoretical frameworks used to guide intervention with families from the disciplines of psychology or social psychology have been traditionally relied on by nurses. These frameworks often target individuals; frameworks are needed that go beyond the individual to the family and community and address social and policy changes needed to alter the social, economic, and environmental conditions under which families must function. Tools are provided for assessing the family and the family within the community. Provided are examples of the extension of family health intervention to larger aggregates, which involves social action to overcome constraints to accessing health services. Non-nursing and community health nursing models of care provided for communities of families are presented and critiqued. The nursing process is applied at the individual, family, and community levels on a home visit. Finally, examples of interventions by the community health nurse at individual, family, and community levels are presented.

Learning Activities

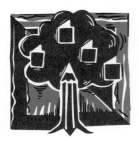

1. With a group of three of your colleagues, each define the term "family." Compare your definitions and list similarities and differences. Develop a list of criteria for being a member of a family.

2. Complete a genogram for your family of origin. What are the high-risk factors in your family history? Current risk factors? Categorize current risk factors into physical, interpersonal, and environmental. Identify needed health education, and determine who needs the education. Identify sources of appropriate screening in the community for the risk factors identified.

3. Complete an ecomap for your current "family," however defined. What is your assessment as to the category of your family as an "open" or "closed" family system? What resources are currently used by your family for mental, physical, emotional, social, and community health? What referrals are needed?

RECOMMENDED READINGS

Austin JK: Assessment of coping mechanisms used by parents and children with chronic illness. Am J Maternal Child Nurs 15:98–102, 1990.

Bomar PJ: Perspectives on family health promotion. Family Commun Health 12:12–20, 1990.

Bomar PJ: Nurses and Family Health Promotion: Concepts, Assessment, and Interventions. Philadelphia, WB Saunders, 1996.

Bushy A: Rural determinants in family health: Considerations for community nurses. Family Commun Health 12:29–38, 1990.

Donnelly E: Family health assessment. Home Healthcare Nurse 11:30–37, 1993.

Francis MB: Homeless families: Rebuilding connections. Public Health Nursing 8:90–96, 1991.

Gennaro S, York R, Brown L, et al.: A sociodemographic comparison of families of very low-birthweight infants: 1982–1991. Public Health Nurs 11:168–173, 1994.

Gilliss CL, Highley BL, Roberts BM, Martinson IM: Toward a Science of Family Nursing. Menlo Park, CA, Addison-Wesley, 1989.

Hall WA: New fatherhood: Myths and realities. Public Health Nurs 11:219–228, 1994.

Lauri S: Health promotion in child and family health care: The role of Finnish public health nurses. Public Health Nurs 11:32–37, 1994.

Reifsnider E: The use of human ecology and epidemiology in nonorganic failure to thrive. Public Health Nurs 12:262–268, 1995.

Seideman RY, Williams R, Burns P, et al.: Culture sensitivity in assessing urban Native American parenting. Public Health Nurs 11:98–103, 1994.

Stetz KM, Lewis FM, Houck GM: Family goals as indicants of adaptation during chronic illness. Public Health Nurs 11:385–391, 1994.

Swanson JM, Swenson I, Oakley D, Marcy S: Community health nurses and family planning services for men. J Commun Health Nurs 7:87–96, 1990.

Weeks SK, O'Connor PD: Concept analysis of family + health = a new definition of family health. Rehabil Nurs 19:207–210, 1994.

Wegner GD, Alexander RJ: Readings in Family Nursing. Philadelphia, JB Lippincott, 1993.

Zotti ME, Siegel E: Preventing unplanned pregnancies among married couples: Are services for only the wife sufficient? Res Nurs Health 18:133–142, 1995.

ADDITIONAL READINGS ON GAY PARENTING

Benkov L: Reinventing the Family: The Emerging Story of Lesbian and Gay Parents. New York, Crown Publishers, 1994.

Bigner JJ, Jacobsen RB: Adult responses to child behavior and attitudes toward fathering: Gay and nongay fathers. J Homosexuality 23:99–113, 1992.

Burke P: Family Values: Two Moms and Their Son. New York, Random House, 1993.

Gold MA, Perrin EC, Futterman D, Friedman SB: Children of gay or lesbian parents. Pediatrics Rev 15:354–358, 1994.

Martin A: The Lesbian and Gay Parenting Handbook: Creating and Raising Our Families. New York, HarperPerennial, 1993.

McIntyre DH: Gay parents and child custody: A struggle under the legal system. Mediation Q 12:135–149, 1994.

Ricketts W: Lesbians and Gay Men as Foster Parents. National Child Welfare Resource Center, Center for Child and Family Policy, Edmund S. Muskie Institute of Public Affairs, University of Southern Maine, 1991.

Tasker F, Golombok S: Adults raised as children in lesbian families. Am J Orthopsychiatry 65:203–215, 1995.

Zeidenstein L: Gynecological and childbearing needs of lesbians. J Nurse Midwifery 35:10–18, 1991.

REFERENCES

Allmond BW, Buckman W, Gofman HF: The Family Is the Patient. St. Louis, CV Mosby, 1979.

American Public Health Association: The Definition and Role of Public Health Nursing in the Delivery of Health Care. Washington, DC, American Public Health Association, 1981.

Anderson MP, O'Grady RS, Anderson IL: Public health nursing in primary care: Impact on home visits. Public Health Nurs 2:145–152, 1985.

Auger JR: Behavioral Systems and Nursing. Englewood Cliffs, NJ, Prentice-Hall, 1976.

Berg C, Helgeson D: That first home visit. J Community Health Nurs 1:207–215, 1984.

Bergman A, Wells L, Bogo M, et al.: High-risk indicators for family involvement in social work in health care: A review of the literature. Social Work 38:282–288, 1993.

Biegel DE, Tracy EM, Corvo KN: Strengthening social networks: Intervention strategies for mental health case managers. Health and Social Work 19:206–216, 1994.

Brewer P, Gadsden V, Scrimshaw K: The community group network in mental health: A model for social support and community integration. Br J Occupat Ther 57:467–470, 1994.

Brooten D, Kumar S, Brown L, et al.: A randomized clinical trial of early hospital discharge and home follow-up of very-low-birthweight infants. N Engl J Med 315:934–939, 1986.

Carpenito LJ: Handbook of Nursing Diagnosis. Philadelphia, JB Lippincott, 1984.

Carter E, McGoldrick M: The family life cycle and family therapy: An overview. In Carter E, McGoldrick M (eds). The Family Life Cycle: A Framework for Family Therapy. New York, Gardner Press, 1980, pp. 3–28.

Carter E, McGoldrick M. (eds): The Changing Family Life Cycle: A Framework for Family Therapy, 2nd ed. New York: Gardner Press, 1988.

Copeland, A: Behavioral differences in the interactions between type A and B mothers and their children. Behav Med 16:111–117, 1990.

Council of Scientific Affairs: Hispanic health in the U.S. JAMA 265:248–252, 1991.

Dawson DA: Report on children with physical, mental, behavioral, and social problems, by family structure, 1988. Family Structure and Children's Health: United States, 1988. (National Health Interview Survey. Vital Health Statistical Series 10. No. 178. DHHS publication No. PHS 91-1506.) Washington, DC, U.S. Government Printing Office, 1991.

Diekelmann N: Primary Health Care of the Well Adult. New York, McGraw-Hill, 1977.

Dreher MC: The conflict of conservatism in public health nursing education. Nurs Outlook 30:504–509, 1982.

Dunn HL: High Level Wellness. Arlington, VA, R. W. Beatty, Ltd., 1961.

Duvall EM: Marriage and Family Relationships, 5th ed. Philadelphia, JB Lippincott, 1977.

Duvall EM, Miller BC: Marriage and Family Development, 6th ed. New York, Harper & Row, 1985.

Erikson E: Childhood and Society, 2nd ed. New York, WW Norton, 1963.

Erkel EA: Conceptions of community health nurses regarding low-income black, Mexican American, and white families: Part 2. J Community Health Nurs 2:109–118, 1985.

Farber B: Family and Kinship in Modern Society. Glenview, IL, Scott, Foresman, 1973.

Flick LH, Reese CG, Rogers G, et al.: Building community for health: Lessons from a seven-year-old neighborhood/university partnership. Health Educ Q 21:369–380, 1994.

Flynn BC, Ray DW, Rider MS: Empowering communities: Action research through healthy cities. Health Educ Q 21:395–405, 1994.

Freeman R: Public Health Nursing Practice, 3rd ed. Philadelphia, WB Saunders, 1963.

Freire P: Education for Critical Consciousness. New York, Continuum Press, 1983.

Friedman MM: Family Nursing: Theory and Assessment, 3rd ed. East Norwalk, CT, Appleton-Lange, 1992.

Gillies LA, Wasylenki DA, Lancee WJ, et al.: Differential outcomes in social network therapy. Psychosoc Rehabil J 16:141–146, 1993.

Glaser B, Strauss AL: Chronic Illness and the Quality of Life. St. Louis, CV Mosby, 1975.

Hanson S, Mischke KB: Family health assessment and intervention. *In* Bomar PJ (ed). Nurses and Family Health Promotion: Concepts, Assessment, and Interventions, 2nd ed. Philadelphia, WB Saunders, 1996, pp. 165–202.

Hartman A: Diagrammatic assessment of family relationships. Social Casework 59:465–476, 1978.

Hartman A: Finding Families: An Ecological Approach to Family Assessment in Adoption. Beverly Hills, CA, Sage, 1979.

Helgeson DM, Berg CL: Contracting: A method of health promotion. J Community Health Nurs 2:199–208, 1985.

Helvie CO: Community Health Nursing: Theory and Process. New York, Harper & Row, 1981.

Jamieson M: Block nursing: Practicing autonomous professional nursing in the community. Nurs Health Care 11:250–253, 1990.

Jamieson M, Martinson I: Comprehensive care built around nursing can keep the elderly at home. Nurs Outlook 33:271–273, 1983.

Johnson R: Promoting the health of families in the community. *In* Stanhope M, Lancaster J (eds). Community Health Nursing: Process and Practice for Promoting Health. St. Louis, CV Mosby, 1984, pp. 330–360.

Jordheim AD: Alternative life-styles and the family. *In* Reinhardt AM, Quinn MD (eds). Family-Centered Community Nursing: A Sociological Framework. St. Louis, CV Mosby, 1982.

Kendall S: Do health visitors promote client participation? An analysis of the health visitor-client interaction. J Clin Nurs 2:103–109, 1993.

Killeen MR: Parent influences on children's self-esteem in economically disadvantaged families. Issues Ment Health Nurs 14:323–336, 1993.

Koepke JE: Health care settings as resources for parenting information . . . physicians' waiting rooms. Pediatric Nurs 20: 560–563, 1994.

Lewis O: The culture of poverty. Sci Am 215:19–25.

Mahon J, McFarland J, Golden K: De madres a madres: A community partnership for health. Public Health Nurs 8:15–19, 1991.

Manley M, Graber A: Coronary prevention program in a community hospital. Heart Lung 6:1045–1049, 1977.

Martinson IM, Jamieson MK, O'Grady BO, Sime M: The block nurse program. J Community Health Nurs 2:21–29, 1985.

Maslow A: Motivation and Personality, 2nd ed. New York, Harper & Row, 1970.

McFarlane J, Fehir J: De Madres a Madres: A community, primary health care program based on empowerment. Health Education Q 21:381–394, 1994.

McGoldrick M: Ethnicity and family therapy: An overview. *In* McGoldrick M, Pearce JK, Giordano J (eds). Ethnicity and Family Therapy. New York, Guilford Press, 1982, pp. 3–30.

Morgan BS, Barden ME: Nurse-patient interaction in the home setting. Public Health Nurs 2:159–167, 1985.

Muecke MA: Community health diagnosis in nursing. Public Health Nurs 1:23–35, 1984.

National Center for Health Statistics: Health, United States, 1994, Hyattsville, MD, U.S. Public Health Service, 1995.

Olds DL, Henderson CR, Tatelbaum R, Chamberlin R: Improving the life-course development of socially disadvantaged mothers: A randomized trial of nurse home visitation. Am J Public Health 78:1436–1445, 1988.

Olson DH, Sprenkle DH, Russell CS: Circumplex model of marital and family systems. I: Cohesion and adaptability dimensions, family types, and clinical applications. Family Process 18:3–28, 1979.

Patrick DL: Health status and use of services among families with and without health insurance. Medical Care 30:941–949, 1992.

Patterson CJ: Children of gay and lesbian parents. Child Development 63:1025–1042, 1992.

Pratt L: Family Structure and Effective Health Behavior. Boston, Houghton Mifflin, 1976.

Puskar KR, Lamb JM, Bartolovic M: Examining the common stressors and coping methods of rural adolescents. Nurs Pract 18:50–53, 1993.

Reilly FE: An ecological approach to health risk: A case study of urban elderly homeless people. Public Health Nursing 11:305–314, 1994.

Riessman CK: The use of health services by the poor: Are there any promising models? Soc Policy 14:30–40, 1984.

Ross MM, Helmer H: A comparative analysis of Neuman's model using the individual and family as the units of care. Public Health Nurs 5:30–31, 1988.

Saluter AF: Marital status and living arrangements: March 1993. *In* Current Population Reports (series P20, No. 478) Washington, DC, U.S. Bureau of the Census, 1994.

Singer BL: Gay & Lesbian Stats: A Pocket Guide of Facts and Figures. New York, New Press, 1994.

Sloan MR, Schommer BT: The process of contracting in community health nursing. *In* Spradley BW (ed). Readings in Community Health Nursing. Philadelphia, JB Lippincott, 1991, pp. 304–312.

Smith JB: Levels of public health. Public Health Nurs 2:138–144, 1985.

Steinglass P: Family systems approaches to alcoholism. J Substance Abuse Treatment 2:161–167, 1985.

Stern PN: Conflicting family culture: An impediment to integration in stepfather families. J Psychosoc Nurs Ment Health Serv 20:27–33, 1982a.

Stern PN: Affiliating in stepfather families: Teachable strategies leading to stepfather-child friendship. West J Nurs Res 4:75–89, 1982b.

Stuart M: An analysis of the concept of family. *In* Whall A, Fawcett J (eds). Family Theory Development in Nursing: State of the Science and Art. Philadelphia, FA Davis, 1991, pp. 31–42.

Swanson JM: Taking the sexual, reproductive, and contraceptive histories. *In* Swanson J, Forrest K (eds). Men's Reproductive Health. New York, Springer, 1984, pp. 342–358.

Teachman JD, Paasch KM: Financial impact of divorce on children and their families. Future Children 4:63–83, 1994.

Von Bertalanffy L: General Systems Theory: Foundations, Development, Applications. New York, George Braziller, 1968.

Von Bertalanffy L: The history and status of general systems theory. *In* Klir G (ed). Trends in General Systems Theory. New York, Wiley, 1972.

Von Bertalanffy L: General systems theory and psychiatry. *In* Arieti S (ed). American Handbook of Psychiatry. New York, Basic Books, 1974, pp. 1095–1117.

Warner M, Ford-Gilboe M, Laforet-Fliesser Y, et al.: The teamwork project: A collaborative approach to learning to nurse families. J Nurs Educ 33:5–13, 1994.

Whall AL, Fawcett J (eds): Family Theory Development in Nursing: State of the Science and Art. Philadelphia, FA Davis, 1991.

Whorton MD: Environmental and occupational reproductive hazards. *In* Swanson J, Forrest K (eds).: Men's Reproductive Health. New York, Springer, 1984, pp. 193–203.

Wright LM, Leahey M: Nurses and Families: A Guide to Family Assessment and Intervention, 2nd ed. Philadelphia, FA Davis, 1994.

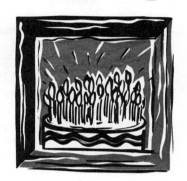

Upon completion of this chapter, the reader will be able to:

1. Identify the major indicators of senior health.

2. Describe the problems associated with aging.

3. Discuss the factors that promote senior health.

4. Coordinate support services for the elderly.

5. Plan appropriate nursing care for seniors in the community.

6. Discuss allocation of resources for senior health.

Olive T. Roen

The first goal for the health of the nation in the year 2000 (Healthy People 2000; U.S. Department of Health and Human Services, 1990) is to increase the span of healthy life. The achievement of this goal will be confirmed by the visibility of active elderly people who continue to make valuable contributions to all aspects of community life. Failure to meet the goal will be demonstrated by the number of elderly people whose life is restricted by physical and mental handicaps before succumbing to a premature death. Nurses working in the community care for the elderly in any state of health that allows them to stay outside the hospital or nursing home.

The goal of health care for the elderly is to maximize the ability to perform activities of daily living (ADLs) rather than to focus on cure of disease. A wise old physician once said that the challenge of aging is to live in symbiosis with one's infirmities. These statements are not meant to imply that no cure should be sought for illness in older people but rather that many diseases associated with aging might be more amenable to compromise than to cure. Health care for the elderly draws on a far wider base than do the more defined protocols of acute care for younger people. Surgery and medication are important, but social disability requires social remedy, much of which is within the competence of the nurse. Health care for elders requires a team approach that includes professionals sometimes not thought of as health care providers. The nurse is the key individual in the coordination of services among the elderly, their families, and community-based services (Neary, 1993).

To introduce the challenges and opportunities of the field, this chapter presents an overview of the elderly population, a discussion of the major age-related problems, and a review of some solutions directed to the goal of an improved quality of life in old age.

MYTHS OF AGING

1. People older than 65 years are old.
2. Most older people are in poor health.
3. Older minds are not as bright as younger minds.
4. Older people are unproductive.
5. Older people are unattractive and sexless.
6. All older people are pretty much the same.

Data from Dychwald K, Flower J. Age Wave. Los Angeles: Tarcher, 1989.

MAJOR INDICATORS OF THE HEALTH OF THE ELDERLY

Demographically, aging is defined by chronological age. As an aggregate, the elderly are considered to be people aged 65 years or older. This aggregate is divided into subgroups. People between the ages of 65 and 74 years are called the "young old" or "younger elderly." (This subgroup may soon include people as old as 84), and those aged 75 and older are called the "older elderly" (U.S. Senate Special Committee on Aging, 1991). People aged 85 years and older are known as the "older ages" (Day, 1993) or the "oldest old" (U.S. Bureau of the Census, 1992a). The "frail elderly" are elderly people who are dependent on others for their day-to-day care. There seems to be a trend away from labeling the different ages to using the ages themselves (e.g., 75+) when referring to specific age groups (U.S. Senate Special Committee on Aging, 1991). It should be remembered that these ages are arbitrary and were originally defined to facilitate the administration of social programs. For example, in Germany in 1884, the age of 65 was determined to be the entrance to old age; that country began its national pension program at a time when far fewer people lived long enough to need provision for retirement. Other nations subsequently followed Germany's lead. Terms are still evolving, and to complicate matters further, people aged 50 to 55 years and older may be called the "older population," especially by advertising and business marketing executives defining their target groups.

Elderly Population in the United States

The aggregate of the elderly is the most rapidly expanding section of the United States population (Fig. 14–1). In 1900, people older than 65 years old made up just 4% of the population. In 1990, this age group accounted for 12.5%, and by 2050, 20.4% of the United States population is projected to be of this age group. The very old will account for the most dramatic increase. In 1900, only 123,000 people, or 0.2% of the United States population, were age 85 or older. By 1990, this group increased to 3.05 million people, or 1.2%, and by 2050, more than 18.9 million people, or almost 5% of the total population, are expected to be in this age group. This increase is due in large part to the increase in births before 1920 and after World War II, the control of communicable diseases, and a recent decrease in mortality among the middle-aged and

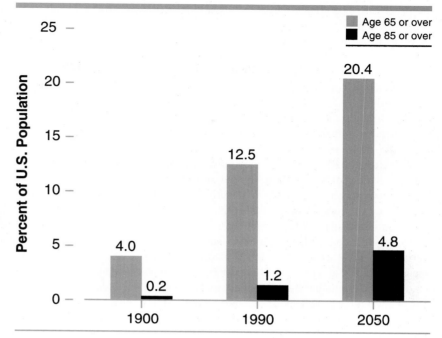

Figure 14–1
Actual and projected elderly population by specified age groups (1900–2050). From Day JC. Population Projections of the United States, by Age, Sex, Race, and Hispanic Origin: 1993 to 2050 (U.S. Bureau of the Census, Current Population Reports, P25-1104. Washington, DC: U.S. Government Printing Office, 1993.)

elderly populations (Day, 1993; U.S. Senate Special Committee on Aging, 1991). The implications of this growth present a great challenge to future government policymakers because the elderly are the greatest users of health services and, with advancing age, are in increasing need of various systems of support.

In 1990, there were more than 31 million people aged 65 years or older in the United States, 13 million aged 75 or older, and 3 million aged 85 or older. California had more than 3 million elderly residents, Florida and New York each had more than 2 million, and there were more than 1 million elderly residents in Pennsylvania, Texas, Illinois, Ohio, Michigan, and New Jersey. There were more than 1 million residents aged 75 and older in both California and New York (U.S. Bureau of the Census, 1992b).

Agricultural states are likely to have a high proportion of elderly residents as younger people move away to seek opportunities elsewhere. The elderly are less likely to move than are other age groups; of those who do move, many seek homes in the South and Southwest for retirement. Typically, they are relatively affluent, well educated, and married. A small but significant number of retirees have begun to move back home, however, to be closer to family members. These countermigrants are an average age of 73 years and are more likely to have incomes below

poverty level. Many are disabled and live in institutions or homes for the aged (U.S. Bureau of the Census, 1992a; U.S. Senate Special Committee on Aging, 1991).

The 1990 Census reported 86.5% of elders to be white non-Hispanic and 13.5% to be minorities. Hispanics make up approximately 3.7% of the present elderly population but are the fastest growing segment. Minorities are projected to represent 33% of the elderly population by 2050 (Day, 1993; U.S Bureau of the Census, 1992b). Age by race analysis of areas with increasing minority populations show most older people are white non-Hispanic, whereas most younger people and children are of another race or ethnic group. This situation demands awareness and cultural sensitivity on the part of planners and providers of all programs and services.

Mortality

Aging has a mortality of 100%. As a species, humans appear to have a natural life span of between 85 and 100 years (Fries, 1980; Hayflick, 1974, 1980), but life always ends in death.

Mortality figures describe the quantity of life. In the United States, life expectancy at birth has increased from 49.2 years in 1900 to 75.7 years for those born in 1992. Life expectancy varies by sex and race; the mortality rate for men exceeds that for women at every stage of life (Fig. 14–2). The tendency of women to live longer than men is true among all ethnic groups, and it is not known whether this is due to biological, environmental, or lifestyle differences. Of racial-ethnic groups, Asian and Pacific Islanders have the greatest life expectancy at birth followed, in descending order, by Hispanics, American Indians (especially women), non-Hispanic whites, and blacks (Day, 1993). After age 85, life expectancy used to be higher for blacks than for whites (U.S. Bureau of the Census, 1992a), but recent data show a slightly longer life expectancy for very old white males (National Center for Health Statistics, 1995). Differences in life expectancy are reduced with decreases in socioeconomic variability; in other words, higher incomes usually mean longer life and better health than lower incomes among all race-ethnic groups. Current trends to a wider gap between rich and poor in the United States (Bradsher, 1995) may result in increases in the difference in life expectancy between people at different socioeconomic levels. More research is needed on other lifestyle variables to determine their impact on longevity.

The leading cause of death for people older than 65 years is heart disease. In 1989 to 1991, the rate of deaths from heart disease was 897.0 per 100,000 people aged 65 to 74 and increased to 6717.3 per 100,000 people aged 85 or older. Cancer is the second leading cause of death in people aged 65 and older, with the largest increase in the 75- to 84-year age group. Death rates from heart and cerebrovascular diseases (the third leading cause of death) have fallen since 1980, whereas death rates from cancer continue to rise. The major acute causes of death are influenza, pneumonia, and accidents; the rates of all three increase with age (National Center for Health Statistics, 1994a).

Morbidity

Morbidity statistics indicate the quality of life. They show where the United States population is on the wellness–illness continuum and can direct the focus of the nurse in pursuit of better health for older people. Most older people in the community describe their health as good to excellent, although many, if not most, of the elderly suffer from one or more chronic and degenerative diseases. Arthritis affects almost half the elderly population, followed in frequency by hypertensive disease. Hearing impairment and heart conditions afflict between one fourth and one third of the elderly. Other disabling conditions are orthopedic impairment, chronic sinusitis, cataracts and other vision problems, and diabetes (U.S. Senate Special Committee on Aging, 1991). Varicose veins, hemorrhoids, constipation, urinary tract diseases, hay fever, corns and calluses, and hernia of the abdominal cavity add to the list of miserable, common conditions.

Many elderly people are hospitalized for acute episodes of chronic conditions, often repeatedly for the same disease. Hospitalization is most often due to cardiac, cerebrovascular, respiratory, or eye diseases

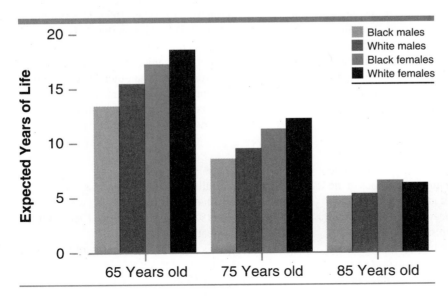

Figure 14–2
Life expectancy at specified ages by sex and race in the United States for 1991. (From National Center for Health Statistics. Trends in the health of older Americans, United States, 1994. Analytic and Epidemiological Studies, Series 3, No. 30, 1995.)

or neoplasms. Fractures (all sites) are an important cause of hospitalization among women older than 75 years. Length of stay in hospitals for sick elderly has decreased for all conditions except pneumonia (National Center for Health Statistics, 1994a). Community and hospital health care systems have a great responsibility to provide services to ensure a smooth transition from hospital to home. Bull (1994) showed that predischarge functional ability and age can predict the need for home care services and suggested that elders who receive visiting nurse services are less likely to suffer hospital readmission.

Only about 5% of the elderly receive nursing home care at any one time, but nursing home residence increases with age (to 24% of people aged 85 years and older) and the loss of ability to provide self-care (U.S. Senate Special Committee on Aging, 1991).

It is interesting to note that older women report occurrences of both acute and chronic conditions more often than do elderly men; the only exception is for conditions that involve limitation of major activity. This apparently inconsistent finding that the longer living female sex is also the less healthy sex is interpreted in three ways. First, the diseases reported by men are more often chronic diseases that cause death, whereas diseases reported by women are more often acute diseases that respond to treatment. The second interpretation is that male morbidity is not fully reported and is actually much greater than the data show. Last, women are considered more likely to seek medical help when ill (U.S. Senate Special Committee on Aging, 1991).

Racial differences in morbidity among elderly people are not sufficiently documented, although more information is becoming available. Almost 47% of blacks and Hispanics aged 65 or older believe that they are in fair or poor health compared with less than 30% of whites who feel this way (Ries, 1990). Much morbidity and mortality is related to socioeconomic factors. Reports from the National Indian Council on Aging in Albuquerque, New Mexico (Hispanic and Indian Elderly, 1989), demonstrate elevated death rates resulting from alcohol abuse, tuberculosis, diabetes, and pneumonia. Socioeconomic factors impact at least the first two of these diseases and possibly all of them.

The former advantage of blacks in life expectancy in the oldest age group is apparent in morbidity data, which show a narrowing health gap with age. Gibson (1994) noted that older whites have a greater increase in rheumatoid arthritis and more deterioration in ADLs

than older blacks. Possible age–race differences in susceptibility to certain diseases or in psychosocial risk factors are suggested.

Two opposing views of morbidity and aging are expressed by Fries (1980) and Schneider and Brody (1983). Fries proposed the ideal that improved health in younger years will continue into old age and compress the degeneration associated with aging into a short period before death. This coincides with the Healthy People 2000 (DHHS, 1990) goals for the United States. Schneider and Brody (1983) surveyed the present scene and suggested that more people will live longer with chronic diseases, which will require increased health care services as the population ages. Fries' view is an optimistic prediction of long-term possibilities, whereas Schneider and Brody's opinion, supported by Callahan (1994), is based on the present reality and the foreseeable future. Taken together, the two opinions form their own continuum and are a useful goal and reference for the health care needs of the elderly as statistics on elderly health accumulate.

Health Behavior and Health Care

Data from the 1985 National Health Survey indicate the elderly may have better health habits than the nonelderly. People aged 65 years and older are less likely than younger people to smoke, be overweight, use alcohol to excess (although alcohol abuse is an often unrecognized problem), and say that stress has contributed to poor health (U.S. Senate Special Commission on Aging, 1991). Many people have used tobacco, alcohol, and other substances when they were younger but cut down or quit as they grew older. Older people are likely to have better eating habits than younger people. The 1985 Health Survey reported that 87% of older people eat breakfast every day and are less likely to eat between meals.

Older people are less likely than younger people to exercise, however; only 40% indicated they walked for exercise (the most common activity), and very few take part in more strenuous activity such as jogging or running. More recent focus on older athletes continuing sports activity (such as tennis and golf tours for professionals no longer competing with younger players) and the growth in scope and participation of the U.S. National Senior Sports Organization (USNSO) (telephone: 314-878-4900) may indicate increased interest in exercise for older people. From the first Senior Olympics in 1987, the USNSO reported that more than 250,000 people were involved in its member games in 1995. Individual and doubles sports, from archery to track and field and triathlon, have categories for men and women by 5-year age intervals from 55 years to 100 and older. The highest age category for team sports such as volleyball is 65 years and older.

After 65 years of life, people do not arrive at the doorstep of old age unscarred but rather as a product of their genes, environment, and lifestyle. Habits, beliefs, attitudes, and values that have accumulated over the years may or may not promote health. Medical visits are expected. In 1991, the elderly made an average of 10.6 visits to physicians compared with fewer than 6 visits for those younger than 65 (National Center for Health Statistics, 1994a).

CHARACTERISTICS OF OLDER PATIENTS

Older patients *are not:*	Older patients *are:*
• Phony	• Punctual
• Well, but worried	• Flexible
• Chronically fatigued	• Polite
• Reckless	• Responsible
• Crybabies	• Postmenopausal

Adapted from Anderson EG. Reflections on a practice going geriatric. Geriatrics 44:91–92, 1989.

The Medicare Current Beneficiary Survey is a continuous, multipurpose survey of a representative sample of the entire Medicare population (the elderly and the disabled population younger than 65 years) living in the community or in institutions (Adler, 1994). From the first round of interviews in 1991, self-reported health status among the Medicare elderly ranged from 41% reporting very good or excellent health to 30% reporting good health and 29% reporting fair or poor health (Fig. 14–3). Those reporting fair or poor health were less likely to have supplemental health insurance than people reporting good to excellent health, although they were more likely to need extra insurance to pay for health care. Women and minorities were less likely to have supplemental insurance, either private or employer sponsored. People reporting poor health have Medicare spending levels about 2.5 times the national average, and people with Medicare only are much less likely to have a regular source for routine health care (either physician's office or clinic) than those with more resources (Chulis et al., 1993). This is very likely to mean that people without insurance that supplements Medicare tend to neglect preventive health care and wait until they are ill before

seeking medical assistance. It may also be related to old friends, education, and income level.

Other Medicare populations with problems of access to care include minorities, residents of urban, high-poverty areas, and residents of health care professional shortage areas (HPSA). These populations neglect preventive services such as Papanicolaou smears and influenza vaccines, rely heavily on hospital emergency rooms and outpatient departments for primary care services, and have longer hospital stays and higher mortality rates (Physician Payment Review Commission, 1994). Obviously, current community health programs are failing to meet the needs of people in these circumstances.

The dental needs of the elderly are neglected. Despite need, the elderly are less likely to visit a dentist than are those younger than 65, usually because of financial reasons. Half of the elderly have no natural teeth, and about half of those with no teeth need dental care to ensure properly fitting dentures. Many of the elderly never visit the dentist. Loss of teeth leads to poor nutrition and causes a change in body image that leads to loss of self-esteem and withdrawal from the important supportive social network (Lebel, 1989). Shay (1994) reported that more older people have their own teeth and visit the dentist, but their dental needs may be very complex because of their dental history plus any disease or disability. The nursing home and homebound elderly with decreased self-care ability need comprehensive dental assessment. A survey of institutionalized and homebound elderly gave similar results for both groups. More than 90% of those surveyed had dental caries, 31 to 50% were not satisfied with their dentures, and almost half had not been to the dentist in more than 5 years (Henry and Ceridan, 1994).

The most common area of monitoring is blood pressure checks. All older people seem to realize that blood pressure is important to health, although the parameters and reasons may not be understood. The advent of blood pressure machines in pharmacies and supermarkets has accelerated and supported this interest. Marion Laboratories estimated that 50% of blood pressure patients do not follow the medical advice they receive, so they made available a guide to wellness—*Why Comply* (1990)—to encourage people to take an active treatment role.

Growing older does not necessarily result in a decline in mental health comparable to that in physical health. Intellectual growth can continue; in the absence of disease, the lack of growth and challenge may

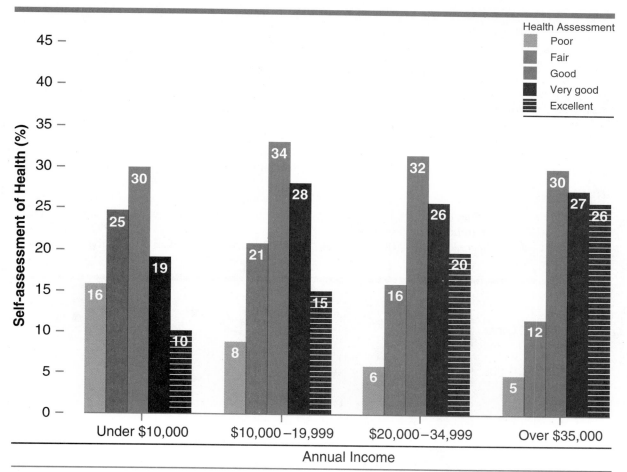

Figure 14–3
Self-assessment of health by income for persons 65 years of age or older (1989). (From National Center for Health Statistics: Current estimates from the National Health Interview Survey, 1989. Hyattsville, Maryland: Vital and Health Statistics, Series 10, No. 176, October 1990.)

predispose to a decline of health and premature death. Elderhostel, the very popular national and international study program for "inquiring minds" older than 55 years, has grown from its beginning in 1975 to an enrollment of 250,000 in 1995 with programs in every state and nearly 50 other countries (Elderhostel, 75 Federal Street, Boston, MA 02110-1941; telephone: 617-426-8056). The American Association of Retired Persons (AARP) sponsors the AARP Online Service on the Internet (accessible through America Online, CompuServe, and Prodigy) for its many members with home computers.

In general, the elderly with mental health problems are neglected. Mental health problems are one of the principal reasons for institutionalization as people grow older. Alzheimer's disease and other dementias

affect 1 in 10 older adults living in the community, ranging from about 3% of people aged 65 to 75 years to 47% of people aged 85 years and older. Suicide, with white males most at risk, is a more frequent cause of death in the elderly than in any other age group. Depression, including depression as a side effect of medication, is described in up to 15% of elderly community residents (U.S. Senate Special Commission on Aging, 1991).

Community mental health resources for the elderly are rarely sufficient to meet needs. Some home health agencies provide psychiatric services for clients with third-party reimbursement. Government programs intended to provide mental health services to the elderly have been weakened and underfunded to the point of being largely ineffective. Even if services are available, many older people may be reluctant to seek them out owing to ignorance of the services offered, distrust, fear of being labeled mentally ill, or a belief that their condition is appropriate for their age. Husaini, Moore, and Cain (1994) found that older people visited their family physician or clergy rather than use mental health services. Women were more likely to seek help from their clergy and through prayer or from their friends and family than were men, who tended to use alcohol and long walks as coping mechanisms.

Income

In 1989, the median income for elderly people living alone was $9422, and families headed by an elderly person had a median income of $22,806 that same year. The median income for elderly whites was $9838, for blacks $5772, and for Hispanics $5978 (U.S. Senate Special Commission on Aging, 1991).

Social Security benefits are the major source of income for the elderly, providing more than half of the total income for the majority of recipients. About 25% of recipients derive almost all of their income from this source. Earnings, interest on savings, and pension plans from other organizations provide other income (U.S. Bureau of the Census, 1992a; U.S. Senate Special Commission on Aging, 1991).

Poverty is most likely to occur in households headed by women and minorities, among individuals not living with relatives, in rural areas, and among the oldest old (U.S. Bureau of the Census, 1992a). Although a substantial number of elderly people live fairly close to

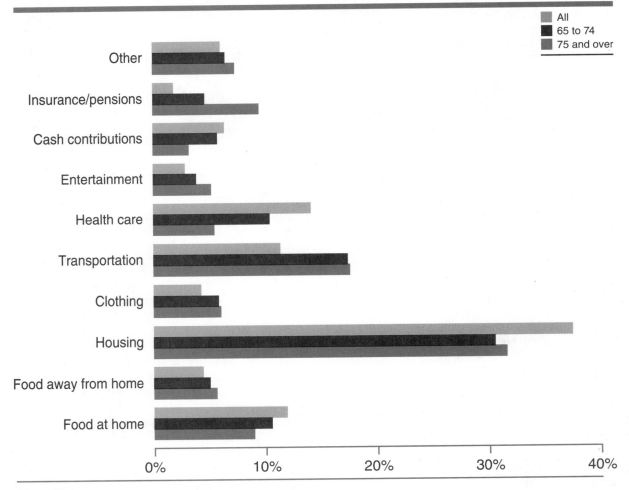

Figure 14–4
Average annual consumer expenditures by type and age. (From U.S. Department of Labor, Bureau of Labor Statistics: Consumer Expenditure Survey, 1990–91. Washington, DC: U.S. Government Printing Office, Bulletin 2425, 1993.)

Table 14–1
Average Annual Consumer Expenditures by Type and Age Group

Variable	All Consumers (%)	Consumers Aged 64–74 (%)	Consumers Aged ≥75 (%)
Food			
At home	$ 2651 (9.0)	$ 2364 (10.5)	$ 1864 (11.8)
Away from home	$ 1620 (5.5)	$ 1102 (4.9)	$ 684 (4.3)
Housing	$ 9252 (31.2)	$ 6849 (30.4)	$ 5871 (37.2)
Clothing	$ 1735 (5.9)	$ 1270 (5.6)	$ 638 (4.0)
Transportation	$ 5151 (17.4)	$ 3906 (17.3)	$ 1765 (11.2)
Health care	$ 1554 (5.2)	$ 2300 (10.2)	$ 2197 (13.9)
Entertainment	$ 1472 (5.0)	$ 841 (3.7)	$ 444 (2.8)
Cash contributions	$ 950 (3.2)	$ 1248 (5.5)	$ 1008 (6.4)
Personal insurance and pensions	$ 2787 (9.4)	$ 1033 (4.6)	$ 268 (1.7)
Other	$ 2145 (7.2)	$ 1432 (6.3)	$ 961 (6.1)
Total	$29,614 (100.0)	$22,564 (100.0)	$15,782 (100.0)

From U.S. Department of Labor, Bureau of Labor Statistics. Consumer expenditure survey, 1990–91. (Bulletin 2425.) Washington, DC: U.S. Government Printing Office, 1993.

the poverty level, most of the elderly are not considered poor. Reduction in family size as children leave home, lower taxes with lower income, and fewer or no work-related expenses may allow relatively more disposable income (Fig. 14–4; Table 14–1).

Many of the elderly want to work after retirement, but they usually prefer part-time work. The companionship of other people and a feeling of purpose may be as important as the extra income. In 1986, age-based mandatory retirement for most workers was abolished, but older people still face discrimination when competing with younger workers for jobs (U.S. Senate Special Committee on Aging, 1991).

Literacy and Education

As an aggregate, the elderly have had less formal schooling than later generations. In 1989, the median education received by the elderly was just over 12 years. More than half of the elderly completed high school, and about 11% reported receiving 4 or more years of college. Among the elderly, whites had achieved higher educational levels than nonwhites. Educational attainment depends on prevailing attitudes and opportunities in various time periods, and the educational achievements of older people increase as more cohorts enter older years (U.S. Senate Special Committee on Aging, 1991).

Education ended at the 8th grade for 21.6% of

people between the ages of 65 and 69 years and 38.8% of people aged 75 years or older (U.S. Senate Special Committee on Aging, 1991). Functional illiteracy, which is the inability to read and write at an eighth-grade level (the level of most newspapers and below the level of most government forms and health promotion material), is present in 20 to 25% of the population as a whole and may be higher in the elderly, especially the oldest old, who have had less opportunity for formal schooling. Nurses must be sure that older people can read the written instructions they are given, or they must find other ways of conveying information.

Marital Status, Relationships, and Living Arrangements

Women live longer than men, so it is not surprising that most older men are married (74% in 1990) and many older women are widowed (49%). Most elderly men live in a family situation, whereas most elderly women, especially those older than 75 years, live alone (U.S. Bureau of the Census, 1992a). A smaller proportion of older Hispanics live alone than blacks or whites, but the trend is for more elderly in all race-ethnic groups to live alone. Living alone increases with age, and about 47% of persons aged 85 years and older live by themselves (U.S. Senate Special Committee on Aging, 1991) (Table 14–2).

Table 14–2
Percent of Persons Living Alone By Age, Sex, Race, and Hispanic Origin: March 1990

Age (Years)	Race-Ethnicity	Men (%)	Women (%)
65–74	White	12.5	33.2
	Black	19.6	35.4
	Hispanic	12.4	22.3
75–84	White	19.3	54.5
	Black	20.9	44.7
	Hispanic	22.8	34.4
85 and over	White	29.8	58.4
	Black	16.0	42.3
	Hispanic	*	*

Persons 85 Years and Older Living Alone	
1980	39.0%
1990	47.0%

*Base less than 75,000 persons

From Saluter AF, U.S. Bureau of the Census. Marital Status and Living Arrangements, March 1990. Current Population Reports, Series P-20, No. 450. United States Government Printing Office, Washington, DC: May 1991.

Alvin Korte warned those at the hearing on Hispanic and Indian elderly (1989) that the family was a fragile resource that was not always available and that the assumption that the elderly were held in high esteem and had strong intergenerational support was a myth. The increasing divorce rate of older people also contributes to the rising number of single elderly who maintain their own households.

However, many of the elderly live in an extended family situation. About 70% have one or more surviving children, 57% live fairly close to at least one child, and most have frequent contact with their child or children. Increasing numbers of the very old are dependent on children who also are elderly. Young family members may find themselves caring for two older generations. This can become an impossible burden, and the larger community may be increasingly called on to provide support.

Most elderly people own their own home, but an increasing number (currently about 25%) rent living space (U.S. Bureau of the Census, 1992a). A significant number of elderly people cling tenaciously to inadequate housing. Many do not have a telephone, which can be a lifeline in case of emergency. About 5% of the elderly live in institutions such as nursing homes or boarding houses.

Religion

As people age, they become more committed to religious beliefs and participate more in church activities. Church membership is claimed by 73% of women and 63% of men older than 50 years, although fewer attend regularly. Women are more likely to attend than men, and attendance increases with age. Overall, 69% of people older than 50 years said their church did a good or excellent job of meeting their personal and family needs. Hispanics tended to be less sure; 31% said their church did only a fair job of meeting their needs (Religion in America, 1990).

Religious institutions have responded well to the needs of older people in their congregations and in the community at large by providing many services to assist them to continue to live at home and participate in community activities. The parish nurse role is expanding steadily (Coldewey, 1993; Mickulencak, 1992). Churches are resources for social networks and, often, safety and reassurance programs and counseling.

PROBLEMS OF THE ELDERLY

Most problems arise from the deterioration of physical or mental abilities possessed in the younger years. Blomquist (1993) stated that happiness in aging is "someplace to live, someone to love, and something to do," which implies the ability to live and function effectively in society and to exercise self-determination. The inability to do these things is perceived as a problem. This section examines the impact made by various disorders on the performance of average ADLs by the elderly in the community.

Difficulties at Home

NUTRITION

Nutrition is a highly complex subject because food serves not merely the body but also the soul. Recommended dietary allowances (RDAs) of nutrients for the elderly are currently controversial. The most recent RDAs for levels of essential nutrients required to meet the nutritional needs of healthy people were set by a subcommittee of the National

Research Council in 1989, but special recommendations were not made for the elderly.

DIETARY GUIDELINES FOR OLDER PEOPLE

The following are recommended dietary allowances for daily intake for moderately active people aged 50 or older:

Nutrient	Women	Men
Calories	1800	2400
Protein	50 g	63 g
Vitamin A	4000 IU	5000 IU
Vitamin C	60 mg	60 mg
Thiamine	1.0 mg	1.2 mg
Riboflavin	1.2 mg	1.4 mg
Niacin	13 mg	15 mg
Calcium	800 mg	800 mg
Iron	10 mg	10 mg
Phosphorus	800 mg	800 mg
Fat	No more than 30% of total calories	
Cholesterol	Not to exceed 300 mg daily	
Sodium	Limit to 1100–3300 mg daily	
Fiber	Limit to 20–30 g daily, not to exceed 35 g	

Data from National Research Council. Recommended Dietary Allowances, 10th ed. (Report of the Subcommittee of the Tenth Edition of the RDAs, Food and Nutrition Board, Commission on Life Sciences.) Washington, DC: National Academy Press, 1989. Sodium recommendation from the American Heart Association; fiber recommendation from the National Cancer Institute.

Testifying before the U.S. House of Representatives Select Committee on Aging (Adequate Nutrition for the Elderly, 1992), Robert York, director of Program Evaluation in Human Service Areas, General Accounting Office, noted that the national nutrition surveys are limited as a source of information on nutrition in elderly people. The National Health and Nutrition Examination Survey (NHANES) III will be the first survey to include people 74 years of age and older. The National Research Council RDA recommendations are based on a sample of healthy adults. They do not provide standards of nutrition for old people or for elderly people with acute or chronic disease, and they do not consider the effects of food and drug interactions.

At the same hearing, Dr. Susan Finn, president-elect of the American Dietetic Association, reported that as many as 50% of older people living alone have specific nutritional deficiencies and that about 24% of all Medicare beneficiaries fall in a high-risk group for inadequate nutrition. Those most at risk are the oldest old, minorities, the poor, and those with Alzheimer's disease or other dementias. The signs of malnutrition are often confused with the signs of aging, and misdiagnosis results in premature mortality and increased cost to the health care system (Adequate Nutrition for the Elderly, 1992).

If food is not appealing and there is no desire to eat, nutrition is not likely to be adequate. Even if prepared meals are delivered, they may not be eaten if food symbolizes family gatherings to a person now living alone or if cultural or religious tradition dictates that the ingredients would have been prepared differently. English tripe and onions cooked with milk is not interchangeable with highly spiced Tex-Mex menudo, and neither would appeal to other ethnic groups unaccustomed to such delicacies.

Loneliness, depression, grief, and anxiety are common reasons for altered eating habits (Walker and Beauchene, 1991). Too many old people exist on coffee and donuts and sink into malnutrition because such food satisfies hunger and is easily available when feelings of low self-esteem sap the energy required for the preparation of more nutritious food.

CASE STUDY: NUTRITION

Mrs. Miller is an 84-year-old widow hospitalized with a history of weakness and weight loss. No organic condition was found that would explain these symptoms. One evening, Mrs. Miller told her nurse she could not shop for groceries any more, but Meals on Wheels delivered a hot meal on Monday, Wednesday, and Friday from which she "kept something back" to eat on the days on which no delivery was made. Mrs. Miller asked for reassurance that her nutrition was adequate.

It is a major challenge for the nurse to identify the nutritional adequacy of food consumed by elderly clients and to piece together the resources available to meet deficiencies in the broad categories of the ability to obtain, prepare, eat, digest, absorb, and eliminate food. If nutritional inadequacy is suspected, request a conference with a registered dietitian. Consistent, good nutrition is probably the greatest single contribution to physical and mental health and gives the greatest return for the money and time invested. Malnutrition resulting from involuntary fasting leads to a delay in any healing process; lowering of the metabolic rate, body temperature, pulse rate, and blood pressure; dry and itchy skin; anemia; ulcerated mouth;

abnormal heart rhythm; erosion of bone mineral; difficulty walking; loss of sight and hearing; speech impairment; coma; and, ultimately, death (Graf, 1981).

DISABILITY

This entire chapter could be written from the perspective of disability. The central theme of senior health is maintaining the mental and physical functional ability to perform the daily activities necessary for a healthy, independent life (Fig. 14–5). Any limit to these activities is a disability.

Disability turns the routine ADLs into time-consuming challenges and is a source of constant irritation because mobility and communication with the outside world are affected. Obvious examples of disability are depression, the breathlessness of emphysema, the residual deficiencies that follow a stroke, the deformities of arthritis and osteoporosis, bladder and bowel incontinence, and the loss of vision and hearing. Many aids have been developed to compensate for these deficiencies; one very common example is the availability of large-print literature to help people see letters and words. Other methods of compensation for

loss of function can be contrived through ingenuity or obtained from medical equipment companies. The Sears (telephone: 1-800-948-8800) catalog of aids for the handicapped is one mail order source.

In 1990, approximately 32% of older people in the community with limitations in ADLs lived with their spouse. Another 35% lived with other people. The remaining 33% lived alone, at risk for institutionalization (U.S. Senate Special Committee on Aging, 1991). In 1990, almost 300,000 people were estimated to live alone who were unable to perform any of the major ADLs (eating, dressing, bathing, toilet, transferring from one place to another). This number will increase with the increase in the older population. Community services are critical for older people (U.S. Senate Special Committee on Aging, 1991).

PROBLEMS OF EVERYDAY LIFE FOR THE ELDERLY

- Opening medicine packages
- Reading product labels
- Reaching items located on high shelves
- Fastening buttons, snaps, or zippers

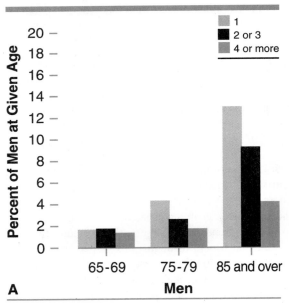

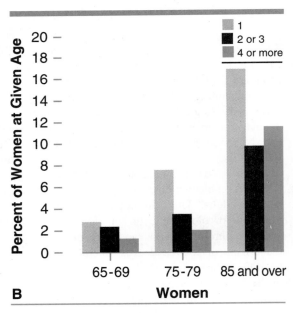

Figure 14–5
A and *B*, Activities of daily living: limitations and difficulties in the noninstitutionalized elderly. (From Leon J, Lair T: Functional Status of the Non-institutionalized Elderly: Estimates of ADL and IADL Activities. DHHS Publication No. [PHS] 90-3462, June 1990. National Medical Expenditure Survey Research Findings 4, AHCPR, Rockville, Maryland: Public Health Service, 1990.)

- Vacuuming and dusting
- Going up and down stairs
- Cleaning bathtubs and sinks
- Washing and waxing floors
- Putting on clothes over one's head
- Putting on socks, shoes, or stockings
- Carrying home purchases
- Using tools
- Accidents or trauma at home going unnoticed by others
- Using the shower or bathtub
- Tying shoelaces, bows, and neckties
- Moving around the house without slipping or falling

Data from Gallup Organization. Survey of New Product Needs Among Older Americans. Princeton, New Jersey, Gallup Organization, 1983.

ACCIDENTS

Reduced sensory perception, increased reaction time, circulatory changes resulting in dizziness or loss of balance, and confusion associated with dementia combine to make the elderly accident prone. Assessment of the environment and intervention to avoid accidents is typical primary prevention in community health care for both old and young clients. Simple measures that prevent accidents include eliminating environmental hazards, reducing the hot water heater setting to 120–125°F, checking the kitchen stove, and providing accessible fire extinguishers near fire hazards and a plan to escape in case of fire. A smoke detector should be installed in every home, but many older houses do not have them.

SOME CAUSES OF ACCIDENTS IN THE ELDERLY

- Altered vision
- Aortic stenosis
- Cardiac arrhythmias
- Diabetes mellitus
- Generalized debility
- Hypothyroidism
- Medication reactions
- Nutritional deficiencies
- Orthostatic hypotension
- Peripheral vascular disease
- Sensory loss

Data from Escher JE, O'Dell C, Gambert SR. Typical geriatric accidents and how to prevent them. Geriatrics 44(5):54–69, 1989.

ACCIDENT PREVENTION AT HOME

Think Accidents
Activities of daily living
Cognition
Clinical findings
Incontinence
Drugs
Eyes, ears, environment
Neurological deficits
Travel history
Social history

- Remove all loose rugs.
- Tack down carpet edges.
- Install secure handrails in the bathroom and wherever else needed.
- Use a nonslip mat in the shower or bathtub.
- Check stairs for stability, uniformity, and safety.
- Eliminate clutter.
- Avoid slippery floors.
- Check the furnace and all heating devices (including the stove) to maintain proper functioning.
- Lower hot water temperatures.
- Label hot and cold water outlets and appliances with directions.
- Install and maintain smoke detectors.
- Check for proper storage of household chemicals, especially flammable substances.
- Increase artificial lighting in all rooms.

Data from Escher JE, O'Dell C, Gambert SR. Typical geriatric accidents and how to prevent them. Geriatrics 44(5):54–69, 1989.

The telephone is literally a lifeline for the elderly not only because help can be summoned directly but also because assistance can be sent if a scheduled call is not answered. Many churches provide a frequent, regular telephone call as a service to people in the area regardless of whether the recipient is a member of that particular congregation. Advance permission is obtained, and provision is made for notifying a third person or entering the home if a call is not answered when expected.

SPECIAL TELEPHONE SERVICES

- Speakerphones for hands-free conversations
- Big-button telephones for easy dialing
- Memory telephones for one-touch dialing
- Telephones compatible with hearing aids

Box continued on following page

- "Signalman" control unit, which flashes a lamp for incoming calls
- Telecommunication Device for the Deaf (TDD) equipment
- PockeTalker listening device to assist listening to television and radio
- Artificial larynx

Information available from AT&T Accessible Communications Products Center, 14250 Clayton Rd, Ballwin, Missouri 63011. Telephone (toll free): 1-800-233-1222.

MEDICATIONS

The elderly are substantial consumers of prescription drugs as well as over-the-counter medications and folk remedies. Because the Food and Drug Administration has not included the elderly in clinical trials, the effect of different drugs on the aging population is unknown, and drug dosage is achieved through trial and error. Little attention is given to possible drug–drug or drug–food interactions.

Even if the most appropriate medications are prescribed, they are often not used as directed. Medications may not be taken unless the person feels ill, they may be overconsumed because of the belief that more is better, they may be taken erratically because of memory loss and lack of a system, or they may never be purchased if money is needed for other things. Monitoring drug therapy in the home is another challenge for community health nurses. Pharmacists and nurses have a common interest in medication compliance and in providing ways to assist elderly people to understand how to take medications. Hussey (1994) recommended tailoring interventions to the individual client, finding success with both verbal teaching and color-coded methods among people with low literacy levels. Mackowiak et al. (1994) surveyed client preference among four devices to assist compliance and found strong preference for simple, easy-to-use devices such as a medication organizer tray.

Alcohol is the drug of choice for older Americans. Elderly alcoholics are the least likely to seek treatment but have the highest rate of treatment success and sobriety after treatment of all age groups. Widowers aged 75 years of age and older have the highest rate of alcoholism in the country. Up to 50% of nursing home residents and up to 70% of older people who were hospitalized in 1991 have alcohol-related problems (Alcohol Abuse and Misuse, 1992). Alcoholism is difficult to diagnose because regular drinking will often be denied. Most at risk are those who suffer loss such as the death of a spouse or other loved ones, loss of employment (including by retirement), or loss of independence. Dependency may stem not only from consumption of the usual alcoholic beverages but also from the considerable alcohol content of some nonprescription sleep aids or "tonics." Alcohol reacts with other drugs and is itself a depressant, although the moderate and appropriate use of wine, beer, and spirits can stimulate the appetite and has a long history of use in medicine, especially in other cultures.

Ten times as many deaths from accidental poisoning occur among the elderly than among all children younger than 15 years (National Center for Health Statistics, 1994b). In the elderly, poisoning results from the combined effect of drugs and alcohol or from an unintentional drug overdose after confusion or forgetfulness. Medications should not be kept by the bedside, outdated medications should be flushed down the drain, and a plan should be devised to assist the client in taking medications only as prescribed. Poisoning prevention education and interventions should be considered when medication instruction is given (Kroner et al., 1993).

THERMAL STRESS

The ability to respond to thermal stress is impaired in the elderly, and emergency care may be needed for heat exhaustion or hypothermia (a core temperature at or below 95°F). A comfortable indoor climate can be maintained through air conditioning or heating. Therefore, the degree of thermal stress is a function of socioeconomic factors (Kolanowski and Gunter, 1983). The frail elderly and the obese are most vulnerable to heat exhaustion, and mortality increases with age, temperature, and duration of heat wave. The frail elderly are also at the greatest risk of hypothermia, which may occur with an environmental temperature of 65°F. Hypothermia may occur after accidents in the elderly, especially if a fall occurs at night when only lightweight nightclothes are worn and the victim is unable to call for help and must wait until someone arrives.

Funding exists to help pay winter fuel bills for low-income elderly, but it is much less frequently available for summer cooling. Local utility companies and human resource offices are good sources of information. If transportation is not a problem, the nearest enclosed shopping mall can provide an agreeable climate as well as social stimulation. This should be seen as a temporary or short-term solution, however, as resources for climate control are identified by discussion with the affected individual, family, or community.

Illness and Hospitalization

PREVENTION: SCREENING

The elderly suffer repeated hospitalization for the exacerbation or loss of control of chronic disease or for symptoms of a new disease. Screening and case-finding programs may control chronic disease processes before they threaten the quality of life and, with clinical progression, become more expensive and difficult to treat. Well-planned and targeted screening programs with a health education component can be valuable tools in disease and disability prevention. However, screening programs have many limitations. Many elderly people in the United States do not have a regular physician and are lost to follow-up as workloads of health care teams increase. There is no reason to screen for problems that are not a health threat to the community if solutions cannot be offered. In many areas of the United States, screening programs may be available, but treatment has not been funded or does not exist. Agency-based screening programs also tend to attract those who are at lowest risk, mobile, motivated, and in the community. Disability, isolation,

and lack of income are the causes or effects of more serious problems and require aggressive programs to identify need effectively.

The National Health Service in the United Kingdom emphasizes annual assessments of all people aged 75 years or older. Concern for staff resources to accomplish this led to a 3-year study using a questionnaire (which focused on functional ability) sent by mail to community residents aged 65 years and older and followed by verification and intervention by a nurse. The study found lower mortality, higher self-rated health status, and reduced duration of hospital stay in the group receiving the questionnaire than in the control group, which received only the usual services. Increased visits to the physician's office were balanced by a lower number of home visits by the physician. The mailed questionnaire with selective follow-up and intervention was recommended as a satisfactory method to influence outcomes and the use of health care resources by elderly people living at home (Pathy et al., 1992). (Note that physicians in the United Kingdom routinely make home visits to people who have difficulty attending their office because of a poor health state. An increased number of visits to the physician's office and reduced home visits may indicate early problem identification or control, which enables people to remain active and improves health status.)

SELECTED POTENTIAL CLINICAL PREVENTIVE SERVICES FOR THE ELDERLY

Immunizations
- Influenza
- Pneumonia
- Tetanus
- Hepatitis B

Screening
- Cancer screening

Breast (clinical examination, mammography)
Colorectal (occult blood stool, sigmoidoscopy)
Cervix and uterus (clinical examination, Papanicolaou smear, endometrial biopsy)
Prostate (clinical examination, ultrasonogram, laboratory tests)
Skin (clinical examination)

- Blood pressure measurement
- Vision examination and glaucoma screening
- Hearing tests

- Cholesterol measurements
- Diabetes screening
- Thyroid screening
- Asymptomatic coronary artery disease (exercise stress test)
- Osteoporosis (developing techniques)
- Dental health assessment
- Mental status–dementia
- Depression screening
- Multiple health risks, appraisal and assessment
- Functional status assessment

Education and Counseling
- Nutrition
- Weight control
- Smoking cessation
- Home safety and prevention of injury
- Stress management
- Appropriate use of medications
- Exercise

From Office of Technology Assessment. The Use of Preventive Services by the Elderly: Preventive Health Services Under Medicare (Paper 2). Washington, DC: Health Program, Office of Technology Assessment, Congress of the United States, 1989.

PREVENTION: IMMUNIZATION

Pneumonia and influenza are two infectious diseases that result in increased mortality in the elderly. Vaccines are available for both diseases and are widely encouraged, especially for the frail elderly. The year 2000 national health objective has a goal of 60% vaccination levels for high-risk persons. In 1993, pneumococcal vaccination in elderly people reached 28%, and influenza vaccination levels reached 52% (Adult Immunizations, 1995).

Whether all elderly persons should be immunized against pneumonia and influenza is an ethical and economic consideration. Immunization itself carries risks, although they are minimal, and the decision of whether to be immunized may be made best by the informed individual. However, in times of epidemic, the cost to society of immunization is far less than the cost of treating these diseases and their associated complications.

IMMUNIZATION SCHEDULE FOR ADULTS AGED 65 AND OLDER

- All persons in this age group should receive influenza vaccine each year. Contraindication: History of allergic reactions to eggs.
- All persons in this age group should receive pneumococcal vaccine. Revaccination should be considered every 6 years.
- All elderly persons should be evaluated for completion of the primary series of vaccination against diphtheria and tetanus and receive booster doses of combined toxoids at 10-year intervals. Contraindication: History of severe reaction to previous dose.
- The lifestyle, occupation, and special circumstances (including travel plans) of older adults should be assessed for consideration of other vaccines.

Recommendations from the National Coalition for Adult Immunization, Bethesda, Maryland, October 1995. The coalition is a network of more than 70 organizations that promote adult immunization, and it issues the Standards for Adult Immunization Practice.

HOSPITALIZATION

In any age group, hospitalization is a major disruption of everyday life for the patient and family. An elderly person can be expected to be weaker and less alert after any hospitalization, and this should be considered by community nurses when planning care. There is a danger that functional decline resulting from hospitalization and bed rest may easily become irreversible, leading to dependency and institutionalization (Creditor, 1993).

Because the U.S. medical model of health care serves acute illness better than chronic conditions, Brown (1990) indicated that many of the problems of the elderly can be attributed to the approach to care. Acute illness sanctions the sick-role behavior pattern and fosters dependency among client populations. These behaviors, which represent coping in a temporary situation, become permanent and inappropriate in chronic disease. Elderly people with serious chronic problems may become socially at risk, avoid medical treatment, reject diagnoses, increase conflict with health care providers, and suffer emotional stress that leads to psychosomatic symptoms.

In line with the attempt made in the 1980s to control health care costs through diagnosis-based prospective payment schedules for Medicare recipients, hospitals are pressured to discharge patients quickly, which means that more severe degrees of illness are now experienced by clients who are at home (Fig. 14–6). Visiting nurses assist not only the client but also the family or household in understanding and complying with required treatment and the management of often complex equipment. This can severely strain the physical, financial, and emotional resources of the family, and the nurse should seek sources of respite care to relieve tension and burnout among family members.

AIDS AND THE ELDERLY

- Ten percent of all persons with AIDS are age 50 or older.
- From 1981 to 1987, 3690 people aged 50 to 59 years and 1419 people aged 60 years and older were diagnosed with AIDS. Between 1993 and October 1995, these numbers had increased to 18,413 and 6513, respectively.

First 500,000 AIDS Cases—United States, 1995. Reported by Division of HIV/AIDS Prevention, National Center for Prevention Services, CDC.

Institutionalization

Institutionalization usually refers to the placement of persons who can no longer care for themselves in a nursing home or care facility from which they are not expected to return to an independent life in the community. Only about 5% of the elderly population

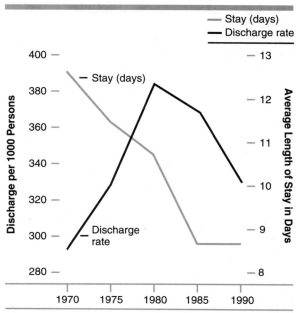

Figure 14–6
Rate of discharges from short-stay hospitals and average length of stay. Study included all persons aged 65 years and older and all conditions from 1970–1990. (From National Center for Health Statistics: National Hospital Discharge Survey. Hyattsville, Maryland: Vital and Health Statistics, Series 13, various reports.)

live in nursing homes, but the proportion increases rapidly with age, from 1% of persons aged 65 to 74 years to 6% of those aged 75 to 84 years and to more than 20% of those aged 85 or older (National Center for Health Statistics, 1995). The use of nursing homes increases as limitations in ADLs increase. Nursing home residents are most likely to be older, female, and white and to have been living alone, with an income below poverty level. Almost 80% of nursing home residents have some type of mental disorder. The most prevalent physical morbidity is cerebrovascular disease (26% of residents), chronic obstructive pulmo-

nary disease (24%), and heart disease (21%) (Hing and Bloom, 1990).

Institutionalization is often a last resort when the care of an aged relative has exhausted a family. Financial and emotional exhaustion may continue. Insurance policies for long-term care are becoming available, but they are expensive and of no assistance to those who are already old. Medicare does not provide for institutionalization, but when resources are spent the resident becomes eligible for Medicaid. The issue of long-term care is of great concern to older people at this time.

Death and Bereavement

Old age is a time of adjusting to loss. In the natural order of things, loss of parents is followed by loss of spouse, siblings, friends, and contemporaries, culminating in one's own death. A new phenomenon is the loss of adult children who have themselves become aged.

The effects of bereavement in the elderly may not be expressed for some months after the death of a spouse and may continue for several years. According to Dimond (1985), the usual view of death as a crisis should be superseded by the concept of grief resolution as a process during which the survivor learns to live without a spouse. Assessment of past experience and coping skills used in adjusting to a previous loss and identification of available support networks will assist in planning for care.

Many of the elderly turn to churches, synagogues, and other religious institutions at this time, and ministers, priests, rabbis, and other religious leaders have much experience in helping people through the grief process. Support groups for widows and widowers are often provided by religious organizations and usually are available for anyone in need. Other resources include secular support groups and private group or individual therapy.

FUNERALS

The usual procedure after death is to notify first the physician, who will sign the death certificate, and then the chosen funeral home. If death occurs at home, regardless of whether expected or unexpected, the police or medical examiner's office must also be notified. This is still true at present even if a hospice is involved in care but may change as the hospice movement expands.

An autopsy is rarely performed for a natural death unless requested by the medical examiner's office.

Many funeral homes are part of national chains, although their image is of individual family operation. Funeral homes and directors are licensed by each state and must comply with regulations set by federal, state, and local regulating

Box continued on following page

agencies. They exist to provide any service a family wants within legal limits. A traditional funeral includes embalming and enhancing the cosmetic appearance of the body, viewing the deceased in the casket, a wake or rosary the evening before burial, and burial in the family-arranged plot. Above-ground entombment may take the place of burial. The funeral home will obtain the death certificate and other necessary papers, place newspaper notices, prepare clergy records, provide automobiles, and coordinate arrangements with the cemetery.

The *average* cost of a traditional funeral in 1995 was about $5500 to $6000 plus $1500 for the purchase, opening, and closing of the grave. Veterans of the armed forces may be buried in military cemeteries without charge for the grave.

Cremation usually is less expensive. A rigid container is all that is required, although a casket can often be rented if viewing is desired. A letter from the medical examiner's office authorizing cremation is usually required in addition to the other papers. Ashes are often interred in urn gardens or may be taken by relatives to scatter elsewhere.

Burial customs vary with religion or ethnic group. Funerals should be conducted in accordance with family wishes to avoid guilt feelings in the survivors. Funeral homes usually lose their association with the survivors after the burial, but personnel are often involved in crisis intervention and may refer survivors to therapy groups or inform such a group of a person in need.

From personal communication with Mr. John Russell, Assistant Manager, Sunset Memorial Park and Funeral Chapel, San Antonio, TX, April 11, 1995.

Community Environment

Assessment of the community for adequacy in meeting the needs of the elderly may produce some surprises. Neighborhoods generally considered highly desirable may not be so for all age groups. While increasing open space and protecting property values, restrictive zoning can result in long distances to grocery stores and a lack of public meeting places, sidewalks, nearby physician offices, and available public transportation (except for taxis). Inner-city residents may fare better than those in middle-class suburbs. Buses, sidewalks, corner shops, community centers, and churches keep the elderly fed and mobile.

Never assume that the wealthy elderly can automatically provide care for themselves. Relying on a maid to shop and prepare meals is not much use if the maid does not arrive for work. Dismissing an unsatisfactory maid and hiring a new maid are traumatic experiences that require a great deal of energy and force a prolonged period of change. Independent wealth can provide a very pleasant situation, however, if someone is available to coordinate and supervise household staff or the staff is sympathetic to the needs of its employers.

Life can present most problems to the middle-class elderly. Often widowed, living alone in a house that has been home for many years but is now difficult to maintain, possibly (if a woman) having had little employment experience but much volunteer involvement in various organizations, they find themselves in a role for which they are unprepared. Their life has

often been directed to helping others, and they are uncomfortable receiving help themselves unless there is the possibility of contributing something in exchange. This may take the form of a cash payment for services provided, which is a satisfactory solution except when there is little money available. Many elderly with a seemingly middle-class lifestyle have become the genteel poor as fixed incomes fall behind inflation and expenses continue to rise, including expenses for health care.

The need for mobility includes driving an automobile even when this has actually become no longer safe. Police, however, are often sympathetic to elderly drivers, especially in small communities in which they are known. The police recognize the importance of mobility and assist as much as possible to keep their residents independent. Talk to police chiefs. Their goal is the smooth running of a community with no unpleasant surprises for residents. They know what happens in the community infrastructure and are very interested to hear about potential problems for community subgroups.

Abuse of the Elderly

Elder abuse is present in all parts of the United States, in private homes as well as other places. It is less likely to be reported than child abuse, but public and professional awareness of the problem is growing with more frequent media publicity and the establishment of shelters for the abused elderly in many communities.

The assessment of elder abuse is often difficult. The

signs of abuse may be subtle and difficult to identify. Time spent observing the interaction between an elderly person and a caregiver and a personal interview alone with the elderly person are necessary parts of the assessment process. A nurse suspecting abuse may be placed in a difficult ethical and legal position if the older person requests that the abuse not be reported (Peirce, 1994). Either from shame or fear, abused elders are less likely to report abuse than are abused persons in other age groups, and the true incidence and prevalence rates of elder abuse are elusive. Abusers are usually experiencing stress, possibly from alcoholism, drug addiction, marital problems, financial difficulty, or personality disorders (Fulmer, 1989).

Abuse generally falls into four categories: physical abuse (which ranges from hours of physical restraint to beating, burning, rape, and murder), psychological abuse (isolation, insult, threat, and fear), financial abuse (theft of money or property), and abuse by neglect (e.g., not providing needed new eyeglasses, dentures, or clean clothes). The majority of states have laws requiring mandatory reporting of elder abuse; most are based on child abuse statutes, and most lack the ability to be enforced. Without federal assistance, inadequate funding is the rule. On the average, states spend about $25 for each adolescent resident but only $2.90 per elderly resident for protective services (Subcommittee on Health and Long-Term Care, 1985).

Fulmer (1994) noted that the direction of thinking about elder mistreatment is related to the unmet needs of the elderly, inadequate care, or caregiver burden. With elder abuse recognized as a problem, future research should examine methods of prevention of the various types of elder mistreatment and identify elders (and caregivers) at risk.

Crime and the Elderly

The difference between abuse and crime is that crime is usually perpetrated by someone to whom the elderly victim has not granted access.

The elderly are the least likely of all age groups in the United States to experience crime, and the rate for personal theft and household crime among people age 65 years and older in 1992 is the lowest in 20 years of records (Office of Justice Programs, 1994).

The elderly are easy targets for crime, however, because physical frailty and mental confusion make them less likely to fight back. The major crime against the elderly is fraud: the promise of large sums of money if a "small deposit" (often equal to life savings) is made. If they are a victim of violent crime, they are more likely than younger people to suffer serious injury, to be attacked by strangers, and to be attacked at or near their home. Older neighborhoods are subject to deterioration before gentrification, and deteriorated neighborhoods usually suffer high crime rates. Elderly residents have often grown old with the neighborhood and do not wish to move from their familiar home regardless of how difficult life has become. However, the regular arrival of Social Security and pension checks and the pattern of movement from mailbox to home to bank invite interference.

It takes a long time for anyone to recover from being a victim of crime, and the elderly do not have much time. Physical injuries in the elderly take longer to heal than in younger people, but the emotional scars may last forever. The fear of being victimized is often enough to precipitate withdrawal, isolation, and depression. Economic and property loss may never be regained.

Security from crime is a major concern of the elderly and an important consideration for builders of retirement complexes. Direct deposit of checks, including Social Security checks, into bank accounts is recommended, transportation and a buddy system for shopping or social activities can be arranged, and education about crime prevention increased. The AARP offers a valuable pamphlet—*Domestic Mistreatment of the Elderly: Towards Prevention—Some DOs and DON'Ts* (Order No. D 12885)—that provides prevention suggestions on individual, family, and community levels.

Families of the Elderly

Most elderly people are usually happily connected with a family unit, but the increasing visibility of elder abuse is directing attention to the family dynamics that occur when the senior members of the family grow old.

Generally, up to the age of 75, most elderly people do more for their children than their children need to do for them (Gelman et al., 1985). If or when physical frailty becomes a problem, however, parent–child roles tend to become reversed, which can be a major source of stress for all. Daughters or daughters-in-law usually become the primary caregivers (Brakman, 1994; Haug, 1985), sometimes at considerable financial as well as emotional cost. Lost wages are compounded by the loss of job-related benefits such as Social Security, a company-related pension, or medical insurance. A direct contribution to national well-being is made by the little-appreciated and unreimbursed caregiver (Nissel, 1984).

Presenting a series of case studies of caregivers of advanced age themselves, Kim and Keshian (1994) noted that, although older caregivers may not have the role conflicts or strain of younger caregivers, their physical capacity is less. Usually, there has been a long relationship between the caregiver and the person cared for, and siblings especially may show amazing mental strength and devotion. Physically, however, they are often very frail and vulnerable, with their own chronic diseases or life-threatening illness, and at great risk for additional health problems from the stress and burdens of caregiving. Community support services should be used to relieve strain. An older caregiver is only one accident or health incident away from institutionalization for him- or herself and the person cared for.

The quality of life for the frail elderly may be substantially increased when care is given by a family member. There is a feeling of being wanted, of comfort, in familiar faces and surroundings (Haug, 1985). There is more freedom and personal control than is possible in any institution. With the increase of home health services, including house calls by physicians, accessible advice and treatment are more easily available, which satisfies both client and caregiver (Zimmer et al., 1985).

For the caregiver, benefits may be of a moral nature, such as the personal satisfaction of fulfilling a family obligation and the avoidance of the guilt of refusing to care for a parent or grandparent. Unfortunately, the benefits for the caregiver can be outweighed by the physical and emotional costs of caring for a sick elder who can only become more dependent until death is seen as a release for everyone (Gelman et al., 1985; Haug, 1985). The caregiver is three times more likely to report symptoms of depression than the recipient of care and four times more likely to report anger. Other expressed feelings include guilt, frustration, and sometimes desperation, as the needs of the elder conflict with and take precedence over the needs of the caregiver (Gelman et al., 1985). Feelings of powerlessness and of being victims of circumstance can affect family caregivers (Davidhizar, 1994). Stress arises from the increased workload; from intrafamily conflicts and social embarrassments caused by the elder's confused behavior; from the increased vigi-

lance, worry, and concern that is the inevitable consequence of being responsible for someone who could hurt him- or herself or others; and from the interference caused by the elderly person's care in the marital, family, work, and community responsibilities of the caregiver (Beck and Phillips, 1983).

Alzheimer's disease is a major cause of caregiver stress. The national headquarters of the Alzheimer's Association (919 N. Michigan Ave, Suite 1000, Chicago, IL 60611-1676; telephone: 312-335-8700) will give information about the disease and family support groups linked with affiliated chapters throughout the United States.

CASE STUDY: JIM C.

Jim C., a 72-year-old man, was admitted to a nursing home suffering from Alzheimer's disease. He was unable to walk, talk, or recognize members of his family. He was kept alive by nasogastric tube feeds. One day his brother went to the nursing home and shot and killed him. The sentence was 10 years' probation, which was terminated after 1 year. Jim's widow still grieves about the manner of his death and the disease that devastated the whole family.

Many families care for their elders with very little outside support and a lack of awareness of existing social programs (Gelman et al., 1985). Family members are often so isolated from support systems that they are not aware such support is needed until they become exhausted. The literature is unanimous in demanding support for caregivers by general public recognition of the problem, extension of existing programs, creation of new programs, and tax credits or financial reimbursement for care given by family members.

In response to obvious need, the provision of case management services for the elderly is a new and rapidly expanding industry. Certification of case managers has been available since 1994 through the Certification of the Insurance Rehabilitation Specialist Commission. Services include the assessment and coordination of care for elderly people who may live some distance from their children. These services are not usually covered by medical insurance but can bring great relief to overstressed family members. Social workers have been pioneers in the case management field, but opportunities exist for gerontological nurses.

For more information, contact the National Association of Private Geriatric Care Managers (655 N Alvernon Way, Suite 108, Tucson, AZ 85711; telephone: 602-881-8008). Case management programs provided by public and nonprofit agencies may be available in some areas.

SUPPORT FOR THE ELDERLY

Major Legislation

Legislation affecting the elderly takes innumerable forms as amendments are added to unrelated bills. The acts discussed here have the most direct impact.

SOCIAL SECURITY ACT

Originally passed in 1935, the Social Security Act has been amended 16 times. It is administered by agencies within the DHHS, including the Social Security Administration and the Health Care Financing Administration. Most employed people are enrolled automatically in the Social Security program, which is financed by contributions from employers, employees, and the self-employed. Part of the Social Security contribution is designated for Medicare, which is the national program of health insurance for the elderly.

Social Security provides four different benefits, two of which are targeted directly to the elderly. Retirement benefits are paid at the full rate to persons retiring at age 65, provided they have met contribution requirements, and at 80% of that rate to persons retiring at age 62. If benefits are not claimed at age 65, an additional 3.5% is added for each year the benefits are not claimed until age 70. A spouse may claim the larger of spousal benefits or any benefits he or she may have earned in his or her own right. Ages when benefits are payable are scheduled to rise to reflect the increasing longevity of the population.

A benefit for survivors is the second provision of social security. Death at any age will bring a one-time "death payment" of $255 plus some income for surviving children younger than a specified age and possible widow or widower benefits from age 60 if claiming on the account of the late spouse or age 50 if totally and permanently disabled. Dependent parents are eligible for survivor's benefits if certain criteria are met.

A third provision of Social Security is disability payments for people unable to work during usual working years.

The fourth Social Security provision is Medicare hospital insurance benefits, which is divided into two parts. Part A is automatic and covers most of the cost of hospital care and certain kinds of care after discharge. The patient must pay a large deductible and copayments. Part B is for medical insurance. If a person elects this coverage, it helps pay for physicians' services, outpatient services, and some other medical items. The monthly premium for Part B is $43.80 as of 1997. In 1996, the premium was reduced from the 1995 premium of $46.10, but the 1997 premium reflects the more usual annual increase.

The elderly poor are eligible for Medicaid coverage of the Part B premiums and the deductibles and copayments if treatment is needed. The criteria vary from state to state and may be obtained from state Medicaid offices. Ask for information about the Qualified Medicare Beneficiary (QMB) program. For people who exceed the QMB limits, options are Medicare supplement (Medigap) insurance policies or joining a health maintenance organization (HMO) or competitive medical plan (CMP), which receives Medicare payments in exchange for providing care.

Managed care (more accurately, managed cost) plans are becoming the dominant force in health care. The Kaiser plan in California has the most experience providing health care in a managed care setting. In other parts of the country, many agencies are competing to attract both Medicare and Medicaid clients. In the Medicare setting, if a Medicare-eligible person joins an HMO, that person will still pay the Part B Medicare premium while the organization receives a contracted amount from the federal government, which is usually about 95% of the amount allocated to an individual. The other 5% remains with the government, helping to reduce the cost of Medicare. The HMO assumes all responsibility for the health care needs of each member, and it is in the interest of the HMO to keep the cost of providing care down by keeping their members healthy instead of having to provide care when members are ill. The managed care industry is largely for profit and is not well regulated at present. There is a concern that current enrollees tend to be fairly young elderly who are reasonably healthy, so that there is not much experience providing profit-making care to a large aged population with more medical needs. Many older, less healthy people have an established relationship with their physician of choice, which they are unwilling to give up to accept an unfamiliar care provider who belongs to an HMO.

The old Medicare system remains in effect to provide familiar care to those who choose it, although the copayments and paperwork of filing claims are a burden. Undoubtedly, the current chaos in the provision of health care will need a few more years to resolve into a more coherent system.

OLDER AMERICANS ACT

Signed into law by President Johnson in 1965, the Older Americans Act established the Administration on Aging within the DHHS. Its purpose is to identify the needs, concerns, and interests of older persons and to coordinate available federal resources to meet those needs. Amendments to the act in 1973 established area agencies on aging to provide local planning and control of programs, which must include nutrition services either as home-delivered meals or in communal settings. Multipurpose senior centers nationwide are sites for not only nutrition programs but also recreational, social, and health programs; housing assistance; counseling; and information services, all mandated by the act (Title III). Other requirements of the act are the development of employment opportunities for low-income elderly by means of the community service employment programs (Title V) and the establishment of programs for training personnel and supporting research (Title VI). Amendments passed in 1984 instruct area agencies on aging to plan for community-based programs to assist older people to remain in their homes and to provide supportive services to persons with Alzheimer's disease and their families. National priority services for the elderly include transportation, home services, legal and other counseling services, and residential repair and renovation programs. The target population is persons older than 60 years with the greatest economic or social needs, especially low-income minorities, but the provisions of the act benefit all older people through response to community needs.

When amending the Older Americans Act, Congress is particularly responsive to the recommendations of the decennial White House Conference on Aging, most recently held in May 1995.

RESEARCH ON AGING ACT

The Research on Aging Act (1974) created the National Institute on Aging within the National Institutes of Health. Its purpose is to conduct and

GOVERNMENT AGENCIES

Almost every federal agency has a local office in addition to state and local agencies. For example:

- Social Security Administration
- Veterans Administration
- Mayor's Office for Senior Citizens
- Area agencies on aging: Each city, county, or state may have a different name for its agencies. Please look under the following listings to cross-reference:
  - Agency on Aging
  - Commission on Aging
  - Council on Aging
  - County Council on Aging
  - Department on Aging
  - Elderly Services
  - Human Services
  - Planning Council on Aging

Check your telephone book or call directory information for national, state, and local agency telephone numbers.

From the National Council of Senior Citizens, 1331 F Street NW, Washington, DC 20004-1171.

support biomedical, social, and behavioral research and training related to the aging process and the diseases and other special problems and needs of the aged. Research goals are to enhance the quality of life, promote health and functional independence, increase understanding and effective treatment of the dementias (including Alzheimer's disease), and develop leadership in working with the aged. The philosophy is to view aging as a fundamental human process about which much more knowledge is needed, with the aim of reducing current rates of morbidity and institutionalization. The National Institute on Aging is a source of grant funding for nurses conducting research on problems of aging.

OTHER LEGISLATION

A maze of legislation has had an impact on people as they age. Two important acts address people still in the work force, but they have implications for options and income available to the elderly. The Age Discrimination in Employment Act (1967) provided workers aged 40 to 65 years with the same opportunities as younger employees for participation in employee benefit plans. In 1978, amendments raised the mandatory retirement age to 70 years, and in 1986 mandatory retirement at any age was abolished for almost all workers.

Employee pension rights in private pension plans were safeguarded by the Employee Retirement Income Security Act (1974), which set minimum federal standards for private plans. The Retirement Equity Act (1984) increased protection for the surviving spouse or former spouse of pension-eligible workers, and the Tax Reform Act (1986) reduced vesting requirements for pension eligibility. These provisions are expected to eventually maintain the income of many elderly women as well as men. Public sector pension plans are subject to a somewhat different set of rules and are a complexity of variables that may leave employees and spouses less claim to benefits.

PROGRAMS FOR THE ELDERLY

Federal programs began with the Social Security Act in 1935. They concentrate on assessing need, planning programs to meet the need, developing program guidelines, implementing funding programs, and evaluating the results. Almost all federal programs are available to all of the elderly without income restriction, but because the poor elderly have the most need, most facilities are located in areas where poorer people have greater access.

Service Agencies:
- Department of Health and Human Services
- Social Security Administration: retirement benefits, survivor benefits, disability, Supplemental Security Income (SSI), guaranteed minimum income
- Health Care Financing Administration: Medicare, Medicaid
- Public Health Service: National Institutes of Health, National Institute on Aging
- Office of Human Development Services: Administration on Aging, Nutrition Program for Older Americans, National Clearinghouse on Aging (information services)
- Department of Agriculture: food stamps, provision of food for nutrition programs
- Department of Housing and Urban Development: planned housing for the elderly; multiunit apartment buildings may include a nutrition site, health clinic, and recreational facilities
- Department of Transportation: Urban Mass Transportation Administration, funding for mass transportation services for the elderly with special needs, reduced fares during off-peak hours on public transportation systems receiving federal funds
- Department of Labor: employment opportunities for unemployed people aged 55 or older; investigates complaints of age discrimination

- Veterans Administration: Serves veterans of the armed forces and dependents of career personnel

Opportunities to Volunteer
- Peace Corps: no upper age limit for healthy volunteers
- Volunteers in Service to America (VISTA): the "domestic Peace Corps," requires a proportion of its volunteers to be older than 55 years
- Retired Senior Volunteer Program (RSVP): volunteers work in the nonprofit agency of their choice for reimbursement of expenses
- Foster Grandparents Program
- Senior Companion Program: low-income elderly are reimbursed with a stipend and some benefits to be a companion to children or adults with special needs
- Small Business Administration: Service Corps of Retired Executives (SCORE); retired business executives assist new small business owners to establish and direct their business

STATES, the original administrative units of the nation, retain responsibility for many programs. In general, they administer and supplement federal programs within the state. Acceptance of federal money means acceptance of federal guidelines for programs. States vary most by the manner in which federal programs are supplemented.

- Department of Human Resources: Medicaid, SSI, and poverty programs of the Social Security Act; food stamps; protective services against abuse, case management, foster care for children and the aged, Medicaid eligibility for institutionalization, information, and referral
- Departments of Health and Mental Health and Mental Retardation: licenses and controls health personnel and facilities, including long-term care facilities and nursing homes; may have special programs for older people

Box continued on following page

- Department on Aging: administers funds provided by the Older Americans Act through designated regional area agencies responsive to local needs

Counties and cities incorporate federal and state programs and may add more of their own. City programs may have strict criteria for eligibility and meet only a fraction of the need. They usually do not receive high priority in the city budget, and services depend on the city tax base and political philosophy. Examples of programs provided include assisted homemaking and job placement, nutrition, transportation, legal, financial, and other types of counseling.

Thousands of other local programs exist, sometimes serving a very limited area. They are sponsored by various professional or service groups, churches, businesses, and individuals, and they provide services such as telephone assistance, home-delivered meals, and adult day care. Funding comes from various sources. Directories that list local resources may be obtained from the United Way, Junior League, Chambers of Commerce, and local religious agencies.

NEW CONCEPTS OF COMMUNITY CARE

Across the country, ways are being devised to meet the needs of the elderly. Four successful programs are presented here.

Nursing Home as Senior Center

Competition in the nursing home industry has inspired programs intended to give the facility greater visibility and deeper roots in the community. This example is based on the Chandler Center, a nonprofit retirement apartment and nursing home complex in San Antonio, Texas. It is an attractive facility conveniently located in an area with a high elderly population. Its philosophy is to be a nursing home without walls, and the target population for its extended programs is the well elderly person who can buy services. The senior center has its own building and staff to coordinate programs. It provides a meeting place and an opportunity for social activities and networking. One program exists to reduce the risk of exploitation for people who need help at home and wish to hire a reliable contractor. The Chandler Center will assist in contacting an appropriate business, which then deals directly with the customer. Other programs are directed toward life enrichment and include the Institute of Lifetime Learning, which provides classes in languages, art, photography, and other subjects of interest to members. Day or vacation trips are organized, exercise and bridge groups meet, and invited speakers talk on topical subjects. Holidays bring special celebrations. Many activities are planned by members themselves, some of whom volunteer regular hours of help. The facility is also a meeting place for church groups and a chapter of AARP. Transportation is arranged for members who need assistance, and lunch is served daily. Meals at home are delivered on request.

Generations Together

Established in 1978 at the University of Pittsburgh Center for Social and Urban Research, Generations Together builds on the affinity of youth and age to develop programs using the strengths of one age group to meet the needs of the other age group in reciprocal relationships. Four distinct intergenerational programs give senior adults the opportunity to assist young people as resources to school teachers and students, as master artists offering their skills to children and youth, as child care aides, and as mentors to high school and university students. A fifth program organizes students aged 14 to 22 to provide direct services to senior citizens in need. Intergenerational child care includes visits by young children to older persons in senior centers or nursing homes. A variety of new demonstration projects are always evolving, and intergenerational activities have developed across the United States to meet community needs. Programs include intergenerational theater, literature discussion, and education of the homebound elderly in subjects such as psychology, politics, and mathematics by adult education students as well as the more usual service projects.

Generations Together develops and investigates the impact of intergenerational programs in settings that are often multicultural and promote mutual growth and learning among youth and the elderly and support the philosophy of the continuity of life. Program assistance and a publication list are available from

Generations Together (811 William Pitt Union, University of Pittsburgh, Pittsburgh, PA 15260).

Mutual Assistance: The Elderly Helping the Elderly

Religious organizations include many elderly persons in their congregations and are aware of their strengths and limitations. In many parts of the country, churches of different denominations are grouping together to combine resources to attack the social problems common to all.

The Jefferson Area Community Outreach for Older People (CO-OP) is a gathering of 11 churches representing most denominations, 1 synagogue, and a retirement community situated in a well-defined area in San Antonio, Texas. The target population is people aged 60 or older who reside within the project area. Religious declaration or affiliation is not required. The purpose of the CO-OP is to promote and encourage independence for older people by establishing a neighborhood network of volunteers to provide mutual assistance, information, and services. A centrally located church provides office space. The CO-OP received a 3-year grant from the Robert Wood Johnson Foundation, but it is now funded by the participating organizations. The CO-OP philosophy is neighbor helping neighbor as needed on a voluntary basis. Services coordinated by the CO-OP include nutrition (home-delivered meals or church lunch programs), transportation, health education (used as a clinical site by nursing students), caregiver support and respite, increased social contact and involvement, counseling, home maintenance assistance, and information and referral. Members of all sponsoring organizations are asked to volunteer their time and talents in the service of those in need. This concept has been very popular, and other groups have begun their own CO-OPs in different geographical sections of San Antonio.

The CO-OP is affiliated with the National Federation of Interfaith Volunteer Caregivers Inc. (P.O. Box 1939, Kingston, NY 12401; telephone: 914-331-1358).

Social–Health Maintenance Organization Demonstration

Developed at Brandeis University's Bigel Institute for Health Policy, this research demonstration project studies the feasibility of providing the elderly with a single prepaid program of preventive, acute, and long-term services by integrating community-based care into the HMO model. Social-HMOs fill three critical gaps in Medicare and private insurance by supplying various long-term, in-home support services to assist members to remain in their homes as well as posthospital home care or nursing home care that goes far beyond current Medicare criteria and 1 to 4 months of custodial nursing home care without restriction on setting or prior hospitalization. Benefits such as hearing aids, eyeglasses, and prescription medications are included.

Four sites (New York, Oregon, Minnesota, and California) enroll volunteer Medicare and Medicaid recipients within their service areas to reflect the local Medicare population by age, sex, marital status, living arrangements, and need for assistance with ADLs. Funding is by a Health Care Financing Administration premium equal to estimated Medicare costs plus a monthly premium from each member similar to the Medicare Part B supplements. The pooling of finances and management of both short- and long-term care services have enabled the sites to break even financially and exceed target membership after 4 years of operation.

The purpose of the project is to provide information for policy and practice decision making for efficient and effective health care for elders. With common screening and assessment tools for the four sites, a 20,000-member data base has become the largest of its kind in the United States, with information on the biopsychosocial supports and needs of an elderly population. Further information is available from the Social-HMO Consortium (Bigel Institute for Health Policy, Heller Graduate School, Brandeis University, Waltham, MA 02254-9110).

APPLICATION OF THE NURSING PROCESS

The nursing process can be used on an individual, family, aggregate, or community level. The principles of assessment, planning, implementation, and evaluation apply to whichever level is required. After some general considerations on the application of the nursing process, an example is given caring for an older person in the community. As happens fairly frequently, this person has no immediate family nearby, and planning emphasizes community relationships.

A theory base applicable to the client's needs should provide the framework within which the nursing process is carried out. Although theories themselves may be very complex, simplified versions distilled from major assumptions can assist the nurse in monitoring the health of the elderly and their responses to treatment. Social theories of aging have developed since the 1950s, usually in response to the concerns of a particular time in U.S. culture. Brown (1990) noted that they may be valid only in certain times and places and that they address specific issues related to aging rather than the experience of aging as a whole. Despite their limitations, theories may provide some guidelines for recognizing problems and planning appropriate care for elderly clients.

Selected Social Theories of Aging

Activity Theory. The key to successful aging is the maintenance of optimal levels of activity from the middle years of life. This theory led to the establishment of many activity centers.

Disengagement Theory. As people age, their needs change from active involvement to withdrawal for contemplation about the meaning of life and impending death. In addition to the withdrawal of the individual from society, there is the withdrawal of society from the aged. This academic theory caused great controversy.

Loss of Major Life Roles Theory. This theory challenged the disengagement theory by claiming disengagement was forced by denying older people societal roles (e.g., mandatory retirement from the work force). This led to the establishment of government programs to provide volunteer and work opportunities.

Continuity Theory. The unique personality and lifelong behavioral characteristics and habits of an individual continue into old age. This theory is an attempt to balance the extremes of the activity and disengagement theories.

Socially Disruptive Events Theory. If life is severely disrupted in a number of ways in a brief period of time (e.g., by retirement, loss of a spouse, and so on), social withdrawal becomes an appropriate response. This response should reverse with time. If disengagement becomes established, however, it becomes difficult to reverse.

Reconstruction Theory. Negative labeling of the elderly by society as well as self-labeling after negative life events led to a view of the elderly as incompetent and helpless.

Age Stratification Theory. This theory assumes that societies are inevitably stratified by age and class. The relative inequality of the elderly at any given time or situation depends on their typical life course experiences and is due mostly to the physical and mental changes that take place and the history of the time (e.g., wars) through which the cohort lived.

Modernization Theory. Loss of social status among the aged is a universal experience in all cultures in which modernization processes, which mostly affect the young and often involve new technology, are occurring.

Assessment

Data collection should be complete and systematic. A standardized form provided by the agency is often helpful, but the nurse must understand the reasoning (theory base) behind the form to be able to adapt it to a situation outside the norm. Two common approaches are the *systems theory* and the *epidemiological triad*. With systems theory, the nurse examines a system, its subsystems and suprasystems, and its relationship with other systems. For example, if the primary focus is on the client as the system, the client's biological, psychological, and social subsystems may be examined as well as the client's suprasystems such as family interaction and neighborhood environment. The nurse is a part (subsystem) of the health care system that has a relationship with the client. The interaction between the client and the health care system provides data for evaluating and planning for desired outcomes. In the epidemiological approach, the host, agent, and environment are analyzed. This method is more easily used for one problem at a time. The client is the host, a particular problem is examined as the agent, and the environment includes all causes of and possible solutions for the problem that affects the host. A third method, which is the one used in the following example, is a problem-solving approach that identifies strengths and weaknesses and compensates for weaknesses. In practice, many theories are used concurrently; the principles of systems theory and the epidemiological triad can be identified in the following case study.

Assessment of the elderly must take into account aging changes, and data must be measured against elderly norms. Assessment categories for the elderly should include nutrition, elimination, activity, medication consumption, body protection, cognitive tasks, life changes, and the environment (Yurick, 1984). Nursing diagnoses stem from validated data.

MENTAL HEALTH OF ELDERS

Positive
- Good relationships
- Friends
- Participation in activities
- Goals for the future
- Enjoyment of life

Negative
- Depression
- Isolation
- Confusion
- Disorientation
- Dementia

Rule out
Poor nutrition
Wrong use of medication
Drug reaction or interaction
Perception of "elderly role"
Illness

More information is available in Aging America, 1988; Caring, August 1989 (entire issue).

Assessment of the family and community of a client follows the same systematic data collection methods. The community nurse is always aware of the health status of both the client's family and the agencies to which clients may be referred (e.g., whether an agency is effective in its stated purpose and has sufficient power, funding, and personnel). As information is gathered on clients and agencies, the larger community is assessed for its strengths and weaknesses. *Community* may be defined on the level that will most benefit the client. For an individual as client, community may be the street of residence, the neighborhood, or the area within the limits of available transportation. If the family is the client, the community will expand to include areas of interest to the family group. If the entire aggregate of the elderly is the client, community will have a national perspective. As the nurse builds a data base on different clients and neighborhoods, strengths and weaknesses of the town, state, and nation become apparent. Many community

nurses eventually pursue health-related issues of personal interest to policymaking levels, developing a wide network of people in all aspects of health care in the process.

Formal nursing diagnoses (e.g., North American Nursing Diagnosis Association [NANDA] diagnoses) are not well developed for use in the community, and nurses should be prepared to devise their own when necessary. Sharing and validating nursing diagnoses with clients also are more complex in the community setting. A nursing diagnosis may be validated with an individual client, but validation may be more difficult for family and community diagnoses because members of each group may have different viewpoints. When making a diagnosis at the family or community level, the nurse should be as objective as possible and seek validation from other agencies or professionals working in the same area as well as from the individual client.

Planning

Planning care also requires a theory base. Maslow's (1970) Hierarchy of Needs and Erikson's (1963) Eight Ages of Man are useful and familiar concepts. It must be remembered that Maslow felt that relatively few people would incorporate survival, security, belonging, and self-esteem needs to reach self-actualization. Realistically, the nurse should set goals aiming for belonging and increased self-esteem after the needs for survival and security are met. Erikson saw the task achievements of the elderly as integrity versus despair. Ego integrity is the comfort and acceptance of self as a unique and valuable being, the completed work of the trials and triumphs of life on an individual, and a sense of fulfillment that brings calmness before death. Despair results from failure to achieve integrity, frustration and anger at the passage of time, and a fear of approaching death.

In community health, it is particularly important for the nurse to set short- and long-term goals that are congruent with the desired outcomes of the client. A community health nurse works in the environment of the client, which adds complexity to the process. The nurse is given power and respect, but patient compliance will not usually be good unless the patient sees some value in outcomes desired by the nurse. The client and the family and environment of the client will control the speed and depth of implementation of the nursing care plan.

Evaluation

Evaluation, as with every other step of the process, is a joint activity of the client and the nurse. It measures movement toward or away from a specified goal and gives dynamic feedback that affects planning and intervention. An elderly person may be slow to achieve progress because of arthritis, frailty, or nutritional status rather than because of deliberate noncompliance. Chronic illness has a long-term time frame, and the standard for evaluation may be the prevention of deterioration instead of the cure of the disease. Community problems may have an even longer time frame, or they may be solved fairly quickly if a general problem affects a small group and the solution is inexpensive.

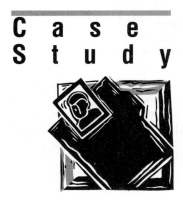

C a s e
S t u d y

Mrs. Darren, a 75-year-old widow, was referred to the community health nurse by her physician, who did not feel she could sufficiently care for herself. Her diagnoses were hypertension, mild congestive heart failure, arthritis, and occasional confusion after transient ischemic attacks. A home visit was made by the nurse. Mrs. Darren lived in a run-down house in an inner-city neighborhood. It was raining and the roof was leaking, and the house had no functioning heat unit. A rat was seen scrambling in the garbage. Mrs. Darren told the nurse that she had no children and her only relative was a sister who lived with her family in another state. She was used to the neighborhood and knew her neighbors, but she was frightened of the teenagers she saw hanging around when she went by bus to the supermarket to cash her Social Security check. She had Supplemental Security Income, Medicare, Medicaid, and food stamps. She ate mostly bread, butter, and coffee, but she enjoyed fried chicken and oranges after going to the supermarket. Constipation was sometimes a problem, so she took a spoonful of laxative every night. She said she did not always remember whether she had taken her medication and held out a small bottle containing an assortment of pills of different colors, shapes, and sizes.

Assessment

With Mrs. Darren as the system, or central planning focus, the nurse identified her biopsychosocial subsystem strengths and weaknesses and looked for actual or potential connections to her family and community suprasystems. Thinking of aging theories, the nurse felt Mrs. Darren was undergoing some forced disengagement because of her physical and social circumstances, which might be reversed if her health could be maintained and her links to the community strengthened. Part of the data gathering process for Mrs. Darren would be to discover her previous pattern of living and her likes and dislikes (using the continuity theory as a basis for planning); the nurse would then assess the community for means to assist Mrs. Darren and then select the available community resources that would be most acceptable to her. On a practical rather than a theoretical level, the nurse also checked with Mrs. Darren's physician regarding the prescriptions and identified the assortment of pills by taking them to the pharmacist who filled the prescriptions.

By means of a problem-solving approach for data gathering, Mrs. Darren's assets were identified as follows:

- Being basically able to care for herself
- Receiving medical treatment
- Receiving income from various sources
- Being accustomed to the neighborhood and knowing her neighbors

Her liabilities were more extensive:

- Inadequate nutrition
- Confusion with medications and improper use of laxatives
- Condition of the house, which was not supportive of health
- Threat of violence in neighborhood and possibility of attack for Social Security money
- Physical impairment resulting from age and illness
- No children or other family living nearby
- Probable progression of confusion
- Possibility of a major stroke at home while unattended

Diagnoses and Planning

Diagnoses and related short- and long-term goals address Mrs. Darren's situation, in which no close family lives nearby. Plans at the three levels of prevention are written for the diagnoses and include suggestions for intervention with families.

Individual   Altered nutrition: less than body requirements, related to difficulty or inability to procure food

Short-Term Goal
- Mrs. Darren will improve her diet to include RDA of nutrients, including fiber and fluids as evidenced by diet recall, and report regular bowel habits without the inappropriate use of laxatives.

Long-Term Goals
- Mrs. Darren will maintain a nutritionally adequate diet through self-care and use of community programs as evidenced by a steady weight and normal tests for nutritional status during physical examinations.
- Inconsistency in medication regimen related to forgetfulness and mild confusion.

Short-Term Goal
- Mrs. Darren will identify medications and know when to take them as evidenced by demonstration to nurse.

Long-Term Goals
- Mrs. Darren will continue to take medications as ordered as evidenced by stabilization of disease processes and intermittent demonstration to nurse.

- Potential for injury related to inadequate housing, possibility of robbery of Social Security money, and aging and progression of disease.

Short-Term Goal
- Mrs. Darren will improve her home to a level allowing healthy habitation, avoid robbery by varying her routine and using banking services, and expand her social network and maintain health care appointments.

Long-Term Goal
- Mrs. Darren will explore sheltered housing for the elderly and continue contact with community health nurse and neighborhood friends.

Family Potential for injury to family unit related to unanticipated loss of interaction with Mrs. Darren because of her declining health and distance of residence

Short-Term Goal
- Addresses of family members are included in Mrs. Darren's record to facilitate emergency contact.

Long-Term Goal
- Mrs. Darren will maintain family contact by mail, telephone, or possible visits.

Community Knowledge deficit of nutritional services related to lack of publicity of available nutritional programs for the elderly

Short-Term Goal
- Identify existing community programs.

Long-Term Goals
- Promote publicity campaign to advertise nutrition services for the elderly in the community.

- Lack of support programs for medication consistency related to unrecognized need.

Short-Term Goal
- Identify existing programs and memory aids for consistency with medication regimen.

Long-Term Goals
- Support community pharmacists in the campaign to increase public awareness of the need to take medications as prescribed.
- Identify and support programs that will assist with provision of prescribed medications for people who have difficulty obtaining prescriptions because of a lack of insurance, money, or transportation or other problems.

- Lack of programs and resources for elderly residents of limited income related to cost of services and competition for limited funds.

Short-Term Goal
- Identify existing programs for the elderly in the community.

Long-Term Goal
- Community groups work together to maximize use of resources.

Intervention

When the nurse discussed the nursing diagnoses and plans with Mrs. Darren, Mrs. Darren agreed with the short-term goals, but she was not sure she wanted to leave her home for other housing or to meet other people through community activities. However, she agreed that she would try to do so.

During the course of the next few visits, the nurse explained basic nutritional principles and helped make a shopping list and menus for 1 week. Together, they developed a plan to assist with medication scheduling. Referrals initiated by the nurse resulted in a greatly improved living situation. A financial advisor from the city's Supportive Services to the Elderly program encouraged Mrs.

Darren to open a bank account for the direct deposit of her checks and showed her how to use it. A home health aide from the same program came for half a day each week to assist with shopping and cleaning. The sanitation department of the health district exterminated the rats, the roof was fixed by the local Area Agency on Aging, and a church-sponsored group painted the house and cleaned the yard. A small heater was purchased from the Salvation Army store, and application was made to the utility company for help with bills during the winter months.

Mrs. Darren was encouraged to talk about her earlier life during the nurse's visits. She had been widowed soon after her marriage when her husband was killed serving with the army overseas, and she had never remarried. She lived in the neighborhood where she grew up, although it had deteriorated over the years. She had worked as a secretary until her retirement for a small company that had paid salaries each week in cash and had no pension plan. She had enjoyed the companionship and the quiet efficiency and routine of the office. Her sister had married a salesman and moved several times. Her sister had four children, all grown now, but Mrs. Darren remembered visits to them when they were small, and they all exchanged letters and cards at Christmas. Mrs. Darren felt pleased with her accomplishments in life but ashamed of the circumstances in which she was now living, and she was reluctant to ask for help from community agencies about which she knew nothing.

With this information, the nurse planned to increase Mrs. Darren's social contacts by introducing her to a structured group that met frequently and offered several activities among which she might find something she enjoyed, and where she would be missed if she were unexpectedly absent. A neighbor was encouraged to invite her to a nutrition site, where she became involved in a domino-playing group. Mrs. Darren allowed her name to be put on the waiting list for an apartment for the elderly, but with the other changes this was no longer a priority, and a decision could be made when an apartment became available.

Evaluation

With the nurse as intermediary and coordinator of community services, Mrs. Darren easily accepted help with the problems related to security and survival. When her home improvements were completed, Mrs. Darren was able to maintain herself more comfortably with the help of the weekly visit from the home health aide. The establishment of orderly routine, the companionship at the nutrition site, and safer financial arrangements increased Mrs. Darren's feelings of belonging and self-esteem. The nurse reduced her home visits to Mrs. Darren but maintained contact with her during her visits to the health clinic for blood pressure checks and preventive health care arranged to supplement and coordinate with her medical care.

Discussion with the home health aide informed the nurse of proposed funding cuts to the city's supportive services to the elderly program , which would result in reduced services. The nurse spoke to the president of the district branch of the professional nurse's association, who notified the state level of the association to monitor funding on the state level and assisted the nurse in working with other local agencies for the elderly to establish a publicity campaign against the proposed funding cuts through letter writing to the editors of local newspapers, speaking at public hearings on the city budget, and speaking at city council meetings. Although funds were reduced, the cuts were much less severe than they would have been without the campaign, and most services were able to continue, although with waiting time increased for admission of new clients.

Levels of Prevention

Primary

Goal
Promote good nutrition

Individual
- Instruct on nutritional needs
- Plan shopping list and menus incorporating any prescribed diet for health problems

Family
- Instruct on nutritional needs of family members by age, sex, or special needs

Community
- Increase nutrition information where food is sold

Goal
Promote safety and prevention of injury

Individual. See Box G: Accident Prevention at Home
- Immunizations as appropriate
- Use of community services for assistance to maintain property and prevent deterioration
- Network of friends and family

Family
- Services of community health nurse or case manager
- Counseling availability
- Respite care availability

Community
- Community education programs for the elderly
- Community health nurse awareness of potential hazards for elderly residents and intervention as needed

Secondary

Goal
Assessment and treatment of nutrition-related disorders

Individual
- Referral for assessment of possible nutrition-related disorders
- Hospitalization or prescribed nutritional supplements for illness resulting from inadequate nutrition

Family
- Referral for nutritional assessment and counseling

Community
- Emergency food supplies

Goal
Diagnosis and treatment of medication-related injury

Individual
- Referral for apparent overmedication or undermedication symptoms
- Drug or food reactions

Family
- Reassessment of understanding of medications

Community
- Twenty-four–hour poison hot line
- Emergency department with 24-hour response
- Medical services

Goal

Response to injury

Individual
- Medical services
- Social services
- Medical alert call systems

Family
- Referral to the appropriate agency

Community
- Emergency housing
- Emergency trauma and medical care
- Police and judiciary system

Tertiary

Goal

Maintenance of improved nutrition

Individual
- Use of community services

Family
- Exchange family recipes.
- Attend home economics classes.

Community
- Campaigns for nutritional awareness and healthy eating
- Healthy snacks in food machines
- Funding of community food services for aggregates or emergencies
- Services providing access to food (e.g., food banks, Meals on Wheels, food stamps)
- Transportation to grocery stores or nutrition services

Goal

Consistency with medications as prescribed and prevention of medication error

Individual
- Written and oral instructions when medications are dispensed, at level of understanding and in language of the client
- Repetition of instructions by client to health care provider

Family
  • Instruction repeated to family member

Community
  • Community education program about understanding medications

Goal

Maintenance of consistency with medications and medication changes

Individual
  • Continued ability to explain current medications as prescribed
  • Stability or progression toward wellness of disease process
  • Use of commercial gadgets to assist memory
  • Home health nurse to give medications if beyond capability of client (e.g., some injections)

Family
  • Ability to explain and assist with medication administration

Community
  • Outreach programs and publicity campaigns
  • Twenty-four–hour availability of pharmacist for consultation

Goal

Maintenance of safe living in the community and delaying the need for long-term care facilities and institutionalization

Individual
  • Safety appliances
  • List of agencies to call for various assistance needs
  • Monitoring by community health nurse

Family
  • Respite care
  • Referrals as needed

Community
  • Housing improvement programs
  • Other programs to assist home living
  • Direct banking services
  • Police surveillance
  • Telephone services
  • Handicapped transportation services
  • Sheltered housing and foster homes for the elderly
  • Retirement communities
  • Nursing homes and long-term care facilities

ALLOCATION OF RESOURCES FOR SENIOR HEALTH

In the case study, many different agencies provided assistance to keep Mrs. Darren functioning adequately in the community, and many more could have been used. The increasing number of older people and their needs for health care are stimulating discussion on the kind of services that should be provided. Netting and Williams (1989) identified four themes concerning ethical decision making in an aging society:

1. Autonomy versus beneficence: the rights, wishes, and competency of a client to accept or refuse professional advice

2. Issues of death, dying, and termination of treatment
3. Allocation of resources in an aging population
4. Family caregiving or the obligation to provide care

Readers are referred to the ethical literature for arguments on these themes. This section is intended only to raise a few questions about the allocation of resources to the elderly.

In a discussion of aggregates and health care, the issue of resource allocation is always in the forefront. Health care, for economic reasons alone, is a limited resource. Questions about the most effective distribution of health care resources among the claims of rival aggregates are issues of "rationing" and social justice.

Callahan (1987) believed that resources should be targeted to the young and that health resources available to people older than 65 years should be limited "first at the level of public policy and then at the level of clinical practice and the bedside." The elderly would be reeducated to become less dependent on medical care and more accepting of a "natural life span" followed by a "tolerable death." In Callahan's view, the elderly should focus on the care of the young and future generations, not on their own cohort. Fry (1988) noted that the content of nursing education would change and that social concerns would take precedence over the individual when planning care for those older than 65 if this philosophy were adopted.

At first glance, this is a repugnant idea that considers the elderly to be disposable, as having outlived their productive value to society, and as now only consuming material resources. Obviously, many people older than the relatively young age of 65 are highly productive and refute such generalization. Aging, however, is very individualistic, and public policy can be a useful scapegoat. For example, cardiopulmonary resuscitation (CPR) is often the entry into high-technology prolongation of a poor quality of life that many elderly fear. Research is establishing guidelines (Clark et al., 1994; Murphy et al., 1989; Podrid, 1989; Schneider et al., 1993) to improve successful CPR rates in the elderly. A national policy limiting CPR to elderly clients with the greatest chance of a successful outcome could be well accepted, reduce legal action against institutional and individual health care providers, and reduce health care costs by using fewer resources.

Because of unmet needs, especially in the areas of long-term care and outpatient support services, organizations advocating for the elderly have worked for a national U.S. health program with universal access to care based on need. As a group, the elderly have already received favored status in access to care by the right to Medicare coverage at the age of 65. With the introduction of prospective payment systems in an attempt to control costs, the elderly have also experienced external control of health care and have been an experimental pilot group in many ways for the general population.

CPR AND THE ELDERLY

- CPR attempts lasting longer than 5 minutes are usually unsuccessful in the elderly.
- CPR is usually unsuccessful in elderly patients with several chronic or acute diseases.
- CPR is rarely effective for elderly patients with cardiopulmonary arrests that are out of hospital, unwitnessed, or associated with asystole or electromechanical dissociation.
- CPR is most successful for an elderly person who functioned independently with a normal mental status before the arrest, had a witnessed cardiac arrest with a vital sign detected at the onset, had ventricular tachycardia or fibrillation, responded within 5 minutes to cardiac massage, and regained consciousness promptly.

Data from Murphy DJ, Murray AM, Robinson MD, Campion EW. Outcomes of cardiopulmonary resuscitation in the elderly. Ann Intern Med 111:199–205, 1989.

RESEARCH ON THE HEALTH OF THE ELDERLY

Topics for research may be identified throughout this chapter. Studies on the elderly and the process of aging are needed in all areas. How can we predict and plan for the welfare of the majority while allowing flexibility for the needs of outliers? Why are the elderly such a diverse group? What causes the different rates of physical and mental aging? How far can we go in defining this aggregate by age alone, or should some other standards be developed? There is an immediate need for studies to show how medication acts in older people and whether drug dosage or frequency should be different.

Different cultural and ethnic attitudes and practices concerning aging must be identified and incorporated into care. As increasingly active groups of the elderly gain increasing autonomy in health care decision making and control of their death and dying (including the right to refuse treatment), there is a danger that not all people will be well served (Kapp, 1989). When individuals are expected to claim the rights they have been given, many less assertive older people, especially those from cultures in which decisions are made within the family rather than by an individual, may not claim the care they need. Health care delivery must be culturally sensitive.

Stein et al. (1984) conducted a study to identify stressors for elderly people living in the community. The participants in this study lived in poor neighborhoods, had a low annual income, and had not completed high school. Immediate economic survival was identified as their utmost concern, specifically related to rising food costs and threatened cuts in Social Security. Fear of having to live in a nursing home, loss of sight, and being robbed were other significant stressors. Concerns about health and disability, with the possibility of increased dependence, caused more distress than did the thought of death. Other concerns related to having to live with children or having lived in the neighborhood for only a short period of time. This last concern may relate to unfamiliarity with the community, lack of peer support, and pervasive change. The authors concluded that their sample as a whole showed a generalized anxiety state about the future, and they suggested that perceived stress for the elderly should be measured in terms of anticipated events or emotions. If this is so, by prolonging uncertainty about the economic future, continued publicity about proposals to lower or tax Social Security benefits, Medicare, and other programs for the elderly is particularly cruel and stressful.

Research is also needed on motivation factors for the recruitment and retention of nurses to care for the elderly as well as the qualities needed to gain satisfaction in what can be a very difficult and challenging field.

ROLES OF THE COMMUNITY HEALTH NURSE

The first role (and duty) of the community health nurse is to be visible in the community and be seen as a resource for health care for everyone. Nurses working with the elderly have the same roles as other community health nurses. At different times, as appropriate, roles include client advocate to the family and health care system, aggregate advocate to the community, educator of client and public, planner, case manager, facilitator, coordinator of care between agencies, observer, data collector, researcher, case finder, and provider of clinical nursing care. Nurses should also seek to be board members of organizations that affect their clients and to be political lobbyists. Given the constraints of working for government agencies on whatever level and within which most community health employment lies, this last may need ingenuity, which is characteristic of community health nurses.

SUMMARY

This chapter has taken a broad approach to the health of the elderly, who form the most diverse and rapidly growing aggregate. Issues that affect the day-to-day life of the elderly are addressed: a functional body rather than the absence of disease; enough money and services to allow enjoyment of life; adequate food, housing, and mobility; the dignity of knowing each life has affected all those whom it has touched; and the respect owed to those who, by nature of advanced age, are closer to the adventure of the end of this life. The purpose of public health is to improve life at all ages for all people, and each chapter in this textbook contributes to that end, which, in effect, is a good life at a good age. The health of the elderly is a function of everything encountered in life—environmental health; occupational health; biological, psychological, spiritual, and social health; men's and women's health; and the history, politics, policy, and future of health—and nurses are major contributors to the entire field of health care. The health of the elderly begins in the prenatal clinic and ends at death, and nurses participate in each step of the way.

ORGANIZATIONS FOR THE ELDERLY

- American Association of Retired Persons (AARP), 601 E St NW, Washington, DC 20049. Telephone: (202) 434-2277.

  Founded in 1958, AARP has more than 33 million members aged 50 or older in almost 4000 local chapters. Members receive *Modern Maturity* magazine bimonthly (the largest circulation magazine in the United States), and the *AARP News Bulletin* 11 times each year. A list of publications is available. AARP is involved in most issues affecting older people and has established the National Resource Center on Health Promotion and Aging to provide information and networking to health professionals across the country.

- Gray Panthers, 2025 Pennsylvania Ave NW, Suite 821, Washington, DC 20006. Telephone: (202) 466-3132.

Founded in 1970 by Maggie Kuhn, Gray Panthers is an organization of people of all ages working together to achieve social justice, to foster the concept of aging as lifetime growth, and to eliminate ageism. It strongly promotes adequate health care for all and has led fights against mandatory retirement and nursing home abuse. Gray Panthers awards grants to academicians, researchers, and creative artists older than 70 years for continued work.

- Older Women's League (OWL), 666 11th St NW, Suite 700, Washington, DC 20001. Telephone: (202) 783-6686.

Formed in 1980 after a White House miniconference on older women and born from the double discrimination of age and sex, OWL's motto—"Don't Agonize—Organize"—could be adopted by nurses. OWL fights for social and economic equity for midlife and older women. Its agenda includes a national universal single-payer health care system, economic security through housing and job access, and pension equity. *Gray Papers* and annual *Mother's Day* reports provide in-depth analysis of key issues. A list of publications and videotapes is available.

- National Council on the Aging (NCOA), 409 3rd St SW, Washington, DC 20024. Telephone: (202) 479-1200.

Founded in 1950, NCOA was the first organization to give a national focus to the concerns of older people. It is an organization of professionals involved in all aspects of work with the elderly and is a national resource for information, training, technical assistance, advocacy, publications, and research on aging. NCOA projects have led to the Foster Grandparents Program, Meals on Wheels, nutrition sites, and the training and placement of older low-income workers; it also has developed intergenerational programs in which the elderly help children. A list of publications is available.

- National Council of Senior Citizens (NCSC), 1331 F St NW, Washington, DC 20004. Telephone: (202) 347-8800.

Formed in 1961 during the struggle to enact Medicare, NCSC is an advocacy organization concerned with preserving and improving benefits for the aged by closely monitoring and initiating legislation. NCSC has strong connections with labor unions and a very active political action committee. Current priorities include a national health program, maintaining access to Medicare-Medicaid, and the rights of legal immigrants in proposed changes in welfare.

- Mature Outlook, Inc., 6001 North Clark St, Chicago, IL 60660-2493. Telephone: 1-800-336-6330.

Part of the Sears organization, Mature Outlook reflects the new image of the elderly as healthy people with time and money to spend and as a legitimate marketing target. For people aged 50 or older, members receive discounts at Sears and a bimonthly magazine.

- U.S. National Senior Sports Organization (USNSO), 14323 South Outer Forty Rd, Suite N300, Chesterfield, MO 63017. Telephone: (314) 878-4900.

Established after the first U.S. National Senior Olympics in 1987, the mission of this not-for-profit organization is to promote fitness and excellence of health of senior adults. Through competition at local and regional games, members may qualify to compete at the biennial national games. Eighteen sports categories include individual, doubles, and team sports with some modified rules and age levels exceeding 100 years.

- Elderhostel, 75 Federal St, Boston, MA 02110-1941. Telephone: (617) 426-8056.

From Cicero to computers, politics to poetry, this nonprofit organization offers inexpensive, noncredit, short-term (typically lasting about 1 week) academic courses hosted by educational institutions around the world. Participants stay in college dormitories or similar commercial sites. Efforts are made to include people with disabilities, and intergenerational programs are offered. Some scholarships are available. Subject interest is usually the only educational requirement.

Learning Activities

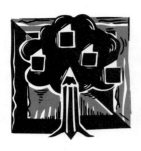

1. As a group activity, review the case history of Mrs. Darren presented in this chapter. Discuss assessment using different theories. What other information would you like to have? What other services may she need (e.g., dentistry)? Where would you find these services in your community? What interventions could have taken place earlier in her life to prevent or delay some of her problems now? What changes should be made in the health system to improve access at all stages of life? What would a comprehensive health system look like?

2. Read your daily newspaper and a weekly news magazine. Keep a scrapbook of articles about legislation that affects the elderly. How many other articles or advertisements highlighted information of specific interest to older people (e.g., products, services, and so on)?

3. Talk to police chiefs in small towns or incorporated cities about the elderly in their communities. Ask what facilities are available for older people. Be prepared to discuss needs and offer solutions. Look for community strengths and weaknesses.

4. Talk to a minister, rabbi, imam, or other leaders of religious organizations. Ask about contributions to the congregation and the community made by elderly members and programs provided for older people. Look for networking of resources.

5. Go to a bookstore and review books describing travel and education opportunities available only to older people. Ask travel agents about their older clients. Are you surprised at the responses?

6. Visit a private retirement community. Talk to the social director, and arrange to interview and record the reminiscences of some residents. Prepare a journal of interviews (and give copies to those interviewed). Do the same in a public-funded housing community for the elderly. Note the similarities and dissimilarities of the stories. Ask your community librarian for local history related by older people.

7. Investigate activity and exercise programs in senior congregate housing. Evaluate (or design and implement) a program for its effectiveness in keeping all residents active and able to live independently.

8. For your eyes only! Answer (in writing) the following questions:

   - What are your personal feelings about growing old?
   - How do you feel when surrounded by elderly people of various physical and mental abilities?
   - What are the positive aspects of aging?
   - What are the negative aspects of aging?
   - Would you want, appreciate, enjoy, or recommend enthusiastically the care available to the elderly in your community? What would you provide if money were no object? What would be your priorities with limited funds? How would you initiate your first priority? Go ahead and try it!

REFERENCES

Adequate Nutrition for the Elderly (hearing before the Select Committee on Aging, House of Representatives, July 30, 1992. Comm. Pub. No. 102-890). Washington, DC: U.S. Government Printing Office, 1992.

Adler GS. A profile of the Medicare Current Beneficiary Survey. Health Care Financing Review 15:153–163, 1994.

Adult Immunizations. MMWR Morb Mortal Wkly Rep 44:741–746, 1995.

Alcohol Abuse and Misuse Among the Elderly. A Report by the chairman of the Subcommittee on Health and Long-Term Care, Select Committee on Aging, House of Representatives, February, 1992. Washington, DC, U.S. Government Printing Office (Comm. Pub. No. 102–852).

Beck CM, Phillips LR. Abuse of the elderly. J Gerontol Nurs 9:97–101, 1983.

Blomquist KB. Prevention: Older adults. In Knollmueller RN, ed. Prevention Across the Life Span. Washington, DC: American Nurses Association, 1993.

Bradsher K. Gap in wealth in U.S. called widest in west. New York Times, April 17, 1995, p. 1A.

Brakman SV. Adult daughter caregivers. Hastings Center Report 24:26–28, 1994.

Brown AS. The Social Processes of Aging and Old Age. Englewood Cliffs, NJ: Prentice Hall, 1990.

Bull MJ. Use of formal community services by elders and their family caregivers 2 weeks following hospital discharge. J Adv Nurs 19:503–508, 1994.

Callahan D. Aging and the goals of medicine. Hastings Center Report 24:39–41, 1994.

Callahan D. Setting Limits: Medical Goals in an Aging Society. New York: Simon and Schuster, 1987.

Chulis GS, Eppig FJ, Hogan MO, et al. Health insurance and the elderly: Data from MCBS. Health Care Financing Review 14:163–181, 1993.

Clarke DE, Goldstein MK, Raffin TA. Ethical dilemmas in the critically ill elderly. Clin Geriatr Med 10:91–101, 1994.

Coldewey LJ. Parish nursing: A system approach. Health Progress 74:54–57, 66, 1993.

Creditor MC. Hazards of hospitalization of the elderly. Ann Intern Med 118:219–223, 1993.

Davidhizar R. Powerlessness of caregivers in home care. J Clin Nurs 3:155–158, 1994.

Day JC. Population Projections of the United States, by Age, Sex, Race, and Hispanic Origin: 1993 to 2050 (U.S. Bureau of the Census, Current Population Reports, P25-1104). Washington, DC: U.S. Government Printing Office, 1993.

Dimond M. Bereavement and the elderly: A critical review with implications for nursing practice and research. J Adv Nurs 6:461–470, 1985.

Erikson EH. Childhood and Society, 2nd ed. New York: Norton, 1963.

Fries JF. Aging, natural death, and the compression of morbidity. N Engl J Med 303:130–135, 1980.

Fry ST. Rationing health care to the elderly: A challenge to professional ethics. Nurs Outlook 36:256, 1988.

Fulmer TT. Elder mistreatment. Annu Rev Nurs Res 12:51–64, 1994.

Fulmer TT. Mistreatment of elders: Assessment, diagnosis, and intervention. Nurs Clin North Am 24:707–716, 1989.

Gelman D, et al. The family: Who's taking care of our parents? Newsweek, May 6, 1985, pp. 61–68.

Gibson RC. The age-by-race gap in health and mortality in the older population: A social science research agenda. Gerontologist 34:454–462, 1994.

Graf JF. Death by fasting. Science 2:18, 1981.

Haug MR. Home care for the ill elderly: Who benefits? Am J Public Health 75:127–128, 1985.

Hayflick L. The strategy of senescence. Gerontologist 14:37–45, 1974.

Hayflick L. The cell biology of human aging. Sci Am 242:58–65, 1980.

Henry RG, Ceridan B. Delivering dental care to nursing home and homebound patients. Dent Clin North Am 38:537–551, 1994.

Hing E, Bloom B. Long-term care for the functionally dependent elderly (National Center for Health Statistics, Vital and Health Statistics, Series 13, No. 104, DHHS Pub. No. [PHS] 90-1765). Washington, DC: U.S. Government Printing Office, 1990.

Hispanic and Indian Elderly: America's Failure to Care (report on a hearing before the Select Committee on Aging, House of Representatives, 101st Congress, Albuquerque, New Mexico, Publication No. 101-730, Part 1). Washington, DC: U.S. Government Printing Office, 1989.

Husaini BA, Moore ST, Cain VA. Psychiatric symptoms and help-seeking behavior among the elderly: An analysis of racial and gender differences. J Gerontol Soc Work 21:177–194, 1994.

Hussey LC. Minimizing effects of low literacy on medication knowledge and compliance among the elderly. Clin Nurs Res 3:132–145, 1994.

Kapp MB. Medical empowerment of the elderly. Hastings Center Rep 19:5–7, 1989.

Kim JJ, Keshian JC. Old old caregivers: A growing challenge for community health nurses. J Commun Health Nurs 11:63–70, 1994.

Kolanowski AM, Gunter LM. Thermal stress and the aged. J Gerontol Nurs 9:13–15, 1983.

Kroner BA, Scott RB, Waring ER, Zanga JR. Poisoning in the elderly: Characterization of exposures reported to a poison control center. J Am Geriatr Soc 41:842–846, 1993.

Lebel JO. Health needs of the elderly. Dent Clin North Am 33:1–5, 1989.

Mackowiak ED, O'Connor TW Jr, Thomason M, et al. Compliance devices preferred by elderly patients. Am Pharm NS34:47–52, 1994.

Maslow AH. Motivation and Personality, 2nd ed. New York: Harper & Row, 1970.

Mikulencak M. The satisfying role of parish nursing. Am Nurse 24:10, 1992.

Murphy DJ, Murray AM, Robinson MD, Campion EW. Outcomes of cardiopulmonary resuscitation in the elderly. Ann Intern Med 111:199–205, 1989.

National Center for Health Statistics. Health, United States, 1993. (DHHS Publication No. [PHS] 94-1232.) Hyattsville, MD: Public Health Service, 1994a.

National Center for Health Statistics. Vital Statistics of the United States, 1990, Vol. II, Mortality, Part A. (DHHS Pub. No. [PHS] 95-110.) Washington, DC: Public Health Service, 1994b.

National Center for Health Statistics. Trends in the Health of Older Americans: United States, 1994. (Analytic and Epidemiologic Studies, Series 3 No. 30.) Hyattsville, MD: Author, 1995.

Neary MA. Community services in the 1990s: Are they meeting the needs of caregivers? J Commun Health Nurs 10:105–111, 1993.

Netting FE, Williams FG. Ethical decision making in case management programs for the elderly. Health Values 13:3–8, 1989.

Nissel M. The family costs of looking after handicapped elderly relatives. Aging Soc 4:185–204, 1984.

Pathy MS, Bayer A, Harding K, Dibble A. Randomized trial of case finding and surveillance of elderly people at home. Lancet 340:890–893, 1992.

Peirce AG. Elder abuse. Imprint 41:59–60, 1994.

Physician Payment Review Commission. Annual Report to Congress. Washington, DC: Author, 1994.

Podrid PJ. Resuscitation in the elderly: A blessing or a curse? Ann Intern Med 111:193–195, 1989.

Religion in America: Approaching the Year 2000. Princeton, NJ: Princeton Religious Research Center, 1990.

The Rich Get Richer Faster (editorial). New York Times, April 18, 1995, p. A14.

Ries P. Americans Assess Their Health: United States, 1987. (Vital and Health Statistics, Series 10, Publication No. 174.) Washington, DC: National Center for Health Statistics, 1990.

Schneider AP II, Nelson DJ, Brown DD. In-hospital cardiopulmonary resuscitation: A 30-year review. J Am Board Fam Pract 6:91–101, 1993.

Schneider EL, Brody JA. Aging, natural death, and the compression of morbidity: Another view. N Engl J Med 309:854–856, 1983.

Shay K. Identifying the needs of the elderly dental patient: The geriatric dental assessment. Dent Clin North Am 38:499–523, 1994.

Stein S, Linn MW, Slater E, Stein EM. Future concerns and recent life events of elderly community residents. J Am Geriatr Soc 32:431–434, 1984.

Subcommittee on Health and Long-Term Care. Elder Abuse: A National Disgrace (Publication No. H2-377). Washington, DC: Select Committee on Aging, Subcommittee on Health, U.S. House of Representatives, 1985.

U.S. Bureau of the Census. Sixty-Five Plus in America. (Current Population Reports, Special Studies, P23-178RU.) Washington, DC: U.S. Government Printing Office, 1992a.

U.S. Bureau of the Census. 1990 Census of Population and Housing. Summary Population and Housing Characteristics, United States. (Publication No. 1990 CPH-1-1). Washington, DC: U.S. Department of Commerce, Economics and Statistics Administration, 1992b March 1992b.

U.S. Department of Health and Human Services. Healthy People 2000: National Health Promotion and Disease Prevention Objectives. (Publication No. [PHS] 91-50213.) Washington, DC: U.S. Government Printing Office, 1990.

U.S. Department of Justice. Office of Justice Programs, Bureau of Justice Statistics. National Crime Victimization Survey. (Publication No. NCJ-147184.) Washington, DC: Author, 1994.

U.S. Senate Special Committee on Aging: Aging America: Trends and Projections. (Publication No. LR 3377 [991]-D12198.) Washington, DC: Department of Health and Human Services, 1991.

Walker D, Beauchene RE. The relationship of loneliness, social isolation, and physical health to dietary adequacy of independently living elderly. J Am Diet Assoc 91:300–304, 1991.

Why Comply: Marion Guide to Wellness. New York, Marion Laboratories, 1990.

Yurick AG. The nursing process and the aged person. In Yurick AG, Spier BE, Robb SS, Ebert NJ, eds. The Aged Person and the Nursing Process, 2nd ed. Norwalk, CT: Appleton-Century-Crofts, 1984, pp. 5–32.

Zimmer JG, Groth-Junker A, McCusker J. A randomized controlled study of a home health care team. Am J Public Health 75:134–141, 1985.

The Homeless

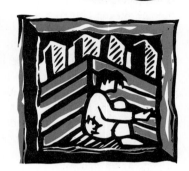

Upon completion of this chapter, the reader will be able to:

1. Discuss two meanings of the term *homeless.*

2. Describe the scope of homelessness in the United States.

3. Analyze factors that contribute to homelessness.

4. Identify major health problems among various homeless aggregates.

5. Discuss access to health care for the homeless.

6. Analyze the health problems of the homeless using upstream thinking and a social justice perspective.

7. Apply knowledge about the homeless when planning community health services for this aggregate.

Diane C. Hatton
Nellie S. Droes

During the 1980s, the number of homeless people surpassed anything seen since the Great Depression (U.S. Department of Housing and Urban Development, 1994). Not only have the numbers of homeless individuals increased, but the demographic profile of this population has changed. Joining the "traditional" homeless predominantly composed of single males are the "new homeless," including families (Wright and Weber, 1987). Projections indicate that in the near future the majority of the homeless in the United States will be single mothers with children (Vladeck, 1990).

The purpose of this chapter is to define homelessness and to describe the scope of this problem. We analyze factors that contribute to homelessness, discuss the consequences of such an existence on health, and describe the health status of various aggregates of the homeless population. We address issues of access to health care and explore conceptual approaches to understanding health among the homeless. Finally, we propose community health nursing strategies for the primary, secondary, and tertiary prevention of homelessness and its associated problems.

DEFINITIONS AND PREVALENCE OF HOMELESSNESS

Many meanings exist for the term *homeless*. Some view the term *home* as a synonym for the place where one's family resides. People without family ties, such as those living in single-room-only hotels (SROs) without family contacts, are, from this perspective, "homeless" (Jencks, 1994). Definitions of homeless, however, usually focus on living quarters and not family ties. For example, in the Stewart B. McKinney Homeless Assistance Act of 1987, the federal government defined "homeless" as

1. "An individual who lacks a fixed, regular, and adequate night-time residence and;
2. An individual who has a primary night-time residency that is:
   - A supervised publicly or privately operated shelter designed to provide temporary living accommodations (including welfare hotels, congregate shelters, and transitional housing for the mentally ill);
   - An institution that provides a temporary residence for individuals intended to be institutionalized; or
   - A public or private place not designed for or ordinarily used as a regular sleeping accommodation for human beings.

3. This term does not include any individual imprisoned or otherwise detained under an Act of Congress or a state law" (U.S. Department of Housing and Urban Development, 1994, pp. 22–23).

Homeless advocates argue that it is also important to consider those who are poor and tenuously housed. This includes those who are without their own shelter but who have "doubled up" with a family member or friend. An estimate at this population is difficult at best.

Demographic Data

Although the homeless are intrinsically difficult to count (Breakey and Fischer, 1990; Jencks, 1994; Lindsey, 1989; Vladeck, 1990), the U.S. Census Bureau has attempted to collect data on the homeless population. On "Shelter and Street Night" or "S-Night" (the evening of March 20 and the early morning hours of March 21, 1990), enumerators counted persons in preidentified locations. Data from the S-Night count revealed 178,638 persons living in emergency shelters for homeless persons, 49,734 persons visible in street locations, and 11,768 persons in shelters for abused women (Fig. 15–1). Further, the breakdown of these data revealed that, in these three categories, males numbered 123,358, 39,255, and 2533, respectively. Females numbered 55,280, 10,479, and 9235, respectively (U.S. Department of Commerce, 1992).

The U.S. Conference of Mayors (1994) provided another source of data on the homeless. Their survey of 30 major cities in the United States revealed that, during 1994, requests for emergency shelter increased

THIRTY MAJOR CITIES INCLUDED IN U.S. CONFERENCE OF MAYORS SURVEY (1994)

Alexandria	New York City
Boston	Norfolk
Charleston	Philadelphia
Charlotte	Portland
Chicago	Providence
Cleveland	St. Louis
Denver	St. Paul
Detroit	Salt Lake City
Kansas City	San Antonio
Los Angeles	San Diego
Louisville	San Francisco
Miami	San Juan
Minneapolis	Santa Monica
Nashville	Seattle
New Orleans	Trenton

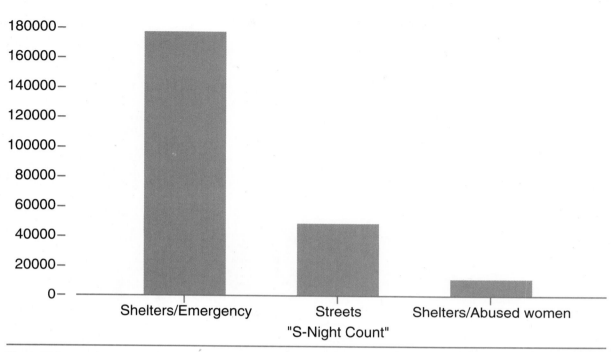

Figure 15–1
U.S. Census data on the homeless population from the "Shelter and Street Night" count. Source: U.S. Department of Commerce, 1992.

overall by 13%. Requests from homeless families increased by 21%, and estimates indicate that one fourth of the requests by homeless families went unmet. Three fourths of the cities indicated that the amount of time people remain homeless increased an average of 9 months overall.

The U.S. Conference of Mayors (1994) survey found that single men made up 48% of the homeless; families with children, 39%; single women, 11%; and unaccompanied minors, 3% (total is greater than 100% as a result of rounding of figures; Fig. 15–2). Ethnic composition of the population reported was as follows: African-American, 53%; white, 31%; Hispanic, 12%; Native American, 3%; Asian, 1% (Fig. 15–3).

Although the data from both the U.S. Census Bureau and the U.S. Conference of Mayors are useful, they have limitations. The count provided by the U.S. Census Bureau is a "point prevalence" count of the total homeless population (i.e., it represents one point in time) (U.S. Department of Housing and Urban Development, 1994). Data from the U.S. Conference of Mayors provides information only on those homeless individuals and families who have sought shelter in 30 major cities during 1994.

To obtain a more thorough understanding, some researchers have attempted to estimate the population from a broader sample and over time. For example, Link and colleagues (1994) sampled persons living in households with telephones and asked subjects whether there was a time in their lives when they considered themselves homeless. The researchers also asked whether subjects had been homeless during the 5-year period between 1985 and 1990. To determine the nature of the homeless experience, interviewers asked whether the subject had (1) slept in a park, abandoned building, street, or train or bus station; (2) slept in a shelter; or (3) slept in a friend's or relative's home because of homelessness. The investigators considered answers of "yes" to either Items 1 or 2 as examples of "literal" homelessness.

The findings indicate that, among the 1507 subjects, the prevalence of homelessness of any type was 14%, and the 5-year prevalence of any type of homelessness was 4.6%. On the basis of these lifetime prevalence rates, the researchers "estimate that about 13.5 million (7.4%) adult residents of the U.S. have been literally homeless at some time during their lives"; and, using

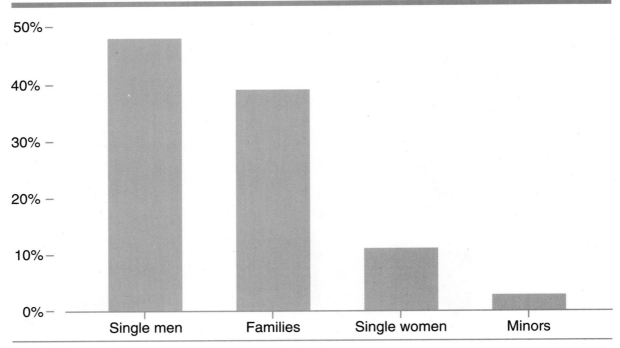

Figure 15–2
Breakdown of persons seeking shelter. Data from U.S. Conference of Mayors 1994.

the 5-year prevalence rates, "5.7 million of these have been homeless" in the span between 1985 and 1990 (p. 1910). Moreover, these figures probably underestimate the problem because the sample excluded households without telephones (about 7% of the U.S. population). The latter may tend to be poor and more likely to experience homelessness. The estimates also exclude those living in institutions such as prisons and mental hospitals; and, again, these individuals are more likely to have experienced homelessness than a domiciled sample.

In sum, the homeless population is difficult to define and to count. However, recent research findings, which attempt to estimate homelessness over time and from a broad sampling of households, have revealed that the magnitude of the problem is greater than thought in the past. Yet, in spite of attempts to count the homeless more accurately, Jonathan Kozol (1988) argued that

we would be wise . . . to avoid the numbers game. Any search for the "right number" carries the assumption that we may at last arrive at an acceptable number. There is no acceptable number. Whether the number is 1 million or 4 million . . . there are too many homeless people in America. (p. 10)

FACTORS THAT CONTRIBUTE TO HOMELESSNESS

Conditions in the larger society that contribute to homelessness include poverty, changes in the labor market, lack of affordable housing, and deinstitutionalization of the mentally ill. In 1992, nearly 37 million Americans were classified as poor. This figure represented 14.5% of the population, a rise from 12.8% in 1989. The value of cash benefits to impoverished families has steadily declined for the past 20 years. In 1992, the value of food stamps combined with Aid to Families with Dependent Children (AFDC) amounted to $14,335, or two thirds of the official poverty threshold (U.S. Department of Housing and Urban Development, 1994).

Changes in the labor market that have consequences for increased joblessness and homelessness include the shift of goods production to services over the past quarter century. Labor markets have also demanded a highly educated work force. The consequences of these economic conditions—decreased job opportunities and extreme poverty—exist in both rural and urban centers (U.S. Department of Housing and Urban Development, 1994).

Lack of affordable housing also contributes to the problem of homelessness. Jencks (1994), in an analysis of the literature, noted that during the 1970s and 1980s, tenants' "rent burdens" rose; this increase occurred not because income fell but because rents have increased at a rate higher than inflation. Between 1974 and 1989, the number of low-income renter households paying more than one half of their income to rent or living in substandard housing or both rose from 3.6 to 5.1 million. A large number of vulnerable persons are at the edge of homelessness: approximately 1.2 million families are on waiting lists to obtain public, subsidized housing (U.S. Department of Housing and Urban Development, 1994).

Another societal factor having consequences for homelessness is the deinstitutionalization of the mentally ill. Rossi (1989) found that one in four homeless persons in a Chicago study had a history of mental illness. Jencks (1994) noted that a series of policies from 1975 to the present contributed to this problem. These policies include the limiting of beds in psychiatric facilities, the end of involuntary commitment, and federal cutbacks for community mental health centers. These policies create a context in which individuals with mental illness have a greater risk of becoming homeless.

Although demographic and economic similarities exist between the homeless and the domiciled extremely poor, the main difference lies in those factors that make it difficult for relatives, and others, to generously provide shelter and support. Especially critical are physical health, mental health, social supports, and criminal convictions or what Rossi (1989) referred to as "vulnerability-enhancing factors."

Jencks (1994) specifically addressed crack cocaine use, a vulnerability-enhancing factor, as a problem in our society and for homelessness. Jencks noted that, among the homeless, this drug is as much of a problem as is alcohol. Heavy use of crack cocaine renders employment problematic, uses money that could otherwise pay rent, and makes it difficult for friends and family to provide shelter. Jencks concluded that "while we have no hard evidence about crack's role in pushing people onto the streets, it clearly helps keep them there" (p. 44).

In sum, not one factor alone forces an individual or family into homelessness. Rather, multiple factors that

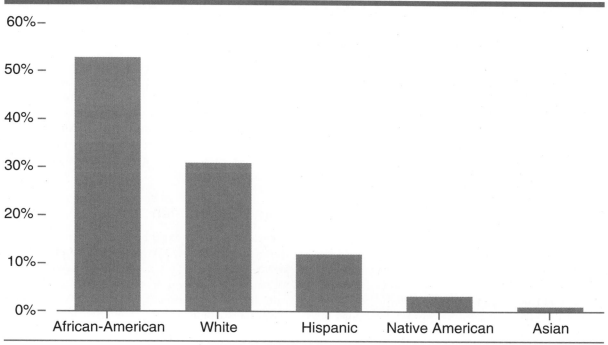

Figure 15–3
Ethnicity of persons seeking shelter. Data from U.S. Conference of Mayors 1994.

reflect conditions in society interact with vulnerability-enhancing factors, found among certain individuals and families, to increase the probability of homelessness. Jencks (1994) noted that "it is a combination of personal vulnerability and political indifference that has left people in the streets" (p. 48).

HEALTH STATUS OF THE HOMELESS

As discussed in Chapter 1, the World Health Organization (WHO) has defined health from a broad perspective. This classic definition, which purports that health is "a state of complete physical, mental, and social well-being and not merely the absence of disease or infirmity" (WHO, 1958, p. 1), is particularly useful when considering the health status of the homeless. For these individuals, there is a continual interaction between these three dimensions—physical, mental, and social—that have enormous consequences for health. Because the boundaries of these dimensions overlap, it is difficult, if not impossible, to address health among the homeless without a concomitant analysis of physical, mental, and social dimensions. We, therefore, address the health status of various homeless aggregates from this broad WHO interpretation. Specifically, the subgroups discussed include men, women, children, and adolescents. Special groups considered are homeless families and homeless persons in the community with mental health and substance abuse problems.

Homeless Men

Reporting on the results of the Health Care for the Homeless Project, Wright (1990b) related that homeless men experience acute physical health problems, respiratory infections, trauma, and skin disorders at higher rates than men in the general population. Chronic disorders—hypertension, gastrointestinal problems, peripheral vascular disease, chronic obstructive pulmonary disease, and seizure disorders—are also more prevalent among homeless populations. In addition, acquired immunodeficiency syndrome (AIDS), tuberculosis, and sexually transmitted diseases (STDs) occur at rates higher than in the general population (Institute of Medicine, 1988).

Many of these acute and chronic conditions are exacerbated by alcoholism, which occurs more frequently among homeless than nonhomeless men. In fact, alcoholism is believed to be the single most prevalent health problem among the homeless. Likewise, serious mental illnesses occur more frequently among the homeless than the general population. In addition, minor emotional problems (e.g., personality disorders) are also found more frequently among homeless than nonhomeless men. Drug abuse, like alcohol abuse, occurs more frequently among the homeless, and there is considerable overlap among alcohol and drug abuse. Men are more likely than women to report alcohol abuse (Glasser, 1994; Institute of Medicine, 1988; Wright, 1990b).

Studies comparing homeless and housed poor persons indicate that homeless adults are more likely to be male and have veteran status than the housed poor. The homeless adults are more likely to be unemployed, or, if employed, the job is temporary or at a low wage and without benefits. Consequently, their income is insufficient to maintain housing costs. Although a lack of monetary resources is a variable directly related to becoming and remaining homeless, additional deficits in social resources contribute to the condition. Many of the homeless have relied on social support from families and friends to provide housing. Homelessness results when both monetary resources and social support are exhausted. In Chicago the average monthly rent in 1985 for an SRO, one of the cheapest types of housing traditionally used by single men, was more than the mean monthly income of homeless adults. Consequently, spending all of one's income on housing would not prevent homelessness (Buckner, 1991; Rosenthal, 1994; Takahashi and Wolch, 1994; Timmer et al., 1994).

As with other homeless subgroups, data from the National Health Care for the Homeless Program in the 1980s provide much of the information available on the health status of the homeless men. Although it is a decade old, it nevertheless stands as one of the major sources of information on the health status of the homeless population.

Homeless Women

Homeless women experience health problems of enormous complexity (Wright, 1990a) and underuse health care services (Adkins and Fields, 1992). These women lack a general or systematic communication with health professionals (Christiano and Susser, 1989) and are unlikely to keep referrals for preventive care (Schlossstein et al., 1991).

Research evidence indicates that homeless women suffer from more acute and chronic health problems than do their housed counterparts (Bassuk and Weinreb, 1993). For example, Wright (1990a) noted that providers found 5.4% of the women in the National Health Care for the Homeless Program to have STDs. STDs were more common in young women than old, and the incidence of STDs in homeless women was about twice that in the ambulatory population in general. Wright also reported that the pregnancy rate among homeless women is surprisingly high. Of the women seen in the National Health Care for the Homeless Program, 10.1% were pregnant. In contrast, a comparable survey of ambulatory care patients in the general population revealed a rate of only 7.1%. Other research suggests that homeless pregnant women are more likely to be younger than their domiciled counterparts, have experienced more serious family disruptions as children, and are less likely to have lived independently (Weitzman, 1989).

Because homelessness entails more than just the loss of a home, there are particular consequences for the mental health of women. Inevitably, homelessness disrupts one's sense of identity and feelings of self-worth and self-efficacy (Buckner et al., 1993). Moreover, considerable stigma accompanies women who are without a home or family in our society (Burroughs et al., 1990). These conditions compound myriad mental health–related problems in this subgroup. For example, North and Smith (1992) found that, of 330 homeless women in a shelter-based sample in St. Louis, 34% met criteria for a lifetime diagnosis of posttraumatic stress syndrome (PTSD) as assessed by the Diagnostic Interview Schedule. Seventy-four percent of the women suffering from PTSD experienced the syndrome before they first became homeless.

Fischer (1991), in a review of epidemiologic studies of the homeless, estimated that approximately 20% of homeless women suffer from alcohol problems and 10 to 20% suffer from drug problems. Studies of homeless women also revealed high lifetime rates of childhood physical and sexual abuse and assault by intimate male partners. Childhood sexual molestation may have a long-term impact on emotions, self-perceptions, social functioning, physiologic well-being, safety, and self-care (Browne, 1993).

Nyamathi and Flaskerud (1992), in a study of black and Hispanic women who were homeless or in drug recovery programs, found complex and multidimensional concerns. Although they did not report the findings of their homeless group separately, the overall

concerns included financial security, lack of social support, discrimination, low self-esteem, loneliness, and helplessness.

In sum, homeless women suffer from the problems that impede many women in the United States, although the problems are likely to be more intense, more frequent, and more apt to occur in concert. Often homeless women have limited education, earning power, and job opportunities and fragmented support networks. Trapped by this lack of economic and social opportunities, they profoundly experience our society's inequities (Bassuk, 1993). Their physical, mental, and social health problems reflect these inequities.

Homeless Children

Reviewing community-based research conducted from 1980 to 1991, Rafferty and Shinn (1991) reported that homeless children are at a disadvantage relative not only to children in the general population but also to other poor children. Homeless women frequently lack prenatal care and sufficient nutrition and are more likely to deliver low-birth-weight infants. The infant mortality rates are higher for infants born to homeless women than for those born to women in public housing. More homeless children experience immunization delays, upper respiratory tract and ear infections, asthma, skin disorders, diarrhea, and anemia than do housed poor children. In addition, more homeless children than domiciled poor children are apt to go without sufficient food because of lack of money.

On the basis of their review, Rafferty and Shinn (1991) indicated that depression and anxiety occur more often among homeless children than among children from poverty groups who are housed. Zima and colleagues (1994) indicated that 37% of homeless children residing in shelters exceeded the cut-off point for depression requiring a psychiatric evaluation, and 28% scored in the borderline clinical range for a serious behavioral problem.

Research findings reveal that when children younger than 5 years are screened using the Denver Development Screening Test (DDST), homeless children are more likely to lack personal and social, language, and gross and fine motor skills than poor housed preschoolers. Among the homeless children, delays in personal and social and language areas occur more frequently than delays in motor skill areas. In other studies using different measurements to assess vocabulary, speech, and gross and fine motor development status, researchers have found both homeless and housed poor children to score poorly (Rafferty and Shinn, 1991).

Notwithstanding the paucity of research on educational achievement of homeless children, Rafferty and Shinn (1991) noted that the few studies undertaken indicate that homeless children score poorly on standardized reading and mathematics tests in comparison to the general school population. A more recent study demonstrated that sheltered homeless children are four times more likely to score at or below the 10th percentile in vocabulary and reading level than children in the general population (Zima et al., 1991). Studies comparing homeless children with housed poor children reveal that homeless schoolchildren are more likely to have repeated grades. Moreover, homeless children miss more days of school than poor housed children. Poor children miss school primarily because of illness; homeless children miss school because of family transience (Rafferty and Shin, 1991).

Most of the research studies related to health status focus on homeless children in emergency shelters. Many of the instruments used to assess developmental and mental health have not been standardized for poor and minority children. It is noteworthy that developmental problems may be underestimated because the DDST is a conservative screening instrument. Assessing the mental health of children is problematic because of the inadequacy of available instruments, the lack of privacy or space to conduct interviews, and parental concerns with daily living rather than the interview. Although care must be taken in generalizing across the studies as a result of frequent small sample sizes, lack of comparison groups, and differences in administration, the studies to date reveal that poor children, in general, face multiple physical, mental, and social problems (Rafferty and Shinn, 1991; Zima et al., 1994).

Homeless Adolescents

An increasing number of adolescents from all sectors of society face serious health problems, including unintended pregnancy, STDs, alcohol and drug abuse, depression, and suicide. Because 20% of persons with AIDS are in their mid-20s, it is most likely that they became infected during their adolescence. Homeless adolescents, however, experience these problems at even higher rates than the general adolescent popula-

tion (American Medical Association, 1992; Forst et al., 1993; U.S. Public Health Service, 1994).

Homeless adolescents experience STDs, physical and sexual abuse, skin disorders, anemia, drug and alcohol abuse, and unintentional injuries at higher rates than adolescents in the general population. Depression, suicidal ideation, and disorders of behavior, personality, or thought also occur at higher rates among homeless adolescents. Family disruption, school failures, prostitution or "survival sex," and involvement with the legal system indicate that homeless adolescents' social health is severely compromised (Cohen et al., 1991; Forst et al., 1993; Reuler, 1991; Smart, 1991; Yates, Pennbridge, et al., 1991).

Homeless adolescents who are pregnant, engage in prostitution, or identify themselves as gay experience more health problems than other homeless adolescents. Pregnant homeless adolescents have more severe mental health problems and use alcohol and drugs more than nonpregnant homeless adolescents. Not surprisingly, they have higher rates of negative pregnancy outcomes than nonhomeless adolescents (Pennbridge et al., 1991).

Runaway or homeless adolescents, female and male, make up a large percentage of all youth involved in prostitution. Many become involved because they need money to live, the source of the term *survival sex.* These adolescents are more likely to have serious mental health problems and to be actively suicidal. Alcohol and drug use occurs at higher rates than among those homeless adolescents not engaged in prostitution. Youths involved in prostitution are more likely to report histories of abuse, both physical and sexual (Yates, Pennbridge et al., 1991).

Rates of attempted suicide are higher among homeless adolescents who are gay identified. A large majority of males involved in survival sex identify themselves as gay or bisexual. Many of these youths are on the streets because of the effects of homophobia and prejudice. Facing problems similar to other homeless adolescents, gay-identified youth face an additional set of problems as a result of the rejection and low self-esteem experienced because of their sexual orientation (Kruks, 1991; Yates, Mackenzie, et al., 1991).

Data on homeless children are scant; however, there are even fewer data on homeless adolescents (Reuler, 1991). A large majority of the studies cited were conducted in metropolitan areas located on the West

Coast. How typical these findings are in other locales is not known. Nevertheless, because adolescents in the general population are at risk, and homeless adolescents are at even higher risk, then the special groups of adolescents, including those who are gay identified, those who are pregnant, and those who are practicing survival sex, present as particularly vulnerable. Health for many of these youths is not only jeopardized but is in double and triple jeopardy.

Homeless Families

Homeless families make up approximately 39% of the homeless population. During 1994, requests for shelter from this aggregate increased 21%, and estimates indicate that 24% of family requests for shelter were not met. In many cases, families seeking shelter have to separate from one another to find accommodations; moreover, they may have to leave the shelter during the day because emergency facilities are often open only in the evening (U.S. Conference of Mayors, 1994).

In a study of 80 families living in shelters in Los Angeles County, McChesney (1992) concluded that homeless families are a heterogeneous group.

Using source of income as a basis, McChesney identified four types of families before homelessness include "(1) unemployed couples, (2) mothers leaving relationships, (3) AFDC mothers, and (4) mothers who have been homeless teenagers" (p. 246). Research indicates that homeless families are predominantly female-headed households and the children usually are preschoolers (Bassuk, 1992).

In a study of homeless and low-income domiciled mothers, Wagner and Menke (1991) reported both similarities and differences between the two groups. Both groups report using similar coping behaviors. However, homeless mothers are "slightly older, have more children to care for, are not as educated, and are less likely to be employed" (p. 82). Additionally, the homeless women have more stressors "in the areas of intra family stress, marital strain, and financial difficulties" (p. 82).

Findings from a study of 80 homeless families in Massachusetts indicate that homeless mothers have had relationships with men characterized by instability, conflict, and violence. Approximately one third leave their parental homes, where family relationships are unstable, and enter relationships with men who batter them. More than 40% of the women noted that

LYDIA

Lydia, standing outside,
waiting to shower
at Rachel's Center for Women.
It is not what she expected,
she says, living on the streets.
Sometimes sleeping on the floor
in an abandoned tire factory
on Tenth Avenue
with three hundred people in one room.
Some on newspapers spread thin to cut the cold,
some on thin mattresses, all on thin soup.
It is not what she expected. It is visible,
this hunger she fights.
For all those years she lived in El Cajon,
wore Calvin Klein slacks, drove her kids
to baseball, she could have been
any one of us.
For all those years she blurred
her husband's insults with Valium,
hunger was what happened just before dinner.
And when he left her, hunger

though she told no one
was what happened
when she couldn't find herself
in the mirror. Hunger all those years
she was draining slowly out
like sawdust trailing from the doll
her daughter once cried for her to fix.
Once, she too had a doll, during the war.
Lydia, born in Krupp, Germany,
down the street from the munitions factory.
She remembers getting dressed, not undressed,
to go to bed, ready to run
from the bombardments. Playing war
with her doll, protecting her from shells.
Taking her brother in hand,
knocking on doors for bread.
It is not, she says, so different
living on the streets.
She knows this war.
It was the bombardments in El Cajon
she couldn't see.

From *Home Sweet Home* by Fran Adler and Kira Corser

their most recent male partner was a substance abuser, and two thirds link battering to alcohol use (Bassuk, 1992).

With their histories of abuse, it is not surprising that some of these mothers may perpetuate the cycle of violence. In the Bassuk study, the Department of Social Services investigated 23% of the mothers for child abuse or neglect or both. Other clinical problems such as mental illness exacerbate these situations. Bassuk reported that 71% of the mothers in her sample had a diagnosis of personality disorder.

In spite of these circumstances, Hodnicki and Horner (1993) reported that homeless mothers describe caring behaviors toward their children, including "sacrificing, struggling with limitations, guarding from harm, and seeking answers" (p. 352). Hodnicki and Horner concluded that the mothers in their study actively sought ways to overcome crises and improve the well-being of their families. Managing children and homelessness is an enormous task for these mothers that has consequences for their health. Anecdotal evidence indicates that homeless mothers rarely tend to their health problems but instead prolong seeking health care until they are so acutely ill that they need emergency treatment (Berne et al., 1990).

The high-risk conditions under which homeless families live "contradict the essence of what we often think of as family life—a stable, secure, and sheltered place for nurturing children" (Hausman and Hammen, 1993, p. 358). We have described the health consequences for children living under these circumstances earlier in this chapter. Moreover, many of the factors that make parents more vulnerable for becoming homeless are also factors that impair their functioning as parents. Homeless families, therefore, deal with a double crisis: the trauma of losing a home as well as the parent's capacity to function as a caregiver (Hausman and Hammen, 1993).

Homeless Persons with Mental Health and Substance Use Problems

A common stereotype of homeless people is that they are alcoholics, mentally ill, or both. Yet estimates of the prevalence of major mental illness and substance use among homeless persons vary widely depending on how researchers define homelessness, the sampling strategy, the interview site, and assessment procedures (Buckner et al., 1993).

In the National Health Care for the Homeless Program, of the 1625 clients known to be mentally ill and who had five or more patient encounters in the first year of the program, 43.7% had a mental illness diagnosed on the first visit; 58.7% were diagnosed as mentally ill on either the first or second visit; and nearly a quarter went undiagnosed until the fifth visit or later (Wright, 1990a). Given this difficulty in diagnosis, research findings too may underestimate mental health problems among homeless subjects if investigators have only one encounter with subjects for data gathering.

On the basis of data derived in the National Health Care for the Homeless Program, 38% of the clients had alcohol problems; 13% had problems with drugs other than alcohol, and 33% had mental illness. By gender, 47% of adult men and 16% of adult women were alcoholic. Psychiatric illness, in contrast, was about twice as common among the women as among the men. The rates of problems with drugs other than alcohol were nearly identical for both genders (Wright, 1990a). In another study, Rossi (1989) found that one in four homeless persons reported at least one episode of hospitalization in a psychiatric institution. The U.S. Department of Health and Human Services (1992), on the other hand, estimated that one third of single homeless adults experience severe mental illness.

Although the estimates of mental illness and substance use problems vary from study to study, the effects of these problems are generally uniform. Specifically, it is difficult for these individuals to find and retain work and housing, form and maintain relationships, and sustain physical and mental health. Moreover, for a sizable proportion of the homeless, severe mental illness exists concomitantly with the problems of alcohol or other drug use, a phenomenon known as "comorbidity" or "dual diagnosis" (U.S. Department of Health and Human Services, 1992). In a review of epidemiologic studies, Fischer (1991) concluded that 10 to 20% of homeless single adults suffer from this combination of a psychiatric disorder and substance use, or comorbidity. These individuals may represent the most vulnerable and the most difficult to treat among the homeless, and they are especially vulnerable to residential instability.

What factors distinguish persons with severe mental illness who are homeless from those who are domiciled? Some suggest that individuals who are mentally ill and have an earlier age of onset of mental illness, co-occurring personality disorders, a history of alcohol or other drug use, physical illness (e.g., AIDS, tuberculosis), a history of childhood disturbances, violent or aggressive behavior, and housing instability are more likely to be homeless. For some, mental illness and substance use cause homelessness; for others, it is the result (U.S. Department of Health and Human Services, 1992).

Popular discussion of the homeless mentally ill focuses considerable attention to the deinstitutionalization of mental patients: the emptying of state mental hospitals beginning in the 1960s. Also it has become considerably more difficult to commit an individual to a psychiatric facility involuntarily. Often homeless persons with severe mental illness come in contact with the criminal justice system, as both offenders and victims. Moreover, some who reside in psychiatric facilities are there because of plea bargaining arrangements negotiated in lieu of being jailed for a bizarre act (Rossi, 1989). For those incarcerated, it is often for relatively trivial and nonviolent offenses (U.S. Department of Health and Human Services, 1992).

Rossi (1989) noted that an important form of chronic mental illness is clinical depression, a painful condition that severely hinders functioning. Findings in his homeless study in Chicago indicate that subjects not only experienced clinical depression but a sense of demoralization (i.e., hopelessness and despair concerning one's prospects). "If the homeless condition can be said to engender mental illness, demoralization appears to be the most likely mechanism through which it has this effect, for the homeless clearly lack even the most common resources that others take for granted" (Rossi, 1989, p. 148).

Most experts generally agree that mental illness alone does not sufficiently explain the prevalence rate of homelessness in most communities. Individual factors contribute to who becomes homeless, but they do not explain why homelessness exists as a major social problem in the first place (Buckner et al., 1993).

ACCESS TO HEALTH CARE FOR THE HOMELESS

Proposing to clarify "access" as it relates to health care services, Penchansky and Thomas (1981) noted that access is a general concept that represents the "degree of 'fit' between the clients and the system" (p. 128). Furthermore, the general term *"access"*

summarizes five specific areas of "fit between the patient and the health care system" (p. 128). These areas are availability, accessibility, accommodation, affordability, and acceptability. After brief definitions, these five factors are used as a framework for exploring problems in accessing health care by (1) persons who are poor but housed, (2) homeless persons in general, and (3) special aggregates of the homeless.

Availability refers to the relationship between the amount (number of providers and facilities) and type of health care services to the amount and type of client needs. *Accessibility* connotes the relationship between the location of the services and the clients' location. *Accommodation* indicates the relationship between how services are organized (e.g., hours of operation, appointment systems) and the client's ability to accommodate to these factors. The client's perception of the appropriateness of these factors is a component of accommodation. *Affordability* refers to the price of provider services or payment requirements and the client's ability to pay. *Acceptability* represents the relationship between the client's attitudes about providers and providers' attitudes about acceptable client characteristics (Penchansky and Thomas, 1981).

Poor but housed persons experience considerable problems related to each of the five access dimensions; however, the primary problem experienced is affordability. Many poor lack any form of health insurance, including Medicaid. Even for those who do meet Medicaid eligibility requirements, the low reimbursement rate discourages or prohibits health care providers from participating. As a consequence of the inability to afford the services of a market-driven system, those who are excluded from the private fee-for-service arrangement must then rely on public hospital systems' outpatient clinics, emergency rooms, and inpatient services. Heavy demands on these less-than-adequate facilities frequently result in less-than-desirable or appropriate accommodations. Long waits for services in overcrowded, uncomfortable settings may discourage persons from seeking care at earlier and hence more easily treated stages of health problems.

Notwithstanding such difficulties, these facilities are frequently situated some distance from the client's shelter or work. Although the innercity resident may access such facilities through a public transportation system, those individuals who reside in rural areas lack such services and must find other resources (relatives, neighbors, friends) or do without health care. Providers in many of the public systems are under considerable stress working in less than optimal conditions, with heavy workloads, and find it difficult to provide care to poor clients who frequently present with complex problems and different cultural and language expectations. Consequently, the clients are prone to find such services unacceptable and fail to present until illnesses are no longer tolerable (Aday, 1992; Institute of Medicine, 1988; Wright, 1990b).

In common with persons who are poor but housed, homeless persons experience considerable difficulty, as outlined previously, in accessing the health care system. However, the homeless face problems over and above those of the housed poor. Eligibility for many services frequently requires forms of documentation that homeless people find difficult to provide because of the exigencies of their homelessness. Lacking secure storage space renders security for personal papers from loss, theft, or elements of the weather problematic. Frequently without access to public transportation because of costs, homeless persons must walk to service sites. Consequently, accessibility is even more problematic for the homeless than for those who are housed and have a relatively more intact system of transportation (e.g., transportation vouchers, relatives, neighbors, friends). Without a permanent mailing address or message center, accommodating a health care system that relies on mailed notification of appointments or results of health care procedures is unlikely. Furthermore, the hours of service may force the homeless to choose between obtaining health care and obtaining food and shelter (Aday, 1992; Institute of Medicine, 1988; Wright, 1990b).

Special aggregates within the homeless population experience additional problems in obtaining health care services. The problems of two groups, the homeless who are chronically mentally ill and pregnant women, are outlined next. Although physical health services available to the poor are inadequate, mental health services are even less available. Given the historic conditions of deinstitutionalization, whereby community-based mental health services failed to materialize, and the current policy, whereby Medicaid reimburses less for mental health services than for physical health services, it should come as no surprise that the need for mental health services for homeless mentally ill clients far exceeds the supply.

The homeless mentally ill also require physical health services. Obtaining such care from these two disconnected and complex systems requires considerable skill in negotiation, skills frequently compromised by the nature of the illness. Notwithstanding the lack of services, the chronically mentally ill, because of the intrinsic nature of their health problems, frequently experience significant problems related to dimensions of accommodation and acceptability. Frequently distrustful of established institutions, the chronically mentally ill find the traditional services provided by mental health agencies inappropriate. Many providers find their bizarre manner of dress, lack of personal hygiene, and inappropriate physical appearance difficult to accept (Aday, 1992; Institute of Medicine, 1988; U.S. Department of Health and Human Services, 1992).

Given the conditions of homelessness in which obtaining food and shelter is preeminent, pregnant homeless women frequently find seeking early prenatal care a lesser priority. Compounding the lower priority are the problems of obtaining prenatal and obstetric care. Some obstetric providers refuse to see or limit the number of women on Medicaid because of low reimbursement rates, complex billing requirements, and increased risk associated with malpractice suits. Consequently, the availability of prenatal and obstetric services is severely compromised. Long waits not only for initial appointments, but at each visit, impose considerable stress in obtaining prenatal care. Many providers find unacceptable the unhealthy lifestyles, the lack of compliance with provider advice, and the failure to keep appointments (Aday, 1992; Curry, 1989; Institute of Medicine, 1988). In sum, multiple complex factors reduce access to health care for this vulnerable, underserved aggregate.

CONCEPTUAL APPROACHES TO HEALTH OF THE HOMELESS

The following discussion provides a conceptual and theoretical framework for exploring health care of the homeless. More specifically, we briefly outline two approaches to the distribution of benefits and burdens: market justice and social justice; provide an explanation of social justice as the absence of structural violence; and discuss upstream versus downstream approaches to the health care of the homeless.

Models of justice provide a blueprint with which to consider the health problems of the homeless.

Beauchamp (1979) distinguished between two types of justice that influence public health policy in the United States: market justice and social justice. Market justice has been the dominant model and purports that people are entitled to valued ends (status, income, happiness) according to their own individual efforts. Moreover, this model stresses individual responsibility, minimal collective action, and freedom from collective obligations other than respect for another person's fundamental rights. In contrast, under a social justice model, all persons are entitled equally to key ends (access to health care, minimum standards of income). Consequently, all members of society must necessarily accept collective burdens to provide for a fair distribution of these ends.

Additional explication of social justice can be found in Galtung's analysis of violence. Distinguishing between physical and structural violence, Galtung (1969) defined violence as "present when human beings are being influenced so that their actual somatic and mental realizations are below their potential realization" (p. 168). In other words, the difference is between the actual and the possible. He further distinguished between physical and structural violence according to whether or not there is a person who acts. Galtung noted that when there is an actor who commits the violence, this is personal or direct violence. In contrast, structural violence is indirect because it lacks an actor. More specifically, the violence is built into the social structure and is displayed as unequal power and consequently as unequal life chances. Stated differently, resources are unevenly distributed (e.g., access to medical services because of ability to pay or because of location). Presence of structural violence is also known as social injustice. Conversely, its absence is social justice.

Butterfield, in this text, discusses McKinlay's (1979) use of the metaphor depicting illness as a river with health workers focused exclusively on pulling people out of the river rather than going upstream to find out the reasons for people being in the river. Hence, the point is that the predominant mode of approaching societal problems is a downstream mode of intervention.

We argue that the market justice model results in a downstream approach to problems and contributes to structural violence. This model holds individuals responsible for their own conditions and negates the responsibility of all individuals and groups to share in the burdens of prevention. In contrast, the social justice model, seeking to reduce through collective action the structural conditions contributing to the problem, supports upstream thinking.

Building on McKinlay's "river" metaphor, we suggest conceptualizing homelessness as the river and the people in the river as the homeless. We purport that governmental and private efforts to address health care problems of homeless have largely focused on "pulling the bodies out of the river of homelessness." Such downstream interventions aimed at treating or alleviating health care problems such as physical disease and mental illnesses are worthy and needed. However, these interventions are far less adequate in alleviating homeless people's social health problems. To improve the social health of the homeless, it is necessary to go upstream and focus on the primary contributors to homelessness itself: lack of access to affordable housing and an adequate income.

Some purport that affordable housing and income support are sufficient to ameliorate homelessness (Timmer et al., 1994). They argued that the homeless are not different from other people in physical and mental health status. The research reviewed here does not support these conclusions; it indicates the homeless have more health problems than the poor who are housed. Although we agree that the primary mode of preventing health problems of the homeless is to prevent homelessness, we also believe that secondary and tertiary types of interventions are necessary.

APPLICATION OF THE NURSING PROCESS

Community health nurses increasingly have contact with homeless individuals and families in a variety of settings, including schools, jails, emergency rooms, community clinics, and shelters. Nurses practicing in these settings have a unique opportunity to address the health needs of this aggregate. The following case study provides an illustration of a community health nurse working with the homeless in a county health department and describes the nursing process at the individual, family, and aggregate levels. Butterfield's use of the "upstream thinking" metaphor facilitates the application of the nursing process to this aggregate. In particular, this metaphor provides a useful perspective for the consideration of primary, secondary, and tertiary prevention with the homeless.

Case Study

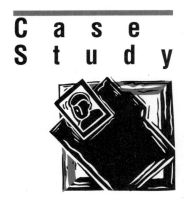

Connie Boiley, a community health nurse working with a county health department, has received a referral from a local homeless shelter. Staff has requested that she assess a client, Ruth Smith, and assist her in adapting to the shelter's communal living situation. The referral form indicates that Ruth is a 29-year-old African-American woman with seven children. Presently, she has only one child, a newborn boy, in her custody. Her other six children either reside with family members or live in foster homes.

Assessment

When Connie visits the shelter, Ruth tells her she has a history of hospitalization for mental health problems. Ruth has difficulty focusing on the topic of conversation and tells Connie she hears voices. Ruth also says that after her infant was born, her obstetrician recommended that she stop all medications because she wanted to breast-feed. Ruth also informs Connie that she has a history of crack cocaine use.

Staff reports that Ruth's behavior is bizarre, and they are unable to manage clients with psychiatric problems in the shelter. Generally, clients who require medications are not allowed to stay because staff are not available to monitor these situations. Staff decided to give special consideration to Ruth because she had a newborn infant. However, difficulties among Ruth, the staff, and other clients have escalated. Connie knows from experience that the community has no other facilities that offer shelter to women who have psychiatric problems and also have children.

Diagnosis

Individual
- Altered health maintenance
- Impaired thought processes

Family
- Impaired home maintenance management
- Alteration in parenting

Community
- Lack of mental health services for women with children

Planning

Connie discusses the priority for managing Ruth's mental health problems with Ruth and the shelter staff. She also consults with colleagues in her community who have experience working with the homeless mentally ill and identifies resources for treatment. Connie explores the community resources for ongoing well-infant care and for family planning services.

Interventions

For evaluation and treatment, Connie refers Ruth to a community mental health agency that provides services to the poor and homeless. Staff facilitates these appointments by assisting Ruth in reestablishing her Medicaid eligibility and by making arrangements for transportation and child care. Connie also works with staff to develop strategies for caring for Ruth and her newborn in the shelter. Ruth attends parenting classes, as do other shelter residents, on a regular basis. Staff clearly identifies expectations for Ruth in the shelter, including household tasks, management of her illness, and care of her newborn. As Ruth adapts to the shelter, Connie also refers her to a community clinic for family planning services and well-infant care.

Evaluation

Connie develops specific guidelines with staff to monitor Ruth's progress in the shelter. Staff, Ruth, and Connie meet on a biweekly basis to review the overall situation and analyze any problems that emerge.

Levels of Prevention

As we noted in the discussion of *Conceptual Approaches to Health of the Homeless,* efforts to address the health care problems of the homeless largely focus on downstream interventions. In Ruth's case, for example, Connie helps pull her body out of the river of homelessness. As McKinlay (1979) argued, providers are so busy pulling the bodies to shore that they have no time to go upstream and see who is pushing them in. To consider an "upstream" intervention, or in this case, primary prevention, community health nurses need to address the primary contributors to homelessness itself (i.e., the conditions in the larger society that contribute to homelessness and the vulnerability-enhancing factors among individuals and families).

Primary Prevention To address the problem of homelessness at this level, community health nurses must deal with the economic and political institutions of our society. Nursing has a long history of responding to public need. The Henry Street settlement nurses provide us with such an example. These nurses saw that their work was different from that of a hospital where infants are cured after they are sick; the Henry Street settlement nurses instead sought to care for infants before they became sick and to keep them well (Portnoy and Dumas, 1994).

Similarly, contemporary community health nurses can work with individuals and families who experience vulnerability-enhancing factors, such as mental illness, substance use problems, violence, and weakened family ties, to prevent homelessness. At an aggregate level, community health nurses play a role by influencing policy that has consequences for homelessness in this country. Rosenheck (1994) summarized the seriousness of homelessness and its implications for public policy action in the following:

Homelessness is a serious public health issue in its own right. In addition, homeless people suffer from associated conditions such as mental illness, alcoholism, tuberculosis, and a substantial excess of deaths. After a decade of trying, we know that emergency approaches to this problem have not worked . . . Homelessness is a symptom of much deeper and more serious changes in American society. How we would reverse these changes is not easy to specify in policy recommendations that are both empirically based and politically acceptable. Effective action is urgently needed in the areas of housing, health care, employment, and education. The alternative of continued social disintegration will have grave consequences for the national health and welfare and makes this a problem on which we cannot turn our backs. (p. 1886)

Secondary Prevention At the level of secondary prevention, community health nurses can work to provide outreach programs for homeless individuals and families. Again, at the aggregate level, the influence on policy for programs for the homeless is critical. Maurin (1990) described how nurse researchers, working with health care providers, can provide research data about the homeless and their health problems to local community leaders to improve the resources available to meet their needs.

Tertiary Prevention At the level of tertiary prevention, the community health nurse can work with clients, such as in the case study of Ruth Smith. In this instance, Ruth's social and mental health problems have escalated. The community health nursing goal is to facilitate management and prevention of further deterioration of her mental illness. At an aggregate level, the community health nurse again works within the political arena to improve resources available to meet the needs of the homeless, particularly those with chronic health problems. Specifically, in cases such as Ruth's, there is a need for facilities that offer housing and psychiatric services to women with children.

RESEARCH AND THE HOMELESS

A number of factors increase the complexity of conducting research among the homeless. The transient nature of the population makes it difficult to locate and maintain study participants. The presence of alcoholism, mental illness, and other acute and chronic conditions can impede data collection procedures, and the researcher may even find it difficult to locate a safe and appropriate place for data gathering. Still, other barriers to data collection include language and cultural differences between researcher and study participant, and often questionnaires and other instruments assume a level of literacy not appropriate for this aggregate. Finally, homeless individuals may be reluctant to participate in research for fear of reprisal or negative consequences that may occur because of information they revealed during a study (Vredevoe et al., 1992).

In spite of these obstacles, investigators have conducted considerable research with the homeless, much of which we have summarized in this chapter. Flagg (1991) noted that these large- and small-scale studies, conducted over the last decade, have provided insight into the extent and causes of homelessness. We have learned that the homeless are diverse, are difficult to count, and have numerous health and socioeconomic needs. Flagg called for a second generation of research (i.e., additional research with a broader perspective) to provide a better understanding of the complex problems facing homeless individuals. In particular, she argued for the use of ethnographic, or qualitative, research approaches that capture the personal and social texture of these individuals' lives.

Nurse researchers, who have expertise in qualitative, ethnographic research methods, have a unique opportunity to conduct these studies, because they can pool their clinical and research perspectives to enhance their work (Schein, 1987). These combined perspectives provide insight into such complex phenomena as family interactions and parenting within an emergency shelter (Droes, 1993; Droes and Hatton, 1991; Hatton and Droes, 1991). In the latter grounded theory study, data analysis revealed a number of family constellations and interactions that have consequences for parenting and health-seeking behaviors. Particularly salient were families in which a male parent dominates the interaction and focused attention on himself for a relatively minor concern rather than on an acutely ill child. Women in these families, moreover, had relatively little voice in the family's health care decision making.

Findings from another qualitative grounded theory study of single women with children living in transitional shelters indicate that for these women too health care decision making was problematic. During in-depth interviews, these women revealed their reluctance both to seek health care and to discuss problems openly with providers. This reluctance stemmed from a variety of reasons, including shame, fear, lack of information, and eligibility for services (Hatton, 1993, 1994, in press). In these instances, shelter staff played a critical role in the identification and management of health needs; yet staff members often had little health-related knowledge and intervened based on their past experiences and intuition. Moreover, they frequently focused attention on health problems such as head lice and chickenpox. They generally did not perceive the importance of dealing with more "invisible" problems, which, from a clinical perspective, had considerably more serious consequences. The latter included tuberculosis and human immunodeficiency virus (HIV) (Hatton et al., 1995).

These qualitative grounded theory studies provided a means to analyze data from the empirical world of the homeless. The findings offer an understanding of the "world of nursing practice" (Chenitz and Swanson, 1986), in this case community health nursing practice. They have, moreover, important implications for designing further research and, more specifically, interventions and client outcomes. How will we creatively design interventions that increase these women's parenting skills and give them a voice in their health care interactions? How will we conceptualize and measure parenting and health care decision making as outcomes? What interventions with shelter staff will provide them with the expertise to deal more effectively with health problems in their settings? How can this expertise be studied? How will we study client outcomes related to staff expertise, such as more effective utilization of health care?

Brooten and Naylor (1995) reviewed the concerns associated with investigating outcomes. Outcomes such as parenting, health care decision making, expertise, and health care utilization can be difficult to measure. Moreover, multiple factors influence these outcomes beyond identified interventions. Such factors include poverty, dysfunctional families, and limited resources. Moreover, nurses do not care for homeless clients in isolation but, instead, work with shelter staff, social workers, physicians, and others. Studies, therefore, with an interdisciplinary focus, in which the perspectives of several disciplines can interact and enhance the process of analysis (Olesen et al., 1990) will provide broader knowledge on which to base our practice.

SUMMARY

Our analysis informs us that homelessness evolves from the interaction of complex factors both at the societal level and among vulnerable individuals. Consequently, these individuals and families find themselves living in the streets, abandoned buildings, other public places, and shelters. Homeless persons are heterogeneous, are difficult to count, and suffer from a variety of complex health problems. Their access to health care is problematic at best, and interventions to deal with this enormous problem represent largely downstream endeavors. Future research with members of this aggregate that explores the complexity of their lives, from a variety of methodologic perspectives, will generate the knowledge necessary for more upstream community health nursing interventions.

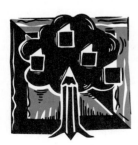

Learning Activities

1. Search a major metropolitan newspaper for articles on the homeless. Compare and contrast the articles with those found in a local newspaper.

2. Make arrangements to serve a meal in a soup kitchen.

3. Interview staff working in a homeless shelter. Inquire about how they manage health problems among their residents.

4. Assess your community to determine what health and social services are provided to the homeless.

5. Attend a governing body (e.g., city council, county board of supervisors) during a discussion of problems related to the homeless.

6. Interview a member of the clergy, a government official, a law enforcement officer, and a hospital administrator about the problem of homelessness in your community.

REFERENCES

Aday LA: At risk in America: The health and health care needs of vulnerable populations in the United States. San Francisco, Jossey-Bass, 1992.

Adkins CB, Fields J: Health care values of homeless women and their children. Fam Community Health 15:20–29, 1992.

American Medical Association: Guidelines for adolescent preventive services. Chicago, AMA, 1992.

Bassuk EL: Women and children without shelter: The characteristics of homeless families. In Robertson MJ, Greenblatt M (eds). Homelessness: A National Perspective. New York, Plenum Press, 1992.

Bassuk EL: Social and economic hardships of homeless and other poor women. Am J Orthopsychiatry 63:340–347, 1993.

Bassuk EL, Weinreb L: Homeless pregnant women: Two generations at risk. Am J Orthopsychiatry 63:348–357, 1993.

Beauchamp DE: Public health as social justice. In Jaco EG (ed). Patients, physicians, and illness, 3rd ed. New York, Free Press, 1979, pp. 443–457.

Berne AS, Dato C, Mason DJ, Rafferty M: A nursing model for addressing the health needs of homeless families. Image J Nurs Sch 22:8–13, 1990.

Breakey WR, Fischer PJ: Homelessness: The extent of the problem. J Soc Issues 46:31–47, 1990.

Brooten D, Naylor MD: Nurses' effect on changing patient outcomes. Image J Nurs Sch 27:95–99, 1995.

Browne A: Family violence and homelessness: The relevance of trauma histories in the lives of homeless women. Am J Orthopsychiatry 63:370–384, 1993.

Buckner J: Pathways into homelessness: An epidemiological analysis. In Rog D (ed). Evaluating Programs for the Homeless: New Directions for Program Evaluation. San Francisco, Jossey-Bass, 1991, pp. 17–30.

Buckner JC, Bassuk EL, Zima B: Mental health issues affecting homeless women: Implications for intervention. Am J Orthopsychiatry 63:385–399, 1993.

Burroughs J, Bouma P, O'Connor E, Smith D: Health concerns of homeless women. In Brickner PW, Scharer LK, Conanan BA, et al. (eds). Under the Safety Net: The Health and Social Welfare of the Homeless in the United States. New York, Norton, 1990, pp. 139–150.

Chenitz C, Swanson J: Qualitative research using grounded theory. In Chenitz WC, Swanson JM (eds). From Practice to Grounded Theory: Qualitative Research in Nursing. Menlo Park, CA, Addison-Wesley, 1986, pp. 3–15.

Christiano A, Susser I: Knowledge and perceptions of HIV infection among homeless pregnant women. J Nurs Midwifery 34:318–322, 1989.

Cohen E, Mackenzie RG, Yates GL: HEADSS, a psychosocial risk assessment instrument: Implications for designing effective intervention programs for runaway youth. J Adol Health 12:539–544, 1991.

Curry MA: Nonfinancial barriers to prenatal care. Women Health 15:85–99, 1989.

Droes N: Family interactions in a homeless shelter: Use of dimensional analysis (abstract) (Communicating Nursing Research 26). Boulder, CO, Western Institute for Nursing, 1993.

Droes N, Hatton D: Family interactions in a homeless shelter. Presented at the meeting of the Western Social Science Association, Reno, NV, 1991.

Fischer PJ: Alcohol, Drug Abuse, and Mental Health Problems Among Homeless Persons: A Review of the Literature, 1980–1990. Rockville, MD, National Institute on Alcohol Abuse and Alcoholism, 1991.

Flagg J: Commentaries. Self identified health concerns of two homeless groups. West J Nurs Res 13:191–192, 1991.

Forst ML, Jonathan H, Goddard PA: A health-profile comparison of delinquent and homeless youths. J Health Care Poor Underserved 4:386–400, 1993.

Galtung J: Violence, peace, and peace research. J Peace Res 16:167–191, 1969.

Glasser I: Homelessness in Global Perspective. New York, GK Hall, 1994.

Hatton DC: Dimensional analysis: Framing a story of self-care among homeless women (abstract) (Communicating Nursing Research 26). Boulder, CO Western Institute for Nursing, 1993.

Hatton DC: Health concerns and self-care among homeless women (abstract) (Communicating Nursing Research 27). Boulder, CO, Western Institute for Nursing, 1994.

Hatton DC: Managing health problems among homeless women with children in a transitional shelter. Image J Nurs Sch (in press).

Hatton DC, Bennett S, Gaffrey EA: Staff perceptions of health problems among homeless women shelter residents (abstract) (Communicating Nursing Research 28). Boulder, CO, Western Institute for Nursing, 1995.

Hatton DC, Droes N: The nature of families and family interaction in a homeless shelter. Presented at the Eleventh Annual Florida VA Nursing Research Conference, Gainesville, FL, 1991.

Hausman B, Hammen C: Parenting in homeless families: The double crisis. Am J Orthopsychiatry 63:358–369, 1993.

Hodnicki DR, Horner SD: Homeless mothers' caring for children in a shelter. Issues Ment Health Nurs 14:349–356, 1993.

Institute of Medicine: Homelessness, health, and human needs. Washington, DC, National Academy Press, 1988.

Jencks C: The homeless. Cambridge, MA, Harvard University Press, 1994.

Kozol J: Rachel and Her Children. Homeless Families in America. New York, Fawcett Columbine, 1988.

Kruks G: Gay and lesbian homeless/street youth: Special issues and concerns. J Adol Health 12:515–518, 1991.

Lindsey A: Health care for the homeless. Nurs Outlook 37:78–81, 1989.

Link BG, Susser E, Stueve A, et al.: Lifetime and five-year prevalence of homelessness in the United States. Am J Public Health 84:1907–1912, 1994.

Maurin JT: Research utilization in the social-political arena. Appl Nurs Res 3:48–41, 1990.

McChesney KY: Homeless families: Four patterns of poverty. In Robertson MJ, Greenblatt M (eds). Homelessness: A National Perspective. New York, Plenum Press, 1992, pp. 245–256.

McKinlay JB: A case for refocusing upstream: The political economy of illness. In Jaco EG (ed). Patients, Physicians, and Illness, 3rd ed. New York, Free Press, 1979, pp. 9–25.

North CS, Smith EM: Posttraumatic stress disorder among homeless men and women. Hosp Community Psychiatr 43:1010–1016, 1992.

Nyamathi A, Flaskerud J: A community-based inventory of current concerns of impoverished and drug-addicted minority women. Res Nurs Health 15:121–129, 1992.

Olesen V, Schatzman L, Droes N, et al.: The mundane ailment and the physical self: Analysis of the social psychology of health and illness. Soc Sci Med 30:449–455, 1990.

Penchansky R, Thomas JW: The concept of access: Definition and relationship to consumer satisfaction. Med Care 19:127–140, 1981.

Pennbridge J, Mackenzie RG, Swofford A: Risk profile of homeless pregnant adolescents and youth. J Adol Health 12:534–538, 1991.

Portnoy FL, Dumas L: Nursing for the public good. Nurs Clin North Am 29:371–375, 1994.

Rafferty Y, Shinn M: The impact of homelessness on children. Am Psychol 46:1170–1179, 1991.

Reuler JB: Outreach health services for street youth. J Adol Health 12:561–566, 1991.

Rosenheck R: Homelessness in America (editorial). Am J Public Health 84:1885–1886, 1994.

Rosenthal R: Homeless in paradise: A Map of the Terrain. Philadelphia, Temple University Press, 1994.

Rossi PH: Down and out in America: The origins of homelessness. Chicago, University of Chicago Press, 1989.

Schein EH: The clinical perspective in fieldwork. Newbury Park, CA, Sage. 1987.

Schlossstein E, St Clair P, Connell F: Referral keeping in homeless women. J Community Health 16:279–285, 1991.

Smart DH: Homeless youth in Seattle. J Adol Health 12:519–527, 1991.

Takahashi LM, Wolch JR: Difference in health and welfare between homeless and homed welfare applicants in Los Angeles County. Soc Sci Med 38:1401–1413, 1994.

Timmer DA, Eitzen S, Talley KD: Paths to homelessness: Extreme poverty and the urban housing crisis. Boulder, CO, Westview Press, 1994.

U.S. Conference of Mayors: A Status Report on Hunger and Homelessness in America's Cities. Washington, DC, U.S. Conference of Mayors, 1994.

U.S. Department of Commerce: 1990 Census of Population. General Population Characteristics, United States, 1990 CP-1-1. Washington, DC, U.S. Government Printing Office, 1992.

U.S. Department of Health and Human Services, National Institute of Mental Health: Outcasts on Main Street: Report of the Federal Task Force on Homelessness and Severe Mental Illness (ADM 92-1904). Washington, DC, Interagency Council on Homeless, 1992.

U.S. Department of Housing and Urban Development: Priority Home! The Federal Plan to Break the Cycle of Homelessness (HUD-1454-CPD[1]). Washington, DC, U.S. Government Printing Office, 1994.

U.S. Public Health Service: Clinician's Handbook of Preventive Services: Putting Prevention into Practice. Waldorf, MD, American Nurses Publishing, 1994.

Vladeck BC: Health care and the homeless: A political parable for our time. J Health Polit Policy Law 15:305–317, 1990.

Vredevoe DL, Shuler P, Woo M: The homeless population. West J Nurs Res 14:731–740, 1992.

Wagner J, Menke EM: Stressors and coping behaviors of homeless, poor, and low-income mothers. J Community Health Nurs 8:75–84, 1991.

Weitzman B: Pregnancy and childbirth: Risk factors for homelessness? Fam Planning Perspect 21:175–178, 1989.

World Health Organization: Chronicle of WHO, 1;1–2, 1947. New York, WHO, 1958.

Wright JD: The health of homeless people: Evidence from the National Health Care for the Homeless Program. In Brickner PW, Scharer LK, Conanan BA, et al. (eds). Under the Safety Net: The Health and Social Welfare of the Homeless in the United States. New York, Norton, 1990a, pp. 15–31.

Wright JD: Poor people, poor health: The health status of the homeless. J Soc Issues 46:49–64, 1990b.

Wright JD, Weber E: Homelessness and health. Washington, DC, McGraw-Hill's Health Care Information Center, 1987.

Yates GL, Mackenzie RG, Pennbridge J, Swofford A: A risk profile comparison of homeless youth involved in prostitution and homeless youth not involved. J Adol Health 12:545–548, 1991.

Yates GL, Pennbridge J, Swofford A, Mackenzie RG: The Los Angeles system of care for runaway/homeless youth. J Adol Health 12:555–560, 1991.

Zima BT, Wells KB, Freeman HE: Emotional and behavioral problems and severe academic delays among sheltered homeless children in Los Angeles County. Am J Public Health 84:260–264, 1994.

Rural Health

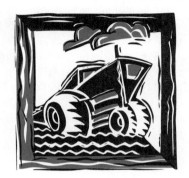

Upon completion of this chapter, the reader will be able to:

1. Discuss the definitions of the term *rural*.

2. Explain why rural populations and geographic areas must be defined as appropriately as possible.

3. Describe features of the health care system and population characteristics common to the rural aggregate.

4. Identify structural barriers to health care.

5. Discuss the impact of structural barriers versus personal barriers on the health of rural aggregates.

6. Describe factors that place farmers and farm families at risk for accidents.

7. Describe the importance of the informal care network to rural health and social services.

8. Describe the unique features of rural community health nursing practice.

9. Apply upstream perspective to health promotion, prevention of illness, and premature death and disability.

Doris Henson
Kathleen Chafey
Patricia G. Butterfield

RURAL UNITED STATES

One in four Americans live in a rural area: approximately 60 million persons living in both farm and nonfarm residences. As this century ends, rural Americans make up 25% of the nation's population, 26% of the nation's children and elderly, and 50% of the nation's poor (Office of Technology Assessment, 1991). Although the urban growth rate has been climbing steeply since about 1890, with urban residents surpassing those in rural areas at about 1920, the actual number of rural residents is greater than anytime in our history (Miller et al., 1994).

When considering the stereotypic rural resident, one often thinks of people living on farms and ranches, people whose livelihood comes from produce, grain, or livestock. However, the 1990 census classified 8% of the rural population (2% of the total U.S. population) as farmers compared with 62% in 1920. In contrast to previous generations, many farms are now sustained by off-farm jobs of one or more family members. Although fewer than 10% of rural dwellers are farmers, agriculture continues to be an important part of the rural and U.S. economy. Agriculture currently generates 17% of the gross national product; by 2005 the figure is projected to be 25%. Although agriculture is one of the fastest growing industries of the 1990s only 40% of the farms currently have the potential for making a profit. Forty percent of farmers and ranchers are older than 65 years, and only 13% of farm property remains in the family for longer than three generations (Kohl, 1995). Changing demographic and economic conditions are moving agriculture from family farm ownership to large agribusiness corporations.

Nonfarm families have always played an important part in the rural community. The ratio of nonfarm to farm residents in rural areas continues to increase in most communities. Traditional nonfarm but rural occupations include mining, government employment, and manufacturing. Located in rural America are 70,000 small- and medium-sized industrial firms (Mayer, 1993). More recent changes have included an influx of retirees and escapees from urban areas who are able, through modern telecommunication and airline travel, to live in rural areas and conduct their business from there (Cordes, 1989).

Definitions of Rural Populations

Multiple definitions of rural populations have been formulated and used to understand characteristics of areas with low population density. The U.S. Census Bureau classifies rural as those people who live in towns with a population of less than 2500 or open country. This definition further delineates the rural population into the subcategories of farm and rural nonfarm. A similar classification developed by the U.S. Census Bureau categorizes counties as metropolitan or nonmetropolitan. Metropolitan counties or "metrocounties" are those that contain an urban population center of 50,000 or more people; all other counties are designated as nonmetropolitan. Nonmetropolitan counties included 2444 of the United States' 3088 counties with a population of approximately 61 million people (1990 Census of the Population). A third classification of interest uses the term *frontier* to delineate geographic areas of fewer than six people per square mile (Elison, 1986). Many counties of the Great Plains and West, including Alaska, are designated as frontier.

A more refined classification scheme arranges residence into one of nine categories; this taxonomy is listed in Table 16–1; categories range from core and fringe areas with a minimum of 1 million people to nonmetropolitan to nonadjacent counties, with the size of the smallest place less than 2500 people (Farmer et al., 1993). Farmer and colleagues used infant mortality data and this nine-category classification scheme to

Table 16–1
Residence Category

1. Core and fringe: 1 million plus

2. Core and fringe: 500,000–999,999 population

3. Core and fringe: 50,000–499,999 population

4. Nonmetropolitan adjacent largest place: 10,000–50,000 population

5. Nonmetropolitan adjacent largest place: 2500–9999 population

6. Nonmetropolitan adjacent largest place: <2,500 population

7. Nonmetropolitan nonadjacent largest place: 10,000–49,999 population

8. Nonmetropolitan nonadjacent largest place: 2500–9999 population

9. Nonmetropolitan nonadjacent largest place: <2500 population

Source: Farmer R, Clark L, and Miller M: Consequences of differential residence designations for rural health policy: The case of infant mortality. J Rural Health 9:17–26, 1993. Used with permission.

show the heterogeneity of rural areas. Infant mortality has been a major health status indicator with high variation by geographic area. Examination by size of residence in two regions of the United States showed mortality for white infants in rural areas adjacent to a population of less than 2500 varied from a high of 9.85 per 1000 in the South to 6.46 per 1000 in the West. This difference is not apparent if a cruder metropolitan versus nonmetropolitan classification is used to view these data. This example explains the complexity of the idea of rural and the importance of selecting an appropriate classification scheme to delineate rural areas. It also provides some insight into the heterogeneity of rural populations and shows why a health status indicator such as infant mortality can be misleading for a particular area. Because of the diversity in rural America, the health status of populations from one aggregate to another and within aggregates can vary.

In summary, the idea of rural is multidimensional; to provide the most useful information, rural populations and corresponding health status indicators should be examined using the most refined classification scheme available. Because of the way data are reported by the government agencies, figures are often not available in these more specific categories.

Rural populations differ because of a complex mix of geographic, social, and economic factors. Although it is true that those who are older, poorer, and less educated are overrepresented in nonmetropolitan areas, that may not be true in all rural areas or for everyone in a given location. When working in rural health care, remembering there are many "rural Americas in rural America" is paramount to a successful community health nursing practice.

COMMUNITY AND STATISTICAL INDICATORS OF RURAL HEALTH STATUS

Rural communities vary along dimensions of economic and cultural resources, employment patterns, population density, relative isolation, age distribution, and ethnic composition. Yet there are commonalities in rural communities when viewed in the aggregate. For example, on the basis of census and health survey data, we know that rural residents are more likely to be white, married, and older than 65 years or younger than 18 years in contrast to their urban counterparts. Additionally, they are also less likely to be employed and less well educated, with incomes that are 75% that of urban dwellers (Office of Technology Assessment, 1990). There are also aggregate differences in the health and lifestyle of rural populations when compared with urban counterparts. For example, rural populations tend to have lower rates of mortality compared with urban populations with two notable exceptions. Infant mortality is slightly higher and deaths from accidents are 40% higher in rural areas. In addition, rural residents have greater levels of injury disability (Office of Technology Assessment, 1990). Interestingly, rural-urban rates of acute health problems are similar. Lifestyle also varies along the rural-urban continuum. Researchers with the National Health Interview Survey concluded that adults in nonmetropolitan areas use seat belts less, are less likely to exercise regularly, have less contact with physicians, and are less likely to use preventive screening (although this trend is confounded by problems of access). Rural residents are also more likely to be obese, smoke more heavily if they do smoke, consume more alcohol than urban people, and far more likely to be exposed to occupational hazards (Office of Technology Assessment, 1990).

Barriers to Health Care

Certain trends constitute economic barriers to receiving adequate health care. First, rural residents have lower income levels, higher unemployment, and higher poverty rates than their urban counterparts. This fact, coupled with employment in industries in economic decline and with low insurance coverage, such as agriculture, forestry, and fisheries, contributes to the increased number of rural families that are uninsured. In addition, although the rural poor are more likely to purchase private insurance, they are much less likely to be covered by Medicaid because farm families tend to be two-parent households. Less than 6% of farm families with incomes below the federal poverty level can qualify for Medicaid (Office of Technology Assessment, 1990).

Regardless of their diverse demographic and geographic attributes, rural groups share unique problems in obtaining health care. There are structural, financial, and personal barriers to accessing health care services, whether in rural or urban environments (Institute of Medicine, 1993). However, rural residents are somewhat unique in the extent to which they experience structural barriers to adequate health care. Availability of services, distance, isolation, low population density, and lack of transportation all contribute to both lack of availability of health care services and lack of access to such services that do exist. This is particularly true for the rural West and other regions that share some or all of its characteristics.

Structural, Financial, and Personal Factors and Health Status

In addition to health concerns related to socioeconomic and geographic patterns, rural (like urban) populations reflect health patterns and problems related to demographic and geographic patterns such as age and gender, occupation, race and ethnicity, and access to health care. These patterns are related to and sometimes confounded by structural, financial, and personal factors. Structural factors may include availability of health information, preventive and illness services, sewage and water systems, and transportation systems. Financial factors often relate to local economic conditions and employment patterns. Population characteristics such as age distribution, size and density, language, culture, and education round out the examples of factors that directly or indirectly affect health and may serve as barriers to availability of services and access to those services that do exist.

Age is an important consideration in planning health care services for rural communities. The elderly, mostly women, often live at or near the poverty level in most rural regions. They tend to be isolated, lack access to health care, and increasingly are the primary caregivers for spouses, even parents who suffer from chronic illness. In contrast, nonmetropolitan areas, particularly those in West, also have higher proportions of the population who are young (younger than 17 years) (Office of Technology Assessment, 1990). Evidence suggests that fetal, infant, and maternal mortality are slightly higher in nonmetropolitan compared with metropolitan areas and that care in the later prenatal stages is problematic. Nonmetropolitan children are involved in farm and highway accidents and deaths and, because of poor insurance coverage, may go without corrective treatment for orthopedic, dental, speech, hearing, visual, and cosmetic problems (Office of Technology Assessment, 1990). Substance use and abuse by youth are problems in rural America. Lisnerski and colleagues (1991) reported on the use of smokeless tobacco by elementary school children in a rural southeastern state. In this study, roughly one third of male first graders had experimented with smokeless

tobacco; by the seventh grade, 70% of these rural males had experimented with or were regular users of smokeless tobacco. Use had to do with "perceived flavor" but was also predicted by "self-concept and presentation to peers" and "family influence." Furthermore, Long and Boik (1993) reported that nearly 60% of rural sixth and seventh graders in their sample reported using alcohol.

Occupation also plays a significant role in rural health, where rates of disabling injuries and injury-related mortality are dramatically higher than in the urban population (Office of Technology Assessment, 1990). In addition to mechanical, chemical, and thermal injuries and high job-related fatalities, farmers are reported to suffer the effects of psychological stress and high suicide rates (Weinert and Burman, 1994). Miners and loggers also work in hazardous conditions and suffer from a variety of acute and chronic problems, including "trauma, respiratory illness, vascular problems and malignancy" (p. 72). To illustrate the magnitude of the problem, the work-related death rate (deaths per 100,000 workers) for the United States in 1990 (private sector only) was approximately 5.5. For the same year in Wyoming and Montana, work-related deaths were 18 per 100,000 workers and 13 per 100,000 workers, respectively.

As mentioned, rural adults (again in the aggregate) exercise preventive behaviors less, have less contact with physicians, and often have less access to care than their counterparts with similar problems in urban areas. Rural cancer patients, for example, experience more late-stage cancers, unstaged at diagnosis, even though rural populations are at lower risk from cancer for most anatomic sites (Monroe et al., 1992). The problem of screening is particularly serious for elderly women. According to National Health Survey data for 1987, 22.6% of elderly white women and 43% of elderly minority women reported never having had a Papanicolaou (Pap) smear. It is also instructive to note that the disparity in numbers of women who reported ever having had a mammogram as of 1990 related both to race (African-American) and income (Calle et al., 1993; Institute of Medicine, 1993).

Problems that affect certain races or ethnic groups are the most illustrative of problems of access in rural health. A 1993 Institute of Medicine study drew attention to the glaring (and growing) disparities in access to health care between white and African-Americans and ethnic minorities. On almost any measure or index (acquired immunodeficiency syndrome, birth weight, blood pressure, cholesterol, cancer, substance use), African-Americans are less healthy than whites, and the disparity is often one exaggerated by rurality and poverty. Johnson and coworkers (1994), for example, concluded that living in a rural area and being African-American significantly increased the likelihood for higher total fat, saturated fat, cholesterol, and sodium intake by children ages 1 to 10 years *regardless* of household income and availability of additional resources for food. Hispanic women and older African-American women have been found to underuse both mammography and Pap smear screening in rural areas. Low income, low educational attainment, and age greater than 65 years were other demographic predictors of women who underuse these screening technologies (Calle et al., 1993). In general, migrant and seasonal farmworkers are primarily nonwhite. Farmworkers tend to be African-American, Hispanic, or Native American in the West and Southwest and African-American or Hispanic in the Southeast. Although the data on farmworkers are not routinely collected, it is evident from records of visits to migrant health centers that this rural population suffers from conditions associated with poor sanitation and overcrowding, pesticide exposure, and problems of pregnancy and early childhood (Office of Technology Assessment, 1990). Migrant and seasonal farmworkers and the rural homeless may be invisible to mainstream community health services, yet they may be most in need of available, accessible health care.

Perhaps no other group illustrates so well the myriad problems that characterize rural health and the difficulties of making health care available and accessible to rural people than Native Americans. The following are excerpts from a special report compiled by faculty and students from the University of Montana School of Journalism entitled "A Health Crisis."

In Montana, Indians die prematurely at a rate almost twice that of the general population. Death rates among Indians as a result of heart disease, cancer, accidents, cirrhosis, suicide and diabetes are higher for Indians than for other citizens of this state.

This terrible toll afflicts Native Americans from the moment of their birth. The state's infant mortality rate for Indian babies is 43 percent higher for Montana Indian infants than for babies born of other ancestry.

Montana Indians live in poverty at a rate three times that of their fellow residents. Half of those Indians who are poor are children and adolescents and they are more than three times more likely to come from homes where a mother is the only parent present. Yet Indians get free health care, so why are they so sick?

Because, as the American Indian Health Care Association found, Indians face significant barriers to getting that health care. Only enrolled tribal members living on a reservation can get full health care benefits supplied by the federal government. And that health care is rationed. Many Indians live long distances from Indian Health Service facilities. That becomes a factor when studies show that more than twice as many Montana Indians than white people have no access to a vehicle. And almost half the Indians in the state are without a telephone. A third of tribal and Indian Health Service facilities in Montana have no emergency and ambulance services, a critical need on Montana's large and rural reservations.

(UNIVERSITY OF MONTANA, SCHOOL OF JOURNALISM, 1993)

It is important to remember that aggregate data reported by the Department of Health and Human Services, for example, or in the special report just quoted must be interpreted with caution. Health status and health care for groups with particular demographic characteristics do vary from area to area even though most may share certain health problems (e.g., diabetes among Native Americans). Furthermore, data reported for rural areas by metropolitan statistical areas (MSAs) are crude. In some rural states, most of the population may live outside MSAs, and many may live in counties that have no health department. Reportable data may be nonexistent or unreliable. Aggregate data should serve as benchmarks against which to direct the nurse's inquiry in assessing local health conditions.

SPECIFIC RURAL AGGREGATES: AGRICULTURAL WORKERS

Agriculture and its commensurate impact on human health is a central focus of rural nursing. Although the proportion of farm to nonfarm families has decreased in the past 20 years, agriculture continues to have a profound impact on the health status of most rural communities. Much of our country's heritage has been strongly associated with agriculture; deep rooted in our history are beliefs that undeveloped land can and should be settled by humans and made productive. The belief of "human's triumph over nature" has evolved considerably in the past century; however, a number of myths about agriculture continue to permeate citizens' beliefs about health and health risks.

The myth of farming as a safe and innately healthful activity has helped perpetuate the notion that farmers and their families, because of their relationship with nature, are in some way protected from the health dangers and threats in contemporary society. In reality, health risks of farming are different, as opposed to less, than those risks encountered in metropolitan areas. Agriculture, along with construction and mining, shares the highest rates of worker fatality of any U.S. industry (U.S. Department of Labor, 1989). Children bear a disproportionally high risk of fatal injury; an estimated 300 pediatric fatalities occur annually (Rivara, 1985). In addition to fatalities, farmers and their families have been found to have excess risks for conditions associated with hearing loss, respiratory illness, nonfatal accidents, and chemical hazards.

Accidents and Injuries

Working in highly variable environmental conditions (i.e., temperature extremes, a wide variety of work tasks, unpredictable circumstances) is associated with an increased frequency of accidents. Farm-related activities are extremely heterogeneous and may vary significantly according to time of year, crop produced, and types of machinery used. In addition to the diversity of agriculture work, farmers are located in geographically isolated areas and often work alone. Together, this constellation of factors places farmers and farm families at increased risk for accidental injury; and, when an accident occurs, farmers are less likely to have timely access to emergency or trauma care than those persons living in nonrural settings.

Agricultural machinery is the most common cause of both fatalities and nonfatal injuries of U.S. farmers according to the National Institute for Occupational Safety and Health (NIOSH, 1992). Tractor-related accidents, particularly rollovers and being run over, are the most frequent events associated with loss of life (Etherton et al., 1991). In addition to these risk events, NIOSH has released an alert, warning of an increase in scalping-type accidents associated with tractor drive shafts that are referred to as power takeoffs (NIOSH, 1994). It is easy to see why accident prevention programs for farm children and families have focused heavily on tractor safety awareness.

Acute and Chronic Illnesses

Several types of farming activities have been associated with higher than expected occurrences of respiratory conditions, both acute and chronic. For example, farmers with chronic exposure to grain dusts, such as grain elevator workers, have been found to have decreased respiratory functioning and generally increased frequency of respiratory symptoms such as cough or phlegm production (Cotton et al., 1989). Occupational asthma and more exotic fungal or toxic gas–related conditions also occur in higher frequency in agricultural versus nonagricultural populations, depending on the nature of work activities (Warren, 1989). Links between farm work and respiratory symptoms are often made by community health nurses, who, in a rural area, are very familiar with farming practices in their community. In such situations, the role of the nurse is to facilitate referrals to an appropriate health provider and to provide support and education for affected persons and their families.

Exposure to pesticides has and continues to be a major area of concern for farmers and their families. From an occupational perspective, farming is unique because the home and the work site are the same. Exposure risks to children and nonfarming spouses may be heightened through farmers' wearing of contaminated clothing and boots into the home during the day. Homes are often located in direct proximity to fields and animal confinement facilities that are sprayed with a variety of pesticidal agents. Nurses employed in rural emergency rooms or ambulatory care settings may be most likely to encounter farmers and others with acute pesticide poisoning. However, in the course of discussions with farmers, ranchers, or other high-risk groups (e.g., nursery workers, tree planters), community health nurses may note a pattern of headaches and nausea that occur at some intervals during planting or spraying seasons. In those instances, the nurse can serve as an important resource by obtaining a careful history of signs and symptoms, the temporal nature of symptom occurrence, and pesticides and personal protection (e.g., respirators, protective clothing) used. In those situations in which the evidence points in favor of pesticide-related illness, appropriate referral and follow-up are imperative to ensure the safety of the affected person and the family.

Signs and symptoms of acute pesticide poisoning are fairly clear and should be recognized by most health providers in rural communities. Although there are exceptions, acute poisoning frequently follows exposure to insecticides, which are classified under the categories of organophosphates or carbamates. These products, which are sold under a wide variety of trade names (e.g., Parathion, Vapona, Sevin, Dursban), poison insects by inhibiting the enzyme acetylcholinesterase, which leads to an accumulation of acetylcholine in the neuromuscular junction (Environmental Protection Agency, 1989). Common symptoms include headache, dizziness, diaphoresis, nausea, and vomiting. If left untreated, affected persons may experience a progression of symptoms, including dyspnea, bronchospasm, and muscle twitching. Deaths are relatively uncommon, but they do occur.

Migrant and Seasonal Farmworkers

Although the discussion of agricultural issues has focused primarily on farmers and farm families, it is important to understand the role of migrant (i.e., migrate to find work) and seasonal (i.e., reside in one place and work when farm labor is needed) farmworkers in agricultural production in the United States and health risks to this population. Each year, an estimated 3 million farmworkers participate in crop planting, weeding, and harvesting activities throughout the United States (Wilk, 1988). Although older references to farmworkers often referred to three "migrant streams," in which workers enter the country through Mexico and migrate north, the present reality is that migrant workers enter the country through a variety of access points in the United States and follow whatever route is necessary to obtain work throughout the season. Seasonal workers are persons who permanently reside in agricultural areas and take on a variety of jobs during picking or harvesting times. For example, a seasonal worker may be employed in restaurant work during the winter but spend his or her summer months picking apples or working in a local apple shed or cannery.

Migrant and seasonal farmworkers make up a vulnerable population in regard to health risks because of their low income and migratory status. They frequently encounter profound physical and cultural isolation in multiple unfamiliar settings. Although most farmworkers are Hispanic, it is inappropriate to assume that all farmworkers speak Spanish or Spanish and English. Depending on the country of origin and home base, workers may speak Creole, any of the Native American languages (e.g., Crow), or be a recent immigrant from eastern Europe, speaking Russian or Croatian. In many rural areas, community health nurses form the central link between farmworkers and health services. Through standing or mobile clinic sites, nurses have established a leadership role in the provision of episodic and preventive services for workers and their families. Lacking access to many types of preventive services, it is not uncommon to have farmworkers present at a migrant clinic site with any of a number of health problems, including severe dental problems, unresolved communicable diseases, or untreated injuries. In addition to the direct provision of care, nurses in many communities have served in important advocacy roles on behalf of farmworkers and have worked to bring down barriers and ensure health care access to workers traveling through their area.

APPLICATION OF RELEVANT THEORIES AND "THINKING UPSTREAM" CONCEPTS TO RURAL HEALTH

Upstream and preventive-oriented approaches have several types of implications for nurses engaged in rural practice settings because of the unique aspects of rural areas. Three avenues for upstream interventions are discussed in the context of health promotion and disease protection in rural communities: (1) attack community-based problems at their roots, (2) emphasize the "doing" aspects of health, and (3) maximize the use of informal networks.

Attack Community-Based Problems at Their Roots

Upstream approaches to community health problems direct the nurse toward seeking an understanding of the precursors (i.e., roots) of poor health within populations of interest. At several levels, in both rural and nonrural communities, individual nurses can be effective forces in uncovering and enhancing community awareness of health-endangering situations. Environmental health issues in rural communities, such as pesticide exposure or health hazards from point-source factory emissions, are more effectively assessed and remediated on a community level rather than on a case-by-case basis. Nurses' involvement in assisting the community to understand health problems in a larger context can be the genesis of change at several levels by those persons most affected. For example, by heightening a community's awareness of sulfur dioxin levels from a local refinery and the relationship of those emission levels to respiratory problems in vulnerable populations, citizens can gain an understanding of the collective rather than individual burden of the refinery on their community's health. Thus, social action on behalf of affected persons can occur by both nurses and other community members.

Emphasize the "Doing" Aspects of Health

There are consistent differences between rural and nonrural residents in regard to conceptualizations and perceptions of health. The central differentiating factor between rural and nonrural groups seems to be the relative importance of "work" and "being able to work" in self-reported definitions of health (Weinert and Long, 1987). Rural persons' conceptualizations have generally emphasized the "doing" aspects of health; in other words, functioning and the performance of daily activities are of fundamental importance in the daily lives of rural persons. The high value placed on "being able to do" by rural persons can provide astute nurses with intervention opportunities at both the family and community levels. Examples of nursing intervention strategies that capitalize on the "doing" aspects of health include the accident prevention programs for both farm and nonfarm children, exercise and nutrition enhancement programs for seniors, and local industry participation in risk reduction programs for workers. A key element of such programs is the recognition that success is fundamentally determined by the active involvement of the population of interest (i.e., 4-H Club children, maids and housekeepers employed in local lodges and hotels) in all phases of program planning and implementation.

Maximize the Use of Informal Networks

A concept somewhat related to the "doing" emphasis with prevention programs in rural communities is the importance of recognizing and using informal networks in the target community. The name given to this type of approach, whether it be titles like "empowerment models" or "community action models," is less important than the actual commitment to soliciting the involvement of informal networks and natural or lay leaders in planning of health interventions. As most persons who have been involved in community empowerment programs will attest, the involvement of lay leaders and community advocates in change is not an easy or direct process. "Turf" issues and collateral agendas can sometimes seem to serve as obstructions rather than facilitators of change. However, the failure to seek community involvement in population-based health interventions will have unfavorable consequences; frequent results of superimposed change (i.e., usually by so-called experts) versus integrated community change are stereotypical program models, which are a poor fit with the dynamics of the community they are intended to serve. Rural change strategies will not be long lived without understanding and maximizing the true investment of community constituencies in their own well-being.

RURAL HEALTH CARE DELIVERY SYSTEM

Current demographic data suggest that 10 million (15.3%) rural dwellers are without a regular source of care, 16 million (21%) are living in communities without adequate primary care providers, and 17 million (23.4%) experience some form of chronic or serious illness (Norton and McManus, 1989). In the past, emphasis in rural illness care has been modeled after that of urban areas. Urban models emphasize specialist providers and in-hospital acute care with many high-tech, expensive procedures. Rural hospitals have found that many cannot compete with the larger facilities in the area. This brief overview discusses where the system has been, and still is typically, and where many community members, providers, and health policy analysts believe it should be directed.

In the 1980s, the focus of attention related to rural health was almost exclusively on rural hospitals. The emphasis focused on how to make hospitals financially viable so they could provide acute care and continue contributing to the economic health of the community. The rural small hospital crisis was examined by health administrators and health policy analysts, who recommended that the community hospital become the community's health center. To many public health professionals, this appeared to be a contradiction of terms. Public health providers are clearly aware that hospitals deliver illness treatment, not health care in the sense of health promotion and proactive disease prevention. A lack of trust between those providers and institutions delivering acute care and those delivering public health has long existed. Public health, with its proactive health policy agenda related to disease prevention, health promotion, and issues of access and availability of community-oriented primary health care, had little in common with cure-oriented hospitals.

In the late 1980s and early 1990s, many hospitals developed wellness programs for community members. However, some increased services beyond wellness programs. For example, at the request of the county government, a small frontier hospital surmounted the barrier between the hospital and public health by taking over basic public health services: home visits, school nursing, and immunization clinics. Nurses employed by the hospital and working in the hospital make school health visits and home visits for prenatal follow-up. The public health orientation served to broaden the hospital's commitment to the people of a frontier county (Clancy, 1992).

Alternative Facility Model

During a 5-year period (1987–1991), 193 rural hospitals closed nationally. Another hospital was often available within 20 miles. However, for populations in frontier counties, there were very real problems with finding basic primary care. In the United States, 11% of rural hospitals are in frontier areas. These hospitals serve a wide geographic area (46% of the total U.S. land area) where 1% of the U.S. population resides. To improve access to care in frontier areas, new rural hospital models are being developed. The first alternative model to be funded from the Health Care Financing Administration was the Montana medical assistance facility (MAF). The medical director is a physician; however, the daily, on-site services are provided by the nurse practitioner or physician assistant. A MAF may hold patients for up to 4 days (Office of the Inspector General, DHHS, 1993). Florida, Washington, and Wyoming have developed model programs based on the MAF idea. Other alternative limited-services facilities are under development (McNeely, 1992).

Health Care Provider Shortages

The shortage of health care professionals is a barrier to delivery of care. In actual numbers, the shortage has been increasing during the last 10 years. Data reported from the 1988 National Sample Survey of Registered Nurses found that of the 1,627,035 active registered nurses 8.7% were practicing in counties with populations less than 50,000, 4.9% in counties between 25,001 and 50,000 in size, 2.9% in counties between 10,001 and 25,000 in size, and 0.9% of the total in counties less than 10,000 in size. The ratio of nurses to population in the small rural areas was less than half the urban areas: 319 versus 726 registered nurses per 100,000 population (Movassaghi et al., 1992). Although approximately 25% of the population lives in nonmetropolitan counties, only 13.2% of patient care physicians and 8.7% of nurses practice in those counties. In addition, the supply of physician assistants

and nurse practitioners has not kept up with the need for their services in rural areas. For example, the percentage of rural physician assistants has dropped from 19.9% in 1989 to 12.9% in 1990 (Ricketts, 1994). Additionally, only about 20% of nurse practitioners practice in rural areas (Akin and Fagin, 1993).

Community-Wide Health Care System

To cope with limited acute care facilities and provider shortages, community members, rural health care planners, and health care professionals are recommending the development of a community-wide health care system, with the hospital as one component. The central focus of this system is community-based care in the form of community-oriented primary care services (COPC) or primary health care (van Hook, 1992).

Primary care is first-line care provided in an office or clinic setting by a provider (physician, nurse, practitioner, physician assistant, mental health counselor, or other health care professional) who takes responsibility for the client's health. A model recommended for adoption in rural communities combines the primary care model with that of COPC. COPC is often called primary *health* care. A primary health care model assumes that providers address the health and illness concerns of not just the group of clients they see in the clinic or office but of the community as a whole using an epidemiologic orientation. Providers integrate aspects of public health, health promotion, and disease prevention into their primary care practice. This model moves the provider's orientation from individual clients in the office or clinic practice to the health of populations. This upstream, or community-oriented, prevention will, for example, help providers focus on a community education program on farm safety as well as provide the immediate cleaning and suturing of a client's hand lacerated by a piece of farm machinery (Butterfield, 1990; Institute of Medicine, 1983).

The formation of a community health care system that includes primary care and a community-oriented primary health care focus may bring to "the country" accessible and affordable illness care. Included in this system is health promotion and disease prevention based on the needs of the community. This model, which brings a holistic and integrated approach to both health and illness care, appears more akin to a nursing model than a medical model (van Hook, 1992). This community approach is seen as a cooperative model as opposed to the market-driven competition-based model. The community oriented model is in concert with the public health philosophy of the best allocation of limited resources and social justice ethic of equitable access to health and illness care.

Rural communities are struggling to define what illness care services they need, want, and can afford. Although outsiders are not always trusted, some communities have successfully brought in trained facilitators to help develop and execute an effective, practical plan for maintaining (or eliminating) local health services. These facilitators have helped communities to determine what kind of service and how much primary care service to put into place. This process, which assists communities in their decision making, is a type of community organization model. This model includes community participation, needs assessment, and leadership training (Amundson, 1993). Because this model focuses on community development, the community health nurses, with their knowledge of community assessment, aggregates, and community involvement strategies, can be an excellent local resource for helping in the planning process. Currently, most of the planning is related to illness care. It is imperative that the community health nurse and other local and state health department personnel be involved so that prevention is an important component as a community-wide health care system evolves. Central to the evolution of a community-wide health care system is community-based care.

COMMUNITY-BASED CARE

In the mid-1990s, the phrase "community-based care" became a popular term for the myriad services provided outside the walls of an institution. In both urban and rural areas, examples of these services include home health care, in-home hospice care, nutrition programs, home visits to high-risk pregnant women, community mental health, and adult day care. The concept of community-based care also includes community participation in decisions about health care services, a focus on all three levels of prevention, and an understanding that the hospital is no longer the exclusive provider of care to the community.

Home Care and Hospice Programs

Home health and hospice programs vary in structure. Larger communities may support a hospital-based

home care agency with a hospice service or a free-standing full-service agency. In sparsely populated rural locations such as those classified as frontier or rural areas with very small towns of a few hundred, these services, if available at all, are often contracted from a larger regional agency. The larger agency may hire a nurse from the local area to provide home health care or hospice services or both. A successful Utah model for hospice service development brings external resources based in a city together with the resources within a small community. The large urban-based facility provides administrative support for local nurses hired to work in the hospice program (Memmott, 1991).

A study by Buehler and Lee (1992) about home care resources as perceived by family caregivers of cancer patients reported that families living in the most rural areas reported fewer formal resources. To improve home care for remote rural cancer patients and support for families, the authors recommend nurse case management and development of local resources, using the county extension services as the bridge for outreach services to the client and families. A partnership between the county health department nurse and county extension service could result in support and information groups and caregiving classes for the important informal network of providers.

Rural Mental Health Care

Reliable up-to-date studies on the prevalence of mental illness in rural dwellers are not available. Several studies have documented that the economic crisis specific to much of the rural population in the 1980s contributed to mental health problems (American Psychological Association, 1995). A lack of understanding of the importance of the diversity in rural America has resulted in research studies that have not examined the differences within the rural population. A simple rural-urban division does not provide discrete information on which to base decisions about the amount of mental illness within various rural groups: the elderly, the poor, and minorities. What is clear is that large sections of rural populations at risk for illness are without mental health care (Wagenfield, 1990).

A survey by the American Psychological Association (1995) found that lack of acceptance and awareness by the residents of both mental health care providers and problems within the rural community is a major barrier for mental health care professionals practicing there. Rural mental health providers face problems similar to those that other primary care providers confront. These problems include a more diverse practice, fewer opportunities for ongoing education, and fewer professionals for consultations than colleagues in an urban practice have.

Emergency Services

Emergency medical services (EMS) in rural areas have become increasingly important with the closure of rural hospitals. Many small rural communities have a volunteer EMS response team but no local hospital or medical clinic. For this reason they are included as a component of community-based care.

Rural EMS teams cover, for the most part, sparsely populated geographic areas. The low population density results in a higher cost per person and lower profit margin, making it unprofitable for private for-profit organizations to locate in these areas. Because of the lack of profit for private organizations, most EMS units are made up of dedicated volunteers from the local community (Garnett, 1991). Because many rural areas are medically underserved, EMS systems have an increasingly important role in decreasing the morbidity and mortality of individuals needing emergency care (Furlow, 1991). Among the problems identified among the rural EMS systems are shortage of volunteers, lower level of training compared with urban providers, training curriculums that often do not reflect rural needs (e.g., farm equipment trauma), lack of guidance from physicians (because of no designated medical responsibility), and lack of physician training and orientation to the EMS system and provider needs. Low population density, large and isolated or inaccessible areas, severe weather, poor roads, and less access to telephone or other communication methods contribute to more difficult public access for emergency care (Office of Technology Assessment, 1989).

Ensuring access to care, especially for geographically isolated populations, is part of the activity of public health (Picket and Hanlon, 1990). Emergency services are an important tertiary prevention component related to protecting the health of the public.

Informal Care Systems

Limited availability and accessibility of formal health care resources in rural areas combined with the traits of self-reliance and self-help of rural residents have resulted in the development of strong rural community informal care and social support networks. Rural residents are more apt to entrust care to established informal networks than to new formal care systems (Weinert and Long, 1987, 1990). One study reported that rural residents sustain a higher level of social health than urban residents. They attributed this social health to the higher level of family and community involvement of rural residents as compared with urban residents (Eggebeen and Lichter, 1993). High level of involvement with community organizations and the family may in turn contribute to the formation and use of informal systems.

Informal care systems or networks include people in a community who have assumed positions of caregiving by their individual qualities, life situations, or social roles. People who are part of the informal care networks may provide support in the form of direct help, advice, or information. They may also serve as a channel of communication within the community (Human Services in the Rural Transition, 1989). Rural residents identify family members, friends, and neighbors as the informal providers of care (Magilvey and Congdon, 1994).

It is important for both institution- and community-based professional health care providers to recognize the strengths and positive contributions of the informal care system. These networks function as a community resource. Therefore, it is especially significant that formal care providers in community-based care identify and combine informal services with formal systems (Weinert and Long, 1987, 1990).

Rural Public Health Departments

The number of local health departments in the United States is about 3200. Some local health departments may be counted in the 3200, but they are not providing full public health services in the sense that they meet the definition of a local health department (Pickett and Hanlon, 1990). Healthy People 2000 (Objective 8.14) sets a goal of 90% for Americans who will be served by a local health department accomplishing effectively the core functions of public health by the year 2000 (U.S. Public Health Service, 1990). The three core functions of public health—assessment, policy development, and assurance—are addressed in Chapter 3. Data collected in 1993 suggest that less than 40% of the American people, urban and rural, are currently served by a local health department that effectively addresses the core public health functions (Turnock et al., 1994).

Many rural counties are either too small to support a health department staffed by adequately trained personnel or have insufficient financial resources to support the needed services. A rural county of less than 10,000 residents cannot support a full-service health department. A sanitarian, nurse, and clerk may be the entire staff of a rural health department. A local physician often serves as a part-time, unpaid health officer (Pickett and Hanlon, 1990). Most of the small health departments are probably in rural poor or sparsely populated counties. Such counties have a small tax base and, therefore, do not have the financial resources to support a full-service local health department. These small rural health departments often can offer only programs funded by federal programs. Few services are funded through local tax dollars.

Managed Care in the Rural Environment

Managed care is one of the most recent changes in the delivery of care in the United States. In rural areas, one of the changes directly related to the expansion of managed care is the development of health care delivery networks with managed care elements. A National Rural Health Association (NRHA) Issue Paper has identified potential benefits and risks of managed care to rural areas. Possible benefits are that managed care has the potential to lower primary care costs, improve the quality of care, and help to stabilize the local rural health care system. Possible risks are also apparent, including probable high start-up and administrative costs and the volatile effect of the presence of large, urban-based for-profit managed care companies (NRHA, 1995). Currently, the effect on the rural care delivery system of the movement of managed care into rural market is not known with any certainty.

LEGISLATION AND PROGRAMS AFFECTING PUBLIC HEALTH

Public health law, legislation, and programs derive their legitimacy from the Preamble to the Constitution, which declares a fundamental purpose of government to be to "promote the general welfare." Furthermore, the Constitution invests Congress with the power "to lay and collect taxes . . . and provide for the common defense and general welfare" (Pickett and Hanlon, 1990, p. 166). Until 1912 and the establishment of the Children's Bureau through the efforts of a public health nurse, Lillian Wald, the federal government was involved in the public's health to a very limited extent,

being primarily concerned with the health of merchant marines and in protecting the public from communicable disease that might be brought to America on board ships carrying immigrants. Maternal and child advocates continued to bring their concerns for the health, welfare, and mortality of mothers and children to national attention. In 1922, in response to concerns about maternal and child care in rural areas, passage of the Sheppard-Towner Act encouraged states to develop programs to address these problems. The act moved federal funding into personal health services for the first time and shifted the orientation of public health "from disease prevention to promotion of overall health" (Institute of Medicine, 1988, p. 66). Grants-in-aid to the states provided incentives to establish the programs and became the model for federal-state partnerships to address particular public health problems until the 1960s, when block grants for federally prioritized public health programs replaced the grants-in-aid program. During the Great Depression, Congress recognized the special health problems in rural areas where hunger and poverty were manifested in alarming increases in infant mortality, the most sensitive index of the overall health of a population. The Social Security Act of 1935, passed during this era, carried the legacy of earlier maternal and child care provisions and added grants-in-aid for public health programs and training of public health personnel. Maternal and child care along with benefits for the poor and elderly were also covered in the Social Security Amendments of 1965, which created direct federal aid to individuals in the Medicare and Medicaid titles of that act.

Health Care Programs Affecting Rural Areas

The Office of Technology Assessment (1990) described four major categories of health care programs that continue to impact the availability and provision of health care services in rural areas. Medicare and Medicaid, of course, benefit rural as well as urban dwellers through individual and programmatic assistance and fund a significant portion of rural health care. When other federal programs that finance or provide direct health care (e.g., Department of Veterans Affairs and Indian Health Service) are added to Medicare and Medicaid, the impact of the federal government on rural health care is substantial indeed.

A second category of federal programs that affect the availability and accessibility of rural health care include federal block grants to the states. The block grants provide states with funding for three major programs: maternal and child health, preventive health and health services, and alcohol, drug abuse, and mental health program administration. Block grants, initiated in the 1960s as a federal-state-local partnership for health, has been marked by shifts in locus of responsibility for funding and struggles for domination in formulating health policy. With every new administration and Congress, the availability of federal funding and the sharing of power between the three levels of government change, making continuity in public health programming and administration profoundly difficult. Furthermore, the burden of providing public services is strained where rural areas have experienced in-migration and other forms of population growth as well as general economic decline. In addition, particularly in the rural West, the cost of delivering services is exacerbated by the problem of low population density, large distances, and a shortage of health care personnel. Furthermore, the trend toward cost shifting from the federal government to the states will, in all likelihood, continue to place an increasing share of the burden on the states as it has with financing health care for Medicaid, where the state contribution has nearly doubled in the past 15 years (Straub and Walzer, 1992).

A third category of federal programs for rural health care services identified in the 1990 Office of Technology Assessment report are those "whose primary purpose is to augment the health resources available to underserved areas and populations" (p. 61). These programs were established through federal legislation and are designed to increase personnel, facilities, and planning resources. Most programs are administered through the U.S. Department of Health and Human Services or the Health Resources and Services Administration (HRSA).

Programs That Augment Health Personnel. Programs such as the National Health Service Corps (NHSC) and the Area Health Education Centers encourage health professionals to practice in health personnel shortage areas (HPSAs) through volunteer, scholarship, and loan repayment programs in the case of the NHSC and by attracting and retaining primary care providers to shortage areas (Office of Technology Assessment, 1990). Other programs attract health professionals to shortage areas through health profession grants to educational institutions, school construction grants, and student assistance programs through traineeships to schools of nursing among others. Special programs are also offered to support programs for advance practice nurses and minority and disadvantaged students preparing for health professions careers (Office of Technology Assessment, 1990).

Programs That Augment Health Care Facilities and Services. Several programs are of particular importance in meeting the public health needs of rural people. One is the community health centers program (CHC), administered by the HRSA of the Public Health Service. CHCs benefit underserved areas and populations by providing primary health care and in some cases supplemental secondary and tertiary health care such as hospital care, long-term home health care, and rehabilitation for rural people. A similar program, also administered by HRSA, is the migrant health centers program (MHC). MHCs must provide the same services as the CHCs and may also offer supplemental services such as environmental health services, infectious disease and parasite control, and accident prevention programs to migrant and seasonal farmworkers and their families. Primary care cooperative agreements facilitate the development of primary care services to HPSAs by health professionals, assist in determining need and planning for primary care services, and attract primary care providers to rural areas.

Special legislation for HPSAs has also created programs to provide acute care facilities and services. The Rural Transition Grants Program, administered by HCFA, helps small rural communities with nonprofit hospitals adjust to changes in clinical practice patterns and in hospital use, shifts from hospital- to community-based care, and changing emergency care delivery patterns.

Programs That Assist with Health Care Policy, Planning, and Research. The Agency for Health Care Policy and Research has included in its mandate health research as well as demonstration and evaluation of the effectiveness of health care services in rural areas (Office of Technology Assessment, 1990). The Office of Rural Health Policy (ORHP) is part of HRSA and serves in an advisory capacity on diverse rural health issues, including availability and access to health professionals and care in rural areas. The advisory committee also offers advice on the prioritization and financing of rural health care services. The ORHP also manages the Rural Health Research Center grant program and serves as a clearinghouse for information about research findings of interest to rural health care delivery (Office of Technology Assessment, 1990).

It is important to keep in perspective the fact that most of the federal programs just listed provide competitive grants for research studies, demonstration and evaluation programs, and training and recruiting of health professionals and, with the exception of CHCs and MHCs, do not provide direct services. Direct health care services to Medicaid recipients and public health programs are increasingly the burden of state and local governments at a time when rural economies are in decline and the demand for services is increasing in many areas. In addition, by almost any indicator, rural residents are less healthy than their urban counterparts. Just under 25% of rural residents experience limitations to major activities because of chronic illness, a substantial percentage consider their health to be only fair or poor compared with 9.3% of metropolitan residents, and accidents are more frequent and more severe (Hicks, 1992).

Until the early 20th century, responsibility for health care policy, programs, and financing was largely a local government matter. With the responsibility shifting from the federal government to the state and from the state to local governments, the extent and quality of public health programming may again come to vary with the ability, and willingness, of citizens to invest increasingly scarce resources in even minimum protections, accessible to all or even most of those who should be its beneficiaries. As an Institute of Medicine study concluded, "despite the huge successes brought about by scientific discovery and social reforms, and despite a phenomenal growth of government activities in health, the solving of public health problems has not taken place without controversy . . . [and] arguments about the scope of public health and the extent of public sector responsibility for health continue to this day" (Institute of Medicine, 1988).

RURAL COMMUNITY HEALTH NURSING

Perhaps a more accurate title than rural community health nursing would be "community health nursing along the rural continuum." At one end of the continuum are nonmetropolitan areas adjacent to a place of 50,000 people and at the most rural end are towns of less than 2500 people and the open country of farms and ranches.

Practice in a rural area may mean working as the only nurse at a health department in a remote western Great Plains frontier county with a population of 6000, at a full-service health department in a town of 50,000, or at a large health department in a rural area next to an urban population. A practice in a rural area adjacent to a large metropolitan area often appears to have more in common with the urban end of the continuum in terms of size of an agency, distance to resources, and availability of resources. For the purposes of this discussion of rural community health nursing, it is assumed that the setting for practice is at the more "rural" end of the continuum.

The following definition illustrates the broad-based, generalist focus of the modern rural community health nurse. Included in the definition is the important geographic and cultural rural environment where the community health practice is located and which helps define appropriate nursing interventions.

Rural nursing is the practice of professional nursing within the physical and sociocultural context of sparsely populated communities. It involves the continual interaction of the rural environment, the nurse, and his or her practice. Rural nursing is the diagnosis and treatment of a diversified population of people of all ages and a variety of human responses to actual (or potential) occupational hazards or actual or potential health problems existent in maternity, pediatric, medical/surgical and emergency nursing in a given rural area.

(BIGBEE, 1993, P. 132)

Nursing Roles in Community Health Practice

The practice of community health nursing in rural communities is broad based and generalist in nature. These strong generalists are the professionals who can move into a selected specialty area or provide care across speciality areas (Turner and Gunn, 1992). Rural community health nurses need a high level of decision making and high-level generalist skills to practice in a setting where there may be little professional support and supervision (Lassiter, 1985). Components of this role include educator, direct care provider, case manager, coordinator, and administrator.

Characteristics of Rural Nursing

Dolphin (1984) reported several positive aspects of rural nursing: the "ability to give holistic care, to know everyone well, and to develop close relationships with the community and with coworkers." Autonomy, professional status, and a feeling of being valued by the agency and community have also been reported as components of positive job satisfaction for rural community health nurses (Davis and Droes, 1993; Dunkin et al., 1992). On the negative side of rural practice are physical and professional isolation, problems related to scarce resource (low salary, fewer positions and personnel), problems within the work environment, role diffusion, and lack of anonymity (Davis and Droes, 1993; Dolphin, 1984; Dunkin et al., 1992; Long and Weinert, 1989; Movassaghi et al., 1992). Components such as "in-depth interpersonal knowledge of clients" (Davis and Droes, 1993, p. 166), a wide variety of work related to both types of skills and range of client problems, and the slower pace of rural life are seen by some nurses as negative characteristics and by others as positive (Bigbee, 1993).

Of those components identified as negative, professional isolation is the one being most actively addressed by agencies and professional organization. Communications and information technology, through distance learning, is moving training and education out to rural nurses. The technology ranges from basic telephone lines to full-motion, interactive, two-way video. Not only does distance learning help currently employed nurses improve skills and network with other nurses, but its presence also assists in attracting new personnel (Crandal and Coggan, 1994; Puskin, 1992).

RESOURCES FOR THE RURAL COMMUNITY HEALTH NURSE

U.S. Office of Rural Health Policy
Parklawn Building, Room 9-05
5600 Fishers La
Rockville, MD 20857
(301) 443-0835

National Rural Health Association
301 East Armour Blvd
Suite 420
Kansas City, MO 64111
(816) 756-3140

National Association for Rural Mental Health
P.O. Box 570
Wood River, IL 62095
(618) 251-0589

National 4-H Council
7100 Connecticut Ave
Chevy Chase, MD 20815
(301) 961-2800

Rural Nurse Organization (RNO)
c/o Regional Services
P.O. Box 248
Spokane, WA 99210-0248
(800) 752-4890, (509) 459-4698

Rural Information Center Health Service (RICHS)
National Agricultural Library
Rm 304
10301 Baltimore Blvd
Beltsville, MD 20705
(800) 633-7701 (nationwide) or (301) 504-5547
Electronic mail through Internet
  (RIC@NALUSDA.GOV)
NAL Bulletin Board (RIC/RICHS Conference)
(301) 504-6510
(Collects and distributes information on rural health, health funding, rural research, and health care delivery)

Rural Information Center (RIC)
National Agricultural Library
Rm 304
10301 Baltimore Blvd
Beltsville, MD 20705
(301) 504-6400
(Information and referral services on a large number of topics important to rural communities)
Resource Guide on Alcohol, Tobacco, and Other Drugs: Rural Communities
U.S. Department of Health and Human Services, Public Health Service, Substance Abuse and Mental Health Services Administration (Publication No. MS416) August 1994.
(800) 729-6686, (301) 468-2600

Videos

Opening Doors: Public Health Nursing in Its 100th Year (1994)
TS Media
16212 Bothell Way SE
Mill Creek, WA 98012
(800) 876-6334
(May be purchased: $178.00 [includes paperback version of same title])

On the Frontier: The Challenges and Rewards of Rural Nursing (1995)
Glaxo Inc.
Research Triangle Park, NC 27709

Rural community health nursing is rewarding and challenging. Services can include prenatal care, infant and child care in clinics and homes, home care of acute and chronic disease, hospice care for all ages, school health, and mental health. The nurse practicing with the autonomy common in rural practice brings to it preexisting knowledge and competency in other clinical specialties. She or he must be a discriminating, consolidated practitioner who can perform general nursing at a level of skill beyond that of the "mile wide, and inch deep" general nursing of a time long gone by. The rural nurse must be an "expert generalist."

Knowledge Base of the Expert Generalist in Rural Community Health Nursing

Personal barriers to health care include cultural, language, attitudes, acceptability, education, and income (Institute of Medicine, 1993). The interaction of personal barriers with structural and financial barriers is complicated and often difficult to understand. For example, the presence of a new primary health provider within easy access in the small town where a family lives does not necessarily mean the family finds this newcomer acceptable. They may prefer to see an established nurse practitioner in a town 40 miles away. In this scenario personal health care preference has caused this family to travel for care although no structural barrier (lack of a local provider) exists.

Health care preferences and health perceptions must be assessed when planning care in order for it to be acceptable to individuals, families, aggregates within the community, and the community as a whole. To know what interventions and implementation strategies are acceptable to an individual, family, or aggregate, the community health nurse must comprehend how health, health care, and illness are understood. Reports of studies are helpful to the nurse as he or she provides care. Understanding and applying this knowledge will decrease personal barriers by making the interventions more acceptable and, therefore, more likely to be carried out with a positive outcome.

Many small rural communities are insular and reluctant to accept assistance from outsiders or outside experts. They often prefer to receive care from someone they know rather than from a provider who is new to the community. Distrust of "outsiders" or "newcomers" has been documented by Weinert and Long (1987). The following examples illustrate this factor. Developing acceptable methods of farm accident information distribution, rural families' resistance to change and to "outside expert" is reported to be a major problem in setting up a primary prevention program about health and safety risks (Posey, 1995). In another example, EMSs being planned in small rural communities were not readily accepted because community members perceived accepting federal money as giving up local control to someone "outside" their local government (Office of Technology Assessment, 1989). Resistance to influence from outside and a preference for close control is shown in these examples. Outsider nurses, physicians, teachers, and ministers can unknowingly pose a threat to the community, especially if they persist in trying to share knowledge (Norris, 1993). The enthusiastic provision of health information by a community health nurse who is new to the county or town can be met with resistance that is unexpected, misunderstood, and discouraging to the nurse.

Independence and self-reliance are characteristics of rural people, and it has been proposed that these are factors influencing their understanding of health and their reaction to illness (Lee, 1985). Rural residents identify themselves as healthy if they can do their usual work. The fact that they may be in pain while working does not result in identifying themselves as ill because they can do the work expected (Weinert and Long, 1987). The ability to function in the work place, be independent, and rely as little as possible on the outside resources are characteristics common in rural populations.

Hardiness is a personality characteristic that influences coping and adaptation when stressful life events occur. Rural families identified as "hardy" are more able to respond to stress as a strengthening experience rather than one that weakens the family. A study about rural family hardiness reported that work, lifestyle, and daily pressures related to occupation play a primary role in the perception of physical ailment and family conflict (Carson et al., 1993). Lee (1991), in a study about hardiness and its relationship to perceived health in rural adults, reported that control and commitment were components of hardiness whose presence predicts positive health. For the nurse, the implications of these findings are, first, that rural clients will react to interventions more positively if they have as much control as possible. Second, commitment to work is very important. Therefore, when planning activities for individuals, families, or communities, consider the importance of the seasonal nature of much of rural America's workers: farmers, ranchers, loggers, firefighters, and forest service workers.

Rural women carry out more traditional roles than do their urban counterparts in relation to marriage and family. They are described as "keepers of the culture" and "carriers of collective healing" (Battenfield et al., 1981). These descriptors relate to role socialization of children (keepers of the culture) and self-care related to health care needs (carriers of collective healing). Most often in rural families the women monitor the health and encourage other family members, especially the men, to seek care (Lee, 1993). Little economic opportunity and few child day care facilities are at least part of the reason rural women continue to carry out their traditional primary responsibility for child care. Economic conditions have caused women to look for employment opportunities. The jobs available in rural areas are fewer for everyone, but especially for women (Bushy, 1990). Community health nurses can be more effective educators and caregivers by recognizing the pivotal role of women in the health care of rural families.

Community and health status indicators, economic factors, and beliefs of rural people influence the community health nurses' practice. Clinical practice is carried out through the application of the nursing process to individuals, families, and groups or aggre-

gates within a community. Within the nurses' practice, both nursing and public health theories are combined to deliver a broad range of services in a number of settings. Integration of information about rural health, rural residents and their communities, community health nursing, and the prevention-oriented "upstream" approach to population-based health into the application of the nursing process can provide direction for holistic nursing care.

APPLICATION OF THE NURSING PROCESS

All three levels of prevention—primary, secondary, and tertiary—are reflected in rural-based practice. These levels of prevention are applied to individuals, families, and aggregates. Because of the generalist nature of the rural community health practice, the nurse has an excellent opportunity to assess health needs of individuals, families, and communities and to help them improve their health at all levels of prevention. The following case study includes short-term individual and family approaches. It also focuses on upstream interventions developed to handle the identified problems. Upstream interventions are population and prevention focused. These interventions deal with political, economic, and environmental factors that are forerunners of health problems.

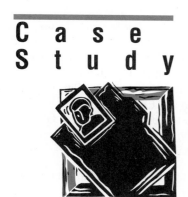

**C a s e
S t u d y**

At 4:30 PM on a hot fall day, registered nurse Mary Fieldson is 40 miles from her office at the county courthouse driving up a rutted, graveled township road. She has just completed her sixth home health visit today. By the time Mary returns home she will have traveled almost 150 miles. Nevertheless, she is enjoying the drive. The rural county of 6000 where she works is the place where she grew up. Today she made a skilled visit to Joe Lingh, the father of a high school friend. Now, on her way home, she is driving through the valley where she once lived. She has recently returned "home" after a 15-year absence to live, work, and raise her 12-year-old daughter. As she approaches the Connelly place, she sees Eliza Connelly standing by the road waving her down. Mary stops to say hello. Mrs. Connelly says, "I called Ruth Lingh and she said you had just left. How is Joe's leg?" Mary is aware that this is a friendly inquiry about a neighbor of 40 years, but she is mindful of the need for confidentiality. Mary tells Mrs. Connelly that Joe is glad to be home from the hospital. Mrs. Connelly then asks whether Mary has heard about her husband's accident Monday evening. He "cut his hand up in the silage chopper and is in the hospital in Spring City," she tells Mary tearfully. "I just knew something was going to happen someday. I worry so much about them working with all that machinery and the men work in the fields alone so much. I feel about ready to fall apart. Thank God Jim [their son] was working with him when it happened!"

Mary has a cup of coffee with Eliza. Eliza is composed but continues to talk about long-standing fears for the safety of her family as they go about the farm work. She asks Mary whether she can stop by and check on her husband, Austin, when he gets home next week. Mary tells Eliza to request a referral from the primary care physician so insurance will pay for the visits if they are covered in the policy. At 5:30 PM Mary begins the drive back to her office in Wolsey, the county seat.

Monday afternoon Mary receives a telephone call from Dr. Lobban, the local primary care physician, who requested skilled nursing visits weekly for Austin for the next 3 weeks to check for infection and to monitor the recovery. Austin will be discharged from the Spring City hospital tomorrow, 6 days after the injury. Dr. Lobban will send over the emergency room records and the hand specialist's discharge summary.

Assessment

The medical records provide the following information. The first finger was severed at the metacarpophalangeal joint (the third joint) and reattached. The second, third, and fourth fingers were severed distal to the proximal interphalangeal joints (between the first and second joints). The severed portions of the second, third, and fourth fingers could not be reattached because they were too badly mangled. At discharge no evidence of infection was evident. The hand was healing well.

The Connelly family provided additional information about the circumstances of the accident. Austin and his son Jim were chopping oats for silage. It was about 6:30 PM. Rain clouds were on the horizon. Jim and Austin were in a hurry to finish before it rained on the grain still left to chop. The silage chopper was not working well. Austin shut it off and hurriedly reached into the inspection hole. The still turning blades caught his right hand, severing the fingers. Jim wrapped his father's hand tightly in his shirt, retrieved the fingers and drove his father to the house 2 miles away. Jim went back to the field to finish up the oats. It had started to rain. Eliza drove her husband 23 miles to the primary care hospital emergency room. The family physician cleaned and dressed Austin's hand, gave him medication for pain, and packed the severed fingers for transport to the hand specialist in Spring City. A family friend and his son drove Mr. and Mrs. Connelly 150 miles to the Spring City hospital, where Austin was admitted and underwent surgery. Eliza drove home with their friend and his son after the surgery. She spoke to Austin by telephone daily and drove to Spring City on Tuesday to bring him home.

On her first home visit Mary assesses the following:

- Individual client, Mr. Connelly, for signs and symptoms of infection, pain control, and functional positioning
- Eliza's comfort level and knowledge of dressing changes and signs and symptoms of infection (she is the primary caregiver)
- Stress and grief processing of all family members
- Ability of family members to provide physical and emotional support during crisis resolution
- Risk-taking behaviors, especially those related to work, of all family members
- Assessment of neighborhood groups and neighbors who can provide support and help the family with the fall harvest work

Diagnosis

Individual
- At risk for infection, pain, and lost of hand function (Austin)
- At risk for grief related to loss of fingers, some use of hand, and decreased ability to do farm work (Austin)
- Anxiety related to ongoing fear for injury of family members (Eliza)
- Stress related to new responsibilities for farm management (Jim)

Family
- At risk for family crisis related to instability caused by the injury

Community
- Inadequate programs for farm injury prevention
- Nonexistent EMS or first response service

Planning

A plan of care is developed at the individual, family, and community levels. At all levels mutual goal setting and contracting are essential if the outcomes are to be positive.

Individual

Long-Term Goal
- Client will experience successful rehabilitation.

Short-Term Goals
- Client will remain free of infection.
- Individual family members will be able to express grief.

Family

Long-Term Goals
- Family will demonstrate coping skills appropriate to crisis.
- Family will identify risky behavior related to farm work.

Short-Term Goals
- Identify support to help with farm work.
- Identify ways to keep in contact with each other when family members are working alone in the fields.

Community

Long-Term Goal
- Program will be established for farm injury prevention education for populations at risk.

Short-Term Goals
- Begin the health planning process to put into place farm injury primary prevention program.
- Explore potential for a volunteer EMS response team.

Intervention

Mutual goal setting between nurse Mary Fieldson and the Connelly's made it possible for them to collaboratively carry out interventions.

Individual Mary taught Eliza how to change dressings and monitor Austin's hand for infection and function. Austin was involved in his care during healing and was able to monitor and manage the pain. He was most concerned about rehabilitation. He especially wanted to know when he could return to work and how disabled he would be. The local physician monitored Austin's progress. With Austin and Eliza present, the local physician consulted with the hand specialist by two-way interactive video conferencing. They were able to confer successfully using video conferencing, thereby eliminating a 150-mile trip to Spring City. The home care physical therapist visited the farm once to set up a program of hand exercises. Austin, who plays the piano, wanted to know if piano playing would be a good exercise. "Playing 'Moonlight Serenade' would sure stretch that right hand," he told the therapist. The physical therapist wrote "play piano q d × 3" as part of the rehabilitation care plan.

Family Mary worked with the family to problem solve ways to finish the fall work. They decided to hire part-time help, and two neighbors furnished a week of full-time help until the crop was harvested. Austin was able to assist his son by being supportive of his ability to make the necessary decisions about the farm management. Austin was also able to participate in the decision making after discharge from the hospital. The family identified the need for more awareness about the dangers of farm work. One change they made right away was the purchase of a cellular phone to take to the field. Eliza felt this would relieve her anxiety about not being able to keep in touch with them and not knowing why they were later than expected for dinner and supper. There was much discussion about the cost of the telephone. Eliza convinced the men that her peace of mind was worth the cost of the telephone and service.

The stress and grief reactions were minimal. Most of the stress centered on getting the fall farm work done and Austin's being able to work again, "the way he is used to doing." The support from neighbors and the rehabilitation program proved to be the interventions that helped them deal with stress and grief.

Community When an accident happens in a small rural community, it brings home the dangerous nature of farm work. People begin recalling their own "close calls" and remembering friends and family members who have been injured. The period when awareness is high is an excellent time to bring people together to discuss accident prevention. During the annual fall 4-H Achievement Days, Mary Fieldson set up an information booth in the exhibit hall and asked for volunteers to plan and implement a farm safety program in the county.

Austin's accident was handled appropriately by the family without EMS intervention. However, there had been other accidents recently that needed trained personnel at the sight to stabilize the injured person and minimize damage during transport to the primary care hospital. Mary's recent home care visits to farm families reinforced for her the need for EMS in these remote areas. She met with the county health department, local physicians, and county commissioners to investigate the feasibility of setting up an EMS.

Evaluation

Individual Individual members of the Connelly family used the home care nurse, physical therapist, and local physician appropriately. The successful healing of Austin's hand and subsequent rehabilitation are evidence of this. Austin has returned to work with minimum disability. During a drop-in visit by Mary 3 months after the accident, Austin treated her to a rousing piano rendition of "Stars and Stripes Forever."

Family With Mary's guidance the family wrote down a list of safety hazards and strategies to improve safety on the farm. Interestingly, one of the items was to wear seat belts when driving in the car and truck. Seat belts were installed in a 40-year-old farm truck still in regular use! A cellular phone was purchased and used to keep Eliza in touch with Austin and Jim in the field. This has proven so successful that several neighbors also bought cellular phones.

The family continued to demonstrate good coping skills as Austin progressed in his rehabilitation. Communication between father and son was excellent after the initial concern that Austin would feel his position as farm manager was being taken over. He was involved with the daily decision making as soon as he returned home from the hospital. The family effectively solved the problem of getting the fall work done by requesting the help of friends and neighbors. Also, they borrowed money from the bank to hire a part-time farm hand until Austin could work again.

Community Mary's information booth at the 4-H Achievement Days attracted the attention of several women from the County Extension Club. As a result of their interest, the club has made farm safety education their service project for the coming year. Development of a volunteer emergency medical first-response team has not progressed because of lack of community interest.

Levels of Prevention

The following are examples from the case study of the three levels of prevention as applied to the individual, family, and community.

Primary Prevention
- Assessment and teaching about farm accident prevention to family
- Initiation of a program of farm safety information at the community level
- Utilization of a cellular telephone to decrease anxiety about family members' location and well-being

Secondary Prevention
- Infection prevention and pain management of injured hand
- Screening at family and community level for farm hazards (a component of the overall primary prevention education program)

Tertiary Prevention
- Rehabilitation of Austin to limit disability
- Assessment and counseling to help family and injured individual cope with stress and grief reactions
- Development (attempted) of an EMS system to facilitate stabilization and safe transport.

RURAL HEALTH RESEARCH

The report of the National Institute of Nursing Research (NINR) Priority Expert Panel, Community-Based Health Care: Nursing Strategies, affirms that typically the rural health research foundation is sparse and studies are infrequently repeated. This situation exists because rural health is not studied as frequently as urban health (NINR, 1995). In order for rural Americans to gain equity in terms of health care cost, access, and quality, high-caliber research must be available to provide an unclouded picture of individuals', families', and communities' health care needs.

Rural research priorities have been identified by nurses working in the rural health field (Bushy, 1991, 1992; Ide, 1992; Long and Weinert, 1989), the National Rural Health Association's (NRHA's) Research Conference (Hersh and van Hook, 1989), and the NINR (1995). Broadly stated, these priorities focus on development of rural nursing theory and refinement of rural nursing practice models, health care policy, rural health care delivery systems, and nursing approaches using community-based interventions directed at the three levels of prevention.

Rural nursing theory and models for practice are in the early stages of development. The work by Long and Weinert (1989) and Weinert and Long (1990) on the development of a foundation for rural nursing theory, although in early evolvement, is helpful in guiding research, rural community nursing practice, and education. This beginning theory work done at Montana State University emphasizes the importance of comprehending the rural resident's definition of health. For example, rural people value the ability to work and are more apt to reject the sick role than are urban residents. If they can do their work, they do not consider themselves to be ill. Concepts related to nursing are identified as lack of anonymity (knowing many people in the rural community in both work and social roles), outsider-insider, and old-timer–newcomer. In relation to the last two concepts of outsider-insider and old-timer–newcomer, acceptance by a rural community of a community health nurse new to the area is less likely than it would be if she or he grew up or had lived in that community for 20 years (Weinert and Long, 1987).

Ide (1992) developed a rural nursing practice model, which includes ideas garnered from current rural literature and needs and priorities synthesized from community health assessments completed by graduate students. This model outlines the ways in which the health status, beliefs, and behaviors of rural dwellers and rural nursing practice are influenced by the rural environment. The extensive discussion of the effects of the rural environment on rural dwellers provides helpful direction to rural community health nurses, teachers, and researchers

for planning health care delivery and initiating scholarly inquiry.

Bushy (1991), in a review of the rural family health literature, identified that more research is needed that addresses the relationship among life events such as marriage, unemployment, business foreclosure, and rural location.

The NRHA research agenda addresses the following specific issues: maternal child health, rural hospitals, alternative delivery systems (health maintenance organizations, managed care), the poor and underserved, the elderly, and primary care. Problems related to research needs and important to all of the specific issues listed were identified as (1) the necessity for standardization of rurality definitions among government agencies that take into consideration the differences of rural populations; (2) the need for secondary data analysis of existing data and reporting of that aggregate data by small geographic regions so that important regional differences are not being obliterated; (3) dilemmas related to recruiting, retaining, and training of health providers in rural communities; (4) the negative effect of professional liability on rural care providers; (5) the obstacles related to transportation—distance, terrain, climatic conditions, poor roads, and no public transit system—on access to health care for rural residents; and (6) outcome measurements of quality health care (Hersh and van Hook, 1989).

The report, Community-Based Health Care: Nursing Strategies, identifies the following three essential topics of research at the primary and secondary intervention levels: unintentional injuries, maternal and child health with a focus on infant mortality, and lifestyle or personal actions that contribute to premature mortality. At the tertiary level of rehabilitation and supportive care, formal and informal support and chronic illness are identified as the two essential subjects of research (NINR, 1995).

Both well-designed qualitative and large-scale quantitative studies are needed to improve the quality of rural research. An important component of rural health research is the collaboration between rural nurses and researchers in describing problems and gathering data. Additionally, and of paramount importance, is the need for research findings to be disseminated to nurses and other rural health care providers in clinical practice (Bushy, 1992). Without that critical link to the clinician in rural practice, research is an academic exercise and does not serve the needs of rural individuals, families, and communities.

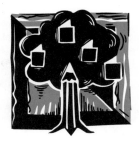

Learning Activities

1. University libraries commonly subscribe to newspapers published within the state. Visit the library, select three to four small town or rural county newspapers, and read them for information about health care activities and concerns related to the health of the individuals, families, and community.

- Report back to your class what you found out about rural health concerns and activities.
- Identify one priority problem that could be researched in the community and has relevance to rural community health nursing practice.

2. Select a rural community health nurse (public health or home care) and conduct an interview in person or by telephone if distance prohibits a face-to-face meeting.

- Identify what the nurse sees as the pros and cons of rural nursing.
- If negative aspects of rural nursing are identified, discuss how the nurse deals with them.
- Ask the nurse to discuss the three highest priority efforts related to his or her rural practice.

3. Choose one of the major causes of morbidity and mortality in rural populations.

- On the basis of the risk factor and natural history, specify interventions for primary, secondary, and tertiary prevention of this disease.
- Identify which of these interventions are examples of upstream thinking.

4. Locate a telephone book or community resource directory from a rural community.

- List and evaluate the resources that are available for prevention, assessment, intervention, and follow-up care for the major cause of mortality and morbidity identified in Learning Activity 3.
- Would it be necessary to go outside the rural town or county for any of the needed resources? Which ones? Where might they be located?

REFERENCES

A Special Report: A Health Crisis. School of Journalism, University of Montana, Missoula, MT, Summer 1993.

Akin L, Fagin C: OP-ED. New York Times, March 11, 1993.

American Psychological Association, Office of Rural Health: Caring for the Rural Community. Washington, DC, American Psychological Association, 1995.

Amundson B: Myth and reality in the rural health service crisis: Facing up to community responsibilities. J Rural Health 9:176–187, 1993.

Battenfield D, Clift E, Graubarth R, (1981): Cited in Bushy A: Rural U.S. women: Traditions and transitions affecting health care. Health Care Women Int 11:503–513, 1990.

Bigbee J: The uniqueness of rural nursing. Nurs Clin North Am 28:131–144, 1993.

Buehler J, Lee H: Exploration of home care resources for rural families with cancer. Cancer Nurs 15:299–308, 1992.

Bushy A: Rural U.S. women: Traditions and transitions affecting health care. Health Care Women Int 11:503–513, 1990.

Bushy A: Rural determinants in family health: Considerations for community nurses. In Bushy A (ed): Rural Health Nursing. Vol. 2, Newbury Park, CA, Sage, 1991, pp. 133–145.

Bushy A: Rural nursing research priorities. J Nurs Admin 22:50–56, 1992.

Butterfield P: Thinking upstream: Nurturing a conceptual understanding of the societal context of health behavior. Adv Nurs Sci 12:1–8, 1996.

Calle EE, Flanders WD, Thun MJ, Martin LM: Demographic predictors of mammography and Pap smear screening in U.S. women. Am J Public Health 83:53–60, 1993.

Carson D, Araquistain M, Ide B, et al.: Hardiness as a mediator of the effects of stressors and strains on reported illnesses and relational difficulties in farm and ranch families. Journal Rural Health 9:215–226, 1993.

Clancy F: Rural Rx. Harrowsmith County Life March/April:31–37, 1992.

Cordes S: The changing rural environments and the relationship between health services and rural development. A Rural Health Services Research Agenda (Special Issue): Conference Summary. Health Serv Res 23:757–784, 1989.

Cotton DJ, Graham BL, Li KLR, et al.: Effects of grain dust exposure on respiratory symptoms and lung function. *In* Dosman JA, Cockcroft DW (eds): Principals of Health and Safety in Agriculture. Boca Raton, FL, CRC Press, pp. 138–143.

Crandall LA, Coggan JM: Impact of new information technologies on training and continuing education for rural health professionals. J Rural Health 10:208–215, 1994.

Davis D, Droes N: Community health nursing in rural and frontier counties. Nurs Clin North Am 28:159–169, 1993.

Dolphin N: Rural health. *In* Logan B, Dawkins C (eds): Family Centered Nursing in the Community. Menlo Park, CA, Addison-Wesley, 1984, pp. 515–531.

Dunkin J, Juhl N, Stratton T, et al.: Job satisfaction and retention of rural community health nurses in North Dakota. J Rural Health 8:268–275, 1992.

Eggebeen D, Lichter D: Health and well-being among rural Americans: Variations across the life course. J Rural Health 9:86–98, 1993.

Elison G: Frontier areas: Problems for delivery of health care services. Rural Health Care, 8:1–3, 1986.

Environmental Protection Agency: Recognition and Management of Pesticide Poisonings, 4th ed (EPA 540/9-88-001). Washington, DC, U.S. Government Printing Office, 1989.

Etherton JR, Myers JR, Jensen RC, et al.: Agricultural machine-related deaths. Am J Public Health 81:766–768, 1991.

Farmer F, Clark L, Miller M: Consequences of differential residence designations for rural health policy: The case of infant mortality. J Rural Health 9:17–26, 1993.

Furlow L: Emergency nursing in rural Texas: A case study. *In* Bushy A (ed). Rural Nursing, vol. 2, Newbury Park, CA, Sage, 1991, pp. 261–269.

Garnett G: Challenges of serving as the director of an emergency medical service in Alaska. *In* Bushy A (ed): Rural Nursing, vol. 2, Newbury Park, CA, Sage, 1991, pp. 251–260.

Hersh A, van Hook R: A research agenda for rural health services. A Rural Health Services Research Agenda (Special Issue): Conference Summary. Health Serv Res 23:1053–1064, 1989.

Hicks LL: Access and utilization: Special populations—special needs. *In* Straub LA, Walzer N (eds): Rural Health Care: Innovation in a Changing Environment. Westport, CT, Praeger, 1992.

Horwitz M, Rosenthal T: The impact of informal care giving on labor force participation by rural farming and nonfarming families. J Rural Health 10:266–272, 1994.

Human Services in the Rural Transition: A Training Packet: Great Plains Staff Training and Development for Rural Mental Health. Lincoln, NE, Department of Psychology, 1989.

Ide B: A process model of rural nursing practice. Texas J Rural Health 38:30–38, 1992.

Institute of Medicine: Community Oriented Primary Care. Washington, DC, National Academy Press, 1983.

Institute of Medicine. (1988). The Future of Public Health. Washington, DC, National Academy of Medicine, 1988.

Institute of Medicine: Access to Health Care in America. Washington, DC, National Academy Press, 1993.

Johnson RK, Guthrie H, Smiciklas-Wright H, Wang MQ: Characterizing nutrient intakes of children by sociodemographic factors. Public Health Rep 109:414–420, 1994.

Kohl DM: Cattlewomen's Column. Times Clarion (Harlowton, MT), April 13, p. 7.

Lassiter P: Rural practice: How do we prepare providers? J Rural Health 1:23–26, 1985.

Lee H: Relationship of Ecological Rurality to Current Life Events, Hardiness, and Perceived Health Status in Rural Adults (Dissertation) Austin, TX, University of Texas at Austin. November, 1985.

Lee H: Relationship of hardiness and current life events to perceived health in rural adults. Res Nurs Health 14:351–359, 1991.

Lee H: Health perceptions of middle, "new middle," and older rural adults. Family Community Health 16:19–27, 1993.

Lisnerski DD, McClary CL, Brown TL, et al.: Demographic and predictive correlates of smokeless tobacco use in elementary school children. Am J Health Promotion 5:426–431, 1991.

Long K, Boik R: Predicting alcohol use in rural children: A longitudinal study. Nurs Res 42:79–86, 1993.

Long K, Weinert C: Rural nursing: Developing the theory base. Scholarly Inquiry Nurs Pract 3:113–127, 1989.

Magilvey J, Congdon J: Circles of care: Rural home care for older adults. Rural Clin Q 4:3–4, 1994.

Mayer LV: Agricultural change and rural America. *In* Gahr WE (ed): Rural America: Blueprint for tomorrow. Ann Am Acad Polit Soc Sci 529:80–91, 1993.

McNeely G: Evaluating alternative rural hospitals models: What are we learning. *In* Walzer L (ed): Rural Health Care. Westport, CT, Praeger Press, 1992, pp. 51–64.

Memmott R: Developing hospice programs in frontier communities. *In* Bushy A (ed): Rural Nursing, vol. 2. Newbury Park, CA, Sage Publications, 1991, pp. 63–75.

Miller M, Farmer F, Clarke L: Rural populations and their health. *In* Beaulieu J, Berry D (eds): Rural Health Services: A Management Perspective. Ann Arbor, MI, AUPHA Press/Health Administration Press, 1994, pp. 3–26.

Monroe AC, Rickett TC, Savitts LA: Cancer in rural versus urban populations: A review. J Rural Health 8:212–220, 1992.

Movassaghi H, Kindig D, Juhl N, Geller J: Nursing supply and characteristics in the nonmetropolitan areas of the United States: Findings from the 1988 National Sample Survey of Registered Nurses. J Rural Health 8:276–282, 1992.

National Institute of Nursing Research: Community-Based Health Care: Nursing Strategies. A Report of the Priority Expert Panel, October 1995. U.S. Department of Health and Human Services, USPH, NIH, Publ #95–3917.

National Institute for Occupational Safety and Health: Alert: Preventing Scalping and Other Severe Injuries from Farm Machinery (NIOSH Publication No. 94-105). Cincinnati, OH, 1994.

National Institute for Occupational Safety and Health, Division of Safety Research: National Traumatic Occupational Fatalities Surveillance System: In House Analyses. Morgantown, WV, 1992.

National Rural Health Association: Managed Care as a Service Delivery Model in Rural Areas. Issue Paper, Kansas City, MO, 1995.

Norris K: Dakota. New York, Ticknor & Fields, 1993.

Norton C, McManus M: Background tables on demographic characteristics, health status, and health services utilization. A Rural Health Services Research Agenda. (Special Issue). Conference Summary. Health Serv Res 23:725–756, 1989.

Office of the Inspector General, DHHS: Medical Assistance Facilities (OEI-04-92-00731). Washington, DC, U.S. Department of Health and Human Services, 1993.

Office of Technology Assessment, Congress of the United States: Rural Emergency Medical Service (Special Report OTA-H-445). Washington, DC, U.S. Government Printing Office, November, 1989.

Office of Technology Assessment, Congress of the United States: Health Care in Rural America (OTA-H-434). Washington, DC, U.S. Government Printing Office. September, 1990.

Office of Technology Assessment, Congress of the United States: Rural America at the Crossroads: Networking for the Future (OTA-TCT-471). Washington, DC, U.S. Government Printing Office. April, 1991.

Pickett G, Hanlon J: Public health: Administration and practice. St. Louis: Times Mirror/Mosby, 1990.

Posey S: Dissemination of farm health and safety information. Poster presented at the 7th Session of the Rural Nursing Conference. Greely, CO, University of Northern Colorado, School of Nursing, 1995.

Puskin DS: Telecommunications in rural America: Opportunities and challenges for the health care system. Extended clinical consulting by hospital computer networks. Ann NY Acad Sci, 670:67–75, 1992.

Ricketts T: Health care professionals in rural America. *In* Beaulieu J, Barry D (eds): Rural Health Services—A Management Perspective. Ann Arbor, MI, AUPHS Press/Health Administration Press, 1994, pp. 85–109.

Rivara FP: Fatal and non-fatal farm injuries to children and adolescents in the United States. Pediatrics 76:567–573, 1985.

Straub LA, Walzer N: Financing the demand for rural health care. *In* Straub LA, Walzer N (eds): Rural Health Care: Innovation in a Changing Environment. Westport, CT, Praeger Press, 1992, pp. 3–19.

Turner T, Gunn I: Issues in rural health nursing. *In* Bushy A (ed): Rural Nursing, vol. 2. Newbury Park, CA, Sage, 1991, pp. 63–75.

Turnock B, Handler A, Hall W, et al.: Local health department effectiveness in addressing the core function of public health. Public Health Rep 109:653–658, 1994.

U.S. Department of Labor, Bureau of Labor Statistics: Occupational Injuries and Illnesses in the U.S. by Industries (Bulletin No. 2379). Washington, DC, U.S. Government Printing Office, 1989.

U.S. Public Health Service: Healthy People 2000: National Health Promotion and Disease Prevention Objectives. Washington, DC, U.S. Government Printing Office, 1990.

Van Hook R: Foreword. *In* Straub L, Walzer N (eds): Rural Health Care. Westport, CT, Praeger Press, 1992, pp. ix–xiv.

Wagenfield MO: Mental health and rural America: A decade review. J Rural Health 6:507–522, 1990.

Warren CPW: Overview of respiratory health risks in agriculture. *In* Dosman JA, Cockcroft DW (eds): Principals of Health and Safety in Agriculture. Boca Raton, FL, CRC Press, 1989, pp. 47–49.

Weinert C, Burman M: Rural health and health seeking behaviors. *In* Fitzpatrick JJ, Stevenson JS (eds): Annual Review of Nursing Research, vol. 12. New York, Springer, 1994, pp. 65–92.

Weinert C, Long KA: Understanding the health care needs of rural families. Family Relations 36:450–455, 1987.

Weinert C, Long KA: Rural families and health care: Refining the knowledge base. J Marriage Family Rev 15:57–75, 1990.

Wilk VA: Occupational Health of Migrant and Seasonal Farmworkers in the U.S.: Progress Report. Washington, DC, Farmworker Justice Fund, 1988.

UNIT 4

Special Needs
of Aggregates

Cultural Diversity and Community Health Nursing

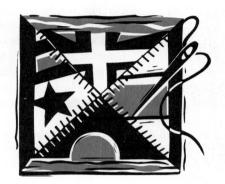

Upon conclusion of this chapter, the reader will be able to:

1. Discuss racial and cultural diversity in U.S. society.

2. Identify the cultural aspects of nursing care for culturally diverse individuals, groups, and communities.

3. Analyze the sociocultural, political, economic, and religious factors that impact on the nursing care of culturally diverse individuals, groups, and communities.

4. Compare health-related values, beliefs, and practices of the dominant cultural group with those of individuals and groups from culturally diverse backgrounds.

5. Apply the principles of transcultural nursing to community health nursing practice.

Margaret M. Andrews

TRANSCULTURAL PERSPECTIVES ON COMMUNITY HEALTH NURSING

The nurse's knowledge of culture and cultural concepts improves the health of the community and groups within it as well as the health of individuals and families. Culturally competent community health nursing requires that the nurse understand the lifestyle, value system, and health and illness behaviors of diverse individuals, families, groups, and communities as well as the culture of institutions that influence the health and well-being of communities. Nurses who have knowledge of and an ability to work with diverse cultures are able to devise effective community interventions to reduce risks in a manner that is culturally congruent with community, group, and individual values.

In the United States, metaphors such as *melting pot, mosaic,* and *salad bowl* have been used to describe the cultural diversity that characterizes the population. Although there is a tendency to identify the federally defined racial-ethnic minority* groups when referring to the cultural aspects of community health nursing, it is important to note that *all* individuals, families, groups, communities, and institutions, including nurses and the nursing profession, have cultural characteristics that influence community health. I believe that community health nurses need to balance cultural diversity with the universal human experience and common needs of all people of the world.

POPULATION TRENDS

By the year 2000, more than one-quarter of the U.S. population will consist of individuals from the federally defined minority groups. By the middle of the next century, minorities will account for 51.1% of the total population. For the first time in U.S. history, minorities will make up a majority of the total population. If current demographic trends continue, the United States will have the following population composition

*The term *minority* is used here because the U.S. Bureau of the Census has reported its data according to the following federally defined minority groups: blacks (African, Haitian, or Dominican Republic descent); Hispanics (Mexican, Cuban, Puerto Rican, and others); Asians (Japanese, Chinese, Filipino, Korean, Vietnamese, Hawaiian, Guamian, Samoan, or Asian Indian descent); and American Indians and Alaska Natives (510 federally recognized tribes). Because the term connotes inferiority and marginalization, members of some groups object to its use.

by the year 2080: Hispanic, 23.4%; black, 14.7%; and Asian and Pacific Islander, 12% (U.S. Bureau of the Census, 1990). At the same time, the American Indian and Alaska Native population is projected to remain at 0.6% or perhaps decrease slightly because of intermarriage. Table 17–1 summarizes the current population composition by race, number, percentage, and percentage of change from 1980 to 1990.

Although the nursing profession has representatives from diverse groups, minorities continue to be underrepresented (Andrews, 1992; Jones, 1992; Rosella et al., 1994). It is estimated that 9%, or 207,000, of the nation's 2.25 million registered nurses come from racial-ethnic minority backgrounds. Estimates for each minority group are as follows: 90,600 black nurses; 30,400 Hispanic nurses; 76,000 Asian and Pacific Islander nurses; and 10,000 American Indian and Alaska Native nurses. Each minority group is distributed differently around the country. Black nurses are more likely to be found in the South, Hispanics in the West or South (especially states bordering Mexico), and Asian and Pacific Islanders in the West or Northeast. American Indian and Alaska Native nurses are found predominantly in states having reservations (U.S. Department of Health and Human Services [DHHS], 1993).

The United States has grown and achieved its success as a nation largely as a result of immigration. Since 1972 more than 10 million legal immigrants have come to this country. The number of immigrants and refugees in the United States is projected to continue to increase. In addition, people from other countries will probably continue to seek treatment in U.S. hospitals, particularly for cardiovascular, neurological, and cancer care, and U.S. nurses will continue to have the opportunity to travel abroad to work in a wide variety of health care settings in the international marketplace. In the course of one's nursing career, it is possible to encounter foreign visitors, international university faculty, international high school and university students, family members of foreign diplomats, immigrants, refugees, members of more than 130 different ethnic groups, and Native Americans from more than 500 federally recognized tribes. A serious conceptual problem exists within nursing in that, without formal preparation, nurses are expected to know, understand. and meet the health needs of culturally diverse individuals, groups, and communities.

Members of some cultural groups, most notably blacks and Hispanics, are demanding culturally relevant health care that incorporates their specific

Table 17–1
Composition of United States Population (1990) and Percentage of Change, 1980–1990

| Population | U.S. Population | | Change from 1980 (%) |
	No.	%	
Total	248,709,873	100	10
Race*			
White	199,686,060	83	6
African-American	29,986,060	12	12
Native American	1,959,234	1	38
Asian and Pacific Islander	7,273,662	3	108
All other	9,804,847	4	45
Hispanic origin†	22,354,059	9	53

*Race does not denote any clear-cut definition of biological stock but rather is a self-classification by people to the race with which they most closely identify.

†Hispanic origin denotes origination of Spanish-speaking people from the Caribbean, Central or South America, Spain, or elsewhere. It is distinct from race; thus, persons of Spanish or Hispanic origin may be of any race.

From the U.S. Bureau of the Census, *General Population Characteristics—Part I: United States Summary,* vol. 1. Washington, DC, U.S. Government Printing Office, 1990.

beliefs and practices. There is an increasing expectation among member of certain cultural groups that health care providers will respect their "cultural health rights," an expectation that frequently conflicts with the unicultural, Western, biomedical world view taught in U.S. educational programs that prepare nurses and other health care providers.

Given the multicultural composition of the United States and the projected increase in the number of individuals from diverse cultural backgrounds, concern for cultural beliefs and practices of people in community health nursing is becoming increasingly important. Nursing is inherently a transcultural phenomenon in that the context and process of helping people involves at least two persons who usually have different cultural orientations or intracultural lifestyles.

HISTORIC PERSPECTIVE ON CULTURAL DIVERSITY

At no other time in the history of nursing have cultures been interacting and communicating with each other more frequently than today. However, nurses have been concerned with the cultural dimensions of care for many years. A brief historic overview of the ways in which nurses have responded to the health care needs of those from various cultural backgrounds follows.

Although the 19th-century concept of culture was limited and thought to be associated primarily with physiologic differences, Florence Nightingale's involvement in the Crimea and her concern with the fate of the Australian aborigines make her the first nurse in modern history to consider cultural aspects of nursing care. Concern for the health care needs of culturally diverse groups is also reflected in early 19th-century U.S. history. In 1870, Linda Richards became the first nurse known to engage in international nursing when, under the auspices of the American Board of Missions, she establisehd a school of nursing in Japan. In the early 1900s, Lillian Wald, Lavinia Dock, and other public health nurses provided nursing care for European immigrants, many of whom resided in low-income tenement houses in New York City.

In the 1960s and 1970s, many racial and ethnic groups, most notably blacks and Hispanics, became increasingly concerned with their civil rights and raised the consciousness of the U.S. public. Influenced by the social and political climate, U.S. nurses responded with growing professional awareness and increased sensitivity to attitudes, values, beliefs, and practices about health, illness, and caring among culturally diverse clients. The nursing profession responded to the sociocultural and historic events of this era with the development of a new subspecialty called *transcultural nursing.*

TRANSCULTURAL NURSING IN THE COMMUNITY

In 1959, Madeleine Leininger, a nurse-anthropologist, used the term *transcultural nursing* to define the philosophical and theoretical similarities between nursing and anthropology. In 1968, Leininger proposed her theory-generated model; in 1970, she wrote the first book on transcultural nursing, *Nursing and Anthropology: Two Worlds to Blend*. According to Leininger, transcultural nursing is "a formal area of study and practice focused on a comparative analysis of different cultures and subcultures in the world with respect to cultural care, health and illness beliefs, values, and practices with the goal of using this knowledge to provide culture-specific and culture-universal nursing care to people" (Leininger, 1978, p. 493). *Culture specific* refers to the "particularistic values, beliefs, and patterning of behavior that tend to be special, 'local,' or unique to a designated culture and which do not tend to be shared with members of other cultures" (Leininger, 1991, p. 491), whereas *culture universal* refers to the "commonalities of values, norms of behavior, and life patterns that are similarly held among cultures about human behavior and life-styles and form the bases for formulating theories for developing cross-cultural laws of human behavior" (Leininger, 1978, p. 491).

Although many nurse-scholars have developed theories of nursing, Leininger's theory of culture care diversity and universality is the only one that gives precedence to understanding the cultural dimensions of human care and caring. Leininger's theory is concerned with describing, explaining, and projecting nursing similarities and differences focused primarily on human care and caring in human cultures. Leininger used world view, social structure, language, ethnohistory, environmental context, and the generic (folk) and professional systems to provide a comprehensive and holistic view of influences in cultural care and well-being. The community health nurse will find the three modes of nursing decisions and actions–culture care preservation and maintenance, culture care accommodation and negotiation, and culture care repatterning and restructuring—useful in providing culturally congruent and competent nursing care (Leininger, 1978, 1991, 1995).

Among the strengths of Leininger's theory is its flexibility for use with individuals, families, groups, communities, and institutions in diverse health systems. Leininger's sunrise model (Fig. 17–1) depicts the theory of cultural care diversity and universality and provides a visual schematic representation of the key components of the theory and the interrelationships among the theory's components.

Although it is beyond the scope of this text to review all the recognized nursing theories from a transcultural perspective, the reader is encouraged to evaulate critically the cultural relevance of a theory before using it in community health nursing. It is especially important to examine the underlying assumptions of theories from a transcultural perspective. For example, those theories emphasizing self-care fail to recognize that many cultures and subcultures value group interdependence, cooperation, and responsibility for others. When clients' cultural values and expressions of care differ from those of the nurse, caution must be exercised to ensure that mutually agreed-on goals have been established.

The term *cross-cultural nursing* is sometimes used synonymously with transcultural nursing. The terms *intercultural nursing* and *multicultural nursing* are also used, as is the phrase *ethnic people of color*. Since Leininger's early work, many other nurses have contributed significantly to the advancement of nursing care of culturally diverse clients, groups, and communities, and some of their contributions are mentioned in this chapter.

Culture

In 1871, the English anthropologist Sir Edward Tylor was the first to define the term *culture*. According to Tylor (1871), culture refers to the complex whole, including knowledge, belief, art, morals, law, custom, and any other capabilities and habits acquired by virtue of the fact that one is a member of a particular society. Culture represents a way of perceiving, behaving in, and evaluating one's world, and it provides the blueprint for determining one's values, beliefs, and practices.

Culture has four basic characteristics.

- It is learned from birth through the processes of language acquisition and socialization.
- It is shared by all members of the same cultural group.
- It is adapted to specific conditions related to environmental and technical factors and to the availability of natural resources.
- It is dynamic.

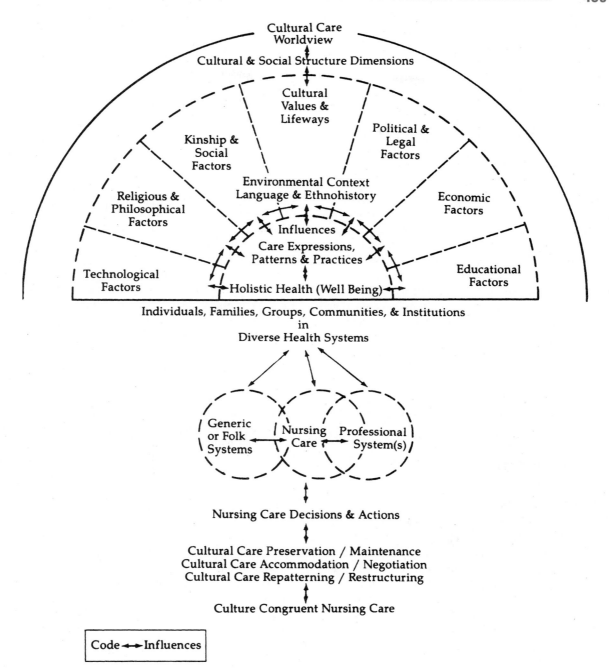

Figure 17–1
Leininger's sunrise model to depict theory of cultural care diversity and universality. (From Leininger MM: Culture, Care, Diversity, and Universality: A Theory of Nursing. New York, National League for Nursing, Publication No. 15-2402, 1991, p. 43.)

Culture is an all-pervasive, universal phenomenon without which no human exists. Yet the culture that develops in any given society is always specific and distinctive, encompassing all of the knowledge, beliefs, customs, and skills acquired by members of the society. Within cultures, groups of individuals share beliefs, values, and attitudes that are different from those of other groups within the same culture. Differences occur because of ethnicity, religion, education, occupation, age, sex, and individual preferences and variations. When such groups function within a large culture, they are referred to as subcultural groups.

The term *subculture* is used for fairly large aggregates of people who share characteristics that are not common to all members of the culture and enable them to be thought of as a distinguishable subgroup. Ethnicity, religion, occupation, health-related characteristics, age, sex, and geographic location are frequently used to identify subcultural groups. Examples of U.S. subcultures based on ethnicity (i.e., subcultures with common traits such as physical characteristics, language, or ancestry) include blacks, Hispanics, Native Americans, and Chinese-Americans; those based on religion include members of the more than 1200 recognized religions such as Catholics, Jews, Mormons, Muslims, and Buddhists; those based on occupation include health care professionals such as nurses and physicians, career military personnel, and farmers; those based on a health-related characteristic include the blind, hearing impaired, or mentally retarded; those based on age include adolescents and the elderly, for example; those based on sex or sexual preference include women, men, lesbians, and gay men; and those based on geographic location include, for example, Appalachians, southerners, and New Yorkers.

Culture and the Formation of Values

According to Leininger (1995), *value* refers to a desirable or undesirable state of affairs. Values are a universal feature of all cultures, although the types and expressions of values differ widely. *Norms* are the rules by which human behavior is governed and result from the cultural values held by the group. All societies have rules or norms that specify appropriate and inappropriate behavior. Individuals are rewarded or punished as they conform to or deviate from the established norms. Values and norms along with the acceptable and unacceptable behaviors associated with them are learned in childhood (Herberg, 1995).

Every society has a *dominant value orientation*, a basic value orientation that is shared by the majority of its members as a result of early common experiences. In the United States, as in other cultures, the dominant value orientation is reflected in the dominant cultural group, which is made up of white, middle-class Protestants, typically those who came to this country at least two generations ago from northern Europe. Because many members of the dominant cultural group are of Anglo-Saxon descent, they are sometimes referred to as WASPs (white Anglo-Saxon Protestants).

In addition to the values identified from U.S. proverbs, the dominant cultural group places emphasis on educational achievement, science, technology, individual expression, democracy, experimentation, and informality (Herberg, 1995).

Although there is sometimes an assumption that the term *white* refers to a homogeneous group of Americans, there is a rich diversity of ethnic variation among the many groups that constitute the dominant majority; origins include eastern and western Europe (Ireland, Poland, Italy, France, Sweden, Russia, and so on) as well as Canada, Australia, New Zealand, and South Africa (origins can ultimately be traced to western Europe). Appalachians, the Amish, and other subgroups are also examples of whites who have cultural roots that are recognizably different from those of the dominant cultural group.

According to Kluckhohn and Strodtbeck (1961), there is a limited number of basic human problems for which all people must find a solution and five common human problems that concern values and norms:
1. What is the character of innate human nature (human nature orientation)?
2. What is the relation of the human person to nature (person-nature orientation)?
3. What is the temporal focus (time sense) of human life (time orientation)?
4. What is the mode of human activity (activity orientation)?
5. What is the mode of human relationships (social orientation)?

Regarding the first question, the innate human nature of people may be good, evil, or a combination of good and evil. Some consider human nature to be unalterable or able to be perfected only through great discipline and effort because they believe life is a struggle to overcome a basically evil nature. For others, human nature is perceived as fundamentally good, unalterable, and difficult or impossible to corrupt. According to Kohls (1984), the dominant U.S. cultural group chooses to believe the best about a person until that person proves otherwise. Concern in the United States for prison reform, social rehabilitation, and the plight of less fortunate people around the world is reflective of the fundamental goodness of human nature, although human nature may also be viewed as a combination of good and evil.

Second, in examining the ways in which our person-nature relationship is perceived, there are three perspectives:

- Destiny, in which the human person is subjugated to nature in a fatalistic, inevitable manner
- Harmony, in which people and nature exist together as a single entity
- Mastery, in which it is believed that people are intended to overcome natural forces and put them to use for the benefit of humankind

Most Americans consider the human person and nature to be clearly separated (an incomprehensible perspective for many individuals of Asian heritage). The idea that one can control one's destiny is alien to many individuals of culturally diverse backgrounds. Many cultures believe that people are driven and controlled by fate and can do very little, if anything, to influence it. Americans, by contrast, have an insatiable drive to subdue, dominate, and control their natural environment (Kohls, 1984).

What does this values orientation have to do with health and illness? Consider three individuals who have been diagnosed with hypertension; each embraces one of the values orientations described. The person whose values orientation is destiny might say, "Why should I bother watching my diet, taking medication, and getting regular blood pressure checks? High blood pressure is part of my genetic destiny, and there is nothing I can do to change the outcome. There is no need to waste money on prescription drugs and health checkups." The person whose values orientation embraces harmony might say, "If I follow the diet described and use medication to lower my blood pressure, I can restore the balance and harmony that were upset by this illness. The emotional stress I've been feeling indicates an inner lack of harmony that needs to be balanced." Finally, the person whose values orientation leads to belief in active mastery might say, "I will overcome this hypertension no matter what. By eating the right foods, working toward stress reduction, and conquering the disease with medication, I will take charge of the situation and influence the course of my disease."

Third, there are three major ways in which people can perceive time. The focus may be on the past, with traditions and ancestors playing an important role in the client's life. For example, many Asians, Native Americans, East Indians, and Africans hold beliefs about ancestors and tend to value long-standing traditions. In times of crisis, such as illness, individuals with a values orientation emphasizing the past may consult with ancestors or ask for their guidance or protection during the illness. The focus may be on the present, with little attention paid to the past or the future. These individuals are concerned with the current situation, and the future is perceived as vague or unpredictable. Nurses may have difficulty encouraging these individuals to prepare for the future, (e.g., participate in primary prevention measures). Last, the focus may be on the future, with progress and change highly valued. These individuals may express discontent with both the past and the present. In terms of health care, these individuals may inquire about the "latest treatment" and the most advanced equipment available for a particular problem.

The dominant U.S. cultural group is characterized by a belief in progress and a future orientation. This implies a strong task or goal orientation. This group has an optimistic faith in what the future will bring. Change is often equated with improvement, and a rapid rate of change is usually viewed as normal.

Fourth, this value orientation concerns activity. Philosophers have suggested three perspectives:

- Being, in which there is a spontaneous expression of impulses and desires that is largely nondevelopmental in nature
- Growing, in which the person is self-contained and has inner control, including the ability to self-actualize
- Doing, in which the person actively strives to achieve and accomplish something that is regarded highly

The doing is often directed toward achievement of an externally applied standard, such as a code of behavior from a religious or ethical perspective. The Ten Commandments, Pillars of Islam, Hippocratic oath, and Nightingale pledge are examples of externally applied standards.

The dominant cultural value is action oriented, with an emphasis on productivity and being busy. As a result of this action orientation, Americans have become very proficient at problem solving and decision making. Even during leisure time and vacations, many Americans value activity.

Finally, consider the cultural values orientations concerning the relationships that exist with others. Relationships may be categorized in three ways:

- Lineal relationships refer to those that exist by virtue of heredity and kinship ties. These relationships follow an ordered succession and have continuity through time.
- Collateral relationships focus primarily on group goals, and family orientation is all important. For example, many Asian patients will describe family honor and the importance of working together toward achievement of a group versus a personal goal.
- Individual relationships refer to personal autonomy and independence. These goals dominate; group goals become secondary.

The social orientation among the dominant U.S. cultural group is toward the importance of the individual and the equality of all people. Friendly, informal, outgoing, and extroverted, members of the dominant cultural group tend to scorn rank and authority, as demonstrated by, for example, nursing students who call faculty members by their first name, patients who call nurses by their first names, employees who fraternize with their employers, and so on. Members have a strong sense of individuality; however, family ties are relatively weak, as demonstrated by the high rate of separation and divorce in the United States. In many U.S. households, the family has been reduced to its smallest unit, the single-parent family.

When making health-related decisions, clients from culturally diverse backgrounds rely on relationships with others in various ways. If the cultural values orientation is lineal, the client may seek assistance from other members of the family and allow a relative (e.g., parent, grandparent, elder brother) to make decisions about important health-related matters. If collateral relationships are valued, decisions about the client may be interrelated with the impact of illness on the entire family or group. For example, among the Amish, the entire community is affected by the illness of a member because the community pays for health care from a common fund, members join together to meet the needs of both the patient and the patient's family for the duration of the illness, and the roles of many in the community are likely to be affected by the illness of a single member. The individual values orientation concerning relationships is predominant among the dominant cultural majority in the United States. Decision making about health and illness is often an individual matter, with the client being the sole decider, although members of the nuclear family may participate to varying degrees.

FAMILY

Despite the alarmingly high rate of divorce in the United States, the family remains the basic social unit. Although there are various ways to categorize families, the following are commonly recognized types of constellations in which people live together in society:

- Nuclear (husband, wife, and child or children)
- Nuclear dyad (husband and wife alone, either childless or no children living at home)
- Single parent (either mother or father and at least one child)
- Blended (husband, wife, and children from previous relationships)
- Extended (nuclear plus other blood relatives)
- Communal (group of men and women with or without children)
- Cohabitation (unmarried man and woman sharing a household with or without children)
- Gay (same-gender couples with or without children)

In addition to structural differences in families cross-culturally, there may be accompanying functional diversity. For example, among extended families, kin residence sharing has long been recognized as a viable alternative to managing scarce resources, meeting child care needs, and caring for a handicapped and/or elderly family member. Sometimes the shared household is an adaptation for survival and protection. In general, families with a culturally diverse heritage include not only a large number of adults but also a larger number of children.

More than half (55.3%) of all black children younger than 3 years are born into single-parent families. Among Puerto Ricans living in the United States, 44% of families are headed by single women. Among black families, grandmothers have the most active involvement with the grandchildren when they live with their single adult daughters. This is not the case in families with two parents or in single-parent families when the grandmother lives in a different household. Thus, black infants are exposed to a variety of other primary care providers and experience very different patterns of social interaction than do their counterparts in the dominant cultural group (Garcia Coll, 1990; U.S. Bureau of the Census, 1990).

In addition to a higher incidence of single heads of household, some cultural groups also have a higher incidence of teenage parents. Both blacks and Hispanics (especially Mexican-Americans and mainland Puerto Ricans) have higher percentages of births to mothers younger than 20 years (24% and 18%, respectively) than do whites (10%). Blacks also have a higher rate of adolescent pregnancy than whites, especially for births to unmarried teenagers. Adolescent pregancies among whites have declined markedly in recent years as a result of sex education programs in schools, availability of contraceptives, and legalization of abortion.

The family constellations associated with teen parenting are unique and provide a special socialization context for infants. Hispanic teen mothers, for example, receive more child care help from grandmothers and peers than do white teen mothers. Among blacks and Puerto Ricans, the presence of the maternal grandmother ameliorates the negative consequences of adolescent childbirth on the infant. Among low-income black families, grandmothers who were more knowledgeable about infant development had adolescent daughters who were more knowledgeable if they were taking care of their infant. In addition, grandmothers are more responsive and less punitive in their interactions with the infant than are their daughters. These data suggest two mechanisms by which three-generational households can have an impact on the infant's development: by influencing the mother's knowledge about development and by providing other more responsive social interactions with infants (Garcia Coll, 1990).

Ethnic families are often characterized as being more conservative in terms of sex roles and parenting values and practices than are white families. For example, traditional Japanese-American and Mexican-American families are family centered, enforce strict gender and age roles, and emphasize children's compliance with authority figures. Thus, infants of culturally diverse backgrounds are involved in different family interactions than are infants from the dominant U.S. cultural group.

Relationships that may seem apparent sometimes warrant further exploration when interacting with clients from culturally diverse backgrounds. For example, the dominant cultural group defines siblings as two persons with either the same mother, the same father, the same mother and father, or the same adoptive parents. In some Asian cultures, a sibling relationship is defined as involving infants who are breast-fed by the same woman. In other cultures, certain kinship patterns, such as maternal first cousins, are defined as sibling relationships. In some African cultures, anyone from the same village or town may be called "brother" or "sister." Certain subcultures, such as Roman Catholics (who may be further subdivided by ethnicity into those who are Italian, Polish, Spanish, Mexican, and so on) recognize relationships such as "godmother" or "godfather" in which an individual who is not the biological parent promises to assist with the moral and spiritual development of an infant and agrees to care for the child in the event of parental death. The godparent makes these promises during the religious ceremony of baptism.

When providing care for infants and children, it is important to identify the primary provider of care because this individual may or may not be the biological parent. Among some Hispanic groups, for example, female members of the nuclear or extended family, such as sisters or aunts, are primary providers of care. In some black families, the grandmother may be the decision maker and primary caretaker of the children.

SOCIOECONOMIC FACTORS

Socioeconomic status (SES) is a composite of the economic status of a family or unrelated individuals based on income, wealth, occupation, educational attainment, and power. It is a means of measuring inequalities based on economic differences and the manner in which families live as a result of their economic well-being.

Most families with racially or ethnically diverse backgrounds have a lower SES than the population at large, with a few exceptions (e.g., Cuban-Americans and subgroups of Asian-Americans). Unemployment is consistently high among Native Americans; most reservations report an unemployment rate of approximately 30%.

Distribution of Resources

Status, power, and wealth in the United States are not distributed equally throughout society. Rather, a very small percentage of the population enjoys most of the nation's resources, primarily through ownership of multibillion dollar corporations, large pieces of real estate in prime locations, and similar assets. Using SES as an indicator of status, power, and wealth, the U.S. population has traditionally been divided into three social classes: upper, middle, and lower. SES may be calculated by considering a wide variety of factors, but it is customarily determined by examining factors such as total family income, occupation, and educational level. In a less formalized examination of SES, factors such as age, sex, material possessions, health status, family name, location of residence, family composition, amount of land owned, religion, race, and ethnicity might be considered.

A disproportionate number of individuals from the racially and ethnically diverse subgroups are members of the lower socioeconomic class, whereas a larger percentage of members of the dominant cultural group (white Anglo-Saxon Protestants) belong to the upper and middle socioeconomic classes. Because the United States has socioeconomic stratification, the idealization of America as the land of opportunity often applies more to members of the upper and middle classes than to those of the lower class. The outcome of social stratification is social inequity. For example, it is well known that school systems, grocery stores, and recreational facilities vary significantly between the inner city and the suburbs.

African-Americans, Hispanic-Americans, and Native Americans experience the most severe economic deprivation of all ethnic groups in the United States. The median income for most European groups who immigrated early in this century nearly equals or has surpassed the dominant group. In 1990 the median income of white families was $36,915; black families, $21,423; and Hispanic families, $23,431. Thus, black families have a median income that is 58% that of whites; Hispanics earn 63% of the median income of whites (U.S. Bureau of the Census, 1992).

In 1990, when husband-wife families were compared, blacks earned 84% and Hispanics earned 69% of the median income of whites. When both husband and wife worked, the gap narrowed even more to 85% for blacks and 74% for Hispanics. When age, education, experience, and other factors are equal to those of white men, the earnings of racial and ethnic minorities and whites become more similar, but the income ratios among the groups still favor whites (U.S. Bureau of the Census, 1992).

Members of racial and ethnic minorities make up a disproportionately high percentage of persons in poverty. Of the white population, 11% fall below the poverty level ($13,359 for a family of four) compared with 32% of the black population and 38% of the Hispanic population. Within the Hispanic population, Puerto Ricans suffer the most (41%) from poverty. Table 17–2 summarizes the percentage of minority populations living below the poverty level.

A study released in 1993 by United Nations Educational, Scientific and Cultural Organization (UNESCO), which compared the standard of living of different nations, clearly showed the difference in the way most whites live compared with blacks and Hispanics. The United States was ranked sixth among the nations in the study. If the data had included only whites, the rank would have been first (instead, first was held by Japan). Blacks would have ranked 31st, the same level as in an underdeveloped country (Gollnick & Chinn, 1994).

For many years, health care settings have been the subject of study and concern regarding distribution of resources, with members of racial and ethnic minority groups clamoring with indignation at the inequalities. As the only industrialized Western nation in the world without a national health care delivery system, the United States provides the best health care to those with the highest SES and the worst health care to those with low SES. Thus, in the United States, the quality of health care is determined largely by one's SES, not by health status.

Education

One of the components considered in determining SES is educational level. Native Americans and Alaska Natives who are at least 25 years old have an average of 9.6 years of formal education; this is the lowest rate for any major U.S. ethnic group. Research suggests that differences between white and Mexican-

Table 17–2
Minority Populations Living Below Poverty Level*

Race	Total	Children Younger than 18 Years	Female Head of Household
Black	32	44	59
American Indian	28	—	—
Hispanic	38	38	57
Asian	13	—	—
White	11	14	32

*Values are expressed in millions.

From U.S. Bureau of the Census Statistical Abstract of the United States, 108th ed. Washington, DC, U.S. Government Printing Office, 1992.

American home teaching strategies can be accounted for by differences in levels of formal schooling rather than by cultural differences or economic indexes. Mothers who had received more years of formal education inquired and praised more often than did mothers with less education. In contrast, the lower the mother's level of formal education, the more often she used modeling as a teaching strategy. Compared with white mothers, Hispanic mothers inquired and praised less often and used modeling, visual cues, directives, and negative physical control more often. These differences disappeared entirely, however, when the mother's or father's educational level was controlled statistically. In contrast, controlling the mother's or father's occupational status did not eliminate the cultural group differences in maternal teaching behavior. These studies contribute to our understanding of the ways in which educational level attained by people from culturally diverse backgrounds affects the didactic aspects of the child-rearing environment (Garcia Coll, 1990).

Lower social class status is associated with differences in parenting behaviors, home environment, and attitudes about health and illness. The caregiving environment of a large percentage of racially and ethnically diverse infants can be a function of culture as much as of SES, and it is probably a combination of the two factors. For example, there are both racial and socioeconomic differences in methods of feeding (breast vs. bottle), use of pacifiers, and age at weaning and toilet training (Garcia Coll, 1990).

The importance of other correlates of SES, such as home language and family size, has also been studied. In a study that measured both the levels and the profiles of performance on measures of various abilities by children from Hispanic and white families of diverse socioeconomic levels, home language backgrounds, and family size, it was found that Hispanic and white children performed equally well when the socioeconomic factors were controlled. However, the combination of low SES and language minority status negatively affected the children's performance in areas such as verbal ability, quantitative ability, and short-term memory.

One reason why blacks and Hispanics suffer from poverty is that they tend to be more visibly segregated than white families. For example, 70% of black households are located in low-income areas, whereas 66% of poor white families live in suburban or rural areas.

CULTURE AND NUTRITION

Long after assimilation into the U.S. culture has occurred, clients from various ethnic groups will continue to follow culturally based dietary practices and to eat ethnic foods. Whenever a new group of immigrants arrives in the United States, it is common to see neighborhood food markets and ethnic restaurants established soon after arrival. Frequently, the ethnic restaurant is a place for members of the cultural group to meet and mingle, and customers from the dominant cultural group may be of secondary interest; thus, food is an integral part of cultural identity that may be even more significant than financial gain.

Nutrition Assessment of Culturally Diverse Groups

Among factors that must be considered in a nutrition assessment are the cultural definition of food, frequency and number of meals eaten away from home, form and content of ceremonial meals, amount and types of food eaten, and regularity of food consumption. Because potential inaccuracies may occur, the 24-hour dietary recalls or 3-day food records traditionally used for assessment may be inadequate when dealing with clients from culturally diverse backgrounds. Standard dietary handbooks may fail to provide culture-specific diet information because nutritional content and exchange tables are usually based on Western diets. Another source of error may originate from the cultural patterns of eating; for example, among low-income urban black families, elaborate weekend meals are frequently eaten, whereas weekday dietary patterns are markedly more moderate.

Although community health nurses may assume that "food" is a culture-universal term, it may be necessary to clarify its meaning with the client. For example, certain Latin American groups do not consider greens, an important source of vitamins, to be food and thus fail to list intake of these vegetables on daily records. Among Vietnamese refugees, dietary intake of calcium may appear inadequate because of the low consumption rate of dairy products common among members of this group. Pork bones and shells, however, are commonly consumed, thus providing adequate quantities of calcium to meet daily requirements.

Food is only one part of eating. In some cultures, social contacts during meals are restricted to members of the immediate or extended family. For example, in some Middle Eastern cultures, men and women eat meals separately, or women are permitted to eat with their husbands but not with other males. Among some Hispanic groups, the male breadwinner is served first, then the women and children eat. Etiquette during meals, use of hands, type of eating utensils (e.g., chopsticks, special flatware), and protocols governing the order in which food is consumed during a meal all vary cross-culturally.

Dietary Practices of Selected Cultural Groups

Cultural stereotyping is the tendency to view individuals of common cultural backgrounds similarly and according to a preconceived notion of how they behave. However, not all Chinese like rice, not all Italians like spaghetti, not all Mexicans like tortillas, and so on. Nevertheless, aggregate dietary preferences among people from certain cultural groups can be described (e.g., characteristic ethnic dishes, methods of food preparation, including use of cooking oils); the reader is referred to nutrition texts on the topic for detailed information about culture-specific diets and the nutritional value of ethnic foods.

Religion and Diet

Cultural food preferences are often interrelated with religious dietary beliefs and practices. As indicated in Table 17–3, many religions have proscriptive dietary practices, and some use food as symbols in celebrations and rituals. Knowing the client's religious practice as it relates to food makes it possible to suggest improvements or modifications that will not conflict with religious dietary laws.

Beyond the scope of this text is the issue of fasting and other religious observations that may limit a person's food or liquid intake during specified times (e.g., many Catholics fast and abstain from meat on Ash Wednesday and each Friday of Lent, Muslims refrain from eating during the daytime hours for the month of Ramadan but are permitted to eat after sunset, and Mormons refrain from ingesting all solid foods and liquids on the first Sunday of each month).

RELIGION AND CULTURE

Although it is impossible to be an expert on each of the estimated 1200 religions practiced in the United States, knowledge of health-related beliefs and practices as well as general information about the religious observances are important in providing culturally competent nursing care. For example, it is important to have a general understanding of the religious calendar, including designated holy days, when planning home visits or scheduling clinic visits for members of a specific religious group. It is also useful to know the customary days of religious worship observed by members of the religion. Although the majority of Protestants worship on Sundays, the sacred day of worship may vary for other religious groups. For example, the Muslims' holy day of worship extends from sunset on Thursday to sunset on Friday, whereas for Jews and Seventh-day Adventists, the day extends

Table 17–3
Dietary Practices of Selected Religious Groups

Religion	Dietary Practice
Hinduism	All meats are prohibited.
Islam	Pork and intoxicating beverages are prohibited.
Judaism	Pork, predatory fowl, shellfish and other water creatures (fish with scales are permissible), and blood by ingestion (e.g., blood sausage, raw meat) are prohibited. Blood by transfusion is acceptable. Foods should be kosher (meaning "properly preserved"). All animals must be ritually slaughtered by a sochet (i.e., quickly with the least pain possible) to be kosher. Mixing dairy and meat dishes at the same meal is prohibited.
Mormonism (Church of Jesus Christ of Latter-day Saints)	Alcohol, tobacco, and beverages containing caffeine (e.g., coffee, tea, colas, and selected carbonated soft drinks) are prohibited.
Seventh-Day Adventism	Pork, certain seafood (including shellfish), and fermented beverages are prohibited. A vegetarian diet is encouraged.

from sunset on Friday to sunset on Saturday. Roman Catholics may worship in the late afternoon or evening of Saturday or all day Sunday. Some religions may meet more than once weekly. In addition to regularly scheduled weekly religious service, most major religions also recognize special days of observance or celebration that last from 1 day (e.g., Christmas, Easter, Rosh Hashanah, and Janamasthtmi) to 1 month (e.g., Ramadan). Some days of commemoration or observation are based on a lunar calendar and some have rotating dates, so it is necessary to consult official information sources such as religious leaders or religious calendars to verify exact dates. It is also important to ask clients what religious practices they follow because individual activity within the religious organization may vary widely.

As an integral component of the individual's culture, religous beliefs may influence the client's explanation of the cause of illness, perception of its severity, and choice of healer. In times of crisis, such as serious illness and impending death, religion may be a source of consolation for the client and family and may influence the course of action believed to be appropriate.

Religion and Spirituality

Religious concerns evolve from and respond to the mysteries of life and death, good and evil, and pain and suffering. Nurses frequently encounter clients who find themselves searching for a spiritual meaning to help explain the illness or disability. Some nurses find spiritual assessment difficult because of the abstract and personal nature of the topic, whereas others feel quite comfortable discussing spiritual matters. Comfort with one's own spiritual beliefs is the foundation to effective assessment of spiritual needs in clients.

Although the religions of the world offer various interpretations to many of life's mysteries, most people seek a personal understanding and interpretation at some time in their lives. Ultimately, this personal search becomes a pursuit to discover a supreme being (e.g., Allah, God, Yahweh, Jehovah, and so on) or some unifying truth that will render meaning, purpose, and integrity to existence.

An important distinction must be made between religion and spirituality. *Religion* refers to an organized system of beliefs concerning the cause, nature, and purpose of the universe, especially belief in or the worship of a god or gods. More than 1200 religions are practiced in the United States. *Spirituality* is born out

of each person's unique life experience and personal effort to find purpose and meaning in life. Suggested guidelines for assessing the spiritual needs of culturally diverse clients are given in Table 17–4.

Prolongation of life, euthanasia, autopsy, donation of body for research, disposal of body and body parts (including fetus), and type of burial may be influenced by religion. You should use discretion in asking clients

---

Table 17–4
Methods of Assessing Spiritual Needs in Culturally Diverse Clients

Environment

Does the client have religious objects in the environment?

Does the client wear outer garments or undergarments that have religious significance?

Are get-well greeting cards religious in nature or from a representative of the client's church?

Does the client receive flowers or bulletins from church or other religious institution?

Behavior

Does the client appear to pray at certain times of the day or before meals?

Does the client make special dietary requests (e.g., kosher diet; vegetarian diet; or diet free from caffeine, pork, shellfish, or other specific food items)?

Does the client read religious magazines or books?

Verbalization

Does the client mention a supreme being (e.g., God, Allah, Buddha, Yahweh, or other), prayer, faith, church, or religious topics?

Is a request made for a visit by a clergy member or other religious representative?

Is there an expression of anxiety or fear about pain, suffering, or death?

Interpersonal Relationships

Who visits the client? How does the client respond to visitors?

Does a church representative visit?

How does the client relate to nursing staff and to roommates?

Does the client prefer to interact with others or to remain alone?

Data from Boyle JS, and Andrews MM: Transcultural Concepts in Nursing Care, Glenview, IL, Scott, Foresman/Little, Brown & Co., 1989.

and their families about these issues and gather data only when the clinical situation necessitates that the information be obtained. Clients and families should be encouraged to discuss these issues with their religious representative when necessary. Before dealing with potentially sensitive issues, it is important to establish rapport with the client and family by gaining their trust and confidence in less sensitive areas.

Developmental Considerations: Childhood

Illness during childhood may be an especially difficult clinical situation. Children as well as adults have spiritual needs that vary according to the child's developmental level and the religious climate that exists in the family. Parental perceptions about the illness of their child my be partially influenced by religious beliefs. For example, some parents may believe that a transgression against a religious law is responsible for a congenital anomaly in their offspring. Other parents may delay seeking medical care because they believe that prayer should be tried first. Certain types of treatment, (e.g., administration of blood or of medications containing caffeine, pork, or other prohibited substances and selected procedures) may be perceived as cultural taboos, which are to be avoided by both children and adults.

Developmental Considerations: Old Age

Values held by the dominant U.S. culture, such as emphasis on independence, self-reliance, and productivity, influence aging members of society. Americans define people at the chronological age of 65 as old and limit their work; in some other cultures, persons are first recognized as being unable to work and then identified as being old. In some cultures, it is the wisdom, not the productivity, of the elderly that is valued; thus, the diminishment of one's activity level and reduction of physical stamina associated with growing old are accepted more readily without loss of status among culture members. Retirement is also culturally defined, with some elderly working as long as physical health continues and others continuing to be active but assuming less physically demanding jobs.

The main task of elderly persons in the dominant culture is to achieve a sense of integrity in accepting responsibility for their own lives and in having a sense of accomplishment. Individuals who achieve integrity consider aging a positive experience, make adjustments in their personal space and social relationships,

maintain a sense of usefulness, and begin closure and life review. Not all cultures value accepting responsibility for one's own life. For example, among Hispanics, Asians, Arabs, and other groups, the elderly are often cared for by family members, who welcome the elderly into their homes when they are no longer able to live alone. The concept of placing an elderly family member in an institutional setting to be cared for by strangers is perceived as an uncaring, impersonal, and culturally unacceptable practice by many cultural groups.

Elderly persons may develop their own means of coping with illness through self-care, assistance from family members, and social group support systems. Some cultures have developed attitudes and specific behaviors for the elderly that include humanistic care and identification of family members as care providers. The elderly may have special family responsibilities (e.g., the elderly Amish provide hospitality to visitors, and elderly Filipinos spend considerable time teaching the youth skills learned during a lifetime of experience).

Elderly immigrants who have made major lifestyle adjustments in the move from their homeland to the United States or from a rural to an urban area (or vice versa) may need information about health care alternatives, preventive programs, health care benefits, and screening programs for which they are eligible. These individuals may also be in various stages of "culture shock," the state of disorientation or inability to respond to the behavior of a different cultural group because of its sudden strangeness, unfamiliarity, and incompatibility to the newcomer's perceptions and expectations (Leininger, 1995).

CROSS-CULTURAL COMMUNICATION

Verbal and nonverbal communication is important in community health nursing and is influenced by the cultural background of both the nurse and the client. Cross-cultural, or intercultural, communication refers to the communication process occurring between a nurse and a client who have different cultural backgrounds as both attempt to understand the other's point of view from a cultural perspective.

Nurse-Client Relationship

From the initial introduction to the client through termination of the relationship, communication is a continuous process for the community health nurse.

Because beginning impressions are so important in all human relationships, cross-cultural considerations concerning introductions warrant a few brief remarks. To ensure a mutually respectful relationship, it is important for the nurse to introduce him- or herself and indicate how the client should refer to the nurse, (i.e., by first name, last name, or title). Having done so, the nurse should ask the client to do the same. This enables the nurse to address the client in a manner that is culturally appropriate and could avoid embarrassment in the future. For example, it is the custom among some Asian and European cultures to write the last name first; thus, confusion can be avoided in an area of extreme sensitivity: the client's name.

One of the major challenges community health nurses face in working with clients from culturally diverse backgrounds is overcoming one's own *ethnocentrism,* which is the tendency to view one's own way of life as the most desirable, acceptable, or best and to act in a superior manner toward another culture. One must also beware of *cultural imposition,* which is the tendency to impose one's own beliefs, values, and patterns of behavior on individuals from another culture.

Space, Distance, and Intimacy

Both the client's and the nurse's own sense of spatial distance is significant throughout the home visit; culturally appropriate distance zones vary widely. For example, nurses may back away from clients of Hispanic, East Indian, or Middle Eastern origin who invade personal space with regularity in an attempt to bring the nurse closer into the space that is comfortable to them. Although nurses are uncomfortable with clients' close physical proximity, clients are perplexed by the nurse's distancing behaviors and may perceive the community health nurse as aloof and unfriendly. Summarized in Table 17–5 are the four distance zones identified for the functional use of space that are embraced by the dominant cultural group, including most nurses. Interactions between clients and nurses may also depend on the client's desired degree of intimacy, which may range from very formal interactions to close personal relationships. For example, some Southeast Asian clients expect those in authority (i.e., nurses) to be authoritarian, directive, and detached.

The emphasis on social harmony among Asian and Native American clients may prevent the full expression of concerns or feelings during the interview. Such reserved behavior may leave the nurse with the

Table 17–5
Functional Use of Space

Zone	Remarks
Intimate zone (0–1.5 feet)	Visual distortion occurs Best for assessing breath and other body odors
Personal distance (1.5–4 feet)	Perceived as an extension of the self, similar to a "bubble" Voice is moderate Body odors are inapparent No visual distortion Much of the physical assessment will occur at this distance
Social distance (4–12 feet)	Used for impersonal business transactions Perceptual information is much less detailed Much of the interview will occur at this distance
Public distance (12+ feet)	Interaction with others is impersonal Speaker's voice must be projected Subtle facial expressions are imperceptible

Data from Hall E: Proxemics: the study of man's spatial relations. *In* Galdston I, (ed): Man's Image in Medicine and Anthropology. New York, International Universities Press, 1963, pp. 109–120.

impression that the client agrees with or understands an explanation. However, nodding or smiling by Asian clients may only reflect their cultural value for interpersonal harmony, not agreement with the speaker. Nurses may distinguish between socially compliant client responses aimed at maintaining social harmony and genuine concurrence by obtaining validation of assumptions. This may be accomplished by inviting the client to respond frankly to suggestions or by giving the client permission to disagree.

In contrast, Appalachian clients traditionally have close family interaction patterns that often lead them to expect close personal relationships with health care providers. The Appalachian client may evaluate the nurse's effectiveness on the basis of interpersonal skills rather than on professional competency. Appalachian clients are likely to be uncomfortable with the impersonal, bureaucratic orientation of most health care institutions. Clients of Arab, Latin American, or Mediterranean origin often expect an even higher degree of intimacy and may attempt to involve the nurse in their family system by expecting participation in personal activities and social functions. These individuals may come to expect personal favors that extend beyond the scope of professional nursing practice and may believe it is their privilege to contact the nurse at home at any time of the day or night for care.

Overcoming Communication Barriers

Nurses tend to have stereotypic expectations of the client's behavior. In general, nurses expect behavior to consist of undemanding compliance, an attitude of respect for the health care provider, and cooperation with requested behavior throughout the examination. Although clients may ask a few question for the purpose of clarification, slight deference to recognized authority figures (i.e., health care providers) is expected. Individuals from culturally diverse backgrounds, however, may have significantly different perceptions about the appropriate role of the individual and family when seeking health care. If you find yourself becoming annoyed that a client is asking too many questions, assuming a defensive posture, or otherwise feeling uncomfortable, you might pause for a moment to examine the source of the conflict from a cross-cultural perspective.

During illness, culturally acceptable "sick-role" behavior may range from aggressive, demanding behavior to silent passivity. Complaining, demanding behavior during illness is often rewarded with attention among Jewish and Italian-American groups, whereas Asian and Native American patients are likely to be quiet and compliant during illness. During the interview, Asian clients may provide the nurse with the answers they think the nurse wants to hear, which is behavior consistent with the dominant cultural value for harmonious relationships with others. Thus, an attempt should be made to phrase questions or statements in a neutral manner that avoids foreshadowing an expected response. Appalachian clients may reject a community health nurse whom they perceive as prying or nosy because of a cultural ethic of neutrality that mandates minding one's own business and avoiding assertive or argumentative behavior.

Nonverbal Communication

Unless one makes an effort to understand the client's nonverbal behavior, it is possible to overlook important information such as that which is conveyed by facial expressions, silence, eye contact, touch, and other body language. Communication patterns vary widely cross-culturally, even for seemingly "inno-cent" behaviors such as smiling and handshaking. Among many Hispanic clients, for example, smiling and handshaking are considered an integral part of sincere interaction and essential to establishing trust, whereas a Russian client might perceive the same behavior by the nurse as insolent and frivolous. Gender issues also become significant; for example, among some groups of Middle Eastern origin, men and women do not shake hands or touch each other in any manner outside of the marital relationship. If the nurse and client are both female, however, a handshake is usually acceptable.

Wide cultural variation exists when interpreting silence. Some individuals find silence extremely uncomfortable and make every effort to fill conversational lags with words. In contrast, Native Americans consider silence essential to understanding and respecting the other person. A pause after a question signifies that what the speaker has asked is important enough to be given thoughtful consideration. In traditional Chinese and Japanese cultures, silence may mean that the speaker wishes the listener to consider the content of what has been said before continuing. The English and Arabs may use silence out of respect for another person's privacy, whereas the French, Spanish, and Russians may interpret it as a sign of agreement. Asian cultures often use silence to demonstrate respect for elders.

Eye contact is among the most culturally variable nonverbal behaviors. Although most nurses have been taught to maintain eye contact while talking with clients, invidivuals from culturally diverse backgrounds may misconstrue this behavior. Asian, Native American, Indochinese, Arab, and Appalachian clients may consider direct eye contact impolite or aggressive, and they may avert their own eyes during the conversation. Native American clients often stare at the floor when the nurse is talking; this culturally appropriate behavior indicates that the listener is paying close attention to the speaker.

In some cultures, including Arab, Hispanic, and black groups, modesty for women is interrelated with eye contact. For Muslim women, modesty is achieved in part by avoiding eye contact with men (except for one's husband) and keeping eyes downcast when encountering members of the opposite sex in public situations. In many cultures, the only women who smile and establish eye contact with men in public are prostitutes. Hassidic Jewish men also have culturally based norms concerning eye contact with women. The male may avoid direct eye contact and turn his head in the opposite direction when walking past or speaking to a woman. The preceding examples are intended to be illustrative but not exhaustive.

Touch

Touching the client is a necessary component of a comprehensive assessment. Although there are benefits in establishing rapport with clients through touch, including the promotion of healing through therapeutic touch, physical contact with clients conveys various meanings cross-culturally. In many cultures (e.g., Arab and Hispanic), male health care providers may be prohibited from touching or examining all or certain parts of the female body. During pregnancy, the client may prefer female health care providers and may refuse to be examined by a man. Be aware that the client's significant other may also exert pressure on health care providers by enforcing these culturally meaningful norms in the health care setting.

Touching children may also have associated meanings cross-culturally. For example, Hispanic clients may believe in mal ojo ("evil eye"): an individual becomes ill as a result of excessive admiration by another. Many Asians believe that one's strength resides in the head and that touching the head is considered disrespectful. Thus, palpation of the fontanelle of an infant of Southeast Asian descent should be approached with sensitivity. It may be necessary to rely on alternative sources of information (e.g., assessing for clinical manifestations of increased intracranial pressure or signs of premature fontanelle closure). Although it is the least desirable option, this part of the assessment may have to be omitted.

Gender

Violating norms related to appropriate male-female relationships among various cultures may jeopardize the therapeutic nurse-client relationship. Among Arab-Americans, a man is never alone with a woman (except his wife) and is usually accompanied by one or more other men when interacting with women. This behavior is culturally very significant, and failure to adhere to the cultural code (set of rules or norms of behavior used by a cultural group to guide their behavior and to interpret situations) is viewed as a serious transgression, often one in which the lone male will be accused of sexual impropriety. The best way to ensure that cultural variables have been considered is to ask the client about culturally relevant aspects of male-female relationships, preferably at the beginning of the

interaction before there is an opportunity to violate any culturally based practices.

Language

When assessing non–English-speaking clients, the nurse may encounter one of two situations: choosing an interpreter or communicating effectively when there is no interpreter.

Interviewing the non–English-speaking person requires a bilingual interpreter for full communication. Even the person from another culture or country who has a basic command of English may need an interpreter when faced with the anxiety-provoking situation of becoming ill, encountering a strange symptom, or discussing a sensitive topic such as birth control or gynecologic or urologic concerns. It is tempting to ask a relative, friend of even another client to interpret because this person is readily available and is anxious to help. However, this is disadvantageous because it violates confidentiality for the client, who may not want personal information shared with another. Furthermore, the friend or relative, although fluent in ordinary language, is likely to be unfamiliar with medical terminology, clinic procedures, and medical ethics.

Whenever possible, a bilingual team member or trained medical interpreter should be used. This person knows interpreting techniques, has a health care background, and understands patients' rights. The trained interpreter also is knowledgeable about cultural beliefs and health practices, can help bridge the cultural gap, and can provide advice concerning the cultural appropriateness of recommendations.

Although the nurse is in charge of the focus and the flow of the home visit or client-nurse interaction, the interpreter is an important member of the health care team. The nurse should ask the interpreter to meet the client before the visit to establish rapport and learn about the client's age, occupation, educational level, and attitude toward health care. This enables the interpreter to communicate on the client's level.

The nurse should allow more time for home and clinic visits with culturally diverse clients who require an interpreter. With the third person repeating everything, it can take considerably longer than interviewing English-speaking clients. It will be necessary to focus on the major points and to prioritize data.

There are two styles of interpreting: line by line and summarizing. Translating line by line ensures accuracy, but it takes more time. Both the nurse and the client should speak only a sentence or two and then allow the interpreter time to interpret. Use simple language, not medical jargon that the interpreter must simplify before it can be translated. Summary translation is faster and is useful for teaching relatively simple health techniques with which the interpreter is already familiar. Be alert for nonverbal cues as the client talks; this can give valuable data. A good interpreter also will note nonverbal messages and communicate those to the community health nurse.

Summarized in Table 17–6 are suggestions for the selection and use of an interpreter.

Although use of an interpreter is ideal, one may find oneself in a situation with a non–English-speaking client when no interpreter is available. Table 17–7 summarizes some suggestions for overcoming language barriers when there is no interpreter.

HEALTH-RELATED BELIEFS AND PRACTICES

One of the major aspects of a comprehensive cultural assessment concerns the collection of data related to culturally based beliefs and practices about health and

Table 17–6
Overcoming Language Barriers: Use of an Interpreter

Before locating an interpreter, be sure that you know what language the patient speaks at home because it may be different from the language spoken publicly (e.g., French is sometimes spoken by aristocratic or well-educated people from certain Asian or Middle Eastern cultures).

Avoid interpreters from a rival tribe, state, region, or nation (e.g., a Palestinian who knows Hebrew may not be the best interpreter for a Jewish client).

Be aware of gender difference between interpreter and client to avoid violation of cultural mores related to modesty.

Be aware of age difference between interpreter and client.

Be aware of socioeconomic differences between interpreter and client.

Ask interpreter to translate as closely to verbatim as possible.

An interpreter who is not a relative may seek compensation for services rendered.

illness. Before determining whether cultural practices are helpful, harmful, or neutral, the nurse must first understand the logic of the belief system underlying the practice and then be sure to grasp fully the nature and meaning of the practice from the client's cultural perspective.

Health and Culture

The first step in understanding the health care needs of clients is to understand one's own culturally based values, beliefs, attitudes, and practices. Sometimes this requires considerable introspection and may necessitate that one confront one's own biases, preconceptions, and prejudices about specific racial, ethnic, religious, sexual, or socioeconomic groups. Second, one must identify the meaning of health to the client, remembering that concepts are derived in part from the way in which members of their cultural group define health. Considerable research has been conducted on the various definitions of health that may be held by various groups. For example, Jamaicans define health as having a good appetite, feeling strong and energetic, performing activities of daily living without difficulty, and being sexually active and fertile. For traditional Italian women, health means the ability to interact socially and perform routine tasks such as cooking, cleaning, and caring for oneself and others. On the other hand, some individuals of Hispanic origin believe that coughing, sweating, and diarrhea are a normal part of living rather than symptoms of ill health, perhaps because of the high frequency of these problems in the clients' country of origin. Thus, individuals may define themselves or others in their group as healthy even though the nurse identifies symptoms of disease.

Defining Illness from a Cross-Cultural Perspective

For clients, symptom labeling and diagnosis depend on the degree of difference between the individual's behaviors and those the group has defined as normal, beliefs about the causation of illness, level of stigma attached to a particular set of symptoms, prevalence of the disease, and meaning of the illness to the individual and family.

Throughout history, humankind has attempted to understand the cause of illness and disease. Theories of causation have been formulated on the basis of religious beliefs, social circumstances, philosophical perspectives, and level of knowledge. The following

Table 17–7
Overcoming Language Barriers When There Is No Interpreter

Be polite and formal.

Greet the client using the last or complete name. Gesture to yourself and say your name. Offer a handshake or nod. Smile.

Proceed in an unhurried manner. Pay attention to any effort by the client or family to communicate.

Speak in a low, moderate voice. Avoid talking loudly. Remember that there is a tendency to raise the volume and pitch of your voice when the listener appears not to understand, and the listener may perceive that you are shouting or angry.

Use any words that you might know in the patient's language. This indicates that you are aware of and respect their culture.

Use simple words, such as "pain" instead of "discomfort."
Avoid medical jargon, idioms, and slang. Avoid using contractions such as "don't," "can't," and "won't."
Use nouns repeatedly instead of pronouns. For example, say "Does Juan take medicine?" instead of "He has been taking his medicine, hasn't he?"

Pantomime words and simple actions while you verbalize them.

Give instructions in the proper sequence. For example say, "First wash the bottle. Second, rinse the bottle," instead of, "Before you rinse the bottle, sterilize it."

Discuss one topic at a time. Avoid using conjunctions. For example say, "Are you cold [while pantomiming]?" "Are you in pain?" instead of, "Are you cold and in pain?"

Validate if the client understands by having the client repeat instructions, demonstrate the procedure, or act out the meaning.

Write out several short sentences in English and determine the client's ability to read them.

Try a third language. Many Indo-Chinese speak French. Europeans often know three or four languages. Try Latin words or phrases.

Ask who among the client's family and friends could serve as an interpreter.

Obtain phrase books from a library or bookstore, make or purchase flash cards, contact hospitals for a list of interpreters, and use both formal and informal networking to locate a suitable interpreter.

section explores some of the more prevalent theories of illness causation.

Causes of Illness

Disease causation may be viewed from three major perspectives: biomedical (sometimes used synonymously with the term *scientific*), naturalistic (sometimes used synonymously with the term *holistic*), and magicoreligious. The first, the biomedical or scientific, theory of illness causation is based on the assumption that all events in life have a cause and effect, that the human body functions more or less mechanically (i.e., the functioning of the human body is analogous to the functioning of an automobile), that all life can be reduced or divided into smaller parts (e.g., the human person can be reduced into body, mind, and spirit), and that all of reality can be observed and measured (e.g., with intelligence tests and psychometric measures of behavior). Among the biomedical explanations for disease is the germ theory, which posits that microscopic organisms such as bacteria and viruses are responsible for specific disease conditions. Most educational programs for nurses and other health care providers embrace the biomedical or scientific theories that explain the cause of both physical and psychological illnesses.

The second way in which clients explain the cause of illness is from the naturalistic, or holistic, perspective, a viewpoint that is found most frequently among Native Americans, Asians, and others who believe that human life is only one aspect of nature and a part of the general order of the cosmos. Individuals from these groups believe that the forces of nature must be kept in natural balance or harmony.

Among many Asians, there is a belief in the yin-yang theory in which health is believed to exist when all aspects of the person are in perfect balance. Rooted in the ancient Chinese philosophy of Tao, the yin-yang theory states that all organisms and objects in the universe consist of yin or yang energy forces. The origin of the energy forces are within the autonomic nervous system, where balance between the opposing forces is maintained during health. Yin energy represents the female and negative forces (e.g., emptiness, darkness, and cold), whereas yang forces are male and positive, emitting warmth and fullness. Foods are classified as hot and cold in this theory and are transformed into yin and yang energy when metabolized by the body. Yin foods are cold, and yang foods are hot. Cold foods are eaten when one has a hot illness, and hot foods are eaten when one has a cold illness. The yin-yang theory is the basis for Eastern or Chinese medicine and is commonly embraced by Asian-Americans.

The naturalistic perspective posits that the laws of nature create imbalances, chaos, and disease. Individuals embracing the naturalistic view use metaphors such as the healing power of nature, and they call the earth "Mother." From the perspective of the Chinese, for example, illness is not seen as an intruding agent but rather as a part of life's rhythmic course and as an outward sign of the disharmony that exists within.

Many Hispanic, Arab, black, and Asian groups embrace the hot-cold theory of health and illness, an explanatory model with its origin in the ancient Greek humoral theory. The four humors of the body—blood, phlegm, black bile, and yellow bile—regulate basic bodily functions and are described in terms of temperature, dryness, and moisture. The treatment of disease consists of adding or subtracting cold, heat, dryness, or wetness to restore the balance of the humors.

Beverages, foods, herbs, medicines, and diseases are classified as hot or cold according to their perceived effects on the body, not on their physical characteristics. Illnesses believed to be caused by cold entering the body include earache, chest cramps, paralysis, gastrointestinal discomfort, rheumatism, and tuberculosis. Illnesses believed to be caused by overheating include abscessed teeth, sore throats, rashes, and kidney disorders.

According to the hot-cold theory, the individual as a whole, rather than a specific ailment, is significant. Those who embrace the hot-cold theory maintain that health consists of a positive state of total well-being, including physical, psychological, spiritual, and social aspects of the person. Paradoxically, the language used to describe this artificial dissection of the body into parts is a reflection of the biomedical-scientific perspective, not a naturalistic or holistic one.

The third major way in which people view the world and explain the causation of illness is from a magicoreligious perspective. The basic premise of this explanatory model is that the world is seen as an arena in which supernatural forces dominate. The fate of the world, and those in it, depends on the action of supernatural forces for good or evil. Examples of magical causes of illness include the belief in voodoo or witchcraft among some blacks and others from circum-Caribbean countries. Faith healing is based on religious beliefs and is most prevalent among selected Christian religions, including Christian Scientists; various healing rituals may be found in many other religions, such as Roman Catholicism, Mormonism (Church of Jesus Christ of Latter-day Saints), and others.

It is possible to have a combination of world views, and many clients are likely to offer more than one explanation for the cause of their illness. As a profession, nursing largely embraces the biomedical-scientific world view, but some aspects of holism have begun to gain popularity, including a wide variety of techniques for management of chronic pain such as hypnosis, therapeutic touch, and biofeedback. Belief in spiritual power is also held by many nurses who readily credit supernatural forces with various unexplained phenomena related to clients' health and illness states.

Culture and Healing

When self-treatment is unsuccessful, the individual may turn to the lay or folk-healing systems, to spiritual or religious healing, or to scientific biomedicine. All cultures have their own preferred lay or popular healers, recognized symptoms of ill health, acceptable sick-role behavior, and treatments. In addition to seeking help from the nurse as a biomedical-scientific health care provider, clients may also seek help from folk or religious healers. Some clients, such as Hispanics or Native Americans, may believe that the cure is incomplete unless healing of body, mind, and spirit is accomplished, although the division of the human person into parts is a Western concept. For example, a Hispanic client with a respiratory infection may ingest antibiotics prescribed by a physician or nurse practitioner and herbal teas recommended by a curandero and also say prayers for healing suggested by a Catholic priest.

A discussion of the variety of healing beliefs and practices used by the many U.S. subcultural groups far exceeds the scope of this chapter. It is important, however, for the nurse to be aware of alternative practices and recognize that, in addition to folk practices, there are many alternative healing practices. Although it is dangerous to assume that all indigenous approaches to healing are innocuous, the majority of practices are quite harmless, regardless of whether they are effective cures.

Folk Healers

There are numerous folk healers. Hispanic clients may turn to a curandero (male) or curandera (female), espiritualista (spiritualist), yerbo (herbalist), or sabador (one who manipulates muscles and bones). Black clients may mention having received assistance from a hougan (voodoo priest or priestess), spiritualist, or "old lady" (an older woman who has successfully raised a family and specializes in child care and folk remedies). Native American clients may seek assistance from a shaman, or medicine man or woman. Clients of Asian descent may mention that they have visited herbalists, acupuncturists, or bone setters. Each culture has its own healers, most of whom speak the native tongue of the client, make house calls, and cost significantly less than healers practicing in the biomedical-scientific health care system. In addition to folk healers, many cultures have lay midwives (e.g., parteras for Hispanic women) or other health care providers who meet the needs of pregnant women.

In some religions, spiritual healers may be found among the ranks of the ordained or official religious hierarchy ranks and are called priest, bishop, elder, deacon, rabbi, brother, sister, and so on. Other religions have a separate category of healer (e.g., Christian Science "nurses" [not licensed by states] or practitioners).

HEALTH, ILLNESS, AND CULTURAL DIVERSITY

Despite the unprecedented explosion in scientific knowledge and the tremendous resources available within the U.S. health care delivery system, members of the federally defined minority groups (i.e., blacks, Hispanics, Native Americans, and those of Asian and Pacific Islander heritage) have not benefited equally or equitably. In response to this lack of equality, Margaret M. Heckler, DHHS secretary in 1984, established the Task Force on Black and Minority Health to examine the nature of the disparities and propose solutions that would result in an overall improvement of health for members of the federally defined minority groups (Heckler, 1985).

Although some progress has been made in improving the overall health status of minorities as a result of the federal program implemented in response to the task force's recommendations, there continues to be a disparity between whites and members of the minority populations.

Since the turn of the century, the overall health status of all U.S. citizens has improved greatly primarily as a result of improved sanitation, better nutrition, and mass immunization, which resulted in a drastic decline in infectious diseases. Since 1960, the U.S. population has experienced a steady decline in the overall death rate from all causes, and remarkable progress is being made in understanding the causes and risks for developing conditions such as heart disease and cancer. The decline in cardiovascular disease mortality from 1968 to 1978 alone improved overall life expectancy by 1.6 years. Advances in the long-term management of chronic diseases mean that conditions such as hypertension and diabetes no longer necessarily lead to premature death and disability, although some individuals do experience both, particularly those from culturally diverse backgrounds (Heckler, 1985). Concomitantly, advances in social and behavior sciences research and methodology have enabled us to understand better the behavioral underpinnings of health, identify effective strategies for disease prevention, maintain treatment regimens, and suggest ways to change behavior in favor of more healthful living habits.

Although tremendous strides have been made in the United States toward improving health and longevity, statistical trends show a persistent, distressing disparity in key health indicators among certain subgroups of the population. In 1991, life expectancy reached a new high of 76.1 years for whites and 71.6 years for blacks, producing a racial gap of 4.5 years. The life expectancy of blacks today was reached by whites in the early 1950s. Infant mortality rates have declined steadily for several decades for both blacks and whites. In 1990, the infant death rate for blacks was 17.6 deaths per 1000 live births; this rate is twice that for whites (8.5 deaths per 1000 live births) and similar to the 1960 rate for whites (20 deaths per 1000 live births) (National Center for Health Statistics, 1991).

Causes of Disease in Minority Populations

In analyzing mortality data from 1979 to 1981, the Task Force on Black and Minority Health identified six causes of death that, in combination, account for more than 80% of the mortality observed among members of the federally defined minority groups in excess of the white population. The Task Force on Black and Minority Health used the term *excess deaths* to express the difference between the number of deaths actually observed in a minority group and the number of deaths that would have occurred in that group if it experienced the same death rates for each age and sex as the white population (Heckler, 1985).

Although the ranking of health problems according to excess deaths differs for each minority population, the six health problems became overall priority issue areas. These six causes of death are cancer, cardiovascular disease and stroke, chemical dependency as measured by deaths from cirrhosis of the liver, diabetes, homicides and accidents (unintentional injuries), and infant mortality.

In addition to excess deaths, special analyses of morbidity and health status indicators for minorities were developed by the Task Force on Black and Minority Health. These indexes included prevalence rates of selected chronic and infectious diseases, hospital admissions, physician visits, limitation of activity, and self-assessed health status. Additional mortality indexes included person-years of life lost, life expectancy, and relative risk of death by cause.

Some factors contributing to the health status of persons from culturally diverse backgrounds are not disease specific but have a bearing on the overall health needs of each minority group. Among those that the Task Force on Black and Minority Health reviewed are demographic data characterizing minority groups, minority needs in education, health professionals, and health care services and financing (Heckler, 1985).

CULTURAL EXPRESSION OF ILLNESS

There is wide cultural variation in the manner in which certain symptoms and disease conditions are perceived, diagnosed, labeled, and treated. The disease that is grounds for social ostracism in one culture may be reason for increased status in another. For example, epilepsy is seen as contagious and untreatable among Ugandans, as a cause for family shame among Greeks, as a reflection of a physical imbalance among Mexican-Americans, and as a sign of having gained favor by enduring a trial by God among the Hutterites.

Bodily symptoms are also perceived and reported in a variety of ways. For example, individuals of Mediterranean descent tend to report common physical symptoms more often than do persons of northern European or Asian heritage. Among Chinese, there is no translation for the English word "sadness," yet all people experience the feeling of sadness at some time

in their life. To express emotion, Chinese clients sometimes somaticize their symptoms; for example, a client may complain of cardiac symptoms because the center of emotion in the Chinese culture is the heart. If the client has experienced a loss through, for example, death or divorce, and is grieving, the client may describe the loss in terms of a pain in the heart. Although some biomedical-scientific clinicians may refer to this as a psychosomatic illness, others will recognize it as a culturally acceptable somatic expression of emotional disharmony.

A discussion of pain follows illustrating the cultural variability that may occur with a symptom of significant concern to nurses.

Cultural Expression of Symptoms: Pain

To illustrate the manner in which symptom expression may reflect the client's cultural background, pain, an extensively studied symptom, is used. Pain is a universally recognized phenomenon and is an important aspect of assessment for clients of various ages. Pain is a very private, subjective experience that is greatly influenced by cultural heritage. Expectations, manifestations, and management of pain are all embedded in a cultural context. The definition of pain, like that of health or illness, is culturally determined.

The term *pain* is derived from the Greek word for penalty, which helps explain the long association between pain and punishment in Judeo-Christian thought. The meaning of painful stimuli for individuals, the way people define their situation, and the impact of personal experience combine to determine the experience of pain.

Much cross-cultural research has been conducted on pain. Pain has been found to be a highly personal experience that depends on cultural learning, the meaning of the situation, and other factors unique to the individual. Silent suffering has been identified as the most valued response to pain by health care professionals. The majority of nurses have been socialized to believe that in virtually any situation self-control is better than open displays of strong feelings.

Studies of nurses' attitudes toward pain reveal that the ethnic background of patients is relevant to the nurses' assessment of both physical and psychological pain. Nurses view Jewish and Spanish patients as suffering the most and Anglo-Saxon–Germanic patients as suffering the least. In addition, nurses who infer relatively greater patient pain tended to report their own experiences as more painful. In general, nurses with an eastern or southern European or African background tend to infer greater suffering than do nurses of northern European background. Years of experience, current position, and area of clinical practice are unrelated to inferences of suffering (Ludwig-Beymer, 1995).

In addition to expecting variations in pain perception and tolerance, a nurse should expect variations in the expression of pain. It is well known that individuals turn to their social environments for validation and comparison. A first important comparison group is the family, which transmits cultural norms to its children.

The anthropologist Zborowski (1969) found that the meaning of pain and behavioral responses to the painful stimulus are culturally learned and culturally specific. Zborowski studied pain in four groups of men admitted to a veterans' hospital. The "old American" patients, defined as third-generation Americans, were found to be unexpressive; they reported pain, but emotional behavior was controlled. Complaining, crying, or screaming was viewed as useless or unnecessary. Both Jewish and Italian men were expressive in their pain response and asked for immediate pain relief by any means possible. Irish men viewed pain as a private event to be endured alone. This group was unemotional and nonexpressive of pain. In addition, when in pain, the old American and Irish groups tended to withdraw socially, whereas the Jewish and Italian groups preferred the company of friends and relatives.

Culture-Bound Syndromes

Clients may have a condition that is culturally defined, known as a culture-bound syndrome. Some of these conditions have no equal from a biomedical or scientific perspective, but others, such as anorexia nervosa and bulimia, are examples of the cultural aspects of illness among members of the dominant U.S. cultural group. Table 17–8 presents selected examples from among the more than 150 culture-bound syndromes that have been documented by medical anthropologists.

CULTURE AND TREATMENT

After a symptom is identified, the first effort at treatment is often self-care. In the United States, an estimated 70 to 90% of all illness episodes are treated first, or exclusively, through self-care, often with significant success. The availability of over-the-counter medications, relatively high literacy level, and influence of the mass media in communicating health-related information to the general population have contributed to the high percentage of self-treatment. Home treatments are attractive because of their accessibility compared with the inconvenience associated with traveling to a physician, nurse practitioner, and pharmacist, particularly for clients from rural or sparsely populated areas. Furthermore, home treatment may mobilize the client's social support network and provide the sick individual with a caring environment in which to convalesce. The nurse should be aware, however, that not all home remedies are inexpensive. For example, urban black populations in the Southeast sometimes use medicinal potions that cost much more than an equivalent treatment with a biomedical intervention.

A wide variety of so-called nontraditional interventions are gaining the recognition of health care professionals in the biomedical-scientific health care system. Acupuncture, acupressure, therapeutic touch, massage, biofeedback, relaxation techniques, meditation, hypnosis, distraction, imagery, and herbal remedies are interventions that clients may use alone or in combination with other treatments.

CULTURAL NEGOTIATION

Although there are subtle differences in the two processes, cultural negotiation and culture brokerage are both considered acts of translation in which messages, instructions, and belief systems are manipulated, linked, or processed between the professional and the lay models of health problem and preferred treatment. In each act, attention is given to eliciting the client's views regarding a health-related experience (e.g., pregnancy, complications of pregnancy, or illness of an infant). Katon and Kleinman (1981) describes negotiation as a bilateral arrangement in which the two principal parties attempt to work out a solution. The goal of negotiation is to reduce conflict in a way that promotes cooperation.

Cultural negotiation is used when conceptual differences exist between the client and the nurse, a situation that may occur for one or more of the following reasons. The nurse and client may be using the same words but have different meanings, apply the term to the same phenomenon but have different

Table 17–8
Selected Culture-Bound Syndromes

Group	Disorder	Remarks
Whites	Anorexia nervosa	Excessive preoccupation with thinness, self-imposed starvation
	Bulimia	Gross overeating, then vomiting or fasting
Blacks	Blackout	Collapse, dizziness, inability to move
	Low blood	Not enough blood or weakness of the blood that is often treated with diet
	High blood	Blood that is too rich in certain components due to ingestion of too much red meat or rich foods
	Thin blood	Occurs in women, children, and the elderly; renders the individual more susceptible to illness in general
	Diseases of hex, witchcraft, or conjuring	Sense of being doomed by spell, part of voodoo beliefs
Chinese or Southeast Asians	*Koro*	Intense anxiety that penis is retracting into body
Greeks	Hysteria	Bizarre complaints and behavior because the uterus leaves the pelvis and goes to another part of the body
Hispanics	*Empacho*	Food forms into a ball and clings to the stomach or intestines, causing pain and cramping
	Fatigue	Asthma-like symptoms
	Mal ojo ("evil eye")	Fitful sleep, crying, and diarrhea in children caused by a stranger's attention, sudden onset
	Pasmo	Paralysis-like symptoms of face or limbs, prevented or relieved by massage
	Susto	Anxiety, trembling, and phobias from sudden fright
Native Americans	Ghost	Terror, hallucinations, sense of danger
Japanese	*Wagamama*	Apathetic childish behavior with emotional outbursts

notions of its causation, and have different memories or emotions associated with the term and its use.

In cultural negotiation, attention is given to providing scientific information while acknowledging that the client may hold different views. If the client's perspective indicates that behaviors would be helpful, positive, adaptive, or neutral in effect, it is appropriate for the nurse to include these in the plan of care. If, however, the client's perspective would result in behaviors that might be harmful, negative, or non-adaptive, the nurse should attempt to shift the client's perspective to that of the practitioner (Herberg, 1995; Spector, 1996).

Because pregnancy and childbirth are social, cultural, and physiologic experiences, any approach to culturally sensitive nursing care of childbearing women and their families must focus on the interaction between cultural meaning and biological functions. Childbirth is a time of transition and a social celebration that is of central importance in any society;

it signals realignment of existing cultural roles and responsibilities, psychological and biological states, and social relationships. Child rearing is also a period during which culturally bound values, attitudes, beliefs, and practices permeate virtually all aspects of life for both the parents and the child (Andrews and Boyle, 1995).

SOLUTIONS TO HEALTH CARE PROBLEMS IN CULTURALLY DIVERSE POPULATIONS

The factors responsible for the health disparity between minority and white populations are complex and defy simplistic solutions. Health status is influenced by the interaction of physiologic, cultural, psychological, and societal factors that are poorly understood for the general population and even less so for minorities. Despite the shared characteristic of economic disadvantage among minorities, common approaches for improving health are not possible; rather, solving problems among minorities necessitates activities, programs, and data collection that are tailored to meet the unique health care needs of many different subgroups. Solutions to health care problems among culturally diverse populations include

- Health information and education
- Delivering and financing health services
- Health professions development
- Cooperative efforts with the nonfederal sector
- Data development
- Research agenda

Health Information and Education

According to the Office of Minority Health (OMH), minority populations are less knowledgeable or aware of some specific health problems than are whites, as demonstrated by the following examples.

- Blacks and Hispanics receive less information about cancer and heart disease than do nonminority groups.
- Blacks tend to underestimate the prevalence of cancer, give less credence to the warning signs, and obtain fewer screening tests and are diagnosed at later stages of cancer than are whites.
- Hispanic women receive less information about breast cancer than do white women. Hispanic women are less aware that family history is a risk factor for breast cancer, and only 25% of Hispanic women have heard of breast self-examination.
- Many professionals and lay persons, both minority and white, do not know that heart disease is as common in black men as it is in white men and that black women die from coronary heart disease at a higher rate than do white women.
- Hypertensive Japanese women and younger men (aged 18–49 years) are less aware of their hypertension than are the nonminority subgroups.
- Among Mexican-Americans, cultural attitudes regarding obesity and diet are often barriers to achieving weight control.

Programs to increase public awareness about health problems have been well received in several areas. For example, the Healthy Mothers/Healthy Babies Coalition, which provides an education program in both English and Spanish, has contributed to increased awareness of measures to improve the health status of mothers and infants. In addition, increased knowledge among blacks of hypertension as a serious health problem is one of the accomplishments of the National High Blood Pressure Education program. The success of these efforts indicates that carefully planned programs have a beneficial effect, but efforts must continue and be expanded to reach even more of the target population and to focus on additional health problems.

PLANNING HEALTH INFORMATION

Sensitivity to cultural factors is often lacking in the health care of minorities. Key concepts to consider in designing a health information campaign include meeting the language and cultural needs of each identified minority group, using minority-specific community resources to tailor educational approaches, and developing materials and methods of presentation that are commensurate with the educational level of the target population. Furthermore, because of the powerful influences of cultural factors over a lifetime in shaping people's attitudes, values, beliefs, and practices concerning health, health information programs must be sustained over a long period. Examples of the ways in which these concepts may be interwoven into health promotion efforts include the following:

- Involve local community leaders who are members of the cultural group being targeted to promote acceptance and reinforcement of the central themes of health promotion messages.
- Health messages are more readily accepted if they do not conflict with existing cultural beliefs and practices. Where appropriate, messages should acknowledge existing cultural beliefs.
- Involve families, churches, employers, and community organizations as a support system to facilitate and sustain behavior change to a more healthful lifestyle. For example, although hypertension control in blacks depends on appropriate treatment (e.g., medication), blood pressure can be improved and maintained by family and community support of activities such as proper diet and exercise.
- Language barriers, cultural differences, and lack of adequate information on access to care complicate prenatal care for Hispanic and Asian women who have recently arrived in the United States. By using lay volunteers to organize community support networks, programs have been developed to disseminate culturally appropriate health information.

- Homicide is the leading cause of death among young black men and one of the leading causes of death for Hispanic men and black women. It is a major contributor to the disparity in mortality rates between these groups and whites. Homicide prevention activities should include strategies such as behavioral modification interventions for handling anger and community-based programs to call attention to the extent and consequences of violence in black and Hispanic communities. In addition, the root cause of the underlying poverty should be examined, and programs to improve the overall financial status of minority groups should be implemented.
- The use of inhalants among young Hispanic and Native American groups should be dealt with through an appropriate and culturally sensitive health education campaign.

Education

Although printed materials and other audiovisual aids contribute to the educational process, client education is inherently interpersonal. The success of an educational effort for clients is often determined by the credibility of the source and is highly dependent on the skill and sensitivity of the nurse in communicating information in a culturally appropriate manner. Education programs are particularly critical and necessary for several health problems with the greatest impact on minority health, such as hypertension, obesity, and diabetes. For example, if diabetics could improve their self-management skills through education, an estimated 70% of complications (e.g., ketoacidosis, blindness, and amputations) could be achieved, thus saving much human misery as well as health care dollars.

Delivery and Financing of Health Services

Innovative models for delivering and financing health services for minority populations are needed. According to community health experts, models should increase flexibility of health care delivery, facilitate access to services by minority populations, improve efficiency of service and payment systems, and modify services to be more culturally acceptable.

The most commonly used indicators of adequacy of health services for a population include distribution of health care providers, but this is an inadequate measurement. The following facts exemplify the problem associated with health services for minorities:

- The disparities in death rates between minorities and whites remain despite overall increases in health care access and use.
- Language problems hinder refugees and immigrants when they seek health care.
- Blacks with cancer postpone seeking diagnosis of their symptoms longer than do whites and delay initiation of treatment once diagnosed.
- A smaller proportion of black women than white women begin prenatal care in the first trimester of pregnancy (63% vs. 76%); this factor is related to the high black infant mortality rate.
- The postneonatal death rate, which constitutes the majority of infant mortality for Native Americans and Alaska Natives, remains high. Postneonatal mortality implies an adverse environment for the infant and is thought to result from problems such as infectious disease, unintentional injury, and a lower rate of use of health care for these acute problems.

Continuity of Care

Continuity of care is associated with improved health outcomes and is presumably greater when a client is able to establish an ongoing relationship with a care provider. The issue is central because many of the major killers of minorities, such as cancer, cardiovascular disease, and diabetes, are chronic rather than acute problems and require extended treatment regimens. Consider the following:

- A higher percentage of blacks and Hispanics than whites report that they have no usual source of health care (29% and 19%, respectively, vs. 13%).
- Refugees are eligible for special refugee medical assistance during their first 18 months in this country. After this, however, refugees who cannot afford private health insurance and are ineligible for Medicaid or state medical assistance may become medically indigent.
- Many Native Americans and Alaska Natives live in areas where the availability of health care providers is half that of the national average, and the Indian Health Service (IHS) is often unable to provide coverage.

Financing Problems

Because of economic inequalities, members of minority groups tend to rely on Medicaid and charity for their health care needs. Elderly minority people are less likely than whites to supplement Medicare with additional private insurance.

- Proportionately three times as many Native Americans, blacks, Hispanics, and certain Asian and Pacific Islander groups as whites live in poverty.
- Proportionately twice as many blacks and three times as many Hispanics as whites have no medical insurance (18% and 26%, respectively, vs. 9%).
- Of those who had no insurance, 35% had not seen a physician during the past 12 months compared with 22% of those who had insurance.

Health Professions Development

Minority and nonminority health professional organizations, academic institutions, state governments, health departments, and other organizations from the public and private sectors should develop strategies to improve the availability and accessibility of health care professionals to minority communities.

- Minorities (and whites) live in communities that do not usually conform to the specific geographic boundaries of political jurisdictions (e.g., states, counties, wards). Minority communities are not evenly distributed and often cross over these geographic boundaries. In contrast, record keeping and other processes for monitoring (and potentially influencing) the availability of health professionals and resources are usually determined by and restricted to these political boundaries.
- The size of a minority population, number of cultural subgroups, and demographic features such as pattern and distribution of minority communities are factors that influence the number of health profession students that each group might be expected to generate and the degree to which a minority group can support a cadre of health professionals in its community. With few exceptions, minorities are underrepresented as students and practitioners of the health professions. Although the number of minority nursing students has been steadily increasing, there still are proportionately more white nursing students.
- Differences in the availability of health personnel resources to minority communities are apparent regardless of the minority group being considered. Communities located in urban-metropolitan areas have significantly more professional resources.

Developing Strategies Within the Federal and Nonfederal Sectors

The OMH (1996) recommends a review of programs having an impact on the actual or potential availability of health professionals to minority communities in an effort to improve collaboration. Activities to improve minority health should involve participation of organizations at all levels: community, municipal, state, and national. The private sector can also serve as an effective channel for programs targeted to minority health projects. National organizations concerned with minorities, such as the National Urban League and the Coalition of Hispanic Mental Health and Human Services Organizations, include health-related issues in their national agendas and are actively seeking effective ways to improve the health of minorities. Organizations such as these have a powerful potential for effecting change among their constituencies because they have strong community-level grassroots support.

Changes in health behavior frequently depend on personal initiative and are most likely to be triggered by health promotion efforts from locally based sources. Community involvement in developing health promotion activities can contribute to their success by providing credibility and visibility to the activities and facilitating their acceptance.

However, not all minority communities have the ability to identify their own health problems and initiate activities to address them. Support from the state and federal governments as well as private sector assistance is needed to assist with identifying and solving health-related problems afflicting the minority community. There are many ways in which assistance may be provided to minority communities, including the use of technical assistance to identify high-risk groups and then help with planning, implementing, and evaluating programs to address the identified needs; specialized community services such as federally or privately funded demonstration projects for infants and the frail elderly; and programs supported by businesses and industries (e.g., health promotion programs organized by unions).

Improving and Using Available Sources of Data

The OMH (1996) recommends that existing sources of health data be improved by including racial and ethnic identifiers in data bases and oversampling selected minorities in national surveys. Analyses such as cross-comparisons from different data sets and specialized studies should be encouraged because they can contribute to understanding the health status and needs of minority populations. Unfortunately, many studies conducted in the past have failed to include data categories for culturally diverse groups and subgroups.

RESEARCH AGENDA

The OMH (1996) recommends that a research agenda be developed to investigate factors affecting minority health, such as risk factor identification, risk factor prevalence, health education interventions, preventive services interventions, treatment services, and socio-cultural factors and health outcomes.

Research on Culture and Community Health Nursing

For further information on current research related to culture and community health nursing, the reader should search library data bases for reports of completed studies in the literature. Electronic bulletin boards also may be valuable when searching for research in progress and for communicating with researchers studying a particular phenomenon of interest. For example, the reader may gain electronic access to the Virginia Henderson International Library and search the most comprehensive listing of nursing research (including dissertations on nursing topics) in the world. In a pilot program, the *American Journal of Nursing* has moderated electronic forums with experts in a variety of nursing specialties, including opportunity to access research experts through the Transcultural Nursing Society. The Transcultural Nursing Society also may be contacted by calling 1-888-432-5470 toll free.

Another electronic bulletin board is available through the University of California, San Francisco in which the reader may communicate with researchers studying cross-cultural nursing phenomena.

Table 17–9 contains summaries of selected research on topics of relevance to community health nurses in providing culturally competent care.

Community Health Nursing and Culturally Diverse Populations

In a study by Bernal and Froman (1987), the degree of self-efficacy among 190 community health nurses caring for Puerto Rican, black, and Southeast Asian clients, the degree of influence of various background variables on the nurses' level of self-efficacy, and the difference in self-efficacy for caring for the three ethnic groups were examined. Using a cultural self-efficacy scale to determine their degree of confidence in caring for the three ethnic groups, the researchers reported that the highest confidence scores were found among community health nurses caring for (in rank order) blacks, Puerto Ricans, and Southeast Asians, but overall the nurses felt very inadequate in providing care to those from ethnically diverse backgrounds.

Low scores were observed on items that included knowledge of health beliefs and practices as well as beliefs about respect, authority, and modesty. Higher scores in using an interpreter correctly were observed. Results suggest that community health nurses do not feel confident about caring for any of the three major ethnic groups. Furthermore, this perceived weakness occurred regardless of the nurses' education and demographic variables.

These results, although disappointing to those who consider cultural aspects of nursing care to be important, are not surprising. They show empirical support for the speculation made by DHHS that nurses are not being provided with the experiences needed to build confidence in the application of community health concepts to the care of culturally diverse populations. The purpose of this chapter is to provide an overview of the various components of culture about which community health nurses need to know in order to provide culturally congruent and competent care to individuals, families, groups, and communities of various cultural backgrounds.

ROLE OF THE COMMUNITY HEALTH NURSE IN IMPROVING HEALTH FOR CULTURALLY DIVERSE PEOPLE

This chapter has provided data detailing the health care problems of culturally diverse individuals, families, groups, and communities. Given the complexity of the problems and the wide variation in incidence and distribution of these problems within specific subgroups, there is no simple method of providing culturally sensitive community health nursing care to all clients.

The following principles may assist the community health nurse when working with culturally diverse clients:

Table 17–9
Selected Research on Culture and Community Health Nursing

Small K, Winans P (1995). Teenage pregnancy: Effects of public health nurse intervention. IHS Care Provider 20:27–27.

Pregnancy for American Indian teenagers carries an increased risk of complications, including low birth weight, pregnancy-induced hypertension, and preterm labor. There also is a potentially negative impact on the social, educational, and emotional development of the teenagers assuming the roles and responsibilities of motherhood. Infants delivered by teenage mothers are at higher risk for developmental delays, neglect, and abuse.

Public health nurses from a southwestern Indian Health Services (IHS) unit working collaboratively with an adolescent health clinic at an Arizona high school provided home services for teenage Indian mothers. The goals of the home services were to provide education about topics such as normal growth and development of infants and parenting skills, to encourage the mother to return to or stay in school, and to follow recommendations for well-child care and immunizations.

Teenage mothers (ages 14–19 years) were placed into two groups. Group 1 (N = 72) served as the nonintervention control group. Group 2 (N = 67) received the intervention, which consisted of home visits by public health nurses at 1- to 2-month intervals during the first year after delivery. Results indicate that enhanced public health nurse intervention decreased the number of repeat pregnancies during the first year after delivery; increased the number of teen mothers who returned to school, finished school, or obtained their graduate equivalent degree; and improved the rate of immunization for their infants. As a result of this study, the same intervention strategy has been incorporated into the entire public health nursing program at the southwestern IHS unit.

Champion VL, Austin JK, Tzeng OCS (1990). Relationship between cross-cultural health attitudes and community health indicators. Public Health Nurs 7:243–250.

This study is based on the premise that improving health standards both in the United States and internationally is a goal for all community health nurses. Using a cultural data set, researchers investigated the relationship between attitudes toward health and indexes of community health. Concepts selected from the data set were I (myself), body, sickness, disease, life, doctor, health, medicine, hospital, nurse, death, and insane. Community health indicators were male and female life expectancy, infant mortality, economic and public health expenditures, and net social progress.

The original sample included 1200 high school males within each of 30 language and cultural communities. Data were derived from informants' ratings of the dimensions of evaluation, potency, and activity for each concept. The results supported the association between attitudes and objective community health indicators. Negative correlations were found between attitudes toward medicine and nurse attitudes toward body and life, indicating that extended contact with health care providers results in negative attitudes toward them. Positive relationships were found between public health expenditures and nurses, indicating that, in countries with more expenditures for community and public health, attitudes toward nurses were more positive.

D'Avanzo CE, Frye B, Froman R (1994). Stress in Cambodian refugee families. Image J Nurs Scholarship 26:101–105.

More than 1 million Southeast Asians from Cambodia, Laos, and Vietnam live in the United States. Rapidly growing and culturally varied, these groups have an increasing need for physical and mental health services. The sources, manifestations, and coping strategies associated with stress experienced by these groups were studied. Interviews with 120 Cambodian women in this comparative descriptive study were conducted to identify their perceptions of stress-related factors confronting families. Memories of the war, financial concerns, language-related communication difficulties, and family problems were frequently cited. Somatic manifestations such as headaches, sickness or sleeping a lot, chest pain, and shortness of breath were the most common physical symptoms. The women in the study perceived themselves as responsible for the emotional equilibrium of their families and yet ineffectual in understanding stress. This research provides useful information for community health nurses providing care for Cambodian refugee families.

Aroian KA (1993). Mental health risks by illegal immigrants. Issues Mental Health Nurs 14:379–397.

Because immigrants are a high-risk population, they are confronted with many adaptive challenges related to extensive changes in lifestyle and environment. Most study participants reported difficulties and distress associated with the illegal immigrant experience. Data analysis revealed that conflicting reports about the illegal immigrant experience reflect the complexity of the immigration phenomenon. A young person who is willing to work without job security may find the experience adventuresome, whereas another may find the same experience stressful. Positive aspects included opportunity for financial benefit. Negative aspects included difficulty finding employment, unsafe or unhealthy working conditions, exploitation by employers, and uncertainty about the future. The findings sensitize community health professionals to the difficulties experienced by illegal immigrants and provide direction for clinical interventions with this high-risk group.

- Conduct a "culturological" assessment (discussed later).
- Conduct a cultural self-assessment.
- Seek knowledge about local cultures.
- Recognize political aspects of culturally diverse groups.
- Increase cultural sensitivity; provide culturally competent care.
- Recognize culturally based health problems.

Culturological Assessment

Because all nursing care is based on a systematic, comprehensive assessment of the client, it is important for the community health nurse to gather cultural data on clients from racially and ethnically diverse backgrounds. A culturological assessment refers to a systematic appraisal or examination of individuals, groups, and communities regarding their cultural beliefs, values, and practices to determine explicit nursing needs and intervention practices within the cultural context of the people being evaluated (Leininger, 1995). The term *culturological* is a descriptive reference to culture phenomena in their broadest sense.

In conducting a culturological assessment, the community health nurse should, therefore, be involved in determining and appraising the traits, characteristics, or smallest units of cultural behavior as a guide to nursing care. Culturological assessments tend to be broad and comprehensive because they deal with cultural values, belief systems, and ways of living now and in the recent past. However, the nurse can learn to appraise segments of these larger areas, such as a particular cultural value, and then relate this finding to other aspects, such as culture practices. Culturological assessments are as vital as physical and psychological assessments. The following section summarizes major data categories pertaining to the culture of clients and offers suggested questions that the nurse might ask to elicit needed information.

BRIEF HISTORY OF THE ETHNIC AND RACIAL ORIGINS OF THE CULTURAL GROUP WITH WHICH THE CLIENT IDENTIFIES

- With what ethnic group or groups does the client report affiliation (e.g., Hispanic, Polish, Navajo, or a combination)? To what degree does the client identify with the cultural group (e.g., "we" concept of solidarity or a fringe member)?
- What is the client's reported racial affiliation (e.g., black, Native American, Asian, and so on)?
- Where was the client born?
- Where has the client lived (country, city) and when (during what years)? (If the client has recently relocated to the United States, knowledge of prevalent diseases in the country of origin may be helpful.)

VALUES ORIENTATION

- What are the client's attitudes, values, and beliefs about birth, death, health, illness, and health care providers?
- Does culture impact the manner in which the client relates to body image change resulting from illness or surgery (e.g., importance of appearance, beauty, strength, and roles in cultural group)?
- How does the client view work, leisure, and education?
- How does the client perceive change?
- How does the client value privacy, courtesy, touch, and relationships with individuals of different ages, of different social class (or caste), and of the opposite sex?
- How does the client view biomedical-scientific health care (e.g., suspiciously, fearfully, or acceptingly)? How does the client relate to persons in a different cultural group (e.g., withdrawal, verbally or nonverbally expressive, or negatively or positively)?

CULTURAL SANCTIONS AND RESTRICTIONS

- How does the client's cultural group regard expression of emotion and feelings, spirituality, and religious beliefs? How are dying, death, and grieving expressed in a culturally appropriate manner?
- How is modesty expressed by men and women? Are there culturally defined expectations about male-female relationships, including the nurse-client relationship?
- Does the client have any restrictions related to sexuality, exposure of body parts, or certain types of surgery (e.g., amputation, vasectomy, and hysterectomy)?
- Are there any restrictions against discussion of dead relatives or fears related to the unknown?

COMMUNICATION

- What language does the client speak at home? What other language does the client speak or read? In what language would the client prefer to communicate with you?
- What is the English fluency level of the client (both written and spoken)? Remember that the stress of illness may cause clients to use a more familiar language and temporarily forget some English.
- Does the client need an interpreter? If so, is there a relative or friend whom the client would like to have interpret? Is there anyone who the client would prefer not to interpret (e.g., member of the opposite sex, a person younger or older than the client, or a member of a rival tribe or nation)?
- What are the rules (linguistics) and modes (style) of communication?
- Is it necessary to vary the technique of communication during the interview and examination to accommodate the client's cultural background (e.g., tempo of conversation, eye contact, sensitivity to topical taboos, norms of confidentiality, and style of explanation)?
- How does the client's nonverbal communication compare with that of individuals from other cultural backgrounds? How does it affect the client's relationship with you and with other members of the health care team?
- How does the client feel about health care providers who are not of the same cultural background (e.g., black, middle-class nurse, or Hispanic of a different social class)? Does the client prefer to receive care from a nurse of the same cultural background, sex, or age?
- What are the overall cultural characteristics of the client's language and communication processes?
- With which language or dialect is the client most comfortable?

HEALTH-RELATED BELIEFS AND PRACTICES

- To what cause or causes does the client attribute illness and disease (e.g., divine wrath, imbalance in hot-cold or yin-yang, punishment for moral transgressions, hex, or soul loss)?
- What does the client believe promotes health (e.g., eating certain foods, wearing amulets to bring good luck, exercise, prayer, ancestors, saints, or intermediate deities)?
- What is the client's religious affiliation (e.g., Judaism, Islam, Pentecostalism, West African voodooism, Seventh-day Adventism, Catholicism, or Mormonism)?
- Does the client rely on cultural healers (e.g., curandero, shaman, spiritualist, priest, minister, or monk)? Who determines when the client is sick and when the client is healthy? Who determines the type of healer and treatment that should be sought?
- In what types of cultural healing practices does the client engage (e.g., herbal remedies, potions, massage, wearing of talismans or charms to discourage evil spirits, healing rituals, incantations, or prayers)?
- How are biomedical-scientific health care providers perceived? How does the client and family perceive nurses? What are the expectations of nurses and nursing care?
- What comprises appropriate "sick-role" behavior? Who determines what symptoms constitute disease and illness? Who decides when the client is no longer sick? Who cares for the client at home?
- How does the client's cultural group view mental disorders? Are there differences in acceptable behaviors for physical versus psychological illnesses?

NUTRITION

- What nutritional factors are influenced by the client's cultural background?
- What are the meanings of "food" and "eating" to the client? With whom does the client usually eat? What types of foods are eaten? What does the client define as food? What does the client believe comprises a "healthy" versus an "unhealthy" diet?
- How are foods prepared at home (e.g., type of food preparation; cooking oils used; length of time foods, especially vegetables, are cooked; amount and type of seasoning added to various foods during preparation)?
- Do religious beliefs and practices influence the client's diet (e.g., amount, type, preparation, or delineation of acceptable food combinations such as kosher diets)? Does the client abstain from certain foods at regular intervals, on specific dates determined by the religious calendar, or at other times?
- If the client's religion mandates or encourages fasting, what does the term "fast" mean to the client (e.g., refraining from certain types or quantities of

foods, eating only during certain times of the day)? For what period of time is the client expected to fast?

- During fasting, does the client refrain from liquids or beverages? Does the religion allow exemption from fasting during illness, and, if so, is the client believed to have an exemption?

SOCIOECONOMIC CONSIDERATIONS

- Who constitutes the client's social network (i.e., family, peers, and cultural healers)? How do they influence the client's health or illness status?
- How do members of the client's social support network define "caring" (e.g., being continuously present, doing things for the client, or looking after the client's family)? What are the roles of various family members during health and illness?
- How does the client's family participate in the client's nursing care (e.g., bathing, feeding, touching, and being present)?
- Does the cultural family structure influence the client's response to health or illness (e.g., beliefs, strengths, weaknesses, and social class)? Is there a key family member whose role is significant in health-related decisions (e.g., grandmother in many black families or eldest adult son in Asian families)?
- Who is the principal wage earner in the client's family? What is the total annual income? (This is a potentially sensitive question that should be asked only if necessary.) Is there more than one wage earner? Are there other sources of financial support (e.g., extended family, investments)?
- What impact does economic status have on lifestyle, place of residence, living conditions, ability to obtain health care, and discharge planning?

ORGANIZATIONS PROVIDING CULTURAL SUPPORT

- What influence do ethnic and cultural organizations have on the client's receiving health care (e.g., Organization of Migrant Workers, National Association for the Advancement of Colored People, Black Political Caucus, churches, schools, Urban League, and community-based health care programs and clinics)?

EDUCATIONAL BACKGROUND

- What is the client's highest educational level obtained? Does the client's educational background

affect the client's knowledge level concerning the health care delivery system, how to obtain the care needed, teaching and learning skills, and any written material that is distributed in the health care setting (e.g., insurance forms, educational literature, information about diagnostic procedures and laboratory tests, and admissions forms)?

- Can the client read and write English, or is another language preferred? If English is the client's second language, are materials available in the client's primary language?
- What learning style is most comfortable or familiar? Does the client prefer to learn through written materials, oral explanation, or demonstration?

RELIGIOUS AFFILIATION

- How does the client's religious affiliation impact health and illness (e.g., death, chronic illness, body image alteration, and cause and effect of illness)?
- What is the role of the client's religious beliefs and practices during health and illness?
- Are there healing rituals or practices that the client believes can promote well-being or hasten recovery from illness? If so, who performs these?
- What is the role of significant religious representatives during health and illness? Are there recognized religious healers (e.g., Islamic imams, Christian Scientist practitioners or nurses, Catholic priests, Mormon elders, and Buddhist monks)?

CULTURAL ASPECTS OF DISEASE INCIDENCE

- Does the client have any specific genetic or acquired conditions that are more prevalent in a specific cultural group (e.g., hypertension, sickle cell anemia, Tay-Sachs disease, or lactose intolerance)?
- Are there socioenvironmental diseases that are more prevalent among the client's specific cultural group (e.g., lead poisoning, alcoholism, acquired immunodeficiency syndrome, drug abuse, or ear infections)?
- Are there any diseases against which the client has an increased resistance (e.g., skin cancer in darkly pigmented individuals)?

BIOCULTURAL VARIATIONS

- Does the client have distinctive physical features that are characteristic of a particular racial group (e.g., skin color or hair texture)? Does the client have any variations in anatomy that are characteristic of a particular racial or ethnic group (e.g., body structure, height, weight, facial shape and structure [nose, eye shape, facial contour], or upper and lower extremity shape)?

- How do anatomic and racial variations affect the assessment?

DEVELOPMENTAL CONSIDERATIONS

- Are there any distinct growth and development characteristics that vary with the client's cultural background (e.g., bone density, psychomotor patterns of development, or fat folds)?
- What factors are significant in assessing children from the newborn period through adolescence (e.g., expected growth on standard grid, culturally acceptable age for toilet training, introducing various types of foods, sex differences, discipline, and socialization to adult roles)?
- What is the cultural perception of aging (e.g., is youthfulness or the wisdom of old age more highly valued)?
- How are elderly persons handled culturally (e.g., cared for in the home of adult children or placed in institutions for care)? What are culturally acceptable roles for the elderly?
- Does the elderly person expect family members to provide care, including nurturance and other humanistic aspects of care?
- Is the elderly person isolated from culturally relevant supportive persons or enmeshed in a caring network of relatives and friends?
- Has a culturally appropriate network replaced family members in performing some caring functions for the elderly person?

Cultural Self-Assessment

Community health nurses can engage in a cultural self-assessment. Through identification of health-related attitudes, values, beliefs, and practices that are part of the cultural baggage brought to the nurse-client interaction, it is possible to better understand the cultural aspects of health care from the perspective of the client, family, group, or community. Everyone has ethnocentric tendencies that must be brought to a level of conscious awareness so that efforts can be made to temper ethnocentrism and view reality from the perception of the client.

Knowledge About Local Cultures

Community health nurses can learn about the cultural diversity characteristic of the subgroup or subgroups that are most prevalent within their communities. Because it is impossible to know about all health-related beliefs and practices of the diverse groups served, it is reasonable to study selected ones. This cultural study may be accomplished by a review of nursing, anthropology, sociology, and related literature on culturally diverse groups; by in-services held at community health agencies, educational institutions in the community, or organizations serving minority groups; by enrolling in courses on transcultural or cross-cultural nursing and medical anthropology; and by interviewing key members of the subgroups of interest such as clergy members, nurses, physicians, and others to obtain information about the influence of culture on health-related beliefs and practices.

Recognition of Political Aspects

Awareness of the political aspects of health care for culturally diverse groups and communities can enable community health nurses to have increased involvement in influencing legislation and funding priorities aimed at improving health care for specific populations. Recognized for their leadership role in community health matters involving culturally diverse groups, community health nurses may be invited by political leaders to participate in political decision making affecting the health of a targeted subgroup. Community health nurses should also be active politically, both individually and collectively, to be able to influence legislation affecting culturally diverse individuals, groups, and communities, and they should offer to serve on key community committees, boards, and advisory councils that impact the health of culturally diverse groups.

Provide Culturally Competent Care

When caring for individuals and families who have culturally diverse backgrounds, the community health nurse can assess, diagnose, implement, and evaluate nursing care in a manner that is culturally congruent, competent, relevant, and appropriate. To provide this culturally appropriate nursing care, it is necessary to be aware of the cultural similarities and differences between the nurse and the client—whether an individual, a family, a group, or a community—and to create a relationship of mutual respect on a foundation of effective cross-cultural communication. A guideline for gathering cultural data has been presented, and this guideline or a similar one may be used for identifying significant areas in which the nurse and client differ. Knowledge about biocultural variations in health and illness is particularly important when conducting cultural assessments.

Recognition of Culturally Based Health Practices

Try to understand the nature and meaning of culturally based health practices of clients, groups, and communities. Once the practices are understood, a determination regarding their appropriateness in a particular context can be made. Generally, it is helpful to decide whether a cultural practice is useful, neutral, or harmful to the client, group, or community. Helpful and neutral practices should be encouraged or "tolerated," whereas harmful practices should be discouraged. The classification of some cultural healing practices is not so easily determined. For example, many Southeast Asians practice coining, which is the rubbing of a coin over body surfaces to expel bad winds that are believed to cause illness such as respiratory disorders. Because coining leaves abrasions on the skin, community health nurses are sometimes faced with an ethical dilemma when coining is practiced on young children; this practice may be construed by some members of the dominant cultural group as child abuse. This practice is not useful, so the decision must be made as to whether it is neutral or harmful.

The argument for the practice being neutral is based on the facts that the abrasions usually heal quickly, no harm is done to the child as a result of the practice, and the practice is meaningful to parents who have much confidence in the healing powers associated with coining.

The argument can also be made that the practice is harmful. The red marks and skin abrasions caused by the coining constitute child abuse because the integumentary system is compromised; thus, the child is placed at increased risk for skin infection. Also, given that the child could require antibiotics or other medication for, in this example, a respiratory disorder, encouraging coining may prevent the child from receiving needed medical intervention and thus delay treatment, which may prove to be harmful.

As a solution, the community health nurse could suggest that parents combine traditional treatment with Western biomedicine; that is, the parents could use coining in conjunction with a biomedical intervention. Therefore, the healing will occur in a manner that has involved the use of both folk and professional health care systems.

Federal Resources

U.S. DEPARTMENT OF HEALTH AND HUMAN SERVICES

Community health nurses will find federal resources for improving the health care of the federally defined minority populations through the U.S. DHHS. Within the U.S. Public Health Service, the OMH and the IHS relate to health promotion, disease prevention, service delivery, and research on minority groups.

OFFICE OF MINORITY HEALTH

The OMH is the unit of the U.S. DHHS that coordinates federal efforts to improve the health status of racial and ethnic minority populations: blacks, Hispanics, American Indians and Alaska Natives, and Asians and Pacific Islanders.

Located within the office of the assistant secretary for health in the Public Health Service, OMH is directed by the deputy assistant secretary for minority health.

Created by a DHHS executive order in 1985, the office and its duties were established in law by the Disadvantaged Minority Health Improvement Act of 1990 (P.L. 101-527), which was signed by President Bush on November 6, 1990. The act requires OMH to carry out certain duties:

- Establish short- and long-range goals and objectives, and coordinate DHHS activities that relate to disease prevention, health promotion, service delivery, and research on the health of minority people.
- Form agreements with other federal agencies that will lead to increased participation of disadvantaged people, including minorities, in health service and promotion programs.
- Create a national minority health resource center.
- Support research, demonstrations, and evaluations of new and innovative models that increase understanding of disease risk factors and support better information dissemination, education, prevention, and service delivery to minority communities.
- Coordinate efforts to promote minority health-related activities in the corporate and voluntary sectors.

- Develop health information and health promotion materials and teaching programs.
- Assist providers of primary care and preventive services in obtaining assistance of bilingual health professionals and other bilingual individuals when appropriate for their service populations.

The act requires OMH to ensure that the services it provides are equitably allocated among racial and ethnic minority groups and that information and services are provided in appropriate language and cultural context.

In carrying out these duties, OMH works closely with each Public Health Service agency and the other operating divisions within DHHS that conduct large-scale health programs and special initiatives intended to improve the health of minority people. It also maintains close liaison arrangements with corporate and voluntary organizations, including a broad range of national and community-based minority organizations, that work with health-related issues.

Initiatives for Improved Minority Health Care

As the focal point for minority health efforts, OMH plays a key role in major initiatives launched by the DHHS secretary and the Public Health Service.

Program Direction 9: Improving the Health of Minority and Low-Income People. DHHS has charted a broad multiyear plan encompassing nine major program directions for the health and social service efforts of the department. Program Direction 9 aims to improve the health of minority and low-income individuals and to reduce disparities in the incidence of premature death, chronic disease, and injuries. OMH works closely with DHHS divisions to monitor the progress in achieving these goals. The two-part strategy, in which all divisions of DHHS participate, involves (1) improving access to health care for minority and low-income persons and (2) reducing the risks of chronic and preventable disease and conditions that disproportionately affect minority and low-income people through expanded biomedical, behavioral, and health services research, prevention, and early detection and treatment.

Healthy People 2000. Progress in achieving national health goals for the year 2000 will depend in large measure on success in improving the health status of special populations, including minority and low-income people and persons with disabilities. Healthy People 2000, the national goal statement for health, includes 49 specific objectives for improvements in minority health status. OMH contributes to this public-private effort by providing technical assistance to states that are working within the Healthy People 2000 framework to prepare and implement their own year 2000 plans for improved minority health.

OMH also chairs an interagency committee, with representatives from each Public Health Service agency and each major division of DHHS, to ensure that agencies and work groups within the department focus efforts on the Healthy People 2000 targets for minority populations.

Grant Programs

The grant programs of OMH have been developed to help communities deal with specific problems such as the high death rates among minority males and the continuing high prevalence of numerous acute and chronic conditions. The grants also have a larger goal—to empower communities both large and small—to help themselves and to overcome the myriad social and health problems facing communities today.

MINORITY COMMUNITY HEALTH COALITION DEMONSTRATION GRANT PROGRAM

OMH provides grants to community coalitions for risk reduction projects that target health problem areas in minority populations. These demonstration grants have provided coalitions with up to 2 years of funding to initiate community designed programs that would address disease risk factors affecting minority populations.

MINORITY HUMAN IMMUNODEFICIENCY VIRUS EDUCATION AND PREVENTION GRANT PROGRAM

OMH provides grants to minority community-based and national organizations for risk reduction projects that target human immunodeficiency virus (HIV) infection and the diseases that often precede or accompany it: sexually transmitted diseases, cervical cancer, and tuberculosis. These education and prevention grants provide minority organizations with up to 3 years of funding to come up with new approaches to prevent and reduce HIV transmission among minority populations.

Minority Male Grant Program. The Minority Male Grant Program was initiated to address the multiple health and human service problems that disproportionately affect minority males. Two components make up the program. *Coalition development* projects address the specific needs of the defined high-risk minority male populations in each community. *Coalition demonstration* grants will go beyond the initial steps of sharing information and developing coalitions to the actual implementation of educational, support, and service programs for high-risk minority males. More than $5.4 million in grants has been awarded to support 97 projects.

Indian Health Service

The DHHS, primarily through the IHS of the Public Health Service, is responsible for providing federal health services to American Indians and Alaska Natives. Federal Indian health services are based on the laws that the Congress has passed pursuant to its authority to regulate commerce with the Indian Nations as specified in the Constitution and other documents.

The Indian Health Program became a primary responsibility of the Public Health Service under P.L. 83-568, the Transfer Act, on August 5, 1954. This act provides "that all functions, responsibilities, authorities, and duties . . . relating to the maintenance and operation of hospital and health facilities for Indians, and the conservation of Indian health . . . shall be administered by the Surgeon General of the United States Public Health Service."

The IHS goal is to elevate the health status of American Indians and Alaska Natives to the highest level possible. The mission is to ensure quality, availability, and accessibility of a comprehensive high-quality health care delivery system providing maximum involvement of American Indians and Alaska Natives in defining their health needs, setting health priorities for their local areas, and managing and controlling their health program. The IHS also acts as the principal federal health advocate for Indian people by ensuring they have knowledge of and access to all federal, state, and local health programs to which they are entitled as American citizens. It is also the responsibility of the IHS to

work with these programs so Indian people will be cognizant of their entitlements.

The IHS has carried out its responsibilities through developing and operating a health services delivery system designed to provide a broad-spectrum program of preventive, curative, rehabilitative, and environmental services. This system integrates health services delivered directly through IHS facilities and staff on the one hand, with those purchased by IHS through contractual arrangements on the other, taking into account other health resources to which the Indians have access. Tribes are also actively involved in program implementation.

The 1975 Indian Self-Determination Act, P.L. 93-638, as amended builds on IHS policy by giving tribes the option of staffing and managing IHS programs in their communities and provides for funding for improvement of tribal capability to contract under the act. The 1976 Indian Health Care Improvement Act, P.L. 94-437, as amended was intended to elevate the health care status of American Indians and Alaska Natives to a level equal to that of the general population through a program of authorized higher resource levels in the IHS budget. Appropriated resources were used to expand health services, build and renovate medical facilities, and step up the construction of safe drinking water and sanitary disposal facilities. It also establishes programs designed to increase the number of Indian health professionals for Indian needs and to improve health care access for Indian people living in urban areas.

The operation of the IHS health care delivery system is managed through local administrative units called service units. A service unit is the basic health organization for a geographic area served by the IHS program, just as a county or city health department is the basic health organization in a state health department. These are defined areas, usually centered around a single federal reservation in the continental United States or a population concentration in Alaska.

A few service units cover a number of small reservations; some large reservations are divided into a number of service units. The service units are grouped into larger cultural-demographic-geographic management jurisdictions, which are administered by area offices. It is estimated that IHS serves one-half of the total American Indian and Alaska Native population in the United States, primarily those residing on reservations.

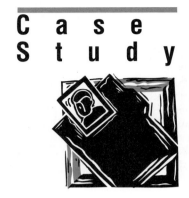

Case Study

Community health nurse Maria Gonzales visits the home of 5-year-old Nguyen Van Nghi, who was recently discharged from the hospital. The pediatrician had diagnosed the child with pneumonia and "suspected failure to thrive" because the child's growth fell below the third percentile on a standard growth chart for height and weight, and he performed poorly on a screening test used to identify developmental delays for 5-year-olds.

Also residing in the home are the child's parents, four siblings, grandmother, aunt, uncle, and three cousins. Although the child's father and uncle speak some English, other members of the household communicate in a language unfamiliar to Maria, which "sounds like Chinese." When Maria approaches the child, he does not look at or speak to her, even when she calls him Nguyen (pronounced "we'en"). During her initial assessment, Maria observes multiple tender, ecchymotic areas with petechiae between the ribs on the front and back of the body, resembling strap marks.

Suspecting child abuse, Maria tells the family that she will return later in the day with an interpreter. She locates an interpreter who speaks Mandarin Chinese and briefs him about her concerns with child abuse.

When Maria and the interpreter return to the client's home, she instructs the interpreter to ask the parents for an explanation of the bruises. The interpreter tells Maria that the family is Vietnamese and cannot understand his Chinese dialect. Both the interpreter and the child's father know a little French and awkwardly manage to communicate.

The interpreter advises the nurse that, in the Vietnamese culture, the person's family name is given first, followed by the middle name and then the first name. Because there are only a few different family names among Vietnamese, it is common practice to call people by their given first name. Nghi's father was confused when the nurse called the child by his last name. Maria also learns that the child is actually 4 years old because the Vietnamese consider a newborn to be 1 year old at birth.

The interpreter explains that a Vietnamese healer has performed *cao gio* (coining) to exude the "bad wind" from Nghi. *Cao gio* is performed by applying a special menthol oil to the painful or symptomatic part of the body and then rubbing a coin over the area with firm, downward strokes. When Nghi's condition seemed to worsen after his hospital discharge, his grandmother convinced his parents that Western biomedicine had failed and that their son required the stronger power of folk healing.

Assessment

Although a systematic and comprehensive cultural assessment is necessary, the community health nurse will find it important to set priorities and focus on selected cultural data categories because they seem most relevant for the Nguyen family at present. After the immediate concerns of a worsening case of pneumonia and potential child abuse are resolved, the remaining data categories of the cultural assessment can be completed. To guide the data collection in an orderly manner, the community health nurse may find it useful to follow Leininger's cultural and social structure dimensions (see Fig. 17–1).

> Gaining skills necessary to address this Vietnamese-American child's health needs will require ability in cultural (sometimes referred to as culturological) assessment. If the community health nurse determines that the agency's assessment instrument is inadequate in cultural data categories, it will be necessary to adopt or adapt published cultural assessment guides (e.g., Andrews & Boyle, 1995; Leininger, 1995).

Technological Factors
- Use of prescription medicines and adherence by family to recommended medical regimen for child's pneumonia
- Use of x-rays for identifying healed fractures in children who may be habitually abused by caregivers

Religious and Philosophical Factors
- Culturally based health-related values, beliefs, and practices pertaining to children
- Yin-yang beliefs and practices concerning health and illness, foods, seasons, organs of the body, and so forth

Kinship and Social Factors
- Family configuration, degree of assimilation, and acculturation; extended family roles and responsibilities
- Sex role–related behavior of parents, siblings, grandmother, aunt, uncle, and cousins
- Children expected to respect and obey adults and others in authority

Cultural Values and Ways of Life
- Cross-cultural communication and use of primary language
- English as a second (or third, fourth, and so on) language
- Normal regression in language skills and stress
- Culturally based child-rearing practices, including expected parent-child relationships and cultural definitions of abuse and neglect
- Cultural value for respecting authority figures, including health care providers
- Patterns of parenting: mothering, fathering, and substitute or surrogate parents
- Identification of primary provider of care and decision-maker for health-related matters affecting the child because this may or may not be the biological parent

Political and Legal Factors
- Cultural fear of authority (which sometimes includes health care providers) resulting from abuse of power by officials during the Vietnam War
- U.S. laws governing child abuse and neglect
- U.S. immigration laws

Economic Factors
- Financial situation of family
- Employment and income of breadwinners in family

- Health insurance
- Cost for cultural healer and folk remedies versus professional Western biomedical practitioners and medical-surgical interventions
- Access to transportation for health care purposes
- Family's ability to afford utility bills, insurance premiums, food, rent and mortgage payments, and other household expenses

Educational Factors

- Parents and other family members
- Correct placement of children in educational settings given cultural conceptualization of age, normal height and weight for children of Asian descent, language, and other sociocultural considerations

Generic or Folk Health Systems

- Role of cultural healers and relationship with families
- Appropriateness of cultural healers as members of health care team
- Folk healing practices in care of child
- Yin-yang beliefs in causation and cure of diseases in children
- Cultural practice of cao gio (coining)
- Interrelationship with Western biomedical practices

Professional Health Systems

- Biocultural variations in normal growth and development
- Use of appropriate growth and development instruments for Asian-American children
- After correction of the erroneous age reported by hospital, reassessment of growth and development based on norms for Asian children
- Reevaluation of pediatrician's diagnosis of failure to thrive

Nursing Care

- Role of community health care nurse in serving ethnic populations
- Overcoming potential barriers to providing culture-congruent and culturally competent nursing care such as ethnocentrism, cultural imposition, cultural stereotyping, cross-cultural miscommunication
- Role of community health nurse in reporting cases of suspected child abuse
- Determining the difference between harmless cultural healing practices, such as coining, and child abuse
- Home health care for Vietnamese-American child with clinical manifestations of respiratory disease
- Health education for child, parents, and other family members

Application of Leininger's Theory of Culture Care Diversity and Universality: Nursing Care Decisions and Actions

To provide culture congruent or culturally competent nursing care for individuals, families, groups, communities, and institutions, the community health nurse will need to review and evaluate all data gathered in the cultural assessment. When making nursing care decisions or actions, nurses will find three options available: cultural care preservation and maintenance, cultural care accommodation and negotiation, or cultural care repatterning and restructuring (Leininger, 1991, 1995).

In the case study, Maria has learned in her assessment that the cultural healing practice called *cao gio* (coining) is responsible for red marks on the torso of a minor child. She must first determine whether this cultural healing practice is helpful, neutral, or harmful to the child.

If the practice is believed to be helpful, Maria may choose cultural care preservation and maintenance (i.e., encourage the family to continue using *cao gio*). If it is neutral—the practice neither helps nor harms the child—she also is likely to choose cultural care preservation and maintenance. If she determines that the practice is harmful (e.g., has concern that the abrasions will become infected or that the practice is preventing the child from receiving biomedical care that will cure the pneumonia), she will choose either cultural care accommodation and negotiation or cultural care repatterning and restructuring. Examples of accommodation or negotiation might include involving the cultural healer as a member of the health care team and suggesting to the family that both *cao gio* and Western biomedical treatments be used to cure the child. Examples of repatterning or restructuring might include asking the family to stop *cao gio* and reporting the case to authorities representing a child protective services agency.

SUMMARY

To provide community health nursing for individuals, groups, and communities representing the hundreds of different cultures and subcultures found in the United States, it is necessary to include cultural considerations in the nursing care. Guidelines for gathering data from clients of culturally diverse backgrounds have been suggested in this chapter and are interwoven throughout the text. Knowledge about culture-specific and culture-universal nursing care is foundational and is an integral component of community health nursing.

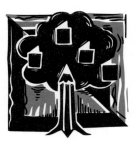

Learning Activities

1. Examine the vital statistics of your community, and compare differences in morbidity and mortality rates for whites and racial and ethnic subgroups. What data are available according to racial and ethnic heritage, and what data would you like to see that are missing?

2. Visit an inner city grocery store, and compare quality, prices, customer services, and variety of products with those of a suburban grocery store.

3. Select a client from your case load who comes from a racially or ethnically diverse background, and conduct a cultural assessment.

4. Interview someone from a racial or ethnic background that is different from your own to determine beliefs about illness causation, use of the lay and professional health care delivery systems, and culturally based treatments.

5. Review your local telephone directory for listings of ethnic restaurants. Dine at one. While dining, notice the type of cultural heritage in restaurant decor and information about the culture available from the menu, placemats, or elsewhere in the restaurant. Ask the owner or manager about the history of the restaurant.

6. Attend religious services at a church, temple, synagogue, or place of worship for a religion different from your own.

7. Interview an official representative (e.g., priest, elder, monk, or bishop) from a religion with which you are unfamiliar. Ask about health-related beliefs and practices, healing rituals, support network for the sick, and dietary practices.

8. Watch primetime television, and note the racial and ethnic diversity that is present during the commercials. During the program, note the role played by racially and ethnically diverse characters. Are they heroes (heroines) or the "bad guys"? What are their occupations, socio-economic status, religions, and lifestyles?

9. Skim a popular magazine for references to racially and ethnically diverse subgroups. What is being written? Is the nature of the article favorable or unfavorable?

REFERENCES

Andrews MM: Cultural perspectives on nursing in the 21st century. J Prof Nurs 8:7–15, 1992.

Andrews, MM, Boyle JS (eds). Transcultural Concepts in Nursing Care. Philadelphia, JB Lippincott, 1995.

Bernal H, Froman R: Confidence of community health nurses in caring for ethnically diverse populations. Image 19:201–203, 1987.

Boyle JS: Culture and the community. *In* Andrews MM, Boyle JS (eds). Transcultural Concepts in Nursing Care. Philadelphia, JB Lippincott, 1995, pp. 323–352.

Garcia Coll CT: Developmental outcome of minority infants: A process-oriented look into our beginnings. Child Dev 61:270–289, 1990.

Gollnick DM, Chin PC: Multicultural Education in a Pluralistic Society, 4th ed. New York, Macmillan, 1994.

Heckler MM: Report of the Secretary's Task Force on Black and Minority Health. Washington, DC, U.S. Government Printing Office, 1985.

Herberg P: Theoretical foundations of transcultural nursing. *In* Andrews MM, Boyle JS (eds). Transcultural Concepts in Nursing Care. Philadelphia, JB Lippincott, 1995, pp. 3–48.

Jones S: Improving retention and graduation rates for black students in nursing education: A developmental model. Nurs Outlook. 40:78–85, 1992.

Katon W, Kleinman A: Doctor-patient negotiation and other social science strategies in patient care. *In* Eisenberg L, Kleinman A (eds). The Relevance of Social Science for Medicine. Boston, D. Reidel, 1981.

Kluckhohn F, Strodtbeck F: Variations in Value Orientations. Evanston, Il, Row, Peterson, 1961.

Kohls LR: Survival Kit for Overseas Living. Yarmouth, ME, Intercultural Press, 1984.

Leininger, M: Nursing and Anthropology: Two Worlds to Blend. New York, Wiley, 1970.

Leininger MM: Transcultural Nursing: Concepts, Theories, Research and Practice. Columbus, OH; McGraw Hill & Enden Press, 1995.

Leininger MM: Transcultural Nursing: Concepts, Theories, and Practice. New York, Wiley, 1978.

Leininger M: Culture, Care, Diversity, and Universality: A Theory of Nursing (Publication No. 15–2402). New York, National League for Nursing, 1991.

Ludwig-Beymer PA: Transcultural aspects of pain. *In* Andrews M, Boyle JS (eds). Transcultural Concepts in Nursing Care. Philadelphia, JB Lippincott, 1995, pp. 301–322.

National Center for Health Statistics: Health, United States, 1990. Hyattsville, MD, U.S. Public Health Service, 1991.

Office of Minority Health, Public Health Service, U.S. Department of Health & Human Services (July/August, 1996). Empowerment zones and enterprise communities. *Closing the Gap*, pp. 1–11.

Rosella J, Regan-Kubinski M, Albrecht S: The need for multicultural diversity among health professionals. Nurs Health Care 15: 242–246, 1994.

Spector R: Cultural Diversity in Health and Illness. Norwalk, CT, Appleton-Century-Crofts, 1996.

Tylor EB: Primitive Culture, vols. 1 and 2. London, Murray, 1871.

U.S. Bureau of the Census: General Population Characteristics—Part 1: United States Summary, vol. 1. Washington, DC, U.S. Government Printing Office, 1990.

U.S. Bureau of the Census: Statistical Abstract of the United States, 1992, 108th ed. Washington, DC, U.S. Government Printing Office, 1992.

U.S. Department of Health and Human Services: Public Health Service, Bureau of Health Professions, Division of Nursing: Fact Sheet: Selected Facts About Minority Registered Nurses. Washington, DC, U.S. Government Printing Office, 1993.

Zborowski, M: People in Pain. San Francisco, Jossey-Bass, 1969.

The African-American Community

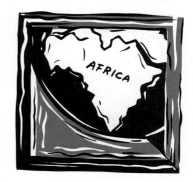

Upon completion of this chapter, the reader will be able to:

1. Identify the impacts of social, economic, and cultural trends in U.S. society on the health of African-Americans.

2. Assess the community health nursing needs of African-American individuals, families, and communities.

3. List the cultural precepts that characterize the African-American world view and identify the cultural strengths.

4. Identify ways in which community health nurses can provide culturally sensitive and culturally competent care for African-American individuals, families, and communities.

5. Analyze the major causes of excess morbidity and mortality among African-Americans and their sociopolitical causes.

6. Propose solutions to the community health problems facing African-American individuals, families, and groups.

7. List the six profiles of African-Americans.

Lucretia Bolin

Special thanks to Margaret M. Andrews for her generous contributions and her expert guidance in the development of this chapter.

To understand and facilitate empowerment in the lives of African-Americans, one needs to understand the history of African-Americans before their arrival in the United States. This intriguing history is often ignored in the teaching of history in general in primary, secondary, and higher institutions of learning. This peculiar absence of information serves to perpetuate distortions and myths about the true contributions of African peoples to historic and contemporary society. Furthermore, contemporary African-Americans live without knowledge of their past, their cultural strengths, and their ancient identity.

AFRICAN-AMERICAN HISTORY

In revealing the history of Africans and African thought and contribution, one begins to understand the significance and impact of sociopolitical, historic, and economic realities, cultural disintegration, and oppression on the lives of African-Americans. It is argued that the traumas endured by Africans forcibly transplanted to the new world sowed the seeds of their contemporary plight.

African history must be looked at anew and seen in its relationship to world history. . . . The hard fact is that most of what we now call world history is only the history of the first and second rise of Europe. The Europeans are not willing to acknowledge that the world did not wait in darkness for them to bring the light. The history of Africa was already old when Europe was born.

(CLARKE, 1991, P. 2)

Africa was not revered as a great civilization with kings and queens, system of thought, technology and science. The ancestors of modern day African Americans and modern day African peoples lived during one of the "longest periods in human development where humanity invented, experimented, and adopted beliefs about the origins and structure of the universe and mankind's nature and role in the universe."

(NOBLES, 1986, P. 20)

Significant distortions in history and knowledge have kept many in the dark, held hostage to falsifications and "scientific colonialism" (Nobles, 1986, p. 19). Scientific colonialism is a process designed to intentionally distort and propagate falsification through modification of fact or suppression. Through scientific colonialism, incorrect or distorted concepts and history are passed along through time. As a result, the purveyors of knowledge inhibit the process of knowing and the knower becomes a prisoner of these false ideas and concepts (Nobles, 1986, p. 19). For many African-Americans, this form of oppression has kept them from knowing and has inhibited them from developing a strong cultural identity in contemporary society.

Ancient African history provides the keys to understanding African value systems. These value systems have been altered and reinterpreted as a result of the diaspora attempt to survive in an alien and hostile environment. However, remnants of Ancient African thought, cultural traditions, and values, which have contributed to the collective's tensile strength and adaptability, are evident.

Before the arrival of the first Africans at Plymouth Rock, there was Pianky, king of Nubia (720 BC); Askia the Great, ruler of Songhay (1444?–1538); Abram Hannibal (1697–1782), a Russian army commander; Joseph Cinque (1811–1879), a revolutionary; Estavanico (?–1539), discoverer of Arizona; Benjamin Banneker (1731–1806), mathematician, inventor, and essayist; Alexander Pushkin (1799–1837), grandson of Abram Hannibal and Russia's greatest poet; and Alexandre Dumas (1802–1870), French playwright who wrote *The Count of Monte Cristo, The Three Musketeers,* and more than 200 volumes of work (Adams, 1972). Lewis Latimer, one of the pioneers working with Thomas Edison, drafted the plans for the telephone. Although Edison originated the principle of the electric light, it was Latimer who designed the filament (Clarke, 1991). All of these individuals were of African descent, and their works attest to the rich and varied contributions of African descendants to theater, science, technology, and government. We know very little about the contributions of other great African descendants. Traditionally, the history of Africans and African-Americans is given credence only as it relates to their plight as chattel slaves in the new world. It is as though Africa and Africans did not exist before their arrival in colonial America.

Early historical documents indicate that Africans first came to the North American continent in 1619, 1 year before the Pilgrims arrived at Plymouth Rock (Bennett, 1962). These early settlers were not slaves but rather free men and women working for their freedom as indentured servants who came to North America for the economic advantages promised by this resource-rich land. Between the time of their 17th-century arrival and 1860, however, more than 4 million Africans were brought to North America, primarily from the West Coast of Africa. Since then, Africans and their descendants have come to the United States from other parts of Africa as well as many Caribbean nations.

Although 19th-century U.S. history reminds us of Civil War efforts to free black slaves, the 20th century will be noted by historians for the struggle of African-Americans to win equal civil rights in virtually all aspects of life ranging from education to recreation. Despite the many legal strides to counter historically suppressive policies and apartheid-like practices, widespread disparities between African-Americans and Euro-Americans prevail. These disparities exist across a wide variety of contexts: serious inequalities exist in health care, such as diminished access to services, lower quality of care, fewer qualified health care providers available to meet the needs of African-American communities, and subtle racial discrimination in determining the allocation of human and material health care resources.

AFRICAN-AMERICANS IN CONTEMPORARY SOCIETY

Sociodemographic Overview

African-Americans in 1990 constituted 12.1% of the U.S. population, up from 11.7% in 1980 (Table 18–1). The African-American population has increased 13.2% versus 6.0% for Euro-Americans and 9.8% for the total population (Current Population Reports, 1991). It is projected that for the year 2000 African-Americans will account for 15% of the total population. An analysis of age composition among African-Americans indicates that 33.1% of the African-American population is younger than 18 years and that 8.2% is 65 years of age or older. An inverse gender phenomenon is reflected in these statistics; males are overrepresented in the 18-year-old and younger cohort and older women are disproportionately represented in the 65-year-old and older cohort.

Rural Versus Urban African-Americans

As shown in Table 18–2, the majority of African-Americans live in metropolitan or urban areas, but significant numbers also reside in nonmetropolitan or rural parts of the country, particularly in the South. The rural and urban lifestyles are markedly different (see Chapter 16).

SOCIOECONOMIC APARTHEID: POVERTY AS A RISK FACTOR

According to the most current data available from the U.S. Bureau of the Census (Current Population Reports, 1991), African-American family income represented 56% of Euro-American family income. The annual median income for white families in 1989 was $35,980, higher than the 1980 level of $23,520, whereas that for African-American families in 1989 was only $20,210, higher than the 1980 level of $14,460 (Current Population Reports, 1991; U.S. Bureau of the Census, 1983). These figures are misleading because they fail to show that African-American family incomes must be used to support more family members and that in more African-American families both the husband and the wife are employed than in white families and they earn disproportionately less than their white counterparts. Furthermore, the U.S. Department of Labor indicated that the majority of female-headed African-American families live below the federally defined poverty level.

Economic deprivation characterizes a significant number of African-American families. One third of the African-American population lives in poverty compared with 12% of the white population. In 1993, more than 10 million (33.1%) of African-Americans were poor. Although 25% of poor African-Americans receive some form of public assistance, only 10% of poor whites receive such aid. African-American families are nearly three times as likely to be poor in comparison with white families. Approximately 45.9% of all African-American children are members of these families. Seventeen percent of white children live in households that are officially defined as poor. African-American families headed by females have the highest poverty rate, compared with African-American married couples and male-headed households (Current Population Reports, 1991; National Center for Health Statistics, 1995).

Poverty statistics reflect employability, education, and opportunity for employment. Overall, the current trend reveals that African-Americans, regardless of gender, are more likely to be unemployed. In 1989 11.8% of African-American men and 10.8% of African-American women in the labor pool were unemployed compared with 4.8% of white men and 4.0% of white women (Current Population Reports, 1991).

Even if African-Americans are employed, there is a great discrepancy in median earnings when contrasted

Table 18–1
Black Resident Population by State for 1990 and 1980

1990 Black Population Rank	State	1990 Black Population	1990 Percentage of State Population	1980 Black Population	1980 Percentage of State Population	Change from 1980 to 1990 (n)	Change from 1980 to 1990 (%)
1	New York	2,859,055	15.9	2,402,006	13.7	457,049	19.0
2	California	2,208,801	7.4	1,819,281	7.7	389,520	21.4
3	Texas	2,021,632	11.9	1,710,175	12.0	311,457	18.2
4	Florida	1,759,534	13.6	1,342,688	13.8	416,846	31.0
5	Georgia	1,746,565	27.0	1,465,181	26.8	281,384	19.2
6	Illinois	1,694,273	14.8	1,675,398	14.7	18,875	1.1
7	North Carolina	1,456,323	22.0	1,318,857	22.4	137,466	10.4
8	Louisiana	1,299,281	30.8	1,238,241	29.4	61,040	4.9
9	Michigan	1,291,706	13.9	1,199,023	12.9	92,683	7.7
10	Maryland	1,189,899	24.9	958,150	22.7	231,749	24.2
11	Virginia	1,162,994	18.8	1,008,668	18.9	154,326	15.3
12	Ohio	1,154,826	10.6	1,076,748	10.0	78,078	7.3
13	Pennsylvania	1,089,795	9.2	1,046,810	8.8	42,985	4.1
14	South Carolina	1,039,884	29.8	948,623	30.4	91,261	9.6
15	New Jersey	1,036,825	13.4	925,066	12.6	111,759	12.1
16	Alabama	1,020,705	25.3	996,335	25.6	24,370	2.4
17	Mississippi	915,057	35.6	887,206	35.2	27,851	3.1
18	Tennessee	778,035	16.0	725,942	15.8	52,093	7.2
19	Missouri	548,208	10.7	514,276	10.5	33,932	6.6
20	Indiana	432,092	7.8	414,785	7.6	17,307	4.2
21	District of Columbia	399,604	65.8	448,906	70.3	−49,302	−11.0
22	Arkansas	373,912	15.9	373,768	16.3	144	0.0
23	Massachusetts	300,130	5.0	221,279	3.9	78,851	35.6
24	Connecticut	274,269	8.3	217,433	7.0	56,836	26.1
25	Kentucky	262,907	7.1	259,477	7.1	3430	1.3
26	Wisconsin	244,539	5.0	182,592	3.9	61,947	33.9
27	Oklahoma	233,801	7.4	204,674	6.8	29,127	14.2
28	Washington	149,801	3.1	105,574	2.6	44,227	41.9
29	Kansas	143,076	5.8	126,127	5.3	16,949	13.4
30	Colorado	133,146	4.0	101,703	3.5	31,443	30.9
31	Delaware	112,460	16.9	95,845	16.1	16,615	17.3
32	Arizona	110,524	3.0	74,977	2.8	35,547	47.4
33	Minnesota	94,944	2.2	53,344	1.3	41,600	78.0
34	Nevada	78,771	6.6	50,999	6.4	27,772	54.5

Table 18–1
Black Resident Population by State for 1990 and 1980 *Continued*

1990 Black Population Rank	State	1990 Black Population	1990 Percentage of State Population	1980 Black Population	1980 Percentage of State Population	Change from 1980 to 1990 (n)	Change from 1980 to 1990 (%)
35	Nebraska	57,404	3.6	48,390	3.1	9014	18.6
36	West Virginia	56,295	3.1	65,051	3.3	−8756	−13.5
37	Iowa	48,090	1.7	41,700	1.4	6390	15.3
38	Oregon	46,178	1.6	37,060	1.4	9118	24.6
39	Rhode Island	38,861	3.9	27,584	2.9	11,277	40.9
40	New Mexico	30,210	2.0	24,020	1.8	6190	25.8
41	Hawaii	27,195	2.5	17,364	1.8	9831	56.6
42	Alaska	22,451	4.1	13,643	3.4	8808	64.6
43	Utah	11,576	0.7	9225	0.6	2351	25.5
44	New Hampshire	7198	0.6	3990	0.4	3208	80.4
45	Maine	5138	0.4	3128	0.3	2010	64.3
46	Wyoming	3606	0.8	3364	0.7	242	7.2
47	North Dakota	3524	0.6	2568	0.4	956	37.2
48	Idaho	3370	0.3	2716	0.3	654	24.1
49	South Dakota	3258	0.5	2144	0.3	1114	52.0
50	Montana	2381	0.3	1786	0.2	595	33.3
51	Vermont	1951	0.3	1135	0.2	816	71.9

The population counts set forth herein are subject to possible correction for undercount or overcount. The United States Department of Commerce is considering whether to correct these counts and will publish corrected counts, if any, no later than July 15, 1991.

Adapted from the U.S. Bureau of the Census. United States Population Estimates by Age, Sex, Race, and Hispanic Origin: 1980 to 1988. Series P-25, No. 1045. Washington DC: U.S. Government Printing Office, 1990; and Current Population Reports: The black population in the United States: March 1990 and 1989. Series P-20, No. 448. Washington, DC: U.S. Government Printing Office, 1991, pp. 1–17.

with those of Euro-Americans. In 1989, the median earnings of African-American men and women were 69% and 98%, respectively, of that of their Euro-American counterparts. African-American women earn comparatively less than African-American men. On the basis of the past rate of progress in integration of African-Americans into the labor force, it will take 90 years for African-American professionals to approximate the proportion of African-Americans in the population (Staples, 1982).

Education

Traditional institutional educational systems have failed the African-American aggregate. The African-American aggregate is struggling with a population that is functionally illiterate secondary to chronic educational failure. Furthermore, those who are capable of navigating traditional institutions tend to take on values and beliefs similar to Euro-Americans. These individuals, socialized into Euro-American culture, fail to grasp at the core the significance of the African-American dilemma. As a result, they fail to develop workable solutions to the problems facing their community. If they do develop solutions, these solutions are born out of Euro-American perspectives and theories. One has to wonder what happens in the psyche of African-Americans socialized in Euro-American educational institutions.

The percentage of African-Americans graduating from high school is lower than that of Euro-Americans. Just over 66% of African-Americans have completed high school compared with 79.9% of Euro-Americans. Disparities in rates of college enroll-

Table 18–2
Percentage Distribution of Whites and African-Americans by Geographic Area, 1990

Geographic Area	Distribution (%)	
	White (N = 206,983,000)	African American (N = 30,392,000)
Total population	84.1	12.3
Northeast	21.1	17.4
Midwest	25.3	19.8
South	31.9	54.3
West	21.7	8.5
Metropolitan areas	76.4	83.8
Nonmetropolitan areas	23.6	16.2

Adapted from Current Population Reports (1991). The black population in the United States: March 1990 and 1989, Series P-20, No. 448. Washington, DC: U.S. Government Printing Office, pp. 1–17.

ment and college completion also exist for African-Americans (Current Population Reports, 1992a). African-American women tend to have completed more education than African-American men. Furthermore, despite much rhetoric about equal opportunities for women in the work place, significant gender bias exists, resulting in women earning much less than men.

College-educated Euro-Americans face fewer barriers to career aspirations than do college-educated African-Americans, who are unemployed as frequently as Euro-American men who have not graduated from high school (U.S. Civil Rights Commission, 1982).

SOCIAL JUSTICE: AN AFRICAN-AMERICAN PERSPECTIVE

Self-Concept, Racism, and Racial Identity

Bridging the great cultural and racial divide requires more than a rudimentary knowledge and understanding of the cultural, historic, and economic realities of African-American life. Cultural sensitivity and cultural competence beyond a level of basic familiarity are tantamount. Cultural sensitivity implies an accep-

tance and understanding of the dynamics that have shaped and altered ancient values and beliefs of African-Americans. To be culturally sensitive suggests that people have an awareness of their own cultural "baggage" and how it affects their interactions and perceptions of African-Americans.

Cultural competence implies that one can effectively use the knowledge of the group and build on the internal strengths to effect positive changes. One does not necessarily need to be an identified member of the aggregate to be culturally competent and sensitive. Understanding the history of Africans before their arrival in the New World promotes cultural sensitivity.

African-Americans share a distinct and unique immigrant history like that of no other group. Their history is distinguished from other immigrant groups in that they

1. Were forcibly transplanted from the continent of Africa
2. Endured the traumatic hardships of chattel slavery, which has affected their contemporary existence in Western society
3. Have had to survive and endure in a hostile and oppressive environment

Although surface similarities and differences are readily apparent, observable and discernible, the dynamic connective factors and forces that give groups wholeness, uniqueness and unity within their own diversity are usually of a different nature and less easily discernible and recognized. Groups are bound together by the intangible, non-material elements of culture.

(BUTLER, 1992, P. 24)

Culture, for African-Americans, helps to define who they are, what they know, what they feel, and what they do. It is these factors that help to distinguish African-Americans from other groups. Contemporary African-American culture and world view are tied to ancient African value systems and philosophy. Therefore, modern-day behavior and thought, which have been altered to survive, reflect ancient African epistemology, cosmology, and ontology. It is the continuation of this African-centered world view that is at the root of the special features of contemporary African-American life.

Ancient African ontologic principles, or the nature of being in the universe, recognize that all things have force or spirit and are interconnected. Humans are but a manifestation of the spirit in a concrete, tangible form. Thus, all things are one. The universe is alive in a multiplicity of forms, and all forms are interconnected through divine spirit. This interconnectedness is made manifest in harmonious and disharmonious patterns between these forces or spirits. All things are striving for harmonious interaction and balance.

Historical forces, in particular the period of slavery, have altered the basic African-centered principles and values. This alteration in ontological, cosmological, and epistemological principles has created a psychological schism within the diaspora. This schism reflects the attempt to achieve and define self-collective identity, and self-determination within the confines of an oppressive environment. The African-American is faced with a peculiar duality of person and consciousness (Fig. 18–1). In seeking to assimilate and to be like those of European descent, African-Americans must struggle with and lose their ancient sense of identity. This has created obvious dilemmas, threats to individual and collective survival, and cultural and community disintegration. Assimilation necessarily creates dissonance because the individual must negate some aspects of him- or herself and accept other false and incorrect perceptions of the group. More specifically, this schism leads some African-Americans to accept covert theories of inferiority.

African-Americans must develop a sense of self in an environment that is often cruel, violent, and indifferent to their existence. They must develop the capacity for self-motivation, initiative, and transcendence in a society whose institutions are often negligent toward their development and well-being. The struggle for identity could easily be considered the major theme of African-American existence (Butler, 1992, p. 26). African-American identity embodies Afrocentric values and ethos, a common cultural

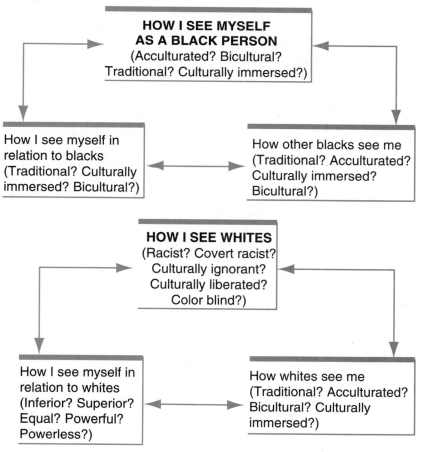

Figure 18–1
Adapted from Butler, JP 1992. Of kindred minds: the ties that bind. *In* Olandi MA, Weston R, Epstein LG (eds): Cultural Competence for Evaluators: A Guide for Alcohol and Other Drug Prevention Practitioners Working with Ethnic/Racial Communities. Rockville, Maryland, U.S. Department of Health and Human Services, Office of Substance Abuse Prevention.

heritage and an emotional bond that is interconnected and interrelated to past generations. These bonds have created a sense of oneness and unity among African-Americans. This unity echoes that the individual is part of a larger whole, and his or her existence is connected to the existence of the whole. Unity is a primary guiding principle of African-American culture and reflects a cultural strength.

Positive self-identity and racial identity for African-Americans are rooted in the conscious awareness of ancient African history, the cultural heritage, and the ability to survive and endure. On the other hand, negative self-identity and racial identity are the result of a negation of African heritage and culture.

The negation of African heritage reflects the process of scientific colonialism. Negative self-identity leads to behaviors that erode the community fabric and cultural and community cohesion and values. Furthermore, negative self-identity contributes to morbidity and mortality and ultimately undermines the strengths that have aided the survival of the group.

African-American identity, past and present, reflects processes of subordination and domination through socialization and contact with an oppressive and violent society. It is through this socialization that African-Americans develop an identity of themselves and of other African-Americans. As a result of this socialization, African-Americans develop a functional sense of inferiority. This process of overt and covert racism and oppression operates within the family, the community, and the society at large. Cress-Welsing (1991) asserted that "this social process of destructive distortion is achieved [in a racist and oppressive social structure] through the imposition, from birth to death, of stressful, negative, and non-supportive social/environmental experience. . . . The negative and stressful experience, which is structured to affect every aspect of life activity, leads to the development of negative self-identity, loss of self-respect and the development of self- and group-destructive behavioral patterns" (p. 244).

Profiles of African-Americans

African-American identity typically aligns along six dimensions or profiles: *the acculturated, the bicultural, the culturally immersed conformist, the culturally immersed Afrocentric, the culturally immersed deviant, and the traditional unacculturated.* These profiles are neither rigid nor fixed. Familiarity with

these profiles is important to understand the diversity within the group and the individual's view of him- or herself.

Acculturated African-Americans tend to resemble Euro-Americans in thought, behavior, and beliefs. They have adopted values and views of the world and of other African-Americans that align with those of Euro-Americans. Thus, they may accept false ideas of African-American inferiority, which is often covertly reinforced in their interactions with Euro-Americans. Acculturated African-Americans have both their human and personal needs met within the Euro-American environment.

Biculturally oriented African-Americans (Bell, 1990) have the ability to move between both the African-American and Euro-American aggregate. They adopt roles and behaviors similar to the group with which they are interacting. Thus, they have unique bilingual ability. They may have tremendous role conflict when interacting in integrated settings, questioning which role to play. Bicultural African-Americans have a strong sense of racial identity and racial pride. The survival needs of bicultural African-Americans are met predominantly within the Euro-American culture, but their personal needs tend to be met within the African-American community.

Culturally immersed conformists (Bell, 1990) have a strong sense of racial pride and identity. Their survival needs are met most often within the Euro-American community, but their interaction with Euro-Americans is limited to the work environment. Culturally immersed conformists meet their personal needs primarily within the African-American community. This group tends to distrust the acculturated African-American.

Culturally immersed Afrocentrics (Bell, 1990, p. 60) have a strong self-identity as African-Americans. Members of this group resemble the acculturated and bicultural only in education. The driving force in culturally immersed Afrocentrics' lives is to "build a powerful and economically independent black community" (Bell, 1990, p. 61).

Culturally immersed deviants (Bell, 1990) represent the group that is often most intimidating to Euro-Americans. They are generally distrustful of Euro-Americans and acculturated and bicultural African-Americans. Members of this group often have value systems that are distinctly opposite of those of Euro-Americans. This group has most of its personal and survival needs met within the African-American community. Some members of this group may be involved in deviant criminal activity, distrustful of organizations, and extremely distrustful of those African-Americans whom they believe have sold out.

Traditional unacculturated African-Americans typically are individuals who have strong spiritual values (Bell, 1990). Members of this group traditionally are older than those of the other subgroups. Members of this group share a sense of pride with acculturated African-Americans with respect to their accomplishments. Their survival needs are met in a Euro-American context, and their human needs are met within the African-American community. They tend to see integration as necessary but do not value assimilation. They are most often the ones who support the ideologies of a color-blind society.

The community health nurse needs to identify the subgroup to which the client belongs. As a general rule and observation, Euro-Americans are most at ease with acculturated African-Americans. Members of this group are most likely to share similar values and ideologies and to deny or ignore the significance of culture and race.

Racism: Redefining It as Violence

According to Amuleru-Marshall (1992) citing Bulhan, "the nature of the historical position of [African-American] people[s] in relation to the fundamental productive and social processes in [Western] society has been characterized as violent" (p. 41). Racism should be redefined as a form of violence characterized by one group's persistent and continuous efforts to dominate and control another. For African-Americans this type of violence manifests as powerlessness, feelings of worthlessness, subjection to ongoing chronic and traumatic stressors, inadequate living conditions, and feelings of rage that are often displaced toward others. The differential exposure or subjection of African-Americans to harm, threats, and differential treatment has been institutionalized and to some extent normalizes racism.

Furthermore, normalization of this type of violence fosters denial, promoting and supporting the political, economic, and interpersonal mechanisms that lead to early morbidity and mortality in the African-American community.

Racism is one of the major recurrent stressors in the lives of African-Americans. Racism—organizational, institutional, and individual—handicaps the lives of African-Americans. It influences and shapes their life experiences over a variety of contexts. The occurrence of disparities across a variety of contexts is linked to the precarious relationship between African-Americans and Euro-Americans. Past and current negative attitudes of Euro-Americans toward African-Americans have contributed to their current social marginality and a lack of structural incorporation in the dominant culture.

According to Cheung (1991), racial discrimination exists, particularly for visible people of color. For many African-Americans, racial discrimination takes the form of socioeconomic segregation. Racial discrimination (i.e., socioeconomic segregation), stated Cheung (1991), "has always denied [African-Americans and other people of color] equal access to social, economic, and political institutions, thereby hampering their [participation] and structural incorporation into the larger society" (p. 593). Blocked opportunities to succeed, achieve, and obtain legitimate goals foster extreme conditions of stress, learned helplessness, and depression at individual and collective levels.

Persistent violence, in the form of racism and disadvantaged conditions, reinforce African-Americans' current position of social marginality. One of the by-products of racial discrimination is continuing and persistent disparities in important indicators of living conditions, particularly in the areas of health, morbidity, and mortality. Furthermore, African-Americans socialized under an oppressive structure struggle with their own issues of internalized racism.

Internalized racism brings with it greater chaos, disorganization, and internal disruption for the aggregate and the individual. Confronted with the duality of self, African-Americans struggle to confront the societal misconception of racial inferiority. To accept the implications of racial inferiority is to accept that one is limited in capacity and potential. Internalized racism is often manifest in within-group rhetoric wherein a caste system based on shade of skin color determines ones inherent value.

The attempt to understand African-American culture and individuals from a Eurocentric philosophical base fails to acknowledge the diversity within the aggregate. Furthermore, there is a failure to accept that Eurocentric theories and strategies are insufficient for an explanation of African-American behavior. What one typically sees is that some African-American behavior is considered pathogenic compared with that of Euro-Americans, which is considered the norm.

What ensues when Euro-American academicians and clinicians attempt to understand one thought system and culture with methods relevant to another is confusion, misunderstanding, inappropriate and incorrect negative perceptions, and faulty theories and strategies that address irrelevant or insignificant factors. These faulty strategies fail to alter negative behavior patterns within the African-American aggregate. When these theories and strategies are unchallenged or uncorrected, they result in a continuation of oppression, racism, and scientific colonialism. Some African-American behaviors are classified as deviant, and interventions are aimed at bringing the behavior of the collective in line with that of Euro-Americans.

African-American Cultural Beliefs

African-American cultural beliefs guide African-American behavior. One would be remiss if one did not understand that contemporary behavior, values, and beliefs of African-Americans reflect a dynamic interplay between the political, social, and economic realities affecting their lives. However, some contemporary behavior such as that exhibited by culturally immersed deviants should not be understood as an expression of African-American culture and values. Such behavior is a response to the forces in play in a hostile environment.

African-American World View and Cultural Precepts

In the traditional African-American community, the world view has been guided by eight cultural precepts that reflect ancient African metaphysics. An awareness of these precepts facilitates cultural sensitivity, provides an Afrocentric framework to guide interventions, and raises our collective understanding of the positive dynamic forces that shape and define values and behaviors of African-Americans.

Consubstantiation: all things have the same essence, which is force and spirit.

Interdependence: all things are interconnected and interrelated.

Egalitarianism: because all things are of the same essence they are in fact the same and equal, and the ideological relationship between all things is harmonious interaction.

Collectivism: the individual is part of a larger whole whose survival is dependent on the collective survival.

Transformation: all things are striving to function at a higher and greater level.

Cooperation: closely tied to collectivism, cooperation is necessary for the transformation and survival of the group.

Humaneness: this guides the individual's relationship and behavior with others to ensure cooperation, collectivism, egalitarianism, cohesiveness, and collective survival.

Synergism: this precept underscores the significance of a cooperative effort that acknowledges the collective effort to be greater than the individual effort in bringing about transformation and change.

Spirituality, the belief in God, has given African-Americans a transcendent meaning to life. Religion and spirituality have provided the aggregate with a framework in which to understand their struggle and plight. African-Americans are an immensely spiritual people. God is the creator of all, and all things are endowed with force and spirit (consubstantiation).

In the practice of spirituality, one finds remnants of the cultural precepts that explain the nuances of African-American behaviors. Vocal expression and oral patterns represent the major form of communication with the African-American community. This is readily apparent in African-American churches and in music and rhythm.

The church service is an exchange that often calls for transformation, collectivism, egalitarianism, and cooperation. The preacher shares his or her force or spirit with the congregation using a highly stylized, lyrical, and rhythmical language. This form of communication, coupled with bodily expressions, communicates that which language alone fails to transmit. The rhythm and vocal expression and intonation set the tone and are used to involve the audience in an affective display of interaction. Expression is encouraged in this interaction to maintain the emotional tone and climate and the interconnectedness between the preacher and the congregation. The preacher is central to this relationship, reflecting the African-American cultural value toward people, who are, in essence, force or spirit. Thus, experiences, phenomena, and information are important as they relate to people. This is typically in opposition to the Euro-American methods of communication and values of individualism.

Within the church, one observes an interactional process of call and response. It is not atypical to hear the congregation engage with the preacher, shouting out "hallelujah," "amen," "thank you, Jesus!" These are not construed as interruptions but rather as affirmations and encouragement. On a deeper level this form of communication serves to maintain the ties between the preacher and the members of the congregation. This is unlike the traditional Euro-American orator-audience scenario in which the orator presents the material and members of the audience patiently wait to respond.

Changing Patterns of African-American Family Life

The African-American family has and continues to struggle against overt and covert forces seeking to undermine its stability. Slavery undermined the stability of family by disrupting child rearing, bonding, and ties between family members. The African slave and his or her offspring responded to these disruptions and premature separations by forming extended kinship clans of individuals who were related to one another by a variety of means.

The African-American family is typically an extended network reflecting the cultural precepts of collectivism, cooperation, and synergism. Members of the family may not necessarily be related by birth or marriage. The family typically has strong kinship ties and shares family roles. Roles are "determined by ability rather than by gender or marital association" (Lassiter, 1994, p. 5).

Marriage reflects a union between networks and extended family, forming a larger network. The network forms the basis of a larger kinship unit that is flexible and adaptable. This flexibility serves to facilitate stability and survival of the family through flexible roles, intergenerational relationships, and child-rearing practices and the transmission of cultural values and expectations through language and behavior.

Married African-Americans face the same economic and cultural forces that undermine the marital stability of the general population. Between 1970 and 1991, the number of individuals who were divorced tripled from 4.3 million to more than 15 million (Current Population Reports, 1992b). There has been a general decline in the percentage of married African-Americans from 1970 (64%) to 1991 (44%). The proportion of divorced African-Americans rose from 4 to 11% in comparison with a rise of 3 to 8% for whites. When the economic aspects are considered, the divorce rate of middle-class African-Americans is lower, because chances for a stable marriage increase in parallel with family income and educational achievement (U.S. Bureau of the Census, 1990).

The strengths of the African-American family are its extended kinship network, sharing of roles, flexibility, and spiritual connectedness. It is not uncommon to find aunts and uncles, grandmothers, and neighbors sharing in the disciplining of children. Children are important. They embody force and spirit and represent the family's ongoing work toward transcendence. Values and behaviors are transmitted to children through intergenerational relationships in which grandparents may play an active and valued role in the network.

The African-American family unit is vitally important in shaping, defining, and socializing its members. The African-American family can begin to prepare the children with skills necessary for self and collective determination through a process of Afrocentric socialization.

ROLES

In recent years, the issue of sex roles has received considerable attention, with the debate centering on female subordination and male dominance and privilege. African-Americans must grapple with both racial discrimination and role identity issues.

African-American men are frequently stereotyped as "irresponsible, criminalistic, hypersexual, and lacking in masculine traits" (Staples, 1988, p. 312). Remember the culturally immersed deviant profile previously mentioned (Cheung, 1991). Although mainstream culture has deprived many African-American men of the economic ability to perform what are considered stereotypic male work roles and functions, most function in a way that gains the respect of their children, peers, and community (Staples, 1988).

African-American women are struggling with issues such as equal pay for equal work, child care facilities, and female parity in the work force. Instead of joining the predominantly white middle-class women's movement, many African-American women have formed their own organizations such as the Welfare Rights Organization, Black Women Organized for Action, and the Black Feminist Alliance.

Relationships between African-American men and women have experienced a unique evolution. Unlike the Euro-American family, which is characterized by a patriarchy historically sustained by the economic dependence of women, the African-American dyad is characterized by more equal roles and economic parity. The system of slavery did not permit African-American men to assume the dominant role in the family constellation. In recent times, lower class African-American women have tended to be the breadwinners (through employment or receipt of government aid), enjoy higher levels of education than their male counterparts, and hold dominant positions in their families. Thus, in African-American families, relationships between men and women depend on sociopsychological factors rather than an economic compulsion to marry and remain married.

Finding and keeping a mate are complicated by a number of psychosocial factors as well as structural restraints. First, there are more African-American women than men, creating high levels of competition among women. Second, although some African-American men are threatened by successful African-American women, further investigation reveals other underlying forces such as the need for security versus the desire for freedom and the quest for monogamous intimacy versus the seduction of sexual variety. The traditional exchange of feminine sexual appeal for male financial support is declining as women are able to define their own status and become economically independent. Research indicates that African-American wives are usually less satisfied with their marriages than are white wives. However, the source of their dissatisfaction is often associated with the problems created by poverty and racism (Staples, 1988).

COMMUNICATION AND LANGUAGE

During the past several decades, there has been increasing literature and interest centering around *black English,* especially its impact on the educational process of African-American children. Smitherman (1977) referred to black English as reflecting "linguistic-cultural African heritage and the conditions of servitude, oppression and life in America."

Black English has been referred to as black dialect, black Creole, soul talk, Afro-American speech, ebonics, and Afro. Regardless of the terminology used, it is a dialect spoken at some time by 80 to 90% of African-Americans and is essentially Euro-American speech with African-American meaning, nuance, tone, and gesture (Smitherman, 1977).

Development of Black English

During the period of slavery, West African slaves from different tribes developed a form of communication,

known as pidgin, to communicate among themselves as well as with whites. Pidgin is a form of communication used when two persons speak two different languages and do not have a common third language *(lingua franca).* Because African languages were not used widely, offspring of the early slaves began to speak English pidgin, which eventually developed into a new language known as Creole. In this language, West African structure and idiom are retained but English words are substituted (Orque et al., 1983; Smitherman, 1977).

Characteristics of Black English

Black English is a highly oral, stylized, rhythmical, spontaneous language. Smitherman (1977) developed an African-American language model that is divided into two aspects: linguistic and stylistic. The linguistic aspect focuses on grammatical structure and word usage, establishing rules of black English.

The stylistic aspect refers to the communication power of black English through various ritual forms or modes that give meaning to the sounds and grammatical structure (e.g., sermon, prayer, spiritual hymns, folk songs, toasts, verbal contests, voodoo curses, and so forth). All of these indicate the power of the spoken word among African-Americans, and many reflect cultural attitudes toward time, nature, the universe, life, death, and evil (Orque et al., 1983; Smitherman, 1973, 1977). African-American communication patterns reflect spontaneity. Spontaneity is a result of the need and necessity to adapt and to be flexible to changing environmental demands. Spontaneity is rooted in historic forces that forced African-Americans to emphasize the spoken word.

African-Americans have a highly developed sense of auditory and listening capacity. They are acutely sensitive to inflections, intonation, and expressions of others. Traditionally, this ability facilitated their adaptability and survival. Slaves were forced to develop highly acute senses and perceptions in order to problem solve. This required great spontaneity and an ability to adapt to internal cues triggered by the expressions, inflections, and behavior of others.

It is important to remember that variations in age, social class, educational level, and locale among African-Americans influence the communicative process. Some African-Americans—the acculturated, the bicultural, and culturally immersed Afrocentrics—are bilingual. Members of these groups move in and out of language patterns depending on the group with whom they are interacting. This underscores the necessity of a thorough cultural assessment to avoid relying on generalizations.

HEALTH BELIEFS AND PRACTICES

Traditional Beliefs About Health and Illness

Traditionally, with regards to health beliefs and health practices, health and illness were viewed as two parts of one unit and connected to the spirit forces. Thus, mind and body were inseparable, and illness was a product of interaction with the environment (Lassiter, 1994). Illness was also the product of disharmony with the environment.

Illness is viewed either as natural or unnatural. Natural illnesses are linked to inappropriate self-care such as exposure to toxins, pollutants, cold, and rain. Unnatural illnesses are the result of forces such as witchcraft, voodoo, or punishment for one's transgressions against others.

Contemporary health beliefs and health practices vary among African-Americans as a function of social class, economics, altered beliefs, and acculturation. Thus, middle-class African-Americans may be less likely to ascribe illness to a theory of hexation or punishment. Traditional unacculturated African-Americans who hold strong religious and spiritual beliefs may view illness as a retribution from God for sins against humanity.

The traditional views of health and illness stem from the African belief regarding life and the nature of being. To many Africans, life is a process rather than a state, and a person is viewed in terms of energy forces rather than matter. All things, whether living or dead, are believed to influence each other. Therefore, humans have the power to influence their own and others' destinies through the use of behavior, whether proper or otherwise, as well as through knowledge of the person and the world. In health, the person is in harmony with nature; illness occurs with disharmony. Traditional beliefs about health are holistic, with mind, body, and spirit being integrally interwoven (Spector, 1986).

Illness, or disharmony, is attributed to a number of sources, primarily demons and evil spirits who act on their own accord. The goal of treatment, from the traditional African perspective, is to remove the harmful spirits from the body of the ill person. Several methods are used by healers.

Sociopolitical Variations in Health and Illness

The health status of African-American peoples is a function of historic and contemporary forces, economics, and unjust power balances. This is painfully evident in the disparities in health status, morbidity, and mortality between African-Americans and Euro-Americans.

Historically, there has been and continues to be a troubling disparity in the health status of African-Americans compared with that of Euro-Americans. Simplistic explanations impute these disparities to perceived genetic differences and inherent inferiority. However, "the evidence suggests that the contribution of genetic susceptibility is relatively small" (Nickens, 1991, p. 27). Adherence to genetic theories and theories of racial inferiority are reminiscent of eugenics. Furthermore, attribution of differences to genetics is oppressive. These troubling disparities continue to exist despite advances in medical technologies and treatments.

Life expectancy for all races climbed to an average of 75.8 years in 1992 (Table 18–3). African-Americans have an average life expectancy of 69.8 years compared with 76.5 years for Euro-Americans (Wegman, 1993). Life expectancy for African-American women was 73.9 years compared with 65.5 years for African-American men.

Major causes of death according to the provisional 1992 mortality rate per 100,000 were heart disease, malignant neoplasms, respiratory diseases, accidents, infectious diseases, diabetes mellitus, suicide, perinatal conditions, homicide and legal intervention, and chronic liver disease (Wegman, 1993).

African-Americans have a higher age-adjusted death rate for all but respiratory diseases and suicide. The major disparities in age-adjusted death rates involve human immunodeficiency virus (HIV) and acquired immunodeficiency syndrome (AIDS) (3.4:1), homicide and legal intervention (6.8:1), and perinatal conditions (2.1:1). The overall age-adjusted death rate for African-Americans compared with Euro-Americans in 1990 was 780.7 versus 486.8 per 100,000. African-Americans have a disproportionately high incidence of hypertensive disease, diabetes, cancer, and glaucoma. One of every four African-Americans has hypertension compared with one of

Table 18–3
Life Expectancy in Years by Race and Sex: United States, Selected Years

Year	All Races Both Sexes	Male	Female	White Both Sexes	Male	Female	Black Both Sexes	Male	Female	Proportion by Which Female Exceeds Male Life Expectancy (%) All Races	White	Black
Average length of life												
1992	75.7	72.3	79.0	76.5	73.2	79.7	69.8	65.5	73.9	9.3	8.9	12.8
1990	75.4	71.8	78.8	76.1	72.7	79.4	69.1	64.5	73.6	9.7	9.2	14.1
1980	73.7	70.0	77.4	74.4	70.7	78.1	68.1	63.8	72.5	10.6	10.5	13.6
1970	70.8	67.1	74.7	71.7	68.0	75.6	64.1	60.0	68.3	11.3	11.2	13.8
1960	69.7	66.6	73.1	70.6	67.4	74.1	63.6	61.1	66.3	9.8	9.9	8.5
1940	62.9	60.8	65.2	64.2	62.1	66.6	53.1	51.5	54.9	7.2	7.2	6.6
1900	47.3	46.3	48.3	47.6	46.6	48.7	33.0	32.5	33.5	4.3	4.5	3.1
Percentage increase in length of life												
1900–1992	60	56	64	61	57	64	112	102	121			
1900–1940	33	31	35	35	33	37	61	58	64			
1940–1992	20	19	21	19	18	20	31	27	35			

Adapted from Wegman ME (1993). Annual summary of vital statistics—1992. Pediatrics 92:747.

every seven whites. African-American men aged 45 to 64 years have a 41% higher mortality rate than white men, and the mortality rate for African-American women is more than twice that for white women. During the past 25 years, the rate of cancer mortality among whites has increased only 5% compared with 26% for African-Americans. Table 18–4 summarizes the annual total and "excess" deaths for African-Americans for selected causes of mortality.

Indicators of Health in the African-American Population

McCord and Freeman (1990) examined excess mortality in Harlem. Age-adjusted rates of mortality, from all causes, was higher for African-Americans living in Harlem than for both Euro-Americans and African-Americans in the United States as a whole. The authors attribute these differences in mortality to poverty, poor housing conditions, chronic psychological stress, substance abuse, and inadequate access to medical care. What is even more distressing than the ratios themselves is that most of the excess mortality among

African-Americans was due to preventable and treatable causes.

When studies controlling for income examine differences in mortality between African-Americans and Euro-Americans, differentials continue to exist. Sorlie and colleagues (1992) studied black-white mortality differences by family income using data from the National Longitudinal Mortality Study. Findings from their data analysis revealed that, regardless of level of income, African-American men and women have higher rates of mortality. Excess mortality was greatest for African-Americans occupying the lowest income group.

Survival rates for African-Americans in later life are greater than those for Euro-Americans. However, elderly African-Americans are more likely to endure greater rates of poverty and illness than their Euro-American counterparts (Johnson, 1991).

In essence, African-Americans are dying earlier in life from preventable and treatable causes. The availability of technology and the strides made against disease have done little to stem the tide in African-American mortality. AIDS and homicide have become leading causes of mortality in the African-American populace. Excess deaths among African-Americans between the ages of 45 and 69 years were mainly the result of cancer, heart disease, stroke, diabetes, and cirrhosis (Nickens, 1991).

CARDIOVASCULAR DISEASE

Heart disease and stroke cause more deaths, disability, and economic loss in the United States than any other acute or chronic diseases, and they are the leading causes of days lost from work. At all ages and for both sexes, cardiovascular and cerebrovascular diseases are major problems for the African-American population.

African-American men are almost twice as likely to die from stroke as are white men, and their death rate from stroke is more than twice that of other minorities. There is also a marked excess of hypertension, a major risk factor for stroke.

Table 18–4
Average Annual Total and Excess Deaths in African-Americans for Selected Causes of Mortality

Variable	Excess Deaths in Males and Females (Cumulative to Age 70)	
	No.	%
Causes of excess death		
Heart disease and stroke	18,181	30.8
Homicide and accidents	10,909	18.5
Cancer	8118	13.8
Infant mortality	6178	10.5
Cirrhosis	2154	3.7
Diabetes	1850	3.1
Subtotal	47,390	80.4
All other causes	11,552	19.6
Total excess deaths	58,942	100
Total deaths, all causes	128,635	
Ratio of excess deaths to total population		42.5
Percent contribution of six causes to excess death		80.4

Adapted from Heckler MM (1985). Report of the Secretary's Task Force on Black and Minority Health. Washington, DC: U.S. Government Printing Office.

Studies show that among 20- to 64-year-old African-Americans there is an excess mortality from coronary heart disease (Kochanek et al., 1994). This is more marked in African-American women than in men. More white men are hospitalized for acute myocardial infarction than are African-American men, possibly because of the higher rate of sudden death in African-Americans before hospital admission or the decreased availability of emergency services such as ambulances and paramedical assistance in African-American communities.

The major risk factors for cardiovascular and cerebrovascular diseases are hypertension, elevated cholesterol levels, smoking, and obesity, factors that can be combated by intensive public health efforts (Brooks et al., 1991).

Hypertension. High blood pressure is much more common among African-Americans, especially men, than in other groups. The mortality rate from cerebrovascular accidents (i.e., stroke) is approximately 51 per 100,000 for African-Americans versus 30 per 100,000 for Euro-Americans (Bernard, 1993). The ratio of end-stage renal disease, a complication of uncontrolled hypertension, is 32.4 per 100,000 for African-Americans compared with 13.9 per 100,000 for the general population. The improved control of hypertension has contributed significantly to the general health of African-Americans, but continued efforts are necessary to increase awareness, treatment, and control of hypertension because a significant excess of hypertension in African-American men and women still exists.

Infant Mortality. In 1992 there was a 5% decline in infant mortality from 1991. The birth rate also witnessed a decline from 1991 to 1992 (16.3 to 16.0) (Wegman, 1993). Although the infant mortality rate decreased in 1992 in both neonatal and postneonatal components, infant mortality, for reasons previously noted, represents an area of public health and community health nursing concern.

African-American females of childbearing age continue to have a higher ratio of infant mortality (2.1:1) in comparison to Euro-American women. The reasons for this disparity in infant mortality are complex but involve socioeconomic variables, such as educational attainment, family stability, and employment status. "Behind these factors lies the specter of [historical and contemporary racism] and oppression" (Wegman, 1993, p. 749).

For African-American women, three components of excess risk for infant mortality exist:

- Increased risk of delivering a low-birth-weight infant (5.7% of white infants compared with 13.5% of African-American infants)
- Increased risk of neonatal death among infants of normal birth weight
- Increased risk of postneonatal death, regardless of birth weight, relative to whites

A focal point in the primary prevention of infant mortality is to improve services designed to help women of childbearing age. High-quality prenatal care is a significant advance toward reducing infant mortality. There was a slight decrease in the numbers of women who had little or no prenatal care from 1989 to 1991 (6.4–5.8%) (Wegman, 1993); yet there continues to be a disturbing pattern in the percentages of African-American women and Euro-American women who had little or no prenatal care. In 1991, 10.7% of African-American women versus 4.7% of Euro-American women, regardless of age, had little or no prenatal care. A slightly larger percentage of African-American female adolescents younger than 15 years had received little or no care. However, a significantly larger gap was evidenced in the 15- to 19-year-old aggregate with regard to little or no prenatal care (13.4% African-American compared with 9.8% Euro-American).

Again, genetic or biological vulnerability contributes little to these discrepancies. Furthermore, on the surface, socioeconomic status seems plausible, but a further examination of what underlies economic disparities moves one to focus on the political and socioeconomic realities of African-Americans. Unfortunately, African-American infants of normal birth weight have a higher rate of neonatal mortality than do white infants. This may reflect the prenatal care received, other health behaviors of the mothers, differential quality of care in hospitals providing routine obstetric care, or other factors. To the extent that deaths occur after the infant is discharged from the hospital, excess deaths may reflect living conditions or inadequate health knowledge and health behavior on the part of the mother and her family.

Postneonatal mortality rates are higher among African-Americans for all major causes of death except congenital anomalies, for which the ratio is 1:1. This finding reduces the validity of explanations for genetic susceptibility and inherent inferiority as relevant factors in neonatal mortality.

The major causes of infant mortality in 1991, with the largest ratio between African-American and Euro-American women, were respiratory distress syndromes (2.6:1), gastrointestinal disease (4.3:1), short gestation and low birth weight (4.4:1), and HIV infection (17.2:1).

The many risk factors associated with poor perinatal outcome among African-Americans that are related to low socioeconomic status include

- Low income and inadequate insurance coverage, which often reduce access to appropriate health care
- Preexisting disease conditions
- Poor nutrition
- Inadequate housing and crowded living conditions
- Limited maternal education
- Stressful work environments
- Disrupted families and lack of social supports
- Problems of transportation and child care, which impede use of services

Furthermore, populations with the worst pregnancy outcomes tend to have more adolescent mothers, more single mothers, and more unintended births.

When many of the social risk factors (education, marital status, trimester of first care, parity, age) are controlled, African-American women still have twice the risk of delivering low-birth-weight infants as do comparable whites.

Childbearing patterns are different for African-American and Euro-American women (Table 18–5). Unintended pregnancy for African-American adolescents of childbearing age is problematic with respect to the viability of the African-American family, the community, and the neonate. Although there are

Table 18–5
Childbearing Patterns of African-American and White Women, 1989

Variable	White (%)	African-American (%)
Age of mother		
<18 years	3.6	10.5
18–19 years	7.2	12.9
Marital status		
Single	19.2	65.7

Adapted from National Center for Health Statistics (1992). Health, United States, 1991. Hyattsville, Maryland: U.S. Department of Health and Human Services.

significant and well-documented disparities in rates of infant mortality between African-American women and Euro-American women, underneath this lies an even larger and self-destructive problem. The "very dynamic that produces the pathological situation wherein children attempt to have and rear children ensures" African-Americans' functional inferiority, which translates into continued oppressed status (Cress-Welsing, 1991, p. 259). In essence, African-American adolescent females are ill equipped and ill prepared to provide and socialize their offspring in a complex society. Furthermore, fecundity is not synonymous with emotional maturity. Efforts to reduce the disparity in infant mortality rates should not be reduced. However, in thinking upstream, a concerted effort must be exercised, within the African-American community, to address, at its roots, the problem of unintended African-American adolescent pregnancy. Even if technology leads to a reduction in the rate of infant mortality, our society must still contend with the emotional and psychosocial development of African-American adolescents.

AIDS and HIV. HIV infection leading to AIDS is the eighth leading cause of death in the United States (Wegman, 1993). Gay and bisexual identified men still account for a significant number of new AIDS cases. However, the rates of transmission have declined in these aggregates and risen in the intravenous drug user group, which comprises a significant number of heterosexual individuals. The drug-sex link has particular importance because it affects a large number of African-Americans, who transmit the virus through sexual contact. Thus, HIV and AIDS are further threatening the integrity and cohesion of the African-American family and community.

African-American men had the highest age-adjusted death rates from AIDS (52.9 per 100,000 population). African-Americans make up more than half of the reported cases of AIDS among those who were heterosexual partners of intravenous drug users. African-American children accounted for more than half of the pediatric AIDS cases, reflecting the higher ratio of postneonatal morbidity previously cited as a primary cause of death.

Infection with HIV constitutes a particularly severe public health problem in African-Americans. In 1991, nearly 32% of all cases reported to the Centers for Disease Control and Prevention were African-American (National Center for Health Statistics, 1992).

An explanation for the rising rates of HIV transmission among African-Americans must be multifactorial, including socioeconomic factors such as unemployment, lack of health insurance, poor overall health, educational disadvantages, and other poverty-related considerations. Furthermore, factors such as late-stage diagnosis and identification leading to short survival time, access to and client retention in clinical trials, and aggregate denial, which fosters high rates of seroprevalence among multiple aggregate cohorts, lead to higher rates of transmission.

As indicated in Table 18–6, AIDS disproportionately affects men and women from culturally diverse backgrounds. For example, more than 72.4% of the women with AIDS are nonwhite; 55.6% are African-American (National Center for Health Statistics, 1992).

Educational programs and nursing interventions must be planned with consideration of the special needs of African-Americans who are at risk for contracting HIV infection and developing AIDS.

Alcohol Problems

Alcohol problems are complex and involve a wide range of medical, social, and legal problems. Although few studies exist on the subject of alcohol and African-Americans, there is evidence that alcohol abuse has a major impact on the health of African-Americans (Heckler, 1985). Using cirrhosis mortality statistics as an indicator of alcohol abuse, the rate of death for African-Americans is twice that for whites.

Overall, drinking patterns among African-Americans are similar to those for the general population, with rates varying greatly by geographic location, sex, and religion. However, African-Americans in the general population experience and endure substance-related health problems to a greater extent than whites (Lee et al., 1991). The consequences of substance-related problems for African-Americans compared with whites appear to be graver in terms of arrests, homicides, unintentional mortality, and accidents. A higher percentage of abstainers and of heavy drinkers is found in the African-American female community than in the white female community (51% vs. 39% and 11% vs. 7%, respectively). African-American and white men have similar drinking patterns. African-American boys aged 14 to 17 years drink less, have consistently higher absten-

Table 18–6
Characteristics of Persons with Reported AIDS, by Year of Report, United States, 1993–1994

Characteristic	1993 Reported Cases		1994 Reported Cases	
	No.	%	No.	%
Sex*				
Male	89,349	83.8	66,095	81.9
Female	17,269	16.2	14,594	18.1
Age group (yr)				
0–4	728	0.7	785	1.0
5–12	214	0.2	232	0.3
13–19	586	0.6	417	0.5
20–29	19,202	18.0	13,198	16.3
30–39	48,380	45.4	36,527	45.3
40–49	27,235	25.5	21,259	26.3
50–59	7596	7.1	6108	7.6
≥60	2677	2.5	2165	2.7
Race/ethnicity†				
White, non-Hispanic	48,058	45.1	33,193	41.1
Black, non-Hispanic	38,455	36.1	31,487	39.0
Hispanic	18,847	17.7	15,066	18.7
Asian and Pacific Islander	771	0.7	577	0.7
American Indian and Alaskan native	348	0.3	227	0.3
Unspecified	139	0.1	141	0.2
HIV exposure category				
Male homosexual/bisexual contact	50,389	47.3	34,974	43.3
History of injected drug use				
Women and heterosexual men	29,792	28.0	21,717	26.9
Male homosexual/bisexual contact	6651	6.2	3853	4.8
Persons with hemophilia	1117	1.0	513	0.6
Heterosexual contact	9793	9.2	8300	10.3
Transfusion recipients	1199	1.1	779	1.0
Perinatal transmission	886	0.8	933	1.2
No risk reported	6791	6.4	9622	11.9
Region				
Northeast	31,094	29.2	25,301	31.4
Northcentral	11,195	10.5	7962	9.9
South	35,611	33.4	28,627	35.5
West	25,328	23.8	16,236	20.1
U.S. territories	3258	3.1	2412	3.0
Total	106,486	100.0	80,538	100.0

*In 1994, two cases were reported in persons for whom sex was unknown.

AIDS = acquired immunodeficiency syndrome; HIV = human immunodeficiency virus.

Adapted from Morbidity and Mortality Weekly Report. Update: Acquired immunodeficiency syndrome—United States—1994. MMWR 44(4):65, 1995.

tion rates, and have consistently lower heavy drinking rates and alcohol-related social consequences than do their white counterparts. African-American males begin to have high rates of heavy drinking and social problems from drinking after the age of 30 years; for white males, heavy and problem drinking is concentrated in the 18- to 25-year-old age group. African-Americans are at disproportionately higher risk for certain alcohol-related problems such as esophageal cancer (10 times the rate of whites) and fetal alcohol syndrome.

Drug-Related Problems

As with alcohol, drug problems are complex and involve the same medical, social, and legal problems. African-Americans, particularly those living in major metropolitan areas, are at greater risk for drug-related problems and their consequences. They have a higher rate of marijuana, cocaine, heroin, and illicit methadone use than do whites. The literature reveals changing trends in drug preference patterns among African-Americans (Harlow, 1990). This shift is heralded by an increase in cocaine-related morbidity and mortality among African-Americans. Harlow (1990) asserted that the rise in cocaine-related mortality was statistically significant when compared with the rates for either whites or Hispanics in 1986 and 1987. This disparity may reflect the use of more dangerous forms of cocaine, like crack, by the members of some African-American communities.

Primm and Wesley (1985) identified aggregate-level factors that may explain the higher incidence of drug- and alcohol-related problems in some African-American communities. These factors are (1) history of racism, which imparts a psychological handicap; (2) poverty, unemployment, and a lack of career and job opportunities; (3) failure of law enforcement officials to eradicate drug trafficking in African-American communities; (4) the allure of and rewards for selling drugs; (5) powerlessness; (6) cultural and economic conditions that favor hustling and reject and devalue menial jobs; (7) social network influences and peer pressure; (8) frustration from confronting racism, discrimination, and rejection; and (9) high levels of stress at both the individual and community levels. To these factors one can add the lack of clear-cut cultural rules and ambiguous, ill-defined norms.

Homicide and Unintentional Injuries

Homicide is a major cause of excess deaths among African-American men aged 25 to 44 years. Homicide accounted for 38% of excess deaths among males and 14% of excess deaths among females younger than 45 years. Violence is the leading cause of death in African-American males aged 15 to 19 years. The rate of violence-related deaths is nine times that for same-aged Euro-American males (DuRant et al., 1994). According to DuRant and colleagues (1994), "violence is not a uniquely racial [phenomenon]" (p. 612); however, its covariation with social factors such as poverty and unemployment, which reflect the lives of many African-Americans, accounts for the excess mortality in this populace. Furthermore, violence among young African-American males and females is correlated with exposure to violence, sense of personal victimization, depression, family conflict, previous exposure to punishment, and self-reported purpose in life. For many African-Americans, these factors reflect the realities of their existence in Western society.

Although African-Americans account for approximately 12% of the total population, they account for 43% of the homicide victims. African-American males have a 1 in 21 lifetime chance of becoming a homicide victim (vs. 1 in 131 for white males). Homicide is the leading cause of death among African-American males aged 15 to 19 years (DuRant et al., 1994). In addition, they are the group most likely to commit homicide. The homicide rate for African-American males is sevenfold that for Euro-American males. The homicide rate for African-American females is 4.2 times that for Euro-American females (Nickens, 1991). This is particularly important for women who may become victims of battering, as in the case of domestic violence. The higher incidence of homicide rates for African-Americans is documented in all regions of the United States. However, these rates are particularly high in major metropolitan cities (DuRant et al., 1994; Heckler, 1985; Nickens, 1991).

Although many of the factors related to homicide are similar in African-Americans and whites, some may be identified more closely with African-Americans occupying lower socioeconomic ranks. For example, both the perpetrator and victim are often found in urban areas characterized by low income; physical deterioration; a high dependence on public assistance; disrupted families; lack of social supports;

ineffective sources of social support; a high proportion of young, single males; overcrowded and substandard housing; low rates of home ownership or single-family dwellings; mixed land use; and high population density (Heckler, 1985; Nickens, 1991; President's Commission on Law Enforcement and Administration of Justice, 1967). More important, homicide brings with it a stigma that makes intervention extremely difficult. Prevention efforts must target the social factors that may play a role in the high incidence of homicide that terrorizes some urban African-American communities.

NURSING CARE OF AFRICAN-AMERICAN INDIVIDUALS, FAMILIES, AND COMMUNITIES: SERVING THE AGGREGATE NEED

Nurses working with African-Americans must be familiar with the variety of problems and barriers that contribute to the health status of this population. The following section targets three areas that account for significant excess morbidity and mortality in African-Americans. Issues, strategies, and examples of culturally relevant and sensitive nursing care are explored.

Infant Mortality

Infant mortality represents a significant threat to existence of the African-American aggregate. Yet a more critical problem exists: unintended pregnancies among African-American adolescents. Finding a solution to the latter necessarily minimizes the significance of the former. African-American adolescent females are often developmentally unprepared for the tasks of raising a child. Primary prevention efforts should target unprotected sexual activity and value systems. The family and the community must redefine the problem of unintended adolescent pregnancy as a genuine threat to group and collective survival. Healthy children must be viewed as a necessary tool in African-American transformation.

Secondary prevention efforts should target those adolescent females who have already endured an unintended pregnancy. Attention should be given to the prevention of additional unintended pregnancies; appropriate sexual behavior; the nature, function, and role of sex in the lives of African-Americans and its potential destructive force to group

survival; and the role of parents in the lives of their offspring.

Homicide

PRIMARY, SECONDARY, AND TERTIARY PREVENTION

In the case of homicide, primary prevention efforts must be directed at those social, cultural, technological, and legal aspects of the environment that perpetuate the extraordinarily high homicide rates among African-Americans. Secondary prevention efforts should be directed to individuals manifesting early signs of behavioral and social problems that are related to increased risks for subsequent homicide. Family violence, childhood aggression, school violence, adolescent violence, and alcohol and drug problems are important focal points for efforts aimed at secondary prevention of homicide. Tertiary prevention is concerned with situations in which a health problem is already well established but efforts can still be made to prevent further disability or death. In relation to homicide, the problems of greatest concern are types of serious violence that occur between eventual victim and perpetrator. Furthermore, redefining violence as a form of racism, both internal and external, and a form of oppression underscores the contributions of sociopolitical factors in the genesis of African-American violence and early morbidity and mortality.

AIDS and HIV Prevention

The U.S. Public Health Service has proposed five strategies to address the issue of AIDS in minority populations (including African-American):

- Expansion of human resources in an effort to control the spread of HIV
- Expansion of the knowledge base, including additional surveys and research studies of AIDS in the African-American community
- Development of culturally appropriate communications through information, education, and outreach programs
- Alleviation of HIV-related discrimination and stigma
- Strengthening of community networks by better collaboration among local, state, and federal governments and community-based organizations and institutions

African-Americans constitute approximately 12% of the total U.S. population but account for an astounding 30% of all diagnosed AIDS cases (Bowser, 1992). There have been significant increases in the number of women diagnosed with AIDS, especially African-American women. Kalichman and colleagues (1993) cited data from the Centers for Disease Control and Prevention indicating that, although women account for only 11% of all AIDS cases, 53% of those women are African-American. This is alarming in light of the fact that as yet there is no cure for HIV and the risk for mortality is high. Furthermore, African-American women are essential to the survival of the African-American community.

Public health efforts show significant promise when framed within the context of an Afrocentric perspective. Such efforts are culturally sensitive and culturally competent, use existing cultural organizations, and reflect the values of the aggregate. Furthermore, AIDS prevention efforts must target the intersecting cohorts (i.e., those with alcohol and drug problems, heterosexual partners, gay and bisexual men and women). AIDS prevention efforts will need to be multifactorial in nature, building on the strengths inherent in the African-American community (i.e., extended family networks, communication styles, and language, which should be interactive and person to person). AIDS prevention efforts should stress individual and collective group survival and transformation. Jemmott and colleagues (Jemmott and Jemmott, 1992; Jemmott et al., 1992) found strong support for decreasing AIDS risk behaviors using the theory of reasoned action. In essence, the theory of reasoned action posits that perceived vulnerability and perceived self-efficacy, coupled with outcome expectancies, influence behavior. AIDS risk reduction interventions may be more effective when working with African-American adolescents when they:

- Are culturally sensitive, relevant, and consistent to the target population
- Focus on increasing perceived risk and perceived self-efficacy
- Target knowledge of AIDS
- Include a skills-building component to enhance perceived self-efficacy
- Focus on altering negative outcome expectancies such as those associated with condom use
- Involve important members of the individual's support network

Public health programs should seek to develop and institute, with the help of the African-American community, programs that at the very least incorporate these elements.

CULTURAL SENSITIVITY

When working with African-American groups or communities, every effort should be made to be culturally sensitive in recommendations and suggestions. It is helpful to have proposed plans for a community project or program reviewed ahead of time by someone familiar with the culture of the population for whom the intervention is intended. The nurse should seek input from African-American nurses or other African-American members of the health care team in terms of cultural content and language.

It must be remembered that socioeconomic factors may be even more significant than racial or ethnic affiliation, so a critique from an African-American colleague from a different socioeconomic class may fail to yield the desired outcome. A middle- or upper-class African-American professional may be unable to relate to the health care needs of lower-class urban or rural African-Americans. Whenever possible, key African-American community-based leaders should be part of the planning, implementation, and evaluation of projects or programs, and it is conventional practice to form an advisory council or board before undertaking major community health projects or programs. If the project or program is likely to impact a culturally mixed population, representatives from each target group should be asked to participate in proportion to their representation in the targeted community.

Cultural sensitivity includes understanding attitudes toward advice from health professionals. If African-American clients appear to be reluctant to follow the nurse's advice, the nurse should explore the possible cultural reasons. The client should not be forced to wear the label "noncompliant." Issues of disharmonic values, language barriers, and mistrust may affect the client's behavior.

When caring for African-American individuals, families, and groups, the nurse must consider the following aspects to be able to give the best nursing care:

- Understand macro- and microlevel historic and contemporary factors that give meaning to and shape the lives of African-Americans

- Conduct a cultural assessment of self and the group to facilitate the nurse's work and facilitate cultural sensitivity and cultural awareness
- Examine the cultural stereotypes held by society and how these affect the holistic health of the aggregate
- Increase knowledge and skills assessment
- Be aware of differences in cross-cultural communication
- Develop cultural sensitivity and cultural competence in working with African-Americans

Cultural Self-Assessment

When caring for African-American individuals, families, and groups, a nurse needs to engage in a cultural self-assessment to identify individual culturally based attitudes and beliefs about African-Americans, race, prejudice, racial discrimination, and related issues. Cultural self-assessment requires considerable self-honesty and sincerity and necessitates reflection on parents, grandparents, and other significant family members and close friends in terms of their attitudes toward African-Americans.

If you are an African-American nurse, how do you feel about caring for other African-Americans? Are there socioeconomic differences between you and the African-American clients in your case load? Do you believe that only other African-Americans can genuinely understand the needs of African-American clients? Could a Hispanic, an Asian, or a Euro-American nurse provide culturally sensitive nursing care to African-American clients as well as you can?

Cultural Stereotypes

A nurse must examine the cultural stereotypes of African-Americans held by other members of the nurse's culture. For example, if the nurse is of Hispanic origin, the nurse must consider what Hispanics, in general, say about African-Americans. The nurse must examine the recent interactions between the two cultures in the local community. Have African-Americans and Hispanics, for example, competed within the community for scarce economic resources, cooperated on a joint venture, or ignored each other? How would these factors impact a nurse's professional interactions with African-Americans? How would a Hispanic community health nurse, for example, be received by an African-American family? What might be the client's cultural stereotypes? How might negative stereotypes of Hispanics influence the professional nurse-client relationship with the African-American family? Some questions are suggested for your self-assessment.

Roles of the Community Health Nurse

Community health nurses working with the African-American aggregate represent an important link between the larger society and the community. The role of the community health nurse may include (1) advocate, (2) educator, (3) social policy analyst, (4) outreach worker, and (5) participant observer.

With respect to working with the African-American aggregate, prevention should attempt to (1) capitalize

---

CULTURAL SELF-ASSESSMENT

- How do your parents, grandparents, other family members, and close friends view people from racially diverse groups? What is the cultural stereotype of African-Americans? Does the cultural stereotype allow for socioeconomic differences (i.e., differentiate lower, middle, and upper classes)? Are all African-Americans the same?
- Have your interactions with African-Americans been positive, negative, or neutral? Do you or significant others in your social network use any derogatory slang words when referring to African-Americans?
- How do you feel about going into a predominantly African-American neighborhood or into

the home of an African-American family? Are you afraid, anxious, curious, or ambivalent?
- What stereotypes do you have about African-American men, women, and children?
- What do you know about African-American culture? What are your stereotypical views about African-Americans; pregnancy, birth, and family planning; child-rearing practices; teen years (e.g., menstruation and sexual practices); adulthood (roles of men and women); old age; and death?
- What culturally based health beliefs and practices do you think will characterize the African-Americans in your case load? How are these different from your own culturally based health beliefs and practices?

on the existing cultural strengths within the community to facilitate functional competence and positive self-identity and (2) seek to modify those environmental and societal factors that continue to threaten the integrity of the aggregate.

As a social policy analyst, advocate, educator, and outreach worker, the nurse's efforts must be directed toward primary prevention. Primary prevention seeks to modify or rectify the causes of symptoms, attacking the problems at their roots. Within-group diversity in the African-American aggregate places some subgroups at higher risk for destructive behavior, early morbidity, and mortality. The goals of primary prevention should reflect the community's concerns, incorporate its cultural strengths, and be culturally congruent and consistent.

Several factors may hinder the nurse's prevention efforts with African-American clients and the African-American community: (1) internal resistance, (2) cultural dissonance, (3) Eurocentrism, and (4) racial-cultural paranoia. Therefore, it is imperative that the community health nurse clearly evaluate the barriers that may undermine any prevention efforts. Evaluation of potential strategies must be preceded by an assessment. As a participant-observer, the community health nurse can enlist members of the community and organizations to identify and define the problems of greatest significance. Gaining entry will be an issue of critical import. Entry can be facilitated by working within the culture and forging an alliance with existing organizations that provide service to the aggregate. Failure to establish credible links will necessarily hinder and minimize the effectiveness of prevention efforts.

Building a therapeutic alliance will be the key to gaining access. A therapeutic alliance implies a relationship of considerable trust. Racial differences alone can invoke a sense of paranoia on the part of the community, which has been victimized by the ongoing inequalities that characterize the lives of the people. Thus, gaining entry and developing a trusting, therapeutic alliance will be central to the success of any prevention efforts.

Primary and secondary prevention can be conducted through community outreach programs that target specific high-risk subgroups such as adolescents and older African-Americans. Outreach can be linked with other community-based programs and can operate within the confines of existing culturally based institutions such as the church.

Prevention programs must rely on the expertise and knowledge existing within the community. Thus, goals should be mutually negotiated between the community health nurse and the community or individual. Prevention efforts, strategies, and goals should be culturally sensitive and congruent with the African-American community.

APPLICATION OF THE NURSING PROCESS IN WORKING WITH AFRICAN-AMERICAN COMMUNITIES

Nurses providing care within the African-American community or directly to African-American clients need to work from both a critical social theory perspective and an Afrocentric perspective. Both perspectives should seek to empower African-Americans. Application of the nursing process incorporates systems theory, critical social theories, and the strengths of African-American culture. Prevention—primary, secondary, and tertiary—is a primary aim of all interventions and, where feasible, is intertwined with process. Finally, exploration of the varied roles of community health nurses is formulated as a template for action.

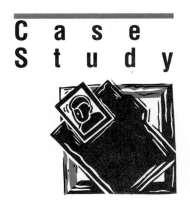

C a s e S t u d y

Anna, a Latina community health nurse, was asked to visit an African-American woman recently diagnosed with AIDS and to develop an HIV-AIDS prevention program targeted toward African-American women. The request for this primary prevention program grew out of the literature and the health department's knowledge of rising HIV-AIDS seroprevalence within the African-American community. Anna's first priority was to perform her own cultural assessment.

Assessment

Although Anna had not experienced the effects of racism directly, other members of her family had endured its pains. Her experience as a woman offered a more parallel scenario for comparison. She noted the numbers of individuals of color with whom she and her family had frequent contact. She asked important members of her social network what they thought about African-Americans. She asked colleagues their thoughts as well. Finally, she wrote down her thoughts, stereotypes, and misperceptions of African-Americans.

The next step for Anna was to assess the African-American women presenting to the women's health clinic at the public health department. Before conducting this assessment, Anna asked African-American colleagues about their perceptions of the problems and issues facing African-Americans. In particular, she inquired about values, beliefs, health practices, male and female roles and relationships, spirituality, and sexuality. She then conducted a focus group with African-American women. She enhanced her knowledge of the African-American aggregate with research pertinent to the prevention program. Further assessment included

- Community organizations that provide HIV-AIDS services
- Risk-taking behaviors
- Clients' social network
- Clients' and families' knowledge of HIV-AIDS disease processes, prevention, and risk-taking behaviors
- Social network configuration and health-engendering or health-threatening behaviors

Using the information gathered from multiple data sources, including the focus group, Anna understood that culture impacts behaviors and perceptions. Furthermore, any prevention program must capitalize on the cultural strengths of the aggregate to effect any lasting change. Data from the focus group provided Anna with an opportunity to make a series of diagnoses.

Diagnosis

Individual
- Lack of perceived risk as related to HIV-AIDS transmission
- Knowledge deficit about the methods of HIV-AIDS transmission
- Potential HIV-AIDS conversion secondary to high-risk sexual behavior

Family-Social Networks
- Inadequate supports for behavior change

Community
- Inadequate community resources to target high-risk behavior
- Knowledge deficit related to culture within existing community health organizations
- Potential conflict secondary to values conflict between existing organizations and the African-American community

Planning

Planning necessitates strengthening the existing community resources and organizations to assist them in addressing the problems of high-risk sexual behavior. Furthermore, planning should focus on the development of interventions that increase women's sense of personal vulnerability to AIDS-HIV infection. Anna incorporated the principles of systems theory with subsystems within the African-American community. Examples of subsystems to be included in the planning include

- Churches
- Community clinics
- Health departments
- Local housing agencies
- Community activists

Planning mandates that Anna derive goals and interventions that are culturally sensitive and culturally competent.

Individual

Long-Term Goal

- Reduce the incidence of early morbidity and mortality in African-American women.

Short-Term Goals

- Reduce the incidence of high-risk behavior.
- Promote increased condom use among sexually active African-Americans.
- Decrease levels of personal susceptibility to AIDS-HIV.

Family

Long-Term Goal

- Social support to enhance family stability and viability will increase.

Short-Term Goals

- Family will identify ways to support health-promoting behaviors.
- Family will discuss behavioral expectations with respect to appropriate sexual behavior.

Community

Long-Term Goals

- Community organizations will be more effective in outreach and earlier identification within the African-American community.
- Community organizations will work from a critical social theory and Afrocentric perspectives.

Short-Term Goals

- Community organizations will conduct more aggressive community outreach within the community.
- Community clinics will offer free, anonymous HIV-AIDS testing, pre- and post-test counseling, and female and male condoms.
- Community organizations will forge links to provide more comprehensive services to the African-American aggregate and women living in the community.
- Community clinics will develop walk-in programs for women with AIDS-HIV.

Interventions

Anna works with several local community health organizations and churches to forge grassroots links. Interventions reflect a mutually negotiated process between the organizations and the community members. Furthermore, interventions are culturally sensitive and competent and are framed from an empowerment stance.

Individuals Women who participated in the focus group specifically indicated a decreased perceived risk of contracting AIDS-HIV. Thus, Anna's intervention focused on increasing perceived personal vulnerability through education and group discussion. Methods to minimize transmission were discussed, and a brief assertiveness training program was instituted within the health department. Some women who expressed an interest in the problem were trained as volunteer community health outreach workers.

Family Examples of interventions with the family include helping them to identify and explore their perception of the family's role. The local church was instrumental in hosting a weekly family night open to the community. The purpose of family night was to bring together the families in the community and to provide a forum for education about community problems, issues, and possible solutions. Other interventions include helping the family (1) identify ways to minimize family stress and (2) utilize community resources.

Community Interventions within the community include mandatory cultural sensitivity training for all community health organizations. Anna will help develop the cultural sensitivity training program using experts within the community. Furthermore, educational programs would be developed that targeted high-risk groups, especially women. Local schools would be required to incorporate in their curricula information about AIDS and HIV, transmission, and prevention. All students would be required to participate in a 10-hour workshop about the effects of oppression, racism, and the nature and significance of culture.

A health fair organized in conjunction with other grassroots organizations, the church, and the schools will be developed. On-site AIDS-HIV testing, counseling, and risk reduction programs will be offered to community participants.

Evaluation

There is a reciprocity among practice, theory, and research. Evaluation is a critical tool of the nursing process. Interventions must be evaluated for their effectiveness in altering risk-endangering behavior, their cultural sensitivity, and their ability to foster greater community integration and stability.

Learning Activities

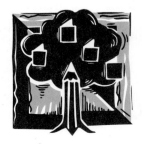

1. Interview an African-American health care professional to ascertain the contextual experience of being African-American. Ask the individual what she or he has experienced both professionally and personally as a result of race.

2. Watch prime-time television and consider the roles of African-American characters. What percentage of the actors are African-American? What message is being conveyed about race?

3. Using the guidelines suggested in Chapter 17, conduct an in-depth cultural assessment of an African-American client.

4. Identify an African-American cultural healer in the community, and schedule an appointment to discuss health beliefs and practices, treatments for various illnesses, and the preparation necessary to become a healer (i.e., how the individual acquired the healing skills).

5. Using census data, identify the number, age, sex, and location of residence for African-Americans in your city or town. Identify the health resources available in African-American neighborhoods, and compare them with those available in predominantly Euro-American areas.

SUMMARY

The problems facing the African-American community can be conceptualized as sociopolitical problems that are rooted in the tenuous relationships between African-Americans and Euro-Americans. The continued struggle for equality and self-determination and the persistent disparities in health, morbidity, and mortality are in reality reflections of our society's unjust power imbalances, cruelty, and inhumanity.

It is imperative to note that we must continue to direct our efforts at improving the health of people of color as our population becomes more and more diverse. Unfortunately, in the foreseeable future, the health status of people of color will continue to be an arena of struggle, conflict, and challenge, as evidenced by the persistent documented disparities. This chapter has presented an overview of the social, economic, and cultural factors that have an impact on the health of African-Americans in contemporary U.S. society.

The major causes of excess deaths for African-Americans have been elucidated, with particular focus on infant mortality, AIDS and HIV, alcohol and drug problems, and homicide. Ways in which community health nurses can provide culturally sensitive, culturally competent, contextually relevant, and meaningful nursing care to African-American individuals, families, and communities have been suggested.

Finally, upstream thinking with regard to many of the problems of the African-American aggregate imputed to poor health practices, socioeconomic status, or race alone serves to justify continuing racial conflict and oppressive practices, failing to attack the unjust power imbalances that prevent African-Americans from full participation and self-determination in Western society. Community health nurses working with African-American clients represent an important link between the often isolated community and the society at large. As a social policy analyst, participant observer, advocate, educator, and outreach worker, the community health nurse has an opportunity to effect change within the aggregate. Any effort must involve the members of the community and the existing organizations. Furthermore, strategies should reflect the cultural strengths and values. All prevention efforts need to be culturally sensitive and congruent with the African-American culture.

REFERENCES

Adams RL: Great Negroes: Past and Present. Chicago, IL, Afro-Am Publishing Company, 1972.

Amuleru-Marshall, O: Political and economic implications of alcohol and other drugs in the African-American community. *In* Goddard, LL: African-American Youth at High-Risk Work Group. An African-Centered Model of Prevention for African-American Youth at High Risk. CSAP Technical Report No. 6, Chapter 3. Rockville, MD, U.S. Department of Health and Human Services, 1992.

Bell P: Chemical Dependency and the African American: Counseling Strategies and Community Issues. Minneapolis, MN. Hazelden Drug Treatment Center, 1990.

Bennett L: Before the Mayflower: A History of the Black American, 1619–1962. Chicago, Johnson, 1962, pp. 1–16.

Bernard MA: The health status of African American elderly. J Nat Med Assoc 85:521–528, 1993.

Brooks DD, Smith DR, Anderson RJ: Medical apartheid: An American perspective. JAMA 266:2746–2749, 1991.

Bowser, B: African-American culture and AIDS prevention: From barrier to ally. West J Med 157(3): 286–289, 1992.

Butler JP: Of kindred minds: the ties that bind. *In* Olandi MA, Weston R, Epstein LG (eds): Cultural Competence for Evaluators: A Guide for Alcohol and Other Drug Prevention Practitioners Working with Ethnic/Racial Communities. Rockville, Maryland, U.S. Department of Health and Human Services, Office of Substance Abuse Prevention, 1992.

Cheung YW: Ethnicity and alcohol/drug use revisited: A framework for future research. J Addict 25:581–605, 1991.

Clarke, JH: New Dimensions in African History: The London Lectures of Dr. Yosef Ben-Jochannan and Dr. John Henrik Clarke. Trenton, NJ, African World Press, Inc., 1991.

Cress-Welsing F: The Isis Papers: The Keys to the Colors. Chicago, Il, Third World Press, 1991.

Current Population Reports: The black population in the United States: March 1990 and 1989 (Series P-20, No. 448). Washington, DC, U.S. Government Printing Office, 1991, pp. 1–17.

Current Population Reports: Educational attainment in the United States: March 1991 and 1990. Washington, DC, U.S. Government Printing Office, 1992a, pp. 1–6.

Current Population Reports: Marital status and living arrangements: March 1991 (Series P-20, No. 461). Washington, DC, U.S. Government Printing Office, 1992b, pp. 1–14.

DuRant RH, Cadenhead C, Pendergrast RA, et al.: Factors associated with the use of violence among urban black adolescents. Am J Public Health 84:612–617, 1994.

Harlow KC: Patterns of rates of mortality from narcotic and cocaine overdose in Texas, 1976–1987. Public Health Rep 105:455–462, 1990.

Heckler MM: Report of the Secretary's Task Force on Black and Minority Health. Washington, DC, U.S. Government Printing Office, 1985.

Jemmott JB, Jemmott LS, Fong GT: Reduction in HIV risk-associated sexual behaviors among black male adolescents: Effects of an AIDS prevention intervention. Am J Public Health 82:372–377, 1992.

Jemmott LS, Jemmott JB: Increasing condom-use intentions among sexually active black adolescent women. Nurs Res 41:273–279, 1992.

Johnson C: The status of health care among black Americans: Address before the Congress of National Black Churches. J Natl Med Assoc 83:125–129, 1991.

Kalichman SC, Kelly JA, Hunter TL, et al: Culturally tailored HIV-AIDS risk reduction messages targeted to African-American urban women: impact on risk, sensitization and risk reduction. J Consult Clin Psychol 61(2):291–295, 1993.

Kochanek KP, Maurer JP, Rosenberg HM: Why did black life expectancy decline from 1984 through 1989 in the United States? Am J Public Health 84(6):938–944, 1994.

Lassiter SM: Black is a color, not a culture: Implications for health care: J Assoc Black Nurs Faculty 5(1):4–9, 1994.

Lee JA, Mavis BE, Stoffelmayr BE: A comparison of problems-of-life for blacks and whites entering a substance abuse treatment program. J Psychoactive Drugs 23:233–239, 1991.

McCord C, Freeman P: Excess mortality in Harlem. N Engl J Med 322:173–177, 1990.

National Center for Health Statistics: Health, United States, 1990, Hyattsville, MD, U.S. Department of Health and Human Services, Public Health Service, 1991.

National Center for Health Statistics: Health, United States, 1991. Hyattsville, MD, U.S. Department of Health and Human Services, Public Health Service, 1992.

National Center for Health Statistics: Health, United States, 1994. Hyattsville, MD, U.S. Department of Health and Human Services, Public Health Service, 1995.

Nickens HW: The health status of the minority populations in the United States. Western J Med 155:27–32, 1991.

Nobles WW: African Psychology: Toward Its Reclamation, Reascension and Revitalization. Oakland, CA, Institute for the Advanced Study of Black Family Life and Culture, 1986.

Nobles WW: Psychological research and the black self-concept: A critical review. J Social Issues 29:11–31, 1973.

Nobels W, Goddard L: An African-centered model of prevention for African-American use at high risk. In Goddard L (ed): Substance Abuse. CSAP Technical Report No. 6. Rockville, MD, U.S. Department of Health and Human Services, 1992, pp. 115–129.

Orque MS, Bloch B, Monrroy LSA: Ethnic Nursing Care: A Multicultural Approach. St. Louis, CV Mosby, 1983.

President's Commission on Law Enforcement and Administration of Justice: The Challenge of Crime in a Free Society. Washington, DC, U.S. Government Printing Office, 1967.

Primm BJ, Wesley JE: Treating the multiply addicted black alcoholic. Alcohol Treat Q 2:155–178, 1985.

Smitherman G: Euro-American English in blackface, or who do I be? Black Scholar 1:32–39, 1973.

Smitherman G: Talkin' and Testifyin': The Language of Black America. Boston, Houghton Mifflin, 1977.

Snow LF: Folk medical beliefs and their implications for care of patients: A review based on studies among Black Americans. Ann Intern Med 81:82–96, 1974.

Sorlie P, Rogot E, Anderson R, et al: Black-white mortality differences by family income. Lancet 340(8815):346–350, 1992.

Spector R: Cultural Diversity in Health and Illness. Norwalk, CT, Appleton-Century-Crofts, 1986.

Staples R: Black Masculinity: The Black Male's Role in American Society. San Francisco, Black Scholar Press, 1982.

Staples R: Black Americans. In Mindel CH, Habenstein RW, Wright R (eds): Ethnic Families in America. New York, Elsevier Science, 1988, pp. 303–324.

Update: Acquired immunodeficiency syndrome—United States—1994. MMWR Morb Mortal Wkly Rep. 44(4):64–67, 1995.

U.S. Bureau of the Census: America's Black Population, 1970 to 1982: A Statistical View, July, 1983 (Series P10/P0P83). Washington, DC, U.S. Government Printing Office, 1983.

U.S. Bureau of the Census: United States Population Estimates by Age, Sex, Race, and Hispanic Origin: 1980 to 1988 (Series P-25, No. 1045). Washington, DC, U.S. Government Printing Office, 1990.

U.S. Civil Rights Commission: Unemployment and Underemployment Among Blacks, Hispanics, and Women. Washington, DC, U.S. Government Printing Office, 1982.

U.S. Public Health Service: Minority issues in AIDS. Public Health Rep 103(suppl 1, rev):91–93, 1988.

Wegman ME: Annual summary of vital statistics—1992. Pediatrics 92:743–755, 1993.

The Mexican-American Community

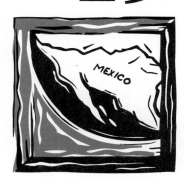

Upon completion of this chapter, the reader will be able to:

1. **Identify the disease and health conditions prevalent among Mexican-Americans.**

2. **Describe two major reasons for the lower health status of a large segment of the Mexican-American community.**

3. **Discuss factors that impede the Mexican-American from receiving health care.**

4. **Describe the folk health system that is unique to Mexican-Americans.**

5. **Apply knowledge of Mexican-American health and culture in planning culturally sensitive nursing care at the individual, family, and community levels.**

Ricardo A. Martinez

There continues to be a lack of empirical data regarding the use of folk medicinal systems, the role of the family in the use of health services, and the role of specific characteristics, such as language, as barriers to health care in the Mexican-American community. This chapter presents traditional Mexican-American concepts and beliefs that are more prevalent in the older segment of the population. Younger, better educated Mexican-Americans may also adhere to traditional values and beliefs, but they may not overtly display them either within the family or publicly.

This chapter focuses on the health needs of Mexican-Americans and implications for community health nursing. Included in the discussion are (1) reactions to illness and its care, (2) unique characteristics of Mexican-American families as they relate to health care, (3) Mexican-American beliefs of disease causation, (4) herbal medicine as it relates to nursing care, and (5) the practitioner's role in integrating culturally relevant factors with health care in the community through improved access, understanding of the bases for lack of health care, language intervention, and health education efforts.

REACTIONS TO ILLNESS: UNDERSTANDING AS A PREREQUISITE

Hispanics are the fastest growing minority in the United States. Typically, they are classified into five subgroups: Mexican-Americans, Puerto Ricans, Cuban-Americans, Central or South Americans, and "other" Hispanics. Use of health care services is affected by perceived health care needs, insurance status, income, culture, and language. Compared with whites, Hispanics are more likely to live in poverty, be unemployed or underemployed, have little education, and have no private insurance. Hispanics are at an increased risk for certain medical conditions, including diabetes, hypertension, tuberculosis, acquired immunodeficiency syndrome (AIDS), alcoholism, cirrhosis, specific cancers, and violent deaths. Disproportionate to their representation in the population, there are few Hispanic health providers, including nurses, emphasizing the need for all medical personnel to be knowledgeable about Hispanic, particularly Mexican-American, health care needs (Anonymous, 1991).

Disease is an ongoing problem that faces every component of a Mexican-American community.

The influence of disease has shaped the destiny of civilizations. The presence of disease has led to the advent of new treatments with an indirect effect of increased life expectancy.

Illness is a social phenomenon as well as a biological reaction. The Mexican-American community's health beliefs and attitudes about disease and illness have a direct effect on perceptions of illness and methods of coping. Each community develops methods and ways of coping that result in medical systems unique to a particular societal group and its culture.

Three categories of beliefs and associated reactions to disease and illness are scientific, nonscientific, and folk medicinal (Gemmill, 1973a, 1973b).

The scientific reaction is characterized by a logical explanation of events in relation to a cause and an effect. The physician learns medical facts that are a compilation of experiments leading to definite clinical application.

The nonscientific reaction stems from the ancient belief that illness may be caused by magic or a supernatural source. A positive side to nonscientific reaction is that illness can be "cured" by magic. In this regard, the reaction to both illness and cure is psychological.

Folk medicine has some basis in the scientific arena. Folk medicine is practiced throughout the world, including all parts of the United States. Within the Mexican-American community, the folk medicinal practice is referred to as *curanderismo*. There are few statistical data confirming the incidence of folk medicine in the country, but anthropologists and sociologists have recognized a strong prevalence in many regions, especially among minority communities.

Traditional medical practitioners may deny the presence of folk medicine. This denial or avoidance response in reaction to minority patient behavior has been called "clinical color blindness" (Gemmill, 1973a, 1973b).

A practitioner who expresses clinical color blindness may also display clinical blindness to patient responses to illness. Unfortunately, patients who do not respond to health care within the practitioner's defined acceptable guidelines may be considered followers of nonscientific medicine.

The practitioner may also be "culturally partially sighted." In this situation, the provider tries to understand the patient's response to health care but is not open-minded, so responses to cultural variation in medical treatment are characterized by overt negative reactions.

The deliberate practitioner is one who is "culturally sighted." A cooperative environment exists between the practitioner and the patient. The goal of adequate health care is achieved regardless of medical beliefs or attitudes.

Nurses caring for patients from ethnic backgrounds may be categorized as culturally blind, but they may progress to culturally sighted if an effort is made to learn about ethnic behaviors in response to modern medical care. Nurses should understand particular folk medicinal systems as well as contributing systems such as families and language patterns. The nurse should also understand that the Mexican-American population has a strong folk medicinal system and that it is also similar in some ways to that of the African-American and Native American cultures.

Postacculturation stress syndrome (PASS) needs to be addressed in order for the health care provider to understand fully the basis for the origin of disease in Mexican-Americans. This syndrome arises as a public health condition that predominately affects minority populations that have attempted to assimilate and become acculturated into the general and dominant population. The primary cause of PASS is the inability to assimilate into the dominant societal group effectively and completely.

The causes for failure of acculturation to the point of experiencing PASS are

- Mistrust of the dominant system
- Lack of job and opportunities to succeed in society
- Prejudice
- Lack of guidance for effective acculturation
- Lack of support from the dominant culture
- Culture shock
- Poverty
- Lack of an acceptable education
- Being from a "vulnerable" population group

Besides being a Mexican-American, individuals are more susceptible to PASS if they are from a "vulnerable" group, such as

- High-risk mothers and infants
- Chronically ill and disabled
- Persons with AIDS
- The mentally ill and disabled
- Alcohol and substance abusers
- Potential suicide or homicide victims
- Abusing families

- Homeless
- Immigrants and refugees

The symptomatology for PASS includes

- Feelings of a lack of self-esteem
- Feelings of a lack of self-worth
- Apathy
- Violence (at home or at the work place or both)
- On-the-job injuries
- Alcoholism
- Gang involvement

PASS can be identified by stage, which is dependent on the individual's level of acculturation, and acculturation continuum (which is related to the level of socioeconomic status, age, and educational level). In Stage I, patients experience apathy and a lack of self-worth and self-esteem, may become involved with gangs, and fail to maintain a job. Stage II patients have problems with alcohol and drug abuse, on-the-job injuries, absenteeism, and self-harm. Stage III patients are violent, have been involved with theft, are chronic drug abusers, and have attempted suicide or self-harm.

Markides and colleagues, in their 1993 study, found that middle-aged men supported an "acculturation stress" model that suggested that stress was higher at the middle of the acculturation continuum. Data from the Hispanic Health and Nutrition Examination Survey (HHANES) were used to examine the influence of acculturation on alcohol consumption among Puerto Rican, Cuban-American, and Mexican-American women. Acculturation was found to be positively related to the frequency of consumption and probability of being a drinker among all three groups. A positive relation was also evident for total drinks consumed among Cuban-American women and volume (drinks per occasion) and total drinks consumed among Mexican-American women (Black and Markides, 1993).

High acculturation has also been associated with higher levels of suicide attempts among Hispanic populations (Vega et al., 1993b). Another study by Vega and colleagues (1993a) demonstrated that family factors are related to the development of attitudes favoring deviant behavior, whereas acculturation conflicts were associated with delinquent behavior among Cuban-American adolescents.

Interventions that may prevent or minimize PASS and also assist the Mexican-American with the acculturation process, and which are related to the various stages of the syndrome, include the following:

1. Stage I
   - Improve the educational status of Mexican-Americans.
   - Provide acculturation "guidance."
   - Provide support from the dominant culture.
   - Increase the number of Mexican-American role models.
   - Provide bilingual education in public schools.
   - Provide diversity training in business and industry.

2. Stage II
   - Provide counseling to Mexican-Americans, including family involvement.
   - Provide training for disadvantaged workers.
   - Provide diversity training in business and industry.

3. Stage III
   - Provide professional counseling and rehabilitation.
   - Provide and improve the correctional systems.
   - Provide professional counseling to the patient and family.

PASS is a public health condition that has not been recognized as a causative factor for many of the psychological, sociologic, and physical ills of Mexican-Americans. Even though the syndrome is global in concept, it appropriately characterizes the stressful condition that Mexican-Americans have endured since the mid-1800s, when northern Mexican territories were annexed into what is now Texas. The stressful condition that is brought on by prejudice, lack of a decent education, and a lasting poverty state results in an unbalanced biopsychosocial state, which requires understanding and attention by the health care provider, including the nurse. The nurse can intervene by listening; by providing useful information so as to decrease mistrust; by providing appropriate referrals to counselors, therapists, and social workers; and by recognizing vulnerable populations.

A BIOLOGICAL PERSPECTIVE: DISEASE PREVALENCE IN THE MEXICAN-AMERICAN COMMUNITY AND ACCESS TO HEALTH CARE

A continuing problem for health care practitioners is the lack of research regarding identification of health differences among minority groups or the prevalence of illness among certain populations.

The complexity of the disparity among minorities in health status has been recognized. For example, Hispanics of Mexican or Cuban origin have low-birth-weight rates not significantly higher than those for the white population despite a lower socioeconomic status. However, there is a clear pattern of less use of preventive services including prenatal care, among adult Mexican-Americans. In addition, Mexican-American children make fewer physician visits and receive fewer vaccinations than do white children (U.S. Department of Health and Human Services, 1986). The question of whether the degree of acculturation has been a determinant in teenage pregnancy has been studied by Reynoso and colleagues (1993). They concluded that acculturated teenagers were younger at the first sexual intercourse, completed more years of schooling, and sought earlier prenatal care. What is interesting is that the degree of acculturation was directly related to the probability of a Mexican-American teenager becoming pregnant (Reynoso et al., 1993). One might speculate on the impact of the closeness of family and holding on to traditional values as a variable for the nonpregnant teenager.

Disease Prevalence: A National Disparity

The first large-scale effort to measure the health of Mexican-Americans was the 1982–1984 HHANES from the National Center for Health Statistics (for a summary, see Lecca et al., 1987). The results of the survey appear to be consistent with the U.S. Department of Health and Human Services (1986) report. In this survey of Southwest Mexican-Americans only 19% of women of child bearing age used oral contraceptive pills. An additional 15% had undergone tubal ligation. Of interest was that these incidence rates were similar to those for the general population. Also of interest is the study's findings that 24% of the mothers surveyed had smoked a mean of 11 cigarettes per day during pregnancy. Infants of these women weighed 101 g less at birth than did infants of nonsmoking mothers and had a low birth weight rate of 8.0% compared with 5.1% for the entire sample of mothers (Wolff et al., 1993).

Vision, hearing, and dental examinations are not a frequent practice among Mexican-American children who failed such examinations. Of these children, at least one third had not had an examination within the past year. Of significance in the survey results was that fewer than 1% of Mexican-American children (4–11 years old) had lead toxicity levels; there may be a continuing decrease in environmental lead exposure.

Also of significance was the increase in cancer screening practices among Mexican-American women. Eight of 10 Mexican-American women (20–74 years old) met American Cancer Society guidelines for periodic Papanicolaou smear. Three of four women met the breast examination guideline of a physician screening (U.S. Department of Health and Human Services, 1986). Some public health educational approaches geared to Mexican-Americans may be successful.

Despite lower socioeconomic status and higher rates of obesity and diabetes, cardiovascular disease rates are lower for Mexican-Americans than for whites (U.S. Department of Health and Human Services, 1986). This was supported in a study by Espino and coworkers (1991), in which data from the HHANES were studied. The authors concluded that there was a higher prevalence of diabetes and a lower prevalence of heart disease and hypertension when compared with the general population. This coincided with results of previous studies (Espino et al., 1991). A 1992 study by the University of Texas Health Science Center at San Antonio found that the prevalence of non–insulin-dependent diabetes was 2.5 times higher among Mexican-Americans than among non-Hispanic white Americans. Among the Mexican-Americans, prevalence followed a sociocultural gradient: 16% in low-income barrios, about 10% in middle-income neighborhoods, and 5% in high-income suburbs in San Antonio, Texas (Mitchell and Stern, 1992).

Another study examined physical, sociodemographic, and psychosocial data of diabetic Mexican-Americans aged 45 to 74 years included in the HHANES. Diabetic Mexican-American women were found to have lower education levels and lower employment rates in comparison with nondiabetics. Glaucoma, retinopathy, and activity limitation were more prevalent in diabetic than in nondiabetic men and women. Diabetic women also had a higher prevalence of hypertension, kidney problems, and cataracts. Among diabetics, duration of diabetes was associated with an increased prevalence of stroke and activity limitation. These findings on the health status of diabetic Mexican-Americans deserve further understanding of the health service needs of this population (Zhang et al., 1991).

Poverty and Health: A Relationship

In a 1987 special report on the results of the National Access Survey from the Robert Wood Johnson Foundation, key indicators of access to health care among minorities were presented (Leon, 1987). Almost one third of Mexican-Americans were without a regular source of health care and had not had an ambulatory visit within 12 months before the survey. Almost one fifth of Mexican-Americans had made an emergency visit within the 12 months before the survey, were without health insurance, and were in fair or poor health. In all of these categories, whites were reported as being better off than the remainder of the population (Leon, 1987). Unlike previous national access surveys, which found that Hispanics were only slightly worse off than the national average, the 1986 National Access Survey found a considerable deterioration in their situation.

Interestingly, a study conducted in 1991 at the University of Texas Medical Branch in Galveston showed that the most significant and consistent predictor of the health status of Mexican-Americans was employment. Less acculturated men had poorer self-assessed health. Married men were more likely to have been hospitalized during the year before the interview, whereas less acculturated women were less likely to have been hospitalized (Markides and Lee, 1991).

Socioeconomic conditions may be seen as both a cause and a result of Mexican-American health conditions. Poor health conditions may affect socioeconomic conditions in three ways:

- By causing an interruption in or termination of employment (especially significant for the head of a household)
- By preventing a person from learning or participating in activities that would increase income and education
- By causing a person to spend a disproportionate amount of income on maintaining health status or reducing disease or injury

Adverse socioeconomic conditions may affect health status in the following ways:

- By subjecting a person to unhealthy environmental conditions (e.g., crowded housing, lack of treated drinking water or proper sewage disposal)
- By depriving a person of the education necessary to understand preventive measures in disease control

and general physical well-being (e.g., lack of knowledge about nutrition, not understanding theory)
- By limiting the care received
- By barring a person from health care services (e.g., through racial discrimination or lack of transportation)
- By leading a person, through ignorance and desperation, to seek types of health care that might ultimately cause self-harm (Lyndon B. Johnson School of Public Affairs, 1979)

In view of the relationships between poverty and health, the socioeconomic status of a large portion of the Mexican-American population in southern Texas indicates that there are many potential health problems. These problems may be summarized as follows:

- The low income of many Mexican-Americans gives them little money for medical services. Lack of funds may require individuals to forgo medical services or reliance on assistance from others (i.e., family, friends, charities, or public funds).
- The lack of formal education among many Mexican-Americans suggests that they are less likely to be aware of or to practice modern preventive health care. In addition, the low income of many, if not most, Mexican-Americans makes the practice of preventive health care difficult.
- Crowded housing and the lack of basic services, such as treated water and proper sewage disposal, result in a greater potential for the spread of communicable diseases among many Mexican-Americans. Lack of these facilities also makes preventive health practices difficult (Lyndon B. Johnson School of Public Affairs, 1979).

Consequently, a system of health care delivery that includes preventive health services and health education and that is designed for relatively well-educated Mexican-Americans with a moderate income probably will not meet the needs of those with a low income. Rather, an appropriate health system must be based on the health risks and health needs of the Mexican-American population and must take into account their age distribution, income, and education.

THE MEXICAN-AMERICAN FAMILY

By the year 2000, Hispanics will outnumber African-Americans and become the majority population (Caudle, 1993). One third to one half of the Mexican-Americans in the Southwest live either below the official level of poverty or immediately above it (Lyndon B. Johnson School of Public Affairs, 1979). The conventional population paradigm in the United States has distinguished between the white majority and the sizable and easily identified black minority. Until recently, much less attention has been paid to Mexican-Americans. The number of Hispanics in the United States, currently 20 million, will increase to 31 million (projected total population, 283 million) by the year 2010. This would translate into 15 million Mexican-Americans by 2010.

Educational opportunities have been so restricted that Mexican-Americans are 3 to 4 years behind the educational levels of the general population. Despite the economic and educational problems, Mexican-Americans continue to demonstrate unique socialization characterized by warmth and closeness, which are the result of the family structure.

Literature that explains economic, educational, and other social characteristics of Mexican-Americans fails to provide a realistic understanding of Mexican-Americans in their daily lives. Some Hispanic writers, such as Octavio Romano-V, lash out at anthropologists and sociologists who present Mexican-Americans as an ahistoric group. Romano-V insisted that, to correct the distortion of Mexican-American history, it is necessary to view Mexican-Americans in the context of a historic culture and an intellectual history instead of the stereotypic, static concepts of a traditional culture and nonintellectual history (Romano-V, 1986).

One way to discuss the Mexican-American family is to differentiate between traditional and nontraditional lifestyles. These characteristics may also be seen in other Hispanic groups or cultures.

Within the traditional framework, the family is seen as a close-knit group in which elders are the decision makers. It is not uncommon to see extended family members living with the nuclear family. All of the members regard the family as the main focus of social identification. Each member is a symbol of the family, and each must help maintain community respect for the family. It is within the family nucleus that one not only is disciplined but also receives love and understanding. This love and understanding permeate outwardly to the extended family of grandparents, uncles, and aunts. If possible, the members of the family live in close proximity to each other and visit frequently. Each is concerned for the other and readily offers assistance when needed. However, family problems are for the family to solve, and "outside" help is seldom sought or desired.

The father is the unquestioned authority of the household. He is hard, unyielding, and strong. He often exemplifies these traits by demonstrating his ability to drink heavily and conquer members of the opposite sex (machismo). The members of his family must show him respect at all times; failure to do so will invoke his wrath, usually in the form of a physical beating. His family is poor, but he provides for them as well as he can because it is his duty as head of the family to look after them (Stenger-Castro, 1978).

The mother is soft, nurturing, and self-sacrificing. Her place is in the home. Her responsibilities are to ensure that the household runs properly and to be in charge of the children's upbringing. She does not openly question her husband's actions. Any pain or suffering she experiences is considered concomitant with being female (Stenger-Castro, 1978).

The children are to be seen and not heard. They are expected to contribute to the running of the household. The girls help their mother with the household chores. The boys find jobs as soon as they are old enough so that they may contribute monetarily to the family. There are usually four or more siblings, and they must remember that the younger children respect the older ones and that the female respects the male. Most find it easier to confide in their mother because their father is someone they respect but do not know very well. Typically, the children will have some schooling; some may finish high school, but they must not forget that their duty to the family takes precedence over personal ambition.

Murillo (1976) pointed out that, because of the close interpersonal ties that exist among family members, the Mexican-American may temporarily forgo job, school, or other activities to meet family needs, which have priority.

The traditional family member is courteous and will demonstrate good manners, which may cause problems in communication. For example, a young Mexican-American boy translating for a white physician may not wish to convey to his mother a question such as "Why did you wait so long to obtain medical care?" or a question regarding her personal status. He may see this as rude or disrespectful.

The nontraditional Mexican-American has adopted acculturative patterns that may be the result of migration into white communities or improvement of educational level or economic status. The Mexican-American maintains characteristics such as close family ties, certain health beliefs, and recreational patterns.

The nontraditional Mexican-American may not engage in the traditional forms of recreation, such as group drinking and conversation, but will still enjoy fiestas, *pachangas,* and *fandangos.* Traditional events such as debuts, or *la quinceanera,* in which 15-year-old girls enter womanhood, are still practiced.

Cultural continuance in families is evident in the ways the members use terms of endearment and address their elders, in the way they behave with their peers, and in the way they use long-tested demeanor when responding to figures of authority. Young Mexican-Americans, some outwardly tough and aggressive and seemingly independent of family ties and restrictions, harbor tender feelings toward their *jefitos* and *jefitas.* Although visible changing characteristics may appear to make contemporary lifestyles unstable and haphazard, the vulnerability of tough gang members is shown during family-oriented gatherings and celebrations, where all indifference and isolation are cast aside when the piñata is broken and "Las Mananitas," a Spanish song traditionally sung at birthdays that symbolizes rejoicing and life, accompanies a family ritual (Enrique, 1980).

It is important for one to remain alert and recognize the ways in which the Mexican-American culture is practiced and kept alive. It is exciting to see a young couple attired in symbolic fashions as they walk with their child, using the word *jita* in addressing the child. Another example of cultural continuance in the health care setting involves nursing interaction with an obstetric patient being first seen for prenatal care. The young Mexican-American patient may be very interested in diet and regular checkups but will explain to the nurse specific folk medicinal habits that have been passed from generation to generation. In the best interest of patient care, the nurse should listen attentively and not be judgmental but rather allow cultural habits to be integrated with modern medical care.

Mexican-Americans are often viewed in a stereotypic manner. What may not be recognized is their unique methods of socialization and their rituals, celebrations, and festivities, which are of both historic and cultural importance. Whether Mexican-Americans are classified as traditional or nontraditional is a matter of individual perception and classification habits. Family loyalty scales and the assimilation processes mark individual differences and degrees of cultural continuance.

BELIEFS OF DISEASE CAUSATION AMONG MEXICAN-AMERICANS

Mexican-Americans typically view health or disease as an area in which God or some other extrahuman force has been influential, either directly or indirectly. Regardless of the causative agent, the explanation as to why the condition happened to the particular individual at a particular time is likely to be sought in the extrahuman realm. A particular cause of an illness may be that of *castigos,* or a punishment. Castigos are sanctions imposed by the supernatural and are used to explain certain conditions of ill health. This source is essentially benevolent and comes from God. The malevolent source, with or without the intermediation of evil, may be in the form of *brujas,* or witches (Clark, 1959). The ultimate source of disease is God, who is said to have placed illness and all other things in the world. Foster (1953) discussed ideas of disease causation that are based on natural phenomena, supernatural or physiologically untrue concepts, magical origins, and emotional concepts. Many recognized and named illnesses are due to a series of emotional experiences.

An important concept within the Mexican-American culture is that of curanderismo, or folk healing. Curanderismo is a complicated system of healing that involves the *curandero,* or healer, who acts as a diagnostician, counselor, or practitioner for many Mexican-Americans. The curandero is usually considered the wisest individual, having derived powers to heal from God.

Mexican-American folk medicine considers three types of causation: empirical, magical, and psychological (Saunders, 1954). In a study of Mexican-Americans in California, Clark (1959) discussed the theory of disease in this population in terms of diseases of "hot and cold" imbalance, diseases caused by dislocation of internal organs, diseases of magical origin, diseases of emotional origin, other folk-defined diseases, and "standard scientific" diseases.

Mexican-Americans can explain etiologic factors associated with disease at two levels: the source of disease at the extrahuman level in its benevolent and malevolent forms (discussed earlier) and provoking agents, which are operative in the daily life processes. The following agents are considered to be provocations (Samora, 1961):

- Food: food that is spoiled; food that does not agree with one; green fruit; food given to one by a bruja; and food to which one is allergic

- Shock: being frightened; receiving unfavorable news, such as news about the death of a loved one
- Accidents of various sorts
- Bodily malfunction: general bodily malfunction; malfunction or displacement of specific organs
- Age: general greater susceptibility to illness with increasing age
- Abuse of the body: overindulgence in eating or drinking; debauchery
- Not taking care of one's self: vague and general acts of omission or commission
- Congenital: being born ill or deformed
- Hereditary: having inherited a tendency toward, or a susceptibility for, certain illnesses
- Contact with the elements: being in drafts; getting the feet wet; night air; too much sun
- Environmental, nonspecific (an illness that is "going around")
- Contact with persons: *mal ojo* ("evil eye") given through admiration; individuals who practice *brujeria* (witchcraft) may hex or bewitch someone; individuals who are *enconosos* (malevolent) may aggravate an illness (this is not the same as causing an illness)
- Occupational causes: lifting heavy objects; working under unfavorable conditions such as excessive heat, dampness, or cold

The germ theory of disease is not recognized by all Mexican-Americans; this may be a function of educational and economic levels.

In a descriptive study conducted in 1978, R.A. Martinez (in an unpublished study) surveyed 50 lower income Mexican-American mothers of preschool-age children about their attitudes toward immunization. Study results indicated that these mothers tend to immunize their children primarily as a prerequisite to enter the public school system. The mothers also believed that immunizing their children would produce fever, which they considered an "illness." They thought that it was in the best interest of the child not to have them go through this unnatural process.

Diseases are classified as being caused by certain factors or having a specific origin. The following sections describe diseases caused by the dislocation of internal organs, by emotions, and by magic.

Diseases Caused by Dislocation of Internal Organs

Caida de la mollera is a disease of infants that occurs when the fontanelle of the parietal or frontal bone of the cranium falls and leaves a "soft spot," which sometimes vibrates during breathing. It usually happens during breast-feeding or as a result of a sudden fall. The infant is usually spoon-fed during the illness (Rubel, 1960). Treatment consists of putting salt on the fallen fontanelle and allowing it to remain for 3 days. As this is done, the curer presses against the roof of the baby's mouth to raise the depression. If not successfully treated, it can lead to "drying up," and death can occur. Normal feeding cannot be resumed until the fontanelle has been raised to its normal position. Along with this ritual, an herbal tea is administered in large amounts (Rubel, 1960).

Empacho is an infirmity of both children and adults that occurs when food particles become lodged in the intestinal tract and cause sharp pains. To treat this illness, the person lies face down on a bed with the back bared. The attending curer lifts a piece of skin from the waist and pinches it, listening for a snap from the abdominal region. Once the nature of the illness is established, this is repeated several times along the spinal column in hopes of dislodging the offending material. Preparations of herbs such as *chichipaste, cascara sagrada, ajenjible* (or *jengibre*) (ginger), and rhubarb as well as drugs like *desempacho* are administered orally to penetrate, soften, and crumble the chunk of food. Empacho is usually not a serious infirmity, and prayer is usually not part of the curing process (Rubel, 1960).

Diseases of Emotional Origin

The mind-body dualism of modern medicine does not exist in traditional medicine. As a result, many physical diseases are tracked to emotional origins and treated psychosomatically.

Bilis, or bile, is a concept brought to Mexico by the Spanish, but it is of Greek origin. Originally, it was based on the ancient belief that the body was composed of four humors. This belief maintains that the humors must remain in balance for a person to enjoy good health. Any highly emotional experience such as anger or fear may cause the humors to become unbalanced, and excess bile may flow into the blood stream, producing a wide variety of illnesses.

In a study of Mexican-Americans in California, Clark (1959) stated,

The term "bilis" is not always used to indicate a disease; sometimes it means simply that a person is nervous or upset about something. In its medical sense, however, bilis is a disorder which is diagnosed and treated like any other illness. Adults are said to be particularly susceptible to it. The illness always comes on after a person becomes very angry, especially if he flies into an uncontrollable rage. A day or two after this fit of anger, the attack occurs. The disorder produces symptoms of acute nervous tension, chronic fatigue and malaise.

(HOLLAND, 1978, P. 104)

Bilis is ordinarily treated with herbal remedies, such as *negrita* and *sauco* (elder tree), that are consumed in the form of teas. Less severe cases are not treated.

Susto, or fright sickness, is another emotion-based illness that is very common in Mexico. All indications suggest that the concept is Indian rather than Spanish in origin.

Almost any disturbing or unstabilizing experience such as an unexpected fall, a barking dog, or an automobile accident may be sufficient to cause susto if part of the self separates from the body. Among Indian groups from southern Mexico, for whom this concept exists in a more aboriginal context, susto is attributed to a spirit loss. With the loss of spirit, cold air rushes in and takes over the body. A case in San Antonio dealt with the traumatic experience of an infant passing through the birth canal as causing susto.

In the early stages, susto is usually accompanied by colic, diarrhea, high temperature, vomiting, and several other symptoms. The person's appetite is lost, and the intestines slowly desiccate and will not allow food to pass through. If not cured in the early stages, the patient suffers long, continuous periods of malaise, listlessness, and loss of appetite (Holland, 1978).

As the disease progresses, the patient is forced to withdraw from active participation in normal family and social activities and remain in bed. Susto is believed to be sometimes fatal.

Traditional curers usually resort to a combination of herbal and magicoreligious devices to treat susto (Holland, 1978). Among Mexican-Americans in Texas and virtually all Mexican Indian and peasant groups, the practitioner calls the spirit back into the patient's body to effect the cure. The illness is treated by brushing the body with *ruda*—an herb that grows in long branches—for nine consecutive nights. The brushing is performed to remove the cold air and allow the spirit that is being summoned to return to the body. This treatment is often accompanied by prayers and burning candles before images of saints in either the home or church.

Diseases of Magical Origin

Mal ojo is assumed to be the magical origin of many illnesses, especially those afflicting children. According to this belief, some people are born with *vista fuerte* (strong vision) with which they unwittingly harm others with a mere glance. One of every set of twins inevitably possesses this power. It is believed that the glance toward a pregnant woman may cause an infant to become ill with fever because the "heat of the pregnancy" damages its tender spirit (Holland, 1978).

An infant with mal ojo sleeps restlessly, cries for no apparent reason, vomits, and has fever and diarrhea. Mal ojo can also be fatal. Mal ojo is treated by rubbing the body with an egg for three consecutive evenings. During this ritual, the healer will chant several prayers. The egg, with the heat captured in the shell, will be broken and left overnight, under the head of the bed. In the morning, if the egg appears to be "cooked," then mal ojo was the cause of the illness.

It is not uncommon for Mexican-American mothers in San Antonio to adorn their children with amulets, which are usually "deer eyes" or *"ojos de venado"* (a legume seed from Mexico), as prevention of mal ojo. In addition, the color red, in the form of either string or yarn, may be tied to the child's wrist for protection. The nurse should not question the parent but rather accept this practice, especially if it is psychologically helping the mother.

Dano, or witchcraft, plays an important part in traditional Mexican disease concepts. Those with close ties to Mexican Indian and peasant cultures are generally credited with greater knowledge of witchcraft than are more assimilated Mexican-Americans. Witches are described as people who sell their souls to the devil in return for the power to harm others through magic (Holland, 1978). Brujeria, or witchcraft, should not be confused with curanderismo, or folk healing.

The Hot-Cold Syndrome

Exposure to excessive heat or cold may be the main cause of illness. Also, certain foods may be thought to cause illness if they generate heat or cold within the body.

Some of the illnesses believed to be caused by cold entering the body are listed next (Currier, 1978):

- Chest cramps: Cold air enters the chest when a person is overheated.
- Earache: A cold draft of air enters the ear canal.

- Headache: The coolness of mist or of the night air, called *aigre,* penetrates the head.
- Paralysis: A part of the body is "struck" by aigre. Stiffness, which is considered to be a partial, temporary paralysis, is ascribed to the same cause.
- Pain caused by sprains: Such "cold pains" are the result of cold entering the damaged part.
- Stomach cramp: When the body is warm and not adequately covered, cold can enter from the air or from a body of water.
- Rheumatism: Cold from some outside source lodges in the afflicted bones.
- Teething: The pain of teething is a "cold pain" that originates in the coldness of the new white teeth that are growing in.
- Tuberculosis: Cold enters the body from water or carbonated beverages, especially when the body is overheated from work or travel.

The following are some of the illnesses believed to be caused by an overabundance of heat in the body:

- *Algondoncillo:* Heat rises from the center of the body to the mouth, causing the gums, tongue, and lips to turn white.
- *Dislipela:* Overexposure to the sun can cause the sun's heat to collect in the skin, resulting in an outbreak of red spots on the hands, arms, or, less often, feet.
- Dysentery: Because it is accompanied by bloody stool and blood is intensely hot, dysentery is classified as a hot disease and may be caused by consuming too much hot food.
- Sore eyes: A person may overstrain the eyes, causing them to "work hard" and thus heat up; alternatively, cold, wet feet can cause the body heat to rise to the head and overheat the eyes.
- *Fogazo:* Heat rising from the center of the body causes the mouth and tongue to break out in tiny red spots. In contrast to algodoncillo, this is not a serious disease.
- Kidney ailments: Any pain in the kidneys is a hot pain; most kidney ailments are accompanied by itching feet or ankles, reddening of the palms of the hands, and fever.
- *Postemilla:* An abscessed tooth results from heat concentrating in the root of the tooth, evidenced by the fact that the abscess releases blood when it bursts.
- Sore throat: Wet feet cause sore throat by driving body heat up into the throat.

- Warts and rashes: Regardless of the cause (a subject on which my informants refused to speculate), these ailments are the result of heat. Warts and rashes are irritating, and irritation is always ascribed to heat and never to cold.

The causes of diseases and the strong beliefs found among Mexican-Americans cannot be ignored and should be taken into consideration by health care providers. Mexican-American clients should not be ridiculed for beliefs of disease causation but rather should be supported in recognizing the existence of disease regardless of the cause. After all, illnesses have some basis for developing, and who is qualified to question the validity of certain beliefs? The underlying importance of recognizing the individual's beliefs is the ability to accept the belief and indirectly begin to educate on "real" causes of illness.

USE OF HERBAL MEDICINE AMONG MEXICAN-AMERICANS

Historically, the most important uses of herbs have been medicinal. For most of history, there have been limited resources for treating injuries and diseases. Plant remedies have been the most continuous and universal form of treatment. Among Mexican-Americans, herbal medicine has strong cultural and historic ties to Indian, Aztec, and Spanish-Moorish societies.

In an extensive study of the healing herbs found in the upper Rio Grande Valley, Curtin (1947)) cited numerous illnesses for which the Mexican population had devised treatment. Although these data are not presented here in great detail, an effort was made to check the *curanderos'* familiarity with the medicines. As expected, the *curanderos* had used the great majority of the herbs described by Curtin for essentially the same symptom complexes.

The use of herbs by Mexican-Americans demonstrates the extent of both their nosologic considerations and their pharmacopoeia. The following is a list of medicinal herbs and the conditions they treat (Martinez, 1978, pp. 262–263):

- Rattlesnake oil *(aceite de vibora)*: rheumatism
- Mineral water *(agua piedra)*: kidney stones
- Garlic *(ajo)*: diphtheria prevention, pain in the bowels, toothache, rabid dog bite, stomach trouble, snakebite, hypertension

- Cottonwood *(alamo sauco)*: swollen gums, ulcerated tooth
- Cottonwood (a different generic herb) *(alamo de hoja redondo)*: boils, broken bones
- Sweet basil *(albahaca)*: hornet bite, colic
- Apricot *(hueso de albaricoque)*: goiter, dryness of the nose
- Camphor *(alcanfor)*: pain, rheumatism, headache, faintness
- Amaranth *(alegria)*: heart trouble, tuberculosis, jaundice
- Alfalfa *(alfalfa)*: bed bugs
- Filaree *(alfilerillo)*: need for diuretic, rheumatism, gonorrhea
- Lavender *(alhucema)*: phlegm, colic, vomiting, menopause
- Licorice *(yerba del lobo)*: clotted blood
- Aster *(cosmose)*: chest congestion
- Parsley *(amis)*: painful shoulders, stomach troubles, colic
- Cocklebur *(cadillos)*: diarrhea, rattlesnake bite
- Wild pitplant *(buchuheat)*: pyorrhea, throat irritation, skin irritation
- Desert tea: headaches, cold, fever, kidney pain
- Scouring brush *(pingacion)*: gonorrhea

In addition, the root immortelle is occasionally ground into powder for upper respiratory infection chest pain, fatigue, and tuberculosis. Spearmint *(yerba buena)* is good for childbirth, newborns with colic, and menstrual cramps. Cupping *(ventosa)* is good for muscle aches and, as a liniment, for the nerves.

A few herbs are used to treat psychiatric conditions, which opens the door for other types of treatment for such conditions. *Yerba del dapo,* an herb in the aster family, is used for *saltido,* or "jumping stomach," which appears to be a nervous kind of stomach disorder. The green plant is formed into a large ball, wrapped in a cloth, and placed on the navel to stop the throbbing. Some herbs are also used as love charms to enhance sexual performance and bring good fortune in the pursuit of love.

The use of herbs in combination with prayer and touch is seen in a variety of rituals associated with folk illnesses such as susto and mal ojo.

Specific herbs or herbal preparations may be used in the treatment of certain chronic conditions such as hypertension, diabetes, arthritis, and some malignancies. Even though few studies have been conducted on the efficacy or effects of these herbal preparations, most herbalists are aware of proper dosages. Nurses usually should allow patients to continue their herbal regimen, but at the same time they should encourage the use of modern medical care and practice.

Ruda is used to "sweep" the person during the ritual for susto. A tea of *cenizo* is administered after the ritual to enhance the warmth needed to draw the spirit back to the person. Yerba buena is administered as part of the ritual for mal ojo. Some herbs with a purgative effect are administered as part of the treatment for empacho.

It would be interesting to trace certain remedies now sold in pharmacies in extract form to the first application in the form of leaf, bark, or root. How have people come by this knowledge? Has knowledge been the result of repeated experimentation or of the coincidental application of the remedy?

In the 1890s, Don Pedro Jaramillo lived in the southern part of Texas near the Mexican village of Los Olmos. Legend says that God bestowed upon Jaramillo the power to *recetar* (prescribe) formulas to cure the sick. Many of his *recetas* included herbs. Because of his popularity and success in helping people, Jaramillo is still recognized as the "saint" of curanderos in Texas.

The use of medicinal herbs continues in modern societies, especially in Mexican-American communities. Stores continue to sell herbs, and their popularity has continued through the practice of curanderismo. Nurses should not be critical of the practice of herbal medicine but rather recognize it as an alternative health care system that supplements modern medical practice.

CULTURAL ADAPTATION TO HEALTH CARE IN THE COMMUNITY

Improving Access

It is well known that Mexican-Americans tend to fall into a lower economic level than the general population.

In 1981, the average income of Hispanic families was 70% that of white families ($16,400 vs. $23,500). One fourth of all Hispanic families lived below the U.S. Bureau of the Census' poverty level (Davis et al., 1983). In 1990, the percentage of all Hispanic families living below poverty level had increased to 28.1% (National Center for Health Statistics, 1992).

Because of a lower economic level, certain conveniences available to other groups, such as transportation, may not be available to Mexican-Americans. Without adequate transportation, problems may arise in relation to access. For example, clinic appointments may be missed or impossible to keep because of inadequate public transportation.

In addition, because some households have no telephones, essential communication such as appointment reminders and contact of ill patients for follow-up care may be a problem.

Use patterns of Hispanics and other low-income persons compared with those of the white population and higher income groups are manifested as follows (U.S. Department of Health, Education, and Welfare, 1979):

- A smaller proportion of Hispanics and low-income patients visit a physician; the average number of physician visits per year is lower among Hispanics but somewhat higher among low-income patients.
- Outpatient department use is greater among nonwhites and low-income patients.
- Short-stay nonfederal hospitalization rates are lower among Hispanics but higher among low-income patients.
- Length of hospital stay is longer for both Hispanics and low-income persons.
- Fewer Hispanics and low-income persons report to a physician versus a clinic as a regular source of care.

Improving access to health care for Mexican-Americans may include making appointment times convenient (e.g., evening and weekend hours), having satellite clinics in the community (close to the population being served), or working through neighborhood associations and churches to provide care and health education.

Mobile vans as portable treatment modules have been used in some communities as a way to improve access. However, in some communities, this may be seen as intimidating or intruding; a permanent facility may be more acceptable (Aranda, 1971).

More than 12% of Americans appear to have particularly serious trouble coping with the conventional health care system and obtaining care when needed. One fifth of Hispanic adults are medically disadvantaged, primarily because of financial problems, lack of health insurance, lack of a regular source of medical care resulting from financial problems, or lack of knowledge as to where to obtain care (Anonymous, 1991).

Reducing Language Barriers and Improving Communication

The most important differences between Hispanic folk medicine and scientific medicine that influence the choice of one over the other are as follows:

- Scientific medicine is largely impersonal.
- Scientific procedures are unfamiliar to the lay person.
- A passive role is played by family members in conventional health care.
- Considerable control of the situation is taken by professional health care providers.

Mexican-American folk medicine is largely a matter of personal relations, familiar procedures, active family participation, home care, and a large degree of control of the situation by the patient or family. Given these differences, it is easy to understand why considerable motivation would be necessary for a Mexican-American to have strong preference for scientific medicine over a system that is more familiar and possibly psychologically more rewarding or at least less punishing (Gemmill, 1973a, 1973b).

Techniques for reducing communication barriers may include recognition that low-income people have a tendency to express positive attitudes about modern health care that may not reflect their true attitudes. Also, to reduce language barriers further, communication between practitioners and patients should be dialogue based rather than one-sided imperatives. This is particularly important because the patient and practitioner may not use the same words for the same meanings of disease processes, even within a similar language (Adams et al., 1992).

In a classic article, Guarnaschelli and associates (1972) reported a case of subdural hematoma occurring in an infant secondary to the manipulations of a folk healer. The curandera had conducted the traditional healing ritual for "fallen fontanelle." The importance of reporting this case is appropriate; however, to label the phenomenon, as occurred in this report, a "variant of the battered child syndrome" was inappropriate. The parents sought treatment from a healer for a disease not recognized by conventional medicine. This could have been considered appropriate behavior in the context of their cultural belief. The parents sought a cure for their child's illness, and the curandera behaved in the accepted manner of the tradition of the art. The injury probably occurred as an accidental complication of the procedure. This may be a good example

of practitioners being "culturally blind" and not understanding the true meaning of folk medicine.

There has been much discussion in the literature regarding the need for bilingual and bicultural health practitioners, especially as a way of gaining the trust and confidence of patients. In addition to the need to transmit information in Spanish, there must be sensitivity in the patient-practitioner interaction. Scherwitz (1980) found that when practitioners spoke in Spanish, the medical recommendations increased in meaningfulness.

IMPROVING HEALTH EDUCATION AND HEALTH COMMUNICATION

According to the U.S. Department of Health and Human Services' report on black and minority health (1986), "health promotion messages and health care to Hispanic groups are most effective when delivered within their social frame of reference, focusing on problems known to exist in the community."

Certain common elements appear to contribute to the success of many health programs:

- Community involvement and outreach
- Program focus on comprehensive services, including disease prevention and health promotion
- Program ability to improve minority access to health services
- Cultural sensitivity to the group being served

Examples of health programs that have been successful in Mexican-American communities include community outreach; hypertension control; maternal and child health care; family planning, health education, promotion, and prevention; bicultural and bilingual health care; and Medicare-Medicaid (U.S. Department of Health and Human Services, 1986). In general, improved access to medical care was cited as a key element of a program's success; however, success was by no means limited to this element.

To develop effective health education programs, health care practitioners and educators need to include in their planning factors related to the homogeneity or heterogeneity of the Mexican-American population; the extent to which socioeconomic status adversely affects Mexican-Americans' access to health care; the influence of demographic and epidemiologic factors in determining their access to the health and medical infrastructures; and the effect of acculturation on the biopsychosocial realms of the Mexican-American.

To this end and as reported by Marin and colleagues (1993), the development of an appropriate research agenda for Mexican-Americans requires progress in three areas: (1) developing an appropriate research infrastructure, (2) increasing the availability of appropriate research instrumentation, and (3) identifying and assigning priority areas. In addition, a Hispanic health research agenda must identify mechanisms for increasing the number of trained Mexican-American researchers and the number of Mexican-American professional staff members at the Department of Health and Human Services. Marin and colleagues recommended that an office of Hispanic health be established within the Office of Minority Health at the Department of Health and Human Services to oversee the implementation of the recommendations made as part of the Surgeon General's National Hispanic Health Initiative.

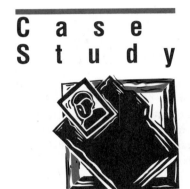

Case Study

Maria Garcia brings her 3-year-old child, Hector, to the hospital emergency department with a high temperature, chills, vomiting, and complaints of flank pain. She is registered at the desk and is questioned as to how payment will be made. Sra. Garcia does not have health insurance for her children. She explains that she will pay cash. The Anglo receptionist demands that a deposit of $25.00 for emergency department services be made before treatment. Sra. Garcia obliges.

Sra. Garcia has two other children, an 8- and a 10-year-old. Her husband is a carpenter, and he spends considerable time traveling to complete contracted jobs.

Sra. Garcia is directed to a waiting room. After 1½ hours of waiting, she is escorted to a treatment room by an Anglo nurse. No communication takes place between the nurse and Sra. Garcia. The nurse asks the mother to hold the child while she takes his temperature. The nurse proceeds to place Hector in a tub of cool water; no explanation is given, and both Sra. Garcia and Hector are wondering what is occurring. Sra. Garcia is alarmed that the nurse is doing this to her child. She strongly believes that his fever and symptoms are the result of being exposed to the cold morning air and that this submersion will only increase his complaints. The nurse begins to ask Sra. Garcia about the child's history. Very little is understood by Sra. Garcia, and the nurse makes no attempt to obtain a translator.

After 30 minutes of being in the tub, Hector is removed; his temperature is retaken. The nurse nods to Sra. Garcia as though she is saying, "He's okay." The nurse then says, "The doctor will be here in a while."

Dr. Williams, a young Anglo physician, walks in and in a very hostile manner asks Sra. Garcia why she had to bring him to the emergency department instead of a physician's office. Sra. Garcia was overwhelmed by his questions and felt guilty about the visit and her failure to bring him to the hospital sooner. Sra. Garcia explained to the physician that she had not had time and that she had been taking Hector to the curandero, who had been giving him some herbal tea to drink.

The physician explained to Sra. Garcia that the child needed to be hospitalized. She stated that she needed to consult with her husband about this and she would return after the decision had been made. The physician could not understand why she had to consult with her husband but agreed to let her go; he stressed the need for the child to be hospitalized.

That afternoon, Sra. Garcia discussed the need for hospitalization with her husband. Mr. Garcia felt that the physician did not know what he was talking about. He insisted that she see Pepito, the curandero, before going back to the hospital. She did, and Pepito concurred that seeking medical attention was probably the proper course of action. After Hector was hospitalized, the family was referred to the local health department for follow-up home visits by a public health nurse.

Study Questions

- Why was communication between Sra. Garcia and the health care professionals a problem?
- What could have been done to explain to Sra. Garcia the purpose of the cool bath?
- Why is the Anglo health care professional considered the ultimate "all-knowing" individual?
- Explain disease causation and lack of knowledge of the germ theory as it impacted the interaction between the health care providers and the Garcia family.
- What significance was there in Sra. Garcia discussing the hospitalization with the husband?
- What significance was there in the Garcias obtaining a curandero's opinion?
- How does the concept of PASS relate to this scenario?

SUMMARY

This chapter presented an overview of the health needs and beliefs of Mexican-Americans and their implications for community health nursing. Major diseases and health conditions prevalent among Mexican-Americans were identified. Socioeconomic and culturally relevant reasons for the status of Mexican-Americans' health were reviewed. The folk health system, including common folk illnesses and herbal medicine unique to Mexican-Americans, was de-

scribed. The need for better cultural adaptation to health care in the community was emphasized, especially by improving access to health care, understanding PASS and its cause and prevention, reducing language barriers, improving communication patterns, and providing health education in a style that is culturally sensitive.

Finally, a case study was presented that serves as a stimulus for the generation of a culturally relevant nursing care plan for a Mexican-American patient.

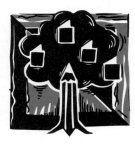

**L e a r n i n g
A c t i v i t i e s**

1. Develop a culturally relevant nursing care plan for this family, including assessment, nursing diagnoses, planning, intervention, and evaluation at the individual, family, and aggregate or community levels, for follow-up by the public health nurse.

2. Categorize these interventions that you generate into primary, secondary, and tertiary levels of prevention.

3. Find where in your community you could (1) take a beginning or advanced course in Spanish; (2) take a course in Spanish specifically designed for health professionals; and (3) refer Spanish-speaking clients to a course in English as a second language.

4. Consider the roles played by Hispanic actors and actresses during prime-time television. What percentage of the actors and actresses are of Hispanic origin? What messages are given about this population?

5. Identify through census data where persons of Hispanic origin reside in your city or town. Locate health care resources in those census tracts and compare them with health care resources available in census tracts populated largely by whites.

6. Locate a curandero, or healer, in the Hispanic community and make an appointment to discuss health beliefs, common illnesses, and their treatments. Ask how the curandero came to be a healer.

REFERENCES

Adams R, Briones EH, Rentfro AR: Cultural considerations: Developing a nursing care delivery system for a Hispanic community. Nurs Clin North Am 27:107–117, 1992.

Anonymous: Hispanic health in the United States. JAMA 265:248–252, 1991.

Aranda RG: The Mexican-American syndrome. Am J Public Health 61:105, 1971.

Black SA, Markides KS: Acculturation and alcohol consumption in Puerto Rican, Cuban-American, and Mexican-American women in the United States. Am J Public Health 83:890–893, 1993.

Caudle P: Providing culturally sensitive health care to Hispanic clients. Nurse Pract 18:40–51, 1993.

Clark M: Health in the Mexican-American Culture. Berkeley, CA, University of California Press, 1959.

Currier RL: The hot-cold syndrome and symbolic balance in Mexican and Spanish-American folk medicine. In Martinez RA (ed). Hispanic Culture and Health Care. St. Louis, MO, CV Mosby, 1978, pp. 138–151.

Curtin LSM: Healing herbs of the upper Rio Grande. Santa Fe, NM: Laboratory of Anthropology, 1947.

Davis C, Haub C, Willette J: U.S. Hispanics: Changing the face of America. Population Bull 38:3, 1983.

Enrique H: Retention of heritage through family ritual. Agenda 10:6, 1980.

Espino DV, Burge SK, Mareno, CA: The prevalence of selected chronic diseases among the Mexican-American elderly: Data from the 1982-1984 Hispanic Health and Nutrition Examination Survey. J Am Board Fam Pract 4:217–222, 1991.

Foster G: Relationship between Spanish and Spanish-American folk medicine. J Am Folklore 66:201–217, 1953.

Gemmill RH: Cultural Differences in Medical Care (Publication No. GR51-240-008-06). San Antonio, TX, Academy of Health Sciences, U.S. Army, 1973a, p. 29.

Gemmill RH: Cultural Variation in Medical Care (Publication No. GR51-240-008-10). San Antonio, TX, Academy of Health Sciences, U.S. Army, 1973b, pp. iii, xii.

Guarnaschelli J, Lee J, Pitts F: Fallen fontanelle: A variant of the battered child syndrome. JAMA 222:1545, 1972.

Holland W: Mexican-American medical beliefs: Science or magic? In Martinez RA (ed): Hispanic Culture and Health Care. St. Louis, MO, CV Mosby, 1978, pp. 99–119.

Lecca PJ, Greenstein TN, McNeil JS: A profile of Mexican-American health: Data from the Hispanic Health and Nutrition Examination Survey 1982–84. Arlington, TX, Health Services Research, 1987.

Leon M: Special Report. The Robert Wood Johnson Foundation Serial Report No. 2. Princeton, NJ, The Robert Wood Johnson Foundation Communication Office, 1987, p. 6.

Lyndon B: Johnson School of Public Affairs. Socioeconomic conditions among Mexican-Americans in South Texas. In Mexican-American Policy Research Project (ed). The Health of Mexican-Americans in South Texas. Austin, TX, University of Texas, 1979, p. 11.

Marin G, Amaro H, Eisneberg C, Opava-Stitzer, S: The development of a relevant and comprehensive research agenda to improve Hispanic health. Public Health Report 108:546–550, 1993.

Markides KS, Lee DJ, Ray LA: Acculturation and hypertension in Mexican-Americans. Ethnic Dis 3:70–74, 1993.

Markides KS, Lee DJ: Predictors of health status in middle-aged and older Mexican-Americans. J Gerontol 46:S243–S249, 1991.

Martinez RA: Hispanic Culture and Health Care: Fact, Fiction, Folklore. St. Louis, MO, CV Mosby, 1978.

Mitchell BD, Stern MP: Recent developments in the epidemiology of diabetes in the Americas. World Health Stat Q 45:347–439, 1992.

Murillo N: The Mexican-American family. In Hernandez CA (ed). Chicanos: Social and Psychological Perspectives. St. Louis, MO, CV Mosby, 1976, pp. 15–25.

National Center for Health Statistics: Health, United States, 1991. Hyattsville, MD, U.S. Public Health Service, 1992.

Reynoso TC, Felice ME, Shragg, GP: Does American acculturation affect outcome of Mexican-American teenage pregnancy? J Adolesc Health 14:257–261, 1993.

Romano-V OI: The anthropology and sociology of the Mexican-Americans: The distortion of Mexican-American history. El Grito II:14–16, 1986.

Rubel A: Concept of disease in Mexican-American culture. Am Anthrop 62:797–799, 1960.

Samora J: Conception of health and disease among Spanish Americans. Am Catholic Soc Rev 22:314–323, 1961.

Saunders L: Cultural Differences and Medical Care. New York, Russell Sage Foundation, 1954, p. 148.

Scherwitz L: The effect of language on physician patient interaction (Publication No. [PHS] 80-3288) (abstract). Washington, DC, Research Proceedings Services, National Center for Health Services Research, Department of Health and Human Services, 1980.

Stenger-Castro EM: The Mexican-American: How his culture affects his health. In Martinez RA (ed). Hispanic Culture and Health Care. St. Louis, MO, CV Mosby, 1978. pp. 23–25.

U.S. Department of Health and Human Services: Report of the Secretary's Task Force on Black and Minority Health: Vol. VIII. Hispanic Health Issues. Washington, DC, U.S. Department of Health and Human Services, 1986, p. 5.

U.S. Department of Health, Education, and Welfare: Health Status of Minorities and Low Income Groups (Publication No. [HRA]-79-627). Washington, DC, DHEW, U.S. Public Health Service, 1979, pp. 11–12.

Vega WA, Gil AG, Warheit GJ, Zimmerman RS, Apospori E: Acculturation and delinquent behavior among Cuban American adolescents: Toward an empirical model. Am J Commun Psychol 21:113–125, 1993a.

Vega WA, Gil AG, Zimmerman RS, Warheit GJ: Risk factors for suicidal behavior among Hispanic, African-American, and non-Hispanic white boys in early adolescence. Ethnic Dis 3:229–241, 1993b.

Wolff CB, Portis M, Wolff H: Birth weight and smoking practices during pregnancy among Mexican-American women. Health Care Women Int 14:271–279, 1993.

Zhang J, Markides KS, Lee DJ: Health status of diabetic Mexican-Americans: Results from the Hispanic HANES. Ethnic Dis 1:273–279, 1991.

Cultural Influences in the Community: Other Populations

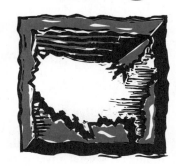

Upon conclusion of this section of chapters, the reader will be able to:

1. Identify a diverse population.

2. Describe three methods of assessing a diverse population within the community.

3. Compare and contrast the three methods of assessing a diverse population within the community.

4. Discuss the theoretical bases for program planning, implementation, and evaluation following the needs assessment of your population.

5. Identify a vulnerable population.

6. Discuss the seven properties of a vulnerable population.

7. Apply two implications for conducting research from the use of the guiding concept—marginalization—to a needs assessment of a diverse population.

Introduction by Janice M. Swanson

The following section contains articles that are reprinted, with the gracious permission of authors and publishers, from professional journals and a book. Each was selected for inclusion for the following reasons:

- To introduce the reader to information about the health status of diverse populations that may be found currently living in communities in the United States
- To introduce students to various approaches to community assessment, interventions, or both with diverse populations
- To stimulate readers' process of critical thinking as they are asked to apply concepts within their local community.

An Introduction to Diverse Populations Who May Be Found Currently Living in Many Communities in the United States. In the following section, the health of several diverse populations is presented, both indigenous and immigrant populations found within the United States: urban American Indians, Alaska Natives, Asian-Americans and Pacific Islanders, and Arab-American women. Finally, the concept of *marginalization* is presented as a guiding concept for the development of nursing knowledge regarding vulnerable populations that values diversity.

An Introduction to Various Approaches to Community Assessment and Interventions With Diverse Populations. Each of the chapters introduces the reader to an approach to community assessment and interventions. In many communities, an assessment of a diverse population may not exist and must be generated by the student in the community. Government vital and health statistics exist largely only for mainstream minority populations. Students in the community may need to assess a diverse population, such as an immigrant group, to determine the health status and needs of the community. Models used to approach an assessment of a population in the community are presented in the following chapters and include (1) the use of routinely reported data (vital statistics and communicable disease reports) (Grossman et al., 1994); (2) extensive manual and computer-based searches of government and private sources of information with specific techniques for uncovering information that is difficult to locate about a diverse community (Chen and Hawks, 1995); (3) conducting a needs assessment, including demographic, ethnographic, and historical information about a population in its social and geographical setting and program planning, implementation, and evaluation based on the needs assessment (Meleis et al., 1993 and Muecke 1983); and (4) the presentation of a concept—marginalization—and its properties (Hall et al., 1994) to sensitize the reader to examine implications for shaping nursing research, theory, and practice related to the health of vulnerable populations.

Stimulating the Process of Critical Thinking Through Application of Concepts Within the Local Community. The student is encouraged to engage in the process of critical thinking by identifying vulnerable populations in the community, developing an approach to assessing the needs of the populations, carrying out the assessment, and engaging in program planning, implementation, and evaluation based on the assessment.

The learning activities listed here can be applied across all the articles and aggregates discussed.

CULTURALLY APPROPRIATE NURSING CARE

A very recent guide to providing culturally appropriate nursing care covers basic information for nurses to help them improve nursing care. Focusing on similarities as well as differences, the guide presents issues related to health and illness, self care, family participation in care, and other topics for 24 distinct cultural groups living in the United States. The guide may be obtained from the UCSF Nursing Press, Box 0608, School of Nursing, University of California, San Francisco, 521 Parnassus Avenue, San Francisco, CA 94143-0608. Lipson JG, Dibble SL, Minarik PA: Culture and Nursing Care: A Pocket Guide. San Francisco: UCSF Nursing Press, 1996.

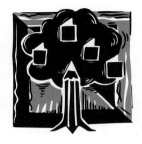

Learning Activities

1. Identify a vulnerable population within your own community; discuss two properties that make this population vulnerable.

2. Identify a diverse population within your community for which traditional health indicators (e.g., longevity, mortality, morbidity, health services usage) are not readily known.

3. Design an approach to assessment of a diverse population within your community; what data are available, and what data would you need to collect that are not available?

4. Conduct an assessment of the diverse population within your community.

5. Based on the needs assessment of the diverse population in your community, design a program plan, an implementation, and an evaluation.

6. List two implications from use of the guiding concept—marginalization—for valuing the diversity in your selected population; state how choice of a relevant design, sampling at the margins, and reflexive involvement of the marginalized persons or groups in your population can be applied in the development of your assessment and program.

REFERENCES

Chen MS Jr, Hawks BL: A debunking of the myth of healthy Asian Americans and Pacific Islanders. Am J Health Promotion 19:261–268, 1995.

Grossman DC, Krieger JW, Sugarman JR, Forquera RA: Health status of urban American Indians and Alaska Natives. JAMA 271:845–850, 1994.

Hall JM, Stevens PE, Meleis AI: Marginalization: A guiding concept for valuing diversity in nursing knowledge development. Adv Nurs Sci 16:23–41, 1994.

Meleis AI, Omidian PA, Lipson JG: Women's health status in the United States: An immigrant women's project. *In* McElmurry BJ, Norr KF, Parker RS, eds. Women's Health and Development: A Global Challenge. Boston: Jones and Bartlett, pp. 163–181, 1993.

Muecke MA: Caring for Southeast Asian refugee patients in the USA. Am J Public Health 73:431–438, 1983.

HEALTH STATUS OF URBAN AMERICAN INDIANS AND ALASKA NATIVES*
A Population-Based Study

David C. Grossman, MD, MPH • James W. Krieger, MD, MPH • Jonathan R. Sugarman, MD, MPH •
Ralph A. Forquera, MPH

Objective.—To use vital statistics and communicable disease reports to characterize the health status of an urban American Indian and Alaska Native (AI/AN) population and compare it with urban whites and African Americans and with AI/ANs living on or near rural reservations.

Design.—Descriptive analysis of routinely reported data.

Setting.—One metropolitan county and seven rural counties with reservation land in Washington State.

Subjects.—All reported births, deaths, and cases of selected communicable diseases occurring in the eight counties from 1981 through 1990.

Main Outcome Measures.—Low birth weight, infant mortality, and prevalence of risk factors for poor birth outcomes; age-specific and cause-specific mortality; rates of reported hepatitis A and hepatitis B, tuberculosis, and sexually transmitted diseases.

Results.—Urban AI/ANs had a much higher rate of low birth weight compared with urban whites and rural AI/ANs and had a higher rate of infant mortality than urban whites. During the 10 years, urban AI/AN infant mortality rates increased from 9.6 per 1000 live births to 18.6 per 1000 live births compared with no trend among the other populations. Compared with rural AI/AN mothers, urban AI/AN mothers were 50% more likely to receive late or no prenatal care during pregnancy. Relative to urban whites, urban AI/AN risk factors for poor birth outcomes (delayed prenatal care, adolescent age, and use of tobacco and alcohol) were more common and closely resembled the prevalence among the African-American population except for a higher rate of alcohol use among AI/ANs. Compared with urban whites, urban AI/AN mortality rates were higher in every age group except the elderly. Differences between urban whites and AI/ANs were largest for injury- and alcohol-related deaths. All-cause mortality was lower among urban AI/ANs compared with rural AI/ANs and urban African Americans, although injury- and alcohol-related deaths were higher for AI/ANs. All communicable diseases studied were significantly ($P < .05$) more common among urban AI/ANs compared with whites. Tuberculosis rates were highest in the urban AI/AN group, but rates of sexually transmitted diseases were intermediate between urban whites and African Americans.

Conclusions.—In this urban area, great disparities exist between the health of AI/ANs and whites across almost every health dimension we measured. No consistent pattern was found in the comparison of health indicators between urban and rural AI/ANs, though rural AI/ANs had lower rates of low birth weight and higher rates of timely prenatal care use. The poor health status of urban AI/AN people requires greater attention from federal, state, and local health authorities.

(JAMA. 1994;271:845–850)

It is generally known that the health status of American Indians and Alaska Natives (AI/ANs) is far below that of other Americans.[1] However, this conclusion is based on statistical reports from the Indian Health Service (IHS), an agency of the Public Health Service, and tribally owned health programs on or near Indian reservations or Alaska Native lands. Little is known about the health status of urban AI/ANs despite the fact that 56% of the AI/ANs identified in the 1990 US Census now reside in urban areas.[2] The IHS was created by Congress and is currently directed to "assure the highest possible health status for Indians and urban Indians and to provide all resources necessary to affect that policy."[3] Congress recently established health status objectives specifically for AI/ANs that are to be accomplished by the year 2000.[3] Funding and politics have restricted most IHS activities to tribal members living on or near Indian reservations or Alaska Native lands.

Very little health information is available regarding AI/ANs in urban areas.[4] Most published studies of urban Indian health are based on data from clinics and hospitals and cannot be generalized to an entire urban AI/AN population.[5] In a comprehensive report on Indian health published in 1986, the Office of Technology Assessment concluded that "the IHS does not collect diagnostic patient care information from urban programs and does not analyze or publish vital statistics or population characteristics for urban AI/ANs except when these data are included with national level data on the reservation states."[6] Since the publication of this report, there have not been any large population-based studies that broadly describe the health status of any urban Indian population.

The purpose of this study was to use available vital statistics and health data to characterize the health status of the AI/AN population in the largest metropolitan county within the state of Washington and to compare its health status with three reference populations. The

---

*Reprinted from JAMA 271(11):845–850, 1994. Copyright 1994 American Medical Association.

comparison populations are the white and African-American populations within the same metropolitan county and the AI/AN population living in rural Washington counties with tribal reservations.

Methods
Site

According to the 1990 US Census, the Seattle, Washington, metropolitan area has the seventh largest concentration of urban AI/ANs in the United States. King County, Washington, is a large metropolitan region with a population of 1,507,319.[2] There are three cities with more than 50,000 residents, the largest of which is Seattle. The 17,305 AI/AN residents comprise 1.1% of the King County population and 21% of the state's AI/AN population. Of the King County AI/AN residents, 1461 (8.4%) reported that they were of Eskimo or Aleut ancestry on the census. Data sets from which numerator data were derived do not allow stratification of Alaska Natives from American Indians. Within King County, there is one small reservation with a tribally operated clinic. The Seattle Indian Health Board, one of 34 nonprofit organizations partially funded by the IHS, operates a comprehensive community-based primary care program that cares for AI/ANs.

Comparison Groups

First, we compared the health status of AI/ANs with that of whites and African Americans within King County. Second, we compared health status indicators of the King County AI/ANs ("urban" AI/ANs) with those of AI/AN residents of rural Washington counties with tribal reservations, a population traditionally served by the IHS. These seven counties are classified by the Washington State Department of Health as "rural" (15 to 100 persons per square mile) or "remote rural" (<15 persons per square mile) counties and have reservation land belonging to federally recognized tribes. King County and the rural reservation counties account for 40% of the state's total AI/AN population. The remainder of the state's AI/AN residents live in other urban/metropolitan counties or rural counties without reservations.

Data Sources

Three main data sources were used to generate numerator data for vital statistics rate calculations. These included birth certificates, linked infant birth and death certificates, and death certificates from 1981 through 1990 from the Center for Health Statistics of the Washington State Department of Health. Communicable disease data were obtained from the Centers for Disease Control and Prevention and the Epidemiology Office of the Washington State Department of Health. Data from the 1980 and 1990 editions of the US Census provided the denominator and socioeconomic data for each of the

comparison groups. Population estimates for urban and rural AI/ANs between 1980 and 1990 were generated by linear interpolation between 1980 and 1990 US Census counts while estimates for urban whites and African Americans were based on Washington Office of Financial Management demographic estimates. These Office of Financial Management estimates were unavailable for all counties in the study, so all AI/AN denominator estimates were derived using linear interpolation. The differences between the two denominator estimates (for the inter-census period) were quite small. The interpolation method gave a slightly higher number for each of the years, with a range of ratios from 1.02 to 1.06. This method consistently exceeded the Office of Financial Management estimate and resulted in a probable underestimate of mortality rates of urban AI/AN residents compared with other races.

We used the post-1989 National Center for Health Statistics definition of race for all infant birth and death rate calculations in the study. The National Center for Health Statistics currently defines an AI/AN birth as an infant born to a mother identified in the birth record as AI/AN, regardless of the father's race. We used linked birth and death certificates for infants, in which the mother's race at birth defines the race at birth and death. Individuals self-report their race to the US Census.

Health Status Measures

The health status indicators used in this study were derived from routinely collected population-based health status data for which race-specific information was available. Mortality rate calculations included infant mortality, age-specific mortality rates in six age groups, cause-specific mortality, and alcohol-associated mortality. To assess alcohol-associated mortality, alcohol-related disease impact software was used.[7] This methodology, developed by the Centers for Disease Control and Prevention, uses the attributable risk from alcohol use for each cause of death to derive a composite rate of alcohol-associated mortality.

Maternal and infant health measures included the proportion at birth of preterm births (<37 weeks' gestational age), of low (<2500 g) and very low (<1500 g) birth weight, of unmarried mothers, of mothers who started prenatal care in the first trimester (on time care) or who had late (third trimester) or no prenatal care, and of mothers who smoked tobacco or consumed alcohol during pregnancy, and the school-age (ages 10 through 17 years) fertility rate. The data source for information on smoking and alcohol use during pregnancy and prenatal care was the birth certificate. Smoking data from 1986 through 1988 were used (question wording on Washington State birth certificates was changed in 1989). Assessment of alcohol consumption was added to the birth certificate in 1989. Maternal drug-use data are not routinely collected on Washington State birth certificates.

Because the AI/AN population is small, only reportable communicable diseases of high frequency were compared. These included sexually transmitted diseases (gonorrhea, syphilis, and chlamydia), tuberculosis, and hepatitis A and hepatitis B. Because detailed data for sexually transmitted diseases were unavailable for rural counties, these data were used for comparisons within King County only.

We used the following *International Classification of Diseases*[8] codes as definitions for cause-specific mortality: heart disease, 391 through 392.0, 393 through 398, 402, 404, 410 through 416, 420–429; cancer, 140–208; unintentional injury, E800 through E949; liver disease, 571; cerebrovascular disease, 430 through 434, 436–438; pneumonia and influenza, 480 through 487; homicide, E960–E969; diabetes, 250; chronic obstructive pulmonary disease, 491, 492, 496; suicide, E950 through E959; and all firearms, E922, E955.0 through E955.4, E965.0 through E965.4, E870, E985.0 through E985.4.

All disease and death rates were age-adjusted to the 1940 US population for two reasons. A recent Centers for Disease Control and Prevention conference on age adjustment concluded that the 1940 US population would continue to be recommended by the National Center for Health Statistics as the standard population for US mortality data (primarily for purposes of comparability to historical national data).[9] Also, IHS uses the 1940 population as the reference in its annual statistical publications, widely cited sources for AI/AN health data; thus, use of the 1940 population will facilitate comparisons. Confidence intervals (CIs) for age-adjusted rates were compiled using the method of Chiang,[10] and CIs for proportional rates were calculated by the method of Fleiss.[11] Three- or 5-year rolling averages were used to assess trends, depending on the frequency of the outcome. Chi-square test for trend was used to determine the statistical significance of rate trends over time.

To determine whether the difference in low–birth-weight rates between urban and rural AI/AN populations could be entirely explained by differences in known behavioral and biologic risk factors, we conducted a logistic regression analysis to determine the model that best explained low–birth-weight variation. The outcome variable was defined as the presence or absence of low birth weight. The main independent variable was whether the birth occurred in an urban or rural location. The covariates included known maternal risk factors for low birth weight, including smoking, alcohol use, adolescent age, prior pregnancies, and the interpregnancy interval.

Results

Socioeconomic Characteristics

Data from the 1990 US Census revealed that, compared with whites, the urban AI/AN population had fewer high

school graduates and higher rates of unemployment and poverty (Table 20–1). However, rural AI/ANs appeared to be the most disadvantaged group in the study. A third of those older than 25 years living in rural counties were without a high school diploma. Unemployment (21%) and poverty rates (35%) were also highest among rural AI/ANs.

Birth Outcomes

The prevalence of low birth weight (<2500 g) was considerably higher among urban AI/ANs compared with urban whites and rural AI/ANs, but was lower than the rate of low birth weight among urban African Americans (Table 20–2). The prevalence of very low–birth-weight (<1500 g) births and premature deliveries shared similar patterns, although only the differences between urban AI/ANs and whites were significant.

Using low birth weight as the dependent variable and urban or rural status as the main independent variable, we found that after adjustment for the interval between births, history of prior pregnancy, adolescent age, use of prenatal care, and maternal smoking, the difference in low–birth-weight risk between the rural and urban groups was no longer statistically significant (odds ratio, 0.90; 95% CI, 0.56 to 1.4; $P = .66$). Thus, it appeared that most of the variation was attributable to differences in risk profiles of each group and not to a community risk or protective factor represented by the urban/rural variable.

Like low birth weight, the infant mortality rate averaged over 10 years was 80% higher among urban AI/ANs than among whites (Table 20–3). Neonatal and postneonatal mortality rates were higher among the urban AI/ANs (data not shown). Infant mortality rates among the urban AI/ANs were not significantly different than those among African Americans or the rural AI/ANs.

Table 20–1
Demographic Characteristics of Study Populations

Characteristic	Urban			Rural AI/AN
	AI/AN*	White	African American	
1990 population	17,305	1,255,339	72,463	15,054
Older than 25 years without high school diploma, %	24	10	21	34
Unemployed, %	8.4	3.7	11.3	21
Below 100% of federal poverty level, %	26	6.1	22	35

*AI/AN indicates American Indian and Alaska Native.

Table 20–2

Prevalence of Risk Factors for Poor Birth Outcomes Among Urban American Indians and Alaska Natives (AI/ANs) Compared With Other Races and Rural AI/ANs

Risk Factors	Average Rates 1988 Through 1990 (Total Births)*			Rural AI/AN (n = 1061)
	Urban			
	AI/AN (n = 994)	White (n = 52,261)	African American (n = 4100)	
Low birth weight (<2500 g)	9.5 (7.7–11.5)	5.0 (4.8–5.2)†	13.0 (12.0–14.1)†	5.6 (4.3–7.2)†
Very low birth weight (<1500 g)	1.6 (1.0–2.7)	0.8 (0.7–0.9)†	2.8 (2.4–3.4)	0.8 (.35–1.7)
Preterm births (<37 wk gestation)	15.9 (13.5–18.6)	8.1 (7.9–8.4)†	17.7 (16.5–19.1)	13.0 (10.9–15.5)
Mother 10–17 y of age	9.1 (7.4–11.1)	1.7 (1.6–1.8)†	9.8 (9.0–10.8)	10.2 (8.5–12.2)
Single mother	59.1 (56.0–62.1)	15.7 (15.7–16.0)†	65.1 (63.6–66.6)†	64.6 (61.6–67.5)
Consumed alcohol‡	20.1 (16.3–24.4)	6.2 (5.9–6.5)†	11.0 (9.5–12.7)†	16.2 (13.5–19.3)
Smoker§	38.2 (34.7–41.7)	20.0 (19.7–20.4)†	33.5 (31.9–35.0)	40.6 (37.5–43.8)
Received first-trimester prenatal care	56.5 (53.1–60.0)	83.9 (83.6–84.2)†	59.2 (57.5–60.8)	64.0 (61.0–67.0)†
Received late or no prenatal care	15.9 (13.5–18.5)	3.4 (3.2–3.6)†	12.7 (11.6–13.9)	10.0 (8.3–12.0)†

*Data expressed as percentage (95% confidence interval). Infant race determined by mother's race on birth certificate. Urban AI/ANs are the reference group for all statistical comparisons.

†Significantly ($P < .05$) different from urban AI/AN rate.

‡Two-year average rates, 1989 through 1990.

§Three-year average rates, 1986 through 1988.

A significant increase in the urban AI/AN infant mortality rate occurred during the decade starting in 1981 (Figure 20–1). Five-year rolling average rates increased consistently every 5-year period from 9.6 per 1000 live births during 1981 through 1985 to 18.6 per 1000 during 1986 through 1990 (χ^2 test for trend, 5.1; $P < .05$). This decade-long trend was not evident among the other county residents or the rural population. The apparent upward trend among African Americans was not significant.

Prenatal Risk Factors for Poor Birth Outcomes

Rural and urban AI/AN mothers shared a similar prenatal risk profile (adolescent age, single marital status, and use of tobacco and alcohol during pregnancy) for poor birth outcomes (Table 20–2). However, urban AI/AN women were less likely than rural AI/AN women to initiate prenatal care in the first trimester (56.5% vs 64.0%; $P < .05$) and more likely to have late (third trimester) or no prenatal care (15.9% vs 10.0%; $P < .05$).

Urban AI/AN mothers had a much higher risk profile in comparison with urban white mothers (Table 20–2). Births among mothers aged 10 to 17 years, mothers who were single, or mothers who used tobacco or alcohol during pregnancy were all more common among AI/ANs. Similarly, the lower rates of first trimester prenatal care and high rates of late (third trimester) or no prenatal care seemed to place AI/ANs at higher risk of poor birth outcomes. This risk profile closely resembled that of African-American mothers across all variables except for prenatal alcohol consumption, where the risk among AI/ANs was significantly higher.

Age-Specific Mortality

Urban AI/AN age-specific mortality rates were higher in almost every age group compared with urban whites. The only exception was among the elderly (older than 65 years), in which the AI/AN rates were lower (relative risk [RR], 0.65; 95% CI, 0.56 to 0.75). The biggest difference was evident in the 25- to 44-year age group, though rates in the 1- to 14-year and 15- to 24-year age groups were nearly twofold higher than among whites. The only significant ($P < .05$) difference between urban AI/ANs and African Americans was in the oldest age group, in which rates for African Americans were higher.

Similarly, a comparison of death rates between urban and rural AI/ANs appeared to demonstrate slightly lower rates among urban AI/AN residents, although only the difference among the elderly (older than 65 years) reached statistical significance (RR, 0.60; 95% CI, 0.51 to 0.72; $P < .05$).

Cause-Specific Mortality

The overall age-adjusted mortality rate among urban AI/ANs was higher compared with whites, but lower compared with African Americans and rural AI/ANs

Table 20–3
Urban American Indians and Alaska Natives (AI/AN) Mortality Rates Compared With Other Races and Rural AI/ANs by Age Group and Cause, 1981 Through 1990*

Mortality Rate	Urban			Rural AI/AN
	AI/AN	White	African American	
Infant (age 0–1 y), 10–y average rate, per 1000 live births (95% CI)†	14.7 (10.6–20.3)	8.0 (7.6–8.4)‡	17.5 (15.3–20.0)	23.2 (18.4–29.2)
Age–specific, y, 10–y average rate per 100,000 popula–tion (95% CI)				
1–14	56 (35–87)	29 (26.4–31.2)‡	39 (29.8–49.7)	62 (42–92)
15–24	162 (121–217)	83 (78.4–86.9)‡	131 (111.2–153.8)	265 (208–337)
25–44	335 (288–389)	127 (123.8–130.6)‡	279 (258.1–302.1)	386 (327–454)
45–64	1122 (992–1269)	693 (682.4–703.9)‡	1303 (1231.8–1378.8)	1092 (950–1255)
65–99	3099 (2685–3573)	4949 (4912.4–4984.9)‡	5158 (4951.3–5373.2)‡	5124 (4650–5643)‡
Total deaths	727	93,048	4525	921
Cause–specific, 10–y age-adjusted (to 1940) rate per 100,000 population (95% CI) All causes	597 (557–638)	473 (469.4–475.5)‡	729 (710.5–748.3)‡	747 (702–791)‡
Alcohol related	149 . . .	82 . . .	105 . . .	182 . . .
Heart disease	141 (120–163)	139 (137.1–140.3)	207 (195.8–217.6)‡	188 (164–212)‡
Cancer	76 (57–92)	127 (124.8–128.2)‡	175 (164.4–185.3)‡	93 (75–110)
Unintentional injury	69 (56–83)	29 (27.6–29.5)‡	39 (34.5–44.4)‡	118 (99–136)‡
Liver disease	50 (37–62)	9 (8.3–9.4)‡	15 (12.0–18.7)‡	44 (31–56)
Cerebrovascular	26 (16–35)	28 (27.7–29.1)	48 (42.5–53.1)‡	56 (42–70)‡
Pneumonia and influenza	22 (14–31)	12 (12.0–12.8)‡	13 (10.2–15.7)	15 (8–22)
Homicide	21 (14–28)	4 (3.8–4.5)‡	30 (25.7–34.0)	20 (12–27)
Diabetes	19 (11–27)	8 (7.8–8.7)‡	30 (25.4–34.3)	20 (12–29)
Chronic obstruc-tive pulmonary disease	18 (10–26)	19 (18.5–19.8)	19 (15.1–22.1)	24 (15–33)
Suicide	17 (10–23)	14 (12.8–14.1)	9 (6.8–11.4)	26 (18–35)
All firearms	15 (9–21)	8 (7.9–8.9)‡	21 (17.3–24.2)	34 (24–45)‡

*CI indicates confidence interval. Ellipses indicate data not available.
†Based on linked birth and death files where mother's race is AI/AN.
‡Significantly different from urban AI/AN rate.

(Table 20–3). Injuries and alcohol-related deaths accounted for the majority of excess mortality among AI/ANs. Urban AI/ANs had significantly ($P < .05$) lower age-adjusted all-cause mortality rates than rural AI/ANs as well as for heart disease, unintentional injury, cerebrovascular disease, and firearm injury. Rates for other specific causes of death (cancer, liver disease, pneumonia and influenza, homicide, suicide, diabetes,

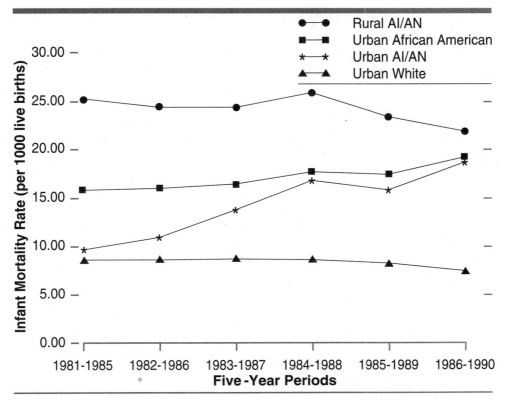

Figure 20–1
Five-year rolling averages for infant mortality trends of urban American Indians and Alaska natives (AI/ANs) compared with other races and rural AI/ANs. Data derived from linked birth and death certificates. Race classified according to maternal race.

and chronic obstructive pulmonary disease) were not significantly different between the groups.

Within the urban county, the most striking differences in cause-specific mortality rates between AI/ANs and whites were for chronic liver disease and cirrhosis, unintentional injury, and homicide. Of the leading causes, only cancer was lower in the AI/ANs compared with whites. Compared with African Americans, the urban AI/ANs had lower all-cause death rates and lower rates from heart disease, cancer, and cerebrovascular disease, but higher death rates from unintentional injury and liver disease.

Communicable Diseases

Among communicable diseases, the prevalence of reported hepatitis A and hepatitis B was higher among urban AI/ANs than among rural AI/ANs, urban whites, and African Americans (Table 20–4). Similarly, urban AI/ANs also experienced a much higher reported prevalence of tuberculosis compared with all three other population groups. Reported prevalence rates of chlamydia, syphilis, and gonorrhea were much higher among

urban AI/ANs compared with urban whites, but considerably lower than rates among urban African Americans. Race-specific rates of sexually transmitted disease were not available for rural AI/ANs.

Comment

The findings of this study confirm the existence of great disparities between the health of AI/ANs and whites living in one large metropolitan area. Urban AI/ANs have poorer health across almost every indicator we examined. The gap appears across almost all age groups and most causes of death. Many of the indicators were similar to those among urban African Americans, a group whose health status has repeatedly demonstrated the health inequities between whites and minorities in the United States.[12]

Our systematic comparison of health status indicators between urban and rural AI/ANs did not reveal a consistent pattern. Our most disturbing finding was the significant decade-long rise of the urban AI/AN infant mortality rate, a trend not shared by any of the other study populations. Rural AI/AN mothers of newborn infants were more likely to have early and adequate prenatal care and were less likely to deliver a low–birth-weight infant than urban AI/AN mothers. This may be a result of access to comprehensive maternal and child health services offered by the IHS that include extensive public health nursing outreach systems. Access to these services in the rural IHS clinics may have led to earlier initiation of and follow-up with prenatal care. Though the earlier use of prenatal care and the lower rate of low birth weight appeared to demonstrate better maternal and infant health in the rural population, rural AI/AN infant mortality (including both neonatal and postneonatal mortality) was not lower in the rural counties. This surprising relationship between low birth weight and infant mortality rates may be a reflection of superior access to neonatal intensive care in the urban county.

The AI/AN mortality rates tended to be higher within the rural counties than within the urban area. The most striking age-specific difference was among the population older than 65 years. The higher rate of unintentional injury fatalities is not surprising since the incidence of fatal motor vehicle crashes is known to be higher in rural areas, especially among AI/ANs.[13] Almost all of the overall mortality difference can be explained by higher rates of the four leading causes of death (heart disease, cancer, injury, and cerebrovascular disease) among rural AI/ANs, compared with their urban counterparts.

Several limitations may have affected the results of this study. Although undercounting of AI/ANs in the census would have the effect of inappropriately increasing morbidity and mortality rates when the census population is used as the denominator, data from the 1980 and 1990 censuses suggest that the problem of undercounting of AI/ANs has diminished in comparison with earlier censuses.[14] Misclassification of race in vital records can result in substantial underestimates of mortality rates among AI/ANs.[15–17] We estimate that this differential misclassification affects mortality data by artificially minimizing some of the true disparity between whites and urban AI/ANs, ie, a conservative bias. We attempted to minimize the effects of racial misclassification for infant mortality rates and the prevalence of birth risk factors by using linked birth and death certificates and the current National Center for Health Statistics designation of race. However, estimates of AI/AN mortality rates for ages beyond infancy were not derived from linked files, raising the potential for significant racial misclassification and underestimation of the AI/AN rates. If misclassification of AI/ANs as other races was less likely to occur in rural areas (perhaps because morticians and coroners are more sensitive to the presence of a large AI/AN population), then urban rates would be selectively underestimated, thus accounting for some of the differences between urban and rural AI/ANs observed in this study. Indeed, in a study of racial misclassification of clients of the Seattle Indian Health Board, almost one third of persons who identified themselves as AI/AN to the clinic while living were classified as other races on death certificates, compared with approximately 12% inconsistent classification among primarily rural, IHS-registered AI/ANs in Washington.[18] Because the direction of this potential bias is known, study conclusions or policy implications should not be significantly affected. Data from birth certificates may be less susceptible to this potential bias.

Table 20–4

Incidence of Communicable Diseases Among Urban American Indians and Alaska Natives (AI/ANs) Compared With Other Races and Rural AI/ANs

Diseases	Urban			Rural AI/AN
	AI/AN	White	African American	
Hepatitis A†	151 (123–178)	42.0 (39.8–44.1)‡	43.4 (34.9–52.0)‡	106 (85–128)
Hepatitis B†	47 (31–63)	10.8 (9.7–11.8)‡	25.3 (18.8–31.9)	25 (14–35)
Tuberculosis§	60 (47–74)	3.0 (2.7–3.3)‡	16.8 (13.5–20.0)‡	20 (12–28)‡
Sexually transmitted diseases‖ Chlamydia	516 (460–573)	255.5 (250.0–261.1)‡	1472.6 (1432.9–1512.2)‡	NA
Gonorrhea	298 (253–342)	81.0 (77.9–84.2)‡	2055.5 (2008.5–2102.5‡	NA
Syphilis	47 (28–66)	4.9 (4.2–5.6)‡	183.7 (166.0–201.4)	NA

*All rates age-adjusted to 1940 US population. NA indicates not available. Data expressed as mean rates per 100,000 population (95% confidence intervals).

†Average rate, 1987 through 1990.

‡Significantly (P < .05) different from urban AI/AN rate.

§Ten-year average rate, 1981 through 1990.

‖Three-year average rate, 1988 through 1990.

In addition to racial misclassification on vital records, several studies in the Pacific Northwest have shown that morbidity rates calculated from registries of cancer,[16] AIDS,[19] end-stage renal disease,[20] and injury[21] may be underestimated among AI/ANs because of racial misclassification. Reporting bias is another potential concern in this study, primarily in the rates of communicable diseases. Care providers in the public sector, where indigent patients are more likely to seek care, may be more likely to report cases of communicable diseases to health authorities than private practitioners. The effect of this bias would be to overestimate the differences noted between whites and urban AI/ANs with respect to communicable diseases such as gonorrhea.

Should urban AI/ANs receive attention as a population with special health needs? More than half of AI/ANs now live in urban areas, but only a few of these areas, such as Albuquerque, NM, Phoenix, Ariz, and Anchorage, Alaska, offer direct IHS services. Title V of the Indian Care Improvement Act of 1976 was the first federal government recognition of the health needs of urban AI/ANs. Despite this recognition, few resources have been allocated to address these needs. The initial 1976 authorization called for a $15 million allocation for urban Indian communities to organize programs to "facilitate access to and, when necessary, provide health services to urban Indian residents."[22] In 1992, only $17 million was appropriated to urban Indian programs in cities where an IHS facility was not present, representing 1% of the total IHS budget. Because eligibility for the full scope of IHS services has been reserved for "persons of descent belonging to the Indian community served by the local facilities and program," it effectively excludes rural AI/AN residents who move to an urban area without an IHS direct care facility, perhaps in search of employment or family reunification.[6] Though the reasons for the presence of large urban AI/AN populations are not completely known, many urban AI/AN residents were coercively relocated from reservations by the federal government to the cities during a period in the 1950s known as the "termination era" in the history of relations between US Indians and whites.[23] This relocation policy separated AI/AN people from tribal land and culture, exposing them to the harsh social and economic conditions of the urban poor. Others migrated to the cities in search of employment and education. Many of these individuals and their families never returned to their reservations. Whatever the reason, many AI/AN people are firmly rooted in the cities.

The allocation of IHS funds to the urban Indian program has been a source of controversy between urban Indian and tribal leaders. Concerned that scarce resources would be redirected from the reservations to the cities, some tribal leaders have opposed the expansion of urban programs. Our data do not support the redirection of funds previously designated for rural AI/ANs living on native lands, since it appears that both populations are vulnerable and in similar great need of health services, epidemiologic surveillance, and prevention activities. The recent drive for health system reform may benefit the health concerns of the urban AI/AN population. Under President Clinton's proposed Health Security Act of 1993 (section 8302), urban AI/ANs will be eligible for the same full health care benefits extended to rural AI/AN residents. Under this plan, all AI/AN enrollees could receive their care in an IHS, a tribal, or an urban Indian facility. Until a solution is reached in the context of health system reform, the responsibility for the health needs of urban AI/ANs must continue to be addressed at local, state, and federal levels in consultation with existing urban Indian programs.

This research was supported by a grant from the Nesholm Family Foundation, Seattle, Wash.

We thank John Kobayashi, MD, MPH, and Ernest Kimball, MPH, for their assistance with the project. We are very grateful to Abraham Bergman, MD, Lawrence Berger, MD, MPH, Thomas Koepsell, MD, MPH, and Steven Helgerson, MD, MPH, for reviewing earlier drafts of the manuscript. We are also deeply indebted to Jim Allen, Cindy Cresap, and Bi-Lan Chiong for their expert technical assistance.

References

1. Rhoades ER, Hammond J, Welty TX, Handler AO, Amler RW: The Indian burden of illness and future health interventions. Public Health Rep 102:361–368, 1987.
2. US Bureau of the Census: 1990 Census of the Population: General Population Characteristics—United States. Washington, DC: US Bureau of the Census; 1990.
3. Pub L No. 102-537: Amendments to the Indian Health Care Improvement Act of 1992.
4. Kramer BJ: Health and aging of urban American Indians. West J Med 157:281–285, 1992.
5. Taylor TL: Health problems and use of services at two urban American Indian clinics. Public Health Rep 103:88–95, 1988.
6. Indian Health Care: Washington, DC: Office of Technology Assessment; 1986. US Dept of Health and Human Services publication OTA-H-290.
7. Shultz JM, Rice OP, Parker DL, Goodman RA, Stroh GJ, Chalmers N: Quantifying the disease impact of alcohol with ARDI software. Public Health Rep 106:443–450, 1991.
8. World Health Organization: Manual of the International Statistical Classification of Diseases, Injuries, and Causes of Death, Based on the Recommendations of the Ninth Revision Conference, 1975. Geneva, Switzerland: World Health Organization; 1977.
9. Reconsidering Age-Adjustment Procedures: Washington, DC: US Dept of Health and Human Services publication PHS 93-1446.
10. Chiang CL: Standard error of the age-adjusted death rate. Vital Stat Special Rep 47:275–285, 1961.
11. Fleiss JL: Statistical Methods for Rates and Proportions. New York, NY: John Wiley & Sons Inc; 1981.
12. Dept of Health and Human Services: Report of the Secretary's Task Force on Black and Minority Health, I: Executive Summary. Washington, DC: US Dept of Health and Human Services; August 1985.
13. Baker SP, O'Neill B, Ginsburg MJ, Li G: The Injury Fact Book. 2nd ed. New York, NY: Oxford University Press; 1992:224.
14. Passel JS, Berman PA: Quality of 1980 census data for American Indians. Soc Biol 33:163–182, 1988.
15. Hahn RA, Mulinare J, Teutsch SN: Inconsistencies in coding of race and ethnicity between birth and death in US infants: a new

look at infant mortality, 1983 through 1985. JAMA 267:259–263, 1992.

16. Frost F, Taylor V, Fries E: Racial misclassification of Native Americans in a surveillance, epidemiology, and end results cancer registry. J Natl Cancer Inst 84:957–962, 1992.

17. Centers for Disease Control and Prevention: Classification of American Indian race on birth and infant death certificates—California and Montana. MMWR Morb Mortal Wkly Rep. 42:222–223, 1993.

18. Sugarman JR, Hill G, Forquera R, Frost FJ: Coding of race on death certificates of patients of an urban Indian health clinic, Washington, 1973–1988. IHS Provider 17:113–115, 1992.

19. Hurlich MG, Hopkins SG, Sakuma J, Conway GA: Racial ascer- tainment of AI/AN persons with AIDS, Seattle/King County, WA 1980–1990. IHS Provider 17:73–74, 1992.

20. Sugarman JR, Lawson L: The effect of racial misclassification on estimates of end-stage renal disease among American Indians and Alaska Natives, Pacific Northwest, 1988–1990. Am J Kidney Dis 21:383–386, 1993.

21. Sugarman JR, Soderberg R, Gordon JE, Rivara FP: Racial misclassification of American Indians: its effect on injury rates in Oregon, 1989 through 1990. Am J Public Health 83:681–684, 1993.

22. Pub L No. 94-437: Indian Health Care Improvement Act of 1976.

23. Prucha FP: Documents of United States Indian Policy. Lincoln: University of Nebraska Press, 1990:237.

A DEBUNKING OF THE MYTH OF HEALTHY ASIAN AMERICANS AND PACIFIC ISLANDERS*

Moon S. Chen, Jr. • Betty Lee Hawks

Abstract

Purpose. To present evidence that the model of healthy Asian Americans and Pacific Islanders (AAPIs) stereotype is a myth.

Search Method. The authors retrieved literature from the National Library of Medicine's compact disk databases (Cancerlit, CINAHL, Health, and MEDLINE), and examined pertinent federal government publications supplemented by the authors' knowledge of other published materials.

Important Findings. This review paper presents three reasons why AAPIs are underserved: (1) the population growth rate has been unusually rapid and recent; (2) data regarding the health status of AAPIs are inadequate; and (3) the myth that AAPIs are model minority populations in terms of their health status was promulgated.

Major Conclusions. The conclusions are as follows: (1) AAPIs are heterogenous with respect to demographic factors and health risk factors; (2) because the current databases on the health status of AAPIs include small sample sizes, both the quantity and quality of these data need to be improved with respect to appropriate gender and ethnic group representation; (3) risk factor and mortality data for AAPIs suggest that the burden of certain preventable diseases, namely, tuberculosis, hepatitis-B, liver cancer, and lung cancer may be higher than those of any other racial and ethnic population. The model healthy AAPI stereotype is a myth. (Am J Health Promot 1995;9[4]:261–8)

Key Words: Asian Americans, Pacific Islanders, Health Status, Epidemiology

Introduction

During the mid-1960s when the nation was experiencing great racial turmoil resulting from the civil rights movement, the media looked for something "positive" to report. The media chose what appeared to be the phenomenal success of Asian Americans, their "hard work, uncomplaining perseverance, and quiet accommodation."[1] Perhaps the motivation was "to discredit the protests for social justice of other minority groups."[1] In any case, the press has continued to portray Asian Americans through such headlines as "Why Asians are going to the head of the class" or "Those Asian American whiz kids."[2] The effects of such media portrayal have been a stereotypical image that has been difficult to correct. This article, as Paul Harvey would

say, is "about the rest of the story" and relates to the image of the model healthy Asian American and Pacific Islander (AAPI).

More specifically, the purpose of this article is to present and discuss three reasons why AAPIs are underserved and to offer recommendations for rectifying underservice. In so doing, the "bottom line" from this review of the literature is that the model AAPI stereotype is a myth.[3, 4] Moreover, considerable needs and challenges face those who wish to serve AAPIs.[5]

Before these three reasons are presented, however, the terms "Asian American" and "Pacific Islander" are first defined. Second, the methodology for conducting this literature review is described. The main body of the paper follows, with a listing and discussion of three reasons why AAPIs are underserved and how they are underserved. The health impact of being underserved is incorporated in the third reason: the myth that AAPIs are healthy minority populations. Finally, recommendations are advanced for increasing the quantity and quality of health research and services for AAPIs.

Definition of Asian, Asian American, and Pacific Islander

The terms *Asian (Asian American)* and *Pacific Islander* are the designations of the Office of Management and Budget according to its Directive No. 15,[5] to differentiate persons into one of five racial/ethnic categories: white, black, Hispanic, American Indian or Alaska Native, and Asian (Asian American) or Pacific Islander.[5, 6] This directive guides all federal record-keeping, collection, and presentation of data, including, for example, such activities of the US Bureau of the Census. Technically, the term *Asian American* refers to those of Asian descent who are US citizens or permanent residents. Individuals may self-designate themselves to be Asian or Pacific Islander just as all residents of the United States at the time of a census count are asked to self-designate their racial or ethnic status. (Return of the household Census surveys is required, but there is not a requirement to complete each item, like the racial/ethnic classification.) The 1990 Census designations of Asian Americans include, but are not limited to, those who self-classify themselves to be Asian Indian, Cambodian, Chinese, Filipino, Hmong, Japanese, Korean, Laotian, Thai, or Vietnamese, or they may become classified as "other Asian."[6]

However, a racial or national origin designation is not equated with within-group homogeneity. For instance,

*Reprinted from American Journal of Health Promotion 9(4):261–268, 1995.

within the population of Asian Indians, major differences exist depending on the geographic (regional) origins of one's ancestors. The diversity of Asian Indians at least equals the diversity of Europeans. In addition, India uses 15 languages on its currency notes, and spoken Asian Indian dialects may exceed 875! Also, residing in the same land space does not equate with use of the same language and being of the same cultural origins. For example, Hmongs may have lived in Laos, but do not consider themselves to be "Laotians."

The term *Pacific Islander* similarly refers to many different populations, ranging from indigenous Hawaiians to Chamorro, the indigenous people of the Mariana Islands (including the island of Guam), American Samoans, and the native peoples of the many other Pacific Islands scattered literally thousands of miles across Oceania. Technically, *Pacific Islanders* refers to those who self-classify themselves to be Native Hawaiian, Micronesian, and Melanesian. Although more detailed classification schemes are available through the US Bureau of the Census, they do not identify the indigenous Hawaiians as "Kanaka Maoli" (the Hawaiian term), which may contribute to undercounts of Native Hawaiians.[7]

Search Methods Used

To adequately cover the health status for the diversity of peoples represented by Asian Americans or Pacific Islanders, we used several sources and literature search strategies. The federal government series of publications most pertinent to discussing health status were manually examined. These series were: (1) the 1985 *Report of the Secretary's Task Force on Black and Minority Health*[8] (hereafter abbreviated as the *Task Force Report*), (2) *Healthy People 2000*[9] and its special report[10]; (3) the National Center for Health Statistics' (NCHS') draft report, *Setting a Research Agenda: Challenges for the Minority Health Statistics Grant Program*,[11] based on the 1991 NCHS workshop of the same title; and (4) the Centers for Disease Control and Prevention's (CDC's) *Morbidity and Mortality Weekly Report* (MMWR) from 1991-November, 1993. Eight articles from the MMWR were identified[12–19] as being specific to the health status of AAPIs. In addition, we examined reference documents related to AAPIs through February, 1994 available from the federal Office of Minority Health Resource Center through February, 1994.

All four of the National Library of Medicine's compact disc read-only memory (CD-ROM) retrievable databases for the professional literature in health were searched. These databases and the corresponding numbers of citations for the terms *Asian American* (includes *Pacific Islanders*) and *health status* were as follows:

1. *Cancerlit,* 1986-February, 1994 (0 citations)

2. *Cumulative Index to Nursing and Allied Health Literature* (CINAHL), 1983–1993 (0 citations)

3. *Health Planning and Administration* (abbreviated as *Health*), 1975-March 1994 (14 citations)

4. *MEDLINE,* the online counterpart to the National Library of Medicine's *Index Medicus,* 1966-March 1994 (3 citations)

The time periods encompassing these literature searches reflected the dates for which the CD-ROM discs were updated.

The small number of articles retrieved through this search strategy suggested a need to use broader citation identification techniques. Therefore, a sample period (1983–1992 for *MEDLINE* and 1983-October, 1992 for *CINAHL*) was explored in greater depth. Adding "or India-ethnology" to capture Asian Indian Americans (as opposed to American Indians or Asian Indians in India) did not appear to significantly alter the number of citations retrieved. Another technique was to increase the specificity of the *Asian-Americans* or *Pacific-Islanders* terms to include: *Asian Indians, Cambodians, Chinese-Americans, Filipinos, Filipino-Americans, Hawaiians, Japanese-Americans, Korean-Americans, Koreans, Vietnamese,* and *Vietnamese-Americans.* A total of 375 citations (334 from *MEDLINE,* 41 from *CINAHL*) were identified from this particular search strategy.

However, after we excluded foreign language articles, articles about Asians or Pacific Islanders in countries other than the United States, articles that dealt with non-lifestyle aspects, and duplicate citations that resulted from articles dealing with more than one ethnic group, the number of articles directly pertinent to elucidating the health status of AAPI dwindled considerably.

Concurrence on the small number of articles on the health status of AAPIs was documented by Kroll and Bradigan's article, "*MEDLINE* search strategies for literature on Asian Americans/Pacific Islanders."[20] They indicated that *MEDLINE* literature citations on the health status of AAPIs have been the fewest of any racial/ethnic minority for as long as the term *Asian American* was introduced as a *MEDLINE* term.[20]

Finally, we reviewed newly published materials (ie, "Special Health Problems of Asians and Pacific Islanders" in *Clinical Preventive Medicine*[21] and *Confronting Critical Health Issues of Asian and Pacific Islander Americans*[22]) and other relevant, refereed articles that have not yet been entered into literature retrieval databases. The new, refereed quarterly journal, the *Asian American and Pacific Islander Journal of Health,* which made its debut in the summer of 1993 was especially pertinent to the literature review. The result is a very current compilation of published materials on the health status of AAPIs.

The theme of underserved populations was used as an

organizing thread for this literature review. In so doing, three reasons emerged as to why AAPIs are underserved, how they are underserved, and the health impact of being underserved. These three reasons are subsequently discussed.

Reasons Why AAPIS Are Underserved, How They Are Underserved, and The Health Impact of Being Underserved

Reason 1: The population growth of AAPIs has been unusually rapid and recent.

Between 1960 and 1970, the population of AAPIs increased by 75.3%,[23] resulting largely from the reclassification of Asian Indians from being white to being Asian Americans. Between 1970 and 1980, the AAPIs increased by 127.5%, and between 1980 and 1990, the AAPIs increased by 108% for a 1990 population of 7.3 million[25] (Fig. 20–2). For three consecutive decades, the percentage growth of the AAPIs' population has far exceeded that of any other US racial or ethnic group.[24, 25] Triple-digit percentage growth for AAPIs has characterized the last two decades. Such unprecedented growth in a single US Bureau of the Census designation was unusually rapid and unanticipated.

The five states that witnessed the largest percentage increases of AAPIs, Rhode Island (245.6%), New Hampshire (219.0%), Georgia (209.9%), Wisconsin (195.0%), and Minnesota (193.5%), are conspicuously not West Coast states nor previously considered major enclaves of an AAPI presence.[24] In fact, 17 non-West Coast states outrank California's 127.0% growth rate among AAPIs.[25] Consequently, many of the public health resources to meet the needs of these AAPI populations were not in place when these population growths occurred.

However, current awareness of these needs means that resources must now be directed toward these underserved populations. The projection is for Asian Americans to increase 356% by the year 2050, making them 11% (41 million) of the US population, compared with 3% (9 million) of the population in 1993.[24–26]

The demographic and health-care characteristics of AAPIs have been previously described by Lin-Fu,[26, 28] and the particular migration and demographic characteristics of Southeast Asian refugees to the United States have been described by others.[29] More recently, the cardiovascular health status of AAPIs has been reviewed,[30] and a 1993 report of the health status of Asian Americans and Pacific Islanders vis-à-vis progress on relevant *Healthy People 2000* objectives was completed.[31] After the detailed 1990 Census data are released, further demographic characterization of AAPIs will be possible. For now though, we conclude that the rather recent, unanticipated, and rapid population growth of AAPIs is one reason why AAPIs are underserved.

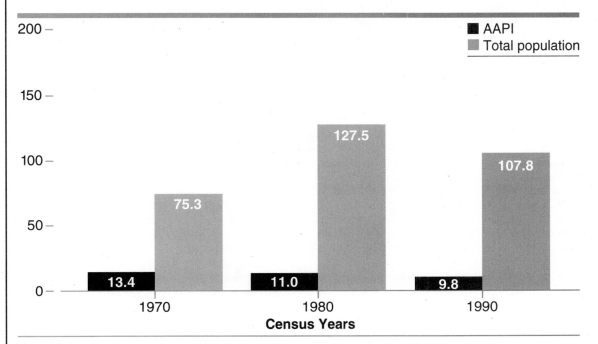

Figure 20–2
Percentage increases since previous census. (Source: U.S. Bureau of the Census, 1983; U.S. Bureau of the Census, 1991.)

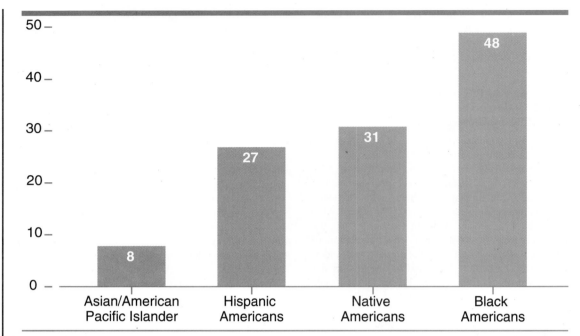

Figure 20–3
Healthy People 2000 objectives for racial/ethnic minorities.

Reason 2: The data regarding the health status of AAPIs are inadequate.

Inadequacies in data to document the health status of AAPIs have been one of the major barriers to harnessing health resources for AAPIs. These inadequacies in data may be classified in terms of (1) the paucity of the data; (2) misclassification of some data; and (3) lack of ethnic specificity of the data. These three factors will be briefly discussed.

First, the health status data on AAPIs are woefully inadequate. For example, Yu and Liu[32] very clearly delineated significant gaps in the federal health statistics collection processes, the limitations in current numerator and denominator data for assessing AAPI health status, and what must be done in the latter part of the 1990s to improve the quality and quantity of the database for AAPIs. They cited the past practice of not even providing the option of *Asian/Pacific Islander* for the National Medical Expenditure Survey and the National Health Interview Survey. They also cited the need for oversampling AAPIs, evidence for the undercount of AAPIs in the 1990 Census, and inconsistent reporting of racial/ethnic origins (eg, between interviewers' observations and respondents' self-report).[32]

One manifestation of the absence of adequate AAPI health data may be noted in the *Healthy People 2000* objectives. *Healthy People 2000* listed 48 objectives targeting black Americans, 31 targeting American Indians/Alaska Natives, 27 targeting Hispanic Americans, but only 8 targeting Asian Americans and Pacific Islanders[9] (Fig. 20–3).

Lack of available baseline data for AAPIs may be a principal reason why relatively few *Healthy People 2000* objectives were formulated with AAPIs specifically in mind and a reason for a 1993 status and commentary on achieving *Healthy People 2000* objectives for AAPIs that was extensively presented elsewhere.[31] The US Public Health Service is conducting a mid-course review of these health objectives and plans to examine new data that may support establishment of additional subobjectives, especially for special populations (eg, racial or ethnic populations).

Another manifestation of the absence of adequate AAPI health data may be seen in two November, 1993 CDC articles. In one article,[17] some Asian/Pacific Islander data were "not reported by number of [health care professional visits] because of insufficient sample sizes." In the other article,[18] AAPI data were not reported "because numbers for other racial/ethnic groups were too small for meaningful analysis."

Second, misclassification of AAPI health data has been documented. In a study of linked infant birth and death records reported by Hahn, Mulinare, and Teutsch,[33] the misclassification of race was greatest for those who were not white or black (43.2%), compared with whites (1.2%) and blacks (4.3%). The misclassification rate was 33.3%,

48.8%, and 78.8% for Chinese, Japanese, and Filipinos, respectively.[33]

Third, the lack of sufficient ethnically specific data is very apparent.[11] Although NCHS has separated Chinese, Japanese, and Filipinos into coding categories, the "other" Asian American category remains very heterogenous with such groups as Asian Indians, Cambodians, Hmong, Koreans, Laotians, Thais, and Vietnamese being lumped together.[11] Preliminary studies suggest that the cardiovascular health profiles of Asian Indians[34, 35] differ from those of other Asian or Pacific Islander groups.[30] Health issues related to "Korean Americans have been generally overlooked until the present time."[36] To neglect ethnic specificity of data or to rampantly aggregate these groups under the rubric of AAPIs can mask enormous heterogeneity of health status changes. Failing to have sufficient ethnically specific data is to grossly misdiagnose the specific health status.

Reason 3: The myth that Asian Americans and Pacific Islanders are model minority populations was erroneously promulgated.

The 1985 *Secretary's Task Force Report on Black and Minority Health* concluded that, "As a group, the Asian/Pacific Islander population in the United States is at lower risk of early death than the White population."[8] However, for the reasons discussed previously in this article, this conclusion is flawed. To its credit, the 1985 *Task Force Report* did state that the National Center for Health Statistics, Bureau of the Census, and the Secretary's Task Force Report all coincided in their probable underestimation of age-adjusted cardiovascular disease mortality rates because of the less frequent reporting of AAPIs on death certificates compared with the Census.[8] Unfortunately, this caveat in interpreting data in the Secretary's *Task Force Report* received little attention, whereas the *Task Force Report's* conclusion that AAPIs are healthier than whites has been cited repeatedly.

However, findings *since 1985* suggest that the health status of AAPIs is really poorer than was initially believed. Studies of the prevalence of chronic disease risk factors document the concerns that the health status of AAPIs will probably deteriorate and that this group will perhaps exceed the mortality rates of other US racial groups in lung cancer and possibly cardiovascular disease in the next 20 years. The following paragraphs cite examples of the higher prevalence of chronic disease risk factors to illustrate chronic disease burdens not discussed in the original *Task Force Report.*

A growing body of evidence supports higher cardiovascular disease and lung cancer death rates in the future based on higher smoking rates among AAPI men. The prevalence of male smoking among Cambodians (55%[9]), Chinese (28%[14, 15]), Filipinos (24%[37]), Hmong (29%[38]), Koreans (36%[37]), Laotians (72%[39]), Native Hawaiians (42%[7, 40]), and Vietnamese (35%,[15] 39%,[41] 42%[16] to

55%[9]) exceeds the total male California smoking rate of 21%.[14] Whereas the overall prevalence of smoking among adults in the United States is declining at an average of 0.5% per year,[9] data documenting this decline among Asian American men are unavailable. Even if this decline were to occur among Southeast Asian men, the prevalence of smoking would still not meet *Healthy People 2000* objectives 3.4 and 16.6 of 15% among people aged 20 and above.[9] If the smoking prevalence rates among Southeast Asian men fail to decline dramatically, mortality because of cardiovascular diseases and lung cancer is likely to rise and may exceed that of any other race or ethnic group. Already, lung cancer death rates for Southeast Asian men exceed those of white men by 18%.[42]

At least two other significant barriers exist for AAPI smokers. First, they are the *least* likely among *all* racial or ethnic populations to see a physician (42.0% did not visit a physician in the last twelve months versus 33.4% for whites).[37] Second, AAPIs have the lowest rates among *all* racial or ethnic groups of having had a doctor ever advise them to quit smoking (33% for AAPIs versus 50% for all races).[43]

On the other hand, the smoking prevalence rates among AAPI women, approximately 10%, are lower than women in general (25%)[44, 45]; however, acculturating influences may bring the level of smoking among AAPI women to increase.[37, 46] Data from California's Proposition 99 study of AAPIs document that smoking rates for younger women, ages 18 to 44, are higher than for older women, ages 45 to 65+.[37] On the other hand, the prevalence of smoking among AAPI men ages 25 to 44 is substantially higher than among AAPI men ages 18 to 24. In fact, the smoking rates for AAPI men ages 25 to 44 are the highest of any of the AAPI age groups.[37] Other challenges facing smoking control among Asian Americans are detailed elsewhere.[42, 47, 48]

An additional respiratory condition affecting AAPIs is asthma.[49] Of concern and deserving further attention is the annually increasing rate of asthma among AAPIs.[49]

Another hazard that adds to future cardiovascular disease mortality rates is the prevalence of elevated blood pressure. In a study conducted among Southeast Asian refugee children in Minnesota, investigators discovered elevated risks of hypertension among Southeast Asian refugee boys vis-à-vis white and black boys. The odds ratios were 1.64 for Vietnamese, 1.84 for Cambodians, 2.69 for Hmong, and 2.89 for Lao. Among girls, only Vietnamese girls had a lower odds ratio (0.39) than their white and black girl counterparts; Lao girls had an odds ratio of 1.45, Hmong girls, 1.49, and Cambodian girls, 2.10.[50] Other investigators have reported that Vietnamese and Cambodians had the lowest awareness of hypertension, lowest medication levels, and lowest control rates among all ethnic groups in California.[51] Non–English-speaking Chinese hypertensives likewise exhibit very high noncompliance with Western prescription antihypertensive medications.[52] Thus the combination of elevated disease rates and failure to take medication may portend higher rates of untreated hypertension for selected Asian American populations than for any other race or ethnic group.

Changing dietary practices pose chronic disease threats to AAPIs. Perhaps the most dramatic changes can be illustrated by the changes in the way Native Hawaiians eat. Before Western contact, Hawaiians were "thin," and the typical Hawaiian diet was high in fiber, high in complex carbohydrates, and very healthy.[53] Today, Native Hawaiians have the highest prevalence of obesity,[7] have the shortest life span among all US ethnic groups,[54] and have the highest death rates caused by cardiovascular disease in the United States.[55] Their overall health is far below that of other population groups.[7]

Similarly, the diets of Asian Americans have changed vis-à-vis the diets of their counterparts in Asia. Compared with either their Asian counterparts or, as in the case of the Vietnamese, before arrival in the United States, dietary changes resulting in elevated risks of cardiovascular diseases or cancer have been documented for Asian Indian Americans,[34, 35] Chinese Americans,[56–60] Japanese Americans,[61] and Vietnamese Americans.[62] Yet the percentage of AAPIs counseled in terms of nutrition was at the same level as that of the population at large (33%).[43] These data may indicate that health providers lack experience in suggesting culturally appropriate dietary changes.

Cancer is the second leading cause of death for AAPIs as a group and is increasing in prominence. Not only will the previously discussed higher risk factors for cancer such as smoking and diet portend higher rates of cancer deaths for AAPIs, but specific instances of higher susceptibility to certain cancers have been documented. For example, the incidence of breast cancer in Hawai'i's (spelling preferred by Hawaiians for their land) Japanese American population is more than twice the rate in Japan and breast cancer deaths among Filipino and Native Hawaiian women are 1.5 to 1.7 times greater than among Caucasians.[63]

Hawai'i has among the highest incidence rates for thyroid cancer in the world and the highest rates of that disease for Chinese men (6.3 per 100,000) and for Filipino women (18.2 per 100,000).[64] Filipinos have the lowest survival rates because of kidney and renal cancer.[65] Chinese have the highest incidence of nasopharyngeal cancer,[8] the lowest survival rates for leukemia, the highest incidence of liver cancer, and the highest liver cancer mortality.[65] These extremely high rates of liver cancer among Chinese men in Los Angeles County are likewise observed among Vietnamese in Los Angeles County.[66]

To more properly address these disparities in health status for AAPIs, we must not only advocate risk reduction behaviors such as smoking cessation and smoking prevention, but also address fundamental barriers to health care. For many AAPIs, these barriers include overcoming linguistic,[47, 68] cultural,[47, 68] socioenvironmental,[47] cognitive,[47] and economic barriers.[47] These barriers may also be ethnically specific.[69]

Common to AAPIs is a lack of knowledge of cancer risk factors and lack of age- or gender-relevant cancer screening practices such as performing breast self-examinations, mammograms, or Pap smears.[14, 70, 71] In the case of liver cancer though, prevention of hepatitis B transmission must also be of high priority.[72] Hepatitis B prevalence rates among AAPIs are the highest of any racial or ethnic group.[74] Hepatitis B is a major risk factor for liver cancer and accounts for up to 80% of liver cancers; approximately 8% to 15% of Asian, African, and Pacific Islander populations are chronically infected with Hepatitis B compared with less than 2% of North Americans; and approximately 50% of women who gave birth to Hepatitis B carrier infants in the United States were Asian foreign-born women.[74]

Another communicable disease threat for AAPIs, particularly the foreign-born and new immigrants is tuberculosis.[19, 75, 76] The risk of tuberculosis for AAPIs was the highest (17.0%) of all racial or ethnic groups and was 9.9 times greater than the non-Hispanic white rate. Currently recommended screening and prevention services are controlling this disease,[19] although vigilance is always warranted.

Parasitic infestations disproportionally affect Southeast Asian refugees compared with the population at large.[77] As many as 80% of Southeast Asian refugees who have been screened were positive for at least one parasite per stool sample. Fifty five percent of the malaria in the United States occurs among Southeast Asian refugees.[77]

Special care to Asian Americans is also warranted for the gamut of genetic and maternal and child health care services. The prevalence of genetic disorders among Southeast Asian refugees as a group is estimated to be 10.3% for hemoglobin E, 8% for alpha-thalassemia-1, 2.3% for beta thalassemia, and 25.2% for G-6PD deficiency,[78] compared with about 10% for Blacks. Children are literally born throughout the period of a woman's reproductive span from mothers being teenagers to age 40 or over.[79] Cambodian women tend to have more previous adverse birth outcomes, short interpregnancy intervals, and a cultural emphasis on a lighter baby.[79] Maternal and child health needs go beyond mere provision of service to the requirement to properly understand the language and cultural backgrounds of the diverse AAPIs being served.[80]

Two noncommunicable but not necessarily chronic health conditions that affect AAPIs are sudden infant death syndrome (SIDS) and sudden unexpected nocturnal death syndrome (SUNDS). In an analysis of Asian SIDS cases in California, investigators determined that the 62 Chinese SIDS cases (1.3 per 1000) were approximately 38 times more likely to occur in Chinese in California than Chinese in Hong Kong and that the most likely Asian groups to experience SIDS correlated with the length of their immigration status.[81] That is, Chinese, being the oldest of the Asian immigrant groups, were most likely to experience SIDS compared with Vietnamese immigrants, who were the most recent immigrant group.[81] On the other hand, SUNDS was more common among the most recent immigrants.[82, 83] In particular, young Southeast Asian male refugees died unexpectedly. Stress and depression may be risk factors.[82]

Finally, though not the least of concerns, is the area of mental health,[22] stress, and post-traumatic stress syndrome being experienced by AAPIs. Just as US military personnel returning from war-torn Southeast Asia experienced mental health problems and post-traumatic stress syndrome, so Southeast Asian refugees have experienced mental health problems and stress. In particular, many Cambodians now in the United States are the survivors of mass violence and torture.[84, 85] To them, the "Killing Fields" was not merely a movie; it was real. At the same time that they show this susceptibility, many Asian Americans are reluctant to use community mental health services.[86] Nevertheless, depression and new coping strategies for stress are needed for many Asian Americans.[87–90]

Conclusions

Three reasons have been presented and discussed as to why AAPIs are underserved. Those reasons are as follows:

1. The population growth of AAPIs has been unusually rapid and recent.

2. The data regarding the health status of AAPIs are inadequate. Where the data are available, AAPIs experience health problems that differ from those of mainstream populations.

3. The myth that AAPIs are model minority populations was promulgated.

A considerable number of literature references provided the documentation for these reasons.

In addition, health concerns not well addressed in the *Task Force Report* were also presented, illustrating some of the more particular and unique health challenges that AAPIs encounter. Based on this review, the evidence that AAPIs are underserved is overwhelming. The model healthy Asian American Pacific Islander stereotype is a myth.

SO WHAT? IMPLICATIONS FOR HEALTH PROMOTION PRACTICE OR RESEARCH

This review seems to indicate that the model healthy Asian American/Pacific Islander stereotype is a myth. These conclusions can be characterized as strong. Based on these findings, practitioners should consider the heterogeneity of the Asian American/Pacific Islander (AAPI) populations and collect as much of the social, cultural, and epidemiologic data in their work with AAPI populations. Researchers should collect ethnically specific data and avoid aggregation of AAPI data in their analyses where possible.

Recommendations

1. Adopt Yu and Liu's[32] agenda for improving the data collection process and data bases to collect more adequate, ethnically specific data relevant to the health of AAPIs.

2. Based on more thorough studies, research and programmatic funds should be made available to address AAPI health concerns in culturally competent ways.

This manuscript has not been subjected to review by Ms. Hawk's organization. The views expressed are solely of the authors and do not necessarily represent the policies of the Office of Minority Health.

References

1. Suzuki B. Asian Americans as the "Model Minority" outdoing whites? or media hype? Changes: the magazine of higher education, (Nov/Dec): 13–9, 1989.

2. Brand D, et al. Those Asian American whiz kids. Time 1989; Aug 31:42–51.

3. Myth of Model Minority Haunts Asian Americans. The Washington Post 1992 June 22.

4. Lin S. Exploding myths about health superiority of Asian Americans. Minority Health Issues for an Emerging Majority: Proceedings of the Fourth National Heart, Lung, and Blood Institute National Forum (June 26–27, 1992), 1993:18.

5. Office of Management and Budget. Directive No. 15: Race and ethnic standards for federal statistics and administrative reporting. In: Statistical Policy Handbook. Washington, DC: Office of Federal Statistical Policy and Standards, US Department of Commerce, 1978:37–8.

6. US Bureau of the Census. 1990 Census of Population and Housing. Summary, Tape File 1, Technical Documentation. Issued March 1991.

7. Blaisdell RK. Health status of Kanaka Maoli (indigenous Hawaiians). Asian American and Pacific Islander Journal of Health 1993; 1(2):116-60.

8. US Department of Health and Human Services. Report of the Secretary's Task Force on Black and Minority Health. Volume 1, Executive summary. Washington, DC: US Department of Health and Human Services, 1985.

9. US Department of Health and Human Services. Healthy people 2000. Washington, DC: US Government Printing Office, 1990.

10. US Department of Health and Human Services, Office of Disease Prevention and Health Promotion. National health objectives: Asian and Pacific Islander Americans. US Government Printing Office, (No date).

11. National Center for Health Statistics. Setting a research agenda: challenges for minority health statistics. Draft report of 1991 NCHS Workshop Proceedings.

12. Centers for Disease Control. Screening for hepatitis B virus infection among refugees arriving in the United States. MMWR 40(45):784–7, 1991.

13. Centers for Disease Control Behavioral risk factor survey of Vietnamese—California, 1991. MMWR 41(5):69–72, 1992.

14. Centers for Disease Control. Behavioral risk factor survey of Chinese—California, 1989. MMWR 41(16):266–70, 1989.

15. Centers For Disease Control. Cigarette smoking among Chinese, Vietnamese, and Hispanics—California, 1989–1991. MMWR 41(20): 363–7, 1992.

16. Centers for Disease Control and Prevention. Cigarette smoking among Southeast Asian immigrants—Washington State, 1989. MMWR 41(45):854–63, 1992.

17. Centers for Disease Control and Prevention. Physician and other health-care professional counseling of smokers to quit—United States, 1991. MMWR 42(44):854–7, 1993.

18. Centers for Disease Control and Prevention. Mortality trends for selected smoking-related cancers and breast cancer—United States, 1950–1990. MMWR 42(44):857, 863–6, 1993.

19. Centers for Disease Control. Screening for tuberculosis and tuberculosis infection in high-risk populations and the use of preventive therapy for tuberculosis infection in the United States. MMWR 39(RR-8):5, 1990.

20. Kroll SM, Bradigam PS. MEDLINE search strategies for literature on Asian Americans/Pacific Islanders. Asian American and Pacific Islander Journal of Health 1:56–62, 1993.

21. Chen A, Ng P, Sam P, et al. Special health problems of Asians and Pacific Islanders. In: Matzen RN, Lang RS, eds. Clinical preventive medicine. St. Louis: Mosby, chap 37, 1993.

22. Zane NWS, Takemchi DT, Young KNJ, eds. Confronting Critical Health Issues of Asian and Pacific Islander Americans. Thousand Oaks, CA: Sage Publications 1994.

23. US Bureau of the Census. 1980 Census population. Vol. I: Characteristics of the population. Chapter A, pp. 1–34, Washington, DC: April, 1963.

24. US Bureau of the Census. 1990 Census Profile: Race and Hispanic Origin. Number 2: June, 1991.

25. Forget Zero Population Growth. US News and World Report. 1992 December 14:18.

26. Lin-Fu JS. Asian and Pacific Islander Americans: An overview of demographic characteristics and health care issues. Asian American and Pacific Islander Journal of Health 1(1):20–36, 1993.

27. US Bureau of the Census. Population projections of the United States, by age, sex, race, and Hispanic origin: 1992 to 2050. Washington, DC: US Government Printing Office, 25:1092, 1992.

28. Lin-Fu, JS. Population characteristics and health care needs of Asian Pacific Islanders. Public Health Rep. 103(1):18–27, 1988.

29. Zaharlick A, Brainard J. Demographic characteristics, ethnicity and the resettlement of Southeast Asian refugees in the United States. Urban Anthropology 16(3–4):327–73, 1987.

30. Chen, MS Jr. Cardiovascular health among Asian Americans/Pacific Islanders: an examination of health status and intervention approaches. Am J Health Promot 7(3):199–207, 1993.

31. Chen, MS Jr. A 1993 status report on the health status of Asian Pacific Islander Americans: comparisons with Healthy People 2000 objectives. Asian American and Pacific Islander Journal of Health 1:37–55, 1993.

32. Yu ESH, Liu WT. US national health data on Asian Americans and Pacific Islanders: a research agenda for the 1990s. Am J Public Health 82(12):1645–52, 1992.

33. Hahn RA, Mulinare J, Teutsch SM. Inconsistencies in coding on racial and ethnic groups. JAMA 267:259–63, 1992.

34. Enas E, Yusuf S, Mehta JL. Prevalence of coronary artery disease in Asian Indians. Am J Cardiol 70:945–9, 1992.

35. Jha P, Enas E, Yusuf S. Coronary artery disease in Asian Indians: prevalence and risk factors. Asian American and Pacific Islander Journal of Health 1(2):163–75, 1993.

36. Koh HK, Koh HC. Health issues in Korean Americans. Asian American and Pacific Islander Journal of Health 1(2):176–93, 1993.

37. Burns D, Pierce JP. Tobacco use in California: 1990–1991. Sacramento: California Department of Health Services, 1992.

38. Bates S, Hill L, Barrett-Connor E. Cardiovascular disease risk factors in an Indochinese population. Am J Prev Med 5(1):15–20, 1989.

39. Levin B, Nachampassack S, Xiong R. Cigarette smoking and the Laotian refugee. Migration World 16:4–5, 1988.

40. Curb J, Aluli N, Kautz J, et al. Cardiovascular risk factor levels in ethnic Hawaiians. Am J Public Health 81(2):164–7, 1991.

41. Jenkins CNH, McPhee SJ, Ha N-T, et al. Cigarette smoking among Vietnamese immigrants in California. Am J Health Promot, 9(4): 254–6, 1995.

42. Coultas DB, Gong H Jr, Grad R, et al. State of the art: respiratory diseases in minorities of the United States. Am J Respir Crit Care Med 149(3):S93–S131, 1994.

43. Progress Report on Chapter 21, Healthy People 2000 to the Assistant Secretary of Health, August 4, 1992.

44. Shelton D, Merritt R, Giovino G, et al. Cigarette smoking among Asian/Pacific Islanders: national estimates, 1987–1990. Presentation at the 1992 American Public Health Association Annual Meeting.

45. Hawks, B. Smoking and smoking-related cancers among Asian and Pacific Islanders. In: Jones L, ed. Minorities and Cancer. New York: Springer-Verlag, 1989.

46. Klatsky A, Armstrong M. Cardiovascular risk factors among Asian Americans. Am J Public Health 81:1423–8, 1991.

47. Chen MS Jr, Guthrie R, Moeschberger M, et al. Lessons learned and baseline data Southeast Asians. Asian American and Pacific Islander Journal of Health 1(2):194–214, 1993.

48. Chen MS Jr. Failing grade given for API anti-smoking efforts. Asian American and Pacific Islander Journal of Health 2(1):67–77, 1994.

49. Wing JS, Anderson BS, Arbeit W, et al. Prevalence of asthma in Hawaii, 1980–1986. Am Rev Respir Dis 143:A272, 1991.

50. Munger RG, Gomez-Marin O, Prineas R, Sinaiko A. Elevated blood pressure among Southeast Asian refugee children in Minnesota. Am J Epidemiol 133(12):1257–65, 1991.

51. Stavig G, Igra A, Leonard A. Hypertension and related health issues among Asians and Pacific Islanders in California. Public Health Rep 103(1):28–37, 1988.

52. Choi E, McGandy R, Dallal G, et al. The prevalence of cardiovascular risk factors among elderly Chinese Americans. Arch Intern Med 150:413–8, 1990.

53. Blaisdell R. Historical and cultural aspects of Native Hawaiian health. In: Ikeda I, ed. Social process in Hawaii. Honolulu: University of Hawaii Press 1–21, 1989.

54. Gardner RW. Life tables by ethnic group for Hawaii, 1980, R & S Report No. 47. Honolulu: Research and Statistics Office, State of Hawaii Department of Health, 1984.

55. Milike LH. Current health status and population projections of native Hawaiians living in Hawaii. Washington, DC: Office of Technology Assessment, April 1987.

56. Pinnelas D, DeLa Torre R, Pugh J, et al. Total serum cholesterol levels in Asians living in New York City: results of a self-referred cholesterol screening. N Y State J Med 92(6):245–9, 1992.

57. Yu H, Harris RE, Gao Y, et al: Comparative epidemiology of cancers of the colon, rectum, prostate and breast in Shanghai, China versus the United States. Int J Epidemiol 20(1):76–81, 1991.

58. Yeung K, McKeown-Eyseen G, Li G, et al. Comparisons of diet and biochemical characteristics of stool and urine between Chinese populations with low and high colorectal cancer rates. J Natl Cancer Inst 83(1):46–50, 1991.

59. Whittemore A, Williams-Wu A, Lee M, et al. Diet, physial activity, and colorectal cancer among Chinese in North America and China. J Natl Cancer Inst 82(11):915–26, 1990.

60. Whittemore A. Colorectal cancer incidence among Chinese in North America and the People's Republic of China: variation with sex, age and anatomical site. Int J Epidemiol 18(3):563–8, 1989.

61. Kagan A, Harris BF, Winkelstein W Jr, et al. Epidemiologic studies of coronary heart disease and stroke in Japanese men living in Japan, Hawaii, and California: demographic, physical, dietary, and biochemical characteristics. J Chron Dis 27:345–64, 1974.

62. Jenkins C, McPhee S, Bird J, et al. Cancer risks among Vietnamese refugees. West J Med 5(1):15–20, 1990.

63. Goodman M. Breast cancer in multi-ethnic populations: The Hawaii perspective. Breast Cancer Res Treat 18(Suppl 1):S5–9, 1991.

64. Goodman M, Yoshirawa C, Kolonel L. Descriptive epidemiology of thyroid cancer in Hawaii. Cancer 61(6):1272–81, 1988.

65. American Cancer Society. Cancer facts and figures for minority Americans. Atlanta: American Cancer Society, 1991.

66. Ross R, Bernstein L, Hartnett N, Bone J. Cancer patterns among Vietnamese immigrants in Los Angeles county. Bry J Cancer 64:185–6, 1991.
67. D'Avanzo C, Barriers to health care for Vietnamese reguees. J Prof Nurs 8(4):245–53, 1992.
68. Chen M, Zaharlick A, Kuun P, et al. Implementation of the indigenous model for health education programming among Asian minorities: beyond theory and into practice. J Health Ed 23(7):400–3, 1992.
69. Seipel MM. Health care strategies for Asian American patients. J Health Soc Policy 1(1):105–46, 1989.
70. Lovejoy N, Jenkins C, Wu T, et al. Developing a breast cancer screening program for Chinese-American women. Oncol Nurs Forum 16(2):181–7, 1989.
71. Pham C, McPhee S. Knowledge, attitudes, and practices of breast and cervical cancer screening among Vietnamese women. J Cancer Ed 7(4):305–10, 1992.
72. Hurie M, Mast E, Davis J: Horizontal transmission of hepatitis B virus infection to United States-born children of Hmong refugees. Pediatrics 89(2):269–73, 1992.
73. Friede A, Harris J, Kobayashi J, et al. Transmission of hepatitis B virus from adopted Asian children to their American families. Am J. Public Health 78:26–9, 1988.
74. Margolis HS, Altern MJ, Hadler SC. Hepatitis B: evolving epidemiology and implications for control. Semin Liver Dis 11(2):84–92, 1991.
75. Centers for Disease Control. Tuberculosis among Asians/Pacific Islanders–United States, 1985. MMWR 36:331–4, 1987.
76. Nolan C, Elarth A. Tuberculosis in a cohort of Southeast Asian refugees. Am Rev Respir Dis 137:805–9, 1988.
77. Hann RS. Parasitic infestations In Nolan WS, Zane DT, Takenchi KNJ, et al, eds. Confronting critical health issues of Asian and Pacific Islander Americans. Thousand Oaks, CA: Sage Publications, 1994.
78. Lin-Fu J. Meeting the needs of Southeast Asian refugees in maternal and child health and primary care programs. MCH Technical Information Series, March 1987, 2–7.
79. Gann P, Nghiem L, Warner S. Pregnancy characteristics and outcomes of Cambodian refugees. Am J Public Health 79(9) 1251–7, 1989.
80. Thomas R, Tumminia P. Maternity care for Vietnamese in America. Birth: Issues in Perinatal Care and Education 9(3):187–90, 1982.
81. Grether J, Schulman J, Croen L. Sudden infant death syndrome among Asians in California. J Pediatr 116:525–8, 1990.
82. Centers for Disease Control. Update: sudden unexplained death syndrome among Southeast Asian refugees-United States. MMWR 37(37):568–70, 1988.
83. Park HY, Weinstein S. Sudden unexpected nocturnal death syndrome in the Mariana Islands. Am J Forensic Med Pathol 11(3): 205–7, 1990.
84. Mollica R, Wyshak G, Lavelle J, et al. Assessing symptom change in Southeast Asian refugee survivors of mass violence and torture. Am J Psychiatry 147(1):83–8, 1990.
85. Boehnlein J. Clinical relevance of grief and mourning among Cambodian refugees. Soc Sci Med 25(7):765–72, 1987.
86. Sue S, Fujino D, Hu L, et al. Community mental health services for ethnic minority groups: a test of the cultural responsiveness hypothesis. J Consult Clin Psychol 59(4):533–40, 1991.
87. Franks F, Faux S. Depression, stress, mastery, and social resources in four ethnocultural women's groups. Res Nurs Health 13:283–92, 1990.
88. Kinzie J, Boehnlein J, Leong P, et al. The prevalence of posttraumatic stress disorder and its clinical significance among Southeast Asian refugees. Am J Psychiatry 147(7):913–7, 1990.
89. Nguyen N, Williams H. Transition from East to West: Vietnamese adolescents and their parents. J Am Acad Child Adolesc Psychiatry 28:505–15, 1989.
90. Flaskerud J, Nguyen T. Mental health needs of Vietnamese refugees. Hosp Community Psychiatry 39:435–9, 1988.

WOMEN'S HEALTH STATUS IN THE UNITED STATES: AN IMMIGRANT WOMEN'S PROJECT*

Afaf I. Meleis • Patricia A. Omidian • Juliene G. Lipson

The Mid East S.I.H.A. Project† is a primary health care/health resource center for Middle Eastern immigrants located in the School of Nursing at the University of California, San Francisco (UCSF). This interdisciplinary project is staffed by faculty and graduate students in the International/Cross-Cultural Nursing and Medical Anthropology Programs at the UCSF and representatives of the Arab-American and Iranian communities of the San Francisco Bay Area. With an emphasis on low-income women, the Project provides health information, cultural and language interpretation, referral services, health promotion workshops, health information, and opportunities for value clarification for immigrants and their families. The Project also serves health care providers by providing cultural interpreters and by giving in-service training on cross-cultural issues and coping styles in illness.

With the support of a Kellogg International Fellowship, the Project developed a series of health education workshops based in the Arab-American community. Called "Being Healthy, Thinking Healthy, Staying Healthy," the workshops were held in the Spring of 1988 at an Arab community center. The focus was on culturally appropriate self-care and health promotion.

The overall goal of the health maintenance/promotion program was to empower women to take responsibility for their own health and that of their families through value clarification and a greater awareness and understanding of their own roles. The program offered a forum for immigrant women to develop skills needed to cope with the difficulties and stressors of living and raising families in a new country, with an emphasis on mastering various roles and coping with new role demands. In addition to affording opportunities for dealing with existing issues related to physical and mental health, the series provided an opportunity to discuss and demonstrate preventive measures with regard to common risk factors in the community. The Arab community participated by choosing the topics, identifying resources and information available in their area, and helping to organize the workshops.

This report describes this series and is intended to provide clinicians with a model for developing and implementing a community-oriented health promotion program based on the health needs of a dispersed ethnic community. It is based on existing health education methods for reaching immigrant and migrant women (Thompson, Harminder, & Mroke, 1986: Ellis, Stoker, & Wood, 1987; Lee & Brentnall, 1986) and on the principle of community participation that is promoted by the WHO/UNICEF 1978 Alma Ata Declaration. Our model conceives health educators as facilitators who help the community to choose its own focus and articulate its own needs and to plan and implement health services to meet these needs. After describing the Arab-American community and its health to provide the context we describe the theoretical framework and the process of program development. The program itself consisted of eight 90-minute sessions on the following topics: raising adolescents, handling stress, self-care, nutrition, AIDS, child safety, employment, and menopause. Attendance varied from 5 to 35 women. The series marked a turning point for health education in the Arab community in that it not only built on previous health education requests but also offered the women a chance to actively plan and participate in a primary health promotion program.

Assumptions and Theoretical Framework

The assumptions on which the program was developed include the following:

1. Language and cultural barriers negatively impact access to health care services. Immigrant women face particular problems locating appropriate services, arranging transportation and dealing with the structure of our complex health and social service systems. Speaking English does not necessarily mean that immigrant women can clearly communicate their needs to health professionals. Mutual understanding is impeded by differences in nonverbal communication style and the different meanings clients and providers attribute to illness. Health and illness are defined in cultural terms and illness is a social event, a social creation that is interpreted within the social network before treatment is sought (Freidson, 1970).

2. Because immigrant women are the conservators of their family's health, their role in health promotion is critical. They make decisions regarding health care use and subsequent actions for all members of the family (Meleis & Rogers, 1987), using cultural definitions to filter information received by health care providers. Immigrant women need opportunities to discuss health topics in an environment that permits clarification of values, identification of options and resources, and the

*Reprinted from McElmurry BJ, Norr KF, Parker RS. Women's Health and Development: A Global Challenge. World Health Organization Global Network of WHO Collaborating Centres for Nursing/Midwifery Development. Sudbury, MA: Jones and Bartlett, 1993.
†The senior author was partially supported by a Kellogg International Fellowship.

range of culturally acceptable choices. Although Western biomedicine places ultimate responsibility for health on the individual, the ability to make choices about one's everyday life is constrained by one's cultural values and limits. When information is presented in a culturally appropriate manner and is accessible and acceptable to the individual, she can better use it to make choices about health and health care.

3. Community members are aware of their community's needs and can communicate these needs when and if given the opportunity to do so. This assumption is based on principles of "community-oriented primary health care" (WHO, 1978; Newell, 1975), in which active community participation provides the groundwork for self-empowerment on a number of levels: individual, family, and community. The proceedings of the WHO conference at Alma Ata stated that "Primary Health Care addresses the main health problems identified by the community, providing promotive, preventive, curative, and rehabilitative services accordingly" (WHO, 1978). Needs are identified and then addressed through mobilization of resources within the community whenever possible. This is an action-oriented process by which the community empowers itself at a local political level (Werner, 1977). Empowerment of individuals occurs within the context of the social group, whether it be family, extended family, or community.

The theoretical framework on which the health maintenance/promotion series was based includes concepts of role, transition, self-care and ethnic identity. A role is:

a designated reciprocity in which an interaction or a social exchange occurs and is seen in terms of relevant other roles. The role that the actor elects to play is derivative of his voluntary actions that are motivated by returns expected, and, indeed, received from others (Meleis, 1975, p. 265).

Women's roles can be analyzed as an aggregation of tasks, sentiments, and goals which are organized in coherent units in response to individual, family, and social expectations, e.g., mother, wife, friend, and health provider. Any changes in expectations, conditions surrounding roles, or symbols within roles cause stress and subsequently may influence health or health-seeking behavior. It is important to consider women's roles in terms of the balance between the stresses and the satisfactions in each. Most immigrant women perceive their role in the context of their families (Meleis & Rogers, 1987); the dominant U.S. emphasis on individualism is not valued.

Transition is a passage from one life condition or status to another and can be developmental or situational. Transition involves both the process and outcome of the passage. A pervasive characteristic is "disconnected-

ness," but its meaning to any individual influences the outcome (Chick & Meleis, 1988). Immigrant women experience role changes in coping with cultural differences in the new country as well as in personal and family development. Transition includes modifying or adding roles when changes occur between the individual and her social network or cultural setting. Value clarification is helpful in allowing the individual to adapt to the new role or roles through knowledge of what the role entails. Role transition involves the acquisition of new knowledge and skills, incorporating value clarification to complete the process (Chick and Meleis, 1988; Swendsen & Meleis, 1978). Self-care focuses on health promotion and disease prevention through education. Fundamental to the workshop series, the self-care model is based on the premise that

individuals have the ability to influence their health and to participate in their health care. Self care is defined here as those activities initiated or performed by an individual, family, or community to achieve, maintain, or promote *maximum* health potential (Steiger & Lipson, 1985).

The workshop series for immigrant women emphasized family and community aspects of self-care and health promotion.

Ethnicity, another component of the model, must be considered when working with immigrant women. Immigrants do not drop their cultural baggage at the entry gate, but pass it on to their children and subsequent generations; thus, we must distinguish between immigrant status and ethnic identity. Ethnic groups are "categories of ascription and identification by the actors themselves" (Barth, 1969) and share such cultural patterns as marriage practices, food styles, and religion, as well as concepts of health and illness. Ethnic identity is a subjective sense of belonging to a group that is distinguishable from other social groups. It includes an answer to the question "who am I?" and feelings about oneself in relation to others.

The Context: Demographics, History and Health

According to the 1980 census, San Francisco's population of 678,974 is 58% white, 13% black, 22% Asian/Pacific Islanders, 0.5% Native Americans, and 7% other. Twelve percent of the white category identified themselves as Hispanic and 0.7% as Middle Eastern (about 4800 individuals). Continuing decline in the city's white and black populations and continuing growth in the Hispanic and Asian/Pacific Island groups is predicted.

In San Francisco, ethnically designed health and social services exist for immigrants in neighborhoods where there are high concentrations of particular groups, e.g., the On Lok Senior Center in Chinatown and the Mission Community Health Center for Hispanics. Arab-

Americans, in contrast, are dispersed and heterogeneous. They come from Egypt, Saudi Arabia, North and South Yemen, the United Arab Emirates, Lebanon, Jordan, Syria, Kuwait, Iraq, and Israel. No services existed to meet their specific culturally based needs until the Mid-East S.I.H.A. Project was established in 1982. Although many Arab-Americans have health insurance, services are often improperly utilized, such as using emergency rooms as primary clinics, or underutilizing private services where co-payment is required (Omidian & Rainey, 1987).

Arabs came to the United States in several waves. The first wave (late 19th Century to WWII) consisted mainly of Christian men who sought economic gain in the New World and who never intended to stay, but eventually settled and brought over wives and other family members (Elkholy, 1966, p. 83), many prominent Bay Area Arab-American families are descended from these early immigrants. Subsequent immigration waves (mid-1940s to present) were associated with changes in the political climate in the Middle East and the establishment of Israel. These immigrants included the intellectual elite and skilled professionals, as well as refugees from the wars in Lebanon. A large number of the most recent immigrants are Moslem (Reizian & Meleis, 1985).

Currently, there are an estimated 2 to 3 million Arab immigrants in the United States. Most came from Israel and the Occupied Territories, Lebanon, North Yemen, Iraq, and Egypt (Meleis & Sorrell, 1981). According to estimates from community leaders, approximately 100,000 Arab-Americans live in the San Francisco Bay Area, and of these, at least 30,000 are Palestinians. These estimates include second and third generations while the census counts only the foreign born. Palestinians, in particular, count all descendants; those from Ramallah keep records, family trees, and directories of all who live in the United States.

Although Arab-Americans maintain many traditional values in the home, in public they are not visually distinguishable from the rest of the population. Cultural patterns and ethnic symbols remain private and are manifested publicly only in times of crises, such as illness and hospitalization.

Some Arab cultural characteristics and values create potential conflict for patients in the United States health care system, such as group rather than individual orientation, the desire to keep some information private, a belief in the primacy of God's Will, and concern for maintaining the family's honor (Lipson & Meleis, 1985). While such values are maintained in various degrees by most Arab-Americans, they are unspoken; however, they affect both patients and their families.

Illness is viewed by Arab-Americans in physical, emotional, behavioral, and spiritual terms (Maloof,

1982). Physical is not separated from psychological, nor is illness defined as a problem with a specific organ system. The experiences of pain and illness tend to be global and generalized (Meleis, 1981; Lipson & Meleis, 1985). A person is considered sick when he or she is no longer able to function or fulfill her or his roles (cf., Apple, 1960; Gallagher, 1976).

Related to the concept of illness are two symbolic categories: 1) the evil eye, and 2) balance of hot and cold. The evil eye is found throughout the Middle East and Latin America. The "eye," which is believed to cause illness, is thought to result from another person's envy or attempting to control the future. Ill effects of the "eye" can be prevented by 1) not attempting to plan for the future; 2) minimizing attention to good fortune, health and children by avoiding direct recognition and compliments; and 3) by calling for God's blessing or touching wood when compliments are made (Sachs, 1983).

Maintaining balance in the body and the environment is another aspect of the Arab view of health. People maintain balance by avoiding sudden changes in temperature and eating a balanced diet according to the season. Hot and cold foods (perceived quality rather than temperature of food) are seen to cause illness when eaten inappropriately or have the ability to bring the body back into balance if properly mixed (Lipson & Meleis, 1985; Maloof, 1982; Meleis, 1981).

In the case of illness, misunderstanding between Arab clients and health providers is due to conflicting expectations: clients expect to be cared for and health providers expect from clients some degree of self-care and share of the responsibility for getting well (Meleis, 1988). Although Arabs perceive their health to be under God's control, they also see Western biomedicine as powerful and expect immediate results from treatment. Self-care models do not make sense in this context. One might observe a person with diabetes drinking cola or a person with asthma smoking; the individual may not understand the relationship between food or smoking and health or think that his fate is determined by God, no matter what he does.

The Western biomedical model assumes a future orientation and a positive attitude toward prevention while some Arab clients have a strictly present orientation. Such value conflicts appear to inhibit the acceptance of health promotion but in reality do not really do so. Self-care is valued, but within a traditional context (protection from the "evil eye" and balancing hot and cold foods). The health promotion program had to consider these beliefs in order to be effective. In short, any health promotion program in an immigrant/ethnic community must incorporate health beliefs and behavior by using the traditional system as the context for introducing new information.

Program

The goal of the program was to empower women to maintain/promote their own and their children's health. At each session women were given a list of community resources and health promotion materials pertinent to the evening's topic in English and Arabic whenever possible. The following sessions were held.

What Are the Barriers to Happiness in America; Handling Life as an Immigrant

The goal of this session was to encourage women to develop skills to deal with stress, particularly as it relates to family relationships. The session provided strategies on how to improve communication in the nuclear and extended family, and cope with family stress and ways to balance Middle Eastern and American ways. The speaker suggested ways to develop a support group when family is not available and answered questions concerning roles of immigrant woman and wife. Coping, time out, and other strategies were reviewed.

Mothering Yourself After Your Child Is Born

This session covered self-care and group-care as ways to improve or maintain participants' own health, just as they would care for family members. The speaker talked about the mother's body having special needs during and after pregnancy, why one might feel tired and depressed after the birth of the last child, and how to relieve back and other kinds of pain. The goal of this workshop was to develop an awareness of self-care methods, and we offered some basic strategies to prevent health problems, such as exercise and breast self-examination.

Child Health and Safety

The goal of this workshop was to develop an awareness of accident prevention, with a special focus on accidents and childhood developmental stages. The topics included potential hazards in the home as they relate to growing children and how to identify dangers by looking at the home from the child's level. Regarding illnesses, the speaker encouraged breastfeeding but described safe ways to bottle-feed and appropriate times to use aspirin. She also taught basic skills to meet some common emergencies such as burns, fevers, and choking.

Adolescence

Information on raising adolescents in the United States has been the most frequently requested topic from the Arab community as well as a concern of social service agencies. This workshop explored the problems teens and parents face and offered suggestions to help parents cope with adolescent children. The adolescent psychiatrist speaker described the developmental phases which occur in the teen years in the United States, what conflicts are normal, and how to keep communication open with the teen.

A goal of this workshop was to provide an opportunity for value clarification. The participants discussed strategies for dealing with their teen son or daughter; the speaker helped mothers understand the teens' conflict between American and Arab cultures and gave some concrete strategies for coping with common situations. The women also received information specific to the cultural context in which they raised their children and had the opportunity to discuss particular problems or concerns with an Arab mental health professional.

Familiar Foods and Balanced Nutrition

This workshop explored nutrition in terms of familiar categories, basing suggestions for healthy changes on the group's dietary patterns and preferences, such as eating fruit and whole grains. The participants discovered that their ethnic foods were essentially very healthy and, with small modifications and portion control, were nutritionally sound. The nutritionist speaker discussed ways of cooking favorite foods and modifying traditional cooking so that it fits special needs and diets. The women left this session with information on how to modify their families' diets in a healthy way without losing the taste and style to which they are accustomed. Those who were on special diets understood more clearly the potential variety of "legal foods" and portion control that allow them to eat familiar food and stay within their program guidelines.

Looking for a Job or Making One of Your Own

Immigrant women deal with a variety of stressors, one of the most difficult being the search for a job. Many women asked such questions as "Where do I start looking?" "What am I qualified to do?" and "How can I work and still be with my family?" The speakers covered these questions and discussed the risks and benefits of owning a business. Women gained an appreciation of the basics of job hunting in California and of the many skills they already have.

This Is Your Body: Lifetime . . . Wellness and Healthy Living

The speaker addressed changes the female body experiences over time, what to expect, and how to cope with some of the changes. The session covered menopause and why every woman needs to begin preparing for it before it arrives. Women gained an understanding of the processes of life changes and the physiological changes women experience, including menopause. Women were able to focus on questions concerning estrogen replacement therapy, bone-loss, and the role exercise plays in maintaining health. They also learned some basic self-care techniques, such as relaxation and breast self-examination.

AIDS: Does It Affect You?

In San Francisco, the issue of AIDS was of particular interest to the Arab community. Women wanted to know what AIDS is, how it spreads, how to keep from getting AIDS, and where could they get information. In this workshop women discussed their fears and gained an understanding of the AIDS epidemic in the United States and what it meant to them. They were reassured that AIDS is not spread through casual contact and given some strategies on how to safeguard their families.

Program Development

The workshop series was developed using a four step process: (a) needs assessment, (b) planning, (c) implementation, and (d) evaluation. In describing each step we describe issues that needed to be resolved and suggest strategies that might be useful for other immigrant communities.

Needs Assessment

The purpose of a needs assessment is to understand the parameters of the community and its concerns. The process involves gathering demographic, ethnographic, and historical information on the population within its social and geographical setting. This information provides the groundwork for understanding the health needs of a community. To accomplish a needs assessment in the Arab community, two issues were apparent—deciding how to define the community and determining the appropriate methods for assessment of community needs. Ways by which communities are usually defined, such as geographical boundaries, professional interests, language, or religion, were not useful. Arabs in the United States are diverse in countries of origin, religion, and language. Therefore, we decided to focus on already established self-proclaimed social groups such as Arab women's associations.

Methods of assessment was the second issue. Demographic data are usually used to predict morbidity/mortality rates in populations for which data are available, such as Hispanics, African Americans and Southeast Asians. However, Arabs in the U.S. are not homogeneous and have not been accurately counted in the census. Neither were the usual epidemiological tools available for preliminary assessment of health care needs of a population, e.g., mortality and morbidity data. Thus, we used a combination of sources, such as key informants, community forums, surveys (Laffrey, Meleis, Lipson, Solomon, & Omidian, 1989), and ethnographic data to obtain information on health needs in the Arab community.

Key informants included community spokespeople and health care professionals, who gave their opinions on health needs and problems in this population. Health providers' opinions included negative or stereotypical attitudes which were probably reflected back in the care of this community. The community forum approach gave community members an opportunity to express their needs directly. The identified needs formed a basis for many of the subsequent workshops. By distributing questionnaires at community lectures (survey approach) we elicited health topics that groups wanted addressed. Some of the needs brought up by community members fell outside of the health education arena, e.g., requests for English as a Second Language (ESL) classes (Lipson & Omidian, 1987; Meleis & Rogers, 1987). However, the combination of methods provided us with a general orientation to the health needs of this community.

At the first workshop, we distributed a questionnaire to get some ideas of participants' health behavior. Of the 25 women who filled out the short initial questionnaire on attitudes toward self-care, 12 answered in English and 13 in Arabic. They came from Palestine, Iraq, Jordan, Lebanon, and Syria. They ranged in age from under 20 to over 40, with the largest number (8) between 26 and 30. Seventy-five percent were married and only one had no children. With regard to breast self-examination, 25% stated they never performed it, yet 36% did it routinely. Fifty percent had never had a pap smear, but 48% had it done routinely. Eighty percent knew their weight.

Planning

The program was planned to address the health needs identified by community members and health care providers. Designed to build on local resources, the planning process utilized weekly meetings with the presidents of five Arab women's organizations, inviting their input on community needs and support in organizing the workshops. This teamwork approach was essential in both planning and implementing the series but was not without difficulty.

In addition to strategies described in the health education literature, we identified the following issues and strategies necessary for success in program planning: work to enhance trust, acknowledge the diversity of the community and avoid alignment with any one segment, and take into account connections with countries of origin. Working with organized community groups had both advantages and disadvantages that relate strongly to the trust issue. Such groups provide quick access and entry into a dispersed community once the leaders are convinced of the value of the program, and through the leaders, the trust of community members is gained. For a community oriented model of health promotion, organized groups also provide a setting that encourages community action because such women's organizations are set up by and for women.

However, working with organized women's groups can be problematic because of distrust between groups, e.g., Christian and Moslem groups. Such distrust slows information dispersal. To reach the greatest number of community members, the factions had to be recognized and incorporated. In the perceptions of Arab women, workshop sponsorship by one group would have prevented members of other groups from attending and destroy the trust of the general Arab population which had been so painstakingly built. For this reason it helped to work with as many different groups and leaders as possible, which reduced polarization caused by political factions. However, our efforts to include all club presidents resulted in slighting one of the larger groups. Consequently, their participation never exceeded two or three women per workshop.

Developing trust, although important in all working groups, is particularly significant in a diverse immigrant population. Among Arabs, trust generally does not extend beyond family and close friends, or to outside institutions. Although we were outsiders, we had gained community trust on one level. The women's club presidents had heard Dr. Meleis speak at Arab gatherings on health issues. They also knew of the S.I.H.A. Project's work in the community. However, we could maintain the trust of the wider Arab community only by recognizing and including different interest groups. In the planning process we constantly confronted religious divisions, national differences, political differences, and even subtle divisions of city/village identification among those who were born in the U.S. Thus, ongoing negotiations were necessary throughout the planning process.

Competition between club presidents required planning to minimize the effects of these differences and foster cooperation. We could never pin down such seemingly simple things as mutually convenient dates for the meeting, because there were frequent conflicts with local gatherings, religious holidays, and holidays imported from the Middle East. When one of us asked a president why dates were not worked out first, she said that no one wanted the responsibility for setting dates and then not keeping them. By leaving the choice of times to someone else, each leader would not feel obligated to attend all meetings or be embarrassed should her members fail to attend.

Maintaining trust necessitated holding the health promotion program on neutral ground to avoid political and religious biases. Community leaders and women's organizations recommended avoiding meeting in any individual woman's house, which would have caused strain on the family or jealousy. In San Francisco, the Arab community, particularly the Palestinians, have a number of formal meeting places. Most of the women's groups used the Arab Cultural Center, and the club presidents encouraged us to use it for the workshop series, as most community members know its location. While it was not entirely neutral, this location was agreeable to the largest number of people.

For immigrants living in a circumscribed area, a good location is the local public library or community center. Churches may operate as central locations for dispersed populations, but they may not be neutral ground for holding a workshop. It is helpful to ask the women where they would prefer to meet and work toward a consensus. Non-community locations in the area may, in the end, be the most appropriate, as no community members would have a stake in them.

The final issue and strategy is acknowledging connections with the country of origin. Current events in the home country affect community members in the host country, because most have families that remain. War, strikes, political upheavals, or natural disasters, as well as religious and secular holidays, have an impact on immigrants. Just after the workshop series began, community attention focused on the strikes in the West Bank and Gaza Strip. Each week there were meetings to discuss the news or talk to people who had just returned from visits, often organized at the last minute. This competition had the greatest single impact on attendance at the health promotion workshops. Workshop participation on particular occasions was reduced because we were unable to anticipate political events in the Middle East or the religious holidays of all the groups involved.

Implementation

In health promotion workshops, community women can actively participate in all levels of implementation. They can choose topics, and translate, type and distribute brochures and health education materials. Leaders can book space in a community hall, organize transportation, and coordinate baby-sitting and children's activities. Invitations can be sent through the organizations or by direct mail. Most importantly, the community should take an active role in evaluating the progress of the workshops. The more involved the community, the greater the impact for empowerment. In our health promotion workshops, the women were the focal point of the process and took charge of organizing the event.

In addition to the nuts and bolts of implementing the workshops, we developed several strategies for success: presence, dialogue, coaching, and empowerment. Presence involved community leadership, S.I.H.A. staff, and the use of Arabic. Presence is the physical and social attendance of both staff and leaders known to the community at large. Presence is, we suspect, what made the difference in participation. In Arab communities in the United States, workshop topics that leaders see as important draw interest and attendance; leadership support is important for garnering community attention, maintaining interest and organizing events. When a group's president did not attend a session, members of her club also stayed away. This meant that the presidents needed to make a firm commitment to the workshop series to maintain attendance. Presence also includes staff attendance at each session; both Meleis and Omidian attempted to attend each session, which demonstrated to the community that we saw the effort as valuable. When Meleis's speaking engagements took her away, fewer people attended. Some women called to inform us that her presence was important to them.

Presence is also symbolized by using the community's language. Whenever possible, we invited Arab speakers with expertise in the workshop topic, as they understand their community's values and symbols, making communication easier and giving a sense of community control. An Egyptian physician volunteered to translate health information materials into Arabic. This emphasis on and recognition of the importance of Arabic, the mother tongue, created a presence of its own. It signaled to the community that we acknowledged the importance of their roots and values. This demonstration is critical to success in an immigrant community in which the people feel misunderstood and often at odds with perceived American values.

The second strategy in implementation was dialogue. There was continuous dialogue among project staff, among project staff and community members and leaders, and among community members and leaders. Two forms of communication were used—written and verbal. Questionnaires were given out at each meeting and by this means all participants were encouraged to state what they learned and what else they would have liked included. These questionnaires became the basis for our evaluation and follow-up and a source of ideas for improving subsequent workshops. In verbal dialogue, the presidents were telephoned weekly to assess the previous meeting and plan the next. Such dialogue helped community members maintain a high level of involvement. We encouraged the organization presidents to seek input from their members and work with us to make needed changes. Concurrently we suggested strategies to maintain community interest. Some leaders waited for our calls on the Monday morning after a workshop, perceiving, correctly, that their opinions were valued and acted upon whenever possible. The dialogue between the women's groups, their presidents and the S.I.H.A. Project staff maintained the excitement and momentum of the series as the weeks progressed. Because the Arab community's attention was divided between Ramadan, Easter or Orthodox Easter, and the political events in the Gaza Strip and West Bank, without the active involvement of and dialogue with the leaders, the series could not have continued.

A third strategy for implementing a health promotion program is coaching. Coaching means orienting speakers to the fundamental goals, rules, and strategies of the event before they come to a session. For the Arab health experts, coaching included a briefing on the age, educational level, and expectations of the audience. In the audience, some spoke little English, others spoke little Arabic, but most were bilingual. This is problematic for any speaker, and thus translators had to be placed in the audience. We also discovered that several Arab-American speakers were not comfortable thinking about professional concepts in Arabic as most had been trained in the United States. Coaching helped the speakers become more comfortable articulating their ideas in Arabic.

As Arabic-speaking experts were not available for every topic, we relied on other experts, some of whom had previously worked with the S.I.H.A. Project. They also needed coaching, not just about the audience age and level of sophistication, but also on more general cultural aspects. For example, the workshop on menopause was led by a nursing faculty member from the women's health clinic at UCSF. Before speaking she wanted to understand Middle Eastern values regarding elderly women and male/female relationships as they relate to support networks for aging women. By gaining some understanding of these cultural norms, she was better prepared to answer questions on coping.

The final strategy involves the concept of empowerment. We conceived of the workshop series as a process of empowerment for immigrant women and their community. Empowerment is the process of learning and development, incorporating self-esteem and social responsibility (Rappaport, 1985). Empowerment cannot be "given;" it is the process whereby the individual internalizes the right to make decisions and accepts the self as the locus of control. We worked with the women to identify and address their health needs in order to empower them in taking responsibility for their own health and that of their families. In creating a forum where their health questions could be addressed, the workshops fostered greater awareness and understanding of (a) their own body's needs and cycles, (b) skills to maintain health, and (c) family and child-rearing issues in the U.S.

Evaluation

Two forms of evaluation are useful in community oriented health promotion programs: terminal and process evaluation. Terminal evaluations help the organizers understand the session's impact on the participants and give an overview of the process, but do not encourage the empowerment that is the basis of our model. Process evaluations are continuous throughout the program, keep it focused on the community's needs, and empower the women by encouraging them to direct the course of the program. Process evaluations provide ongoing information to the organizers at a participatory level, ensuring that the sessions are being conducted at the right information level for the audience. They also provide speakers with feedback about their own teaching and alert the staff to the level of coaching needed by speakers. Evaluations also serve to maintain a sense of continuity for the women involved, allowing issues raised to be explored further.

Process evaluations were written and verbal. As mentioned previously, the workshop series started with a short survey of attitudes toward self-care, which included questions about weight and breast self-exams. Each session was followed by a short questionnaire in Arabic and English to see what women learned, what they wanted to learn, and what they saw as important, and elicited their opinions on how to improve the series. This question, although not always answered, was a means to encourage participation and dialogue and increased the women's participation in designing programs that meet their needs.

Verbal process evaluations occurred each week when the project coordinator called various women in the different organizations to obtain their reactions and to ask what needed to change after each session. In general, the women were positive about the workshops and appreciated the efforts made to organize them. The only consistent suggestion for change was to help the women obtain better child care so that they would not have to bring children to the workshops. Even with children being watched by others downstairs, they came into the meeting room to visit their mothers and many women complained. A specific complaint concerned the presence of the man who videotaped the first session. Because we intended to use videotapes in other areas of the country, it would have been worthwhile to hire a woman to tape the sessions properly. Finally, some women thought that the topics were too sweeping to be useful and they would have liked more time to ask questions.

On the written evaluation forms, participants provided responses to the following questions:

What skill/strategy will you take home from this workshop? The women listed strategies that could enhance health or well-being or prevent illness in themselves or their family members. From the menopause session the women listed the need for awareness of vitamins and calories, exercise, proper nutrition, and positive and negative aspects of estrogen replacement therapy (ERT). Regarding self-care, they listed as important breast self-exam (BSE), exercise, relaxation, taking care of one's self, and breaking large goals into smaller ones. The stress session yielded planning and communication, self-acceptance, and resources. Regarding child safety they listed prevention, diseases, e.g., ear infection, and how to deal with small accidents. Communication was the skill noted after the adolescence session. On employment, self-esteem and knowing your own abilities were the skills noted. And finally, on nutrition, they stated "how we can eat Arab foods." We indirectly rated the usefulness and popularity of the sessions by the number of strategies noted. The three sessions that earned the most comments were menopause (7 of 12), self-care (21 of 21), and adolescence (9 of 12 responses).

What information did you need that was not covered in the workshop? The women wanted more general sessions on self-care, stress, and AIDS. There were specific requests for information that probably reflected individual needs on which there was no consensus. They requested the following specific information:

1. Self-care: post-partum, headaches, marriage and health, more on physical and psychological health;
2. Stress: communication with husbands, marriage within immigrant communities, and communication in general;
3. Child care: information on how to handle children from 6 to teen, child abuse, divorce and premature babies, how to do CPR, strep throat, constipation, baby-sitting, e.g., who can they leave their children with, and breast-feeding;
4. Adolescence: lying, more detailed information on individual cases, and societal effect on teens;
5. Employment: finding the right job (more details), employment interview requirements, daily life of working mothers, and specific companies;
6. AIDS: how to treat it, prevention, and condoms.

How can we improve this workshop for you? On the whole, this question generated positive feedback. The women stated that the workshops were presented professionally and included useful information. They suggested more workshops, longer sessions with more opportunity for questions and answers, and improved advertisement. Some suggested involving husbands in some of the workshops, particularly the stress and adolescent sessions. One woman requested a second session on adolescents to which fathers are invited; another stated that fathers need this information more than mothers do.

Finally, speakers were asked for written feedback on the sessions. In general, all speakers thought that the evening's topic was significant to the audience, except for the topic of menopause, which was too narrow; the speaker suggested adding nutritional issues, exercise, and anti-smoking. All speakers thought that the handouts were appropriate and one commented positively on the consumer focus. Most speakers observed that the women were interested in the topics, were lively contributors to the discussions, and were pleasant.

Conclusion

The health promotion series encouraged the women to gather, as they would have done in the Middle East, without the men around. We were surprised by the strong community cohesiveness among the participants and observed relationships similar to those maintained in the Middle East, where women turn to each other for support and not, as many Americans do, to such external resources as clinics and self-help groups. In the meetings women asked questions, visited with old friends and met new ones, learned self-care techniques, and discussed a broad range of issues. Although the sessions were structured, each meeting also dramatically illustrated the importance of nonstructured dialogue. Someone always asked for more information, and many called the Project the following week to discuss issues that had been highlighted at the workshop. New skills introduced (often related to mental health and well-being) included health maintenance issues. Classes were requested on improving or acquiring skills in entrepreneurship, job seeking/interviewing skills and techniques, and when necessary, self-empowerment through English language acquisition.

Once the workshops were organized, a high level of commitment from community members was needed for all the women to travel to a central location for the sessions. While the workshops were planned for low income women with limited English skills, from a dispersed ethnic community, this initial series was attended by middle and upper income women with varied educational levels.

To date, the Project has realized its goals. In needs assessment, planning, implementation, and evaluation, the health promotion workshops encouraged community control and empowerment through dialogue, negotiation, presence, and trust. Realizing that the consequences of empowerment could be stressful, we encouraged the women to utilize traditional support systems. We also made referrals where needed for culturally sensitive counseling.

The success of this health promotion workshop series demonstrates that the principles of primary health care are effective in urban settings with a diverse and scattered ethnic community. It is only through community participation and ownership of the series that effective health education could be carried out.

References

Apple D: How laymen define illness. Journal of Health and Human Behavior, 1:219–225, 1960.

Barth F: Ethnic groups and boundaries. London: George Allen and Unwin, 1969.

Chick N, and Meleis, AI: Transitions: A nursing concern. In P. C. Chinn (Ed.), Nursing research methodology: Issues and implementation (pp. 237–257). Rockville, Md.: Aspen Publications, 1986.

Elkholy A: The Arab American family. In CH Mindel & RW Haberstein (Eds.), Ethnic families in America. New York:, Elsevier North-Holland, Inc., 1976.

Ellis M, Stoker L, Ward T: Health education package for women of non-English-speaking background. N.S.W. Department of Health, Southern Metropolitan Region, 1987.

Freidson E: The lay construction of illness. In Profession of medicine: A study of the sociology of applied knowledge (pp. 278–301). New York: Dodd, Mead & Co., 1970.

Gallagher E: Lines of reconstruction and extension in the Parsonian sociology of illness. Social Science and Medicine 10:207–218, 1976.

Kieffer C: Citizen empowerment: A developmental perspective. Prevention in Human Services, 3(2–3):9–36, 1984.

Laffrey S, Meleis AL, Lipson J, Solomon M, Omidian P: Assessing Arab-American health care needs. Social Science and Medicine 29:877–883, 1989.

Lee I, Brentnell R: Cultural awareness for health professionals: A training manual. Sydney: Multicultural Centre, Sydney College of Advanced Education, 1986.

Lipson JG, Meleis AI: Issues in health care of Middle Eastern patients. Western Journal of Medicine 139:854–861, 1983.

Lipson J, Omidian P: Afghan refugees: Community needs and care. Paper presented at the 13th Transcultural Nursing Society Conference, Miami, Florida, 1987.

Maloof P: Maternal-child health beliefs and practices among Palestinian-Americans. Paper presented at the American Anthropological Association 81st Annual Meeting, Washington, DC, 1982.

Meleis AI: Role insufficiency and role supplementation: A conceptual framework. Nursing Research 24:264–271, 1975.

Meleis AI: The Arab American in the health care system. American Journal of Nursing 81:1180–1183, 1981.

Meleis AI: The sick role: A symbolic interaction perspective. In Hardy ME, Conway ME (Eds.), Role Theory: Perspectives for Health Professionals (2nd ed.). San Mateo: Appleton and Lange, 1988.

Meleis AI, Jonsen A: Ethical crises and cultural differences. Western Journal of Medicine, 138:889–893, 1983.

Meleis AI, Rogers S: Women in transition: Being versus becoming or being and becoming. Health Care for Women International 8:199–217, 1987.

Meleis AI, Sorrell L: Arab American women and their birth experiences. American Journal of Maternal Child Nursing 6:171–176, 1981.

Milio N: Public participation in planning for personal health services. In Jain SC, Paul JE (Eds.), Policy Issues in Personal Health Services. Rockville, MD: Aspen Publication, 1983.

Newell K: Health by the people. Geneva: World Health Organization, 1973.

Omidian P, Rainey P: All my kids are sick: Afghan and Yemeni women. Paper presented at the annual meeting of the American Anthropological Association, Chicago, Illinois, 1987.

Rappaport J: The power of empowerment language. Social Poll 16(2):15–21, 1985.

Reizian A, Meleis AI: Arab-Americans' perceptions of and responses to pain. Critical Care Nurse 6(6):30–37, 1985.

Sachs L: Evil eye or bacteria: Turkish migrant women and Swedish health care. Stockholm: Stockholm Studies in Social Anthropology, 1983.

Steiger N, Lipson J: Self-care nursing: Theory and practice. Bowie, MD: Brady Communications Company, 1985.

Swendsen L, Meleis AI, Jones D: Role supplementation for new parents—A role mastery plan. The American Journal of Maternal Child Nursing 3:84–91, 1978.

Thompson P, Harminder S, Mroke M: O.A.S.I.S. health education for immigrant women: A manual and resource guide. Vancouver: O.A.S.I.S., 1986.

Viviano F, Silva S: The new San Francisco. San Francisco Focus Magazine, pp. 64–73, 1986.

Warheit G, Bell R, Schwab J: Needs assessment approaches. (DHEW Publication No. (ADII). 79–472). Washington, DC: National Institute of Mental Health, 1979.

Werner D: Where there is no doctor: A village health care handbook. Palo Alto: The Hesperian Foundation, 1977.

World Health Organization. Primary Health Care: Report of the International Conference on Primary Health Care, Alma Ata, USSR. Geneva: World Health Organization, 1978.

SOUTHEAST ASIAN REFUGEES
Marjorie A. Muecke

It has been over a decade since this article was originally published and in that time the numbers of refugees from Southeast Asia accepted for resettlement in the United States has declined, such that only 33,214 Vietnamese and far fewer of the other groups were admitted in 1995. The case of refugees from Southeast Asia is the same worldwide; only 330,000 of the world's documented 15 million refugees have fled Cambodia, Laos, or Vietnam, and almost all of them were displaced within Asia.[41] Further, since the early 1980s governmental interest in refugee resettlement has been waning: the United States is no longer among the 25 top-ranking countries for either the largest number of refugees or the highest ratio of refugee population to total population.

Some of the examples provided in this article pertain to the mutual disorientation of newcomers and hosts toward each other and, therefore, may no longer pertain to Southeast Asian-Americans today. However, the point of the article—the painful mismatch between persons from Third World countries and U.S. society and the discomfort that this mismatch entails for both the refugee and the host—pertains to refugees coming into the United States for permanent resettlement in the 1990s.

Whereas the highest numbers of asylum applicants come from Central America, the highest asylum approval rates are for Bosnians, Somalies, Sudanese, and Burmese. There are close to half a million applications for asylum waiting to be processed. Countries of origin of those accepted for resettlement in the United States are predominantly from the former Soviet Union followed by Vietnam, Iraq, Iran, Ethiopia, Liberia, Bosnia, Rwanda, and Somalia.

In the past 6 years, over 500,000 refugees from Southeast Asia have settled in the United States.* Some 90% of them are under 45 years of age. Consequently, their first contacts with our health care system are usually through obstetrics, pediatrics, and emergency rooms. Whereas the first wave of Southeast Asian refugees in 1975 was generally well educated and familiar with Western ways, most of those arriving in the past 3 years have had little or no formal education and have led self-subsistent lives in rural and remote hill areas. Many of the recent arrivals have stayed in refugee camps for 3–5 years. Health problems such as tuberculosis, anemias, and dental and gum disease are much more prevalent among them than the first wave of refugees.[3]

This paper aims to ease the frustrations that physicians, nurses, and dentists commonly report in trying to work with the less-Westernized refugees and to promote refugee patients' adherence to health care plans. The focus is upon explaining behavior patterns and health care expectations that are common among Southeast Asian refugee patients. Disease conditions that are prevalent among this population are not discussed because they are treated in available literature.[3–20]

The author's areal focus in medical anthropology is mainland Southeast Asia.[21, 22] She is a volunteer at the Seattle-King County Health Department's Refugee Screening Clinic; works with refugees in her teaching of undergraduate and graduate nursing and anthropology students at the University of Washington, Seattle; and consults extensively with health care professionals working with refugees. Many of the observations that follow are based upon personal experience.

Background

The refugees have fled from three countries of mainland Southeast Asia: Cambodia, Laos, and Vietnam. The French held suzerainty over these countries from the late 19th century to 1954 and grouped them together under the label "Indochina." The French coined the term "Indochina" in a superficial attempt to unify the disparate groups in the area by emphasizing their heritage of Indic and Chinese influences. French control ended with the Geneva Agreements in 1954 and, with it, the political basis for the use of the term. To refer to the refugees as Southeast Asians is accurate but somewhat misleading in that the refugees have fled none of the countries of *insular* Southeast Asia, nor any of the mainland Southeast Asian countries of Burma, Malaya, Singapore, and Thailand. Nevertheless, "Southeast Asian" is used in this paper because we possess no other more accurate designation of this diverse group of refugees.

Although the refugees have only three national origins, they represent a wide variety of ethnic, language, and religious groups (Table 20–5). The extent of conversion to Christianity among the different groups has yet to be

---

*From 1975 to December 1981, 565,757 refugees from Southeast Asia entered the United States.[1] While the United States has accepted more refugees from Southeast Asia than any other country, on a per-capita basis (number of Southeast Asian refugees per national population), the United States ranks third after Australia and Canada, and in terms of per-capita financial contributions to international refugee aid agencies, the United States ranks 12th.[2] The People's Republic of China and France rank second and third after the United States in terms of the total number of Southeast Asian refugees accepted for resettlement (265,588 and 71,931, respectively, as of April 30, 1981).[1]

This article is reprinted from the American Journal of Public Health, April 1983, Vol. 73, No. 4. © 1983 American Journal of Public Health. We thank Dr. Muecke and the American Journal of Public Health for allowing us to reprint the article.

Table 20–5
Major Ethnic, Language, and Religious Identifications of Southeast Asian Refugees, by Country of Origin and Urban, Rural, or Hill Residential Background

Country of Origin	Urban, Rural, or Hill Background	Ethnic Group	Primary Language*	Religion
Cambodia	Rural	Cambodian (or Khmer)	Cambodian	Theravada Buddhism
	Urban (rural)	Cham	Cham	Islam (Sunni sect)
	Urban	Chinese	Teochiu, Cantonese†	Confucian-Taoism-Mahayana Buddism; Roman Catholicism
	Urban	Vietnamese	Vietnamese	(Same as Chinese)
Laos	Rural (urban)	Lao, Lu	Lao	Theravada Buddhism
	Rural	Thai Dam	Thai Dam; Lao	Animism‡
	Urban (rural)	Chinese	Chinese†	Mahayana Buddhism
	Hill	Lao Theung	Khmu; T'in; Lamet; Lao	Animism
		Hmong (or Meo or Miaw)	Hmong	Animism; some Christianity
		Mien (or Man or Yao)	Mien	Animism
Vietnam	Urban or rural	Vietnamese	Vietnamese	Confucian-Mahayana Buddhism-Taoism; Roman Catholicism
	Urban	Chinese	Cantonese†	(Same as Vietnamese)

*Many refugees are fluent in more than one language.

†A variety of dialects/languages are spoken by the ethnic Chinese refugees, including the following: Teochiu (from Swatow), Cantonese, Hakka, Halnanese, Fukien, Hokkien, Toi Sanese, and among the educated, Mandarin.

‡Although there are myriad interpretations of animism, they all involve the belief that anthropomorphic spirits may reside in organic material such as rice, trees, or earth, and can influence or determine human events and well-being.

studied. Folk medical practices are less likely to be carried out by Christian than non-Christian refugees. Relationships among the different groups vary and often reflect a long history of sociopolitical conflict. Refugees in the United States generally choose first to be with their own ethnic group, second with Americans, and last with refugees from other groups.

Four characteristics of refugees distinguish the Southeast Asian refugees from other Asian groups who have resettled in the United States through immigration:

- They have come to the United States by second, not first choice; their first choice was almost invariably to return to their native country if its political and economic conditions were similar to those that existed before the 1975 changes of government.
- They have come to the United States with little preparation, scant belongings, and no nest of compatriots to greet or help them.
- There is no realistic option for them ever to return to their homeland.
- They are survivors. Although statistics are not available, it is commonly estimated that for every refugee resettled, one died in flight.

Caring For Southeast Asian Refugee Patients

Most Southeast Asians who come to the United States are likely to know some diseases that are recognized by Western medicine. The diseases they know, however, are often ones with which U.S. health personnel are unfamiliar because they are rarely seen in the United States, e.g., cholera, leprosy, malaria, smallpox, or tuberculosis. Complicating the poor cross-cultural correspondence of knowledge of disease, such medical basics as the germ theory and principles of anatomy and physiology are foreign to Southeast Asians who have not been educated, and there is no surgical tradition in Southeast Asia.

Nevertheless, when inconvenienced by sickness, most Southeast Asian refugees want to go to a doctor. Some common problems that they pose are that they rarely seek care when they are asymptomatic and few are familiar with our appointment system: some regard the most convenient doctor as the closest one not requiring an appointment and accepting medical coupons, i.e., a hospital emergency room. To cope with these and related problems, general guidelines follow for working with partially English-speaking Southeast Asian refugee patients who are in the early stages of integrating into U.S. culture.

The most important caveat is to seek the refugee patient's opinion whenever possible. This is necessary because cultural patterns are not predictive at the level of the individual and because the cultural orientations that the refugees have brought with them are undergoing rapid change. Not only are ethnic variations in practices, beliefs, and reactions common, they are complicated by variations in rural-versus-urban background, sex, and educational experience of the individual, as well as by group and individual variations in patterns of adjustment to life in the United States. There is also a tendency, particularly among refugees sponsored by Americans and among converts to Christianity, to renounce traditional religious and medical beliefs and practices. This is associated with the expectation of appearing less different from, and therefore more acceptable to, Americans. As such, it is an example of Goffman's "passing" in order to hide the stigma of being a refugee.[23]

The First Encounter

A quiet, unhurried but purposeful demeanor is a part of normal professional decorum that is particularly reassuring to Southeast Asians because it symbolizes characteristics that are highly valued among them, such as wisdom, good judgment, and dignity.

When the patient is accompanied by relatives, addressing at least the initial conversation to the oldest of the group shows appropriate respect for elders; this person is also usually the ultimate decision maker for the patient.

Naming systems vary by ethnic group and can be very different from the Western system, fomenting consternation among record keepers. The surname is often placed first and may be a clan name (Hmong, Mien) or dynasty name (Vietnamese) rather than a family name (Table 20–6). Among most groups except the Lao, the woman does not change her family (clan or dynasty) name at marriage. Among some groups, an individual may take additional names at certain points of the life cycle. Many refugees, however, are changing their names to conform to U.S. practice. Because of this and the wide ethnic variation in name systems, it is best to ask the patient what he or she wants to be called. To initiate contact, it is usually appropriate to address adults by title (Mrs., Mr., Dr.) plus first (given) name (see Table 20–6).

Provider attempts to obtain information through medical, health, and fertility histories of the less well educated Southeast Asian patient tend to be unproductive. This is because in Southeast Asia, medical patients are rarely told the names of their illnesses, of the medicines given, or of the diagnostic procedures performed on them; consequently, they rarely know what was done for them or why. Furthermore, refugee patients from rural or hill areas or with little formal education are not accustomed to the Gregorian calendar used in the West. Their methods for calculating ages may vary by up to 2 years from our method of counting birth as day 1. In addition, fertility

Table 20–6

Selected Common Characteristics of Southeast Asian Naming Systems by Ethnic Group

Ethnic Group	Usual No. of Names Per Person	Common Surnames	Husband and Wife Share Surname	Example of a Name 1 = given name, 2 = middle name, 3 = surname
Cambodian	2	Chak, Chep, Samroul, San, Sok, Som, Vuthy	No	3　　1 Sovann Loeung
Chinese*	3	Chan, Chau, Ha, Lau, Lee, Lieng, Ly, Ong, Pho, Tang, Vuong	No	3　2　1 Wang Din Wah
Hmong	2–4	Chang, Fang, Hang, Khang, Lee, Lor, Ly, Moua, Thao, Xiong, Vang, Vue, Yang	No	3　　1 Vang Koua
Lao	2	(varied: usually 3–5 syllables)	Yes	1　　　　3 Thongsouk Vongkhamkaew
Mien	2–4	Saechan, Saechao, Saelau, Saelee, Saelui, Saephan, Saetau, Saetang, Saetem, Saezulai	No	3　　1 Saeteun MuiChua
Vietnamese	3–4	Cao, Dinh, Hoang, Le, Luu, Ly, Ngo, Nguyen, Phan, Pho, Tran	No	3　2　1 Nguyen thi Canh

*In Chinese publications, the family name precedes the given name (usually hyphenated): Chen Tai-chien or Chen, Tai-Chien. But in American and British journals, a Chinese name is usually anglicized and transposed: Tai Chien Chen or Chen, T. C. (see Council of Biology Editors Style Manual, 3d Ed., 1972, p. 156).

histories are likely to underreport pregnancies and fetal losses because many people in Southeast Asia do not consider the fetus human, and some do not consider the newborn human until the baby is 3 days old (Hmong, Lao) or even older.

Interpreters

If the patient does not speak English easily, trained bilingual interpreters should be sought to ensure accurate two-way flow of information at the key decision-making points in the health care process, i.e., for history taking, when prescribing and evaluating diagnostic or therapeutic procedures that are new to the patient, and before any change in management, as from the intensive care unit to the medical floor in a hospital or from parenteral to oral medication. Without a trained bilingual interpreter at such points, intentions to provide for the patient's informed consent are thwarted, patient safety is jeopardized, and patient's noncompliance to medical regimen is likely.[24] Ideally, the interpreter should be bilingual and bicultural, treated as a colleague, and chosen both for competence in the language foreign to the health care professional and for familiarity with biomedicine.

When speaking through an interpreter, watching the patient (rather than the interpreter) will enable you to pick up behavioral cues. If the patient's responses do not fit your comment, check that you have made your meaning clear to the interpreter. Sometimes it will take an interpreter much longer to say in a Southeast Asian language what has just been said in English; this is often the sign that a cultural as well as a linguistic translation is being made. Sometimes the interpreter may appear to answer for the patient; this may be because he or she knows the information sought from having been that patient's interpreter on previous occasions.

If trained interpreters or bilingual health care providers are not made available for work with non- or partially English-speaking patients, the health care agency may be failing to meet the requirement of Title VI of The Civil Rights Act of 1964 for the provision of equal access to care, regardless of national origin.* Resettlement agencies (commonly called "VOLAGS" for "voluntary agencies") can provide information on the availability of interpreters in local areas. Each refugee's initial resettlement in the United States is organized by a VOLAG so the refugee should know the name of his or her VOLAG.†

---

*All agency recipients of federal funds, including Medicare, are subject to the stipulations of Title VI.

†The VOLAGS are American Council for Nationalities; American Fund for Czechoslovak Refugees; Buddhist Council for Refugee Rescue and Resettlement; Church World Service; International Rescue Committee; Iowa Refugee Service Center; Lutheran Immigration and Refugee Service; Tolstoy Foundation, Inc.; United Hias Service, Inc.; US Catholic Conference (USCC); World Relief Refugee Service; and Young Men's Christian Association. All but USCC are headquartered in New York.

Whether speaking through an interpreter or directly with a patient who is not sufficiently functional in English, ambiguity of meaning can be minimized in the following ways[25]:

- Using basic words and simple sentences and using nouns rather than pronouns
- Paraphrasing words that carry much meaning (e.g., "workup") in order to be precise about the specific meaning intended
- Avoiding use of metaphors, colloquialisms, and idiomatic expressions
- Learning and using basic words and sentences in the patient's language; this induces the patient or interpreter to take greater care in making their use of language accurate
- Inviting correction of your understanding of the matter at hand ("Am I understanding you correctly that . . .?")

Informed Consent

Obtaining a Southeast Asian refugee patient's informed consent prior to undertaking a medical procedure is difficult because cultural differences in health-related concepts often cannot be simply translated linguistically and because values of biomedicine might conflict with those of the patient's culture.[26] From an uninformed Southeast Asian perspective, diagnostic tests are baffling, inconvenient, and often unnecessary. Procedures such as circumcision or tonsillectomy, which biomedicine considers simple, are generally unknown. Any invasive procedure is frightening and may be believed to have long lasting and multiple effects. The prospect of surgery can be terrorizing. There is a great fear of mutilation that stems from widespread beliefs (among non-Christians) that souls are attached to different parts of the body and can leave the body, causing illness or death. This fear of mutilation extends through death, so that few Southeast Asians consent to autopsy unless they know and agree with the reasons for it in their own case.

Ensuring that a patient gives or withholds adequately informed consent to procedures guards his or her legal and ethical rights and can also prevent iatrogenic psychological distress and promote patient adherence to the medical regimen.[27] However, a belief that verbal statements in and of themselves can cause the event described to occur lingers among some peoples from Southeast Asia. As a result there is a tendency to avoid discussing problems, risks, and dangers. Explanations about why necessary procedures are recommended should be made routinely. For example, once the patient understands that the body continuously produces its own blood, that red blood cells live only 120 days, and that blood drawn from patients is used to help assess their physical status, the patient will usually consent to blood drawings for laboratory analysis.

However, the difficulties in achieving truly informed consent can be large. Reducing the number of procedures performed to a minimum is desirable. In some cases, cultural considerations may have to supersede usual policy for obtaining informed consent. For example, if the group to which the patient belongs believes that at death grandparents and parents become ancestors who should be worshipped and obeyed and who shape the well-being of living descendants, the children of the patient for whom a decision about terminating active intervention needs to be made may have difficulty consenting to terminate care. Such consent would be equivalent to contributing to the death of an ancestor, i.e., of one who would shape the survivors' fates.

The "Passive Obedient Patient"

Southeast Asians generally expect health professionals to be experts in diagnosis, treatments, and medications. Consequently, they tend not to contribute as much information as health care professionals want or consider essential.[28] According to many Southeast Asian cultural traditions, authority figures should not be questioned or opposed directly so as not to offend or embarrass them openly; they may, however, be discreetly disobeyed "behind their backs." That is, the passive obedience may be a culturally adaptive and sanctioned illusion of conformity. However, among some refugees in the United States, the tendency to passivity around authority figures is compounded by fear and ignorance of our legal system: suspicion that divulging personal information, as for a medical history, could jeopardize their legal rights is common. When the health problem is severe or complex, it may be useful to ask an intermediary who is close to the patient (e.g., VOLAG caseworker or the sponsor) to assist. Sometimes a refugee patient considers the doctor or nurse to be of such exalted status that the patient could do nothing other than obey.

The better a refugee patient understands reasons for a health professional's inquiries, the more direct and complete the responses tend to be. However, gaps in cross-cultural meaning may preclude refugees' understanding of medical rationales. The interpretation of organic signs and symptoms is not isomorphic across cultures[29, 30]: points of major concern to health professionals may be irrelevant (exact age, medical or fertility history, causes of relatives' deaths) or unfamiliar (allergy, depression, virus, names of medications) to refugee patients. Values between two cultures may conflict (prolong life versus relieve suffering). The Southeast Asian refugee patient often copes with uncertainty and authority in a way—passive obedience—that is consonant with cultural heritage but frustrating to the norms of biomedicine. The refugee can protect self-esteem by

concealing, through passivity, his or her own ignorance. The refugee believes that he or she can protect the health professional's status by concealing disagreements or incomplete understandings, i.e., by appearing obedient or compliant. Asking the patient to explain the issue at hand can reduce the illusional aspect of the patient's passive-obedient behaviors.

The "Noncompliant Patient"

Two common causes of failure to adhere to the medical or nursing regimen reiterate the need for bilingual and bicultural trained interpreters or for the assistance of refugee advocates or caseworkers: 1) the patient's misunderstanding of the medical regimen (e.g., taking the antimalarials chloroquine or Fansidar for a fever, as fevers in hill areas were commonly associated with malaria) and 2) the patient's inability to carry out behaviors that are prerequisite to observance of the medical regimen, such as locating and getting to the referral site or using the telephone to report new medical or nursing problems.

Ethnographic and clinical evidence suggest that noncompliance among Southeast Asian refugee patients is associated with the following patient perceptions: 1) cessation of symptoms, 2) inconvenience of observing the regimen, and 3) lack of cultural precedent for the regimen. Therefore, to help prevent noncompliance, the rationale(s) for continuing treatment after cessation of symptoms (or despite the absence of symptoms, as in prophylactic isoniazid treatment or antihypertensive therapy) should be made explicit to the patient. The patient should also be asked whether the patient knows of a cultural precedent for the proposed prescription and what there is about carrying it out that would be difficult for the patient. If the patient identifies no cultural precedent for it or identifies one that the patient values negatively or identifies barriers to its implementation, the necessity for the regimen should be reconsidered. If still indicated, special efforts should be made to assist the patient in adhering to the regimen.

Constraints of Body Image

Notions of body image that are widespread among Southeast Asians but uncommon among Americans include reverence for the head, dispassionate acceptance of the female breast as the natural means for infant sustenance, and extreme privacy of the lower torso. The human head is regarded as the seat of life and therefore as highly personal, vulnerable, honorable, and untouchable except by close intimates. Procedures that invade the surface or an orifice of the head tend to frighten Southeast Asians with the thought that the procedures could provide exits for one's life essence. This is particularly true for infants on whom a scalp vein is used for intravenous lines because infants are considered at high risk for loss of life and because the lines are close to the soft fontanel from where it is believed that the soul may take easy exit. Explanation of the rationales for the procedures in question is necessary to allay undue anxiety.

Although breast-feeding in public is commonplace among rural and hill populations of Southeast Asia, the refugees quickly observe that it is unusual in the United States. Most refugee women prefer to bottle-feed their infants in the United States because of its perceived convenience and conformity to American norms.

The area of the body between the waist and knees is almost never exposed, even in privacy, by anyone other than young children. The loose hospital gown or physical examination of the genital area consequently can be deeply humiliating and unnerving to the Southeast Asian patient. Pelvic examinations of unmarried Southeast Asian women should not be undertaken routinely. When there is medical indication for a pelvic examination, the woman may want her husband to be present; if possible, the practitioner, and interpreter if one is needed, should both be female.

Social Supports

To be alone is frightening to many Southeast Asians. Offering to involve the patient's family as much as possible during the diagnostic and treatment program can help put them at ease; scheduling an entire family for care simultaneously can promote understanding and adherence as well. Different cultures dictate that different persons accompany the patient; e.g., at childbirth, a Chinese woman should have her mother-in-law in attendance, and a Hmong woman, her husband to bathe the newborn; for infants and children, either parent may assume what Americans term a mothering role.

Adult Southeast Asians are generally more comfortable with health care providers of their own sex rather than the opposite sex. This is particularly true for young and unmarried women.

If the option exists when making staff assignments or referrals for a Southeast Asian patient, ask if the patient would prefer an Asian service provider; often the patient would prefer a Filipino, Korean, or Japanese to an American even if the health care provider cannot speak a Southeast Asian language. However, because of political differences, persons from Laos and Cambodia might prefer not to have a Vietnamese nurse or physician.

Many non-Christian and non-Muslim Southeast Asians wear strings around their wrists and amulets on necklaces, ankle bands, or clothes. Although simple in appearance, such accoutrements can carry deep sacred and social meanings for the sick person and family. The wrist strings are believed to prevent soul loss, which in Laos and Cambodia is thought to cause illness. In a commonly practiced ritual, a soul-caller, respected elders, and kin symbolically bind the sick person's soul in the body by tying strings around the wrists (and, for infants, the neck, ankles, or waist). The strings thus signify both the spiritual wholeness and social support of the sick person. The soul-calling, wrist-tying ritual is also performed to bolster the strength of the ritualee in the face of major change, as at marriage or leaving home. If the strings or amulets must be removed for medical purposes, an explanation of the need to do so usually brings the patient's consent; some might want to keep the removed item.

Medication

Southeast Asians tend to define their health problems in terms of physical symptoms and to seek symptomatic treatment. They also tend to express emotional disturbances somatically; doing so enables them to avoid the heavy stigma that mental illness carries among Southeast Asians.[23, 31]

The main reason most refugees from Southeast Asia go to a doctor is to get medicine for a symptom. They usually believe that Western medicine is very powerful and cures quickly. If they go to a doctor when sick and do *not* receive medicine, they are likely to feel cheated. Once given medicine which they find effective, however, they might reason, "Since I forgot to take one yesterday, I'll take two today," or, "If one pill is good, two are better." While most are familiar with the beneficial effects of Western medicine, few understand the risks of overdosages or underdosages.[28, 32] This is related to the fact that all kinds of medicines were imported from the West and were widely available over the counter in Southeast Asian cities and towns. They were popular for quick relief of acute symptoms and usually self-administered by a people who could not read the foreign language in which the package instructions were written.

Underlying this conviction about the powerfulness of Western medicine to cure, however, is an anxiety that Western medicine might not be appropriate for Eastern people. Not only is the belief widespread that Asian bodies, diets, and behaviors are different from American, but also there is the, at times, perplexing knowledge that according to the Chinese "hot-cold" theory most Western medicines are classified as "hot," while most Southeast Asian herbal medicines are "cool." Such contradictions and uncertainties tend to heighten the Southeast Asian patient's concern about drug-induced idiosyncratic and side effects. Their concern often results in self-management of prescribed as well as over-the-counter medication. Prescriber efforts to explain the reason(s) for set dosages will increase the safety of the patient's tendency to self-medicate.

Traditional Self-Care Practices

Southeast Asians have traditionally dealt with illness through self-care and self-medication. When illness occurs in the United States, they practice self-care longer before seeking professional care than do Americans. This is related to their having had access to most drugs over the counter at low cost in Southeast Asia, to having had few hospitals and physicians, and to the high cost of Western medical care. Four major forms of self-care that are commonly performed by refugee patients in the United States are offerings to spirits, dermabrasive techniques, maintenance of hot-cold balance, and use of herbal medicines.

Theories of supernatural etiology and cures of illness are widespread among non-Christian Southeast Asians. Traditional treatment of illness includes a focus on the supernatural agent as well as on the body of the sick person. For example, among non-Christian Hmong, illness is interpreted as a visitation by spirits. It is commonly believed that a child becomes sick when its spiritual parents try to take it back; treatment consequently involves placation of the spiritual parents, and this may be done by offering them chicken at an altar in the home.[33] When sickness occurs in other persons, the head of household administers herbal remedies, having grown the herbs in a home garden. If sickness persists, a shaman may be called to enter a trance in order to communicate directly with offended spirits and to negotiate for the return of the sick person's soul; the negotiation is usually accompanied by a sacrifice of a pig or a chicken.

Because of the pervasive influence of China on the development of the peoples of Southeast Asia, Chinese medical tenets and practices have influenced the belief systems of most people from the area—the medical texts of Mien shamans were even written in Chinese. Chinese folk remedies that are widely practiced among the Vietnamese, Khmer, Hmong, and Mien (but not significantly among the Lao) include modifications of acupuncture, massage, herbal concoctions and poultices, and the dermabrasive practices of cupping, pinching, rubbing, and burning.

The dermal practices are the most common among the refugees (regardless of religion) but the least known by Americans. The dermal methods are perceived as ways to relieve headaches, muscle pains, sinusitis, colds, sore throat, coughs, difficulty breathing, diarrhea, or fever. In *cupping,* a cup is heated and then placed on the skin; as it cools, it contracts, drawing the skin and what is believed to be excess energy or "wind" or toxicity into the cup; a circular ecchymosis is left on the skin. *Pinching* and rubbing produce bruises or welts on the site of treatment; pinching may be at the base of the nose, between the eyes, or, like rubbing, on the neck, chest, or back. *Rubbing* involves an insistent rubbing of lubricated skin with a spoon or a coin, in order to bring toxic "wind" to the body surface.[34, 35] A similar remedy is *burning*— touching a burning cigarette or piece of cotton to the skin,

usually the abdomen, in order to compensate for "heat" lost through diarrhea. These measures all produce changes in the skin and can be misread as signs of physical abuse by persons who are not sufficiently informed to make the differential diagnosis of cultural self-care.[36] The practices present a threat to the physical integrity of the person only if that person has a blood clotting disorder. They nurture the person's sense of being cared for and sense of security in being able to do something about disturbing symptoms. There is sound psychosociocultural reason to allow, or even support, these practices among the Indochinese.[35]

The above remedies are related to Chinese theories of health as a state of balance among the different components of the body and of the body with its environment. Illness prevention and treatment involve modification of food intake in order to maintain or restore equilibrium by rebalancing the body's component parts. Therapeutic adjustment of the diet requires consideration of the hot or cold nature of foods, cooking methods, and the person's ailment. The qualities hot and cold, like the polarities of energy called yin and yang, must be kept in balance to ensure health. Although the rules for classifying foods as hot or cold are difficult to decipher and seem to vary by informant,[37, 38] most fruits and vegetables, along with fish, duck, and other things that grow in water, are cold, and most meats, sweets, coffee, and spicy condiments, such as garlic, ginger, and onion, are hot. Hot foods and beverages are thought to replace and strengthen one's blood; consequently, after surgery and childbirth, hot drinks are preferred, and cold drinks, jello, and juices are avoided. Many refugees in the United States have organic medicines for a wide variety of problems from impotence to mental illness and may take them simultaneously with prescribed medications. The Hmong and Chinese are particularly skilled herbalists.

Death and Depression

Southeast Asian and biomedical reactions to death often differ in two ways. First, the biomedical drive to prolong life conflicts with the general Southeast Asian preference for quality of life over length of life because of the expectation of less suffering in one's next reincarnation. Because of this expectation, they may seem to "give up" on relatives who are severely injured but survive an accident or on infants requiring intensive care because they were born prematurely. Second, almost all Southeast Asians want themselves and their relatives to die at home rather than in the hospital. At home they know they can give or receive the comfort of loved ones, comfort that they do not expect in the hospital. Furthermore, most believe that the spirit of a person who dies away from home is unhappy and so will cause trouble to the survivors long afterward.

Perhaps the greatest threat to refugee health is depression. It is related to the pervasive and overwhelming losses and changes that refugees have experienced in a relatively short time. These may leave the refugee confused and disoriented for years afterward.[39, 40] Compounded with the sorrow and homesickness is the insecurity of isolation from their past and present environments. And on top of these are the role reversals, intergenerational conflicts, and reduced social status that commonly occur within each refugee ethnic group in the United States. Refugees, in general, are vulnerable and afraid in the United States. Because the health care system is one of the few culturally sanctioned sources of institutional support for them (the other sources—church and school—are not available for all refugees) and because their access to informal U.S. social life is extremely limited, many adult refugees can be expected to seek care and attention on a long-term basis from health care providers.

References

1. Refugee Reports. Washington, D.C., American Council for Nationalities Service, pp. 3, 4, 8, 1982.
2. 1981 World Refugee Survey. New York, U.S. Committee for Refugees, Inc., pp. 40–41, 1981.
3. Catanzaro A, and Moser RM: Health status of refugees from Vietnam, Laos, and Cambodia. JAMA 247:1303–1307, 1982.
4. Intestinal parasites (editorial). MMWR 347:28–29, 1979.
5. Wiesenthal AM, Nickels MK, Hashimoto KG, et al: Intestinal parasites in Southeast Asian refugees: Prevalence in a community of Laotians. JAMA 244:2543–2544, 1980.
6. Malaria—US 1980. MMWR 26:413–415, 1980.
7. Trenholme GM, and Carson PE: Therapy and prophylaxis of malaria. JAMA 240:2293–2295, 1978.
8. Follow-up on tuberculosis among Indochinese refugees. MMWR 29:47–53, 1980.
9. Tuberculosis among Indochinese refugees—US 1979. MMWR 29:383–384, 389–390, 1980.
10. Tuberculosis drug resistance found among Indochinese. Refugee Rep 2:4, 1981.
11. Follow-up on drug resistant tuberculosis. MMWR 29:602–604, 609–610, 1980.
12. Viral hepatitis type B. MMWR 29:1–3, 1980.
13. Hepatitis B associated with acupuncture—Florida. MMWR 30:1–3, 1981.
14. Centers for Disease Control: Health status of Indochinese refugees. Natl Med Assoc 72:59–65, 1980.
15. Skeels MR, Nims LJ, and Mann JM: Intestinal parasitosis among Southeast Asian immigrants in New Mexico. Am J Public Health 72:57–59, 1982.
16. Yankauer, A: Refugees, immigrants, and the public health (editorial). Am J Public Health 72:12–14, 1982.
17. Peck RE, Chuang M, Robbins GE, and Nichaman MZ: Nutritional status of Southeast Asian refugee children. Am J Public Health 71:1144–1148, 1981.
18. Erickson RV, and Hoang GN: Health problems among Indochinese refugees. Am J Public Health 70:1003–1006, 1980.
19. Feldstein B, and Weiss R: Cambodian disaster relief: Refugee camp medical care. Am J Public Health 72:589–594, 1982.
20. Davis JM, Goldenring J, McChesney M, and Medina A: Pregnancy outcomes of Indochinese refugees, Santa Clara County, California. Am J Public Health 72:742–744, 1982.
21. Muecke MA: Health care systems as socializing agents: Childbearing the North Thai and Western ways. Soc Sci Med 10:377–383, 1976.
22. Muecke MA: An explanation of "wind illness" among the Northern Thai. Cult Med Psychiatry 3:267–300, 1979.
23. Goffman E: Stigma: Notes on the Management of Spoiled Identity. Englewood Cliffs, New Jersey, Prentice-Hall, 1963.
24. Kline F, Acosta FX, Austin W, et al: The misunderstood Spanish-speaking patient. Am J Psychiatry 137:1530–1533, 1980.
25. Werner O, and Campbell DT: Translating: Working through interpreters and the problem of decentering. In Naroll R, and Cohen R, eds.: A Handbook of Method in Cultural Anthropology. New York, Columbia University Press, pp. 398–420, 1970.
26. Kunstadter P: Medical ethics in cross-cultural and multicultural perspective. Soc Sci Med 14B:289–296, 1980.
27. Miller IJ: Medicine and the law: Informed consent I–IV. JAMA 244:2100–2103, 2347–2350, 2556–2558, 2661–2662.
28. Tran, Minh Tung: Indochinese Patients: Cultural Aspects of the Medical and Psychiatric Care of Indochinese Refugees. Washington, DC, Action for South East Asians, pp. 54–72, 1980.
29. Kleinman A: Patients and Healers in the Context of Culture. Berkeley, California, University of California Press, 1980.
30. Leslie C: Medical pluralism in world perspective. Soc Sci Med 148:191–195, 1980.
31. Dunn FL: Traditional Asian medicine and cosmopolitan medicine as adaptive systems. In Leslie C, ed: Asian Medical Systems: A Comparative Study. Berkeley, California, University of California Press, pp. 133–158, 1976.
32. Tran, Minh Tung: The Vietnamese refugees as patients. In A Transcultural Look at Health Care: Indochinese With Pulmonary Disease. Rockville, Maryland, The Lung Association of Mid-Maryland, pp. 26–40, 1980.
33. Chindarsi N: The Religion of the Hmong Njua. Bangkok, The Siam Society, 1976.
34. Golden S, and Duster, MC: Hazards of misdiagnosis due to Vietnamese folk medicine. Clin Pediatr 16:949–950, 1977.
35. Yeatman GW, and Viet, Van Dang: Cao gio (coin rubbing): Vietnamese attitudes toward health care. JAMA 244:2748–2749, 1980.
36. Yeatman GW, Shaw C, Berlow MJ, et al: Pseudobattering in Vietnamese children. Pediatrics 58:616, 1976.
37. Breakley G, and Voulgaropoulos E: Laos Health Survey: Mekong Valley 1968–1969. Honolulu, The University Press of Hawaii, p. 41, 1976.
38. Wu, Duh: Traditional Chinese concepts of food and medicine in Singapore. Singapore, Institute of Southeast Asian Studies, 1979.
39. Charron DW, and Ness RC: Emotional distress among Vietnamese adolescents: A statewide survey. J Refugee Resettlement 1:7–15, 1981.
40. Smither R: Psychological study of refugee acculturation: A review of the literature. J Refugee Resettlement 1:58–63, 1981.
41. U.S. Committee: World Refugee Survey 1996. Washington, DC, Author, pp. 4, 5, 7, 1996.

PROMOTING HEALTH IN DIVERSE COMMUNITIES: APPLYING THE CONCEPT OF MARGINALIZATION

In the United States, we live in a very diverse, mobile society. Sometimes the task of making care culturally competent seems like an impossible job. The more closely we look at diverse communities, the more we realize that each person is uniquely affected by a matrix of social, political, and economic influences that have health implications. How can we "walk in someone else's shoes" when there are so many differences?

In this section, the concept of marginalization is introduced, and its properties are explored to provide guidance for nursing in diverse communities. Marginalization is one way of theoretically summing up some of the common experiences of marginalized persons and groups, those whose lives are somehow different from what is believed to be the normative "center" of society. This section does not begin to account for all cultural differences among clients, nor does it explain all the intracommunity patterns of difference. Rather, it is intended to provide nurses with some basic properties and principles from which to draw implications for more informed, culturally competent, and politically conscious care.

MARGINALIZATION: A GUIDING CONCEPT FOR VALUING DIVERSITY IN NURSING KNOWLEDGE DEVELOPMENT*

Joanne M. Hall, RN, PhD • Patricia E. Stevens, RN, PhD • Afaf Ibrahim Meleis, PhD, FAAN

This article explicates marginalization as a guiding concept for the development of nursing knowledge that values diversity. The seven key properties of marginalization as it applies to the domain of nursing are (1) intermediacy, (2) differentiation, (3) power, (4) secrecy, (5) reflectiveness, (6) voice, and (7) liminality. Through examination of each of these properties, the relationship between marginalization and vulnerability is clarified, and by this means the relevance of marginalization of health is established. The implications for shaping future nursing research, theory, and practice related to the health of diverse populations are discussed. Key words: diversity, marginalization, minorities, research, theory.

The future of nursing depends on the ability of the discipline to reach out to diverse communities and to meet the health needs of those most vulnerable. This article offers a conceptual direction for the development of nursing knowledge that will strengthen this ability. The authors draw from their individual and collaborative programs of research and theory development about vulnerable populations,[1-10] as well as from the critical and feminist social sciences literature, to introduce the concept of marginalization; identify and describe its key properties; propose its relationship to the concept of vulnerability; and discuss its implications for shaping future nursing research, theory, and practice related to the health and health care of diverse populations.

In the past decade, nursing has clearly identified the health of vulnerable groups as a priority.[10-14] There are, however, a number of constraints to knowledge development regarding vulnerable groups. These groups are often hidden, stigmatized, lacking access to services, and mistrustful of the research process. Previous research has tended to ignore or pathologize many of these groups, with the result that extant health-related knowledge is most representative of the needs of Euro-American, middle-class males. For instance, biomedical researchers have frequently excluded women under the assumption that the menstrual cycle and pregnancy are "deviant" processes that confound results. Similarly, in general population surveys, findings from ethnic and racial groups other than Euro-Americans have often been deleted from the analysis, or arbitrarily grouped within an "other" category, because their numbers failed to meet statistical requirements.

With recent federal directives mandating inclusion of women and members of underrepresented ethnic and racial groups in research, these patterns of sampling are starting to change. But problems remain in terms of how data from these samples are analyzed. When findings from underrepresented groups are included, the analysis may not adequately capture the distinctiveness of their experiences if research questions have been posed from norm-based reference points that contain unexamined gender and cultural biases.[15, 16] Including members of vulnerable groups within traditional research designs does not in and of itself provide adequate information about how health services need to be structured to meet their needs, nor does it reliably reveal health strengths and practices indigenous to these groups.[17] Access to care and culturally competent nursing decisions for vulnerable populations require conceptual frameworks and research methods that recognize and incorporate gender, sexual orientational, racial, cultural, social, political, and economic diversity.[18, 19]

Traditional approaches to knowledge development that depend on assumptions of homogeneity, normality, and statistical reliability rather than accurate, coherent reflections of diverse human experience have limitations in generating culturally competent models of care. Large-scale quantitative studies tapping randomized national samples provide aggregate-level data that can inform nursing about general trends, but such data are of limited value in developing interventions for individuals, social networks, and diverse cultural communities. As a practice discipline, nursing requires means of inquiry that are durable and flexible enough to be applied in circumstances where statistical measures are unwieldy, too sweeping in their generalizations, nonspecific to the question at hand, or too economically burdensome in their requirements. By incorporating the concept of marginalization as basic to empirical and theoretical activities, nurses can build understanding about the complex linkages between vulnerability and health. As a guiding concept, marginalization promises knowledge development that is well grounded, cogent, justifiable, relevant, and meaningful to the diverse groups nurses serve.

Concept Definition and Distinction

Marginalization is a concept emerging from a focus on the characteristics, functions, and meanings of margins— that is, borders or edges. *Margins* are defined as the peripheral, boundary-determining aspects of persons, social networks, communities, and environments. Margins are established in several ways: in contrast to a

---

*Reprinted from Advances in Nursing Science 16(4):23–41, 1994.
Copyright © 1994 Aspen Publishers, Inc.

central point, according to the separations they maintain between the internal and external, or as distinctions between the self and others. From this perspective, persons are viewed as relatively different from the norm or as cast out to varying degrees from the societal "center" to its periphery. *Marginalization* is defined as the process through which persons are peripheralized on the basis of their identities, associations, experiences, and environments. *Marginality* is therefore defined as the condition of being peripheralized on these bases.

Marginalization is distinguishable from other related processes. Marginalization may involve gender, racial, political, cultural, or economic oppression. Marginalization and oppression are not equivalent terms, however. Although marginalization and oppression are frequently concurrent processes, marginalization can be viewed as inclusive of oppression, incorporating aspects of experience beyond power imbalances. In another sense, it is more specific than oppression, because it points to a particular set of dynamics through which oppression is concretized: those having to do with boundary maintenance. *Alienation* often accompanies marginalization, but this term is narrowly focused on the subjective experience of not belonging and so is less inclusive than the concept of marginalization. *Stigmatization* refers to the marking of "outsiders." Stigmatization is an aspect of marginalization, although it is not always present in every instance. For example, one may have a marginalizing experience, such as a myocardial infarction, which is not necessarily socially stigmatizing. *Segregation* refers to the physical separation of social groups but does not emphasize the notion of living at the edge that marginalization implies. These related concepts illuminate aspects of marginalization without necessarily replacing the unique perspective marginalization offers as a lens through which to view nursing phenomena.

Properties of Marginalization

The seven key properties of the concept of marginalization as it applies to the domain of nursing are (1) intermediacy, (2) differentiation, (3) power, (4) secrecy, (5) reflectiveness, (6) voice, and (7) liminality. Through examination of each of these properties, the relationship between marginalization and vulnerability will be clarified, and by this means the relevance of marginalization for health will be established.

Intermediacy

The first property, intermediacy, is the essence of marginalization. *Intermediacy* is defined as the tendency of human boundaries to act both as barriers and as connections. Intermediacy refers to the quality of "betweenness." This property can be illustrated by considering the human body as an organism with a center and an outermost boundary, the skin, which is also its most extensive sensory system. The skin is the periphery that acts as a barrier against the environment by protecting the center and as a connection to the environment by informing the center of conditions affecting survival. The human immunodeficiency virus (HIV) crisis has underscored the implications for maintaining the integrity of physiologic boundaries and reinforcing them via artificial barriers.

At the interpersonal level, margins mediate the physical and emotional safety of individuals as they interact with others. Psychic and emotional boundaries maintain integrity, uniqueness, autonomy, and value of the self in relation to others as well as offer opportunities for social connection.[20, 21] Integral to the process of shaping these personal boundaries are individual perceptions, intellectual abilities, and cultural influences, including gender role expectations, religious beliefs, and ethnic values. For example, investigation of US women's self-definitions suggest that they maintain more open boundaries than do men, viewing themselves as more contiguous with, and responsible for, significant others.[22]

These observations indicate that margins are indeed intermediate, protecting and containing in some circumstances, connecting and extending in others. A logical nursing approach to health promotion is to view persons as having interrelated immunologic, physical, and social boundaries, any or all of which might be sites for intervention. Viewing persons and health from the standpoint of margins highlights the person–environment interface, which is consistent with nursing's perspective and germane to holistic and culturally grounded aspects of wellness, illness, and healing.

Differentiation

Differentiation, the second property of marginalization, is defined as the establishment and maintenance of distinct identities through boundary maintenance. "Mainstream" society is depicted as at the center of a community, and those relatively excluded from power and resources are at the periphery.[23–26] Diversity of identities increases with physical and social distance from the center. Experiences at the center are hypothetically homogeneous, normative, and predictable. Distinctions in identity and experiences of oppression "repel" individuals outward from the center. The edge is thus an experiential

> "Mainstream" society is depicted as at the center of a community, and those excluded from power and resources are at the periphery. Diversity increases with physical and social distance from the center.

place in which peripheralized persons are distinct and isolated not only from the center, but also from one another. Their diversity is more palpable and more consequential.

Differentiation has two aspects, the diversity of identity that is found at the periphery and the potential for stigmatization of those identities that differ from the center. In Western societies, the center of a community is the seat of hierarchical power and the conceptual location of the homogeneous "majority." People who differ from those at the center, or from the projected image of those at the center, are forced outward. It is through pressing those viewed as "outsiders" toward the periphery that the majority defines itself.[27] The marking or stigmatization of outsiders thereby provides the center with its identity.[28, 29] By assigning negative values to marginalized persons and groups, those at the center reinforce their sense of belonging and belief in a singular, moral "reality." The dynamics of scapegoating has a long history in which selected "victims" who symbolically embody the sins of the majority are driven out of the societal center.[30] The scapegoats in centuries past— heretics, witches, and madmen—were ostracized, tortured, and sometimes executed to complete the ritual. Modern-day scapegoats include persons of color, gay men, lesbians, addicts, illegal immigrants, and persons infected with HIV.

Differentiation is a property of marginalization that takes into account not only the diversification of identity occurring among racial, social, and cultural groups, but also the varying degrees and types of peripheralization that occur within these groups. There is significant variability in acculturation and accommodation within immigrant groups, for example.[31] In another instance, persons of mixed race may be stigmatized by the groups their heritages represent. Conversely, lighter skinned persons of color may be more highly favored because they have access to opportunities proffered by the dominant Euro-American group.[32] Stigmatization is thus seen as a fluid, complex process; identities are given meaning and value according to their proximity to the centers and margins of relevant reference groups. The property of differentiation conveys that marginalization creates distinctions within distinctions, a multiplicity of identities that shift with varying political, economic, and social circumstances.

From a postmodern theoretical perspective, it can be argued that the societal center is empty, because no individual actually fits the projected image completely.[25] This perspective has been useful in countering hegemonic theories. Nevertheless, postmodernism is still predominantly the product of male European theorists; its rhetoric does not nullify the real existence of a powerful group at the center that continues to enforce policies from a central cultural and political position. The impact of these policies remains clearly visible in the daily lives of those at the periphery of the society.[33] In other words, it is indisputable that some people continue to be differentiated and peripheralized on the basis of visible marks, such as race, gender, appearance, and presence of disability; practices, such as religion, occupation, and sexual behavior; cultural identities, such as sexual orientation and ethnicity; associations, such as political affiliation and national origin; stigmatized illnesses and addictions; and social and economic statuses.

Power

The property of *power* is defined as influence exerted by those at the center of a community over the periphery and vice versa. Authority and control that flow from the center outward are demonstrations of hierarchical power. Innovation and resistance originating from those at the margins to affect the center are demonstrations of horizontal power. Cultural change is an oscillating movement from center to periphery and back again.[34] Innovations in political action, music, visual arts, fashion, humor, and language illustrate how those at the societal center frequently must look to the periphery for creative, original approaches. In a profit-based economy, those at the periphery depend on technologic and economic sustenance from the center. The center, in turn, depends on the periphery for labor, consumption of its products, and new ideas.

Inquiry and intervention often consider only the movement of power and knowledge from center to periphery, reducing marginalized persons to entities in need of "development"—that is, "welfare," education, and technical assistance. Some marginalized individuals are able to garner a measure of hierarchical power, usually only to the degree that they compensate for or conceal their differences from the dominant cultural images and refrain from appearing powerful in their own right. Inequities in political, economic, and social resources are the basis for hierarchical power that sustains rulers, entrepreneurs, and bureaucracies at the expense of least-ranking groups, including residents of inner-city neighborhoods, Native Americans, unskilled laborers, low-income single mothers, children, and the homeless.

The power of the center depends on a relatively uncontested authority; visibility of marginalized populations presents a significant challenge.[25] The current debate about lifting the ban on sexual minorities in the military is a case in point. On one hand it seems a moot point, since gays and lesbians have always been in the military but have remained hidden as such. On the other hand, the integration of publicly acknowledged gays and lesbians into the military becomes a linchpin issue as it allows new counterimages to invade traditional hierarchical definitions of power as exclusively male and heterosexually identified. These counterimages are a source of horizontal power.

Horizontal power is that which is exerted by the marginalized in resistance to the hegemony of the center. It is often best expressed in solidarity among marginalized persons, coalitions of diverse subgroups who challenge underestimations of their influence and prerogatives. Rather than rejecting, ignoring, or trying to destroy difference, these efforts at valuing diversity enrich movements for social change. Relating across human differences as equals creates power.[35]

A great deal of knowledge is situated at the margins. Subordinated groups create knowledge that enables them to resist oppression.[17] Of necessity, they know a great deal about their oppressors' ways of thinking; the converse is seldom true. For example, domestic workers are intimately familiar with their employers' needs and habits, while their employers may not even know the names of the workers' children or where they live.[36] Heterosexual people are often shocked to learn details of gay and lesbian subculture that has thrived in their cities for decades unknown to them. Gay men and lesbians have no such lack of knowledge about straight culture. Survival depends on the ability of the marginalized to at least emulate or mouth the values of the dominant culture. Beyond survival, knowledge about the dynamics and details of those at the hierarchical center can be a source of horizontal, liberating power for the marginalized. Thus, marginalization not only results in deprivation and powerlessness, but also can provide a locus of resistance and empowerment as well as the possibility for overturning oppressive, hierarchical power dynamics.[36]

Secrecy

A fourth property of marginalization is secrecy. *Secrecy* is defined as confining information to establish interpersonal bonds, maintain trust, and avoid betrayal. Secrecy both creates and characterizes marginalized social groups and environments.[37] Secrecy can be a means to coalition and protection for the marginalized as well as a process contributing to their marginalized status. While marginalized groups often have more knowledge about their oppressors' ways of thinking and being than is conversely true, the exclusion of those marked as outsiders by the center is often accomplished by withholding specific information from them that could increase their access to resources.[38] Those at the edges are often stymied by bureaucratic red tape because they do not know the "secrets" or shortcuts that insiders are privy to. Also, if members of marginalized groups do not have some modicum of influence over schools, media, and other cultural institutions, they cannot make their perspectives known outside their groups.[17]

Because the marginalized are often suspected of betraying the mainstream, they are forced to use secrecy, to hide their identities or activities, for survival. For instance, on the basis of identity alone, gay men and lesbians, Jews, and communists have all been investigated and blacklisted as traitorous groups in the United States.[39] Helping organizations such as social services, scientific research institutions, and public health departments reach out from the center to the periphery to encourage marginalized people to disclose their secrets,[40] to trust that their interests will be served.[41] But by design, many of these organizations are then forced to use the information they have gathered to betray the marginalized, as in cases of "welfare fraud," medical studies that reinforce racist assumptions, and health databases used to discontinue insurance coverage of individuals at risk.[37] "Passing" is a common form of secrecy used by immigrants, refugees, gay and lesbian persons, Jewish persons, and those espousing suspect political ideas.[42] They keep their identities secret by imitating majority appearances or behaviors, sometimes even including the fabrication of false names and personal histories. Passing should be understood not as an intention to mislead or defraud others, but as a means of protection and evasion of dangers associated with being discovered as an outsider.

Activities considered morally taboo at the societal center occur in marginalized environments under the cloak of secrecy. Marginalized environments include locations characterized by economic destitution; joblessness; physical dangers; social isolation; increased illness; and lack of access to health care, police protection, and other resources. Examples are areas near the borders of countries, abandoned urban slums, and streets where predatory adults locate runaway youths for sexual exploitation. In these borderlands, the potential for violence and illegal activity is escalated because the inhabitants have been betrayed and secreted away by the center. Those at the societal center who have power, property, and mobility exercise their privilege to engage marginalized people in exploitive ways while escaping the dangers and limitations of living in marginalized environments. The pace of exchange in illicit goods and services, such as narcotics, pornography, and the labor of sex workers and undocumented immigrants, is accelerated by the stark conditions in these fringe areas.

In locales of extreme conflict, boundaries are drawn more tightly and bonds are intensified via secrecy and intense loyalty. Social bonds are concretized in a worldview of "us against the world." Betrayal of one's peers in such groups is highly unacceptable. Interpersonal bonds forged in prisons and combat situations are examples of this intensified connection to peers. Perhaps a less obvious example is that of an African American, low-income lesbian couple who survive ostracism from both the Euro-American lesbian community and the general African American community through a fierce commitment to one another and a narrowing of their social world. Conditions of secrecy can thus create intense relational bonds among members of marginalized groups and reinforce profound distrust of others, contributing to subsequent social isolation and privatization of individual experience.

Reflectiveness

As a consequence of stigmatized differentiation, disempowerment, and secrecy, marginalized persons have subjective experiences that distinguish them from more centrally located community members. The inner worlds of marginalized persons mirror the contradictions and pressures external to themselves and create the necessity for continual, purposeful introspection. Marginalized persons live "examined lives" out of necessity. The property of reflectiveness connotes both of these qualities, mirroring and introspection. *Reflectiveness* is defined as the fragmenting and conflicting psychic effects on marginalized persons of discrimination, privatization, isolation, invisibility, and fragmentation and the interior work that is required to understand and compensate for these effects.

A case in point is the plight of children who go through the marginalizing experience of being physically or sexually abused. They may take flight interiorly, compartmentalizing or dissociating negative experiences, sometimes to the extent that they develop alternate personalities to cope with the contradictions and pain they experience.[43] Such abuse, so well privatized and kept secret, can lead to a profound sense of isolation and inner fragmentation that may persist into adulthood. A substantial amount of psychic energy is bound up in internal processes that are needed to cope with and eventually to heal from such trauma.

> The inner worlds of marginalized persons mirror the contradictions and pressures external to themselves and create the necessity for continual, purposeful introspection.

Persons marginalized on the basis of race or sexual orientation, for instance, internalize their own identities as well as the negative, stereotypic mainstream images of members of their categories,[44, 45] which results in another kind of inner fragmentation, a splitting of the self-image.[46] This conflict regarding self-worth requires conscious, introspective effort to resolve, usually with the help of supportive others and the embracing of empowering, positive counterculture images. The experiences of internalized sexism, racism, and homophobia and their resolution are not often accounted for in theories of

human growth and development, identity formation, and health promotion. Nevertheless, these processes occupy significant life space and time for members of marginalized groups. Lorde provided an eloquent example:

Women of color in America have grown up within a symphony of anger, at being silenced, at being unchosen, at knowing that when we survive, it is in spite of a world that . . . hates our very existence outside its service. And I say symphony rather than cacophony because we have had to learn to orchestrate those furies so that they do not tear us apart. We have had to learn to move through them and use them for strength and force and insight within our daily lives. Those of us who did not learn this difficult lesson did not survive. And part of my anger is always libation for my fallen sisters.[26 p. 119]

Those with hidden stigmatizing features and those who have limited mobility and access to others like themselves may have only stereotypes against which to compare themselves. Paradoxically, even those with visible attributes that make them different, such as skin color, can still be invisible. Invisibility, in this case, is the experience of not being seen or of being seen as an object.[33] The media reflects central images. The occasional Asian American, Latino, gay, or lesbian character in a film is often presented in a negative light, so that youths from these subgroups internalize very limited views of these persons.[47–49] Marginalized persons can feel like "the only one" who has transited particular stigmatizing experiences. If they do not come to develop knowledge of the heterogeneity within their category, they retain a sense of self-uniqueness that compounds their sense of isolation.[20]

Persons who embody several boundaries by virtue of multiple stigmas, cultures, or marginalizing experiences can feel even more displaced, more in between than those clearly in one group or another.[8, 50–52] For example, the Latina refugee who is addicted, is HIV positive, and has a history of incest, experiences the alienating effects of gender, racial, social, and traumatic marginalization. The net result of these processes is a sense of profound delegitimization—that is, the sense of being an outsider in almost any group.[26] With the capacity to introspect can come the understanding that this sense of alienation is neither imagined nor a result of personal failure.

Marginalized persons not only have experiences that are distinct from those at the center, but also interpret reality differently. That is, they have particular standpoints about the ways in which they are oppressed. The capacity for reflecting on one's marginality is empowering in the sense that one can strategize more effectively with increased awareness of specific conditions of discrimination, isolation, privatization, and oppression. Reflectiveness can be a double-edged sword, however. The political consciousness it engenders increases the chances of survival and success. Yet those who have the ability to be reflective, but who lack sufficient social support and resources for addressing the fragmentation and isolation that they discover, may feel their marginalization even more intensely.

Voice

Marginalized persons and groups have ways of communicating that distinguish them from those at the center. Hierarchical power from the center, however, forces majority concepts to be expressed in the majority language, resulting in the devaluing of other voices. Marginalized persons and groups are thus silenced within the dominant stream of communication. Within this silence, however, are other forms of expression created and used by the marginalized. *Voice,* as a property of marginalization, is defined as the languages and forms of expression characterizing marginalized subcultures. Voice encompasses types of talk and ways of telling. Three examples of marginalized talk are "mixed talk," "back talk," and "new talk." A common way of telling is narrative.

As central concepts and terms become less applicable and meaningful, marginalized persons and groups "mix talk" in their attempts to understand their own experience and exert their own power. Words from the center are transformed and reframed by the marginalized, creating a powerful counterlanguage, a "language of refusal" that resists through preservation of collective cultural memories.[36] Biculturalism and bilingualism facilitate exchange, which is the currency of value in many marginalized environments. Hybrid words and creolized or mixed languages, such as Pidgin, Tex-Mex, and Chicano forms of Spanish, meet the needs for cooperation and negotiation that are essential for survival. Speakers of mixed talk are in odd positions, however; theirs is a border language not fully validated by the centers of any of the cultures it mixes.[53]

Those at the center exert power through "misnaming."[35] For example, the tension between Euro-Americans and African Americans is sometimes called the "race issue," as if color differences are inherently problematic. From the standpoint of African Americans, the appropriate term is "racism"; the problem is not skin pigmentation, but domination of one group by another. To counter misnaming and other forms of exploitation, people reclaim words previously used to oppress, such as "queer" and "black," to reappropriate power and create intellectual and cultural space. "Back talk"[54] involves speaking to central, hierarchical authority from the standpoint of equality, questioning oppressive customs and cultural expectations. The marginalized are not expected to speak as equals to their "superiors" at the societal center, giving this type of talk the empowering element of surprise.

Marginalized experiences often lack precedents and do not correspond with frames of reference proffered by mainstream media, so marginalized persons coin new words to describe their experiences. "New talk" is also needed to achieve palpably intense expressions for painful qualities of marginalized experiences, to create an escape from them, or to compensate for having to speak in a language that is not one's own.[55] Sometimes new terms and symbols are incorporated into mainstream, central language, but usually the depth of their meanings remains enigmatic to those outside the particular subculture in which they were created. Subcultural argot, as a type of neologistic language development, thus maintains boundaries and secrecy and helps to preserve the safety of marginalized persons.

When the languages of marginalized groups have been barred from public and written discourse, their members construct and preserve experience in the form of storied knowledge: individual and collective counternarratives.[56] By relating actual episodes and mythic stories,[57] storytellers preserve the history of the group, provoke exchange of ideas, and meet political goals. A narrative is not a passive account of reality, but a form of mediation.[52] Through telling stories, narrators transact with an audience, changing the power relationship.[58] In fact, individual narratives take on collective significance because the experiences of marginalized persons occur in charged, narrowed contexts, so that each event is magnified and immediately politically significant.[55]

If culture does indeed change through oscillation between center and periphery, the narratives of those at the margins contain valuable information. Experiences at the margins represent aspects of the future and the past that are usually repressed in accounts emanating from the societal center. The stories marginalized people tell can thus illuminate histories that explain present conditions of the larger society and suggest a range of future possibilities for development.

Liminality

As a property of marginalization, liminality captures the sense of living and perceiving at the edge.[59, 60] *Liminality* is defined as altered and intensified perceptions of time, worldview, and self-image that characterize and result from marginalizing experiences. Marginalization has a liminal quality in that it carries crucial consequences for human development, maintenance of self-esteem, and health promotion and restoration. The extremity of marginalizing situations clarifies the stakes involved. The loss of comforting, stabilizing identities during serious illness is a case in point. In such a transitional period, when individuals face life-and-death contingencies or irreversible changes in their lifecourse, they are likely to feel isolated from the societal center, if only for a limited period of time. But time is perceived in relation to the meanings attached to pressing concerns. Perceptions of the world and one's place in it may shift radically during illness, along with previously well-established priorities. Healers such as nurses are often present during these kinds of marginal, transitional experiences.[61] As witnesses to and facilitators of transitions, nurses are intermediaries between persons and their experiences, having both access to and influence on the perceptions and meanings attached to them.

Transitional experiences are often related and always have health implications.[62] They create openings, ruptures in the daily fabric of existence, in which new awareness can be gained and new strategies incorporated.[63, 64] Health transitions may also be openings for further marginalization, with negative outcomes. For example, individuals who test positive for HIV may experience rejection by family and friends, loss of health insurance, depression, and ultimately a sense of hopelessness and depersonalization if their support needs are not met.

Marginalization, Vulnerability, and Health

Marginalization has health implications that can best be understood by explicating its relationship to the concept of vulnerability. Exploring the properties of marginalization exposes the linkages between vulnerability and health for those living at the edges of society and suggests that the health consequences of marginalizing experiences result not only from the perceptions of marginalized persons, but also from the contingencies of their environments.

Vulnerability is defined as the condition of being exposed to or unprotected from health-damaging environments.[10] One can be physically, psychologically, socially, and economically vulnerable to sources of illness. Vulnerability has negative and positive implications, as expressed in its two major aspects of risk and resilience. *Risk* is the increased potential for developing illness as a result of disproportionate exposure to damaging environmental factors. *Resilience* incorporates the capacities gained from person-environment interactions that foster survival.[65, 66] Resilience includes not only genetic predispositions and learned abilities of persons, but also factors in their surroundings that enhance well-being. Many persons and groups who face adversity due to marginalization develop durable individual and collective survival strategies in relation to their environments that differ from tactics used by those at the societal center.[23] They may also have personal or social characteristics that enhance their chances for successful development, health maintenance, and recovery, despite constraints. There is significant variability, however, in resilience among marginalized persons across adverse circumstances. Strategies, supports, and skills that are effective in one environment, at one stage of development, in response

> There is significant variability in resilience among marginalized persons. Strategies, supports, and skills that are effective in one environment are not always effective in other circumstances.

to one type of marginalization are not always effective in other circumstances.

Each of the properties of marginalization carries elements of risk and resilience that have health consequences. Intermediacy suggests that interpersonal barriers may be obstacles as well as sources of protection. Differentiation implies that diversity can be stigmatized by the central "majority" while honored and celebrated by members of one's group. Power refers to the negative impact of domination as well as the creative forces of coalition and solidarity. Secrecy involves fear of betrayal and exclusion via tight interpersonal bonding, yet also preserves trust and a sense of belonging. Reflectiveness reveals how social processes engender internal fragmentation, an awareness that can be demoralizing or empowering, depending on whether there is adequate support from others. Voice carries implications of being silenced and misunderstood as well as the possibility for positive, powerful expression. Liminality characterizes experiences that are often fraught with danger and yet may be invaluable opportunities for change and insight.

Although nurses often focus on risk in dealing with vulnerable populations, resilience is an important aspect of marginalization, because it fosters understanding of how individuals and groups creatively maneuver and use resources at hand to avoid illness and to maximize their chances for survival.[67] The health of those who are marginalized is relevant to that of the whole community, because marginalized persons comprise a community's most at risk, but perhaps most resilient, members. Without knowing the health-related responses of the marginalized, community health assessments will be sorely inadequate in estimating communicable and toxic disease threats and in suggesting solutions to problems stemming from social alienation, economic deprivation, and political repression. Access to health resources is only part of the struggle for marginalized persons. They must also have the political and economic resources to ensure their basic needs and the social legitimation and respect necessary to make decisions affecting their health.

Implications for Nursing Research, Theory, and Practice

As a nursing concept, marginalization implies a deliberate focus on functions of boundaries; peripheralized persons; environments at the borders; and liminal, transitional human experiences, especially as each of these relates to health and illness. This focus creates a unique lens through which to view nursing phenomena. By examining the margins, nurses can gain knowledge about the whole that has previously been unavailable to us. With marginalization as a guiding concept, inquiry can more accurately explicate the health and health care of diverse populations, because it helps us to avoid universalizing empirical and clinical approaches and impresses on us the need to approach members of marginalized groups with an ear to their experiences and an eye to their struggles.

Questions From the Margins

The source and focus of questions for inquiry are uniquely shaped if one takes the perspective of the marginalized. Who are the people at the margins, and what risks do they face? What questions are relevant to those who have had little voice in shaping health sciences research? How might problems be renamed and reconceptualized according to the experiences of those who exist far from the societal center? What problems do specific marginalized individuals and groups identify regarding their own health? How do borders and boundaries function in relation to illness? Does life at the edge protect or expose? What interiorized perceptions and environmental contingencies guide marginalized persons as they make decisions about health behaviors? What strategies are most durable, and what environmental resources are most effective for marginalized persons in terms of health promotion, avoidance of illness, and recovery? How do hierarchical power dynamics affect the health of stigmatized groups? How does betrayal by the center become manifest in the daily experiences of marginalized youths? What factors contribute to survival and resilience in marginalized environments?

Marginalized persons are seldom directly consulted about their opinions and experiences, largely because most research models depend on hierarchical power dynamics in which predetermined information is elicited from representative "subjects" under conditions that are designed to "control for" variables considered extraneous or confounding. Such processes constrain participants and mold the findings to fit the conceptual framework of the researcher. Members of marginalized groups often avoid participation in research because they find the atmosphere and conduct of research to be adversarial, lack an investment in the research questions, or mistrust researchers' motives.[17] Questions about the genetic patterns of sickle cell disease, for example, are not equally valued by scientists and those affected by the disease. The latter are probably more concerned about access to services, pain relief, and improvements in daily functioning. These client-

oriented questions seem very much within the realm of nursing inquiry.

While many marginalized communities are asking for research that is "traditional" enough to be persuasive to policymakers and program funders, they want more-inclusive, participatory methodologies. One key to success in knowledge development with diverse populations is to invite marginalized people to talk at length about the health problems they face, the obstacles that block their access to health care and other resources, and what they believe is needed to remedy their situations. While this seems almost too simple to be efficacious, the truth is that it is rarely done in research or practice in any discipline.

Relevant Design

Designs for inquiry also change when one is guided by the concept of marginalization. Knowledge development is no longer restricted to traditional research, but includes individual therapeutic alliances, group forums, storytelling, participatory research, political action, and any other means by which understanding is expanded and theory is developed by engaging marginalized persons and groups in the process. Research is a communal endeavor, and the knowledge it yields is public property. This means that professional researchers and clinicians should synchronize their efforts with the needs and prerogatives of marginalized persons and refrain from unilaterally imposing preselected projects and solutions.[68]

As Collins said, "One cannot use the same techniques to study the knowledge of the dominated as one uses to study the knowledge of the powerful."[17(p751)] She suggested that it requires more ingenuity to examine the standpoint of marginalized persons, who have had to create independent ways of knowing and doing to survive outside the center. Traditional research methods often force members of marginalized groups to objectify themselves, displace their own motivations, and confront researchers who have more social, economic, and professional power than they. Studies of incidence and prevalence of various diseases, for instance, target marginalized groups, but often only as reservoirs of infection and danger, stigmatizing them in the process. One example is research about violence that emphasizes the high rates of homicide among young men of color without a thorough understanding of the contexts and conditions of these young men's lives. Stigmatizing stereotypes about marginalized groups can persist in spite of empirical results, as in studies of female sex workers and the HIV epidemic in the United States. An increased prevalence of the virus has not been supported in the data, yet the nearly indestructible stereotype that these women are dangerous disease carriers has persisted.[69]

It is the authors' contention that microscopic descriptions of experiences at the margins hold the promise of capturing the specificity, scope, and variability of health-related phenomena in ways that measures of central tendency simply cannot. Seldom are those at the margins studied in their own habitats, from their own perspectives, as experts on their own lives. Research that aims to describe marginalized persons uncovers not only needs but also strengths and innovative strategies for survival that such persons and their social networks create. For example, studies demonstrating how individuals thrive despite stigmatizing illness yield important information about basic health-maintenance strategies. Because of the harsh conditions at the periphery, workable health-promoting strategies developed there are likely to be stable and also potentially effective for those existing nearer the center.

Language is of critical importance in the design of inquiry. Language about the processes of research and theory as well as language expressing the content of findings should be meaningful and understandable to both researchers and consumers. Using rigid methods of data collection, such as forced-choice questionnaires or highly structured interview formats, may be a way of silencing marginalized people. This is especially true when the terminology used reflects researchers' preconceived notions about what is relevant. For example, researchers might draw blank stares if they ask low-income women what their concept of "wellness" is. On the other hand, such persons may have a lexicon of their own terms that are relevant to the concept of wellness, such as "surviving," "getting through," and "listening to your gut feelings." Theory development should use language that functions as a bridge between the substantive knowledgebase of the discipline and actual contexts of health-related phenomena, achieving a necessary level of abstraction without losing the diversity, intensity, and particularity of marginalized experiences.

Sampling to Enhance Diversity

The casting of probability-based statistical nets over communities may fail to recognize heterogeneity at the boundaries and the increasing differentiation of experiences from center to periphery. Statistical methods assume that persons are analogous to identical "cells" in a grid that can be accurately accessed through randomization, a process ensuring that each cell has an equal chance of being tapped. Communities are less like grids and more like unique organisms, exhibiting diverse characteristics and processes in each of their parts. Communities are not oceans of identical fish to be snared in random sampling nets. Communities are made up of many interacting subcultural groups, which in turn comprise unique individuals situated in particular contexts.

The care taken in choosing where to sample the tissue for a biopsy is analogous to planning research that respects persons and communities in their organicity and complexity.[70] Microscopic margins of biopsied tissue samples provide comprehensive information about the whole body—that is, the nature of illness, its extent, and even its outcome. In another analogy, even small changes

> The casting of probability-based statistical nets over communities may fail to recognize heterogeneity at the boundaries and the increasing differentiation of experiences from center to periphery.

in peripheral structures of the body, such as size, shape, color, texture, and movement of extremities, can reveal central functions. Likewise, sampling at the margins can be informative about the health of the whole community. But special efforts need to be made to represent the diversity at the margins, which is greater than at the center. This may require overrecruitment of various marginal subgroups using a theoretically sound scheme to adequately explore "bites" of the heterogeneous edges versus the homogeneous center.

Innovative approaches including time and resources for building trust, collaborating with community members, and power sharing are needed for research and knowledge development with groups who have had to construct layers of secrecy to protect themselves and with those who participate in highly stigmatized activities. Conventional approaches to preserving the safety and confidentiality of research participants may not be adequate for specific marginalized groups. In these cases, protective strategies must be carefully designed and incorporated at each phase of the research process.

Reflexive Involvement

Reflexive involvement refers to establishing and maintaining solidarity with the marginalized throughout the knowledge development process. Research, theory, and practice with marginalized persons and groups can be obstructed by a lack of trust, understandable in the light of secrecy, stigmatization, and other dynamics associated with marginalization. Investigators can feel betrayed when marginalized persons conceal information or fail to comply with their instructions. Marginalized persons can feel betrayed when research findings are not disseminated and used to improve their daily lives, but are instead used to justify repressive policies. They can also feel betrayed when health services are inaccessible, culturally incongruent, or abruptly withdrawn after the research project is ended. Marginalized persons resent the "rip and run" practice of extracting data to support the theoretical interests and career advancement needs of researchers without a reciprocal process. Reflexive involvement makes nurses accountable for providing participants with the opportunity to speak freely in their own words, the power to affect the design of investigations and interventions, and compensation for individual and community involvement.[70–72]

The properties of marginalization ought to be viewed not as obstacles to the research process, but rather as elements of a framework for assessing the safety, sensitivity, relevance, and empowering capacity of a given approach to inquiry. Establishing trust is not merely an interpersonal issue. It involves changing the images of research and institutional health care practice that are etched in the minds of marginalized groups through a long history of exploitation, exclusion, and misrepresentation. In fact, these images cannot really be changed until the structures that perpetuate them are changed.[73]

The fragmenting and isolating effects of stigma, secrecy, and mistrust require nurses' compassionate, partisan commitment to the interests of marginalized groups.[68] To develop knowledge with marginalized persons and groups who have been so frequently silenced within the dominant stream of communication, nurses need to identify and investigate other forms of expression that they have created and used. Knowledge may be gained through emotions rather than words, verbal performance rather than text, political action rather than cognitive appraisal, or behaviors of a daily life of work and caring rather than answers to standardized questions.

Marginalized people often tell through stories, theorize through narratives.[74] Eliciting and analyzing narratives, therefore, provide a channel of communication between the marginalized and the community as a whole. Such inquiry not only constitutes research, but also functions as mediation. Telling one's story without the language constraints inherent in questionnaires and structured interviews is empowering for marginalized persons, because it overcomes the invisibility and silencing they are so familiar with. Most narratives not only relate actual experiences, but also convey interpretive reflections on those experiences. Narratives therefore represent processes of self-inquiry that allow for the sharing of power in research and practice.[75]

• • •

Knowledge development includes all of the processes that generate theory to guide nursing practice. Theory should not be a collection of static concepts generated from within the discipline, accounting only for majority-based, norm-referenced observations. Theory should have currency as vivid, substantive reflections of the full spectrum of human experience from margin to center.[76] Marginalization as a guiding concept provides direction for scholarship that embraces this diversity and requires the revision of extant models of inquiry as well as promotion of entirely new methods. The concept of marginalization, as it has been explicated here and related to the larger concept of vulnerability, breaks new ground for nursing from which we can conduct future inquiry about the health of complex, culturally diverse communities.

References

1. Hall JM: Alcoholism recovery in lesbian women: a theory in development. Sch Inq Nurs Pract 4(2):109–122, 1990.
2. Hall JM: An exploration of lesbians' images of recovery from alcohol problems. Health Care Women Int 13(2):181–198, 1992.
3. Hall JM: How lesbians recognize and respond to alcohol problems: a theoretical model of problematization. ANS 16(3):46–63, 1994.
4. Hall JM, Stevens PE, Meleis AI: Developing the construct of role integration: a narrative analysis of women clerical workers' daily lives. Res Nurs Health 15(6):447–457, 1992.
5. Meleis AI: Community participation and involvement: theoretical and empirical issues. Health Serv Manage Res 5(1):5–16, 1992.
6. Meleis AI: Theory testing and theory support: principles, challenges and a sojourn into the future. In: Neuman B, ed. Research with Neuman's System Model. Norwalk, Conn: Appleton & Lange. 1994, pp. 447–457.
7. Stevens PE: Marginalized women's access to health care: a feminist narrative analysis: ANS 16(2):39–56, 1993.
8. Stevens PE: Protective strategies of lesbian clients in health care environments. Res Nurs Health 17:217–229, 1994.
9. Stevens PE: HIV prevention education for lesbians and bisexual women: a cultural analysis of a community intervention. Soc Sci Med 39:1565–1578, 1994.
10. Stevens PE, Hall JM, Meleis AI: Examining vulnerability of women clerical workers from five ethnic/racial groups. West J Nurs Res 14:754–774, 1992.
11. American Nurses' Association: Cabinet on Nursing Research. Directions for Nursing Research: Toward the 21st Century. Kansas City, Mo: Author: 1985.
12. Meleis AI: Directions for nursing theory development in the 21st century. Nurs Sci Q 5(3):112–117, 1992.
13. Oberst MT: Nursing in the year 2000: setting the agenda for knowledge generation and utilization. In: Sorensen GE, ed. Setting the Agenda for the Year 2000: Knowledge Development in Nursing. Kansas City, Mo: American Academy of Nursing: 29–37, 1986.
14. U.S. Department of Health and Human Services: Healthy People 2000: National Health Promotion and Disease Prevention Objectives. Washington, DC: Author: 1990. U.S. Dept of Health, Education, and Welfare publication PHS 91-50213.
15. Smith A, Stewart AJ: Approaches to studying racism and sexism in black women's lives. J Soc Issues 36(3):1–15, 1983.
16. Zambrana RE: A research agenda on issues affecting poor and minority women: a model for understanding their health needs. Women Health 12(3–4):137–160, 1987.
17. Collins PH: The social construction of black feminist throught. Signs J Women Culture Society 14:745–773, 1989.
18. American Academy of Nursing: Expert panel report: culturally competent health care. Nurs Outlook 40:277–283, 1992.
19. Stevens PE: Who gets care? Access to health care as an arena for nursing action. Sch Inq Nurs Pract 6(3):185–200, 1992.
20. Frable DES: Being and feeling unique: statistical deviance and psychological marginality. J Pers 61(1):85–109, 1993.
21. Markus H: Self-schemata and processing information about the self. J Pers Soc Psychol 35:63–78, 1977.
22. Gilligan C: In a Different Voice: Psychological Theory and Women's Development. Cambridge, Mass: Harvard University Press: 1982.
23. Anzaldua G, Moraga C, eds: This Bridge Called My Back: Writings by Radical Women of Color. 2nd ed. New York, NY: Kitchen Table Press: 1987.
24. Derrida J: Writing and Difference. Chicago, Ill: University of Chicago Press: 1978.
25. Ferguson R: Introduction: invisible center. In: Ferguson R. Gever M, Minh-ha T, West C, eds. Out There: Marginalization and Contemporary Cultures. Cambridge, Mass: MIT Press: 9–18, 1990.
26. Lorde A: Sister Outsider. Freedom, Calif: Crossing Press; 1984.
27. Becker H: Outsiders. New York, NY: Free Press; 1963.
28. Goffman E: Stigma: Notes on the Management of Spoiled Identity. Englewood Cliffs, NJ: Prentice Hall; 1963.

29. Jones EE, Farina A, Hastorf AH, Markus H, Miller DT, Scott RA, French R: Social Stigma: The Psychology of Marked Relationships. New York, NY: W.H. Freeman; 1984.

30. Szasz T: The Manufacturer of Madness: A Comparative Study of the Inquisition and the Mental Health Movement. New York, NY: Delta; 1970.

31. Meleis AI, Lipson JG, Paul S: Ethnicity and health among five Middle Eastern immigrant groups. Nurs Res 41(2):98–103, 1992.

32. Hurtado A: Relating to privilege: seduction and rejection in the subordination of white women and women of color. Signs J Women Culture Society 14(4):833–855, 1989.

33. Wallace M: Modernism, postmodernism and the problem of the visual in Afro-American culture. In: Ferguson R, Gever M, Minh-ha T, West C, eds. Out There: Marginalization and Contemporary Cultures. Cambridge, Mass: MIT Press: 39–50, 1990.

34. Ferguson R, Gever M, Minh-ha T, West C, eds: Out There: Marginalization and Contemporary Cultures. Cambridge, Mass: MIT Press; 1990.

35. Lorde A: Age, race, class and sex: women redefining difference. In: Ferguson R, Gever M, Minh-ha T, West C, eds. Out There: Marginalization and Contemporary Cultures. Cambridge, Mass: MIT Press: 281–288, 1990.

36. Hooks B: Marginality as site of resistance. In: Ferguson R, Gever M, Minh-ha T, West C, eds. Out There: Marginalization and Contemporary Cultures. Cambridge, Mass: MIT Press: 241–244, 1990.

37. Akerstrom M: Betrayed and Betrayers: The Sociology of Treachery. New Brunswick, NJ: Transaction Publishers; 1991.

38. Simmel G, Wolff K. trans: Secrets as creators of social bonds. In: Wolff K, ed. The Sociology of Georg Simmel. New York, NY: Free Press: 307–355, 1964.

39. Adam BD. The Survival of Domination: Inferiorization and Everyday Life. New York, Elsevier: 1978.

40. Foucault M; Hurley R, trans: The History of Sexuality: Vol One. An Introduction. New York, NY: Random House; 1978.

41. Harding S: Introduction: Is there a feminist method? In: Harding S, ed. Feminism and Methodology. Bloomington, Ind: Indiana University Press; 1987:1–14.

42. Ponse B: Identities in the Lesbian World: The Social Construction of Self. Westport, Conn: Greenwood Press; 1978.

43. Herman JL: Trauma and Recovery. New York, NY: Basic Books; 1992.

44. Memmi A: Dominated Man: Notes Toward a Portrait. New York, NY: Orion; 1968.

45. Nungesser LG. Homosexual Acts, Actors, and Identities. New York, NY: Praeger, 1983.

46. Bhabha HK: The other question: difference, discrimination and the discourse of colonialism. In: Ferguson R, Gever M, Minh-ha T, West C, eds. Out There: Marginalization and Contemporary Cultures. Cambridge, Mass: MIT Press: 71–88, 1990.

47. Rofes EE: "I Thought People Like That Killed Themselves": Lesbians, Gay Men and Suicide. San Francisco, Calif: Grey Fox Press; 1983.

48. Russo V: The Celluloid Closet: Homosexuality and the Movies. New York, NY: Harper & Row; 1987.

49. West C: The new cultural politics of difference. In: Ferguson R, Gever M, Minh-ha T, West C, eds. Out There: Marginalization and Contemporary Cultures. Cambridge, Mass: MIT Press: 19–38, 1990.

50. Hall JM: Alcoholism in lesbians: developmental, symbolic interactionist and critical perspectives. Health Care Women Int 11(1):89–107, 1990.

51. King DK: Multiple jeopardy, multiple consciousness: the context of a black feminist ideology. Signs J Women Culture Society 14:42–72, 1988.

52. Minha-ha T: Cotton and iron. In: Ferguson R, Gever M, Minh-ha T, West C, eds. Out There: Marginalization and Contemporary Cultures. Cambridge, Mass: MIT Press: 327–336, 1990.

53. Anzaldua G: How to tame a wild tongue. In: Ferguson R, Gever M, Minh-ha T, West C, eds: Out There: Marginalization and Contemporary Cultures. Cambridge, Mass: MIT Press: 203–212, 1990.

54. Hooks B: Talking back. In: Ferguson R, Gever M, Minh-ha T, West C, eds. Out There: Marginalization and Contemporary Cultures. Cambridge, Mass: MIT Press: 337–340, 1990.

55. Deleuze G, Guattari F: What is a minor literature? In: Ferguson R, Gever M, Minh-ha T, West C, eds. Out There: Marginalization and Contemporary Cultures. Cambridge, Mass: MIT Press: 59–70, 1990.

56. Personal Narratives Group, eds: Interpreting Women's Lives: Feminist Theory and Personal Narratives. Bloomington, Ind: Indiana University Press; 1989.

57. Britton BK, Pellegrini AD, eds: Narrative Thought and Narrative Language. Hillsdale, NJ: Erlbaum; 1990.

58. Todd AD, Fisher S, eds: Gender and Discourse: The Power of Talk. Norwood, NJ: Ablex; 1988.

59. Hallstein AL: Spiritual opportunities in the liminal rites of hospitalization. J Religion Health 31(3):247–254, 1992.

60. Van Gennep A: The Rites of Passage. Chicago, Ill: University of Chicago Press; 1960.

61. Turner V: Forest of Symbols: Aspects of Ndembu Ritual. Ithaca, NY: Cornell University Press; 1967.

62. Chick N, Meleis AI: Transitions: a nursing concern. In: Chinn PL, ed. Nursing Research Methodology: Issues and Implementation. Rockville. Rockville, Md: Aspen Publishers: 237–257, 1986.

63. Miles M: Towards a methodology for feminist research. In: Bowles G, Klein RD, eds. Theories of Women's Studies. Boston. Mass: Routledge & Kegan Paul: 117–139, 1983.

64. Stanley L, Wise S: Breaking Out: Feminist Consciousness and Feminist Research. Boston, Mass: Routledge & Kegan Paul: 1983.

65. Garmezy N, Masten AS: Stress, competence and resilience: common frontiers for therapist and psychopathologist. Behav Ther 17(5):500–521, 1986.

66. Rutter M: Psychosocial resilience and protective mechanisms. Am J Orthopsychiatry 57(3):317–331, 1987.

67. O'Brien ME: Pragmatic survivalism: behavior patterns affecting low-level wellness among minority group members. ANS 4(3):13–26, 1982.

68. Stevens PE, Hall JM: Applying critical theories to nursing in communities. Public Health Nurs 9(1):2–9, 1992.

69. Corea G: The Invisible Epidemic: The Story of Women and AIDS. New York, NY: HarperCollins; 1992.

70. Hall JM, Steven PE: Rigor in feminist research. ANS 13(3):16–29, 1991.

71. Anderson JM: Reflexivity in fieldwork: toward a feminist epistemology. Image J Nurs Sch 23(2):115–118, 1991.

72. Oakley A: Interviewing women: a contradiction in terms. In: Roberts H, ed. Doing Feminist Research. London, England: Routledge & Kegan Paul; 30–61, 1981.

73. Clare J: A challenge to the rhetoric of emancipation: recreating a professional culture. J Adv Nurs 18:1033–1038, 1993.

74. Christian B: The race for theory. Feminist Stud 14(1):67–79, 1988.

75. Mishler EG: Research Interviewing: Context and Narrative. Cambridge, Mass: Harvard University Press; 1986.

76. Hooks B: Feminist Theory: From Margin to Center. Boston, Mass: South End Press; 1984.

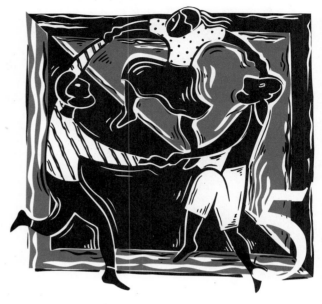

Special Needs in Community Mental Health

Violence in the Community

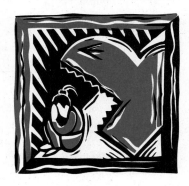

Upon completion of this chapter, the reader will be able to:

1. Describe the concept of community violence.

2. Identify long-term effects of violence on our society.

3. Identify the effect of guns on the problem of violence.

4. Identify at risk populations for violence and the role of public health in dealing with the epidemic of violence.

5. Analyze assessment data to determine the risk of abuse.

6. Describe the role of the nurse in primary, secondary and tertiary prevention of violence.

7. Identify protection measures necessary for nurses working in situations where violence is prevalent.

Ann C. Watkins

The purpose of this chapter is to explore violence in the community from a public health perspective as it relates to individuals, families, and communities. Included in this chapter are discussions of (1) the effects of violence on society in terms of mortality and morbidity; (2) homicide and suicides of younger and younger individuals; (3) the effect of guns on the mortality and morbidity of assaults; (4) the effect of violence on children, youth, women, and the elderly and public health interventions to stem the tide of violence; (5) the role and responsibilities of the community health nurse in dealing with victims of violence; and (6) issues to help ensure safety of community health workers.

A man is shot dead outside of a business by a gunman who does a "victory dance" over the body. A drive-by shooting just as school is over leaves 3 children dead on the playground and 12 children injured. A 30-year-old man, angry and despondent about the breakup of a relationship with a 20-year-old woman, shoots her, her mother, and her 13-year-old brother with an assault rifle and then kills himself. A mother suffocates her 2-week-old twins because she cannot stand to hear them cry and she does not know what to do for them. A young police officer planning to be married in a month stops a car for speeding and is shot dead in his police vehicle by the driver who shouts obscenities. A truck packed with explosives is detonated outside of a federal office building killing scores of infants, children, and adults and injuring almost 500 people. These are just six examples of the violence that surrounds us in our communities today. Violence has been declared a public health epidemic by three surgeon generals, Koop, Novello and Elders, and the president of the United States has declared that violence is a worse health problem for women and children than cancer. In dealing with this epidemic from a public health perspective, we must accept the fact that violence is a learned behavior and so can be changed and prevented (Belloni et al., 1991).

Violence is the intentional use of physical force against another person or against oneself, which either results in or has a high likelihood of resulting in injury or death. Violence includes suicidal acts as well as interpersonal violence such as rape, assault, child abuse or elder abuse. Fatal violence results in suicides and homicides.

(Rosenberg et al., 1992, p. 3071)

Violence is used to refer to a particular class of behaviors that cause injuries or death. In public health, injuries from violence are referred to as **intentional** injuries.

The reasons for the amount of violence in our society are complex. "Alvin Toffler in his book *Powershift* identifies violence or the threat of violence as one of the three fundamental sources of all human power, the other two are money and knowledge. Of the three, violence is the lowest form of power because it can only be used to punish" (Koop and Lundberg, 1992, p. 3075). Many social and economic factors, such as poverty, racism, disintegration of the family, peer pressure, and absence of positive values, contribute to violence (Novello, 1991). Violence is a pervasive topic in television and motion pictures. Research at the Family Television Research and Consultation Center has demonstrated a link between violence in television shows watched by children and heightened aggressive behavior. Watching violent behavior on television makes it harder for children to distinguish between reality and fantasy. Access to firearms is easy, and even children are carrying guns to elementary school to protect themselves. Gang involvement makes violence inevitable (Mitchell et al., 1991). A high level of violence is associated with the sale of crack cocaine to the poor in our cities. Killings, either execution style or drive-by shootings, are not unusual as a remedy for a drug deal gone sour.

Anger abounds in our society among individuals who have not been taught ways to control or deal with anger in a nonaggressive fashion. Mercy (1993) stated that violence is increasingly used by adolescents and children as a means of resolving conflicts. There have been many studies over the years that link abuse during childhood with violent behavior later in life. Many children in our society are brutalized by a parent or parents or witness one parent being beaten by the other. Research supports the idea that children who experience violence in childhood may grow up to become child or spouse abusers or kill another person. A study of adult male prisoners convicted of first-degree murder found that two thirds had experienced "continuous, remorseless brutality during childhood" (Mason, 1991).

HISTORY OF ABUSE

Violence is not limited to our century. Humans have dealt with other humans violently since the beginning of time. Cain killed his brother Abel because of jealousy and anger. Infanticide, or the killing of unwanted newborn children, has been practiced throughout history. Sickly or deformed children, a twin, a girl, or simply one too many in the family often were left to die from exposure or some other means. It was not until early in the fifth century that infanticide was condemned. That did not protect children, however, in many societies. Children, especially first-born children, were often sacrificed for religious reasons. Children were seen as the property of the father, and he could do with them what he pleased.

Corporal punishment has consistently been used as a means of controlling children through the ages. Beethoven, who created beautiful music that has endured through the centuries, whipped his piano pupils with a knitting needle if they made mistakes. When Louis XIII was a child, he was whipped upon arising in the morning for the mistakes he had made the previous day. A schoolmaster in Germany kept track of the discipline he administered to his pupils during his career. He recorded 911,527 strikes with a stick, 124,000 lashes with a whip, 136,715 slaps with his hand, and 1,115,800 boxes on the ear (DeMause, 1975). Truly not an enviable record!

Even the nursery rhymes that are read to small children seem to condone violence against them. Consider this nursery rhyme from Mother Goose:

There was an old woman who lived in a shoe,
She had so many children she didn't know what to do.
She gave them some broth without any bread
And whipped them all soundly and sent them to bed.

Wife beating was legal in the United States until 1824. Wives were seen as chattel of their husbands and could be beaten for such offenses as "nagging too much." It was not until the 1960s with the civil rights movement that the problem of assault against women began to be explored in America. Marital rape was not considered an offense in the United States until 1980.

Abuse of the elderly is also a problem that is not unique to this century. In preindustrial Europe, it was common for legal documents to be drawn to allow the elder parent to continue to sit at the family table and use the front door. The problem is of greater magnitude today because persons are living longer so that there are more elderly.

SCOPE OF THE PROBLEM
Homicide

America is the most violent country in the industrialized world (Blow and Gest, 1993). U.S. Surgeon General Antonia Novello reported in 1991 that the United States had the highest homicide rate of any Western industrialized country. The number of deaths by violence and unintentional misuse of firearms in the United States exceeded the combined total of the next 17 nations (U.S. Department of Health and Human Services [USDHHS], 1990). Homicide became the 10th leading cause of death among all age groups. Former Surgeon General C. Everett Koop reported in 1992 that 1 million U.S. inhabitants die prematurely each year as the result of intentional homicide or suicide.

Certain populations are at greater risk for death by homicide. These include young people, women, and African-American and Hispanic males. The population of the United States is 12% African-American; however, African-Americans constitute 50% of all murder victims, and statistics from 1990 reveal that in 93% of cases, African-Americans were killed by other African-Americans (Elders, 1994).

Homicide of Youths. Homicide is the second leading cause of death among Americans 15 to 24 years old and the leading cause of death among 15- to 34-year-old African-American males. This homicide rate is eight times greater than for whites of comparable age. The homicide rate for children and adolescents has more than doubled in the last 30 years (Novello et al., 1992). Not only are children being killed, but younger and younger children are increasingly committing murder (Ruttenberg, 1994). Criminal homicide arrest rates increased 140% for 13- to 14-year-old boys; 217% for 15-year-old boys; 158% for 16-year-old boys; and 121% for 17-year-old boys between 1985 and 1991. In a news conference, the Council on Crime in America warned that because of the skyrocketing rise in violent crime among teenagers and because the number of 14- to 17-year-old males will increase by 23% by 2005, governments must start now to attach more importance to preventing young people from becoming criminals (Butterfield, 1996).

Homicide of Women. According to Dannenberg and colleagues (1994), homicide is the fourth leading cause of death from injury among females. The rate is substantially higher among African-American females than white females in all age groups. Homicide is the leading cause of death from injury and also the leading cause of death from all causes in African-American women ages 15 to 34 years. Murder-suicide is another form of violence against women. One half to three fourths of murder-suicides in the United States involve a male who abused and murdered his girlfriend or wife and then committed suicide (Loring and Smith, 1994).

Suicide

The suicide rate in the United States has tripled; suicide is the eighth leading cause of death in all age groups. Suicide is common in younger and younger age groups and in certain populations. The rate of suicide among 10- to 14-year-old adolescents increased 120% between 1980 and 1992 according to the Centers for Disease Control (MMWR, 1995). Suicide is the third leading cause of death for those aged 15 to 34 years and the second leading cause of death for 15- to 24-year-old Native Americans, and these rates are growing (Novello et al., 1992). Guns are used in 60% of teen suicides and are the leading method used by this age group. The Centers for Disease Control reported that if a gun is in the home the odds that potentially suicidal adolescents will kill themselves doubles. Violence against women is also responsible for high rates of female suicides and suicide attempts. Fifty percent of all African-American women and 25% of all white women who attempt suicide do so to escape domestic violence (Sassetti, 1993).

As the age of suicide has changed, so has the cause. The cause of suicide before 1980 was depression when the predominate victim was a white older male. Suicide among youth no longer totally fits the depression profile. It is more likely an impulsive act as a result of trouble at home, in school, or with the police. That, combined with weapons in the home, creates a deadly combination (Rosenberg and Fenley, 1991).

Suicide is the leading cause of death in jail populations where the victim is usually an unmarried white male in young adulthood (USDHHS, 1990). Seventy-five percent of these victims were arrested for nonviolent offenses; 27% of the offenses are related to drugs or alcohol. More than half of these victims were intoxicated when first incarcerated. High-risk times for suicide are immediately after admission, after adjudication when the inmate is returned to the jail facility, after hearing bad news regarding themselves or their family, or after some type of humiliation or rejection. Those inmates who are severely depressed are also at greater risk.

Assault

Each year an estimated 650,000 women are raped, and 1.5 to 2.5 million children and 700,000 to 1.1 million elderly Americans are abused or neglected (Novello,

1991). Each year more than 500,000 Americans visit emergency rooms as a result of a violent injury (Blow and Gest, 1993). Houk and Warren (1991) reported that assault, primarily in the context of marital or dating relationships, is a major source of injury among African-American females. It has been reported that 22 to 35% of all women seeking treatment in emergency rooms are abused. Annual estimates of the impact of injuries from family violence on health care are 21,000 hospitalizations that total 99,800 days; 39,000 physician visits and 28,700 emergency room visits for a total medical cost of $44,393,700 (Loring and Smith, 1994).

Impact of Guns

Surgeon General C. Everett Koop (Koop and Lundberg, 1992) reported that from 1960 to 1980 the U.S. population increased by 26%, but the homicide rate caused by guns increased 160%. In 1990, comparison of death by handguns in the United States with other industrialized nations showed the following:

Australia, 10 deaths
Sweden, 13 deaths
Great Britain, 22 deaths
Japan, 87 deaths
Switzerland, 91 deaths
United States, 10,567 deaths

When the 1990 rates are compared with those of 1992, the number of homicides from handguns in the United States rose to 13,200; Canada had 128, Japan had 60, and the United Kingdom had 33 (Gibson, 1995). Cotton (1992) reported that during the 1980s almost three times as many people died from gunshot wounds as died from acquired immunodeficiency syndrome, and guns killed more than five times the number of Americans killed during the Vietnam War. For the first time in the history of the Texas, firearms killed more people in 1991 than did motor vehicle crashes. On an average day, more than 700 Americans are shot; 30 of them are children (Novello et al., 1992); and 65 of those shot die (Blow and Gest, 1993).

The death rate from gunshot wounds varies with age groups. It is the leading cause of death among people aged 15 to 24 years. Three of four homicide victims and two of three suicide victims die of gunshot wounds. More than 50% of the victims are younger than 25 years, and 85% are males.

Guns are present in nearly half of homes in the United States, and one in three of those is a handgun.

Handguns are of particular concern, and although they account for about one third of all firearms in the United States they account for two thirds of all firearm-related deaths (Cotton, 1992). Dannenberg and others (1994, p. 137) stated that "many public health professionals believe that the widespread private ownership of firearms is a major contributor to the high homicide rates in the United States compared to other countries." People may feel that they need a handgun in their home for protection; however, statistics show that a handgun kept in a home is 43 times as more likely to be used to commit suicide, to commit criminal homicide, or to unintentionally kill someone as compared with killing someone while defending oneself (Dannenberg et al., 1994).

Guns do not cause violence, but they greatly raise the severity of the health consequences (Rosenberg et al., 1992). Major trauma centers report that between 20% and 25% of nonfatal gunshots wounds cause permanent neurological impairment. The violence produced by guns is more severe and also is more likely to lead to death instead of just injury.

The cost of violence from guns is enormous. The cost per person of firearm-related fatalities is the highest of any injury-related death, averaging $373,000 per death, much of which comes from lost potential earnings of disproportionately young victims. Hospital costs for treating patients with firearm injuries in Washington, DC, hospitals were $20.4 million in 1989, according to a 1994 study by Ozmar. Eighty-five percent of the cost of hospital treatment of firearm injuries is unreimbursed care (Elders, 1994). At San Francisco General Hospital, 86% of hospital costs from firearm injuries are paid by taxes (Cotton, 1992). The cost of intentional injury nationally is estimated to amount to $24 billion of the total annual national injury costs.

As lethal weapons proliferate, this final decade of the 20th century is likely to be characterized by ever-increasing violence that will supplant drugs as a major public health problem and social concern.

(Marwick, 1992, p. 2993).

VIOLENCE OF AGGREGATES
Youth-Related Violence

Violence is taking a toll on youth as an aggregate population. Violent crimes among youth are increasing, and crimes such as homicide, rape, robbery, and aggravated assault are much more prevalent among adolescents than among adults (Mercy, 1993). Mercy reports that almost 50% of the nonfatal crimes of violence in the United States in 1989 were committed by offenders between 12 and 24 years of age, and teenage victims named their attacker as an acquaintance almost twice as often as adults did.

The average age of both homicide offenders and victims has grown younger and younger in recent years. Most of the increased homicide rates among our youth are attributable to death caused by firearms. Mason (1991) reported that homicide is the second leading cause of juvenile injury death and is second only to motor vehicle crashes. Gunshot wound is the cause of death about 75% of the time. Table 21–1 lists risk factors for youth-related violence.

Violence among youth exists across our country and is not a problem just of minority communities and inner cities, but it is more concentrated there (Belloni et al., 1991). It puts a disproportionate burden on minority communities. In 1992 a Social and Health Assessment was conducted on 6th, 8th, and 10th graders in New Haven, Connecticut. Seventy-four percent of those surveyed felt unsafe in their home, neighborhood, or school, and 40% had witnessed a shooting or stabbing during the previous year. Psychologically, the result of chronic fear of violence is the necessity to accommodate the threat and lack of safety into the psychological development of the youth. This adaptive pattern then becomes normalized, expected, and reasonable. The results of such normalization will be to sustain the climate of violence (Gibson, 1995).

Shooting or killing someone has even become the symbol of a new rite of passage and the bestowing of manhood in some parts of our country (Ozmar, 1994). Minority youth are particularly impacted, and violence among them is both a large and complex problem. The toll of homicide and assault among young minority men, both African-American and Hispanic, is well known. However, the toll of rape, sexual assault, and spousal abuse upon young minority women is generally underreported by both the victims and the media.

Violence is increasingly used by adolescents and children to handle disputes. Many children are not taught nonviolent ways of resolving differences. Mason (1991) reported that fighting is a prominent cause of injuries among high school students and often precedes homicides. Studies have indicated that homicide or suicide by youths is almost always an impulsive act that is immediately regretted. Unfortunately, in the case of suicide, the impulsive act destroys

Table 21–1
Risk Factors for Youth-Related Violence*

Risk Factor	Comment
Poverty	The most closely correlated risk factor with youth violence is low family income.
Repeated exposure to violence	Children in inner city neighborhoods are often exposed to chronic and extreme violence, enough that inner city children often exhibit the same symptoms of posttraumatic stress as children living in war-torn countries.
Drugs	Not only does a pharmacological connection exist between aggressive behavior and consumption of drugs and alcohol, but there is also a financial connection between the drug trade and violence.
Easy access to firearms	About 50% of all households in the United States own a gun.
Unstable family life	Seventy percent of juvenile offenders come from single-parent homes. Single-parent homes correlate with elevated rates of school dropout, which in turn correlates with elevated violent crime rates.
Family violence	Juvenile delinquency has been found to correlate with a history of childhood abuse and neglect.
Delinquent peer groups	Gangs are using ever-more lethal weapons to engage in increasingly violent behavior.
Media violence	By the time a child reaches seventh grade, he or she has witnessed 8000 murders and more than 100,000 other acts of violence on television. Witnessing violence increases both short- and long-term aggression, desensitization, and fear in children.

*Multiple risk factors have a cumulative effect.
Adapted from Ruttenberg H: The limited promise of public health methodologies to prevent youth violence. Yale Law 103:1885–1912, 1994.

one life and in homicide it destroys two lives. A news report told of a gang war that has been ongoing almost a year. It has now claimed five lives, including one grandmother who was standing in her yard and was shot accidentally. The cause of the war was an incident where a member of one gang accidentally stepped on the shoe of a member of another gang.

Many young people have become immune to violence. They believe that they are invincible. There is tremendous peer pressure to experiment with guns, and their impulsiveness and immaturity results in tragedy which changes their lives forever.

Domestic Violence

Domestic violence can be described as *a pattern of coercive behaviors that are perpetrated by someone who is or was in an intimate relationship with the victim.* These behaviors include battering resulting in injury, psychological abuse, and sexual assault. These acts result in progressive social isolation, deprivation, and intimidation of the victim. Abuse is repetitive and

often escalates in frequency and severity. The repetition and severity of aggression are aided by the fact that the victim is readily available, the amount of time at risk is high, and assaults can be carried out in private (Boyer and Fine, 1992).

Battering, spousal abuse, wife abuse, and domestic violence are terms used to describe violence within an intimate relationship. Partners do not need to be married; violence may begin in casual or dating relationships. Violence is directed against women by men 90 to 95% of the time; however, it may also be directed by women against women in lesbian relationships and in a small percentage of cases by women against men. It cuts across all ethnic, racial, socioeconomic, and educational lines and affects 2 to 4 million women in the United States every year. Surveys vary in their reports on the incidence, but it is estimated that domestic violence may affect one fourth of all American families. Domestic violence is a crime; however, it is the least reported crime in our country.

Domestic violence is the single greatest cause of injury to women. A woman is beaten in our country every 10 to 12 seconds. Twenty-two to 35% of women seeking emergency treatment do so as the result of a battering incident (Loring and Smith, 1994). Sexual abuse occurs in almost half of the battered population. The majority of women in a study by Campbell (1989) reported that their husbands believed it was their right to have sex whenever they wanted. Women reported that they were subjected to forced intercourse when they were ill or had recently given birth. They also reported forced anal intercourse, being hit, burned or kicked during sex, or forced to have sex with animals or while their children were watching (Campbell and Alford, 1989). Violence often increases in frequency and severity. The *FBI Uniform Crime Report* states that 42% of abused women ultimately are killed by their male partners (Stein, 1994).

Abuse During Pregnancy. Abuse frequently begins during pregnancy. The reported incidence of battering during pregnancy varies. Gelles' study in 1975 found that 25% of the women victims were beaten while they were pregnant. Research during the 1980s by Walker, Stacey, Shupe, Fagan, Stewart, and Hansen reported an incidence between 40% and 60% (McFarlane and Parker, 1994). The Surgeon General's 1986 Workshop on Violence recommended that all pregnant women be screened for abuse because pregnancy was such a high-risk period for battering.

Battered pregnant women report blows to the abdomen, injuries to their breasts and genitalia, and sexual assault (Helton et al., 1987). The results of such violence are spontaneous abortion, stillbirths, and preterm deliveries. Parker and associates, McFarlane, and Soeken, (1994) analyzed danger assessment scores and compared abused pregnant women and abused nonpregnant women. Women abused during pregnancy had significantly higher danger assessment scores and were deemed at greater risk for medical complications of pregnancy, delivery of lower birthweight infants, and homicide. Pregnancy does not exclude women from the danger of beating. In fact, pregnancy may increase stresses within the family and provoke an attack.

The Abusive Pattern. The cycle theory of violence was developed by Walker (1979) and explains a common abusive pattern of violence containing three phases: tension, explosion, and contrition. During the **tension** phase, there may be minor battering incidents in which the woman attempts to cope by using techniques that may have been successful before. The second and most dangerous phase is the **explosive** phase. It is inevitable as tension builds and is characterized by rage out of control. Walker reported that *the man cannot seem to stop even if the woman is severely injured.* After the attack is over, shock and disbelief occur in both the batterer and the victim. Unless the injury is severe, usually no medical help is sought. However, if the police are called, it is usually during this phase. The last phase is one of **loving kindness and contrition** by the batterer where he attempts to make up for his behavior with pleas and promises (Fig. 21–1).

The objective of the abuser is to exert power and control over his victim. The Domestic Abuse Intervention Project in Duluth, Minnesota, has developed a wheel of violence that depicts the types of power and control that are used. This includes emotional abuse and intimidation, minimizing, denying and blaming,

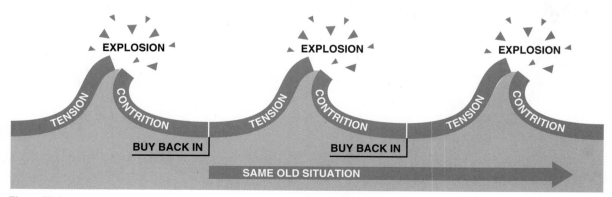

Figure 21–1
Wave pattern of violence. (Redrawn based on cycle of violence from The Battered Woman. By Lenore E. Walker. Copyright © 1979 by Lenore E. Walker. Reprinted by permission of Harper Collins Publishers.)

coercion and threats, isolation, economic abuse, and using children, economics, and male privilege. Figure 21–2 depicts the power and control wheel.

Effects of Abuse. The effects of repeated battering have been compared to those seen in posttraumatic stress disorder. Posttraumatic stress disorder is described in the *Diagnostic and Statistical Manual of Mental Disorders* as "a serious threat to one's life or physical integrity" or "a serious threat or harm to one's children" (Browne, 1993). Stress characterizes the lives of women in relationships with violent mates. On the list of stressor categories, ongoing physical or sexual abuse is number 5 in the extreme stressor category. The only higher category is number 6 and includes captivity as a hostage or in concentration camps.

When subjected to repeated abuse, a woman experiences a variety of responses, including shock, denial, confusion, withdrawal, psychological numb-

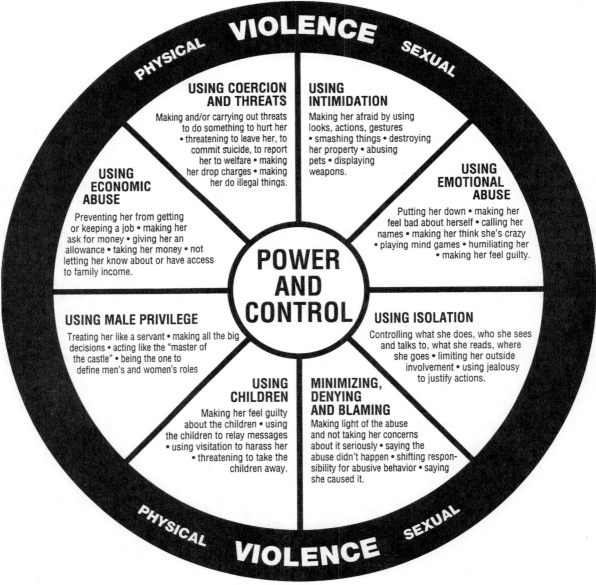

Figure 21–2
Domestic Abuse Intervention Project, 206 West Fourth Street, Duluth, Minnesota 55806. Used by permission.

ing, and fear. She lives in anticipatory terror and often suffers chronic fatigue and tension, disturbed sleeping and eating patterns, and nightmares. In the long term, this results in emotional numbing, extreme passivity, and helplessness (Browne, 1993).

Fear and helplessness are the primary reasons many women do not readily leave an abusive situation. The legal system is cumbersome, and often women who seek help by restraining orders or other judicial means find that there may not be real safety in such methods. Other factors that keep a woman in an abusive situation are culture, religion, and economics. Frequently, women who leave the abusive situation face serious economic problems and may fall into poverty. The most dangerous time for the woman is when she leaves. She is more likely to be killed at this time than any other time in the relationship.

Hiraki and Grambs (1990), in their work with women who are beaten, identified those women who are the *most likely to leave* a battering situation. These include women (1) who have resources such as money, friends, family, and support; (2) who have power (a job, credit cards, status outside the family); (3) with no children; (4) who were not abused as children; (5) who did not see their mothers beaten; (6) involved in battering situations that are frequent or severe; (7) whose partner begins to beat children in the family.

Child Abuse

There are four basic types of child abuse: (1) physical abuse; (2) child neglect, both physical and emotional; (3) emotional maltreatment; and (4) sexual abuse.

Physical abuse is an intentional injury inflicted by other than accidental means on a child by another person. The most common type of physical abuse is beating with an instrument. This can cause cuts, bruises, burns, and fractures. The type of physical injury varies only with the imagination of the adult. Parents often select a method to meet what they see as the disobedience of the child. This may produce a patterned injury, which is one that gives some clue to how the child was injured (Mittleman et al., 1987). Thus, a child who walks where he is not supposed to might have his feet dipped in scalding water and the burns would cover the stocking area of the foot. A child who touches a light cord or light plug might be beaten with it producing a looped or linear pattern. A child who plays with matches or the stove might have his hand placed in the flame. A crying child or one who

talks back might have hot pepper or Tabasco sauce poured into his mouth or might be suffocated with a pillow.

Male children are more likely to be abused than female children. Young children from ages 2 to 5 years are often the most frequently injured. Infants are in the greatest danger of severe injury or death because of their small size in contrast to the size of the punishing adult.

Shaken baby syndrome is an example of abuse where a blow is not struck. Shaking can cause trauma at the brain stem–spinal cord junction, and the morbidity and mortality for this injury are high. Serious and potentially permanent damage may occur, which includes retinal hemorrhages, spinal cord injuries and brain damage because of hemorrhage and contusions. Rotational forces of the head during the shaking episode is thought to be the mechanism of injury (Monaco and Brooks, 1994). This type of injury is usually inflicted by men, the spouse or boyfriend of the mother. The next most likely person to inflict this type of injury is a female babysitter (Wolfner, Gelles, 1993).

Child neglect is negligent treatment or maltreatment of a child by a person responsible for the child's welfare. The term includes both acts and omissions on the part of the responsible person and includes failure to provide a loving environment in which a child can thrive, learn, and develop. Physical neglect entails the failure to provide for basic needs. These include needs for safety, food, clothing, and shelter. In addition, failure to provide for the health needs of a child can also be construed as neglect. Emotional neglect is similar to emotional maltreatment in that results can be observed in the child. Its cause, however, is the lack of sensitivity and love shown by the parent for the child. The results are equally detrimental to the child.

Emotional maltreatment is willfully inflicting on a child unjustifiable mental suffering, causing the child to be emotionally damaged. The behavior evident in the child may demonstrate a substantial impairment in a normal range of performance and behavior such as an overly compliant or passive child or the child who is very aggressive and apt to fly into a rage. These children frequently do not progress with the normal rate of physical, intellectual, and emotional development. Because emotional abuse is almost always done in the home and is not witnessed by others and because the symptoms displayed by the child can occur in children who are not abused, treatment of these children is very difficult. Examples of emotional abuse include locking a child in a closet for a prolonged period of time, tying a child to a bedpost, or engaging in bizarre acts of torture. Subtle abuse might include name calling such as "you're stupid," "you're a slut," "you're bad or evil." Name calling can destroy a child's self-concept.

Sexual abuse is any sexual activity between an adult and a child including use of a child for sexual exploitation, prostitution, or pornography. Incest is the term used for sexual relations between close family members such as father-daughter, mother-son, or siblings within the family. Sexual abuse often involves a person known to the child, a relative or friend. It may occur over a prolonged period of time, and threats to the child may be used to ensure secrecy. Sexual abuse has many long-term consequences. A study by Boyer and Fine (1992) showed that two thirds of pregnant adolescents had been sexually abused. Sexual abuse can cause low self-esteem, psychiatric illness, depression, suicide ideation, drug and alcohol addiction, negative sexual esteem and sexual maladjustment, delayed developmental processes, and planned pregnancy to escape from an abusive situation. Table 21–2 describes physical and behavioral indicators of child abuse and neglect.

Child abuse is a socially learned behavior and is generational. Wolfner and Gelles conducted the second national violence survey in 1993. They concluded that a psychosocial diathesis-stress model can best explain the incidence of child abuse in certain families. In this model, there is a socially learned or constitutional predisposition for violence. When this is combined with a stress, violent behavior is likely to occur. This model can be compared to an allergy to pollen. The allergy exists in the individual, but it is not manifested until exposure to the pollen. Then sneezing and other allergic signs will occur. This model helps explain that, although abuse crosses all socioeconomic, educational, racial, and cultural lines, the youngest, poorest, most socially isolated, and economically frustrated caretakers, and therefore the most stressed, are the most likely to act violently toward their children (Wolfner and Gelles, 1993). Because violence can be socially learned (by having been abused as a child by a parent; by witnessing abuse inflicted on another person, usually the mother; by witnessing violence as a response to conflict in the media and on the streets), responding violently can also be unlearned.

Abuse of the Elderly

The exact number of abused elderly is not available because elder abuse is significantly underreported, even more so than child abuse. However, estimates indicate that from 1 to 10% of the elderly population suffers some form of maltreatment, and 2 million cases of elder abuse in family settings were reported during 1989 (Ramsey-Klawsnik, 1993). The most likely victims of elder abuse are elders in poor health, poor women of advanced age who suffer physical and mental impairments, and those living with others rather than those living alone. The perpetrator of the abuse can be a relative or family member who is living with the elderly person, a relative or family member who is visiting an elder who lives at home, or a caregiver. Research suggests that the most common abuser is a relative, particularly an adult child, and that elder abuse tends to escalate in incidence and severity over time.

When an elderly person can no longer care for himself or herself because of physical or mental infirmities of age, what happens to that person may depend on whether there are relatives who can provide care or whether the person has financial resources to purchase care in his or her own home, in a retirement home, or in a residential care facility. If none of these possibilities exist, the elderly person may continue to live alone. This may be an unsatisfactory way of dealing with the problem because of safety issues. The caregivers often become the adult children, nieces, or nephews or another relative of the elderly person. This generation of individuals in their 40s, 50s, and 60s are often called the "sandwich generation," who begin by caring for their children on one end of the time frame and end by having to provide care for their parents on the other end of the time frame.

Care of an aging parent may require more sacrifice and commitment than did care for children. When providing care for children, their dependency on the caregiver usually lessens as the child grows older. However, when caring for an aging parent or relative, they become more and more dependent and may become cognitively or physically impaired, which may be a factor in the likelihood of abuse. The elder may not know who they are or they may suffer changes in personality that make it very difficult for their adult children to care for them. They may need to be lifted, which may be difficult for someone not used to lifting. They may need assistance walking,

Table 21–2
Physical and Behavioral Indicators of Child Abuse and Neglect

Physical Indicators	Behavioral Indicators
Physical Abuse	
The skin is the largest and most frequently injured organ system. It may show	Wary of adult contacts
• Unexplained bruises and welts in various stages of healing that may form patterns	Apprehensive when other children cry
• Unexplained burns by cigars or cigarettes or immersion burns (socklike, glovelike, or on buttocks or genitalia)	Constantly on the alert for danger
• Rope burns	Extremes of behavior; aggressiveness or passive and withdrawn
• Unexplained lacerations or abrasions	Frightened of parents
Skeletal injuries	Afraid to go home
• Unexplained fractures in various stages of healing; multiple or spiral fractures	Report injury by parents
• Unexplained injuries to mouth, lips, gums, eyes, or external genitalia	
Physical Neglect	
Hunger	Begging or stealing food
Poor hygiene	Alone at inappropriate times or for prolonged periods
Poorly or inappropriately dressed	Delinquency
Lack of supervision for prolonged periods of time	Stealing
Lack of medical or dental care	Early arrival and late departure from school
Constant fatigue, listlessness, or falling asleep in class	Reporting no caretaker
Sexual Abuse	
Difficulty in walking or sitting	Negative self-esteem
Torn, stained, or bloody underwear	Inability to trust and function in intimate relationships
Genital pain or itching	Cognitive and motor dysfunctions
Bruises or bleeding from the external genitalia, vaginal, or anal areas	Deficits in personal and social skills
Venereal disease, especially in preteens	Bizarre, sophisticated, or unusual sexual behavior or knowledge
Drug and alcohol abuse	Delinquency or runaway
Developmental delays	Suicide ideation
Teen pregnancy	Reporting of sexual assault
Emotional Maltreatment	
Failure to thrive	Behavior extremes from passivity to aggression
Lags in physical development	Habit and conduct disorders (sucking and biting to antisocial behavior and destructiveness)
Speech disorders	Neurotic traits
Developmental delays	Attempted suicide

toileting, or eating, which takes time that the caregiver may not feel they have. Another factor that can come to bear on an aging parent is the care they gave their children when they were young. If they were abusive to their children, the adult child may use the elder's dependency as an opportunity to finally respond in an abusive manner to them.

All of these factors cause stress that may lead to abuse. This is especially true in families in which violence is a response to stress. Stress in the primary caretaker can be caused by the needs of the elderly person exceeding the family's ability to meet them as well as personal stresses of the caretaker such as the interference with their job, illness, or other family problems.

There are five commonly described types of abuse

Table 21–3 Indicators of Possible Elder Abuse	
Physical Indicators	**Behavioral Indicators**
• Any injury that has not been cared for properly • Any injury incompatible with the history • Lack of care for injuries • Evidence of inadequate care • Evidence of inadequate or inappropriate administration of medicine • Poor skin hygiene • Absence of hair, or hemorrhage beneath the scalp • Signs of confinement (tied to furniture, bathroom fixtures, locked in room)	• Fear • Withdrawal • Depression • Helplessness • Resignation • Hesitation to talk openly • Implausible stories • Confusion or disorientation • Ambivalence, contradictory statements not caused by mental dysfunction • Anger • Denial • Nonresponsiveness • Agitation, anxiety
Family-Caregiver Indicators	**Financial Indicators**
• Will not let the elder speak for himself or herself or see others without presence of the caregiver • Aggressive behavior • Attitude of indifference or anger • Blaming the elder for things beyond his or her control such as incontinence • Problems with alcohol or drugs • Conflicting accounts of incidents by the family and victim • Unwillingness or reluctance to comply with service providers in planning for care of elder • Indications of inappropriate sexual relationship • Withholding security and affection • Lack of amenities such as grooming items, clothing when the estate can afford to buy it	• Unusual activity in bank accounts • Activity in bank accounts that is inappropriate to the elder • Concern by relatives that too much money is being spent for the care • Refusal to spend money on the care of the elder • Power of attorney given when the elder is unable to give a valid power of attorney • Recent will change when the elder is incapable of making a will • Recent acquaintances expressing undying affection for a wealthy elder • Recent change of title of house in favor of a "friend" when the elder is incapable of understanding the nature of the transaction • Isolation of elder from old friends and family so that the elder becomes alienated from those who care about him/her so he/she becomes overly dependent on the caretaker • Promises of lifelong care in exchange for willing or deeding of all property or money to the caretaker • Checks and documents signed when the elder cannot write • Missing personal belongings such as art, silverware, jewelry • Placement outside the home not commensurate with the financial ability of the elder • Signatures on checks that do not resemble the elder's signature

Adapted from Carlton L: Elder Abuse Prevention Protocol. San Francisco, San Francisco Task Force, 1983.

and neglect of the elderly: (1) physical abuse is the purposeful infliction of physical pain or injury or unnecessary physical restraint; (2) psychological-emotional abuse includes verbal assault, threats, provoking fear, or isolation; (3) sexual abuse is unwanted sexual contact; (4) physical neglect is the withholding of personal care, food, medications, or medical care or the lack of supervision, withholding companionship, or intimidation or humiliation; and (5) financial exploitation, theft, and misuse of money or property.

A helpless elderly adult is in the same vulnerable position as an abused child. Someone must become aware of the problem in order for her or him to receive help. Lists of possible indicators help the professional become aware of possible abusive situations. None is conclusive in itself; however, they alert the professional to the need for further careful and full assessment. Table 21–3 lists the indicators of possible abuse of the elderly.

THE PUBLIC HEALTH PERSPECTIVE

Dealing with violence has traditionally been the responsibility of the criminal justice system in the United States. However, violence has been named a **public health epidemic** in the United States. Violence has tremendous impact not only on morbidity and mortality but also on quality of life and health care resources. Violence is a problem of such magnitude that it has reached beyond criminal justice methods of protecting the public. Dr. William Foege, director of the Carter Center at Emory University, observed that "public health is in the business of continually redefining the unacceptable." This has been true in controlling infectious diseases such as polio and smallpox; it can also be true in interpersonal violence. Public health focuses on prevention. It is a systematic, upstream thinking approach, seeking to ensure health for all and using core public health functions to determine the causes, create policy and programs to ameliorate the problem, and institute assurance measures to monitor and evaluate those programs and policies for their effect.

In 1990, the USDHHS Public Health Service released *Healthy People 2000*. This national effort, involving more than 10,000 people, including expert working groups, national organizations, all state health departments, the Institute of Medicine, and the National Academy of Sciences as well as the Public

Health Service, developed the report with Objectives for the Year 2000 to aid policymakers to invest in the identified priority areas to improve the health of the people of the United States. Section 7 in the report deals with violent and abusive behavior and 18 Year 2000 objectives related to reduction of violence have been identified. These are divided into objectives for health status, risk reduction, and services and protection and focus on six areas: homicide and assaultive behavior, domestic violence, child abuse, sexual assault, suicide, and firearm injury (USDHHS, 1990). Table 21–4 lists the Year 2000 objectives related to violent and abusive behavior.

Public health has many resources that can be mobilized that are practical and time tested and that work. Rosenberg and coworkers (1992) identified three public health methods that should be the approach to violence prevention. The first is health event surveillance; the second, epidemiological analysis; the third, intervention design and evaluation focused on a single, clear outcome. These public health methods have been used with a wide degree of success on not only infectious diseases but other health problems as well (Mercy, 1993). The challenge that faces public health is the fact that violence intertwines with many other problems such as poverty, unemployment, social injustice, racism, drugs, and so on. All of these are major social problems that have no easy remedies.

PREVENTION OF VIOLENCE IN THE COMMUNITY

The nurse who cares for victims of violence must be a skilled clinician with good assessment skills who is knowledgeable about the problem and resources available in the community. The nurse may also be in a position of dealing with individuals and families before abuse has occurred. She or he can educate families in the care and nurturing of family members, growth and development of children, and needs of the elderly. Components of a comprehensive program to reduce violence in the community are found in Table 21–5.

Primary Prevention

The goal of primary prevention is the promotion of optimal parenting and family wellness. Education plays a major part of primary prevention—from education of children in grade schools regarding healthy family life and nonviolent methods of conflict resolution to education of professionals to increase

Table 21–4
Year 2000 Objectives Related to Violent and Abusive Behaviors

Health Status Objectives

- 7.1 Reduce homicides to no more than 7.2 per 100,000 (Baseline 8.5).
- 7.2 Reduce suicides to no more than 10.5 per 100,000 people (Baseline 11.7).
- 7.3 Reduce firearm-related deaths to no more than 11.6 per 100,000 people from major causes (Baseline 14.6 in 1990).
- 7.4 Reduce to less than 22.6 per 1,000 children the rising incidence of maltreatment of children younger than age 18 (Baseline 22.6).
- 7.5 Reduce physical abuse directed at women by male partners to no more than 27 per 1,000 couples (Baseline 30).
- 7.6 Reduce assault injuries among people aged 12 and older to no more than 8.7 per 1,000 people (Baseline 9.7).
- 7.7 Reduce rape and attempted rape of women aged 12 and older to no more than 108 per 100,000 women (Baseline 12.0).
- 7.8 Reduce by 15 percent the incidence of injurious suicide attempts among adolescents aged 14 through 17.

Risk Reduction Objectives

- 7.9 Reduce to 110 per 1,000 the incidence of physical fighting among adolescents aged 14 through 17 (Baseline 137 incidents per 1,000 high school students per month).
- 7.10 Reduce to 86 per 1,000 the incidence of weapon carrying by adolescents aged 14 through 17 (Baseline 107 incidents per 1,000 high school students per month).
- 7.11 Reduce by 20 percent the proportion of people who possess weapons that are inappropriately stored and therefore dangerously available.
- 7.12 Extend protocols for routinely identifying, treating, and properly referring suicide attempters, victims of sexual assault, and victims of spouse, elder, and child abuse to at least 90 percent of hospital emergency departments.
- 7.13 Extend to at least 45 states implementation of unexplained child death review systems (Baseline 33 states).
- 7.14 Increase to at least 30 the number of states in which at least 50 percent of children identified as neglected or physically or sexually abused receive physical and mental evaluation with appropriate follow-up as a means of breaking the intergenerational cycle of abuse (No baseline data).
- 7.15 Reduce to less than 10 percent the proportion of battered women and their children turned away from emergency housing due to lack of space (Baseline 40 percent).
- 7.16 Increase to at least 50 percent the proportion of elementary and secondary schools that teach nonviolent conflict resolution skills, preferably as a part of comprehensive school health education (No baseline data).
- 7.17 Extend coordinated, comprehensive violence prevention programs to at least 80 percent of local jurisdictions with populations over 100,000.
- 7.18 Increase to 50 the number of states with officially established protocols that engage mental health, alcohol and drug, and public health authorities with corrections authorities to facilitate identification and appropriate intervention to prevent suicide by jail inmates.

1995 Addition

- 7.19 Enact in 50 states and the District of Columbia laws requiring that firearms be properly stored to minimize access and the likelihood of discharge by minors (Baseline zero states in 1993.)

From U.S. Department of Health and Human Services: Healthy People 2000. Washington, DC, U.S. Department of Health and Human Services, Public Health Service, 1990.

their awareness of the problem of violence and facilitate case detection and provision for early treatment. Community services are needed so that there is a place to provide care for families before serious injury occurs to any member. Nurses can be in the forefront in communities and act as an advocate for those in need of services. The nurse can work in the community to educate citizens about the problem of violence, potential causes of violence, and the com-

munity services that are necessary to serve those in need. Reduction of violence in the media and control of handguns and assault weapons are also essential.

Primary prevention of abuse against women must begin at a societal level, helping to change attitudes toward violence and toward women. It should include education of children that no one has the right to beat another person. Children who are in abusive families and witness their mothers being beaten are at particular

Table 21–5
Components of a Comprehensive Program to Reduce Violence for Individuals, Families, and the Community

Individuals	Family	Community
Primary Prevention—Goal: Promotion of Optimal Parenting and Family Wellness		
• Family life education in schools, churches, and communities • Educating children on methods of conflict resolution • Birth control services for sexually active teens • Child care education for teens who babysit • Preventive mental health services for adults and children • Training for professionals in early detection of violence	• Parenting classes in hospitals, schools, and other community agencies • Provision of bonding opportunities for new parents • Referral of new families to community health nurses after early discharge from the hospital for follow-up services • Social services for families	• Community education concerning family violence • Reduction of media violence • Development of community support services such as crisis lines, respite placement for children, respite care for families with dependent elderly members, shelters for battered women and their children • Handgun control
Secondary Prevention—Goal: Diagnosis of and Service for Families in Stress		
• Nursing assessment for evidence of family violence in all health care settings • A well thought-out safety plan for victims • Knowledge of legal options to help ensure safety • Shelter or foster home placement for victims	• Social services for individuals or families • Referral to self-help groups in the community • Referral to community agencies that provide services for victims	• All health professionals skilled in assessment of violence and equipped with protocols for dealing with the victim to help ensure their safety • Hospital emergency rooms and trauma centers with 24-hour response, reporting, case intake, coordination with legal and medical authorities, coordination with voluntary agencies who have services, coordination with social services departments for provision of services • Death review teams to review deaths from injury, especially for infants and children • Public authority involvement, by police, district attorneys, and courts • Epidemiological tracking and evaluation of violence • Handgun control
Tertiary Prevention—Goal: Reeducation and Rehabilitation of Violent Families		
• Empowerment strategies for battered women • Professional counseling services for individuals	• Parenting reeducation—formal training in childrearing • Professional counseling services for families • Self-help groups	• Foster homes, shelters, and care for the elderly • Public authority involvement • Follow-up care for known cases of abuse • Gun control

risk. Boys are at risk to grow to adulthood and abuse women with whom they have an intimate relationship. Girls are at risk for developing low self-esteem and ending up in an abusive relationship. Primary prevention must focus on stopping the generational aspect of abuse.

Primary prevention for the prevention of child abuse must include education about parenting. In a nation in which people are educated to perform many varieties of skills, we are yet to value the education to be a parent. Individuals become parents by being handed a child. That does not necessarily qualify them for the responsibility. Classes for parents should focus on more than preparation for labor and physical care for the baby. The realities of parenthood, the effect of fatigue on a new mother, the need for support from a significant other or family member, and fears and questions of the new parents must be addressed. This has become much more difficult because mothers and infants are being discharged from the hospital early, some within 6 hours of delivery. Nurses in the hospital are no longer in the position of having sufficient time to assist a mother in caring for the newborn. There must be follow-up by hospitals and/or public health agencies to ensure that the new parents can adequately care for their infant. This is especially true of any person deemed to be in the high-risk category: teenage mothers, mothers without supportive others, or women who have a history of spousal abuse.

Support for caregivers can help in primary prevention of abuse of the elderly. Education about the needs of the elderly and the need for respite care for the caregiver should be available to middle-aged citizens as they face the care of aging parents. Just as a parent does not know all about parenting simply by having a baby, so an adult who may not have had intimate contact with anyone of advanced age needs to be educated about the developmental processes and needs of the aging.

Secondary Prevention

The goal of secondary prevention in a comprehensive program is to provide diagnosis of and service to families in stress that facilitates early diagnosis and treatment. Safety of family members is critical. Family violence does not occur just from 9 to 5 during weekdays. Around-the-clock assistance is crucial. There must be access to legal options for women who have no money. Shelters may be available to offer sanctuary to a victim and to shield a woman and her children from danger. A shelter can temporarily provide safety while the woman plans for her future. However, in 1993 there were only 1300 shelters in existence in the 3200 counties in the United States (Velsor-Friedrich, 1994). Public health surveillance is important to obtain accurate numbers for intentional injuries of all individuals. Death review teams can play an important part by reviewing cases of death from injury to determine whether the injury was intentional or unintentional. Removing guns from the hands of children and violent individuals is also an important facet in reducing deaths from violence.

Secondary prevention begins with assessment of a victim who is battered. The time that provides a consistent opportunity for assessment of women is during pregnancy. This is the one time in a woman's life that she may access the health care system on a regular basis. Women should be alone when they are interviewed about battering. They should be asked in a matter of fact way, and the health care provider should not show shock or dismay at their response. A simple three-question abuse assessment screen has been developed by the Nursing Research Consortium on Violence and Abuse. The three questions should be asked of **all** women at **each visit.** If the woman responds yes to the questions about physical battering, she should be handed a pencil and allowed to mark the areas on the body where she has been injured. If the nurse observes injuries, careful and detailed charting should be done. Table 21–6 provides the abuse assessment screening tool that was developed by the Nursing Research Consortium on Violence and Abuse. It may be reproduced and used in assessing women in a wide variety of settings.

Once the existence of a violent situation is known, the victim must be helped to plan for her safety. She may not be ready to leave her situation; however, it is wise to explore her options with her and help her plan ahead. She should have knowledge of legal options and how to access them. She should be asked about what resources she has, including friends and family, and if she could enlist their support if needed. Some states that have mandatory reporting laws for spousal abuse have developed protocols for nurses who deal with the victims. Review of these protocols can help the nurse become familiar with the questions to ask the client and the suggestions she should make to help the woman make a safety plan. A safety plan is essential in providing comprehensive care. It should be discussed with a woman in privacy and placed in the woman's hands if that is safe to do. Table 21–7 is a sample of a safety plan that can be used to help a woman explore her options.

Secondary prevention of child abuse begins with the discovery that the child has suffered from dysfunctional parenting or has been injured. The community health nurse in the home or school may be the one to discover the injured child and institute the report to child protective or emergency services. The nurse can continue to support and educate the parent even though a report must be made. A crucial aspect of providing help and complying with medicolegal requirements is precise charting of the nurse's assessment when a child has been abused. The nurse should fully and completely record what she *actually* observes and refrain from opinions and interpretations. Because documentation may be used in court proceedings that may have direct bearing on the child's welfare, this is especially important.

In secondary prevention of abuse of the elderly, the focus of the nurse should be on the client and his or her needs. The needs of the family, community, and property should not take precedence.

In all care of the elderly, trust in the nurse is an important part of treatment. A single nurse working

Table 21–6
Abuse Assessment Screen

1. WITHIN THE LAST YEAR, have you been hit, slapped, kicked, or otherwise physically hurt by someone? YES NO

   If YES, by whom? _____

   Total number of times _____

2. SINCE YOU'VE BEEN PREGNANT, have you been hit, slapped, kicked, or otherwise physically hurt by someone? YES NO

   If YES, by whom? _____

   Total number of times _____

MARK THE AREA OF INJURY ON THE BODY MAP. SCORE EACH INCIDENT ACCORDING TO THE FOLLOWING SCALE: SCORE

1 = Threats of abuse including use of a weapon _____

2 = Slapping, pushing; no injuries and/or lasting pain _____

3 = Punching, kicking, bruises, cuts, and/or continuing pain _____

4 = Beating up, severe contusions, burns, broken bones _____

5 = Head injury, internal injury, permanent injury _____

6 = Use of weapon; wound from weapon _____

If any of the descriptions for the higher number apply, use the higher number.

3. WITHIN THE LAST YEAR, has anyone forced you to have sexual activities? YES NO

   If YES, by whom? _____

   Total number of times _____

Developed by the Nursing Research Consortium on Violence and Abuse. Readers are encouraged to reproduce and use this assessment tool.

with the client over a long period of time can promote the most favorable climate for improved care. It takes time to gain an elderly client's confidence and to build a trusting relationship. As long as the client can make decisions, he or she should be allowed to. The nurse should also work with all family members or caregivers who provide care for the elderly client and help promote healthier relationships. Stress is a contributing factor to abuse. Helping the caregiver deal with their stress by finding respite care, a home health aide,

---

Table 21–7
Planning for Safety

You can choose to leave or to stay with an abusive person. It is your choice, and your choice alone. We all have the right to say and do what we want and to feel safe all the while. Also, we all have the right to want to save an important relationship. We have the right to protect ourselves and our children while we maintain the relationship.

If You Choose to Leave

Here are some things to consider as you plan to leave the abuser.

Support We all need support people. Do you have people in your life who want to help you and who are able to help?

	Yes	No
Parents?	❑	❑
Brothers and/or sisters?	❑	❑
Friends?	❑	❑
Other relatives?	❑	❑
Counselors?	❑	❑
Support group members?	❑	❑
Others? (specify)	❑	❑

Have these people helped you with past difficulties? Under what circumstances do you think you could call on them for help? What kinds of help do you think you could ask from them?

Basic Survival Needs We all have different ideas about where and how we want to live. Do you have a plan that suits you?

	Yes	No
Do you have a place to live?	❑	❑
Do you have furniture?	❑	❑
Do you have money for food?	❑	❑
Do you have medical care?	❑	❑
Do you have a regular income that is large enough to live on?	❑	❑
Do you have transportation?	❑	❑
Do you have safe, reliable child care?	❑	❑

If you answer no to any question, how would you solve that problem? Can your support people help?

Legal Protection Abusers use different threats to control victims. Many use divorce and custody battles, continued violence, and manipulation. Do you have a plan to deal with these potential problems?

	Yes	No
Will the abuser use legal battles?	❑	❑
Will he try to steal the children?	❑	❑
Will he abuse you if he finds you?	❑	❑
Do you need a restraining order?	❑	❑
Do you need a lawyer?	❑	❑

If you answer yes to any of these questions, how can you solve these problems? Can your support people help?

Table 21–7
Planning for Safety *Continued*

If You Choose to Stay

Here are some things to consider as you plan to return to your partner.

Support   We all need support people. Do you have people in your life who want to help you and who are able to help?

	Yes	No
Parents?	❏	❏
Brothers or sisters?	❏	❏
Friends?	❏	❏
Other relatives?	❏	❏
Counselors?	❏	❏
Support group members?	❏	❏
Others? (specify)	❏	❏

Have these people helped you with past difficulties? Under what circumstances do you think you could call on them for help? What kinds of help do you think you could ask from them?

Basic Survival Needs   We all need a safe place to go in a crisis. Do you have a plan you can carry out?

	Yes	No
Do you have a safe place to go?	❏	❏
Do you have money or a way to get money?	❏	❏
Do you have transportation or a way out?	❏	❏

If you answer no to any question, how would you solve that problem? Can your support people help?

Legal Protection   Abusers use different threats to control victims. Do you have a plan for handling legal problems?

	Yes	No
Do you recognize when he is getting abusive?	❏	❏
Will you get out while you are still safe?	❏	❏
Do you know how to get a restraining order?	❏	❏
Will you call the police for protection?	❏	❏
Do you need a lawyer?	❏	❏

If you answer no to any question, how would you solve that problem? Can your support people help?

From Mid-Valley Women's Crisis Service, P.O. Box 851, Salem, Oregon 97308. Used by permission.

or counseling may help. Most elderly victims live with the offender and are dependent on them; consequently, to help the victim the nurse must also help the offender deal with the stresses that are causing or contributing to the abuse. The caregiver may also have problems such as mental illness or drug or alcohol abuse. Until these problems are dealt with, as long as the elderly person remains in the home, the abuse will most likely continue.

The right to privacy should be respected as should confidentiality. However, in states in which there are mandatory reporting laws for abuse of children, women, or elders, the nurse **must** comply with the law.

Tertiary Prevention

The goal of tertiary prevention is to provide rehabilitative services to violent families. Because of the responsibility to report assault, there will necessarily be involvement of a social service agency or local law enforcement members if an injury has resulted in a report. There may be prosecution and punishment of the abuser or court-ordered removal of the victim from the family situation. Professional counseling services as well as self-help groups can be helpful to the family. Long-term follow-up and supervision may be necessary as in any rehabilitative situation. Tertiary care may take place in shelters or mental health settings and may involve both physical and mental health care.

Tertiary prevention is aimed at rehabilitation of a woman who has been severely beaten. When dealing with an abused woman, the nurse should focus on the person first and not the problem. Accepting the woman as she is and developing a trusting relationship is important in order for the patient to confide in the nurse. Resources within the community should be made available to the patient. Bulletin boards in community health clinic waiting rooms can list telephone numbers of crisis lines and shelters. Nurses can carry cards in their pockets with referral numbers and give them to women they are concerned about to keep for reference. Long-term care is necessary for a battered woman. Maintaining contact with the individual and continuing support is essential for therapeutic nursing intervention. Support in the woman's ability to make decisions, even small ones, can help empower the woman. Empowerment is necessary in order for her to have the strength to change her conditions.

Tertiary care for a victim of child abuse usually involves a family involved in the court system. The family may be referred to the community health nurse by the courts. The nurse may work with the parents while the child is out of the home in foster care after severe abuse, and when a child is replaced with their family the nurse may provide ongoing care and supervision.

Tertiary prevention is important for children and adolescents who were sexually abused. Psychotherapy is necessary to resolve chronic emotional problems that result from sexual abuse. These can be numerous and include anxiety, anger, attacks of hysteria, and somatic complaints such as headaches, abdominal distress, and concern with the genitourinary tract in younger children. Older girls may have increased substance abuse, sexual deviance involving promiscuity, pregnancy, and prostitution. They may be truants or run away from home.

Tertiary prevention may continue in the treatment of the adult woman who was sexually abused as a child. Nurses dealing with gynecological care of adult women and nurses who are providing mental health nursing care especially may be involved with patients who have a history of sexual abuse in their background. Depression is a common complaint as are chronic complaints of sleep disorders. These women often experience anxiety and low self-esteem and may have chronic sexual problems dealing with fear of intimate relationships. Self-destructive behavior and substance abuse may also be evident. Problems of this magnitude need extensive treatment. The first step to receiving treatment is the discovery of the problem. It is here that nurses play an important role. After discovery of the problem, the patient should be referred to a mental health professional for long-term assistance. The nurse should remain available and in a supportive relationship with the patient.

Many obstacles may be present for the nurse in tertiary prevention of abusive situations in the elderly. These include the reluctance to report abuse, the necessity for establishing a trusting relationship with the client, and ambiguous indications or lack of verifiable evidence. There are few clear indicators of elderly abuse. An additional factor is the fact that the client is an adult and as such should be able to control his or her affairs as much as he or she is able to. An adult should be able to live out his or her life in the manner he or she chooses freely and safely. Care should not overly restrict the individual's freedoms. Just as care is not forced on a battered woman, care should not be forced on an elderly adult. However, the elderly who because of senility cannot make informed choices may need similar protection an abused child would have. More research is necessary to develop appropriate care for our elderly citizens.

THE SAFETY OF THE HEALTH PROFESSIONAL

The nurse is not immune from danger in the work place. During recent years there have been increasing numbers of attacks on individuals at their place of work. In some cases this is a random attack, in other cases a particular individual is sought, attacked, and possibly killed. "Homicide was the third leading cause of occupational death among workers in the United States between 1980 and 1988 and the leading cause of fatal occupational injuries among women from 1980 to 1985" (Simonowitz, 1993, p. 1).

Identifying risk factors may offer some protection to the worker. Simonowitz (1993) identified three

Table 21–8
Safety Issues for the Caregiver

Plan Ahead

1. Know the area you are visiting.
2. Schedule the visit ahead of time and get the correct address, directions, and information about who will be in the home.
3. Tell the office where you will be and check in regularly.
4. Carry a small amount of money, change for pay telephones, and keep other items to a minimum.
5. Dress for function and mobility and wear a name tag.
6. The vehicle you drive should be in good repair, have a full gas tank, and emergency equipment. Always carry two sets of car keys.

Approaching the Home

1. Notice the environment, animals, fences, activity, indicators of crime, places where you could go for assistance if necessary.
2. Walk with confidence and maintain a professional attitude.
3. Listen for signs of fighting before knocking. If you hear sounds of fighting, leave!
4. Do not enter a home if you suspect an unsafe situation.

In the Home

1. Be aware of who is in the home and what is going on. If there are angry people in the home, use your professional and social skills. Do not expect the client to protect you.
2. Note the exits and sit between the client and an exit of the home. Be prepared to leave quickly if the situation changes suddenly.
3. If someone in the home is violent, leave and call 911.

Handling a Tight Situation

1. Don't show fear; control your breathing.
2. Speak calmly and in a soothing manner. Be assertive but not aggressive.
3. Repeat the reason for your visit, and find a reason to leave.

Leaving the Home

1. Take all of your belongings and keep your car keys in your hand.
2. Watch for cars following you when you leave. Don't stop. If you feel you are in danger, go to the nearest police station or well-lighted business and ask for help.

Trust Your Instincts. Never Forget Your Own Safety.

Adapted from the *Public Health Nursing Domestic Violence Protocol*, Oregon Public Health Association and the Washington State Public Health Association, 1993.

risk factors: (1) the environment, (2) work practices, and (3) the victim and perpetrator profile that are applicable to the situation of the nurse in dealing with violence in the family and community. The nurse who works in the community must be very aware of her environment because a health care worker making home visits has little control over conditions of the community or the home. The nurse will sometimes find herself in homes where violence is the rule. The greatest protection for the nurse is in careful work practices. Many involve common sense; others involve careful preparation. Preparing

for the home visits, keeping the office aware of where she is at all times, and having emergency equipment such as a cellular telephone or a communication device is helpful. The third risk factor is the victim and perpetrator profile. Knowledge of previous violence by a member of a household may be the best indicator of the future potential for violence in that family. Interviewing a victim of violence, where the secrecy is broken, may put the nurse at risk if the perpetrator is on the premises or should return suddenly. Table 21–8 offers safety tips for public health nurses.

DIAGNOSIS

Nursing Diagnoses for Victims of Abuse

There are many NANDA nursing diagnoses that can be related to the victim of abuse. Most of the diagnoses are psychologically oriented and deal with feelings and coping abilities. Physically oriented diagnoses will necessarily vary with the type of injury.

Psychologically Oriented Nursing Diagnoses
Anxiety
Family Coping: Disabling
Family Process: Alteration in
Hopelessness
Knowledge Deficit
Powerlessness
Posttrauma Response
Social Isolation
Thought Processes: Alteration in
Violence: Potential for

Physically Oriented Nursing Diagnoses
Injury: Potential for
Impairment of Skin Integrity

SUMMARY

Violence is a common occurrence in our society. It affects individuals from birth to death, in families, and in communities. Violence is used too commonly in our society to solve problems and to deal with stress and frustration. Violence at home, in the neighborhood, and at school affects countless num-

bers of children in this country who live in fear for their lives. The proliferation of handguns in the United States has contributed to violence, often ending in death.

The problem of violence can be generational. If the behavior is not stopped, it can continue into the next generation where the battered often becomes the batterer. This self-perpetuating cycle causes indescribable pain to children, women, and elderly, who are the primary victims. The abuser is also a victim and the ultimate victim is society, who must care for the results of violent acts.

Violence has been declared a public health epidemic. National objectives for reducing violence have been identified. The efforts of public health have been mobilized to help stop this epidemic and bring healing to the nation. Health for all includes freedom from intentional injuries caused by violence. The core public health functions of needs assessment and surveillance, policy development, and assurance are useful methods of combating this epidemic.

The public health nurse can be a crucial member of the team fighting violence. Commitment to caring about the problem is a first step. Careful assessment of all clients for evidence of injury is a second step. Teaching alternate methods of dealing with stress, improved parenting relationships, and considerate care of the elderly is the essence of primary prevention. If an upstream approach of discovering the problem and then preventing it from occurring is used, ultimately the generational cycle will be broken and society as a whole will be stronger and more caring.

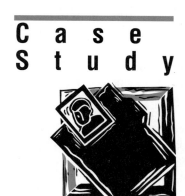

Case Study

Jenny J., a 23-year-old pregnant woman, is being seen for her first prenatal visit at a health department clinic. On physical examination, she is noted to have a black left eye with a conjunctival hemorrhage. She has bilateral bruises on her upper arms that appear to reveal the imprint of fingers. There are a number of bruises on both legs, and her right knee is swollen.

At the conclusion of the physical examination, the Abuse Assessment Screen was administered. Jenny responded that she had been hit, slapped, or kicked and physically injured by someone on numerous occasions in the past year. The perpetrator is her boyfriend, who is the father of the baby. She reports that he is very unhappy about her pregnancy, and the abuse has increased since the pregnancy became known. The body map reveals injuries to many parts of Jenny's body. Jenny's boyfriend has a handgun in the home and has threatened to take her life.

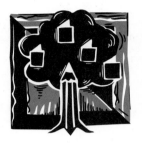

Learning Activities

1. Develop a nursing care plan for Jenny. Include interventions that could actually be used in the community in which you live.

2. Determine your professional responsibilities in your state by securing a copy or reviewing the reporting laws for child abuse, battering of women, spousal rape, and abuse of the elderly.

3. Using the telephone directory, find three community agencies (public or private) in your community that provide help for victims of violence. Make a list of the telephone numbers to keep in the pocket of your uniform.

4. Call a child abuse warm line or hot line in your community and ask them what services they provide.

5. Call a battered women's shelter and determine the procedure in securing shelter placement for a battered woman and her children.

6. Visit a respite center for the elderly, and observe the clients and the activities that are provided for them. What behaviors do you observe that would contribute to stress in the caretaker?

7. Follow the newspapers for 1 month and clip articles that deal with violence. Determine how many individuals were killed or injured during that period in incidents of violence. How many of them were gun related, and what type of weapon was used?

REFERENCES

Belloni MA, Blumenthal D, Bracy P, et al.: Public Health Reports 106:244–264, 1991.

Blow R, Gest E: A social disease: Violence. Mother Jones 18:26–29, 1993.

Boyer D, Fine D: Sexual abuse as a factor in adolescent pregnancy and child maltreatment. Fam Plann Perspect 24:4–12, 1992.

Browne A: Violence against women by male partners. Am Psychol 48:1077–1087, 1993.

Butterfield F: Crime panel fears new wave of violence. San Francisco Chronicle, January 6, 1996, p. A7.

Campbell J: Women's responses to sexual abuse in intimate relationships. Health Care Women Int 10:335–346, 1989.

Campbell J, Alford P: The dark consequences of marital rape. Am J Nurs 89:946–949, 1989.

Center for Disease Control: Suicide Among Children, Adolescents, and Young Adults—United States, 1980–1992. MMWR vol 44, No 15, 1995.

Cohen S, Lang C, Wilson-Brewer R, et al.: Forum on youth violence in minority communities: Setting the agenda for prevention. Public Health Rep 10:269–277, 1991.

Cole C, Finnie D, May B, et al.: Public Health Nursing Domestic Violence Protocol. Oregon Public Health Association. Washington State Public Health Association, 1993.

Cotton P: Gun-associated violence increasingly viewed as public health challenge. JAMA 267:1171–1173, 1992.

Dannenberg A, Baker S, Li G: Intentional and unintentional injuries in women. Ann Epidemiol 4:133–139, 1994.

DeMause L: Our forebears made childhood a nightmare. Psychol Today 9:85–86, 1975.

Elders J: Violence as a public health issue for children. Childhood Educ 70:260–262, 1994.

Gibson CM: Answers to violence. Yale Med 30:3–20, 1995.

Helton A, McFarlane J, Anderson E: Battered and pregnant: A prevalence study. Am J Public Health 77:1337–1339, 1987.

Hiraki S, Grambs M: Volunteer manual on marital violence. Available from Battered Women's Alternatives, Pacheco, CA, 1990.

Houk V, Warren R: Public Health Rep 106:225–229, 1991.

Koop C, Lundberg G: Violence in America: A public health emergency. JAMA 267:3075–3076, 1992.

Loring M, Smith R: Health care barriers and interventions for battered women. Public Health Rep 109:328–338, 1994.

Marwick C: Guns, drugs threaten to raise public health problem of violence to epidemic. JAMA 267:2993, 1992.

Mason J: Prevention of violence: A public health commitment. Public Health Rep 106:265–269, 1991.

McFarlane J, Parker B: Abuse During Pregnancy: A Protocol for Prevention and Intervention. March of Dimes, 1994.

McFarlane J, Parker B, Soeken K, Bullock L: Assessing for abuse during pregnancy. JAMA 267:3176–3178, 1992.

Mercy J: Youth violence as a public health problem. Spectrum J State Government 66:26–31, 1993.

Mitchell M, Prothrow-Stith D, Cohen L, et al.: Panel discussion. 1: Lessons learned—The community experience. Public Health Rep 106:237–242, 1991.

Mittleman R, Mittleman H, Wetli C: What child abuse really looks like. Am J Nurs 87:1185–1188, 1987.

Monaco J, Brooks W: The critical care aspects of child abuse. Pediatr Clin North Am 41:1259–1269, 1994.

Novello A: Violence is a greater killer of children than disease. Public Health Rep 106:231–234, 1991.

Novello A, Shosky J, Froehlke R: A medical response to violence. JAMA 267:3007, 1992.

Ozmar B: Encountering victims of interpersonal violence. Crit Care Nurs Clin North Am 6:515–523, 1994.

Parker B, McFarlane J, Soeken K: Abuse during pregnancy: effects on maternal complications and birthweight in adult and teenage women. Obstet Gynecol 84:323–328, 1994.

Ramsey-Klawsnik H: Recognizing and responding to elder maltreatment. Pride Inst J Long Term Home Health Care 12:12–20, 1993.

Roper W: The prevention of minority youth violence must begin despite risks and imperfect understanding. Public Health Rep 106:229–232, 1991.

Rosenberg M, Fenley M: Violence in America: A Public Health Approach. New York, Oxford University Press, 1991.

Rosenberg M, O'Carroll P, Kenneth E: Let's be clear; violence is a public health problem. JAMA 267:3071–3072, 1992.

Ruttenberg H: The limited promise of public health methodologies to prevent youth violence. Yale Law J 103:1885–1912, 1994.

Sassetti M: Domestic Violence. Primary Care Clin Office Pract 20:289–303, 1993.

Simonowitz J: Guidelines for Security and Safety of Health Care and Community Service Workers. San Diego, CA, Medical Unit, Division of Occupational Safety and Health, Department of Industrial Relations, 1993.

Stark E: Focus: Managing care for victims of violence discharge planning with battered women. Discharge Planning Update 14:1–7, 1994.

Stein A: Will health care reform protect victims of abuse? Treating domestic violence as a public health issue. Human Rights 21:16–19, 1994.

U.S. Department of Health and Human Services: Healthy People 2000. Washington, DC, U.S. Department of Health and Human Services Public Health Service, 1990.

Velsor-Friedrich B: Family violence: A growing epidemic. J Pediatr Nurs 9:272–274, 1994.

Walker LE: The Battered Woman. New York, Harper & Row, 1979.

Wolfner G, Gelles R: A profile of violence toward children: A national study. Child Abuse Neglect 17:97–212, 1993.

Mental Health

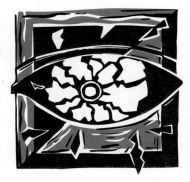

Upon completion of this chapter, the reader will be able to:

1. Describe the concept of aggregate mental health.

2. Describe how the nursing process is applied to promote the mental health of individuals and families in the community.

Mary E. Allen

This chapter explores the concept of aggregate mental health as it relates to individuals and families in the community. The components of mental health for individuals include the absence of mental disease, normality of behavior, adjustment to environment, unity of personality, and correct perception of reality (Jahoda, 1955). Individuals do not function as isolated beings in this society; each individual is part of a network. That network may be a family or some other group to which the individual belongs (e.g., a group of single or widowed senior citizens who live in a common dwelling). Networks create systems. Family and group systems network through lines of communication, through human bonds, and, as subsystems of communities, through societal norms.

When individuals experience mental illness, abnormal behavior, environmental maladjustment, disunity of personality, and altered perceptions of reality, the family or group to which the individual belongs is also affected. In many cases, the family or group may even enhance or intensify individual experiences. For example, alcoholism has been referred to as a family disease even though there may be only one alcoholic family member. The effects of alcoholism on a community manifest themselves through the noncontributions of the alcoholic to society as well as through the personally detrimental behaviors exhibited by the codependent significant others. For example, adult children of alcoholics can suffer the influence of growing up in a codependent family system for generations to come. It is important in situations of this type that the nurse plan interventions with emphasis on primary, secondary, and tertiary prevention. Primary prevention is implemented before the onset of an illness; secondary prevention is more appropriately used after the onset of a particular illness. The focus of tertiary prevention is more rehabilitative in nature.

Families and other groups within a given community system collectively form an aggregate. *Aggregate mental health* may be defined as the degree to which families and groups contribute to enhance or intensify individual interaction along the mental health–mental illness continuum within a given environment.

COMMUNITY MENTAL HEALTH MOVEMENT

Historic Evolution

In general, the practice of psychiatry can be viewed in terms of three phases. The first phase of psychiatry, in which it is viewed as an independent science, began near the end of the 18th century and heralded a new empathic attitude toward mental illness. The second phase began approximately 100 years later as a result of the development of psychoanalysis by Sigmund Freud. The third phase hallmarked the coming of community psychiatry (Bellak, 1964). Community psychiatry differs from hospital-based psychiatry in that the emphasis is on practice in the community rather than treatment in institutional settings, and it acknowledges the importance of offering services within the context of community values, norms, and agencies.

Before 1960, the majority of mentally ill persons received treatment in isolation from their home communities. Having to travel great distances for treatment contributed to the difficulty of achieving mental health promotion and maintenance. The establishment of the Community Mental Health Centers Program of the National Institute of Mental Health (NIMH) was an attempt to alleviate some of these problems. The passing of appropriate legislation was the next step.

Legislation

A number of political forces contributed to the Community Mental Health Centers Construction Act of 1963. There was public concern about the quality of mental health care; leadership of mental health agencies was supportive of public concern; and a national mental health establishment was being maintained through federal fiscal support (Foley, 1975). The Community Mental Health Centers Amendments of 1975 and the Community Mental Health Centers Construction Act of 1963 provided for the establishment of community-based therapeutic centers to replace custodial mental institutions. Figure 22–1 summarizes these important events and legislation (Dowell and Ciarlo, 1983).

The NIMH identified the essential elements of comprehensive community mental health services:

- Inpatient services
- Partial hospitalization or at least day care service
- Outpatient services
- Emergency services provided on a 24-hour basis and available within at least one of the three services listed previously
- Consultation and educational services available to community agencies and professionals

The goals of community mental health as a concept

History of Community Mental Health Movement

1963	Funding of Community Mental Health Centers (CMHC) program through National Institute of Mental Health
1963	CMHC Construction Act provided establishment of centers to replace custodial mental institutions
1975	CMHC amendments increased the number of essential services from 5 to 12
1978	Report of task panel on CMHC's assessment
1980	Community Mental Health Systems Act
1981	Omnibus Budget Reconciliation Act and repeal of Community Mental Health Systems Act

Figure 22–1
History of community mental health.

have been questioned (Amesbury, 1983; Lowery and Janulis, 1983). Financial cutbacks have impeded the development of the concept (Goplerud et al., 1983) with resultant program disintegration (Hagar and Kincheloe, 1983). Several questions raised about the goals of community mental health relate to implementation of the concept. For example, who is the patient? Who is the therapist? What is the therapeutic process? What is the goal? What is the theory? What is the role? The answers to many of these questions will depend on whether the patient is an individual, family, or aggregate; the profession of the therapist; the adopted school of thought for therapy; and the existence of a prevention, promotion, or maintenance goal. Program disintegration results when these questions are not adequately addressed by the treatment team of the community mental health center. Continuity of care is then lost, and the patient suffers. Figure 22–2 delineates nine goals that have been used as the basis for organizing information about community mental health centers (Dowell and Ciarlo, 1983).

Of great importance is the evaluation of community mental health program effectiveness (Dowrick, et al., 1992; Miller and Duffey, 1993). Particularly relevant to evaluation for the nurse working in the area of community mental health are discussions of intervention effectiveness (Hellwig, 1993; Brooker, 1984); role

function (Trimbath and Brestensky, 1990; Haylett and Rapoport, 1964); and emerging trends, issues, and problems of community psychiatric nurses (Duffy, 1993; Dowd, 1989).

FACTORS CONTRIBUTING TO THE MENTAL HEALTH OF AGGREGATES

Environmental Factors

Environmental factors can influence the mental health of aggregates. An objective of the Healthy People 2000 initiative is to "establish and monitor the plans of 35 states to define and track environmental diseases"(U.S. Department of Health and Human Services [DHHS], 1990). Environmental diseases include lead poisoning, other heavy mental poisoning, pesticide poisoning, carbon monoxide poisoning, heat stroke, hypothermia, acute chemical poisoning, methemoglobinemia, and respiratory diseases triggered by

Goals of Community Mental Health

1. Increase the range and quantity of public mental health services.

2. Make services equally available and accessible to all.

3. Provide services in relation to the existing needs in the community.

4. Decrease state hospital admissions and residents.

5. Maximize citizen participation in community programs.

6. Prevent development of mental disorders.

7. Coordinate mental health–related services in the catchment area.

8. Provide services as efficiently as possible.

9. Provide services that reduce suffering and increase personal functioning.

Figure 22–2
Goals of community mental health.

environmental factors such as asthma. Several of these diseases have potentially serious consequences for the cognitive status of affected individuals. When aggregates are exposed to toxicants, the functioning of entire communities is hindered, if not halted.

Biological Factors

Aggregates are composed of holistic individuals whose physical health and mental status are intricately woven. The Healthy People 2000 initiative (U.S. DHHS, 1990) proposed objectives to ensure that health-related dimensions of physical activity that encompass key physiologic and physical mechanisms become part of individuals' regular behavioral patterns. Evidence exists for the multiple health benefits of regular physical activity. Specifically related to mental health are the benefits of regular physical activity to assist individuals to manage depression and anxiety. The Healthy People 2000 objective to "increase community availability and accessibility of physical activity and fitness facilities" focuses on aggregates. A related objective to "increase the proportion of worksites offering employer-sponsored physical activity and fitness programs" also focuses on aggregates.

Social Factors

It is estimated that more than 20 million adults living in communities in the United States are severely incapacitated from mental disorders, not including substance abuse–related disorders; and almost twice that number have experienced at least one diagnosable disorder (Regier et al., 1988). The incidence of mental disorders within a community has social implications for aggregates. According to Healthy People 2000 (U.S. DHHS 1990), psychosocial interventions can improve psychologic well-being during stressful life conditions via enhancing social supports systems and the strengthening of individual interpersonal, psychological, and physical resources. The following Healthy People 2000 objectives have implications for the positive enhancement of social factors: (1) "reduce to less than 35 percent the proportion of people aged 18 and older who experienced adverse health effects from stress within the past year"; (2) "increase to at least 30 percent the proportion of people aged 18 and older with severe, persistent mental disorders who use community support programs"; (3) "reduce to less than 10 percent the prevalence of mental disorders among children and adolescents"; (4) "decrease to no

more than 5 percent the proportion of people aged 18 and older who report experiencing significant levels of stress who do not take steps to reduce or control their stress"; (5) "increase to at least 40 percent the proportion of worksites employing 50 or more people that provide programs to reduce employee stress."

ASSESSMENT OF AGGREGATE MENTAL HEALTH

An ideal conceptual framework for the assessment of aggregate mental health includes components reflecting the application of systems theory, the nursing process, and a theoretical approach for the analysis of groups and families. These components provide the groundwork for a thorough assessment of the degree to which subsystems of families and groups contribute to enhance or intensify individual interaction along the mental health–illness continuum within a given environment, such as a catchment or service area.

Nursing Process

Nurses use the tools of the nursing process— assessment, nursing diagnosis, planning, intervention, and evaluation—in their work with aggregates. The application of the nursing process is facilitated by good observational skills and the use of therapeutic communication techniques. Work with aggregates necessitates an ability to look beyond the individual client and consider the family or groups of which that person is a member, the client's environment, and the society as a whole. The nursing process serves as the organizing framework. The nurse's beliefs about humankind, society, nursing, mental health, and the environment, in addition to the application of existing relevant theoretical frameworks, serve as a guide for the placement of substantive material within the organizing framework.

Work with aggregates is facilitated by the application of a theory of group development. Direct patient care of individuals who are members of families and groups involves interaction in small groups. The usual size of a small group ranges from 2 to 10 members (Shaw, 1971). Small groups tend to be more predictable than large groups. To aid in nurses' understanding of all groups, a wide variety of theoretical perspectives may be applied. Among the most common approaches to the analysis of groups are the psychoanalytical approaches, focusing on unconscious processes in group behavior; symbolic interactionism, focusing on meaning and identity in group behavior; systems analysis, examining exchange and equilibrium in group behavior; and theories that focus on temporal relationships in group behavior (Sampson and Marthas, 1981). A more eclectic theoretical approach that uses several of the common approaches to group analysis may be used to achieve the desired outcomes.

Role of the Community Mental Health Nurse

The role of the community mental health nurse working with aggregates may be defined in terms of educator, practitioner, and coordinator of services. As educator, the nurse instructs individuals, families, or groups through community organization about various aspects of preventive mental health, treatment of mental illness, and community management of individuals who are mentally ill and who yet function in the community. For example, the management of chronically mentally ill persons may cause disequilibrium for a particular community system. Providing education programs on the causes, symptoms, and treatment for chronicity may serve to dispel myths about this population. In addition, group and family education provides a ready support network for the exchange of ideas related to disease management and an arena for the ventilation of shared feelings about chronicity and its impact on group and family networks.

As practitioner, the nurse works directly with individuals, groups, and families through the formation of a therapeutic relationship. For the master's-prepared advanced practitioner, provision of individual, group, and family therapy facilitates the mental health of aggregates by collaborative identification of those dynamics that contribute to, intensify, or enhance the individual's experience with the environment and the mental health–illness continuum.

The following list represents examples of reasons for referral to community mental health nurses:

- Discharge follow-up
- Assessment
- Drug monitoring
- Crisis intervention
- Parent education
- Preventive work

As a coordinator of services, the community mental health nurse not only functions as a referral source but also makes referrals to the following groups of professionals:

- Social work
- Psychology
- Psychiatry
- Occupational therapy
- Physical therapy
- Speech therapy
- Health departments

Mental illness may be accompanied by a wide variety of related health problems. As one of the few professionals who visits clients in community settings, such as the home or a halfway house, the nurse is in an excellent position to assess the physical and psychosocial status of the client and the environment.

Tools of Assessment

Commonly identified phases of any therapeutic relationship are the initial phase, or orientation, working phase, and termination phase. At the initial phase, the client and nurse get to know each other. An assessment is made to identify the needs of the client, and a contract is formulated to identify the responsibilities of both nurse and client in achieving the desired goals. At this stage, the nursing diagnosis reflects the mutually identified problems and needs of the client, whether individual, family, group, or community.

During the working phase, the client and nurse may actively become involved in the following activities:

- Identifying systemic patterns of behavior that are causing disequilibrium
- Identifying intrapersonal, interpersonal, and other system components interactions that may be detrimental to mental health
- Exploring ways to modify dysfunctional behavioral and environmental patterns
- Testing new and modified patterns for effectiveness
- Identifying problematic client-nurse-system boundary issues

Termination is the final phase of the therapeutic relationship. At the beginning of a relationship, termination is discussed in terms of the length of time the nurse plans to work with the client on the formulated contract. Ideally, time boundaries are built into therapeutic contracts through long- and short-term goal statements. During the termination phase, the nurse and client summarize the outcomes of the relationship. The extent of goal achievement is explored, and plans for continuity of care are identified.

Boundary issues that may be problematic in thera-peutic relationships can stem from excessive dependency on the part of the client or nurse, ineffective communication patterns, role ambiguity on the part of the client or nurse, and resistance to change.

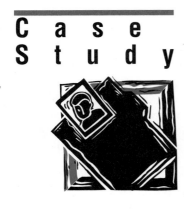

C a s e
S t u d y

At 9:02 AM on April 19, 1995, the Alfred P. Murrah Federal Building in Oklahoma City, Oklahoma, was destroyed by bombing. Multiple lives—men, women, and children—were lost, survivors of the explosion were traumatized, and significant others were plunged into a state of grieving. The blast was felt across the state. The personal accounts of more than 1000 survivors, rescuers, nursing staff, medical staff, counselors, volunteers, and children have been shared (Irving, 1995). The residual effects of this tragedy remain in the hearts and minds of those left behind. Nursing played an important role during the disaster relief efforts. On the day of the bombing, nurses assisted in rescue efforts by caring for the injured and dying. Nurses set up on-site triage units, administered tetanus shots to rescue workers, provided mental health counseling, served as supplemental hospital staff for emergency care, provided support to families, assisted temporarily displaced homeless persons, and cared for victims' significant others and fellow disaster workers. At this very moment, the postdisaster work of public health nurses, pediatric nurses, critical care nurses, medical-surgical nurses, psychiatric–mental health nurses, gerontologic nurses, nurse practitioners, and clinical nurse specialists continues.

Assessment

Assessment of aggregates in community mental health first involves identification of the community systems that make up the aggregate and the boundaries of those systems. The boundaries may be cultural, ethnic, geographic, socioeconomic, or religious. A community study can assist the nurse in assessing a particular community system and the degree of interaction with other systems. When examining this case, questions related to identification of the following areas should be addressed:

Mental Health–Illness Problems Within the Community

- How is mental health defined by the family and members of the community?
- How is mental illness defined by the family and members of the community?
- Are people with psychiatric or mental health problems rejected or accepted by the community?
- How is rejection and acceptance exhibited by the community?
- Is the family labeled as abnormal or deviant by the community?
- What political or socioeconomic views support the acceptance or rejection of the family labeled as abnormal or deviant?
- What is the influence of culture, ethnicity, religion, and socioeconomic status on the prevailing definition of mental health or illness in terms of normality, adjustment to environment, unity of personality, and perception of reality?

Diverse Perspectives

- How do the subsystems of consumers, health care professionals, other professionals, government officials, law enforcement groups, business owners, and civic groups describe this family within the context of community?

Resources and Contributions of Various Groups

- What are the characteristics of the community environment?
- What age, sex, race, and family groupings are represented?
- To what degree are space and territoriality issues for the community?
- What is the relationship among income, occupational, and educational level groupings; strengths and concerns; and resulting mental health and illness?
- What community resources exist for this family, and where are they located?

Weaknesses or Neglected Areas

- How and by whom are family problems solved?
- What is the family's decision-making process?
- Do all individuals in the family have a mechanism for expressing concerns?
- How effective is the mechanism?

Possible Points of Intervention

- How are nurses received by the family?
- If change is warranted, to what degree does the family system resist change?
- What groundwork must be laid before change can occur?
- Who are the power brokers within the family?
- Will power, tradition, or norms be affected by change?
- Who will benefit or suffer most from the change?

Evaluation of Intervention Effectiveness

- To what extent were long- and short-term goals met?
- Have problematic and dysfunctional patterns within the family system changed as a result of nursing intervention?
- To what extent did collaboration with other health professionals occur?
- Was a professional relationship maintained within ethical and legal boundaries?
- What is the longitudinal effectiveness of the nursing intervention?

When deciding whom to assess, the nurse may choose a deductive approach. When initially introduced to a community system with community as client, the nurse will want to use an approach to assessment starting with the more global concept of community working toward the individuals, families, and groups that make up that community. This deductive approach would start with a community study, with the end result being, for example, a mental health prevention education program. A program of this type could lead to the identification of groups at high risk for mental illness, of families in crisis, and of individuals having difficulty coping with activities of daily living.

With an inductive approach, the nurse is introduced to the community system through work with an individual as client. The individual is the identified person who has the problem. Assessment of the individual client will necessitate identification of the family, groups, and community to which the person belongs and subsequent assessment of those components.

Diagnosis

Aggregate Versus Individual Diagnoses Nursing diagnosis is the identification of the actual or potential human responses to illness and factors that maintain the responses. Nursing diagnoses are not always illness oriented and, in the absence of illness, may be used to identify client strengths or positive responses to the human condition and the factors that maintain those responses.

Nursing diagnoses for more than one individual, such as a family, group, community, and aggregate, may be content-level or process-level nursing diagnoses. Content-level nursing diagnoses arise from a first-level assessment of the family, group, community, and aggregate and are a direct or indirect result of the initial assessment of individual content and subsequent determination of its meaning for the system components. Process-level nursing diagnoses arise from a second-level assessment of the system components and reflect the more abstract and dynamic responses of the family, group, community, or aggregate to the process.

Examples of Aggregate Diagnosis

I. Nursing diagnosis
   A. Individual nursing diagnosis—content level
      1. Decreased ability to perform activities of daily living related to depression secondary to posttraumatic stress disorder
      2. Decreased ability to perform activities of daily living related to mental confusion secondary to posttraumatic stress disorder
      3. Decreased ability to cope related to feelings of helplessness and hopelessness
   B. Family nursing diagnosis
      1. Content level—decreased ability to perform shared activities of daily living related to complicated bereavement
      2. Process level—potential family crises related to decreased equilibrium
   C. Community nursing diagnosis
      1. Content level—lack of understanding related to inadequate information about manmade disasters
   D. Aggregate nursing diagnosis
      1. Content level—lack of systematic programs for community education related to inadequate disaster planning among community systems and lack of funds

Through the process of induction, a diagnosis is made for each system component, culminating in an aggregate diagnosis. Note that the content-level diagnoses specially relate to the individual content of loss of personal control. The process-level diagnosis is more conceptually abstract and dynamic.

Planning Mental Health Promotion Activities

Mutual Goal Setting Mutuality in goal setting through collaboration with the agent and clientele is extremely important. The needs of the clientele must be clearly identified before formulation of nursing diagnoses and development of long- and short-term goals. The therapeutic relationship with clients is initiated during the contracting phase. If mutuality is built in early in the relationship, a good base will have been provided for the working and termination phases. No matter how confused, chaotic, or dysfunctional a family or group may appear, the individuals in those subsystems must be allowed to share in developing the plan of care.

In the case study, after individual and family diagnoses are validated with family members, examples of long- and short-term goals are as follows:

Individual

Short-Term Goals
- The client will verbalize feelings about the disaster.
- The client will maintain current level of coping mechanisms in the face of disaster.

Long-Term Goals
- The client will experience the resolution stage of grieving.
- The client will regain predisaster level of biological, psychosocial, and spiritual functioning.
- The client will have increased ability to cope as evidenced by verbalizing feelings of being more in control.
- The client will identify ways to decrease feelings of anxiety associated with the disaster when they occur.
- The client will identify at least three ways to control impending feelings of depression associated with the disaster.

Family

Short-Term Goals
- The family will identify specific ways to cope with loss.
- The family will maintain a state of equilibrium as evidenced by recognition and utilization of system support services as necessary.

Long-Term Goals
- The family will exhibit an increased ability to perform shared activities of daily living as evidenced by an ability to discuss present roles and duties and to redefine those roles as necessary.
- There will be a decreased potential for family crisis as evidenced by members' verbalizations of feeling more in control.

Community

Short-Term Goals
- Information will be disseminated to individuals, families, and groups in the community about the differential effects of natural disaster versus manmade disaster.
- Disaster debriefing information will be provided to individuals, families, and groups in the community.

Long-Term Goal
- There will be increased community understanding of the disaster as evidenced by active participation in community education programs.

Aggregate

Short-Term Goals
- Existing programs within various communities will be identified.
- Existing community programs will be coordinated to eliminate duplication of services.

Long-Term Goal

- Systematic programs will be established for populations in crisis as evidenced by collaborative efforts of local, state, and federal planning bodies with ongoing evaluation of progress toward meeting the needs of the population

Intervention

It is a good idea for the nurse to keep in mind alternative interventions if those originally planned are not successful. If rationales for interventions are carefully researched with an identification of why the intervention should work, there is a higher probability that the intervention will work.

A multitude of factors could determine why some interventions work in one situation and not in another. These influencing factors could be related to demographic or environmental variables or to individual personality characteristics. Whatever the influencing factors, they must be taken into consideration before the interventions are implemented. Figure 22–3 presents examples of interventions for this case at the primary, secondary, and tertiary levels of prevention.

Evaluation

Components The problems associated with the measurement of community mental health nursing intervention have been identified in the literature (Brooker, 1984). Evaluation is the process for determining the extent of goal achievement in addition to the ongoing judgments about nursing effectiveness as interventions are implemented. Self-awareness involves a continuous examination of the extent to which the nurse's personality characteristics contribute to, intensify, or enhance the therapeutic relationship with the client. Self-evaluation through self-awareness is also part of the evaluation process.

Just as aggregates are multidimensional, so must be the evaluation by the nurse. Evaluation takes into consideration the system components of individual, group, family, and community. Evaluation of the following main points of nursing intervention are commonly considered in community mental health nursing (Brooker, 1984):

- Health education
- Drug supervision
- Supportive and practical help
- Counseling
- Psychotherapy
- Family therapy
- Behavior therapy
- Referral

In addition, for aggregates, the following areas merit evaluation:

- System equilibrium
- Homeostatic mechanisms
- Degree of change (positive, negative, openness, and closeness)
- Degree of networking (between-system components and within-system components)

Primary Prevention   **Goal:** Increased understanding of chronic disease

Individual	Family	Aggregate
Establish baseline level of knowledge	⟶	⟶
Establish learning capabilities	Identify family member(s) to receive education	Identify groups to target for education activities
Discuss application of learned knowledge to typical situations that could be encountered	⟶	⟶

Secondary Prevention   **Goal:** Increased ability to perform activities of daily living

Individual	Family	Aggregate
Establish baseline data on current level of performance for activities of daily living for impaired client	Identify with the family system the activities of daily living with which the impaired client will need assistance	Identify resources within the community that could offer supportive services to the family system
Model and role play facilitative communicative techniques	⟶	⟶

Tertiary Prevention   **Goal:** Adherence to prescribed medication regimen

Individual	Family	Aggregate
Discuss factors that contribute to the inability to adhere to the medication regimen	Discuss strategies that family can use to increase adherence by the impaired member	Satisfy the agency or institution that dispenses medication for the family and explore compliance aids with them

Figure 22–3
Example of interventions at primary, secondary, and tertiary prevention levels.

RESEARCH IN MENTAL HEALTH

Kane CF, DiMartino E, Jimenez M. (1990). A comparison of short-term psycheducational and support groups for relatives coping with chronic schizophrenia. Arch Psychiatr Nurs 4:343–353.
Kane et al. (1990) explored the differences between two short-term multifamily group intervention programs for relatives of hospitalized chronic schizophrenics in a nonequivalent comparison group design. A psychoeducational intervention consisted of interactive instructional activities, and the support group intervention consisted of nonstructured discussions. The analysis of covariance on adjusted posttest means indicated a differential treatment effect for depression and satisfaction for the psychoeducational groups. The authors' findings suggest that the process of a support group may not be compatible with a short time frame.

Taft LB, Barkin RL. (1990). Drug abuse: Use and misuse of psychotropic drugs in Alzheimer's care. J Gerontol Nurs 16: 4–10.
Taft and Barkin (1990) explored the use and misuse of psychotropic drugs in care for Alzheimer's patients. The authors noted that family caregivers often report feelings of guilt associated with administering psychotropic drugs and may attribute the use of these to their own inability to cope. As noted, the role of the nurse is to establish and monitor therapeutic goals, to assess the incidence and severity of predictable side effects, and to provide a safe, supportive environment that reduces the need for pharmacologic interventions.

SUMMARY

The purpose of this chapter was to explore the concept of mental health as it relates to groups of individuals and families in the community. The concept of aggregate mental health was described as was the application of the nursing process to promote the mental health of individuals within families and groups in the community.

L e a r n i n g
A c t i v i t i e s

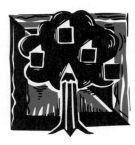

1. Conduct a community study of the catchment or service area in which you live. Include the following:
   - An identification of mental health problems within the community
   - Diverse perspectives on relevant issues (e.g., interviews with consumers and their families, professionals of health care, other professionals, government groups, police and law enforcement groups, business and civic groups)
   - An identification of resources and the contributions of various groups to the coping strengths of the community related to mental health and other community concerns
   - An identification of weaknesses or neglected areas for mental health and other community concerns
   - An identification of possible points of intervention in community action
   - An identification of areas for further study

2. Repeat this study for an area in which a selected client resides.

REFERENCES

Amesbury WH: The comprehensive mental health system: Is it achievable. Perspect. Psychiatr. Care 21:31–33, 1983.

Bellak L.(ed): Handbook of Community Psychiatry and Community Mental Health. New York, Grune & Stratton, 1964.

Brooker CG: Some problems associated with the measurement of community psychiatric nurse intervention. J Adv Nurs 9;165–174, 1984.

Dowd TT: Ethical reasoning: A basis for nursing care in the home. J Commun Health Nurs 6:45–52, 1989.

Dowell DA, Ciarlo JA: Overview of the Community Mental Health Centers Program from an evaluation perspective. Commun Mental Health J 19:95–128, 1983.

Dowrick C, Graham-Jones S, Stanley I: Mental health in the community. Med Educ 26:145–152, 1992.

Duffy J: Psychiatric home care. Home Healthcare Nurse 11:22–28, 1993.

Foley HA: Community Mental Health Legislation. Lexington, MA, DC Heath, 1975.

Goplerud EN, Walfish S, Apsey MO: Surviving cutbacks in community mental health: Seventy-seven action strategies. Commun Mental Health J 19:62–76, 1983.

Hagar L, Kincheloe M: The disintegration of a community mental health outpatient program, or off the back wards into the streets. Perspect Psychiat Care 21:102–107, 1983.

Haylett CH, Rapoport L: Mental health consultation. *In* Bellak L. (ed): Handbook of Community Psychiatry and Community Mental Health. New York, Grune & Stratton, 1964, pp. 319–339.

Hellwig K: Psychiatric home care nursing: Managing patients in the community setting. J Psychosoc Nurs 31:21–24, 1993.

Irving C (ed): *In Their Name.* New York, Random House, 1995.

Jahoda M: Toward a social psychology of mental health. *In* Kotinsky R, Witmer HL (eds). Community Programs for Mental Health. Cambridge, MA, Harvard University Press, 1955, pp. 296–322.

Lowery BJ, Janulis D: Community mental health and the unanswered questions. Perspect Psychiatr Care 21:156–158, 1983.

Miller MP, Duffey J: Planning and program development for psychiatric home care. JONA 23:35–41, 1993.

Regier DA, Boyd JH, Burke JD, et al.: One-month prevalence of mental disorders in the United States: Based on five epidemiologic catchment area sites. Arch Gen Psychiatry 45:977–986, 1988.

Sampson EE, Marthas, M: Group Process for the Health Professions, 3rd ed. New York, John Wiley, 1981.

Shaw ME: Group Dynamics: The Psychology of Small Group Behavior. New York, McGraw-Hill, 1971.

Trimbath M, Brestensky J: The role of the mental health nurse in home health care. J Home Health Care Pract 2:1–8, 1990.

U.S. Department of Health and Human Services: Healthy People 2000: National Health Promotion and Disease Prevention Objectives. Washington, DC, Public Health Service, 1990.

Substance Abuse

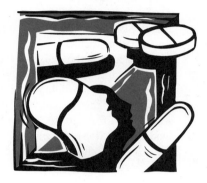

Upon completion of this chapter, the reader will be able to:

1. Discuss the historic trends and current conceptions of the cause and treatment of substance abuse.

2. Describe the current social, political, and economic aspects of substance abuse.

3. Identify issues related to substance abuse in various populations encountered in community health nursing practice.

4. Detail the typical symptoms and consequences of substance abuse.

5. Apply the nursing process to substance abuse problems presented in a case study.

6. Assess and describe the needs of special populations of substance abusers.

Erika Madrid
Joanne M. Hall
Lucretia Bolin

Perhaps no other health-related condition has as many far-reaching consequences in contemporary Western society as does substance abuse. These consequences include a wide range of social, psychological, physical, economic, and political problems. Substance abuse costs of health problems and disability are approximately $240 billion annually (Robert Wood Johnson Foundation, 1992; Rice, 1993; Rice et al., 1990). More deaths, illnesses, and disabilities are attributed to substance abuse than to any other preventable health condition in the United States. Substantiating this is that liver disease is the ninth leading cause of death in the United States; alcohol abuse is the cause of cirrhosis of the liver in one half of the cases. Additionally, drug-related deaths are increasing, particularly among male substance abusers; the fastest growing cause of drug-related deaths is attributed to acquired immunodeficiency syndrome (AIDS) (Horgan, 1993).

Looking at the social consequences of substance abuse, many offenders commit crimes while under the influence of drugs or alcohol or both. At least half of the people arrested for homicide, theft, and assault had used illicit drugs near the time of their arrest (Horgan, 1993).

Men, women, children, adolescents, and the elderly are among those directly affected by substance abuse problems because of the effect of addictive substances on their bodies. Infants are born addicted to alcohol, stimulants, or opiates and are at risk for developmental problems because of their exposure in utero (Chasnoff, 1992). Indirect social effects of substance abuse include relationship conflicts, divorce, spousal and child abuse, as well as child neglect (Campbell and Landenburger, 1995; Murphy et al., 1991; Scherling, 1994; Straus and Gelles, 1990). In spite of good intentions, many local and national efforts to change the situation often are inadequate and ineffective.

In the past, alcoholism and drug addiction were considered problems of the urban poor, and they were virtually ignored by society as well as by most health professionals. Because substance abuse problems now pervade all levels of U.S. society, awareness has increased. Community health nurses, in particular, must be aware of substance abuse, a problem that is also frequently intertwined with other medical and social conditions.

This chapter focuses on assisting community health nurses to recognize substance abuse in their clients and in the larger community in which they function. Historic trends, conceptions of the cause, and treatment of substance abuse are reviewed along with the most common symptoms of these disorders. Nursing interventions appropriate for assisting substance abusers are also suggested to provide the community health nurse with tools for addressing these problems.

HISTORIC TRENDS IN THE USE OF ALCOHOL AND ILLICIT DRUGS

During this century, the fluctuations in the use of alcohol and illicit drugs have been influenced by shifts in public tolerance and political and economic trends. Alcohol use has enjoyed more social acceptance in general than other drug use. Alcohol consumption in the United States was higher during World Wars I and II and decreased during Prohibition and the Great Depression. More recently, alcohol use was highest during 1980, when the states lowered the drinking age to 18 years. Lawmakers became alarmed at the increased rate of drinking as well as the increased number of alcohol-related deaths among 18- to 25-year-olds after the lowering of the drinking age limit, and they reversed the decision. Alcohol use declined again during the 1980s after the minimum drinking age was raised back to 21 years. The recent decrease in alcohol consumption has also been attributed to the shift in beverage preference away from distilled spirits to wine and beer, which have less ethanol content (NIAAA, 1992).

Like that of alcohol, the history of illicit drug use has been influenced by public attitudes and governmental policies. Although 19th-century physicians prescribed morphine for a large variety of ailments, new awareness of the addictive properties of cocaine and opiates at the beginning of the 20th century led to their increased government regulation. The Harrison Narcotic Act of 1914 and other subsequent laws lessened the medical profession's control of the use of addicting drugs because they specified under what conditions the physician could prescribe these drugs: only in the course of general practice, not specifically to maintain an addiction (Brecher, 1972). This limitation of the physician's power to prescribe and dispense addictive drugs, as well as restrictions on the importation of narcotics, limited the supply of these drugs until the 1950s and 1960s. At that time, as a result of an increase in illegal drug trafficking, heroin use became a problem in the inner city. By the 1970s, influenced by increased availability and a change to a positive attitude toward drug use in the younger segments of society, the use of heroin and other illicit drugs had spread beyond urban drug subcultures to the general population. Alarmed by the social and personal consequences of this change, public tolerance decreased, and prevention and treatment programs were given more attention and resources. After peaking in 1979, illicit drug use decreased again among most segments of the population during the 1980s and early 1990s. Although the use of marijuana and other drugs has declined, there continues to be concern over the impact of cocaine and its more accessible derivative crack or "rock" cocaine on adolescents and young adults (Substance Abuse and Mental Health Services Administration [SAMHSA], 1993).

To combat the concerns of the physical, social, and psychological impact of drug abuse and dependence, federal drug policy has emphasized law enforcement and interdiction to reduce the supply of illicit drugs. In spite of the large amounts of money spent toward this goal, this strategy has been less than effective. Trends have shown renewed interest in prevention and treatment efforts to decrease the amount of illicit drug use in the society and lessen its impact (Westermeyer, 1992).

PREVALENCE OF SUBSTANCE ABUSE

The U.S. National Household Survey on Drug Abuse (Substance Abuse and Mental Health Services Administration [SAMHSA], 1992) reported that 11.1% of the general U.S. population used illicit drugs in the past year (5.5% in the month before the survey) and 64.7% used alcohol in the past year (20% consumed it once a week or more). Marijuana was the most commonly used illicit drug: 32.8% of the population reported they had used marijuana in their lifetime, and 4.4% were current users. Psychoactive prescription drugs and cocaine were the next most commonly used drugs in 1992. Approximately 11.6% of the household population surveyed reported that they had used one or more prescription-type psychotherapeutic drugs for nonmedical purposes in their lifetime, and 11% had used cocaine in their lifetime. Approximately 0.6% used cocaine in the month before the survey. Other illicit drugs were used by fewer than 8% of the household population in a lifetime and fewer than 1% within the month before the survey. Roughly 1% of the household population reported having ever used heroin (0.9%) or crack cocaine (1.4%) in their lifetime (SAMHSA, 1992).

Demographic correlates in the 1992 SAMHSA survey showed some regional, gender, and racial differences related to individuals having ever used substances over their lifetimes. People living in the West had the greatest percentage of lifetime drug use at 46.6% compared with 34.9% for those in the Northeast, 32.6% for those in the North Central region, and 33.1% for those in the South. Whites showed the greatest percentage of lifetime drug use at 37.7% compared with blacks at 33.6% and Hispanics at 29.2%. Lifetime alcohol use ranged from 85.5 to 75.2%. Alcohol use within the last month ranged from 39.8 to 52.9%; blacks in the South had the lowest percentages and whites in the Northeast and the West had the highest percentages.

Studying specifically gender differences related to drug use, the 1992 SAMHSA Household Survey reported that (1) 41% of males have ever used illicit drugs during their lifetime compared with 31.7% of females and (2) 7.1% of males used illicit drugs during the month before the survey compared with 4.1% of females. The 26- to 34-year age group had the highest prevalence of drug use, a change from previous surveys in which prevalence was highest in the 18- to 25-year age group. Marijuana use was more common among women and opiate addiction was less common. In fact, women represented only 50% of the opiate addict population but had more serious social, economic, and personal consequences than their male counterparts.

Studies confirm that there are distinctly different indicators for alcohol problems in women (Schmidt et al., 1990). Overall, women have tended to be predominantly light drinkers, with abstinence increasingly common in women older than 50 years. The heaviest drinking occurs in middle-aged women (ages 35–54 years). Women with lower socioeconomic status drank less than higher status women, and divorced, separated, never married, and cohabiting women drank at greater levels than married women (Wilsnack et al., 1984). In the 1992 Household Survey, 29.7% of men and 11.5% of women consumed alcohol once a week or more (SAMHSA, 1992).

CONCEPTUALIZATIONS OF SUBSTANCE ABUSE

Conceptualizations of substance abuse and dependence are related to historic trends and have often changed over the years for political and social reasons more than for scientific ones. Some conceptualizations focus on the phenomenon of addiction, manifested by compulsive use patterns and the onset of withdrawal symptoms when substance use is abruptly stopped. Other views focus on the problems resulting from the substance use itself, regardless of whether an addictive pattern is present. Problematic consequences of substance abuse include intoxication, psychological dependence, relational conflicts, employment or economic difficulties, legal difficulties, and health problems (Cahalan, 1988). For example, addiction need not be present for individuals to experience legal consequences of illicit drug use, driving while intoxicated, or alcohol- or drug-related domestic violence. Drawing fine distinctions among ideas of dependence, addiction, and abuse concerning substance use may seem irrelevant if there is evidence that the substance use has become problematic (Widiger and Smith, 1994). On the other hand, broadly labeling all habitual or compulsive behavior patterns as "addiction" or "dependence" may obscure the fact that very specific interventions may be needed for each separate "addictive problem," such as overeating, gambling, and so on (Jaffe, 1990).

Definitions

The term *substance abuse* came into common usage in the 1970s. Earlier conceptualizations generally focused on either alcoholism or drug addiction as singular addictive disorders. More currently, the most consistent trends in substance abuse theories are the identification of core commonalities occurring in a variety of different substance use or compulsive behavior syndromes (Marlatt et al., 1988) and an emphasis on relapse prevention that may include moderate use goals as well as abstinence (Larimer and Marlatt, 1990).

There remains debate about how substance use and abuse should be defined and what substances should be included under this heading. Traditional conceptualizations of substance abuse focus solely on alcohol and illicit street drugs. Other conceptualizations include prescription medications such as tranquilizers or analgesics as abusable substances (Table 23–1). In eating disorders like bulimia and compulsive overeating, food is viewed as the abused substance.

In addition to varying in their abuse potential, substances vary in their degree of potential harm to those who use them as well as to others in the immediate environment. Tobacco is an example of a substance that is considered unsafe to both the smoker and those who inhale the secondhand smoke in the environment.

Integrating the various opinions regarding the diagnosis of substance abuse, the American Psychiatric Association (APA), in its most recent diagnostic manual (1994), has classified substance use disorders as either dependence or abuse. The APA focused on psychoactive substances that affect the nervous system: alcohol, amphetamines, cannabis, cocaine, caffeine, hallucinogens, inhalants, nicotine, opioids, phencyclidine, sedatives, and hypnotics or anxiolytics. Substance use disorders can also be categorized as being in partial or full remission.

The criteria for the diagnosis of dependence include a cluster of cognitive, behavioral, and physiologic symptoms that indicate continued use of the substance in spite of significant substance-related problems. A pattern of repeated, self-administered use exists that results in tolerance, withdrawal, and compulsive drug-taking behavior, frequently accompanied by a craving or strong desire for the substance. These symptoms of dependence are similar for most categories of substances except they are less prominent in some (Table 23–2).

A diagnosis of substance abuse, in contrast, indicates a maladaptive pattern of substance use, manifested by recurrent and significant adverse consequences related to repeated use of a substance, and may be viewed as a precursor of substance dependence. These adverse consequences include failure to fulfill major role obligations, repeated use in physically hazardous situations, multiple legal problems, and recurrent social and interpersonal problems (Table 23–3).

Etiology of Substance Abuse

Substance abuse has had an impact on virtually every aspect of individual and communal life and has, therefore, been addressed by many institutions and academic fields. As a result, many theories have been developed to explain the cause and scope of these problems and to offer solutions. Some theories address individual physiologic, spiritual, and psychological factors. Others deal with social influences involving family, ethnicity, race, access to drugs, environmental stressors, economics, political status, culture, and sex roles.

In many theories, a combination of factors is cited as the underlying impetus for substance abuse, but no

Table 23–1
Classification of Commonly Used and Abused Substances

Substance	Desired Effect	Possible Withdrawal Symptoms
CNS depressants		
Alcohol Barbiturates Sedative-hypnotics Tranquilizers	Euphoria, disinhibition, sedation	Anxiety, irritability, seizures, delusions, hallucinations, paranoia
CNS stimulants		
Amphetamines Cocaine Nicotine Caffeine	Euphoria, hyperactivity, omnipotence, insomnia, anorexia	Depression, apathy, lethargy, sleepiness
Narcotics-opioids		
Codeine Meperidine and acetaminophen (Demerol) Hydromorphone (Dilaudid) Fentanyl Heroin Methadone Morphine Opium Oxycodone (Percodan)	Euphoria, sedation	Anxiety; irritability; agitation; runny nose, watery eyes; chills, sweating; nausea and vomiting; diarrhea; tremors; yawning
Hallucinogens		
Mescaline LSD PCP STP/MDA (Ecstasy) Psilocybine (mushrooms)	Hallucinations, illusions, heightened awareness PCP: violent dissociative effect	Depression
Cannabis		
Marijuana Hashish, THC	Relaxation, euphoria, altered perceptions	Restlessness, insomnia, anxiety
Inhalants		
Gasoline Toluene acetate Cleaning fluids Airplane cement Amyl nitrate	Euphoria	Restlessness, anxiety, irritability

CNS = central nervous system; LSD = lysergic acid diethylamide; PCP = phencyclidine; STP = 2,5,dimethoxy,4,methyl amphetamine; MDA = methylene-dioxy-phenyl-iso-propanolamine; THC = tetrahydrocannabinol.

Adapted from Faltz B, Rinaldi J: AIDS and Substance Abuse: A Training Manual for Health Care Professionals. San Francisco, Regents of the University of California, 1987, p. 23. Used with permission.

single factor or agent has been verified as causative of substance abuse as a general phenomenon (Peele, 1985). Therefore, depending on the etiologic framework used, a variety of interventions have been devised to deal with the problem, but not all of them address the purported cause of the problem as defined by the framework.

Although disease-oriented, medical model theorists have defined alcoholism as a loss of control over drinking or an individual malfunction, the cause of the

Table 23–2
Diagnosis of Psychoactive Substance Dependence

A maladaptive pattern of substance use leading to clinically significant impairment or distress as manifested by three (or more) of the following occurring at any time in the same 12-month period:

1. Tolerance, as defined by either of the following:
   a. A need for markedly increased amounts of the substance to achieve intoxication or desired effect
   b. Markedly diminished effect with continued use of the same amount of the substance

2. Withdrawal, as manifested by either of the following:
   a. The characteristic withdrawal syndrome for the substance
   b. The same (or closely related) substance is taken to relieve or avoid withdrawal symptoms

3. Substance is often taken in larger amounts or over a longer period than intended

4. A persistent desire or unsuccessful efforts to cut down or control substance use

5. Much time is spent in activities necessary to obtain the substance, use the substance, or recover from its effects

6. Important social, occupational, or recreational activities are given up or reduced because of substance use

7. Substance use is continued despite knowledge of having a persistent or recurrent physical or psychological problem that is likely to have been caused or exacerbated by the substance

Specify if with or without physiologic dependence (tolerance or withdrawal)

Adapted with permission from the Diagnostic and Statistical Manual of Mental Disorders, Fourth Edition. Copyright 1994, American Psychiatric Association.

disease of alcoholism remains ambiguous (Brown, 1969; Jellinek, 1960; Keller, 1972). The genetic risk factor for alcohol problems appears to be modest (Naegle, 1988; Peele, 1986; Valliant, 1983). Genetic theories alone do not account for why certain ethnic, sex, or socioeconomic groups have a high incidence of problem drinking and alcoholism (Cahalan and Room, 1974). Currently, medical model theories view addiction as the result of a biogenetic predisposition in vulnerable individuals combined with stressors in their environment (B.C. Wallace, 1990; J. Wallace, 1990).

The medical models of alcoholism and other substance abuse conditions also tend not to provide an understanding of commonalities among addictive behaviors (e.g., excessive drinking, gambling, eating, drug use, and sexual behavior). In reality, cross-addiction or polydrug use is increasingly prevalent compared with abuse of a single substance (O'Donnell et al., 1976). More studies point to the presence of both automatic and nonautomatic factors in addictive behavior (Tiffany, 1990). Thus, specific biological medical models are giving way to multicausal models. In the biopsychosocial model, addiction is thought to develop from an interplay of many factors. Risk factors interact with protective factors to develop a predisposition toward drug or alcohol use. This predisposition is next influenced by exposure to the substance, availability, and the quality of the first experience of use (pleasant or unpleasant). Continued availability of the substances and a social support system that enables or supports their use are also necessary. All these factors combine to determine whether addiction develops and is maintained.

Another conceptual change regarding substance abuse is the increasing focus on not only persons who are using substances but also persons who are in close interactional proximity to these individuals. The concepts of co-alcoholism, codependency, and the constellation of difficulties faced by the adult children of substance abusers exemplify how addiction can be viewed as a more global relational pattern. Adherents

Table 23–3
Diagnosis of Psychoactive Substance Abuse

A. A maladaptive pattern of substance use leading to clinically significant impairment or distress as manifested by one (or more) of the following occurring within a 12-month period:
   1. Recurrent substance use resulting in a failure to fulfill major role obligations at work, school, or home
   2. Recurrent substance use in situations in which it is physically hazardous
   3. Recurrent substance-related legal problems
   4. Continued substance use despite persistent or recurrent social or interpersonal problems caused or exacerbated by the effects of the substance

B. The symptoms have never met the criteria for substance dependence for this class of substance.

Adapted with permission from the Diagnostic and Statistical Manual of Mental Disorders, Fourth Edition. Copyright 1994, American Psychiatric Association.

of this view observe that characteristic dysfunctional behavior patterns develop in those having significant, continual interaction with a substance abuser. These response patterns may become very problematic for the significant others and result in depression, excessive caretaking of others, emotional repression, and development of their own compulsive patterns regarding work, food, spending, alcohol, and other drugs (Haaken, 1990). Care should be taken, however, to consider gender and cultural factors so as not to pathologize individuals as "codependent" for simply meeting societal expectations of caring behaviors.

Addiction can be seen on a larger scale as a consciousness or propensity in communities, which then becomes exaggerated by the interaction of cultures and social structures (Saleebey, 1986). This extension of the concept of addiction to "uncontrolled consumption" beyond alcohol or drug use per se treats it as a social and political problem rather than as an individual or familial problem (Wilson-Schaef, 1987).

Sociocultural and Political Aspects of Substance Abuse

In the community health sphere, substance abuse problems are not always easy to identify. The consequences of the sale and use of crack cocaine in an inner city African-American neighborhood may be apparent through media attention. However, the silent ravages of alcohol abuse among elderly women are much less a focus of attention. Nurses must, therefore, incorporate the sociocultural and political dimensions of these phenomena, being critical of media trends.

Although there are subcultures with different norms, the dominant culture drinking norms in the United States are permissive (Pattison, 1984). Many traditional ceremonial, symbolic substance use patterns have been overshadowed by the influences of urbanization, consumerism, and mass culture. The consumption of mood-altering substances has become separated from family and food activities and is undertaken for the "use value" of a particular drug (i.e., what it can "do" for the individual). Past cultural definitions of these practices are inoperative, leaving a void regarding social expectations. These cultural conditions create ambiguity in determining clearly when a substance abuse problem exists. Each subculture may socially define abuse in a different way.

A particular drug experience can be understood as an ongoing interaction between the individual's subjective mood and the actual pharmacologic effects of the drug. This interaction does not take place in a vacuum; rather, the expectations of what drugs will do are shaped by the culture of the user and involve the adoption of roles that are learned from more experienced users and reinforced by other social groups, including health care providers in some cases (Montagne and Scott, 1993).

Substances are also given economic value and are bought and sold as commodities in a variety of social arenas. The ways in which drugs, including medications and alcohol, are produced and distributed among the various segments of the population are determined largely by economic, cultural, and political conditions. For example, the economic realities of the poor Colombians and Peruvians who rely on the growth and production of the coca leaf for financial survival can be understood as a confluence of larger society-level and individual-level factors. These individuals are involved on the fringes of the drug trade because of their financial survival needs. Coca leaf production is a valuable enterprise that brings needed resources to the individual and the family. The drug trade has become more lucrative for some, raising their societal status as well as giving them access to valued commodities. This process can enhance one's sense of power in a society that makes every attempt to disempower the collective and keep power in the hands of a selected few. Among urban poor minority youth in the United States, the fact that drug trafficking often precedes drug use underscores the felt need for economic power and sensation seeking among these youth (Greenberg and Schneider, 1994).

On the cultural level, these changes in power can have other consequences on the subgroups within the society who attain this new status. A group without cultural values or with competing cultural values suffers from chaos and disorganization. Unable to draw on its cultural strengths, neither the group nor its members can survive. Competing value systems lead to cultural disintegration and a sense of powerlessness and hopelessness. The group becomes susceptible to pernicious forces that further threaten the survival of the culture and the group's ability to survive. Political forces that are intricately interwoven with the society-level forces are in operation. Unable to organize or to determine a collective direction because of confounding values, the group and its members are separated and disempowered. The history of cocaine abuse and dependence among people of color is a good example of how these conditions are interrelated.

Crack Cocaine Epidemic

Once touted as a drug of great medicinal and religious significance, cocaine has become known as a highly potent and addictive substance. Cocaine abuse was perceived as a problem of epidemic proportions, with the 1980s being called the "decade of cocaine." The Senate Judiciary Committee's study of cocaine abuse (National Institute on Drug Abuse, 1990) conservatively estimated that 2.2 million Americans use cocaine at least once a week.

The availability of cocaine increased dramatically during the 1980s. This increase began shortly after a change in drug control laws in the early 1970s that placed greater control on prescription drugs and focused less on street drugs. Trends regarding use demonstrated that the densely populated areas, especially western and northeastern regions of the United States, had a higher prevalence of cocaine use than other areas (Abelson and Miller, 1985). One major consequence of increasing accessibility of cocaine and prevalence of its use was a 200% increase in deaths as well as a 500% increase in admissions to government treatment facilities between 1976 and 1986 (Gold et al., 1986).

Cocaine is a powerful stimulant that can be inhaled, injected intravenously, or smoked. The newest form of cocaine (crack) is relatively inexpensive and has thus made cocaine available to the adolescent, young adult, and poor populations. This development has led to a greater number of complications and greater societal awareness of the pernicious effects of cocaine and other substance abuse. Reports in the literature and the media document a cocaine abuse crisis of unparalleled proportions precipitated by the underlying issues of poverty, unemployment, community disintegration, social and psychological isolation, and depression. The crisis was and still is particularly evident in some African-American communities of major U.S. metropolitan areas.

Gross (1988) wrote that "nothing in the history of substance abuse has prepared us for the devastation that is caused by crack cocaine. Crack has destroyed entire communities by engulfing families in the web of crack sales or use. Parents who have teenage sons and daughters who have become entrepreneurs by selling crack are unable to refuse the help that this new wealth . . . brings" (p. 1). Crack is rapidly accelerating the destruction of the economically disenfranchised living in poor urban neighborhoods.

Crack cocaine has also been implicated in a number of medical complications such as seizure, stroke, myocardial infarction, psychosis resembling schizophrenia, and death. Even more alarming is the relationship between what Fullilove and Fullilove (1989) called "intersecting epidemics" (p. 146). The association between crack use as "chemical foreplay" and unprotected sexual interaction has resulted in a rising prevalence of sexually transmitted diseases (STDs), in particular human immunodeficiency virus (HIV) infection. Bowser (1989) cited the common practice of bartering unsafe sex for drugs as a factor contributing to the rise in STD prevalence in adolescent and young adult African-Americans. These youths are literally bartering their lives for crack cocaine.

Typical Course of Addictive Illness: Focus on Cocaine

Perhaps the best approach to understanding the behavioral course and patterns of addictive illness is to view it on a continuum from initiation to dependency. It is, however, necessary to note that not all who initiate drug or alcohol use will progress in a linear fashion to dependency or display behaviors commonly associated with dependency. Data from surveys of high school seniors reveal that there is no clear evidence that all who use cocaine or other substances will progress to behaviors diagnostic of addiction. This supports the idea that addiction, or dependency, is not a unitary phenomenon with a single isolatable cause but rather the result of the multiplicative interaction among a host of variables.

Genetic and environmental vulnerabilities play important roles in the progression from initiation to continuation, transition, abuse, and, finally, addiction and dependency. No one ever plans to become dependent or addicted, and most people do not wish to be labeled as such. Individuals often describe a progression that began with socially mediated use. Such use appears to meet usual expectations and occurs in the context of social interactions. For some, the substance and setting will be reinforcing, priming the individual for a pattern of use. For others, the experience will be unpleasant enough to prevent further use. In the case of cocaine, the drug produces such strong feelings of euphoria, alertness, control, and increased energy that future use, particularly where access is easy, is quite enticing (Daigle et al., 1988).

The continuation stage of substance abuse is a subsequent period in which substance use persists but does not appear to be detrimental to the individual. In cocaine abuse, continued use often occurs in a binge pattern (Gawin, 1988). Individuals are able to exercise some control over use, but use becomes more frequent. Use during this stage is not seen as problematic by either the individual or the social network.

However, drugs like cocaine are thought to be primary reinforcers that act on "reward pathways" within the brain. Evidence for this view comes from animal studies in which the animal with unlimited access will self-administer cocaine until exhaustion or death (Gawin, 1988; Rowbotham, 1988). This reinforcement phenomenon suggests that a sizable portion of the human population is at risk for cocaine addiction. Perhaps we have witnessed so few cocaine-related fatalities in the past because of the high cost and illicit nature of the drug. However, crack is rapidly attenuating this effect; many crack users state that they "use until the money runs out or the drug runs out."

A critical point is the transition from substance use to substance abuse. There may be evidence to both the users and their social networks that the use of the substance is having adverse effects. During this stage, users may begin to use more often and in more varied settings. Rationalizations for use are commonly constructed during this stage to deny the seriousness and consequences of the substance use.

The social network may also play a role in allowing the substance abuse to continue. Spouses may call work to report that their partner is "sick." Social network members may compensate for the fact that the student is absent from school, the car payment is late, or an important appointment is canceled or forgotten. These distress signals are quite common but often go unrecognized. One of the main reasons for this is that periods of use may be interspersed with periods of abstinence. This reinforces the individual's, and often the significant other's, perceived sense of control over the substance use, control that is, in fact, illusory.

The changes in the neural norm and the resultant reinforcement play a significant role in the progression, in susceptible individuals, from abuse to dependency. In cocaine, heroin, and alcohol dependency (addiction), abstinence symptomatology plays a significant role in the progression from use to abuse and to dependency and addiction. Gawin (1988) discussed abstinence symptoms in the cocaine abuser as depression, lethargy, and anhedonia (inability to feel pleasure). In the genetically and environmentally primed individual, these symptoms determine the pattern of withdrawal from the drug. The marked depression experienced by the user when off cocaine, which resembles clinical depression, is contrasted with the recalled euphoria produced by the use of the drug. These factors, coupled with associational cues, help to initiate the vicious cycle of binge use with increased craving and continued self-administration to relieve symptoms.

The development of addiction or dependency is marked by changes in both behavior and cognition. There is an increasing focus on the substance and a narrowing of interests, social activities, and relationships. The process of becoming dependent or addicted requires the individual to negate evidence or information that may challenge the behavior or the rationalization of the behavior. There is a preoccupation with the substance and its procurement during this stage,

---

TYPICAL COURSE OF ADDICTIVE ILLNESS: STAGES IN CONTINUUM FROM INITIATION TO DEPENDENCY

I. Initiation
   A. First use of the substance
   B. Exposure frequently through family or friends
II. Continuation
   A. Continued more frequent use of substance
   B. Usually social use only with no detrimental effects
III. Transition
   A. Beginning of change in total consumption, frequency, and occasions of use
   B. More than just social use with beginning of loss of control
IV. Abuse
   A. Adverse effects and consequences to substance use
   B. Rationalizations for continued use and denial of adverse effects present in user and significant others
   C. Unsuccessful attempts at control of use
V. Dependency/addiction
   A. Physical or psychological dependence, or both, on the substance marked by behavioral and cognitive changes
   B. Preoccupation with the substance and its procurement despite negative consequences
   C. Narrowing of interests, social activities, and relationships to only those related to the substance use

even in the face of negative consequences. Intervention in this negative, self-destructive downward spiral of the addiction stage is paramount. Although we have outlined the process of cocaine addiction, dependency on other substances, such as alcohol or narcotics, usually takes a similar course.

MODES OF INTERVENTION

As a result of the numerous theories about substance abuse, there are a wide variety of intervention strategies. At the community level, legislative measures have limited access to potentially addictive pharmaceuticals and illicit street drugs. The growing social demand for smoke-free environments in public buildings, restaurants, airplanes, and similar areas exemplifies how perceptions of tobacco and its risks have changed over the past 50 years. Alcohol taxes, zoning schemes for liquor outlets, a legal drinking age, and legal sanctions on driving while intoxicated are other examples of community efforts to prevent or contain substance abuse.

Educational programs administered through schools and penal institutions have also developed to prevent or foster early recognition of substance abuse. Television and radio have provided public service communications about the risks of substance abuse and the availability of treatment for these problems.

The formation of national associations, such as the National Council on Alcoholism, and the establishment of federal research entities, such as the National Institute on Drug Abuse and the National Institute on Alcohol Abuse and Alcoholism, have facilitated centralized efforts in the areas of education, research, and treatment. At the state level, there have also been legislative provisions to fund substance abuse treatment and rehabilitation.

Prevention

In keeping with our philosophy of "thinking upstream," our actions as community health nurses and client advocates should be geared toward primary prevention. Primary prevention in the community includes working with community gatekeepers to identify high-risk situations and potential problems that threaten the integrity of the community and its inhabitants. Community health nurses may choose to work with community-based organizations and community leaders to develop education programs that help to maintain cultural and community integrity. A community assessment can help to identify macro- and microlevel factors that predispose individuals to high-risk behavior such as alcohol and drug problems.

Prevention is a critical tool in minimizing the impact of alcohol and drug problems on contemporary society. The word "minimizing" suggests a reduction in harm, not abatement or amelioration. In this chapter we ascribe to a view that acknowledges society's continued preoccupation and flirtation with potentially lethal and noxious substances for the purpose of achieving an altered state. This practice is well documented throughout history. Most individuals will never come to the attention of health care providers. However, others, those with a biopsychological and environmental vulnerability, should be targeted with preventive efforts at every level.

On the federal level, prevention efforts have been overshadowed by the ongoing "war on drugs." A significant amount of fiscal resources has been allocated to law enforcement, interdiction, crop eradication, and harsh, punitive laws to prosecute drug users and manufacturers. Debate continues to be waged as to the cost-benefit ratio of drug legalization or decriminalization (Grinspoon and Bakalar, 1994; Kleber, 1994). Supporters for legalization and decriminalization (Grinspoon and Bakalar, 1994) argue that to do so would lead to a reduction in crime and would move the drug problem out of the realm of moral failings of individuals toward more humane treatment and approaches.

Opponents argue that decriminalization and legalization of drugs would do little to abate crime related to drug manufacture, sales, and use (Kleber, 1994). It would, in fact, lead to more crime because decriminalization and legalization of drugs such as heroin and cocaine are used in an escalating pattern requiring the individual to direct more energy and effort toward procurement. Children would be able to purchase what were typically expensive drugs such as cocaine if drugs were societally sanctioned and subsidized. Finally, Kleber (1994) argued that until society can effectively deal with the pernicious effects of two lethal but legal drugs (i.e., alcohol and nicotine) the argument for adding more is difficult to accept and to justify.

No doubt legalization and decriminalization would have some effect on society's drug problem, but in which direction? Prohibition did not solve the alcohol problem, and its impact on the culturally dry drinking norms of African-Americans has been well documented in the literature (Kleber, 1994).

Programs like needle exchange, although controversial because they challenge the morality of traditional society and appear to support the proponents of legalization and decriminalization, have had some success. Needle exchange programs may not lead the intravenous drug user down the path of abstinence, but they do, in fact, serve to break the link in the deadly chain of AIDS transmission and exposure (Bowersox, 1994). Other prevention efforts should target susceptible aggregates (i.e., women, adolescents, people of color, and the aging population). Prevention must seek to reduce the potential harm and morbidity and mortality associated with alcohol and drug problems.

Prevention efforts in the African-American community and in other communities of color have produced results that are less than dramatic. This is perhaps for the same reasons that treatment programs are criticized: failure to incorporate culturally sensitive and appropriate interventions and strategies. The demand for ethnic-specific focused prevention and treatment reflects the growing awareness that Euro-American treatment strategies are failing to minimize the problems of alcohol and drugs in communities of color. The demand for culturally specific approaches is evidence that previous approaches and the assumptions that underlie them are insufficient for understanding and explaining the behavior of people of color. Until this fundamental fact finds acceptance in the general public, prevention and treatment efforts will continue to yield dismal results for certain susceptible aggregates. Successful prevention efforts are usually not focused solely on alcohol and drug abuse but are community controlled and work toward improving individuals' general competencies, communication skills, and self-esteem (Montagne and Scott, 1993).

Nurses may be the first to identify or suspect an alcohol and drug problem in the clients and families with whom they are working. The key to identifying alcohol and drug problems is to maintain a high index of suspicion. Substance use patterns should be routinely assessed by nurses in all care contexts when client histories are performed. The client history is a critical assessment and screening tool that can be used to identify those at risk. The history is the most valuable source of information. Using current knowledge and theory about etiologic process and risk factors should help to identify those individuals predisposed to alcohol and drug use.

Treatment

There are two main types of treatment programs: inpatient and outpatient. Each of these programs may or may not include a detoxification component. Treatment programs also differ in other ways: they may be voluntary versus compulsory and pharmacologically based versus drug free (Brown, 1985). Although treatment in general is intricately tied to the concept of recovery, specific treatment approaches are guided by disciplinary philosophy. Thus, there are a variety of (sometimes contradictory) treatment approaches and models, as determined by the composition of staff and the philosophical approach (social vs. psychological vs. medical models) to substance abuse problems. Most recently, emphasis has been on matching clients to treatment modes to improve success rates (U.S. Department of Health and Human Services, 1990).

Inpatient treatment isolates individuals from the external world and provides an opportunity to focus only on the substance abuse issues. Outpatient treatment, on the other hand, is appropriate for those who do not require such structure and protection; it is best suited to those with strong supportive social networks and high levels of motivation to recover.

Other types of treatment settings include the therapeutic community, which is a semistructured environment offering a supportive network of other recovering individuals. The classic example of a therapeutic community is that of Synanon, a society developed to reorient addicts to be socially productive (Olin, 1980). The therapeutic community helps to integrate the individual slowly into mainstream society and has had some success with long-term narcotics users.

The necessity and type of treatment are determined by the severity of the individual's alcohol or drug problems as well as pertinent cultural factors. The assessment process is, therefore, of primary importance and begins with an accurate social and medical history. The history taking begins with more general questions about lifestyle, employment, relationships, and self-perception. This general line of questioning permits the development of a therapeutic relationship with the client (Nilseen, 1994).

A therapeutic relationship based on trust is essential to collecting information about high-risk socially deviating behavior such as drug and alcohol use. The assessment should then proceed to ascertain at-risk behavior patterns and stressors. The interviewer asks about dietary practices, prior health problems, allergies, hospitalizations, including psychiatric disorders, and family history of such problems, including drug- and alcohol-related problems. This general line of questioning can be followed by more specific questions about injurious behaviors such as smoking, drinking, and illicit drug use. This ordering of questions moves from the more societally sanctioned to societally disapproved behavior, from the general to the more specific. Positive responses to questions about drug and alcohol use should be probed in a nonjudgmental but direct way for pattern, frequency, and timing.

Screening tools such as the CAGE test are simple and brief and can be incorporated in the interview and history. A positive response to any of the CAGE questions does not constitute a diagnosis of alcohol or drug dependence but should raise a high index of suspicion and mandate further investigation (Mayfield, et al., 1974).

The physical examination is another valuable tool in evaluating the client for potential or actual alcohol and drug problems. Although at-risk clients may not have physical signs of alcohol and drug problems and may even deny obvious consequences of such, certain physical findings warrant further investigation. Complaints such as vague, nonspecific abdominal pain, insomnia, depression, chronic fatigue, back pain, chronic anxiety, and night sweats require more intensive investigation. Clients with hypertension unaccounted for by specific pathogenesis or refractory to pharmacotherapeutic intervention should be questioned about heavy alcohol consumption. Spider angiomata on the thorax or face may be the result of long-term alcohol use. Laboratory tests may yield no clues to drug or alcohol use. However, certain laboratory findings in the absence of other etiologic agents may increase the index of suspicion. An elevated mean corpuscular volume and liver function test when coupled with hypertension, tachycardia, and brisk reflexes may point to active abstinence symptomatology.

Brief intervention strategies frequently begin with information about the effects of alcohol and drugs and a discussion of the solutions to substance abuse–related problems. This initial educational approach can defuse frequently encountered barriers to intervention. These barriers include shame, denial, guilt, fear, and the client's erroneous perceptions and attitudes about alcohol and drug problems. Presenting information

and solutions in a nonjudgmental and clear fashion may help to minimize defensiveness. Reframing interventions within the context of health maintenance or health promotion and education can be less threatening. Confronting myths about alcohol and drug problems may help clients to change their attitudes and thus minimize the potential for serious consequences. Ambivalent clients may respond to education and decide to abstain from or seek treatment. Other clients, however, even when confronted with legal, financial, physical, and psychological consequences, may resist offers of treatment. Therefore, the clinician needs to continue to work with the client and involve important members of the social network to remove internal and environmental barriers and move the client toward a place of readiness for change and treatment (Hall, 1994). Sometimes fear of discrimination in group settings and logistic problems such as lack of child care are part of the resistance to treatment. Clients from marginalized groups may not trust health care providers because of past negative experiences (Hall, 1993; Stevens and Hall, 1990).

At the local level, a major proportion of the total effort has been invested in detoxification, residential, and, more recently, outpatient treatment programs. Detoxification is best described as a short-term treatment intervention designed most often to manage acute withdrawal from the substance. Detoxification involves medical management to attenuate the untoward side effects of the substance and to help stabilize the client.

Addressing acute withdrawal symptoms is of utmost importance, particularly in the case of the cocaine abuser who may experience extreme depression with suicidal ideation. Such feelings may cause the individual who is withdrawing from treatment to begin the vicious cycle of abuse again. Alcohol detoxification may have life-threatening medical consequences. Thus, detoxification is one of the most crucial periods in the recovery process. Some detoxification programs are not medically supervised but instead are administered by volunteer recovering addicts who offer social support. Clinicians should be aware of the level of services offered in any detoxification program to make appropriate referrals.

Outpatient and inpatient treatment programs vary but usually include group and individual therapy and counseling, family counseling educational techniques, and socialization into 12-step mutual self-help groups. Some of these programs have also used disulfiram (Antabuse) therapy, methadone maintenance, hypnosis, occupational therapy, psychoanalysis, confrontation, assertiveness training, cognitive therapy, blood alcohol level discrimination training, and other behavior modification approaches. Because relapses are common, most efficacious treatment programs have incorporated some form of relapse prevention as a part of the healing process (Annis, 1990; Marlatt and Gordon, 1986).

Mutual self-help therapeutic groups like Alcoholics Anonymous (AA), Cocaine Anonymous, and Narcotics Anonymous are believed by many to be an essential component of the recovery process. These groups prescribe a program of introspection and personal growth with social support to maintain long-term abstinence. The programs endorse the disease concept of addiction, accept loss of control as its hallmark, and advocate total abstinence. Drug addiction and alcoholism are thus believed to be chronic in nature, with acute periods of symptom exacerbation occurring with relapses to substance use. Treatment programs that demand total abstinence as the basis of recovery form a strong therapeutic alliance with mutual help groups. Many substance-abusing clients find mutual help groups to be of great benefit to them, but health care professionals should be aware that these groups vary in their composition, and some clients may choose to be only marginally involved or not at all.

Some important points to remember regarding treatment are as follows:

1. Treatment should be tailored to the specific needs of the individual because not all addicts and alcoholics are the same.
2. Treatment should stress the importance of family or significant other interaction and attempt to engage important social network members in the process.
3. Treatment is not recovery but rather part of the recovery process and experience. As such, treatment programs must address the aftercare needs of the client to maintain the gains made in treatment.
4. A comprehensive treatment approach will recognize the multifaceted nature of dependence and addiction and attempt to address these multiple influences within the course of the treatment and after discharge.

Having a substance abuse problem does not mean that problems are always attributable to the addictive difficulty. Many substance-abusing clients also have other psychiatric problems, such as schizophrenia, depression, bipolar affective disorders, dissociative disorders, and posttraumatic stress syndrome. These require specialized attention and warrant a case management approach. Likewise, many of these clients have chronic medical problems. Currently, an abundance of research links childhood abuse with later substance abuse problems (Brown and Anderson, 1991; Miller et al., 1987; Windle, 1994).

Research on treatment programs demonstrates that some treatment is better than no treatment but has not established significant differences in the rate of effectiveness of particular kinds of treatment programs (Miller and Hester, 1980; Sobel, 1978). Treatment evaluation depends also on the criteria used to measure effectiveness and the period of time over which the assessment takes place.

Examples of criteria that have been used are

- Number of days abstinent
- Number of days without negative consequences of substance use
- Employability or work attendance
- Self-image improvement
- Spouse's assessment of client's functionality
- Regular attendance at 12-step groups
- Compliance with follow-up appointments
- Absence of overt psychiatric symptoms, such as depression or anxiety
- Self-reports of progress
- Evidence of personal satisfaction and growth

It is clear that treatment programs vary and that certain programs will be more culturally appropriate and effective than others for particular aggregates of individuals.

Pharmacotherapies

In the search for a panacea for the treatment of those susceptible to drug and alcohol problems, several pharmacotherapeutic adjuncts to formalized treatment have been discovered. This section is a brief primer on pharmacotherapies currently used by treatment providers. Good clinical judgment and patient motivation should guide the use of any pharmacotherapy. Current pharmacotherapies include either those drugs used to assist in the initiation and maintenance of abstinence or those drugs used as a substitute for illegal drug use.

Disulfiram (Antabuse) is widely used as an adjunct to formal treatment in those individuals with recalcitrant alcohol problems refractory to treatment. Disulfiram, when combined with alcohol, produces the classic disulfiram ethanol reaction (DER) (i.e., flushing, tachycardia, nausea, headache, chest tightness, and chest pain). The DER is a dose-dependent response and is highly variable. The DER is thought to be the result of a disturbance in alcohol metabolism. According to Banys (1988), "most symptoms can be attributed to increased levels of circulating acetaldehyde" (p. 246). The DER typically begins within minutes after alcohol consumption. Significant risks of the DER are cardiovascular symptoms of tachycardia, hypotension, dysrhythmia, and shock. Thus, preexisting cardiac disease is an absolute contraindication. Emergency treatment of the DER is symptomatic. Disulfiram is not a complete form of treatment of alcohol problems. A select group—those who are relapse prone, those who have supportive networks, and those who have histories of abstinence—may benefit from short-term use. Requests for disulfiram, in the absence of treatment and supportive relationship, should not be granted.

Naltrexone, also known as Trexan or ReVia, was first synthesized in 1965 (Kleber, 1985). Naltrexone is a long-acting narcotic antagonist currently used as an adjunct in the treatment of opiate dependence. It blocks the effects of opiates via competitive binding but does not block the effects of other substances such as benzodiazepines, cocaine, or alcohol. Most recently, the National Institutes on Alcohol Abuse and Alcoholism (Gordis, 1995) released preliminary findings of a study detailing naltrexone's use in alcohol-dependent clients. Preliminary information indicates that naltrexone reduces craving, rates of relapse to alcohol, and severity of alcohol-related problems. Other clinical studies are ongoing.

Methadone and buprenorphine deserve special mention as therapeutic aids in drug and alcohol treatment. The use of methadone, a long-acting oral opioid, continues to be debated. This debate reflects philosophical commitments to abstinence versus sanctioned use. For a select group of opiate-dependent individuals, methadone has facilitated their return to normal functioning. Traditionally, methadone has been used either as a detoxifying agent or a maintenance drug. As a detoxification agent, methadone is dispensed over a 21-day period in a tapering dose. Dosage is dependent on the degree of opiate withdrawal symptoms present. Dose reduction typically occurs gradually over a 1- to 2-day period. Methadone maintenance is more controversial because the individual remains dependent on the drug, which is dispensed under medical supervision as part of a treatment program. Maintenance may minimize or abate illegal activity, eliminate the infection hazards of injection drug use, reduce social disruption typically seen with opiate use, and facilitate

increased levels of functioning. A myth about maintenance programs is that methadone produces a euphoric "high" and is, therefore, merely a legal substitute for heroin.

Buprenorphine is an opioid angonist-antagonist that has been used in the treatment of opiate-dependent clients and those with concurrent cocaine dependence (Mello et al., 1993). Buprenorphine does not produce severe withdrawal, an advantage over methadone, on abrupt cessation. Its antagonist component helps to reduce the possibility of lethal overdose (Mello et al., 1993). Preliminary clinical studies as reported by Mello and colleagues (1993) support the use of buprenorphine in reducing the frequency of heroin and cocaine self-administration.

Opiate withdrawal produces classic symptoms such as sweating, anxiety, hypertension, piloerection, increased gastrointestinal motility, diarrhea, and tachycardia because of long-standing central nervous system depression (Clark and Longmuir, 1985). Clonidine, or Catapres, has been successfully used in opiate detoxification. Although clonidine has not been approved by the U.S. Food and Drug Administration for this purpose, the drug is frequently used to assist in detoxification. Clonidine attenuates signs of active opiate withdrawal by reducing sympathetic tone and outflow as well as decreasing peripheral vascular resistance, heart rate, and blood pressure. Oral clonidine or transdermal clonidine patches and nonsteroidal agents assist in detoxification. On an outpatient basis, the client using clonidine should be monitored closely for signs of clonidine overdosage including hypotension, dry mouth, and fatigue. As is true of disulfiram, the use of clonidine alone is insufficient as a treatment modality for those with opiate dependence. Social, behavioral, and cognitive interventions should accompany pharmacotherapies.

Other Approaches

Substance abuse problems are socially defined and frequently imputed to sufferers who are not complaining about their substance abuse (Szasz, 1985). Furthermore, the substance abuse treatment system has increasingly taken on social welfare and criminal justice tasks (Weisner, 1983). In this sense, substance abuse differs from many other health-related problems. Most states have laws pertaining to involuntary treatment of substance abusers. Employers and families are often enlisted to assist or coerce the identified client into accepting treatment. This aspect of substance abuse as a health concern raises some crucial questions for health care providers in terms of the encroachment of therapeutic intervention on individual rights to privacy, informed consent, and self-determination (Peyrot, 1985).

On the individual level, substance abuse is dealt with in a number of ways, depending on the cultural and educational background and resources of the person, the attitudes of significant others, the degree of invasiveness of the effects of the substance use, and the visibility of alternatives. Some research has shown that a small percentage of individuals who recognize a harmful pattern of substance use are able to stop using the substance or to achieve a controlled, nonpathologic pattern of use (Biernacki, 1986). There are those who, because of the impact of an important life change such as completion of education or getting married, appear to change from excessive use to social use of alcohol. Interventions have been developed to assist some individuals in achieving moderation (Larimer and Marlatt, 1990).

Nevertheless, significant numbers of people exhibit serious problems related to their use of mood-altering substances. These individuals are usually not able to stop or control their use without outside intervention. Historically, in U.S. society, the stigma against addicts and alcoholics has ensured that substance abuse problems are usually not recognized before they have become severe or chronic. In the case of alcohol, research on the ability of identified problem drinkers to return to social alcohol use is still inconclusive. Consequently, most scientists and health care providers advocate abstinence from alcohol as a cornerstone of recovery. Moderate or social use of illicit drugs is usually not considered because of the serious criminal implications involved.

Abstinence is difficult to maintain on a long-term basis (after 1 year). Therefore, an important area of continuing research is relapse prevention, a behavioral approach that aims to prepare the client for the relapse situation in the hope of preventing it or minimizing its negative impact on the entire recovery process (Marlatt and Gordon, 1986). The relapse prevention model can be applied to alcohol, drug, and behavioral addictive problems such as overeating and compulsive gambling and can have either controlled use or abstinence as its goal. In relapse prevention, cognitive reframing, role-playing, and plans for coping with negative mood states are done in preparation for meeting the challenge of craving and potential relapse.

Mutual Help Groups

Mutual help groups are associations that are voluntarily formed, are not professionally dominated, and operate through face-to-face supportive interaction focusing on a mutual goal. Many mutual help groups exist, and they are usually organized by recovering substance abusers or those recovering from compulsive behavior patterns. The first of these was AA, which was founded in 1935. Initially, a small group of Euro-American male alcoholics found a way to stay sober one day at a time through meetings with others like themselves. The early AA members developed 12 steps to guide the recovery process (Kurtz, 1979). The process can be summarized as follows:

- Admission of defeat and surrender to a power higher than one's self
- Inventory of past shortcomings and strengths
- Spiritual practices (prayer and meditation)
- Willingness to change
- Making amends
- Extension of this process to all of one's life (Brown, 1985; Kurtz, 1979)

AA has been popularly viewed as relatively successful. Because it is nonprofessional and is an ongoing source of assistance, it is an invaluable resource to the community. However, not all of those with alcohol problems find AA to be comfortable, culturally relevant, and socially supportive. Predominantly in large cities, women, people of color, gay men, and lesbians with alcohol problems have formed their own AA groups as well as other mutual help organizations for social support in recovery. Because of the realities of social discrimination and regional variation in customs, AA should not be considered a universal form of assistance for alcohol problems. However, it is surprising how many individuals from diverse social backgrounds find acceptance and support in AA.

Other 12-step programs have developed through adaptation of AA's approach to similar addictive problems. Narcotics Anonymous, Gamblers Anonymous, Debtors Anonymous, Cocaine Anonymous, Overeaters Anonymous, and Sex and Love Addicts Anonymous are examples. Because they became organized more recently than AA, these groups may not be as well known or as widely available and may not exhibit as much diversity among their membership as does AA. The 12 steps have also been applied to the syndromes of compulsive behavior and other difficulties experienced by the children, partners, and close associates of substance abusers. Al-Anon, Codependents Anonymous, and Adult Children of Alcoholics are examples of these groups. Although these groups initially had a predominance of female members, the trend is moving toward participation by equal numbers of men and women.

In general, 12-step meetings follow one of the following formats:

- Uninterrupted talks by one or more speakers about "what it was like, what happened, and what it is like now"
- Discussion in which each person at the meeting has the opportunity to speak briefly
- Some combination of the first two options

The customs shaping the actual format and sequence of the meeting vary according to group size, region of the country, ethnic and sex composition, and other cultural biases of the members. AA meetings are not standardized.

At least two mutual help groups have developed in response to their founders' negative experiences in AA or their failure to succeed in AA. Women for Sobriety was organized to replace or augment AA for women who tend to find AA inappropriately ego diminishing and often sexist in its literature and customs (Kirkpatrick, 1978). Secular Sobriety Groups were organized to meet the needs of atheists, agnostics, and others who are unable to accept the concept of or to depend on a "higher power" in their recovery from alcohol problems (Christopher, 1988).

Other mutual help groups that do not follow the 12 steps are available for a variety of addictive problems. Some of these, such as Weight Watchers, require monetary commitment, unlike AA, which has no required dues or fees. Others have more involvement by professionals, such as Recovery Incorporated, which offers support to psychiatric clients. Any of these groups might also be considered resources for selected persons with substance abuse problems.

The organization and proliferation of mutual help groups may be one of the most important social developments of the 20th century. The groups make up the most important human and ideologic resource readily available to communities for the purpose of managing substance abuse. In the future, mutual help groups may begin to address prevention as well as become more involved with professional and government entities in the war on substance abuse. An example of such involvement can be seen in neighborhood organization strategies, such as "Fighting Back," devised by those whose immediate environment has become highly unsafe, flooded with illicit drugs, and subject to the effects of gang warfare (Robert Wood Johnson Foundation, 1992). In this scenario, recovery has been redefined as the communal reclamation of living space through collective action; this is often achieved one building and one block at a time. These actions are important examples of how substance abuse can be responded to as a collective rather than as an individual problem.

MODES OF INTERVENTION FOR SUBSTANCE ABUSE

Individual and Family Levels

- Education
- Treatment: detoxification, inpatient, outpatient, residential
- Mutual help groups (e.g., Alcoholics Anonymous, Narcotics Anonymous, Cocaine Anonymous, Al-Anon, Narcanon)

Community Level

- Law enforcement measures to limit access and distribution of addictive substances (street drugs)
- Alcohol taxes, zoning schemes for liquor outlets
- Legal drinking age and legal sanctions on driving while intoxicated
- Education programs at schools and penal institutions
- Television and radio public service communications concerning the risks of substance abuse and the availability of treatment

State and Federal Levels

- Formation of national associations such as the National Council on Alcoholism
- Establishment of federal research entities such as the National Institute on Drug Abuse and the National Institute on Alcohol Abuse and Alcoholism to centralize research, education, and treatment efforts
- Legislative provisions at the state level to fund substance abuse treatment and rehabilitation

SOCIAL NETWORK INVOLVEMENT
Family and Friends

The social network of the substance abuser can either be quite influential in helping the individual alter behavior or aid and abet the substance abuser in self-destruction. There is evidence for both positive and negative effects of social support in either mitigating or supporting the behaviors of substance abusers (Cronkite and Moos, 1980; Hall and Havassey, 1986; Jackson, 1954; Steinglass, 1985).

There is also evidence, particularly in the aggregate of adolescents and young adults, that substance use and abuse often occur in the context of social interactions. Alcohol and other substances may be used by adolescents as a social lubricant during an often-troubled developmental period (Abelson and Miller, 1985; O'Malley et al., 1985). Family treatment is considered essential in substance abuse because the family can be instrumental in enabling the continuation of substance abuse through protection and support of the individual during both using and inactive using time. In addition, the family has suffered the effects of the substance abuse emotionally, socially, economically, physically, and spiritually. For the substance abuser to return to an environment supportive of recovery, the family's wounds must be acknowledged and treated.

A term that deserves particular attention is *codependency*. Codependency is a common but ambiguous term and is used differently by various disciplines and segments of the lay population. Perhaps its most comprehensive definition is that by Subby (1984): codependency is "an emotional, psychological and behavioral condition that develops as a result of an individual's prolonged exposure to, and practice of, a set of oppressive rules; rules which prevent the open expression of feelings as well as the direct discussion of personal and interpersonal problems" (p. 26).

Codependency is actually a newer term for an interactional pattern that was recognized long ago by investigators (Jackson, 1954). There are definite and identifiable patterns of interaction that describe the alcoholic or addicted family system. Other researchers (Stanton et al., 1978; Steinglass, 1985) supported the existence of these patterns in the family of the substance abuser and alcoholic. These behaviors help to maintain the family in a pattern that supports substance abuse and addiction.

There are mutual help groups for addressing codependency that are founded on the principles of AA and provide opportunities to discuss the issues germane to the alcoholic or addicted family system or network. Families participating in treatment should also be encouraged to participate in these mutual help groups.

Codependency cannot be concretely defined the same way in each culture. Cultures and ethnic groups vary in the degree to which individuals are expected to anticipate the needs of others and care for them. The danger in applying a rigid definition of codependency in all cases is that it might unfairly and inappropriately be labeled as a disease in some cultures that value interdependency over individualism (Haaken, 1990).

The nurse needs to identify the important members of the social network for each client and the ways in which these individuals provide support for the client. The nurse must also recognize that the concept of family refers not only to nuclear families but also includes alternative family systems. Whatever the constellation of family, significant others should be included in the treatment and intervention. Substance abuse, addiction, and recovery do not occur in a vacuum, and many relapses are precipitated by interpersonal conflicts.

Effects on the Family

Substance abuse has been called a family disease because it affects the entire family system, with potential adverse, psychological, and physical consequences for the family members in addition to the abuser (Bekir et al., 1993; Bradshaw, 1988). Family theorists view families, whether the traditional nuclear form or an alternative, as social systems that try to stay in balance (Minuchin, 1974; Satir et al., 1975). They see families as either functional or dysfunctional depending on how well they fulfill the social tasks expected of them by our society. Substance-abusing families are frequently observed to be dysfunctional in clinical terms. However, cultural and political factors should also be considered because families may have developed these patterns for historic reasons rather than as the effects of substance abuse.

A functional family system is open and flexible and allows its members to be free to be themselves. In the nuclear family model, the parents model intimacy for the children, differences are negotiated, boundaries are clear, and communication is consistent and clear. In functional family systems, whether the traditional nuclear family or other nontraditional forms, there is trust, individuality, and accountability among family members. All family members are able to have their needs met in a reasonable way.

On the other hand, dysfunctional families are closed systems with fixed, rigid roles. In the case of substance abuse, a major purpose of the system is to deny the substance abuse of the affected family member and keep this shameful family secret. When a parent is the substance abuser, there may be only the appearance of intimacy between the parents. Generally, ego boundaries between the family members are weakened or nonexistent, with enmeshment of the members and an intolerance of individual differences. Rules are rigid, and communication is unbalanced, either always conflictual or always superficially pleasant. Children may be caught up in a "role reversal" in which they act as caretakers of their parents.

All family functions are centered around the substance abuser, accommodating or compensating for the abuser's behavior (Brown, 1988). The individual needs of the other family members often go unmet. Denial is central to functioning of the family system. The spouse gradually takes over the functions of the substance abuser and control of the family. The children are cast into various roles in their struggle for survival in this environment, such as hero, junior parent, scapegoat, "little princess," peacemaker, or caretaker.

Adult children of these dysfunctional families often carry these roles and coping mechanisms into adult life. Many become substance abusers or partners of substance abusers. The children of alcoholics have been found to be 3.5 times as likely to experience alcoholism (Cotton, 1979; National Institute on Alcohol Abuse and Alcoholism, 1985). They are also more likely to develop problematic behavior patterns that can have serious consequences in their adult lives (Woititz, 1983). Frequently, they have difficulties with intimacy and parenting. Many have lifelong problems with depression and anxiety as well as physical illnesses often associated with depression and anxiety, such as ulcers, colitis, migraine headaches, and eating disorders (Beattie, 1987).

In addition to these psychological burdens that substance abuse places on families, there are the financial burdens related to medical costs, loss of income from job difficulties or unemployment, and the financial losses attributable to divorce. Additionally, spousal violence and child abuse and neglect are strongly associated with substance abuse (Horgan, 1993).

Professional Enablers

Health care professionals have also contributed to the initiation and continuation of substance abuse and dependency in various ways. One obvious way is the physician's role in prescribing psychoactive medications. The medical model advocates the treatment of symptoms by medication, and the relief of pain, anxiety, and insomnia are no exceptions. The addictive potential of narcotic analgesics and antianxiety agents is often ignored if quick symptom relief is the main goal. Long-term goals for the treatment of the medical problems and nonmedication management of pain and anxiety are more thoughtful approaches that could be used.

Also physicians and nurses are often the first to see the physical effects of the substance abuse and are in an excellent position to intervene. By focusing on the health consequences of the substance abuse, they can often form trusting relationships, provide information, and refer patients to the appropriate treatment. Too often, this opportunity is missed because of the health care professional's reluctance to bring up this taboo subject. This reluctance may be based on professionals' inability to examine their own drinking or drug-taking behaviors or those of significant others or on misconceptions and moral judgments of clients.

In the past, many psychiatrists and psychotherapists have focused on the reasons why the person uses substances rather than on the dependency itself. The assumption was that insight would lead to a change in behavior. This approach has usually not proved to be effective, especially if the psychiatrist is concurrently prescribing other potentially addictive antianxiety medications or hypnotics. Complete abstinence from all mood-altering medication is a more effective model for preventing the cross-addiction common in substance abusers (i.e., substituting one substance for another, such as a benzodiazepine for alcohol). Exceptions to this approach are patients with serious medical conditions requiring pain medication and those who also have a second psychiatric disorder, such as schizophrenia, depression, or bipolar affective disorder, which requires medication. Recovering substance abusers often need support when they also must take medication for these conditions, because their recovering peers may condemn the use of any medication, placing the client in a no-win situation. Caregivers have become more aware of signs of substance abuse in clients. Some providers are willing to begin therapy with a non-abstinent client under the stipulation that if no therapeutic gains are being made, the client will be referred for treatment or the caregiver will withdraw services. Clients who lack social support may succeed using this strategy, which allows the formation of a trusting relationship before taking the "leap" to abstinence. Clinical wisdom and research continue to point toward more tailored, individualized approaches to substance abuse (Hall, 1993).

VULNERABLE AGGREGATES

Substance abuse problems viewed from a community perspective clearly affect some populations more severely. Some groups are more susceptible to experiencing substance abuse problems, may tend to deteriorate more quickly in the process, or may have fewer sources of support for recovery compared with the traditional comparison group of middle-class, Euro-American, heterosexual men. These groups are, therefore, called "vulnerable aggregates," and they require special attention in terms of prevention, intervention, and rehabilitation strategies. The current resources for prevention, treatment, and mutual support may not be flexible enough to meet the needs of various vulnerable aggregates who are at risk of experiencing substance abuse problems and are often excluded or alienated from services by policies, provider attitudes, economic constraints, and social isolation.

Most often, substance abusers are young men aged 18 to 35 years, only a portion of whom actually experience lifelong patterns of addiction. African-Americans, Hispanics, and Native Americans are thought to be especially at risk, although some Euro-American ethnic groups, such as Irish-Americans, are also more likely to experience problems, especially with alcohol (Day and Leonard, 1985). A complex web of factors, including ethnic practices, religious beliefs, economic conditions, availability of options and alternatives, and physiologic susceptibility, influences the incidence and type of substance abuse that will be involved in each of these groups of men. For example, gay men have some unique difficulties, such as social ostracism and hostility, to face in adolescence as well as in adulthood.

Adolescents

Adolescence is a period of transition and social stress in which substances are often used for the first time. Substance abuse patterns may be established at this time because of the combined influences of peer pressure, the physiologic immaturity of the user, social role pressures, a risk-taking orientation, and, frequently, the lack of other recreational alternatives. Experimentation often begins early; by Grade 8, 70% have tried alcohol, 10% have tried marijuana, 2% have tried cocaine, and 44% have smoked cigarettes. By Grade 12, 88% have used alcohol, 37% have used marijuana, 8% have used cocaine, and 63% have smoked cigarettes. Because cigarettes and alcohol are tried before illicit drugs such as marijuana, hallucinogens, or cocaine, they are considered "gateway drugs" and are increasingly the focus of prevention efforts. The younger the age for the initiation of drug or alcohol use, the more likely heavy use will exist when the individual becomes older (Horgan, 1993).

Polydrug use characterizes the large majority of adolescent alcohol abusers; marijuana and cocaine are used most frequently. This use appears related to the phenomenon of sensation seeking and the disinhibiting effects of the substances (Martin et al., 1993).

Overall, there has been a decline in the use of drugs by adolescents, especially among the middle class. Adolescent substance abusers are more receptive to treatment than ever and are effectively using AA and other self-help modalities. Among poor socioeconomic groups, however, there may be minimal or no access to affordable care. The adolescents in these groups tend to face multiple problems related to social and family conditions and especially need effective treatment. There has been a decrease in funding for substance abuse treatment by insurance and other third-party payers in general, with less availability of resources. This, unfortunately, comes at a time when the problems of adolescent substance abusers are becoming more complex.

Adolescent substance abuse is viewed more as a behavioral problem rather than a disease because it is so often tied in with developmental issues, especially the task of forming an identity. Adolescents entering treatment now tend to present with more problems that complicate the process of forming an adequate identity than in previous years. Problems such as severe learning disorders, borderline personality disorders, and physical, sexual and emotional abuse and neglect are common. These problems faced by the adolescent substance abusers are frequently related to inadequate parenting and the presence of alcoholism or other addictions in family members (Morrison et al., 1993).

Past prevention efforts for adolescents have focused on drug education with a simplistic abstinence philosophy ("Just say no") that has been neither realistic nor as effective as originally hoped. A more practical approach emphasizes harm reduction as a goal rather than elimination of substance use and advocates using low-risk behaviors (e.g., not sharing needles). Increasingly, drug education in schools is focusing on the choices of adolescents and the consequences associated with these choices (O'Connor and Saunders, 1992). Negative parental attitudes toward illicit drug use, absence of substance-abusing role models, and the existence of an extended family support system are also deterrents against illicit drug abuse, especially in high-risk minority group adolescents (Gfroerer and de la Rosa, 1993).

Elderly

Elderly men and women are considered vulnerable to substance abuse problems because of diminished physiologic tolerance, the increased use of medically prescribed drugs, and the effects of cultural and social isolation that characterize industrial and postindustrial society. Alcohol and drug abuse is the third leading health problem among Americans 55 years of age and older and constitute 10% of cases in geriatric mental health facilities. Although the overall prevalence of alcohol abuse in the elderly population is 10%—the same as in the younger population—the health consequences are worse and the use of effective interventions is more limited (King et al., 1994).

Illicit drug use is not currently common among the elderly but is expected to increase as young and middle-age addicts grow older. Prescription drug abuse, however, is common among elderly women, especially narcotic analgesics, sedatives, and hypnotics. The elderly of both sexes use many over-the-counter medications that may have synergistic or interactive effects with their other medications (Seibert, 1990). Professionals contribute to prescription drug problems when they fail to ascertain all the medications an elderly person is already taking before prescribing more. The complicated medication schedules required by many elderly patients demand full alertness to avoid inadequate doses or self-administered, unintentional overdoses (Seibert, 1990).

Part of early intervention efforts is adequate assessment and diagnosis, which is difficult with the elderly because they do not manifest the problem in the same ways as younger substance abusers. Moos and colleagues (1994) identified these points to remember in assessing the elderly for substance abuse problems:

- One third of the elderly alcoholics do not have onset of symptoms until after age 60 years.
- There is a wide fluctuation in symptoms over time with elderly substance abusers in contrast to younger substance abusers, who experience more consistent and immediate symptoms.
- Elderly substance abuse is more frequently associated with medical, psychiatric, and social problems or dysfunction.

Women

Women make up the vulnerable aggregate that has received the most attention relevant to substance abuse in the past three decades. This attention has been in response to the fact that women had been relatively neglected in substance abuse research. Within the population of women, there are smaller aggregates who are thought to be more severely affected by substance abuse problems (Johnson, 1987); these aggregates include women of color, low-income or no-income women, and working-class women whose increased risk stems from economic, social, and cultural factors. Lesbians are another aggregate of women in whom substance abuse is suspected to be prevalent because of its association with stigmatization and social isolation (Hall, 1994). Women who were sexually abused as children not only are more susceptible to substance abuse problems in adolescence and adulthood, but face many more distressing consequences in substance abuse treatment and recovery (Hall, 1996b).

Many chemicals affect the bodies of women more quickly and destructively than they do men. Drug-dependent women report frequent physical and medical problems; many of these problems are related to their reproductive systems (Sutker, 1981). Also alcoholism appears to have a more rapid progression in women than in men. Women tend to experience symptoms of alcoholic hepatitis and cirrhosis sooner than men in part because they metabolize alcohol at a different rate. Women have higher blood alcohol levels relative to body weight than do men, and estrogen has been shown to be able to change the rate of alcohol metabolism (Vourakis, 1983). Because of these occurrences, it is important to identify problem drinking and drug use early in women before they experience serious consequences.

Substance abuse during pregnancy is a serious health concern because of its effect on the mother and the developing fetus. Nationally, drug use among pregnant women increased steadily from 1980 to 1988 but then appeared to level off (Dicker and Leighton, 1994). The estimated current prevalence of substance abuse among pregnant women is an average of 11% of this population; cocaine is the most frequently abused drug (Jessup, 1992). Excessive alcohol use during pregnancy continues to have long-term developmental consequences on the newborn (Sampson et al., 1994). Problems in pregnant teenagers who are substance abusers are even more complicated than for older women (Trad, 1993).

Women who engage in the abusive pattern of cocaine (crack) use who become pregnant are usually unable to stop their drug use without treatment. Cocaine use during pregnancy is associated with increased risk of spontaneous abortion, premature delivery, and abruptio placentae (Burkett et al., 1990; Mena, 1990). Infants who have been addicted to cocaine in utero are hyperirritable, subject to seizures, possibly at increased risk for sudden infant death syndrome, and extremely difficult to care for. Long-term learning disabilities, behavioral problems, mental retardation, and physical handicaps are other potential consequences for children of cocaine-using mothers (Snyder, 1985). It is important, however, to consider that mothers using crack cocaine do make efforts to protect their children from negative consequences and try to care for them adequately (Kearney et al., 1994).

Getting the pregnant woman into treatment and managing her withdrawal needs to be a top priority but is frequently problematic (Finkelstein, 1993; Jessup, 1992). Social and psychiatric issues complicate the process as well as the pregnant substance abuser's fear of punitive legal actions (Horne, 1993). Besides this fear, the addiction itself often interferes with getting adequate or any prenatal care. Also worrisome is that the high-risk behavior associated with the addiction increases the chances of both the mother and the infant becoming HIV positive.

People of Color

"Thinking upstream" necessitates the examination of causes rather than symptoms alone. This is especially true in the phenomenon of substance abuse.

People of color pose special challenges for the health care professionals working in the field of substance abuse and dependency. For purposes of clarification, people of color constitute a diverse aggregate that includes African-Americans, Latinos and Latinas, Asian and Pacific immigrants, Afro-Caribbean immigrants, and other darker skinned peoples. Although this section focuses on the problems and peculiarities affecting the lives of African-Americans, these same problems can be extrapolated to the lives of other peoples of color, who face similar issues of covert and overt cultural oppression. These vulnerable aggregates are particularly susceptible to the effects of substance abuse and dependency because of their often-oppressed positions in the greater society. Under the strain of poverty, oppression, underemployment, decreased job opportunities, macro- and microlevel aggressions, and ongoing racism, some members of these aggregates find the escapism of substance abuse a preferable alternative to confronting the realities of a hostile and oppressive environment.

Theories of stress, social causation, and oppressed status all argue in favor of institutionalized racism as a factor in the generation of mental illness and alcohol and drug problems in these special aggregates (Dawkins, 1988). Socioeconomic, political, and historic realities have forced some people of color into the illegal drug trade as a means of economic survival. This has altered cultural and community-level values, resulting in an acceptance of high-risk behavior. These sociopolitical and historic realities place people of color at a greater risk for alcohol and drug problems.

Oppression is, in fact, violence in its subtlest form. Bulhan (1985) argued that violence is manifested in any process, condition, or relationship whereby any individual, group, or community inhibits either covertly or overtly or constrains the psychological, physical, or social well-being of others. He further explained that there are four specific types of violence; institutional, intrapersonal, interpersonal, and sociostructural. Sociostructural violence is manifested in oppression, racism, and other constraints on the individual's and the group's ability to actualize potential or self-determination. He argued that the most vivid example of ongoing sociostructural violence is the continuation of disparity in morbidity and mortality between African-Americans, as well as other people of color, and Euro-Americans.

Sociostructural violence has hampered the ability of people of color, in particular African-Americans, to maintain cultural, community, and spiritual integrity.

These problems confronting our society are the remnants of chattel slavery and are reflected in ongoing, but baseless, debates about the significance of skin color as evidence of intellectual, spiritual, physical, and psychological inferiority. Alcohol and drug problems as cultural phenomena are symptoms of this sociostructural violence in the lives of people of color. The implications of alcohol and drug problems in the lives of people of color are clear: continued dissolution of cultural and community integrity, chaos, hostility, and ultimately physical destruction. Patterns of African-American drug-related male homicide support this position. The "chemical slavery" (Amuleru-Marshall, 1993, p. 25) of drug and alcohol abuse is but a symptom of a deeper and persistent problem plaguing our race-conscious society: the problem of cultural domination, oppression, and ongoing sociostructural violence against people of color.

In working with ethnic and racial minorities, it is important for the health care professional to recognize the sociopolitical and socioeconomic factors that form the context of substance use, abuse, and dependency. These same factors will have an impact on help seeking, treatment, and outcome. Cultural sensitivity to the needs and issues germane to these vulnerable aggregates is a prerequisite to successful intervention and treatment.

Critics warn that traditional Euro-American substance abuse treatment modalities negate the ethnoracial minority experiences (Dawkins, 1988; Primm and Wesley, 1986; Ziter, 1987). Thus, treatment approaches geared toward a white society may be inappropriate or less effective for people of color. Regarding the African-American aggregate, Ziter (1987) explained that, because of the institutionalized racism and oppression in U.S. society, the environment for recovery may be contextually and experientially different than that of Euro-Americans, just as the environment that contributed to the initial abuse was different.

In the African-American community, there are several barriers to treating the substance abusing or addicted individual:

- Ongoing sociostructural violence and the history of racism and the psychological handicap it creates on the individual's self-esteem and awareness
- Poverty, underemployment, and unemployment
- Increased availability and accessibility of both drugs and alcohol within the community

- Cultural and community disintegration, which has altered traditional Afrocentric values and behaviors
- Allure and economic rewards of selling drugs
- Inadequate social support system for recovery as an alternative lifestyle and a tool of sociopolitical empowerment for the communities of color, especially African-Americans
- Low self-esteem, internalized racism, anger, and frustration
- A unique and violent "immigrant experience" as slaves

Both external and internal constraints combine to cause and promote alcohol and drug problems within this aggregate of people of color. Chemical slavery is a powerful tool in the arsenal of cultural oppression.

Studies have identified that socioeconomic factors and social support have positive effects on treatment and outcome. Racial and ethnic minorities may represent a sizable portion of the U.S. population that is economically disenfranchised. Limited financial resources may limit alternatives to public treatment settings, which are often understaffed, underfunded, and filled to capacity, with long waiting lists.

Even if the individual completes treatment, returning to the original social environment may undermine any gains made within the treatment setting. Environmental cues and conditioned reinforcement for continued drug and alcohol use may be extremely powerful. The person of color may return to an environment of nonsupport characterized by continued use by important members of the individual's social network. The individual needs a well-coordinated aftercare program that addresses these issues.

The African-American recovering from alcohol and drug problems may return to a community that is rife with conflict and chaos; the culture may be spiritually disintegrating and marred by ongoing sociopolitical violence in the form of intra- and interpersonal racism and oppression. One often feels, without genuine support, a great sense of frustration, isolation, and hopelessness, which characterizes many communities of color. Thompson and Simmons-Cooper (1988) explained that "it becomes a challenge to be an OK individual in an environment where the prevalence of alcohol and drugs is highly visible, provides lucrative rewards and is tolerated within the community" (p. 29).

Recovery ideologies and programs may create an air of conflict and confusion and be in disharmony with the culture of the greater African-American community. As a result, African-Americans in recovery from substance abuse feel alienated and isolated. In early recovery, these feelings may be counterproductive to continued behavioral change and abstinence. Participation in groups such as AA may offer some support, but the African-American may sense or be told that the discussion of underlying issues of racism and oppression is perceived as irrelevant or inappropriate by the AA group. This further increases the individual's sense of isolation.

The treatment of ethnic and racial minority aggregates (people of color) poses special challenges related to the individuals seeking treatment. The health care professional's value system will be challenged as well. Treatment providers must recognize that these vulnerable aggregates will encounter a host of barriers that will make treatment and long-term recovery extremely difficult. Some of these barriers are embedded in the historic and sociopolitical fabric of U.S. society and support the current conditions of racism and oppression. Other factors will be internal to the aggregate. To ignore the significance of either will lead to ineffectiveness in engaging the individual in treatment and promoting long-term recovery. The dilemma confronting people of color and treatment provider alike is deciding what culturally sensitive and appropriate elements need to be incorporated in a program.

For African-Americans, recovery built on Afrocentric values conceptualizes alcohol and drug problems as a "cultural-political disorder imposed on African-American communities [and other communities of color] as a social control mechanism to maintain Euro-American [dominance]" (Rowe and Grills, 1993, p. 256). Effective treatment and recovery must emphasize empowerment, which is an essential necessity that facilitates African-Americans' self-determination and cultural survival. Recovery is reframed as consciousness raising, a tool of empowerment for people of color.

Programs and providers must, if they are to work from the public health perspective of thinking upstream, examine larger macrolevel issues that increase the susceptibility of people of color to alcohol and drug problems. Cultural domination by Euro-Americans and cultural disintegration as a result of this domination must be addressed. To this end, many have called

for a drastic philosophical change in the way current treatment programs operate (Rowe and Grills, 1993; Smith et al., 1993).

African-American–centered treatment and prevention frameworks have been developed to address the deficits of contemporary programs. These programs incorporate Afrocentric value structures with the intent of empowering the African-American community to "alter the fundamental cultural and political power imbalances" that give a superior position to the person of European ancestry (Rowe and Grills, 1993, p. 26).

Bolin (1995), in an unpublished manuscript, posed the question, "Is Alcoholics Anonymous culturally sensitive to the needs of people of color?" The current demand for an Afrocentric framework suggests that the answer may very well be no. An Afrocentric prevention and treatment framework such as the African-American Extended Family Project (AAEFP), located in San Francisco, is a model that attempts to address some of the deficits of traditional 12-step programs and formalized treatment. Like other Afrocentric models, AAEFP is the direct result of the forward thinking of such notable scholars and clinicians as David Smith, the founder of the Haight Ashbury Free Clinics, and Dr. Peter Bell, an African-American addictions specialist. AAEFP incorporates some of the fundamental strengths of the African-American value systems: family, spirituality, collective culture, and racial consciousness.

The program questions tenets of 12-step programs such as AA, particularly the concept of powerlessness and anonymity, both for the individual and the collective group. Although AAEFP makes use of AA, it has developed its 10 "terms of resistance" (Smith et al., 1993, p. 103), which echo some of the fundamental aspects of the 12 steps of AA. More specifically, African-Americans, because of historic and contemporary sociostructural violence, have felt and endured a tremendous sense of powerlessness as it relates to self-determination and individual and collective change. Western epistemological ideologies stress individualism, which clashes with the Afrocentric values of family, community, and collective survival. The terms of resistance attempt to reframe abstinence and sobriety, not as ends in themselves but as tools of empowerment that are necessary for living in a hostile and violent environment (Smith et al., 1993).

Recovery at AAEFP occurs within the context of the extended family with a shift away from powerlessness and anonymity to self-determination, personal responsibility, collective consciousness, and community survival. Alcohol and drugs are conceptualized as direct blocks to opportunities for participation in the larger social system, further encapsulate and isolate the community and the individual, and support the negative valuations levied by a racist and oppressive society. Programs such as AAEFP do more to address the macrolevel issues than traditional programs by expanding the conceptualization not only of alcohol and drug problems but of recovery as well. This conceptualization of recovery as empowerment may be more meaningful to people of color than a definition of recovery as "returning to the mainstream."

Other Aggregates

Substance abuse is considered the most common psychopathologic problem in the general population. Within this category is a smaller aggregate of persons with one or more psychiatric diagnoses in addition to substance abuse itself (dual diagnosis). A study of individuals with alcohol- or drug-dependence problems in the community found that 47% also had an additional psychiatric diagnosis (Helzer and Pryzbeck, 1988). These persons may be difficult to locate, lack understanding of how the two problems compound one another, be socially isolated, be possibly unemployed, and be less readily identified by health care providers, who fail to realize that both problems may coexist (Westermeyer, 1992).

Treatment and integration of these dual-diagnosis persons into 12-step groups are often complicated when the need for the individual to take prescribed psychotropic medications is perceived as prescription drug abuse or as the substitution of one addiction for another. Special attention and flexibility are needed in meeting the needs of the dual-diagnosis aggregate, and such strategies are largely still in the developmental phase. Childhood maltreatment, including verbal, physical, emotional and sexual abuse and neglect, frequently lead to the development of a wide array of difficulties in adulthood. Substance abuse is one of the most common of those aftereffects. Approximately one in four girls and one in six boys are sexually molested before age 18 (Hall, 1996b; Van der Kolk, et al., 1996). Therefore, substance abuse prevention and treatment should address these issues. Caution

should be taken, however, to avoid forcing the disclosure of a traumatizing event in a group setting (Hall, 1996a).

In assessing the risks for substance abuse and the extent of its impact in the real life of the community, it should be noted that frequently there are several bases for the vulnerability occurring in one individual or group. The adolescent, the low-income Hispanic male, the lesbian African-American mother receiving public assistance, and the Native American family living on reservation land are all facing multiple sources of oppression and vulnerability that contribute to an increased potential for substance abuse.

Special attention must be focused on the impact of the HIV epidemic and its relationship to substance abuse. Substance abusers are at increased risk of HIV-related health deficits in the following ways:

- Substances may cloud judgment, leading to high-risk sexual practices involving exchange of body fluids (e.g., sex without use of appropriate barriers such as condoms).
- Intravenous drug use may involve the sharing of hypodermic needles.
- Chronic substance use (e.g., alcohol, heroin, amphetamines, nicotine, cocaine) impairs the immune system so that infection by HIV or by other pathogens that increase the chances of HIV infection is facilitated.
- Substance abuse may hasten physical and mental deterioration from the condition of seropositivity to an AIDS diagnosis and, eventually, the terminal phase.
- Chronic substance abusers generally have fewer supportive relationships available to them in the process of coping with the hardships that accompany HIV illness.
- Persons facing a stigmatizing, terminal, debilitating illness in themselves or a significant other are more prone to experience substance abuse problems in an attempt to cope with distress.

Last, substance abuse among health care professionals can also no longer be ignored. Physicians, nurses, dentists, and pharmacists are vulnerable to substance abuse; commonly they abuse alcohol or narcotics (Bissell and Haberman, 1984; Talbott and Wright, 1988). Health care professionals are assumed to be "immune" to dependency because of their knowledge of medications. Yet their increased access to drugs, belief in pharmaceutical solutions, and work-related stress place them at increased risk for substance abuse (Haack and Hughes, 1989; Shore, 1987). They are generally not addicted to street drugs, but instead gain access to drugs through their work settings by diverting medications for their own use or through abuse of drugs obtained by prescription. Through drug theft or when the effects of their substance abuse impair their professional functioning, these health care professionals come to the attention of state regulatory boards (Madrid, 1994).

Most states have rehabilitation programs for health care professionals that consist of treatment and monitoring, during which they are allowed to retain their professional licenses. Despite their usually favorable recovery rate, it is difficult to get this population into treatment because of the denial and shame related to their substance abuse. However, the threatened loss of their professional license to practice may be a good motivator to break through their denial of the problem and encourage them to seek treatment (Sullivan and Handley, 1992).

SEXUALLY TRANSMITTED DISEASES AND SUBSTANCE ABUSE

There is an increased risk for STDs (e.g., HIV-related illness, herpes, genital warts, syphilis) among substance abusers for the following reasons:

1. Substances may cloud judgment, leading to high-risk sexual or drug practices involving exchange of body fluids (i.e., sex without appropriate barriers such as condoms).
2. Intravenous drug use may involve the sharing of hypodermic needles.
3. Chronic substance abuse impairs the immune system so chances of infection are increased.
4. Substance abuse may hasten the physical and mental deterioration of HIV-related illness.
5. Chronic substance abusers generally have fewer supportive relationships available to them to help in coping with severe illness.

NURSING PERSPECTIVE ON SUBSTANCE ABUSE

Beginning with the Civil War, a substance abuse problem with which nurses were confronted but for which they had few solutions was patient addiction to medically prescribed narcotic analgesics such as codeine and morphine. Nurses often felt implicated in the development of these problems because of their role in administering these drugs at close intervals to patients in acute pain. A craving for the euphoric effects of the drug developed that persisted after the need for analgesia had ceased.

Nurses have also encountered substance abuse in clients whose health problems are clearly related to alcohol abuse, such as cirrhosis of the liver, heart disease, neurologic syndromes, and nutritional deficits. Unfortunately, in the past, alcohol problems were often not addressed in these health encounters because of the stigma of alcoholism and the lack of effective treatments (Sullivan et al., 1994).

The nursing literature did not clearly address substance abuse as a nursing problem until the late 1960s and not as a significant problem until the 1970s. Before this, substance abuse was usually viewed as a moral problem or, if it involved illicit drugs, as a legal problem.

In the past decade, nursing has become more involved in the spectrum of compulsive behavior problems, including substance abuse. The American Nurses Association Cabinet on Nursing Research (1985) asserted that substance abuse is a health problem of concern to nurses. A specialized organization, the National Nurses' Society on Addiction (NNSA), has been established with the philosophy that abuse of alcohol and other drugs, eating disorders, sexual and relational addiction, and compulsive gambling, working, and spending are closely related behavior patterns. Additionally, educational course work related to alcohol and drug abuse is now recommended for inclusion in general nursing school curricula (Naegle, 1994).

Nursing Diagnosis

The NNSA has been developing nursing assessment and interventions for the dependent client and has published two volumes of nursing care plans (1989, 1990). These plans adapt the nursing process to help individuals with various types of substance abuse and dependencies and physical or psychological problems associated with this abuse.

The nursing diagnoses from these volumes are based on four types of human responses to addictive disease: biological, cognitive, psychosocial, and spiritual. Common nursing diagnoses for clients with substance abuse and dependency problems (NNSA, 1989, 1990) are as follows:

- Alteration in comfort related to withdrawal symptoms
- Self-care deficits
- Hopelessness and depression related to substance abuse
- Powerlessness related to loss of control over use
- Knowledge deficit about addictive disease
- Dysfunctional family processes
- Alteration in self-concept and self-esteem
- Noncompliance related to denial of addictive disease
- Sleep pattern disturbance
- Anxiety
- Alteration in nutrition (less than body requirements)
- Social isolation
- Spiritual distress
- Ineffective individual coping
- Altered growth and psychosocial development
- Potential for violence
- Sensory-perceptual alterations related to withdrawal of the substance

Another concern that may be associated with women's alcohol problems is rape trauma syndrome. Women with histories of rape, sexual abuse, or childhood sexual trauma may experience heavy or problematic patterns of alcohol or other drug use as a means of compensating for posttraumatic stress symptoms in their daily lives (Bass and Davis, 1988; Covington and Kohen, 1984; Hurley, 1991; Schaefer and Evans, 1987).

Community Health Nurses and Substance Abusers

The problem of substance abuse is so widespread that it affects every community and its inhabitants in varying degrees; the community health nurse is frequently concerned and involved with substance abusers or their significant others. Substance abuse nursing interventions with clients and their caregivers are necessary to ensure the success of other health interventions. Ignoring substance abuse problems frequently leads to lack of progress and clients' inability to carry out needed health practices. This is especially frustrating for the community health nurse and the other professionals who have collaborated on a comprehensive plan to allow an

individual with a serious health problem to remain at home and avoid placement in an institution, for example.

Substance abuse or dependence either contributes to or complicates the course of many other illnesses and injuries. It is often a direct cause of falls and automobile accidents. Particularly in the elderly, falls and fractures may be related to alcohol consumption. Prescription medications, such as narcotic analgesics, tranquilizers, and hypnotics, can also contribute to mental status changes and impair judgment in the elderly. In high-crime, high-poverty areas, gunshot injuries may be secondary to involvement in illegal drug trade, burglaries, and robberies. Domestic violence injuries frequently occur when one or more family members are intoxicated.

Substance abuse can sometimes have lethal consequences when it occurs simultaneously with certain health problems such as STDs (e.g., AIDS), mental illness, pregnancy, and the medical problems of the elderly. Drug or alcohol use in someone with an STD, in particular AIDS, contributes to impaired judgment and the likelihood of unsafe sexual practices (i.e., sex without use of barriers such as condoms). In persons who are mentally ill, it can precipitate the onset and complicate the course of the illness. In depressive disorders, alcohol or drug use is frequently the factor that tips the scale toward a completed suicide. Alcohol or drug use during pregnancy has adverse consequences, as documented by the problems of the fetal alcohol syndrome infant and the crack cocaine syndrome infant, and can contribute to a stillbirth.

Attitude Toward Substance Abusers

Although alcoholics and drug addicts are frequently recipients of nursing care in hospitals and community settings, nurses have historically had ambivalent attitudes toward them (Naegle, 1983; Sullivan and Handley, 1993). As part of the larger culture, nurses may reflect the attitude that substance abuse is a stigmatizing, immoral behavior and, as a result, have difficulty providing care to these individuals. The moral view of substance abuse implies that individuals choose to become sick, injured, or addicted.

Strong negative feelings that conflict with nursing's humanistic stance may also stem from personal experiences. Being the emotionally or physically abused spouse or child of a substance abuser can have lasting effects on nurses' attitudes toward substance-abusing clients. On the other hand, alcohol or drug use by nurses to relieve stress or self-medicate dysphoric states may lead them to overidentify with the patient and deny the severity of the client's substance abuse.

Frequently, substance abusers are difficult clients in health care settings (Endicott and Watson, 1994; Faltz and Rinaldi, 1987). When intoxicated, they may be obstreperous, uncooperative, and antisocial. When not intoxicated, they may exhibit none of these negative behaviors or may be manipulative and demanding, using flattery or intimidation to hide drug-seeking behavior. Although nurses may initially be warm and understanding, once aware of manipulative attempts, they may have difficulty maintaining an accepting, nonjudgmental attitude. Realizing that recovery from substance abuse often comes very slowly can help nurses feel less pressured to get patients into treatment and be more able simply to raise consciousness by presenting the facts about addictive illness and leave the decision making to the client.

Nursing Interventions in the Community

How can community health nurses assist individuals, families, and groups experiencing substance abuse problems? First, they can provide an accurate assessment, which includes a family history and specific questions about personal drug and alcohol use (Fortin, 1983; Seibert, 1990; Sullivan et al., 1994). They can be alert to environmental cues in the home that indicate substance abuse, such as empty liquor and pill bottles. An indication of prescription medication abuse is the patient's involvement with several physicians from whom narcotic analgesics and tranquilizers are obtained. This type of assessment can help with case finding and referral for treatment, even though the individual may have initially denied the existence of a substance abuse problem.

Denial of substance abuse or dependence may range from completely blocked awareness of the entire problem to partial disavowal of the detrimental effects of the substance use and abuse. One of the primary tasks of intervention and treatment with the substance-dependent individual is to increase the individual's awareness of the problem. Family and significant others can assist with this process by being more

honest and direct with the individual about the detrimental effects of the substance abuse, especially as it has an impact on significant relationships. Before this occurs, the significant others have to overcome their own denial of the problem and its associated shame and guilt. Referrals to community education programs on substance abuse and dependence and mutual help groups such as Al-Anon and Narcanon are interventions most useful to family and significant others.

The community health nurse may also include the social network to get the person into treatment. Although individuals who are forced to enter treatment may not be willing to admit the severity of the abuse or may lack awareness, they can still benefit from exposure to the treatment program and eventually begin recovery from their dependency. Experiencing serious health consequences related to the dependency may constitute "hitting bottom" for the individual and may break through denial or collusion on the part of the family. The concept of hitting bottom is particularly important: this is not a mysterious process but rather consists of myriad interacting forces that bring the individual to a point of despair that paradoxically becomes a window of opportunity for intervention. Behavioral prescriptions for abstinence will be ineffective if the cognitive structure that permits the behavior to continue is not also challenged. Therefore, capitalizing on "cracks in the cognitive accounting system" is essential.

The trust that develops in a caring nursing relationship can support disclosure of substance abuse problems and decrease denial in the client or family members. A realistic and positive attitude toward the person with substance abuse can provide families with hope. The nurse needs to have knowledge that recovery is possible and that community resources are available to help with that recovery. One of the primary roles of the community health nurse in helping substance abusers is to facilitate contact with helping agencies such as local treatment programs or mutual help groups. Collaboration with the client's physician is helpful should medical detoxification be necessary.

The other traditional community health nursing roles and interventions are also appropriate to use with substance abusers. Examples are as follows:

- Health teaching regarding addictive illness and addictive effects of different substances

- Providing direct care for abuse- and dependence-related medical problems
- Counseling clients and families about problems related to substance abuse
- Collaborating with other disciplines to ensure continuity of care
- Coordinating health care services for the client to prevent prescription drug abuse and avoid fragmentation of care
- Providing consultation to nonmedical professionals and lay personnel
- Facilitating care through appropriate referrals and follow-up

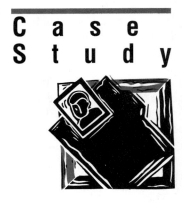

Case Study

Application of the Nursing Process

Evelyn Weaver, a 72-year-old widow, was referred to the Visiting Nurse Association for follow-up after hospitalization for a seizure and fall she experienced in her home. Her hospital discharge diagnoses were ethyl alcohol abuse, seizure disorder, hypertension, and bruises and contusions on her left arm and leg. Her discharge medications were phenytoin sodium (Dilantin), 900 mg orally at bedtime; one multivitamin orally every day; hydrochlorothiazide, 50 mg orally every day; and methyldopa (Aldomet), 250 mg orally every day.

Mrs. Weaver has lived alone in a two-bedroom house in a middle-class suburb for the 10 years since her husband's death. Until 4 years ago, her daughter lived nearby with her two children and she visited frequently. However, after a bitter divorce, the daughter and the children moved several hundred miles away and visited only once or twice a year. Mrs. Weaver also had a married son in the area. He paid her bills once or twice a month but otherwise had minimal contact and appeared to be angry at her because of her alcohol abuse. Mrs. Weaver's occupation had been primarily a homemaker and mother, and she tended to be socially isolated. She stopped driving after her last automobile accident, infrequently saw her two elderly cousins in town, and was not involved in any local community organizations.

Assessment

Individual The visiting nurse performed an in-home nursing assessment of the client, and information was obtained through the nursing interview and physical assessment. Mrs. Weaver admitted to an alcohol abuse problem but tended to minimize its severity. She reported that she had stopped drinking for 2 days on her own and then had a seizure. She denied any past alcohol treatment such as counseling or AA meetings and said she was not interested in any now. She was abstinent from alcohol since her discharge from the hospital and thought that she would remain that way. She admitted to some loneliness and social isolation. She also reported sleep disturbances (i.e., difficulty falling asleep and staying asleep) and decreased nutritional intake with loss of appetite. She denied other psychoactive medication use, such as hypnotics, narcotic analgesics, or tranquilizers (benzodiazepines). She agreed to a social work referral to investigate attendant care and Meals on Wheels to help her.

Family Telephone contact between the nurse and the client's daughter revealed that the daughter was very concerned about her mother. She denied that alcohol abuse was her mother's problem but thought that poor nutrition and health practices were the cause of the hospitalization. She was anxious for the social work referral to get attendant care to assist her mother in the home.

It took several calls and messages before the nurse was able to speak with the client's son. He said his mother was an alcoholic and that he had tried unsuccessfully in the past to get her to stop drinking. He was unwilling now to do more than visit her twice a month to pay her bills. He lived 1 hour away by car.

Community   The middle-class suburb in which the client lived had no alcohol treatment services especially geared for the elderly. AA meetings and private substance abuse counselors were available, but none of them were willing to make home visits and deal with an elderly, homebound client. The local senior center had no programs or education involving substance abuse and refused to allow AA meetings to be conducted in their building because they thought that their clients would be offended. The client's physician was aware of her alcohol abuse problem but did not know how to help her. Referral to an inpatient program for substance abuse was not possible because Mrs. Weaver refused to go.

Diagnosis

Individual

- Altered cardiovascular status secondary to hypertension
- Altered neurologic status secondary to alcohol withdrawal seizures
- Knowledge deficit about addictive disease and effects of alcohol abuse
- Sleep pattern disturbance
- Alteration in nutrition (less than body requirements)
- Social isolation
- Ineffective individual coping related to inability to adjust to role of widow and maintain involvement in community activities
- Knowledge deficit about the effects and side effects of all of her medicine

Family

- Knowledge deficit about addictive disease and effects of excessive intake of alcohol
- Knowledge deficit of treatment approaches available for alcohol abuse and the recovery process
- Alteration in family process secondary to poor communication and denial of alcohol abuse in client

Community

- Knowledge deficit in senior center staff regarding the prevalence of alcohol abuse problems in the elderly population and adverse health effects of alcohol consumption in the elderly
- Knowledge deficits in community agencies that assist alcohol abusers (local AA and counselors) regarding the need to make home visits and provide services geared to the elderly

Planning

Planning for Mrs. Weaver's care involved collaboration among her family, her physician, the agency's social worker, and the community alcohol treatment resources. Health teaching and counseling were the main approaches used in assisting the client and her family directly. Indirect approaches involved networking with community agencies and supervising other caregivers.

Intervention

Individual

- Nursing visits two to three times weekly initially to monitor the client's medication issues or problems as related to maintaining abstinence or medication dosing, cardiovascular status, neurologic status, and nutritional status
- Social work referral to set up attendant assistance in the home and Meals on Wheels
- Health teaching regarding addictive illness, effects of excessive alcohol intake on the body, alcohol withdrawal seizures, no-added-sodium diet, and effect of medications
- Health teaching about all of the client's medications, their effects and side effects, and the necessity of following recommended dosing schedules
- Referral for alcohol treatment counseling and AA meetings when the individual is receptive

Family

- Continued contact with the client's daughter and son to involve them in her care
- Health teaching to the family on the course and treatment of addictive illness and the adverse effects of alcohol abuse on the client and the family as related to functioning, cohesion, and communication
- Role modeling by the visiting nurse of the use of clear, direct, and nonjudgmental communication about the client's alcohol abuse problems

Community

- List of local and national referral resources for clients with substance abuse problems made available to physicians, with a particular focus on resources providing services for older or elderly substance abusers
- Health teaching to community groups (e.g., senior center, AA fellowship, substance abuse counselors) regarding the prevalence of alcohol abuse in the elderly population and treatment and counseling approaches useful with this aggregate
- Collaboration with community organizations that provide outreach for homebound elderly to assist in identification and referral
- Establishment of a referral network (i.e., telephone hot line) of concerned older or elderly recovering individuals

Evaluation

Initially, interventions proceeded smoothly. Mrs. Weaver obtained attendant help for 2 hours three times weekly and also received Meals on Wheels. The visiting nurse filled her Medi-Set weekly. The attendant ensured that the client took her medications and ate her meals and assisted Mrs. Weaver with personal care. Mrs. Weaver remained abstinent from alcohol during this time but refused any treatment or counseling for her alcohol abuse problem. However, after about 3 weeks, she was rehospitalized after falling again at home. She was diagnosed with phenytoin toxicity; this occurred because she had surreptitiously been taking extra phenytoin at night to help her sleep.

After a few days, Mrs. Weaver was discharged from the hospital, and the case was reopened by the Visiting Nurses Association. Private attendant care and Meals on Wheels were also reinstated. This time, the physician discontinued the phenytoin and prescribed disulfiram (Antabuse) with the understanding that the client receive alcohol counseling. The client did follow-up with the counseling referrals given to her by the visiting nurse, but her social situation did not change. She remained very isolated and refused AA involvement.

A third hospitalization occurred within a few weeks when Mrs. Weaver ingested alcohol in combination with the disulfiram. She became physically ill and required treatment. After this last hospitalization, the daughter decided to take action. She moved her mother, despite her initial resistance, into a retirement community that provided meals and social activities. The visiting nurse continued to follow the case in the new setting.

Initially, the client was angry and isolative at her new home. This changed after an attendant was hired to assist her with personal care and get her involved with the social activities at the community. The visiting nurse also set up medical follow-up with a new physician because she had moved too far away from the previous physician and informed the physician of the client's past medical and alcohol abuse problems. The situation remained stable for several weeks as a result of Mrs. Weaver's continued abstinence from alcohol. The visiting nurse continued to remain active in the client's care by arranging for aftercare, focusing on providing goal-specific social support for abstinence and general support for addressing the client's concerns and issues, particularly as related to feelings of isolating loss and transitions. Occasional lapses were framed as an opportunity for increasing the client's level of awareness about substance abuse–related problems and their cause.

Levels of Prevention

Primary
- Involves health teaching to individuals and groups on risk factors, early symptoms of substance abuse, adverse health and social consequences, addictive disease process, and treatment services available
- Need to gear educative approaches especially to the more vulnerable aggregates (e.g., adolescents, minorities, mentally ill, women, and elderly)

Secondary
- Involves screening and early treatment approaches aimed at minimizing health and social consequences of substance abuse
- Involvement of physicians, nurses, and other health care professionals in various health care settings in this process
- Use of various screening and assessment tools as well as referrals to treatment services and mutual help organizations

Tertiary
- Involves more direct approaches (e.g., detoxification and inpatient or outpatient treatment) to halt the physiologically damaging effects of the substance abuse (e.g., liver disease, organic mental deficits, gastritis)
- Frequent use of medications to treat the symptoms of substance abuse–related disorders or as part of aversion therapy (e.g., disulfiram)
- Services provided by medical practitioners, treatment services, and mutual help organizations; generally advocate abstinence from the substance and improving the individual's health status

This case study illustrates the possible complexity and frustration involved in helping the substance abuser. Significant others and the medical community must be involved to assist the nurse in interventions. Often, the social situation, living situation, or social acquaintances also must change to maintain long-term recovery. However, with patience, persistence, and a caring, nonjudgmental attitude, the nurse can be effective in getting clients with substance abuse problems into recovery and improving their health status.

Intervention is effective if nurses believe that addiction treatment and recovery are possible and know the community resources available to aid with this process.

NATIONAL OFFICES OF MUTUAL HELP OR RESOURCE ORGANIZATIONS

Al-Anon Family Groups
P.O. Box 862, Midtown Station
New York, NY 10018-0862
(212) 302-7240.

Alcoholics Anonymous
P.O. Box 459, Grand Central Station
New York, NY 10163
(212) 686-1100

Drug Abuse Information and Treatment
Referral Line:
(800) 662-HELP

Drug and Alcohol Nursing Association, Inc.
660 Lonely Cottage Drive
Upper Black Eddy, PA 18972-9313
(610) 847-5396

National Clearinghouse for Drug and Alcohol Information: Information Services
P.O. Box 2345
Rockville, MD 20852

National Council on Alcohol
12 W 21st St
New York, NY 10010
(212) 206-6770

National Institute on Alcohol Abuse and Alcoholism
16-105 Parklawn Building
5600 Fishers La
Rockville, MD 20857

National Institute on Drug Abuse
10-05 Parklawn Building
5600 Fishers La
Rockville, MD 20857

National Self-Help Clearinghouse
City University of New York
33 West 42nd St
New York, NY 10036

Women for Sobriety Inc.
P.O. Box 618
Quakertown, PA 18951
(215) 536-8026

SUMMARY

This chapter has attempted to provide an overview of the complex, multifaceted phenomenon of substance abuse and its manifestations in the community. The focus has been on the social, economic, and political as well as health-related aspects of substance abuse. Substance abuse was related to the more general concept of addictive behaviors, not just those related to drug or alcohol abuse.

From the review of the various etiologic theories, it is clear that there is no one causative factor in the development of the problem. Consequently, there is no one treatment approach to apply to all substance abusers. Cocaine addiction was presented in detail to illustrate the progression of substance use to abuse and dependency. Cocaine addiction is also a relevant example of the strong economic and social factors present in the development of dependency that must be taken into account in the recovery process.

A discussion of vulnerable aggregates focused on women, adolescents, the elderly, and people of color. Resources for prevention and intervention at the individual, family, and community levels were outlined. Also a case study applied the nursing process at these different levels.

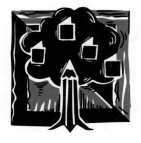

Learning Activities

1. Attend several local open Alcoholics Anonymous, Narcotics Anonymous, or Cocaine Anonymous meetings, and share your impressions with your classmates.

2. Attend a local open Al-Anon, Narcanon, or Adult Children of Alcoholics meeting, and share your impressions with your classmates.

3. Visit a local treatment center that provides detoxification, inpatient, or outpatient treatment, and determine their treatment philosophy and the types of services they provide to patients and their families.

4. Visit a treatment program for women, and determine how the particular needs of this population are assessed and addressed.

5. Learn about the local community college or high school's drug and alcohol education programs.

6. Contact your county or city's mental health services or substance abuse treatment services, and obtain a list of local treatment and education resources.

REFERENCES

Abelson HI, Miller JD: A decade of trends in cocaine use in the household population. *In* Kozel NJ, Adams EH (eds): Cocaine Use in America (NIDA Research Monograph No. 61). Rockville, MD, National Institute of Drug Abuse, 1985, pp. 35–49.

American Nurses Association Cabinet on Nursing Research: Directions for Nursing Research: Toward the Twenty-first Century. Kansas City, MO, American Nurses Association, 1985.

American Psychiatric Association: Diagnostic and Statistical Manual of Mental Disorders, 4th ed. Washington, DC, American Psychiatric Association, 1994.

Amuleru-Marshall O: Political and economic implications of alcohol and other drugs in the African American Community. *In* Goddard LL (ed). An African-Centered Model of Prevention for African American Youth at High Risk. Rockville, MD, Substance Abuse and Mental Health Services Administration (SAMHSA), 1993, pp. 23–33.

Annis HM: Relapse to substance abuse: Empirical findings within a cognitive-social learning approach. J Psychoactive Drugs 22:117–124, 1990.

Banys P: The clinical use of disulfiram (Antabuse): A review. J Psychoactive Drugs 20:243–260, 1988.

Bass E, Davis L: The Courage to Heal: A Guide for Women Survivors of Child Sexual Abuse. New York, Harper & Row, 1988.

Beattie M: Codependency No More: How to Stop Controlling Others and Start Caring for Yourself. New York, Harper & Row, 1987.

Bekir P, McLellan T, Childress A, Gariti P: Role reversals in families of substance misusers: A transgenerational phenomenon. Int J Addict 28:613–630, 1993.

Biernacki P: Pathways from Heroin Addiction: Recovery Without Treatment. Philadelphia, Temple University Press, 1986.

Bissell L, Haberman P: Alcoholism in the Professions. New York, Oxford University Press, 1984.

Bolin L: Culturally Sensitive Substance Abuse Treatment for African-Americans. Unpublished manuscript, 1995.

Bowersox J: Needle-exchange programs show promise for AIDS prevention. NIDA Notes, 5:8–9, 1994.

Bowser BP: Crack and AIDS: An ethnographic impression. J Nat Med Assoc 81:538–540, 1989.

Bradshaw J: Bradshaw on the Family: A Revolutionary Way to Self-Discovery. Deerfield Beach, FL, Health Communications, 1988.

Brecher E: Licit and Illicit Drugs. Boston, Little, Brown, 1972.

Brown GR, Anderson B: Psychiatric morbidity in adult inpatients with childhood histories of sexual and physical abuse. Am J Psychiatry 148:55–61, 1991.

Brown R: Vitamin deficiency and voluntary alcohol consumption. Q J Stud Alcohol 30:592–597, 1969.

Brown S: Treating the Alcoholic: A Developmental Model of Recovery. New York, Wiley, 1985.

Brown S: Treating Adult Children of Alcoholics: A Developmental Perspective. New York, Wiley, 1988.

Bulhan H: Frantz Fanon and the psychology of oppression. New York, Plenum Press, 1985.

Burkett G, Yasin S, Palow D: Perinatal implications of cocaine exposure. J Reprod Med 35:35–42, 1990.

Cahalan D: Understanding America's Drinking Problem: How to Combat the Hazards of Alcohol. San Francisco, Jossey-Bass, 1988.

Cahalan D, Room R: Problem Drinkers Among American Men. New Brunswick, NJ, Rutgers Center for Alcohol Studies, 1974.

Campbell JC, Landenburger K: Violence against women. *In* Fogel CI, Woods NF (eds): Women's Health Care: A Comprehensive Handbook. Thousand Oaks, CA, Sage, 1995, pp. 407–425.

Chasnoff IJ: Cocaine pregnancy and the growing child. Curr Probl Pediatr 22:302–321, 1992.

Christopher J: How to Stay Sober: Recovery Without Religion. Buffalo, NY, Prometheus, 1988.

Clark HW, Longmuir N: Clonidine transdermal patches: A recovery oriented treatment of opiate withdrawal. Calif Soc Treat Alcohol Other Drug Dependence 13:1–2, 1985.

Cotton NS: The familial incidence of alcoholism: A review. J Studies Alcohol 40:89–116, 1979.

Covington SS, Kohen J: Women, alcohol and sexuality. Adv Alcohol Substance Abuse 4:41–56, 1984.

Cronkite RC, Moos RH: Determinants of post treatment functioning of alcoholic patients: A conceptual framework. J Consult Clin Psychol 48:305–316, 1980.

Daigle RD, Clark HW, Landry MJ: A primer on neurotransmitters and cocaine. J Psychoactive Drugs 20:283–295, 1988.

Dawkins MP: Alcoholism prevention and black youth. J Drug Issues 18:15–20, 1988.

Day N, Leonard K: Alcohol, drug use and psychopathology in the general population. In Alterman A (ed): Substance Abuse and Psychopathology. New York, Plenum Press, 1985, pp. 15–44.

Dicker M, Leighton EA: Trends in U.S. prevalence of drug-using parturient women and drug-affected newborns, 1979 through 1990. Am J Public Health 84:1433–1439, 1994.

Endicott P, Watson B: Interventions to improve the AMA discharge rate for opiate addicted patients. J Psychosocial Nurs 32:36–40, 1994.

Faltz B, Rinaldi J: AIDS and Substance Abuse: A Training Manual for Health Care Professionals. San Francisco, Regents of the University of California, 1987.

Finkelstein N: Treatment programming for alcohol and drug-dependent pregnant women. Int J Addict 28:1275–1309, 1993.

Fortin M: Community health nursing. In Bennett G, Vourakis C, Woolf D (eds): Substance Abuse: Pharmacologic, Developmental and Clinical Perspectives. New York, Wiley, 1983, pp. 209–223.

Fullilove MT, Fullilove RE: Intersecting epidemics: Black teen crack use and sexually transmitted diseases. J Am Med Women's Assoc 44:146–153, 1989.

Gawin FH: Neuropharmacology of cocaine: Progress in pharmacotherapy. J Clin Psychiatr 49(suppl):11–15, 1988.

Gfroerer J, de la Rosa M: Protective and risk factors associated with drug use among Hispanic youth. J Addict Dis 12:87–107, 1993.

Gold MS, Washton AM, Dackis CA, Chatlos JC: New treatments for opiate and cocaine users but what about marijuana? Psychiatr Ann 16:206–214, 1986.

Gordis E: Letter to colleagues. Washington, DC, U.S. Department of Health and Human Services, National Institute on Alcohol Abuse and Alcoholism, 1995.

Greenberg M, Schneider D: Violence in American cities: Young black males is the answer, but what is the question? Soc Sci Med 39:179–187, 1994.

Grinspoon L, Bakalar JB: The war on drugs: A peace proposal. N Engl J Med 330:357–360, 1994.

Gross S: Report on Crack. Paper presented to the San Francisco Health Commission, San Francisco, 1988.

Haack M, Hughes T (eds): Addiction in the Nursing Profession: Approaches to Intervention and Recovery. New York, Springer, 1989.

Haaken J: A critical analysis of the codependence construct. Psychiatry 53:397–406, 1990.

Hall JM: What really worked? A case analysis and discussion of confrontational intervention for substance abuse in marginalized women. Arch Psychiatr Nurs 7:322–327, 1993.

Hall JM: How lesbians recognize and respond to alcohol problems: A theoretical model of problematization. Adv Nurs Sci 16:46–63, 1994.

Hall JM: Geography of childhood sexual abuse: Women's narratives of their childhood environments. Adv Nurs Sci 18:29–47, 1996a.

Hall JM: The pervasive effects of childhood sexual abuse in lesbians' recovery from alcohol problems. Subst Use Misuse 31:225–239, 1996b.

Hall SM, Havassey BE: Commitment to abstinence and relapse to tobacco, alcohol and opiates. In Tims FM, Leukefeld CG (eds). Relapse and Recovery in Drug Abuse (NIDA Research Monograph Series No. 72). Rockville, MD, National Institute on Drug Abuse, 1986, pp. 118–135.

Helzer JE, Pryzbeck TR: The co-occurrence of alcoholism with other psychiatric disorders in the general population and its impact on treatment. J Stud Alcohol 49:219–244, 1988.

Horgan C. Substance Abuse: The Nation's Number One Health Problem, Key Indicators for Policy. Institute for Health Policy, Brandeis University. Princeton, NJ: The Robert Wood Johnson Foundation, 1993.

Horne M: Babies Born on Crack Cocaine: Maternal Drug Abusers under Seige. In Proceedings of the Second National Conference on Preventing and Treating Alcohol and Other Drug Abuse, HIV Infection, and AIDS in Black Communities: From Advocacy to Action (CSAP Prevention Monograph 13). Rockville, MD, Center for Substance Abuse Prevention, 1993, pp. 101–111.

Hurley DL: Women, alcohol and incest: An analytical review. J Studies Alcohol 52:253–268, 1991.

Jackson JK: The adjustment of the family to the crises of alcoholism. Q J Stud Alcohol 15:562–586, 1954.

Jaffe JH: Trivializing dependence. Br J Addict 85:1425–1427, 1990.

Jellinek EM: The Disease Concept of Alcoholism. New Haven, CT, Hillhouse Press, 1960.

Jessup M: Drug Dependency in Pregnancy: Managing Withdrawal. Sacramento, CA, California Department of Health Services, Maternal and Child Health Branch, 1992.

Johnson E: Substance abuse and women's health. Public Health Rep 102:42–48, 1987.

Kearney MH, Murphy S, Rosenbaum M: Mothering on crack cocaine: A grounded theory analysis. Soc Sci Med 38:351–361, 1994.

Keller M: On the loss of control phenomenon in alcoholism. Br J Addict 67:153–166, 1972.

King C, van Hasselt V, Segal D, Hersen M: Diagnosis and assessment of substance abuse in older adults: Current strategies and issues. Addict Behav 19:41–55, 1994.

Kirkpatrick J: Turnabout: Help for a New Life. Dubuque, IA, Kendall-Hunt, 1978.

Kleber HD: Naltrexone. J Substance Abuse Treat 2:117–122, 1985.

Kleber HD: Our current approach to drug abuse: Progress, problems and proposal. N Engl J Med 330:361–364, 1994.

Kurtz E: Not God: A History of Alcoholics Anonymous. Center City, MN, Hazelden Educational Services, 1979.

Larimer ME, Marlatt GA: Applications of relapse prevention with moderation goals. J Psychoactive Drugs 22:189–195, 1990.

Madrid E: Substance Abuse Among Nurses: Occupational and Personal Risk Factors. Dissertation Abstracts International (University Microfilms No. 9502636), 1994.

Marlatt GA, Baer JS, Donovan DM, Kivlahan DR: Addictive behaviors: Etiology and treatment. Annu Rev Psychol 39:223–252, 1988.

Marlatt GA, Gordon JR: Relapse Prevention: Maintenance Strategies in the Treatment of Addictive Behaviors. New York, Guilford Press, 1986.

Martin C, Arria A, Mezzich A, Bukstein O: Patterns of Polydrug Use in Adolescent Alcohol Abusers. Am J Drug Alcohol Abuse 19:511–521, 1993.

Mayfield D, McLeod G, Hall P: The CAGE questionnaire: Validation of a new alcohol screening instrument. Am J Psychiatry 36:1121–1123, 1974.

Mello NK, Mendelson JH, Lukas SE, et al.: Buprenorphine treatment of opiate and cocaine abuse: Clinical and preclinical studies. Harvard Rev Psychiatry 1:168–183, 1993.

Mena M: Perinatal substance abuse: An overview. Calif Hospital 4:27–33, 1990.

Miller BA, Downs WR, Gondoli DM, Keil A: The role of childhood abuse in the development of alcoholism in women. Violence Victims 2:157–172, 1987.

Miller WR, Hester RK: Treating the problem drinker: Modern approaches. *In* Miller WR (ed): The Addictive Behaviors: Treatment of Addiction, Drug Abuse, Smoking and Obesity. New York, Pergamon Press, 1980, pp. 11–141.

Minuchin S: Families and Family Therapy. Cambridge, MA, Harvard University Press, 1974.

Montagne M, Scott DM: Prevention of substance abuse problems: models, factors and processes. Int J Addict 28:1177–1208, 1993.

Moos R, Brennan P, Mertens J: Diagnostic subgroups and predictors of one-year re-admission among late-middle-aged and older substance abuse patients. J Studies Alcohol 55:173–183, 1994.

Morrison M, Smith D, Wilford B, et al.: At war in the fields of play: Current perspectives on the nature and treatment of adolescent chemical dependency. J Psychoactive Drugs 25:321–330, 1993.

Murphy JM, Jellinek M, Quinn D, et al.: Substance abuse and serious child mistreatment: Prevalence, risk and outcome in a court sample. Child Abuse Neglect 15:197–211, 1991.

Naegle M: The nurse and the alcoholic: Redefining a historically ambivalent relationship. J Psychosocial Nurs Mental Health Serv 21:17–25, 1983.

Naegle MA: Theoretical perspectives on the etiology of substance abuse. Holistic Nurs Pract 2:1–13, 1988.

Naegle M: The need for alcohol abuse-related education in nursing curricula. Alcohol Health Res World 18:154–157, 1994.

National Institute on Alcohol Abuse and Alcoholism: A Growing Concern: How to Provide Services for Children From Alcoholic Families (DHHS publication No. ADM 85-1257). Washington, DC, U.S. Government Printing Office, 1985.

National Institute on Drug Abuse: Third Triennial Report to Congress: Drug Abuse and Drug Research III. Rockville, MD, U.S. Department of Health and Human Services, 1990.

National Nurses Society on Addiction: Nursing Care Planning with the Addicted Client, Vol. I. Skokie, IL, National Nurses Society on Addictions, 1989.

National Nurses Society on Addiction: Nursing Care Planning with the Addicted Client, Vol. II. Skokie, IL, National Nurses Society on Addictions, 1990.

Nilseen O, Cone H: Screening patients for alcohol problems in primary health care settings. Alcohol World: Health and Research 18:136–139, 1994.

O'Connor J, Saunders B: Drug Education: An Appraisal of a Popular Preventive. Int J Addictions 27:165–185, 1992.

O'Donnell JA, Voss HL, Clayton RR, et al.: Young Men and Drugs: A Nationwide Study (NIDA Research Monograph 5). Rockville, MD, National Institute on Drug Abuse, 1976.

Olin W: Escape from Utopia: My Ten Years in Synanon. Santa Cruz, CA; Unity Press, 1980.

O'Malley PM, Johnston LD, Bachman JG: Cocaine use in America. *In* Kozel NJ, Adams EH (eds): Cocaine Use in America (NIDA Research Monograph 61). Rockville, MD, National Institute on Drug Abuse, 1985, pp. 50–75.

Pattison EM: Sociocultural approaches to the problem of alcoholism. *In* Galanter M, Pattison EM (eds): Psychosocial Treatment of Alcoholism. Washington, DC, American Psychiatric Press, 1984, pp. 69–96.

Peele S: The Meaning of Addiction: Compulsive Experience and Its Interpretation. Lexington, MA, Lexington Books, 1985.

Peele S: The implication and limitations of genetic models of alcoholism and other addictions. J Stud Alcohol 47:63–76, 1986.

Peyrot M: Coerced voluntarism: The micropolitics of drug treatment. Urban Life 13:343–365, 1985.

Primm BJ, Wesley JE: Treating the multiply addicted black alcoholic. Alcohol Treat Q 2:155–178, 1986.

Rice D: The economic cost of alcohol abuse and alcohol dependence: 1990. Alcohol World: Health and Research 17:10–12, 1993.

Rice D, Kelman S, Miller L, Dunmeyer S: The Economic Costs of Alcohol and Drug Abuse and Mental Illness: 1985. San Francisco, Institute of Health and Aging, University of California at San Francisco, 1990.

Robert Wood Johnson Foundation: Substance Abuse (Annual Report). Princeton, NJ, Robert Wood Johnson Foundation, 1992.

Rowbotham MC: Neurological aspects of cocaine abuse. West J Med 149:442–448, 1988.

Rowe D, Grills C: African-centered drug treatment: An alternative conceptual paradigm for drug counseling with African-American clients. J Psychoactive Drugs 25:21–33, 1993.

Saleebey D: A social psychological perspective on addiction: Themes and disharmonies. *In* Watts TD (ed): Social Thought on Alcoholism: A Comprehensive Review. Malabar, FL, Robert E. Krieger, 1986, pp. 25–38.

Sampson P, Bookstein H, Barr H, Streissguth A: Prenatal alcohol exposure, birthweight, and measures of child size from birth to age 14 years. Am J Public Health 84:1421–1429, 1994.

Satir V, Stachowiak J, Taschman H: Helping Families to Change. New York, Jason Aronson, 1975.

Schaefer S, Evans S: Women, sexuality and the process of recovery. J Chem Depend Treat 1:91–120, 1987.

Scherling D: Prenatal cocaine exposure and childhood psychopathology: A developmental analysis. Am J Orthopsychiatry 64:9–19, 1994.

Schmidt C, Klee L, Ames G: Review and analysis of literature on indicators of women's drinking problems. Br J Addict 85:179–192, 1990.

Seibert J: Understanding chemical abuse and dependency in the elderly. J Home Health Care Pract 2:27–31, 1990.

Shore J: The Oregon experience with impaired physicians on probation: An eight year follow-up. JAMA 257:2931–2934, 1987.

Smith DE, Buxton ME, Bilal R, Seymour RB: Cultural points of resistance to the 12-step recovery process. J Psychoactive Drugs 259:97–108, 1993.

Snyder S (ed): Cocaine: A New Epidemic. New York, Chelsea House, 1985.

Sobel LC: Critique of alcoholism treatment evaluation. *In* Marlatt GA, Nathan PE (eds): Behavioral Approaches to Alcoholism. New Brunswick, NJ, Rutgers Center for Alcohol Studies, 1978, pp. 166–182.

Stanton MD, Todd TC, Hemp DB, et al: Heroin addiction as a family phenomenon: A new conceptual model. Am J Drug Alcohol Abuse 5:125–150, 1978.

Steinglass P: Family systems approaches to alcoholism. J Substance Abuse Treatment 2:161–167, 1985.

Stevens PE, Hall JM: Abusive health care interactions experienced by lesbians: A case of institutional violence in the treatment of women. Response Victimization Women Children 13:23–27, 1990.

Straus MA, Gelles R: Physical Violence in American Families. New Brunswick, NJ, Transaction, 1990.

Subby R: Inside the chemically dependent marriage: Denial and manipulation. *In* Subby R (ed). Codependency: An Emerging Issue. Deerfield Beach, FL, Health Communications, 1984.

Substance Abuse and Mental Health Services Administration (SAMHSA), Office of Applied Statistics: National Household Survey on Drug Abuse: Population Estimates 1991 (DHHS Publication No. [ADM] 91–1732). Rockville, MD, U.S. Department of Health and Human Services, Public Health Service, 1992.

Substance Abuse and Mental Health Services Administration (SAMHSA), Office of Applied Statistics: National Household Survey on Drug Abuse: Population Estimates 1992 (DHHS Publication No. [SMA] 93-2053). Rockville, MD, U.S. Department of Health and Human Services, Public Health Service, 1993.

Sullivan E, Handley S: Alcohol and drug use in nurses. Ann Rev Nurs Res 10:113–125, 1992.

Sullivan E, Handley S, Connors H: The role of nurses in primary care: Managing alcohol abusing patients. Alcohol World: Health and Research 18:158–161, 1994.

Sutker P: Drug dependent women: An overview of the literature. *In* Bescher G, Reed B, Mondanaro J (eds): Treatment Services for Drug Dependent Women, Vol. I. Rockville, MD, National Institute on Drug Abuse, 1981, pp. 25–43.

Szasz T: Ceremonial Chemistry: The Ritual Persecution of Drugs, Addicts and Pushers. New York, Anchor Press, Doubleday, 1985.

Talbott G, Wright C: Chemical dependency in health care professionals. Occup Med: State Art Rev 2:581–591, 1988.

Thompson T, Simmons-Cooper C: Chemical dependency treatment and black adolescents. J Drug Issues 18:21–31, 1988.

Tiffany ST: A cognitive model of drug urges and drug use behavior: Role of automatic and non-automatic processes. Psychological Rev 97:147–168, 1990.

Trad P: Substance abuse among adolescent mothers: Strategies for diagnosis, treatment and prevention. J Subs Abuse Treat 10:421–431, 1993.

U.S. Department of Health and Human Services. Seventh Special Report to the U.S. Congress on Alcohol and Health. Washington, DC, U.S. Public Health Service, 1990.

Valliant GE: The Natural History of Alcoholism: Causes, Patterns and Paths to Recovery. Cambridge, MA, Harvard University Press, 1983.

Van der Kolk BA, McFarlane AC, Weisaeth L (eds): Traumatic Stress: The Effects of Overwhelming Experience on Mind, Body and Society. New York, Guilford Press, 1996.

Vourakis C: Women in substance abuse treatment. *In* Bennett G, Vourakis C, Woolf D (eds): Substance Abuse: Pharmacologic, Developmental, and Clinical Perspectives. New York, Wiley, 1983.

Wallace BC: Crack cocaine smokers as adult children of alcoholics: The dysfunctional family link. J Substance Abuse Treat 7:89–100, 1990.

Wallace J: The new disease model of addiction. West J Med 152:502–505, 1990.

Weisner C: The alcohol treatment system and social control: A study in institutional change. J Drug Issues 13:117–133, 1983.

Westermeyer J: Substance use disorders: Predictions for the 1990's. Am J Drug Alcohol Abuse 18:1–11, 1992.

Widiger TA, Smith GT: Substance use disorder: Abuse, dependence and dyscontrol. Addictions 89:267–282, 1994.

Wilsnack S, Wilsnack R, Klassen A: Drinking and reproductive dysfunction among women in a 1981 national survey. Alcohol Clin Exp Res 8:451–457, 1984.

Wilson-Schaef A: When Society Becomes an Addict. San Francisco, Harper & Row, 1987.

Windle M: Substance abuse, risky behaviors and victimization among a US national adolescent sample. Addiction 89:172–182, 1994.

Woititz JG: Adult Children of Alcoholics. Deerfield Beach, FL, Health Communications, 1983.

Ziter ML: Culturally sensitive treatment of black alcoholics. Natl Assoc Social Workers 12:130–135, 1987.

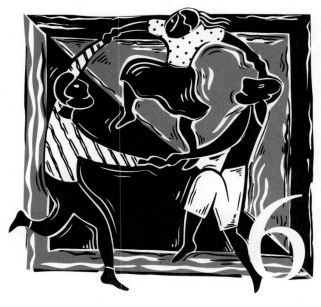

6

Special Service Needs

Communicable Disease

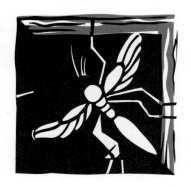

Upon completion of this chapter, the reader will be able to:

1. Discuss the routes for transmission of communicable diseases.

2. Identify the protocols for notifiable diseases within the Centers for Disease Control Monitoring and Surveillance System and explain why the system is important.

3. List three communicable diseases currently causing high morbidity in the United States, and identify their epidemiological indicators, including racial-ethnic disparity.

4. Specify the immunizations required by law in the United States, for what ages, and discuss their efficacy.

5. Discuss the prevalence and risk factors involved in the acquisition of human immunodeficiency virus–acquired immunodeficiency syndrome and other sexually transmitted diseases and identify methods for control.

6. Explain the difference among prevention, control, elimination, and eradication of communicable diseases.

Della J. Dash
Vera Labat

As the world becomes a more sophisticated and technologically advanced international network, increasing control can be asserted over many types of communicable diseases. Throughout history, epidemics have been responsible for the annihilation of entire groups of people, but there has existed the capacity to greatly reduce the alarming rates of morbidity and mortality caused by many of these infectious diseases. However, the recent emergence of new pathogens and the reemergence of old pathogens are creating formidable challenges for infectious disease control workers worldwide. Immunization, accomplished through the use of vaccines, may be one of the most important medical discoveries yet, providing a method to protect large aggregates of people through a simple, cost-effective preventive health measure. Entire generations can be prevented from experiencing painful death and debilitating deformity through the facilitation of universal immunization coverage of vaccine preventable diseases.

Although global eradication campaigns have been in process for decades, malaria and other vector-borne communicable diseases, polio, and measles continue to cause significant mortality in most developing countries. Treatments exist for many sexually transmitted diseases (STDs), yet syphilis and gonorrhea continue to be global problems. From 1988 to 1992, the United States experienced a measles epidemic. In 1993, it experienced a doubling of pertussis cases (6087 cases) in comparison with the number of cases reported during 1992 (3264 cases), whereas the 1994 figure dropped to 3484 cases, nearly matching that of 1992 (Centers for Disease Control and Prevention, 1994a). With routine administration of childhood immunization practices, why are diseases like pertussis demonstrating a periodic resurgence? These are some of the questions to be answered in this chapter.

In the last 150 years, major advances have been made in hygienic practices through the design of water and sanitation facilities, which greatly contribute to the prevention of communicable diseases. At the 1990 World Summit for Children, the global goal of safe water and sanitation for all families by the year 2000 was agreed upon (United Nations Children's Fund [UNICEF], 1994). In the United States, the U.S. Environmental Protection Agency (EPA) is responsible for the establishment and enforcement of standards for water quality control. Chemical treatment and filtration methods are used for disinfection of drinking water supplies. Simple preventive measures like these, which we take for granted in our "developed" nation,

are the foundation for protecting the public's health from waterborne diseases and their sequelae. Unfortunately, because of economic and political disparities, people most likely to suffer from water-borne infections are often those living in developing countries who are without access to a safe water supply and sanitary means of excreta disposal. As the percentage of Americans living below the poverty level continues to increase, inequities in access to public health measures appear in growing proportions and are responsible in part for the increases in preventable communicable disease rates in the United States. Additionally, climatic changes, global warming, ecological instability, industrial development, floods, earthquakes, and human behaviors play a role in the environmental, social, and host interaction that create new opportunities for emergent pathogenic outbreaks.

To further control communicable diseases, health care reform in the United States is urgently needed. More attention must be given to maximizing opportunities for immunizing children and adults in the primary health care setting. Emphasis must be placed on preventive care, which in the long run is much more cost effective. Interdisciplinary working relationships among those charged with the surveillance, monitoring, and prevention of communicable diseases (such as epidemiologists, climatologists, entomologists, and virologists) will also play an important role in reforming health care. Affordability for primary prevention is the key to a sustainable health care system, but it must be accomplished without compromising quality of care. If this new design in primary prevention is successful, the eradication of many communicable diseases could be accomplished, producing a healthier environment for us all.

Two thirds of all employed nurses in the United States today are currently working in hospital settings (Moses, 1994). However, projections for the future of nursing, based on cost-containment and disease prevention health policies, place nurses in ambulatory care and other community-based health care settings. In these areas, they will be better able to meet the health needs of the communities in which they work by initially applying a community-based health profile, followed by the provision of health education outreach efforts and disease prevention programs designed specifically to meet the health needs of each community served. Community health nurses do not work alone but rather are part of a multidisciplinary team working together with the community. School nurses ensure vaccination of students, occupational health nurses keep industry safe for employees, STD clinic nurses provide health education and reporting of notifiable diseases, and nurse epidemiologists monitor surveillance systems and interpret data for appropriate planning of future interventions. It is important for each discipline to follow through with its role to provide the most comprehensive and effective care for the aggregate concerned.

This chapter discusses transmission, immunity, prevention, defining and reporting, control, elimination, and eradication of communicable diseases. Vaccine-preventable diseases, vaccines for travelers, and STDs are detailed. The chapter concludes with the application of the nursing process to a case study of the assessment, diagnosis, planning (short and long term), intervention, evaluation, and prevention (primary, secondary, and tertiary) of an epidemic at the individual, family, and community levels.

THE COMMUNICABLE DISEASE SPECTRUM

Transmission of communicable diseases can occur via direct, indirect, and airborne routes in individuals, in families, and within other aggregates and in populations. For transmission of disease to occur, there must be a host portal of entry and a microbe source or reservoir. These two criteria are different and very specific for each individual class of pathogens; and unfortunately, there are many possible routes for the spread and acquisition of communicable diseases in humans. Resistance and vulnerability, which change over time, impact whether a host becomes infected after exposure to a circulating pathogen. Environmental conditions such as crowding, pollution, nutritional status, natural disasters, deforestation, and industrialization also influence the transmission of communicable diseases (see Chapter 26). Individual and herd immunity can be enhanced through active immunization for protection against many communicable diseases. *Herd immunity* states that those not immunized will be safe if at least 80% of the population has been vaccinated (see Immunity). However, children need to be up to date and age-appropriately immunized for immunogenic coverage to be as high as possible. Assessments of childhood immunization coverage have been helpful in estimating low immunization rates.

Between 1959 and 1986, the U.S. Immunization Survey annually estimated national vaccination cov-

erage rates. Once discontinued in 1986, the National Health Interview Survey conducted by the Centers for Disease Control and Prevention (CDC) National Center for Health Statistics assumed the responsibility for producing quarterly and annual reports of national, state, and local immunization coverage statistics. These report results are shared with the World Health Organization (WHO).

In 1978, the WHO sponsored the Alma Ata Conference, which closed with the declaration of "health for all people by the year 2000." This ambitious global agenda emanated from the WHO, UNICEF, and other organizations that had the political will, the ideological commitment, and a sense of accountability for the cost of human morbidity and mortality in both the developing and the developed world. The conference gave public health workers from all over the globe an increased sense of direction as well as a vision of shared goals.

WHO and UNICEF have also sponsored global goals for international public health priorities, including eradication of specific communicable diseases. Previously responsible for the eradication of smallpox in 1977, other diseases are now being targeted for global control, elimination, and eradication by the end of this century.

In line with these global initiatives, the U.S. Public Health Service (USPHS) launched the National Health Promotion and Disease Prevention Objectives entitled "Healthy People 2000," which focused on achieving the goal of completing all seven types of routine childhood immunizations (diphtheria-tetanus-pertussis [DTP], oral polio vaccine [OPV], mumps-measles-rubella [MMR]) repeated at recommended intervals (4:3:1) for 90% of all children by their second birthday by the year 2000. The Childhood Immunization Initiative (CII) was established to facilitate by 1996 the increase of antigen-specific vaccinations to 90% coverage of all 2-year-olds. Additional coverage rates have been added for both *Haemophilus influenzae* type B (Hib) and hepatitis B (Hep B) vaccines, increasing the number of routine vaccines to 9. Additionally, chickenpox (varicella) and hepatitis A vaccine are now available. Adult immunizations are requiring an increased focus because pneumococcal disease is the number one killer of persons of all the vaccine-preventable diseases, and influenza is the second highest killer. Pneumococcal disease causes more than 40,000 deaths per year in the United States and an excess of 40,000 deaths per year occur from flu epidemics (CDC, 1995a).

It is important to identify the reasons why we choose to protect the public against communicable diseases, because these reasons have a substantial impact on the implementation of public health programs, both nationally and internationally. Application of a community-based health profile can assist in developing preventive public health programs designed to interrupt or prevent the transmission cycle from occurring and provide an assessment of the risk factors that impede health and increase the likelihood of transmission. Analysis of the underlying environmental, socioeconomic, political, educational, employment, and health factors should be considered when promoting the development of interventions for disease prevention and surveillance designed specifically for health promotion of the individual, family, and aggregate.

TRANSMISSION

Communicable diseases do not occur in a vacuum, but are the result of an interaction among a host (e.g., a person), an infectious agent (e.g., a bacterium), and the environment (e.g., a contaminated food supply),

known as an epidemiological triad (see Chapter 5). Communicable diseases can be transmitted vertically or horizontally (Gordis, 1996). Vertical transmission occurs between parent and offspring when the infection is passed via placenta, milk, contact with the vagina during birth, or sperm. Horizontal transmission occurs in either a direct manner (as in person-to-person contact) or indirectly (through a common vehicle such as contaminated food or water, through a vector, such as arthropods [ticks or mosquitoes], or via airborne route, such as contaminated droplets in the air). Some of the modes of transmission and communicable diseases are shown in Table 24–1.

Direct transmission implies the immediate transfer of an infectious agent from an infected host or reservoir to an appropriate portal of entry in the human host through physical contact. Uninterrupted person-to-person contact is responsible for the transmission of many communicable diseases, including scabies, measles, and STDs such as gonorrhea.

Indirect transmission is the spread of infection through vehicle fomites, animals, and vectors that carry a parasite or pathogen to a suitable portal of entry in the human host. Vehicle-borne or contaminated fomites can be any inanimate object, material,

Table 24–1
Examples of Types of Transmission for Various Communicable Diseases*

Direct	Indirect	‡Fecal-Oral	Airborne
Candidiasis	Arthropodborne viral diseases	Amebiasis	Meningococcal meningitis
Herpes	Lyme disease	*Giardiasis*	Mumps
Mononucleosis	Tetanus	*Escherichia coli*	Common cold
Syphilis	Onchocerciasis	*Campylobacter*	Rubella
Gonorrhea	Rabies	Hepatitis A	Pertussis
Ebola	Rocky Mountain spotted fever	Salmonellosis	Psittacosis
Cryptosporidiases	Diphtheria	Cholera	Influenza
Leprosy†	Taeniasis	Typhoid fever	Measles
Trachoma	Botulism		Tuberculosis
Viral warts	Dracunculiasis		Legionellosis
Chickenpox	Plague		
Yaws	Schistosomiasis		
	Yellow fever		
	Malaria		

*As communicable diseases, these diseases can occur in the individual, in the family, or in other aggregates or populations.

†Exact mode of transmission not clearly understood.

‡Transmission may be person to person or animal to person.

or substance that acts as a transport agent for a microbe. Reproduction of the infectious agent may take place on or in the vehicle before the transmission of the pathogen. Substances such as food, water, and blood products can provide indirect transmission through ingestion and intravenous transfusions. Foodborne diseases may include viruses, bacteria, parasites, and enterotoxins. Botulism is an example of an indirectly transmitted foodborne enterotoxin disease. Animal and vectorborne transmission can be communicated through biological and mechanical routes. The mechanical route involves no multiplication or growth of the parasite or microbe within the animal or vector itself. Biological transmission occurs when the parasite grows or multiplies inside the animal, vector, or arthropod, such as with arthropodborne viral diseases, including hemorrhagic fevers, viral fevers, and viral encephalitides. The modes of transmission from animals to humans vary considerably and may include biting, spitting, spray from urine, and fecal-oral transmission, among others. Tetanus is an example of indirect mechanical transmission via soil carried by an animal, which then contaminates a human through a wound or bite. Transmission from a vector to the human host is usually through a bite or sting. Malaria is an example of indirect biological transmission from a mosquito vector to a human host.

Fecal-oral transmission can be both direct and indirect. It can occur through the ingestion of water supplies that have been fecally polluted, by consumption of contaminated food, and through engagement in oral-genital sexual activity. Polio virus is spread through fecal-oral transmission.

Airborne transmission occurs mainly through aerosols and droplet nuclei. The time frame in which an airborne particle can remain suspended greatly influences the virility and infectivity it can possess. The size of the particle can also play an important role in how long it remains airborne and how successful it will be at penetrating the human lung. Aerosols are defined as extremely small solid or liquid particles that may include fungal spores, viruses, and bacteria. When inhaled into the lungs, they are responsible for many infections, including fungal diseases such as cryptococcosis and histoplasmosis. Droplet nuclei, such as the spray from sneezing, travels approximately a meter but usually not further before the droplets fall on the ground. Within this distance, contaminated droplets may make direct contact with an open wound or with a mucus membrane, including eye conjunctiva, nose, or mouth, or they may be inhaled into the lung. Measles virus is propagated through the inhalation of contaminated droplets.

IMMUNITY

Immunity can be described as "protection from infection." There are several different kinds of immunity, each providing resistance to any of a number of specific infectious diseases. *Natural immunity* is an innate resistance to a specific antigen or toxin. *Acquired immunity* is derived from actual exposure to the specific infectious agent, toxin, or appropriate vaccine. *Active immunity* is present when the body can build its own antibodies that provide protection from a bacterial or other antigenic substance, such as the introduction of a vaccine or toxoid. *Passive immunity* implies the temporary resistance that has been donated to the host through transfusions of plasma proteins, immunoglobulins, and antitoxins or from mother to neonate transplacentally; passive immunity lasts only as long as these substances remain in the blood stream.

These various types of immunity provide protection against the transmission of many communicable diseases and are available for use in the fight against local endemic disease as well as in the control of global pandemics and epidemics.

The concept of herd immunity, in which those not immunized will be safe if at least 80% of the population has been vaccinated, is especially true for the transmission of diseases that are found only in the human host and that have no invertebrate host or other mode of transmission. Thus, without the presence of a virgin population to infect, the organism will be unable to live.

Primary vaccine failure is the failure of a vaccine to contribute any level of immunogenicity, and can be caused by a break in the cold chain that renders vaccines ineffective. Additionally, a certain portion of persons receiving vaccine never seroconvert and thus are not protected from the communicable disease. *Secondary vaccine failure* is the waning of immunogenicity after eliciting an initial immune response that fades over time, often present in immunosuppressed patients. Both types of vaccine failures can be elicited by the lack of age-appropriately immunized children and by those who are not up to date in their immunization schedules.

PREVENTION

Primary, secondary, and tertiary levels of communicable disease prevention have been developed to define public health actions for individuals, families, and aggregates (Table 24–2). Please refer to Chapter 1 for definitions and examples of primary, secondary, and tertiary prevention.

For example, the individual child must be taught hand washing and toileting to prevent fecal-oral contamination and subsequent illness from ascariasis infection; the family must know proper personal and household hygiene to protect itself against the invasion of disease-carrying rodents and vectors such as rats and fleas infected with plague; and the community must provide a safe water supply and waste disposal system to prevent epidemics of cholera.

Personal hygiene, environmental sanitation, and safer sexual practices represent the easiest and most cost-effective methods for prevention of transmission of many parasitic and bacterial infectious disease. This includes the availability of potable water. A potable water system is represented by the lack of high numbers of coliforms, which are the bacterial parts used to measure fecal contamination of water supplies. The percentage of coliforms found in the water usually represents the level of contamination from bacteria, amoebas, nematodes (worms), viruses, and other disease-spreading organisms. These organisms are responsible for the direct spread of infection of many waterborne diseases such as *Giardia,* intestinal worms, hepatitis, diarrhea and dysentery, cholera, and typhoid fever. During the 1990 World Summit for Children, it was decided that the global provision of safe water and sanitation facilities for all families was achievable and should be targeted for the year 2000.

Airborne transmission can be extremely difficult to control as air quality deteriorates with growing urban and suburban populations producing pollution at uncontrollable rates. In the United States, the EPA is responsible for the establishment and enforcement of standards for air quality control. These standards are designed to ensure that the public health is protected. The use of air conditioners and atomizers can cause particles to remain in the air for long periods of time, and it is therefore important to have intact and reliable

Table 24–2
Levels of Prevention of Communicable Diseases

Affected Population	Level		
	Primary	Secondary	Tertiary
Individual (AIDS)	Education Change sexual behavior/ other high-risk practices	Screening for AIDS in at-risk populations Reporting Early diagnosis and treatment	HIV drugs Maintain health Prevent conversion from HIV to AIDS Prepare for dying
Family (malaria)	Sleeping under bed net Protective clothing (long-sleeved shirts and long pants) Insect repellents Eliminate mosquito-breeding stagnant water/spraying of ponds	Reporting Immediate diagnosis and treatment of infected individuals	Prevent mosquito feeding on infected individuals Appropriate treatment using correct drugs to prevent further drug resistance
Aggregate (measles)	Education Measles vaccination Documentation	Screening for unimmunized individuals Early diagnosis and treatment Reporting Control of spread (epidemics)	Treatment of disease Epidemic measures

AIDS, acquired immunodeficiency syndrome; HIV, human immunodeficiency virus.

air filtration systems in all public buildings, surgical suites, and rooms reserved for isolation patients.

UNIVERSAL BLOOD AND BODY FLUID PRECAUTIONS

To prevent and control the transmission of diseases found in blood and body fluid, the CDC has developed a set of universal precautions (Table 24–3). Infected persons may have no signs or symptoms or not have any knowledge of their conditions; therefore, all persons are assumed to be infectious and treated as such by health care workers, especially in emergency situations (CDC, 1988).

DEFINING AND REPORTING

The CDC (CDC, 1996b) lists 52 infectious diseases that are designated nationally notifiable by the Council of State and Territorial Epidemiologists in conjunction

Table 24–3
Universal Blood and Body Fluid Precautions

The Department of Labor, Occupational Safety and Health Administration, established guidelines on occupational exposure to bloodborne pathogens in 1991 (Rekus, 1991). These guidelines state that workers are to consider any contact with blood or body fluid as hazardous. These guidelines, which followed others (e.g., CDC, 1988), give ways exposure to bloodborne diseases to workers can be minimized:

- Special training and education programs
- Use of protective equipment such as gloves, gowns, eye protection, and face masks
- Hand washing after each patient contact
- Proper handling and disposing of sharps
- Engineering control such as special sharps containers and safety cabinets for biologicals
- Programs of immunization such as hepatitis B vaccine for employees
- Proper contaminated waste disposal
- Use of disinfectants
- Proper labeling and signs

Adapted from Centers for Disease Control: Universal precautions for prevention of transmission of HIV, hepatitis B virus, and other bloodborne pathogens in health care settings. Morb Mortal Wkly Rep 37:377–382, 387–388, 1988; Rekus JF. Bloodborne Pathogens, Washington, DC: Federal Register, Occupational Safety and Health Administration, Department of Labor, 1991.

with CDC (Table 24–4). These classifications of diseases are defined according to confirmed cases, probable cases, laboratory-confirmed cases, clinically compatible cases, supportive laboratory results, epidemiologically linked cases, and, last, a diagnosis that meets the clinical case definition. Standardizing definitions of diseases is important for local, state, national, and global public health surveillance teams because it provides a baseline for comparison of data and monitoring of epidemiological trends across the country and around the world. Screening, intervention, control, and eradication programs can readily be designed and implemented based on the data collected from adherence to this set of case definitions. Not all nationally notifiable diseases are reportable in every state or territory, however. Data in the table, unless otherwise noted, are transmitted to the CDC via the National Electronic Telecommunications System for Surveillance. Cases of infectious diseases are reported by geographical region, state, and for the nation each week in the CDC's *Morbidity and Mortality Weekly Report (MMWR)*. Weekly and cumulative totals of communicable disease and information on prevention and control are presented as well. Other topics include occupational and environmental hazards and unusual cases and outbreaks of disease. The *MMWR* can be found in medical libraries, at local health departments, at infection control departments in hospitals and medical centers, and in many community-based organizations.

CONTROL

Control of a communicable disease is the reduction of incidence or prevalence of a given disease at any point in time. The WHO's Expanded Programme on Immunizations (EPI) is a global attempt to control morbidity and mortality for six of the major childhood vaccine preventable diseases, with each country adapting these guidelines as necessary. In 1994, the USPHS launched the CII with the same overall objective.

At the World Summit for Children, the WHO, UNICEF, and several other international health organizations established several mid-decade goals for the global control of specific diseases by the end of 1995 (UNICEF, 1994). These included the achievement of 80% immunization coverage (with the six basic immunizations, including bacille Calmette-Guérin [BCG], OPV, DPT, and measles) in all countries; 80% use of oral rehydration therapy (ORS) to control

Table 24–4

National Notifiable Diseases Surveillance System*

Acquired immunodeficiency syndrome	*Haemophilus influenzae,* invasive disease	Rabies, animal
Anthrax	Hansen disease (Leprosy)	Rabies, human
Botulism†	Hantavirus pulmonary syndrome	Rocky Mountain spotted fever
Brucellosis	Hemolytic uremic syndrome, post-diarrheal†	Rubella
Chancroid†	Hepatitis A	Salmonellosis†
Chlamydia trachomatis, genital infection	Hepatitis B	Shigellosis†
Cholera	Hepatitis, C/non-A, non-B	Streptococcal disease, invasive, group A†
Coccidioidomycosis†	HIV infection, pediatric	*Streptococcus pneumoniae,* drug resistant†
Congenital rubella syndrome	Legionellosis	Streptococcal toxic-shock syndrome
Congenital syphilis	Lyme disease	Syphilis
Cryptosporidiosis	Malaria	Tetanus
Diphtheria	Measles	Toxic-shock syndrome
Encephalitis, California	Meningococcal disease	Trichinosis
Encephalitis, eastern equine	Mumps	Tuberculosis
Encephalitis, St. Louis	Pertussis	Typhoid fever
Encephalitis, western equine	Plague	Yellow fever†
Escherichia coli O157:H7	Poliomyelitis, paralytic	
Gonorrhea	Psittacosis	

*Although varicella is not a nationally notifiable disease, the Council of State and Territorial Epidemiologists recommends reporting of cases of this disease to Centers for Disease Control and Prevention.

†Not currently published in the weekly tables.

Information from Centers for Disease Control and Prevention: Notice to Readers, Changes in national notifiable diseases data presentation. Morb Mortal Wkly Rep 45:41–55, 1996.

dehydration from diarrheal disease, including health education for increased breast-feeding; and reduction of measles morbidity by 90% and measles mortality by 95% (UNICEF, 1994).

ELIMINATION

The process of elimination of a communicable disease involves controlling it within a specified geographical area such as a single country, an island, or a continent and reducing the prevalence and incidence to eventual eradication.

At the World Summit for Children, the WHO, UNICEF, and several other international health or-

ganizations established several mid-decade goals for the global elimination of specific diseases and conditions by the end of 1995 (UNICEF, 1994). These included the elimination of poliomyelitis from Europe and the Western Pacific; measles from the English-speaking Caribbean; and neonatal tetanus, vitamin A deficiency (and related blindness), and iodine deficiency disorders (goiter and cretinism) globally.

Several diseases or their clinical manifestations are also targeted for elimination by the year 2000: poliomyelitis, which has been virtually eliminated from Latin America; leprosy, which is defined as less than one case per 10,000 population; and measles on the European continent. Only one disease, onchocerciasis, has been targeted for elimination by the year 2007 and that is limited to the Americas.

ERADICATION

The International Task Force for Disease Eradication (ITFDE) defines eradication as reducing the incidence of a disease worldwide to zero as a function of deliberate efforts, with no need for further control measures (CDC, 1993a).

Smallpox, eradicated in 1977 and certified by WHO in 1980, was the first vaccine-preventable disease to be globally eradicated (CDC, 1991). Thus, the smallpox vaccine is no longer administered anywhere in the world. Many factors contributed to this public health success, including the mode of transmission of the disease (directly transmitted), the isolated geographical distribution of the infection, the ease of administration of the freeze-dried vaccine, the establishment of an effective surveillance system, the increase of national and international political will, and tremendous community participation.

Since the accomplishment of this public health success, the WHO and other public health forums and organizations around the world have rallied together to target additional diseases for global eradication. In 1989, the CDC established the ITFDE, with the delegated responsibility of defining and applying epidemiological and political criteria to a select group of communicable diseases to establish probability and prioritization for further global eradication campaigns.

Subsequent scientific feasibility and political will were defined (Table 24–5) and applied in depth to 30 selected diseases out of a potential register of 94 communicable diseases. One noncommunicable disease was included as a control. The results were separated into four categories: (1) six diseases that could be eradicated; (2) seven diseases with elimination of selected aspects possible; (3) nine diseases not now eradicable; and (4) six diseases not eradicable (CDC, 1993a) (Table 24–6).

At the World Summit for Children, WHO, UNICEF, and several other international health organizations established one mid-decade goal and one year-2000 goal for global eradication: eradication of dracunculiasis by the end of 1995 and poliomyelitis by the year 2000 (UNICEF, 1994). To date, there are 21 dracunculiasis-endemic countries globally: 18 in Africa, 1 in the Middle East (Yemen), and 2 in Asia

Table 24–5
Criteria for Eradication

Epidemiology

1. Human host only; no host in nature
2. Easy diagnosis; obvious clinical manifestations
3. Limited duration and intensity of infection
4. Natural lifelong immunity after infection
5. Highly seasonal transmission
6. Availability of vaccine and/or curative treatment

Political Will

1. Substantial global morbidity-mortality
2. Cost effectiveness of campaign and eradication
3. Integration of eradication with additional public health variables
4. Eradication imperative over control measures

Information obtained from the Centers for Disease Control: Recommendations of the International Task Force for Disease Eradication. Morb Mortal Wkly Rep 42:1–38, 1993.

(Pakistan and India). Pakistan is thus far the only country to have succeeded in eliminating the disease. The region of the Americas is the only area to have eliminated indigenous poliomyelitis, accomplished in 1991 (CDC, 1994b).

VACCINE-PREVENTABLE DISEASES

Relatively few children die annually in the United States from vaccine-preventable diseases compared with the number of children who die from these diseases in developing countries. Because of the virulency and reemerging patterns of these diseases, which can cause major outbreaks, emphasis must be placed on continuous control and prevention through active vaccination programs for aggregates and populations.

The American Academy of Pediatrics (AAP), the Advisory Committee on Immunization Practices (ACIP), and the American Academy of Family Physicians (AAFP) recommend that all children in the United States complete the routine 4:3:1 schedule of childhood vaccines by the age of 18 months, including four doses of diphtheria and tetanus toxoids and pertussis (DTaP) vaccine; three doses of a live, attenuated oral (OPV) or an injectable, inactivated poliovirus vaccine (IVP); and one dose of MMR vaccine. Three to four doses of Hib conjugate vaccine and three doses of hepatitis B vaccine (Hep B) have been added to the schedule, increasing the number of routine childhood vaccines to nine (CDC, 1996a).

Table 24-6
Recommendations for Disease Eradication: Categories and Results

Eradicable Diseases

Dracunculiasis (guinea worm)	Rubella
Poliomyelitis	Taeniasis/cystercosis (pork tapeworm)
Lymphatic filariasis	
Mumps	

Possible Elimination of Selected Aspects of Disease

Hepatitis B	Rabies
Iodine deficiency disorders*	Trachoma
Neonatal tetanus	Yaws and endemic treponematoses
Onchocerciasis (river blindness)	

Not Now Eradicable

Ascariasis (roundworm)	Measles
Cholera	Pertussis (whooping cough)
Diphtheria	Rotaviral enteritis
Hookworm	Schistosomiasis
Leprosy	(bilharziasis)

Not Eradicable

Amebiasis	Enterobiasis
Bartonellosis	American trypanosomiasis
Clonorchiasis	Varicella zoster

*Iodine deficiency disorders comprise the only noncommunicable disease included in this study.

Information obtained from the Centers for Disease Control: Recommendations of the International Task Force for Disease Eradication. Morb Mortal Wkly Rep 42:1–38, 1993.

Varicella has been recommended also, and hepatitis A vaccine is now available.

The National Health Promotion and Disease Prevention Objectives entitled "Healthy People 2000" focuses on achieving the goal of completing all seven routine childhood immunizations (4:3:1:[DTP:OPV:MMR]) for 90% of all children by their second birthday by the year 2000. As a precursor, the CII will facilitate by 1996 the increase of antigen-specific vaccinations to 90% coverage of all 2-year-olds.

In a 1991–1992 study of vaccine coverage of preschool and school-age children in the United States, a mean of 87% complete vaccine coverage of children had been achieved by age of school entry; coverage rates of children younger than 2 years (mean of 44%) were very low compared with the year 2000 goal (Zell et al., 1994). However, coverage rates for 1993 show progress toward the 1996 CII goal and the year 2000 national health objectives (CDC, 1994c).

Compliance with routine vaccination schedules remains one of the greatest problems for global immunization programs, with high dropout rates that leave many children only partially protected, reducing overall coverage rates that would otherwise contribute to herd immunity.

This section contains comprehensive information on vaccines from the ACIP and includes vaccine types, storage, transport, handling, administration and routes, dosages, spacing, hypersensitivity, documentation, vaccine-related injuries, and additional sources of vaccine information. The 10 childhood vaccine-preventable communicable diseases are discussed in detail, including presentation, complications, transmission, incubation, current statistics, risk groups, diagnosis, treatment, vaccination, and control and possible eradication activities.

Vaccines

As the rate of vaccine-related research advances, it becomes more important for periodical consultation with current sources of information regarding immunizations. Recommendations, policies, and procedures concerning immunization information are governed internationally by the WHO and nationally (in the United States) by the Committee on Infectious Diseases of the AAP and the ACIP of the USPHS. The recommended schedule for immunization of healthy infants and children by the ACIP, AAP, and AAFP is listed in Table 24–7. Occasionally, there are differences in opinions regarding the information from these agencies, and it is therefore extremely important to thoroughly consider the population involved when interpreting these recommendations and procedures. The cost of fully vaccinating a single child should include the total number of doses, the equipment and personnel necessary for administration, the cold chain system, and the surveillance system for ensuring that the child is fully immunized.

Table 24–7
Recommended Childhood Immunization Schedule United States, July–December 1996

Vaccine	Birth	1 mo	2 mos	4 mos	6 mos	12 mos	15 mos	18 mos	4–6 yrs	11–12 yrs	14–16 yrs
Hepatitis B*	Hep B-1		Hep B-2		Hep B-3					Hep B*	
Diphtheria, tetanus, pertussis†			DTP	DTP	DTP	DTP³ (DTaP at 15+ m)			DTP or DTaP	Td	
H. influenzae type b‡			Hib	Hib	Hib‡	Hib‡					
Polio§			OPV§	OPV	OPV				OPV		
Measles, mumps, rubella‖						MMR			MMR‖ or	MMR‖	
Varicella zoster virus vaccine¶						Var				Var¶	

Vaccines are listed under the routinely recommended ages. Open bars indicate range of acceptable ages for vaccination. Shaded bars indicate *catch-up vaccination:* at 11–12 years of age, hepatitis B vaccine should be administered to children not previously vaccinated, and varicella zoster virus vaccine should be administered to children not previously vaccinated who lack a reliable history of chickenpox.

Approved by the Advisory Committee on Immunization Practices, the American Academy of Pediatrics, and the American Academy of Family Physicians.

Infants born to hepatitis B surface antigen (HBsAg)-negative mothers should receive 2.5 µg of Merck vaccine (Recombivax HB) or 10 µg of SmithKline Beecham (SB) vaccine (Engerix-B). The second dose should be administered ≥1 mo after the first dose.

Infants born to HBsAg-positive mothers should receive 0.5 mL hepatitis B immune globulin within 12 hr of birth, and either 5 µg of Merck vaccine (Recombivax HB) or 10 µg of SB vaccine (Engerix-B) at a separate site. The second dose is recommended at 1–2 mo of age and the third dose at 6 mo of age.

Infants born to mothers whose HBsAg status is unknown should receive either 5 µg of Merck vaccine (Recombivax HB) or 10 µg of SB vaccine (Engerix-B) within 12 hr of birth. The second dose of vaccine is recommended at 1 mo of age and the third dose at 6 mo of age. Adolescents who have not previously received three doses of hepatitis B vaccine should initiate or complete the series at the 11–12-yr old visit. The second dose should be administered at least 1 mo after the first dose, and the third dose should be administered at least 4 mo after the first dose and at least 2 mo after the second dose.

†DTP may be administered at 12 mo of age, if at least 6 mo have elapsed since DTP3. DTaP (diphtheria and tetanus toxoids and acellular pertussis vaccine) is licensed for the fourth and/or fifth vaccine dose(s) for children aged ≥15 mo and may be preferred for these doses in this age group. Td (tetanus and diphtheria toxoids, adsorbed, for adult use) is recommended at 11–12 yr of age if at least 5 yr have elapsed since the last dose of DTP, DTaP, or DT.

‡Three H. influenzae type b (Hib) conjugate vaccines are licensed for infant use. If PRP-OMP (PedvaxHIB [Merck]) is administered at 2 and 4 mo of age, a dose at 6 mo is not required. After completing the primary series, any Hib conjugate vaccine may be used as a booster.

§Oral poliovirus vaccine (OPV) is recommended for routine infant vaccination. Inactivated poliovirus vaccine (IPV) is recommended for persons with a congenital or acquired immune deficiency disease or an altered immune status as a result of disease or immunosuppressive therapy, as well as their household contacts, and is an acceptable alternative for other persons. The primary three-dose series for IPV should be given with a minimum interval of 4 wk between the first and second doses and 6 mo between the second and third doses.

‖The second dose of MMR is routinely recommended at 4–6 yr of age or at 11–12 yr of age, but may be administered at any visit, provided at least 1 mo has elapsed since receipt of the first dose.

¶Varicella zoster virus vaccine (Var) can be administered to susceptible children any time after 12 mo of age. Unvaccinated children who lack a reliable history of chickenpox should be vaccinated at the 11–12-yr-old visit.

Source: Centers for Disease Control and Prevention: Immunization Action News 3(5):1, 1996c. Recommended childhood immunization schedule United States, July–December 1996. MMWR 45:635–638, 1996a.

CAUTION IN GIVING IMMUNIZATIONS

Caution must be taken when giving any immunization. The most recent recommendations regarding which immunization to give, to whom, how, and how they are to be transported, stored, and administered must be obtained from the Centers for Disease Control and Prevention in Atlanta, Georgia. Information about the most recent immunizations should be transmitted from the CDC to state health departments, from state health departments to local health departments, and from local health departments to physicians and other professionals working in primary care and other health facilities.

Vaccine efficacy is dependent on many factors, which are detailed in the following section. When policy recommendations are not followed, the public health system is jeopardized along with all of its constituents. A breakdown in this chain can leave children unimmunized, workers unprotected, and surveillance systems vulnerable to incomplete or inaccurate information. Additional information on vaccines can be obtained from the sources listed in Table 24–8.

Types of Immunization

Vaccination is the administration of a vaccine or toxoid, which confers active immunity by stimulating the body to produce antibodies or antitoxins. Immunization is a broader term that includes not only *vaccines* for active immunity but also passive immunogenic solutions such as *immune globulins* and *antitoxins*. This section deals exclu-

Table 24–8
Additional Sources of Vaccine Information

1. American Academy of Pediatrics. Active and passive immunization. *In* Peter G, Ed. 1994 Red book: Report of the Committee on Infectious Diseases, 23rd ed. Elk Grove Village, IL: American Academy of Pediatrics, 1994, pp 1–67.

2. Benenson AS. Control of Communicable Diseases in Man, 16th ed. Washington, DC: American Public Health Association, 1995.

3. General Recommendations on Immunization, ACIP. Morb Mortal Wkly Rep 43(RR-1), 1–38, 1994.

4. Health Hints for the Tropics, 11th ed. American Society of Tropical Medicine and Hygiene, 1992.

5. Official Manufacturer's Package Inserts or Physicians' Desk Reference, 50th ed. Montvale, NJ: Medical Economics, 1996.

6. Health Information for International Travel: CDC prints an annual publication and has a telephone hotline—(404) 332-4559.

7. CDC National Immunization Program, Telephone (404) 332-4553, Atlanta, GA: *Immunization National Resource Directory.*

8. National Vaccine Injury Compensation Program
   Health Resources and Services Administration, Parklawn Building, Room 8-05
   5600 Fishers Lane
   Rockville, MD 20857
   Telephone: (800) 338-2382 (24-hour recording)

9. Vaccine Adverse Events Reporting System (VAERS), 24-hour recorded telephone message: (800) 822-7967.

10. Guide for Adult Immunization (1994), American College of Physicians. Telephone: (800) 523-1546.

11. National Coalition for Adult Immunization (NCAI)
    4733 Bethesda Ave, Suite 750
    Bethesda, MD 20814
    Telephone: (301) 656-0003.

12. Werner D. Where There is No Doctor: A Village Health Care Handbook. Palo Alto, CA: The Hesperian Foundation, 1977.

13. Werner D, Bower B. Helping Health Workers Learn. Palo Alto, CA: The Hesperian Foundation, 1987.

Table 24–9
Type of Vaccine

Vaccines	Description
Live Attenuated	
Viral	Measles, mumps, rubella, polio, yellow fever, vaccinia, varicella
Bacterial	BCG Bacille Calmette-Guérin
Recombinant	Typhoid
Inactivated	
Viral	Influenza, polio, rabies, hepatitis A
Bacterial	Pertussis, typhoid, cholera, plague
Subunit (fractional)	Hepatitis B, influenza, acellular pertussis
Toxoid	Diphtheria, tetanus, botulism
Recombinant	Hepatitis B
Polysaccharide	
Inactivated subunit vaccines	Pneumococcal, meningococcal, *Haemophilus influenzae* type b

Source: Centers for Disease Control: *Epidemiology and Prevention of Vaccine-Preventable Diseases.* Atlanta: Centers for Disease Control and Prevention, Public Health Services, 1995; pp. 173–197.

sively with vaccines, except in the cases of diphtheria and tetanus, for which antitoxin is administered as part of the treatment for infection, and rabies, for which an immune globulin is used for treatment.

Vaccines can be prepared in several ways. They may be suspended in many types of solutions; protected with preservatives, stabilizers, or antibiotics; or may be mixed with adjuvants, which are used to increase immunogenicity (Table 24–9). Vaccines can be live and attenuated, or they may be killed (inactivated), with the virulence removed, leaving only the antigenic property necessary to stimulate the human immune system to produce antibodies. Types of inactivated vaccines include toxoids and polysaccharide vaccines. Inactivated conjugate vaccines with a chemically linked polysaccharide and protein, and the genetically engineered "recombinant" vaccines, are also now being administered. Inactivated vaccines can be parts of (fractions or subunits) or whole "killed" bacteria or viruses. Immune globulins and antitoxin are solutions that contain antibodies from human or animal blood and are introduced into a patient to provide passive protection without initiating the immune system to produce an immunogenic response.

Vaccine Storage, Transport, and Handling

Vaccines should be safely stored, transported, and handled at all times. Deviation from standard practice can be deleterious to the efficacy of vaccines. Storage information for routine childhood vaccines is important. A cold chain is a system used to ensure that vaccines are kept below 4°C from the time they are manufactured until they are used for vaccination. There are many levels of a cold chain, including locations at the national, regional, and local areas to be served, and lapses in the degree of refrigeration can occur at any of these levels as a result of factors ranging from bad roads and weather conditions to poor power supplies or faulty thermometer readings. The importance of a cold chain must be stressed here as any improper storage that allows the vaccines to be exposed to higher or lower temperatures, thus causing them to lose their potency and rendering them completely useless. This becomes an extremely difficult job when attempting to distribute vaccines in rural areas and in developing areas that do not have access to electricity or cold storage and where the vaccine may be distributed by bicycle or on foot. Many vaccine failures can be blamed on improper vaccine storage, causing the loss of vaccine efficacy. Because of the fluctuation in electricity in many areas, solar- and kerosene-powered refrigeration systems have been designed and distributed, particularly in rural areas in the developing world. Proper operation and maintenance of these systems are essential. Several methods are available for ensuring that the appropriate temperature has been maintained throughout vaccine transport and storage, including liquid crystal thermometers, dial thermometers, recording thermometers and digital thermometers, ice pack indicators, shipping indicators that change color if the temperature exceeds or falls below the recommended level, freeze-watch indicators, and 3-M cold chain monitors (Cutts and Smith, 1994). (For information about storage and transport of vaccines, see CDC, 1994n.)

Vaccine Administration and Routes

Vaccines are designed with specific types of administration needs. If administration routes and procedures are not strictly adhered to, vaccine efficacy can be adversely affected. Sterile technique should be used to ensure that both the vaccinator and the vaccinee are protected from infection. Once the needle is inserted, the plunger should be pulled back to ensure that no blood is present, which would be evidence of needle insertion directly into a blood vessel. If so, the needle should be withdrawn and changed, and a new site selected for administration, with the same procedure followed.

Needle size is important for the administration of vaccines. The needle size and angle of the bevel should be selected based on the site of administration (e.g., intramuscular, subcutaneous) and the size of the patient (adult or child). If more than one vaccine is being administered simultaneously, different anatomical sites should be used.

Vaccine Dosages

It is important to administer the specific dosage of a vaccine recommended in the package insert because a deviation may cause alterations in vaccine efficacy. For a summary of dosage information, consult the manufacturer's package insert or the *Physicians' Desk Reference.*

For international dosage information, refer to the WHO EPI Program. For Americans vaccinated outside of the United States, especially in developing countries, recommendations of the ACIP should be consulted.

Vaccine Spacing

Wherever possible, all children should be age-appropriately immunized and kept up-to-date using the recommendations of the ACIP (see Table 24–7), to avoid age-related complications or interference with the immune response. Clinically stable premature infants should adhere to the same schedule as term infants.

The recommended number of injections for any one immunobiological substance should be administered according to ACIP recommendations. An interruption in the schedule does not require that the entire series begin again. However, if injections are administered at less than the recommended intervals, they should not be counted as part of the primary series of immunization. Booster doses as recommended are essential and necessary to maintain the body's antibody level at a protective level.

Live, attenuated vaccines can be administered simultaneously with inactivated vaccines because no specific alteration in immunogenicity has been proven. Many vaccines can be administered simultaneously without contraindication; however, yellow fever and cholera vaccines should not be administered at the same time; at least 3 weeks should elapse between the administration of one and the other.

Vaccine Hypersensitivity

Although most individuals immunized do not experience adverse effects, occasionally allergic reactions are experienced ranging from mild local inflammation to severe systemic responses, including anaphylaxis. Reactions can be due to vaccine components such as eggs, egg proteins, antibiotics, preservatives, and adjuvants. Patient allergies should be considered before administration of specific vaccines. For additional precautions and contraindications, the vaccine package insert should be consulted as well as the latest instructions from the Centers for Disease Control and Prevention (CDC, 1994o).

Fever is not a contraindication for vaccination where the risk of infection is high or the chance for revaccination unreliable. Where the probability is high that a patient will return for vaccination after a moderate to severe fever subsides, it is recommended to wait to avoid any confusion between a vaccine side effect and an unknown underlying cause.

Pregnancy is not a contraindication for immunization using vaccines, antitoxins, or immune globulins. However, unless the risk of infection is very high, live vaccines, including MMR, should be avoided wherever possible.

Immunocompromised patients should not receive live vaccines, including OPV. If polio vaccination is recommended for an immunocompromised patient or household member, then IPV should be administered. MMR is recommended for human immunodeficiency virus (HIV)–infected persons. Killed or inactivated vaccines can be given, but they may not produce an optimal antibody response.

Vaccine Documentation

Legal documentation of vaccinations is important for both the individual and the provider for future administration and for follow-up of hypersensitivity reactions. Both individual and provider immunization records should be maintained. For each patient immunized, the health care provider is responsible for maintaining accurate records, including patient name, dates immunized, vaccine type, vaccine manufacturer, vaccine lot number, and the name, title, and address of the person administering the vaccine. Individual records should be kept by the patient and should include dates vaccinated, vaccine type, all allergies or hypersensitivities, doses, administration route and site, vaccine manufacturer, vaccine lot number, and the name, title, and address of the person administering the vaccine.

Reporting Adverse Events and Vaccine-Related Injuries

Health care providers must report specific postvaccination adverse events to the Vaccine Adverse Events Reporting System, which has a 24-hour recorded telephone message (1-800-822-7967). Information and reporting forms are available in both the Food and Drug Administration (FDA) Drug Bulletin and the *Physicians' Desk Reference.*

In 1988, the National Vaccine Injury Compensation Program became effective as a result of the National Childhood Vaccine Injury Act passed in 1986. This system provides assistance for individuals and families who experience a vaccine-related injury, including disability and death. Additional information regarding the program can be obtained from the following address and telephone number.

National Vaccine Injury Compensation Program
Health Resources and Services Administration
Parklawn Building, Room 8-05
5600 Fishers Lane
Rockville, MD 20857

Telephone: (800) 338-2382 (24-hour recording)
(301) 443-6593
For individuals filing a claim, the following address should be used:
Clerk of the U.S. Court of Federal Claims
717 Madison Place
NW Washington, DC 20005
Telephone: (202) 219-9657

VACCINE NEEDS FOR SPECIAL GROUPS

Adolescents and Young Adults

After the 1989–1991 measles epidemic in the United States, it was recognized that an adolescent immunization schedule was needed to provide routine vaccination of the second MMR for those children who did not receive it at school entry and to ensure that this age group also received the recommended 10-year doses of tetanus and diphtheria toxoids, adsorbed (Td). The ACIP, in its 1995 recommendations establishing the adolescent schedule, added universal administration of the hepatitis B series and the varicella (chickenpox) vaccines to the schedule for unvaccinated youths who have no documented history of vaccination of the disease (see Table 24–7). It is hoped that this practice will reduce the morbidity and mortality of hepatitis B and shingles in the adult and elderly populations.

Outbreaks of measles cases on college and university campuses in the recent past have alerted health care workers that there is a need for a routine assessment of immunization status across all age groups. Because many colleges and universities across the United States are requiring some minimal level of proof of immunizations before enrollment for new student entries, particularly for MMR, some form of immunization assessment will become a routine standard of practice for these young adults preparing to enter colleges and universities.

Adult and Elderly

Although immunization programs in the United States have greatly reduced the morbidity and mortality among children, vaccine-preventable diseases continue to cause thousands of hospitalizations and deaths in the American adult and elderly populations. The National Vaccine Advisory Committee in January 1994 adopted a report that called for the U.S. adult immunization status to reach the USPHS adult immunization goals for the year 2000 (National Vaccine Advisory Committee, 1994). The recommendations set forth were the following: (1) Increase the demand for adult vaccination by improving provider and public awareness; (2) ensure that the health care system has an adequate capacity to deliver vaccines to adults; (3) ensure adequate financing mechanisms to support the expanded delivery of vaccine to adults; (4) monitor and improve the performance of the nation's vaccine delivery system; and (5) ensure adequate support for research (National Vaccine Advisory Committee, 1994).

To support these goals, the CDC recommended that a preventive health care visit for the 50-year-old adult be routinely scheduled (CDC, 1995a). Missed immunization opportunities for this age group often occur during the office visit for "acute" or "chronic" health problems. This preventive health visit will have three immunization goals:

1. To assess the current immunization status
2. To administer the Td if indicated
3. To determine whether the adult has risk factors (e.g., cardiovascular, pulmonary, kidney, metabolic blood disorders) that would suggest the need for pneumococcal and influenza vaccinations.

Recent outbreaks of diphtheria in the former Soviet Union and the emergent drug-resistant pneumococcal bacteria give urgency to the implementation of this midlife immunization assessment and practice. Additionally, it will reduce the risk of the adult acting as a potential "carrier" and "spreader" of these diseases to susceptible persons.

The elderly, 65 years and older, account for 90% of the annual 20,000 to 40,000 deaths in the United States from active influenza and pneumonia disease. Many of these deaths are premature and preventable, especially when there are highly effective influenza and pneumonia vaccines available, and the cost of the vaccines and their administration are reimbursable by Medicare. The CDC has estimated that $4.6 billion a year can be attributed directly to medical care cost for influenza alone. There are at least 200,000 cases of invasive pneumococcal disease occurring across all age groups each year in the United States. An estimated 57 million people fall into the high-risk groups needing influenza or pneumococcal vaccines.

The vaccines can be administered simultaneously at the same visit, because those individuals needing both vaccines share common risk group factors. Additionally, the emergence of serious new drug-resistant

pneumococci gives an urgency to the need for the susceptible groups to be immunized and protected from this group of bacteria.

MAJOR GROUPS AT RISK OF SUFFERING MOST FROM INFLUENZA:

- Persons 65 years of age and older
- Residents of nursing homes and other chronic care facilities housing persons of any age with chronic medical conditions
- Adults and children with chronic disorders of the pulmonary or cardiovascular systems, including children with asthma
- Adults and children who have required regular medical follow-up or hospitalization during the preceding year because of chronic metabolic diseases (including diabetes mellitus), renal dysfunction, hemoglobinopathies, or immunosuppression (including immunosuppression caused by medications)
- Children and teenagers (6 months to 18 years of age) who are receiving long-term aspirin therapy and therefore may be at risk for Reye's syndrome after influenza
- Adults of any age with HIV infection or AIDS

Adapted from Centers for Disease Control. Immunization Action News 10(1), 1994.

Immunosuppressed

There are significant groups of people in the United States who are in some altered or compromised immune state. Severe immunosuppression status can occur for various health conditions: leukemia, lymphoma, HIV infection, AIDS, congenital immunodeficiency, radiation, general malignancy or therapy with alkylating agent, large doses of corticosteroids, or antimetabolites. For the severe immunosuppressed person, live viruses or bacteria vaccines can pose serious threats to the individual's health. The killed or inactivated vaccines are not problematic and can follow the same recommended administration schedule as for the healthy person. The individual's physician has the responsibility to determine to what degree the person is immunosuppressed. (For recommendations of use of vaccines in immunocompromised persons, see CDC, 1993d.)

Pregnancy

Vaccination risk during pregnancy is largely a theoretical issue according to the ACIP (CDC, 1994j). The tetanus-diphtheria toxoid combination vaccine is the only vaccine routinely indicated for susceptible pregnant women. However, the potential risk should never outweigh the known immunization benefits for a pregnant woman when (1) the risk of exposure to the natural disease is high; (2) special risk to the mother or fetus from the infection is present; and (3) harm is not likely to occur from administration of the vaccine.

The MMR vaccine is contraindicated when pregnancy is known, even though there are no cases on record of congenital rubella syndrome or abnormalities in infants born to mothers who received the vaccine while pregnant. Live virus vaccines, OPV, and yellow fever vaccine are not recommended during pregnancy, but can be administered and are recommended for susceptible pregnant women who live in areas or may travel to areas where there is a high risk of exposure to these natural diseases. Inactivated virus and bacteria vaccines or toxoids are not contraindicated immunizations during pregnancy. Hepatitis B, influenza, and pneumococcal vaccines are recommended for at-risk pregnant women and the immune globulin preparations have no known risk for the fetus.

VACCINE-PREVENTABLE DISEASES

Diphtheria

Diphtheria is an acute bacterial disease most commonly affecting the upper respiratory tract, including the nose, tonsils, larynx, and pharynx. Associated lesions are caused by the release of a cytotoxin, and present as a patch or patches of inflammation surrounding a grayish membrane. Complications may result in severe swelling of the neck, thrombocytopenia, neuritis, and myocarditis. The case fatality rate is 10 to 15% of all infections. It is transmitted through direct contact with an infected individual, with an incubation period of 2 to 5 days, and occasionally longer (Benenson, 1995). Globally, diphtheria continues to persist as a major cause of morbidity and mortality, especially in children younger than 5 years. However, in the United States, only 14 cases of diphtheria have been reported since 1990 (CDC, 1994d), with only one case reported in 1994.

General susceptibility exists for unimmunized individuals, while those previously immunized have waning protection for approximately 10 years after vaccination. A carrier state exists for diphtheria, and those identified should be immediately treated. Diag-

nosis is made through bacteriological culture of nasal and throat secretions from lesions. Treatment for diphtheria is twofold. First is the administration of a single dose of equine antitoxin followed by a full course of antimicrobial therapy. Strict isolation should be maintained for patients of toxigenic strains of pharyngeal diphtheria (American Academy of Pediatrics, 1994). Immunization with diphtheria toxoid is available in both monovalent diphtheria toxoid (Td) used only for adults and children older than 7 years and will usually promote the formation of antibodies against the toxin for approximately 10 years. Combined preparations, including diphtheria and tetanus toxoids (DT) for boosters every 10 years of life after the initial immunization series of diphtheria, tetanus toxoids, and pertussis vaccine (DTP or DTaP) used for routine childhood immunization, provide good antibody response. (For recommended schedule, see Table 24–7). These immunizations may cause soreness at the site of injection, and fever may appear for 1 to 2 days. Where pertussis immunization is contraindicated, DT should be used for the regular childhood schedule. No contraindications exist for diphtheria toxoid. The DTP is now available in a combined preparation with Hib (CDC, 1996d). There are two DTaP vaccines licensed in the United States: Tripedia (Connaught) and Acel-Imune (Lederle). Acel-Imune is FDA approved only for the fourth and fifth doses of the series in infants older than 15 months. On July 31, 1996, the FDA approved Tripedia for use in infants and young children for the initial first four doses of the routine diphtheria, tetanus, and pertussis vaccination series. Neither vaccine has FDA approval for a combined preparation with the Hib vaccine.

Diphtheria has been classified as "not now eradicable" by the ITFDE (CDC, 1993a) because although it is found only in the human host, it is difficult to diagnose, and only a multiple-dose vaccine is currently available. Therefore, WHO has determined that control of diphtheria should be continued by including DTP in the global EPI schedule.

Caution: **Hib** should not be confused with **influenza types A, B, and C.** Hib is a bacterial infection commonly found in children younger than 5 years, whereas influenza types A, B, and C are viral infections commonly found in persons 65 years of age and older (see following respective sections). Distinctive types of vaccines are available to prevent each disease.

Haemophilus Influenzae Type b

Haemophilus influenzae type b (Hib) is an acute invasive bacterial infection that can affect multiple organ systems (Benenson, 1995). Hib is not to be confused with influenza types A, B, and C (see later), which are viral diseases. Hib-associated illnesses include meningitis, epiglottitis, otitis media, pneumonia, arthritis, and cellulitis. These illnesses may present with fever, lethargy, vomiting, meningeal irritation, decreased mental status, stiff neck, bulging fontanelle in infants, swelling of the epiglottis, respiratory distress, skin lesions, and ear infections. Complications are serious and include septic arthritis, life-threatening airway obstruction, fulminating infection, and death. Hib occurs worldwide and is the major cause of bacterial meningitis in children younger than 5 years in developing countries. During the early 1980s the United States experienced an annual case rate of about 20,000. There has been a noticeable decline in Hib cases with the licensing of the conjugate Hib vaccines and an aggressive targeted immunization campaign for children younger than 5 years. In 1993, only 1419 Hib cases were reported in the United States. The disease is not commonly found in individuals older than 5 years; the attack rate peaks at 6 to 7 months of age, and two thirds of all cases are found in children younger than 18 months. Living in a large, poor, overcrowded household, having a low educational level, attending day care, having a chronic disease, having a school-age sibling, and being a racial minority are risk factors that increase the chances of exposure to Hib.

Hib is transmitted by droplets from nasal and oral secretions during the infectious period. The incubation period is unknown but is assumed to be short, 2 to 4 days. Persons are considered communicable for as long as the organisms are present in the nose and throat discharges. Diagnosis is made by identifying organisms from blood or spinal fluid. Treatment usually requires hospitalization and an immediate 10- to 14-day course of antimicrobial therapy with chloramphenicol or an effective third-generation cephalosporin. Ampicillin is no longer used as the first-line initial drug of choice because of commonly found ampicillin-resistant strains of bacteria. Individuals are considered noncontagious 24 to 48 hours after effective drug treatment begins. For prophylaxis, rifampin should be given to all household contacts if all contacts younger than 4 years are not fully immunized against Hib disease; this same rule applies to contacts in day care classrooms.

Five conjugate Hib vaccines are currently licensed for use in the United States (see Table 24–7 for vaccine schedules). Two DTP-HIB vaccine combinations are currently available for the first three doses of the initial series at 2, 4, and 6 months. The ACIP recommendations to replace DTP with DTaP and FDA approval of the DTaP vaccine use for the initial series in infants will require that the two vaccines again be administered separately until the FDA approves a DTaP-Hib combination, when DTaP is used for the primary series. Only whole cell DTP can be used in combination with Hib.

Adverse reactions to the vaccines are uncommon; swelling, redness, and pain at the site of injection have been reported. The vaccines are contraindicated for children with moderate or severe illnesses and for persons who experience anaphylaxis after a dose of a specific Hib conjugate vaccination. The same precautions and contraindications apply to the use of the combination DTP-Hib as are applied to those for the single-component DTP and Hib vaccine.

Hepatitis A and B

Viral hepatitis exists in several forms, which are very different from one another and include hepatitis A (infectious), B (serum), C (parenteral), D (delta viral), and E (enteric). Vaccines are now available for both hepatitis A and B.

HEPATITIS A

Hepatitis A virus (HAV) is an acute viral infection that presents with fever, anorexia, and general malaise followed by jaundice, which lasts a couple of weeks. Rarely it can last several months and has a very low fatality rate. It is transmitted through fecal-oral contamination of food and water and has an incubation period of 15 to 50 days (average, 25–30 days). HAV is endemic in many developing countries. In the United States, child care centers have become the source of many epidemics; although in children the virus is usually asymptomatic, they easily infect the adults in and around these centers. Between 1984 and 1994, the annual number of case reports for HAV has remained relatively static at approximately 23,000, with the exception of 1989 during which 35,000 cases were reported (CDC, 1994d). With the introduction of new hepatitis A vaccines, it is expected that the incidence of HAV will decline over the next decade, given a decrease in the vaccine cost and an increase in availability of vaccine for those most at risk. The two-dose vaccination series is recommended for those considered at high risk: persons traveling to or living in a country of endemicity; communities experiencing an outbreak or that have a high endemic incidence rate; persons with chronic liver disease; persons who use illicit intravenous or oral street drugs; American Indian or Alaska Natives; persons with occupational risks such as caretakers in institutions for the developmentally disabled, laboratory workers who handle hepatitis A virus, handlers of primate animals, and staff of child day care centers; and males having sex with other males.

Susceptibility is general and no carrier state exists. HAV is diagnosed through the presence of serum antibodies. No specific treatment is recommended. There are two inactive hepatitis A vaccines licensed for use in the United States: Vaqta (Merck) and Havrix (SmithKline) (CDC, 1995a). The vaccines are not FDA approved for use in children younger than 2 years, and the vaccination schedule for children 2 to 18 years of age varies with the vaccine. Both Merck's Vaqta and SmithKline's Havrix have a two-dose pediatric preparation scheduled to be given 6 to 12 months apart. SmithKline has a three-dose Havrix preparation; the first two doses are given 1 month apart and the third 6 to 12 months after the second dose. The vaccine may cause soreness at the site of injection.

Contraindications for HAV vaccination include a hypersensitivity to any component in the vaccine or a previous hypersensitive reaction after HAV vaccine administration. Pregnancy is not a contraindication; however, breast-feeding mothers should use the vaccine with caution.

HAV is not presently targeted for eradication because of the ease of spread, the high cost of the vaccine, and the lack of current political will resulting in part from the low fatality rate.

HEPATITIS B

Hepatitis B virus (HBV) is a viral infection of insidious onset that ranges from asymptomatic illness to generalized nonspecific symptoms such as anorexia, nausea, and vomiting followed by jaundice and occasionally resulting in fulminant fatal hepatitis. It is transmitted through direct contact with contaminated blood and body secretions, transplacentally, and through sexual intercourse and has an incubation period of 45 days to 6 months (average, 90 days). HBV is endemic worldwide, with an estimated incidence of infection ranging between 70 and 90% in the developing world, and a carrier prevalence rate of 8 to 15%. The serological markers for HBV in persons without a history of acute infection suggest that it is extremely common to have subclinical cases of disease (Sherlock, 1990). Undetected acute subclinical cases of HBV infection could include as many as two thirds of all adult cases and most neonatal cases (Hollinger et al., 1990). During 1994, approximately 11,000 cases of HBV were reported in the United States. There are approximately 300 million hepatitis B surface antigen (HBsAg) carriers worldwide, many of whom have no clinical signs of disease. It has been estimated that in the United States at least 15,000 people become carriers (approximately 23% are neonates) every year (Hollinger et al., 1990). This carrier status of chronic disease is extremely dangerous because severe damage to the liver may be occurring without obvious symptomatology to the patient (Sherlock, 1990). Eighty percent of all cases of primary liver cancer are due to HBV (Maynard, 1990). It is estimated that 6 months after infection with HBV approximately 90% of adults and 2% of infants and children experience clearance of serum HBsAg. The remainder of these children will become carriers for life, will continue to spread infection, and will have increased risk of mortality from chronic liver disease and hepatocellular carcinoma.

General susceptibility exists for unimmunized individuals; the period of immunogenicity for those who have been vaccinated is currently unknown because of the fairly recent licensing of the first HBV vaccine in 1982. Diagnosis of acute and chronic illness and presence of immunity after vaccination is made through serological presence of HBsAg and antibodies to HBsAg (anti-HBs), respectively. Total antibody to hepatitis B core antigen (anti-HBc) represents those with an acute or past HBV infection (not immunization), whereas hepatitis Be antigen (HBeAg) identifies infected individuals at increased risk for infecting others. Antibody to HBeAg (anti-HBe) specifies those carriers who are at low risk for transmitting infection. No treatment currently exists for HBV, although interferon-α has demonstrated limited effectiveness in combating chronic infection of the liver from adult-acquired HBV infections. Enteric precautions should be applied for all patients with a hepatitis infection. In the United States there are two types of hepatitis B inactivated virus vaccines licensed for general use. Both are prepared from recombinant deoxyribonucleic acid (DNA) and bakers' yeast; the original vaccine produced from plasma is no longer used. The HBV vaccine has been added to the routine childhood immunization schedule in the United States. (For recommended schedule, see Table 24–7.) It is extremely important to continue effective implementation of the current programs for vaccination of all pregnant women who are seropositive for HBsAg, which indicates carrier status, and to provide all of their newborn infants with hepatitis B immune globulin and hepatitis B vaccine at birth. These neonates should then be followed up at 1 and 6 months with boosters to complete this series. Non–follow-up with the second and third inoculations can inhibit the success of seroconversion; therefore, strict programs for follow-up must be established. There will always be a small percentage of persons who do not seroconvert, even after three doses. However, if everyone received the series, then this small cohort would be protected through herd immunity. Vaccination with HBV vaccine may cause soreness at the site of injection. Plasma-derived vaccine is preferred for dialysis and immunocompromised patients. No contraindications exist for HBV vaccination.

Several factors contribute to the success of a worldwide and a national eradication program for hepatitis B. In 1988, the cost for three doses of the vaccine in the United States was $62.04 (American dollars). By 1993 the price was reduced to $22.80 (American dollars). Further cost reduction is necessary if affordability is to be achieved for developing countries. The second prohibitive factor is the presence of a carrier status with this disease. As long as there are carriers (300 million worldwide) (Ghendon, 1990), this disease can never be eradicated, only controlled. For eradication, there must be universal immunization of infants and adolescents (Alter et al., 1990). This can be accomplished by requiring 100% coverage with the hepatitis B vaccine as part of the regular WHO-EPI immunization schedule for all infants and children. Universal screening of all blood and its components is also necessary to prevent further transmission.

Influenza Types A, B, and C

Influenza is an acute viral respiratory infection that may be confused with the common cold or other common respiratory illnesses. Influenza, a viral disease, also must not be confused with Hib, a bacterial disease (see prior section on Hib). Influenza has three types, including A, which is responsible for most outbreaks on an epidemic scale worldwide; B, responsible for regional outbreaks such as the recent outbreaks in the United States; and C, which is less common and usually results in mild illness. These viruses have the ability to frequently change their antigenic make-up, type A more so than types B and C, which are more stable. Type A is susceptible to antigenic shifts on a regular basis, possibly because of genetic redesign between animal and human hosts (Wiselka, 1994). Until a few years ago, type A was exclusively responsible for most pandemics of influenza around the world, causing a high mortality rate in susceptible groups, including the elderly. Antigenic drifts are minor antigenic changes that are responsible for annual epidemics and regional outbreaks. Epidemic and pandemic outbreaks occur periodically throughout the world as a result of these antigenic shifts and drifts. Because strains of the viruses change from year to year, influenza vaccines are prepared annually on the basis of a prediction of the type that will be prevalent that year. Thus, influenza vaccinations are given in the early fall before the "flu" season.

Influenza affects the respiratory tract and presents with a dry cough, fever, headache, myalgia, sore throat, and other generalized symptoms of malaise. Complications range from pneumonia, otitis media leading to hearing impairment, meningitis with febrile convulsions, and Reye's syndrome, with exacerbation of conditions such as myocarditis, resulting in death. Influenza is highly infectious and is passed from one individual to another through droplets or direct contact with infected mucous secretions, either wet or dried, and has an incubation period of 1 to 5 days. Infection from one type of influenza provides little or no protection against other types or subtypes. The peak transmission season for influenza activity in the United States usually occurs from November through February and is responsible for periodic outbreaks throughout the country, especially in schools, nursing homes, and the work place. For the 1993–1994 season, deaths from influenza and pneumonia represented 9.2% of total deaths (CDC, 1994e).

Groups with the highest risk for complications from influenza include the elderly, individuals of all ages with underlying health problems, children and adolescents on aspirin therapy who are at risk for Reye's syndrome, and health care workers and others in close contact with individuals at high risk (CDC, 1994f). Diagnosis of influenza is accomplished through laboratory viral isolation, serological testing, antigen detection, and gene amplification. The FDA has approved the drug amantadine for treatment of influenza in both adults and children. For adults only, a second drug, rimantadine, has been approved for treatment.

A vaccine is currently available for the control of influenza. It is a multivalent vaccine for influenza types A and B that contains several viral subtypes that are exchanged annually depending on the viral strains expected to be prevalent during the upcoming influenza season. Depending on how closely that match is achieved, immunogenicity can be very high. Individuals with known anaphylactic hypersensitivity to eggs should not receive the annual influenza type A vaccination. Pregnancy is not a contraindication for influenza vaccination except during the first trimester (Benenson, 1990). Chemoprophylaxis for influenza is also an option for individuals in whom vaccination is contraindicated, and the same two drugs used for treatment have also been approved for preventive use. Swelling, redness, and pain at the site of injection are the most frequent side effects, followed infrequently by fever, malaise, myalgia, and other systemic symptoms.

Because of the worldwide spread of influenza, the possibility of an animal host, the shifting serotypes, and the high infectiousness of the disease, it is not currently feasible to consider eradication of influenza. However, as new and improved vaccines become available and additional control measures are established, substantial reductions in influenza-related morbidity and mortality may be achieved.

Measles

Measles is an acute viral infection that presents with fever, cough, conjunctivitis, Koplik's spots on the buccal mucosa, and a red rash that begins on the face and becomes generalized. Measles can progress into severe complications, including pneumonia, diarrhea, encephalitis, and death. It is highly infectious and is transmitted through droplets and direct contact with nasal secretions of an infected person, with an average incubation period of 10 days from exposure to onset of fever. WHO estimates that 45 million cases of measles occur worldwide every year, resulting in approximately 1.1 million deaths of infants and children (Global Programme for Vaccines of the World Health Organization, 1994). Between 1963 and 1989, the United States experienced a declining incidence of measles cases. From 1989 to 1991, a resurgence of measles occurred, resulting in a fivefold increase from the early 1980s (Smoak et al., 1994). In response to this epidemic, a two-dose measles vaccination schedule was introduced for preschool-age children; measles vaccine was also administered to school-age children, adolescents, and young adults (regardless of

previous vaccination status), resulting in less than 700 indigenous cases in 1994 (CDC, 1994a).

In the developing world, infants below the recommended age for vaccination—9 months—are the group most at risk for measles and its sequelae. Factors that contribute to this early susceptibility include underlying malnutrition, vitamin A deficiency, and HIV infection. In the United States, current measles incidence is due primarily to unvaccinated inner city infants and vaccine failure of appropriately vaccinated school-age children. Risk factors for vaccine failure include a young age at vaccination (before 15 months of age when residuals of maternal antibodies interfere with vaccine virus replication), poor vaccine handling, and the presence of an upper respiratory tract infection at the time of vaccination (Orenstein et al., 1994). Diagnosis of measles is confirmed by tissue culture of nasopharyngeal secretions. There is no specific treatment for measles. Three measles vaccines are currently available and include a monovalent measles live virus vaccine, a combined measles-rubella (MR) vaccine, and a trivalent measles-mumps-rubella (MMR) vaccine.

MMR vaccine is a combined vaccine of live, attenuated measles, mumps, and rubella viruses and is the vaccine of choice for routine vaccination globally because it provides approximately 95% seroconversion for measles in age-appropriate vaccinated children, which is 15 months. For children living in developing countries or highly endemic areas, the age for vaccination can be as early as 6 months. However, a one-dose schedule administered at a very early age will provide only limited control, not elimination of measles. For further information on developing countries, consultation with WHO-EPI and national health policies is necessary for individual country regimens. (For recommended schedule, see Table 24–7.) The live, attenuated measles vaccine may cause malaise and fever that can occur as long as 12 days after inoculation and may have a 1- to 3-day duration. Measles vaccine–related encephalopathy is rare, occurring in less than 1 in 1 million children. MMR is contraindicated for pregnant women. Persons who have experienced an anaphylactic reaction to neomycin or to eggs should not be immunized using MMR because it contains a small amount of neomycin and is prepared using chicken embryo cell cultures (CDC, 1994g). There are no other contraindications for measles vaccine.

In 1990, at the World Summit for Children, the World Declaration on the Survival, Protection and Development of Children established the following two global goals for measles: (1) the reduction of measles cases by 90% by 1995 and (2) the reduction of measles deaths by 95% by 1995 (Orenstein et al., 1994). Thus, the control of measles has been established as a global target. However, if the goal becomes eradication of measles, then, although it is epidemiologically possible (humans are the only host, and there are no subclinical cases of measles—every case is 100% visible), also needed will be additional political will, financial support for mass campaigns, and scientific feasibility with the production of a suitable vaccine for infants under 1 year of age.

Mumps

Mumps is an acute systemic viral disease that presents with fever and painful swelling of the salivary and parotid glands. Complications may range from meningoencephalitis to permanent hearing impairment and, in postpubescent males, orchitis but rarely sterility. Mumps is transmitted through droplets and direct contact with saliva of infected individuals, with an incubation period of 12 to 25 days. Since the beginning of mumps reporting in the United States, there has been a steady decline in the number of cases reported annually. However, in 1987, a fourfold increase in cases was experienced, with numbers falling every year since (CDC, 1994d), with an all-time low of less than 1400 cases reported in 1994 (CDC, 1994a).

Susceptibility is general with lifelong immunity obtained from vaccination and from previous exposure with subsequent apparent or inapparent infection. Diagnosis of mumps is based on isolation of virus from oral and throat spray, urine, and spinal fluid. Skin tests for mumps virus are not reliable. Treatment for mumps is supportive only. Mumps vaccines include both a monovalent live, attenuated mumps virus vaccine, and a trivalent live, attenuated MMR virus vaccine.

MMR vaccine is a combined vaccine of live, attenuated measles, mumps, and rubella viruses and is the vaccine of choice for routine vaccination globally because it provides approximately 95% seroconversion for mumps. (For recommended schedule, see Table 24–7). The mumps vaccine may cause a mild fever a few weeks after inoculation. It is recommended that this vaccine be given after the age of 12 months and before the age of 12 years to reduce the chance of serious side effects. Respiratory isolation is necessary for confirmed cases of mumps. MMR is contraindicated in pregnant women. Persons who have experienced an anaphylactic reaction to neomycin or to eggs should not be immunized using MMR because it contains a small amount of neomycin and is prepared using chicken embryo cell cultures (CDC, 1994g). There are no other contraindications for mumps vaccination.

Humans are the only reservoir for the mumps virus, and lifelong immunity is established with infection and vaccination. Eradication of mumps is considered probable by the ITFDE, by using MMR and linking eradication activities with mass campaigns for measles (CDC, 1993a).

Pertussis

Pertussis, or "whooping cough," is an acute bacterial infection that begins with an upper respiratory cough and proceeds into a paroxysmal stage of coughing, ending in vomiting. Complications include seizures, pneumonia, encephalopathy, and death. It is transmitted through direct contact with respiratory secretions of an infected individual and has an incubation period of 7 to 10 days. During 1993, the United States experienced an 82% increase in the number of reported cases of pertussis compared with 1992 and the highest number of cases reported since 1967. Of the 5000 reported cases for which age was known, 45% were infants and 20% were 1 to 4 years old. It has been suggested that the recent increase in pertussis is neither from a reduction of vaccine antigenicity nor from a decline in vaccine coverage, but is perhaps due to the transmission in the home from older children and adults with waning immunity to young susceptible infants with precarious immune status (CDC, 1993c).

Unimmunized and partially immunized children younger than 5 years are highly susceptible to complications of pertussis infection. Diagnosis is confirmed by a positive culture of nasal or throat secretions. Treatment with antimicrobials is effective only before the paroxysmal stage of disease when it may lessen the severity of infection. Prophylaxis should be given to all exposed persons, regardless of vaccination status. Several types of pertussis vaccines are currently available in the United States.

The killed pertussis vaccine is either monovalent or combined with tetanus and diphtheria toxoids (DTP). In 1993, the United States licensed several new combined vaccines, including acellular DTaP for children at risk for seizures, and Tetramune, which combines diphtheria and tetanus toxoids with pertussis and Hib vaccines (CDC, 1993b).

Tripedia DTaP (Connaught) is now FDA approved and licensed for the first three doses of the initial series for infants and young children. This new recommendation and approval come as a result of case-control studies showing lower rates of the common adverse effects of the pertussis vaccine: prolonged crying, slight to moderate to high temperature, drowsiness, redness and soreness at the injection site, and irritability. In addition, good clinical efficacy of about 80%, the same as the whole cell pertussis vaccine, has been reported. The routine DTP immunization series continues to consist of five doses of the vaccines. The vaccines are interchangeable and can be given for any dose of the series. The only exception is Acel-Imune (Lederle), which is approved and licensed for use only after 15 months of age. Individuals who have valid DTP contraindications and who have experienced severe reactions to any of the three vaccines should not receive further doses. There is no single acellular pertussis vaccine available, and the pertussis vaccine is not recommended for children older than 7 years (for recommended schedule, see Table 24–7).

Pertussis disease is not now considered eradicable by the ITFDE because of the large numbers of cases worldwide, the early age of infection, the high infectiousness of the disease, and the multidose vaccination schedule.

Polio

Poliomyelitis is an acute enterovirus that occurs in three types, all of which can cause paralysis. Symptoms may range from inapparent illness to severe paralysis or death. It is transmitted through airborne droplets and fecal-oral contamination, with an incubation period ranging from 7 to 21 days. Globally, over the last 6 years, reported cases of polio have declined by more than 70%. In 1993, worldwide distribution was as follows: 15% of global cases were reported from the African region, 25% from the Eastern Mediterranean region, 2% from the European region, 45% from the Southeast Asia region, 13% from the Western Pacific region, and 0% from the region of the Americas (CDC, 1994b).

Groups most at risk for contracting poliomyelitis include all persons not previously vaccinated, those who have been previously vaccinated but are now immunosuppressed, and individuals experiencing vaccine failure who enter an endemic area. Diagnosis of poliomyelitis is made through isolation of the virus from fecal or oropharyngeal specimens. Treatment of poliomyelitis is supportive only. There are two types of poliomyelitis vaccines: prepared by either live or killed virus.

The live vaccine is a trivalent live, attenuated virus vaccine (OPV) used for primary inoculation of infants and children. Once swallowed, the vaccine attaches to the cellular mucosal lining of the intestines, where it colonizes and then enters the blood stream to stimulate an antibody response. Antigenicity with three doses of OPV or IPV is 95%. (For recommended schedule, see Table 24–7.) A report from the Institute of Medicine, National Academy of Sciences, states that the risk of vaccine-associated paralytic (VAP) disease occurring from a first dose of OPV is about one case per 500,000 inoculations, and for subsequent doses, approximately one case per 12 million (Stratton et al., 1994). If there is a substantial risk of exposure to a pregnant woman who has not been previously immunized, she should receive OPV (CDC, 1994g) because there is an increased risk of paralytic polio associated with pregnancy (Benenson, 1995). The live vaccine is contraindicated for immunosuppressed persons. Diarrhea is not a contraindication for administration of OPV.

IPV and enhanced-potency IPV (EIPV) contain inactivated viruses of all three serotypes and are used in many parts of the world. Although with IPV and EIPV the cost is slightly higher than OPV and the administration is parenteral rather than oral, there seems to be no risk of VAP disease. However, anyone recently immunized with either OPV or EIPV may excrete revertive wild-type viruses in stool for up to 60 days. Studies have demonstrated that the risk of VAP disease is reduced by administering EIPV for the first dose and then OPV for subsequent doses. In 1990, Israel introduced a combined schedule of IPV and OPV, with no reported cases of VAP disease identified since (Abraham et al., 1993). Levels of seroconversion are similar with both vaccines; thus, many countries, including the United States, are now considering a combined schedule of both EIPV and OPV (Swartz, 1993–1994).

On September 16, 1996, the director of the CDC accepted the ACIP's recommendations for a change in the polio vaccination schedule (CDC, 1996d). To reduce effectively the number of vaccine-related paralytic cases of polio each year, studies have shown that the use of IPV for the first two doses followed by two doses of OPV offer the same level of clinical efficacy as the three-dose OPV while substantially reducing the number of cases of VAP disease. This change will require an increase in the number of injections infants will need on a visit to the physician's office or clinic;

the polio vaccination series will be more expensive and the duration of the immunity will be unknown; however, those are a small price to pay if the change can eliminate the 8 to 10 VAP cases per year.

In 1988, WHO declared the goal of global eradication of poliomyelitis by the year 2000. This is achievable if a high level of coverage, greater than 80%, with OPV and or IPV can be maintained, national vaccination days (especially in developing countries) are routinely facilitated, and stringent global surveillance systems are sustained. WHO estimated that the external cost of eradicating poliomyelitis in U.S. dollars is $1.1 billion (CDC, 1993a).

Rubella

Rubella is often a mild viral disease that presents with a maculopapular rash. Whereas children may be relatively asymptomatic, adults may experience fever, headache, and malaise. Complications may include encephalitis and thrombocytopenia. Transmission is through droplets or direct contact with respiratory secretions of an infected individual, with an incubation period of 14 to 23 days. In 1989–1991, there was a resurgence of rubella in the United States, which peaked in 1991 with 1401 cases, occurring mostly among religious groups who refused vaccination. In 1992–1993 the lowest number of cases ever were reported—160 and 190 cases, respectively—followed by a slight increase in 1994 with a total of 219 cases reported (CDC, 1994h).

The fetuses of pregnant women who are exposed to natural infection or vaccination are at high risk for congenital defects. Diagnosis of rubella is based on culture of virus from nasal specimens. Treatment for rubella is supportive only. Rubella vaccines are prepared in monovalent and trivalent forms.

One dose of monovalent live, attenuated rubella virus vaccine provides 99% seroconversion and is available where the trivalent MMR is not recommended. MMR vaccine is a combined vaccine of live, attenuated MMR viruses and is the vaccine of choice for routine vaccination globally because it provides approximately 90% seroconversion and subsequent lifelong immunity. (For recommended schedule, see Table 24–7.) MMR vaccine may cause malaise and fever for as long as 12 days after inoculation and may have a 1- to 3-day duration. Both MMR and monovalent rubella vaccine are contraindicated for pregnant women. Persons who have experienced an anaphylactic reaction to neomycin or to eggs should not be immunized using MMR because it contains a small amount of neomycin and is prepared using chicken embryo cell cultures. However, monovalent rubella vaccine can be safely administered to persons with egg allergies (CDC, 1994g). Rubella vaccines should not be administered to immunosuppressed patients, immunodeficient patients (except HIV), or individuals who have received blood or immune globulin during the past 3 months (American Academy of Pediatrics, 1994). There are no other contraindications for rubella vaccination.

Rubella has been identified as an eradicable disease by the ITFDE (CDC, 1993a). Criteria include the availability of the immunogenic MMR vaccine, although the impact of rubella in developing countries is currently unknown.

Tetanus

Tetanus, or lockjaw, is an acute neurological illness caused by an anaerobic bacterium that produces an exotoxin in the portal of entry in the human host. Tetanus presents with gradually worsening neurological symptoms, including painful muscle contractions and spasms. The leading complication from tetanus is death. Tetanus is transmitted indirectly through contamination of a wound or portal of entry with tetanus spores, usually from soil or contaminated fomites. The incubation period ranges from 1 to 20 days. During 1993, neonatal tetanus was responsible for approximately 515,000 neonatal deaths worldwide. In the United States, 36 cases of tetanus were reported for the same year (CDC, 1994j).

Newborns in the developing world are at increased risk for neonatal tetanus because of the use of contaminated razor blades for cutting the umbilical cord after birth. Anyone previously unimmunized is at risk for contracting tetanus. Diagnosis is confirmed clinically because the bacterium is rarely found in wound cultures. Treatment for tetanus involves administration of tetanus immune globulin (TIG), preferably human. In areas where TIG is not available, equine tetanus antitoxin can be used. Antibiotics may also be given. Supportive care is essential. Tetanus toxoid is available in several forms.

Tetanus toxoid is available as a monovalent vaccine (Td) and in combined forms, including diphtheria and tetanus toxoids and pertussis vaccine (DPT and DTaP), as well as Hib (Tetramune). Tetanus toxoid provides lasting immunity for approximately 10 years; however, if a wound occurs or a person is entering a high risk area between 5 and 10 years after vaccination, then it is recommended that an additional dose of Td be administered. Pregnant women who have not received a booster within the last 10 years should receive routine immunization with Td. (For a recommended schedule, see Table 24–7.) Common side effects experienced after routine inoculation include soreness at the site of injection and possibly fever for 1 to 2 days. Contraindications to tetanus toxoid include a previous anaphylactic reaction to this vaccine. There are no other contraindications for tetanus toxoid vaccination.

Tetanus is controlled through the use of universal immunization. WHO has declared the elimination of neonatal tetanus as a global goal by the end of 1995. Eradication is probably not possible because spores are routinely found broadly in the environment.

Varicella (Chickenpox)

Varicella is a highly contagious viral disease with a variable onset (Benenson, 1995). Varicella may present with a sudden mild fever and malaise, or the only sign may be a rash. Varicella is a herpes simplex virus (HSV) of the same type that causes shingles (herpes zoster). The rash is progressive, changing from maculopapular to vesicular, and forming a crust or scab. The skin lesions, which may range between 250 and 500, tend to be more numerous on covered parts of the body. They can also be found on membrane tissue of the cornea, conjunctiva, respiratory tract, vagina, and oropharynx. They tend to be very pruritic, and scratching can cause the most common complication: secondary bacterial infection. Complications are low in healthy children. Immunocompromised, susceptible adults and infants whose mothers develop the disease 5 days before or 2 days after delivery are most likely to have serious complications such as encephalitis. Transmission is by droplet infection from respiratory tract secretions, direct contact with vesicular fluid, or maternal infection during pregnancy.

Latent acute reinfection can occur, usually in adulthood as shingles from the virus and persistent dormant presence in the sensory nerve ending (ganglia). The rate of shingles transmission is lower than that of varicella, but the susceptible person acquires chickenpox. The incubation period ranges from 10 to 21 days, usually 14 to 16 days after exposure. In infected persons, the virus is considered communicable from 1 to 2 days before and up to

6 days after the rash erupts or until the lesions are crusted. Both the incubation and communicable periods may be prolonged in immunocompromised persons.

Approximately 150,000 to 200,000 cases of varicella occur yearly in the United States. Ninety percent of the cases occur in children younger than 15 years. Susceptible adults who contract the disease have a more severe disease course and a higher case fatality rate, usually from viral pneumonia. Although adults represent only 2% of cases, they account for 50% of the approximately 90 deaths per year. Cases peak in the winter and each spring.

All individuals not previously infected are universally susceptible to varicella worldwide. Diagnosis is usually made by direct observation of the skin lesions, and laboratory tests are not routinely required. The vidarabines drugs adenine arabinoside, Ara-A, and acyclovir (Zovirax) provide effective treatment for varicella infections. Varicella-zoster immune globulin, when administered within 96 hours of exposure, can modify or prevent the disease in susceptible persons.

The live, attenuated varicella vaccine, Varivax (Merck), was approved and licensed by the FDA in March 1995 and is now available in the United States for routine childhood vaccination in children 12 to 18 months of age. This includes use as catch-ups in children 2 to 12 years old and in susceptible persons with high-risk exposure to severe illness themselves or likely to be exposed to persons at high risk of severe illness. The vaccine, developed in the 1970s in Japan, has a 70 to 90% efficacy rate in preventing any lesions, and the "breakthrough" cases are mild. (For recommended schedule, see Table 24–7.) The vaccine can be given simultaneously with all other vaccines; however, if it is not given on the same day as the MMR, at least 4 weeks should elapse between the administration of the two vaccines. Common side effects include pain, soreness, redness, and swelling at the injection site and a less frequent varicella-like rash at the site or elsewhere on the body. The vaccine is contraindicated for persons with severe allergic reactions to neomycin, who are pregnant, have moderate to severe illness, who are immunocompromised, and who have a recent history of receiving a blood product. The vaccine is extremely fragile, and an absolute cold chain temperature of −15°C (+5°F) from manufacturer to vaccinee must be maintained at all times. Varicella has not been classified as "not now eradicable" by the ITFDE.

VACCINES FOR INTERNATIONAL TRAVEL

For individuals traveling outside of the United States into regions endemic for specific infectious diseases, vaccination is recommended. Additional vaccines are available, and, depending on the area, the season, and the likelihood of exposure, each vaccine should be considered. It is important for those traveling abroad to obtain the most current recommendations from the Office of Overseas Travel at the CDC through their telephone hot line—(404) 332-4559—or annual publication, *Health Information for International Travel.*

International Certificates of Vaccination, printed by WHO on heavy yellow paper, can be obtained from any physician administering vaccinations, including health departments, and should be carried at all times with a passport while traveling abroad.

In this section, the eight major vaccine-preventable communicable diseases that place international travelers at risk are covered in detail, including presentation, complications, transmission, incubation, current statistics, risk groups, diagnosis, treatment, vaccination, and control and possible eradication activities.

Cholera

Cholera is a toxin-producing acute enteric bacterial infection that can be asymptomatic or can cause grave illness. Cholera presents as profuse watery diarrhea, vomiting, and dehydration. Complications of cholera include severe dehydration, leading to acidosis, circulatory collapse, convulsions, coma, and death. Transmission of cholera occurs through the fecal-oral route, usually from ingestion of fecally contaminated water or food, and has an incubation period of a few hours to 5 days. Since 1965, fewer than 27 cases of cholera have been reported annually in the United States. However, in 1992, an outbreak of cholera (103 cases) occurred. Since then, the number of annually reported cases has returned to the pre-epidemic level of less than 32 cases (CDC, 1994d).

Groups in poor hygienic environments are at higher risk for outbreaks of cholera. Diagnosis of cholera is made through culture of stool. Treatment of cholera involves immediate oral fluid rehydration therapy using oral rehydration solution (ORS); parenteral transfusion should be used for patients in shock. Antimicrobials may be used to shorten the duration and intensity of illness. One cholera vaccine is currently available.

The cholera killed whole cell vaccine is available worldwide; however, WHO has recommended that it no longer be required for entrance into any country because of its limited usefulness. In highly endemic areas, the cholera vaccine provides 3 to 6 months protection for 50% of individuals vaccinated, but this excludes areas where new strains of cholera (not covered by this vaccine) have appeared. The cholera vaccine may cause soreness at the site of injection, fever, headache, and malaise. There are no contraindications for administration of the cholera vaccine; however, it should not be used for control of epidemics or management of contacts of cases.

Although no animal host exists for cholera, the organism can exist in the environment for years. Because of newly appearing strains of cholera and the poor efficacy of the existing vaccine, cholera is considered a disease that is not now eradicable. However, control measures for disease prevention, including improved environmental, personal, and food hygiene, should be continued.

Japanese Encephalitis

Japanese encephalitis (JE) is an acute inflammatory arbovirus. It can be asymptomatic or can present with fever, headache, and disruptions to the central nervous system. Complications may include hepatitis, polyarthritis, convulsions, paralysis, and death. JE is transmitted through the bite of infected mosquitoes, and it has an incubation period of 5 to 15 days. The People's Republic of China, Korea, Japan, Southeast Asia, the Indian subcontinent, and parts of Oceania report approximately 50,000 cases of JE annually from epidemic and sporadic occurrences. The prevalence of the disease is higher in rural areas. There have been only 11 cases among U.S. citizens since 1981, 8 of which involved military personnel and their dependents.

Anyone who has not been previously infected and is traveling to or residing in an endemic area is at risk for JE infection. JE is diagnosed through differentiation in serological examination or by using virus isolation techniques. No specific treatment is available for JE. There is currently one JE vaccine (JEV) available.

The JEV is an inactivated virus vaccine developed from infected mouse brain tissue. The vaccine may cause soreness at the site of injection. The JEV is contraindicated for pregnant women.

JE is not considered an eradicable disease at present because of the existence of animal hosts, the low political will, and the endemic proportions of the disease (CDC, 1993a). Control of JE is possible with immunization of infants and children in endemic areas and control of the mosquito vector population.

Meningococcus

Meningococcal meningitis is an acute bacterial infection that may be asymptomatic or can present with fever, headache, stiff neck, nausea and vomiting, and often a maculopapular or petechial rash. Complications may include shock, coma, and death. Transmission is through airborne droplets or direct contact with an infected individual or carrier, and the incubation period ranges from 2 to 10 days. About 3000 to 4000 cases of *Neisseria meningitides* occur annually in the United States, and it is the second most common cause of bacterial meningitis. Multiple serogroups cause endemic and epidemic disease. There has been no major epidemic in the United States since 1946, only episodic local outbreaks. The serogroups vary in the percentage of cases presenting yearly: serogroup B, 50 to 55%; serogroup C, 20 to 25%; serogroup W-135, 15%; serogroup Y, 10%; and Serogroup A, 1 to 2%.

Children younger than 5 years are at greatest risk for contracting meningococcal meningitis because susceptibility decreases with age. Diagnosis is made through culture of blood and cerebrospinal fluid. Treatment includes high doses of antibiotics parenterally administered. A multivalent vaccine is currently available.

The meningococcal vaccine is a quadravalent vaccine composed of serotypes A/C/Y/W-135. The vaccine is effective for adults; however, serotype C is poorly immunogenic in children. Routine immunization is not recommended; however, those entering high-risk areas with epidemic outbreaks, including pregnant women, should consider vaccination. Pregnant women should not otherwise be vaccinated. Side effects from vaccination may include soreness and swelling at the site of inoculation for 1 to 2 days. There are no contraindications for this vaccine.

Although humans are the only host and a vaccine exists for meningococcal meningitis, the possibility for eradication at present is low for many reasons, including the presence of asymptomatic carriers, the existence of several serotypes, the occurrence of drug resistance during treatment (Woods et al., 1994), the epidemic tendencies of the disease, and the low level of political will. However, the meningococcal vaccine should be used for the control of epidemics.

Plague

Plague is a serious zoonotic bacterial infection that may be asymptomatic or present with fever and painful swollen lymph nodes (bubonic) that may suppurate, specifically around the area of the flea bite. Complications include dissemination throughout the body, including the meninges. Secondary pharyngeal and pneumonic plague are of importance because of direct human transmission and a fatality rate of 50% in untreated cases. Transmission of bubonic plague is through the bite of an infected flea that has fed on a contaminated rodent, often a rat, or through direct contamination with the infected drainage of a purulent bubo. Airborne droplets from an infected individual are responsible for transmission of pharyngeal or pneumonic plague. The incubation period is usually 2 to 6 days. During 1993, the United States reported 10 cases of human plague, with one fatality, from four western states. In general, peridomestic transmission is increasing, especially through domestic cats (CDC, 1994i).

Susceptibility is general, but those living in crowded and unhygienic conditions and individuals working in areas where plague is endemic are at increased risk. Diagnosis of bubonic plague is made through culture of cerebrospinal fluid, blood, and aspirate from infected buboes and from sputum for pharyngeal and pneumonic plague. Treatment includes the immediate use of antibiotic therapy. Both live and killed vaccines are available.

The vaccine in general use is an inactivated whole cell bacterial preparation that has fairly high efficacy for several months, after which boosters are required. Side effects may include soreness at the site of injection. No contraindications are noted for this vaccine.

Although current political will is fairly high, plague is not now considered an eradicable disease by the ITFDE because of the presence of large reservoirs of wild rodents, infectivity of fleas for months after contamination, and existence of multiple forms of the disease. Control measures should focus on suppression of wild rodent and flea populations, especially in urban and periurban areas where crowded human conditions exist (CDC, 1993a).

Rabies

Rabies is a zoonotic viral disease that usually presents with progressive central nervous system involvement, including anxiety, dysphagia, and convulsions. The most common complication from rabies is death. Rabies is directly transmitted through the bite of an infected animal to a human host, with an incubation period ranging from a few days to more than 1 year. In the developing world, cases of rabies from dogs who are chronic excretors have become more common, leading to the possibility of a chronic carrier state for rabies, which has been rarely documented in the United States (Dutta, 1994). Since 1977, the United States has experienced an increasing raccoon rabies epizootic, which has elevated the risk for subsequent human infections. In 1990, raccoons became the leading species in which rabies was detected in the United States (CDC, 1994k). Between 1980 and 1994, 19 human rabies cases have been reported in the United States. Bats have played an increasing role in transmission of rabies to humans over the last several years (CDC, 1994l).

Susceptibility for contracting rabies is general. However, individuals living or working in areas with a high risk of exposure, including spelunkers, may be at increased risk for rabies infection. The long incubation period of rabies often makes the initial diagnosis difficult because of the relative distance of the episode of transmission from the onset of clinical symptoms. Definitive diagnosis can be made through isolation of virus in cerebrospinal fluid or saliva and through antibody detection in serum and cerebrospinal fluid of unvaccinated individuals; however, early diagnosis does not usually alter the treatment or prognosis of rabies. Treatment of rabies begins with immediate and thorough cleansing, with soap and water, of bite wounds or mucous membranes that have possibly become contaminated with saliva from an infected animal. Immediate passive immunization should be administered using rabies immune globulin (RIG). The patient should also receive active immunization with either human diploid cell vaccine (HDCV) or rabies vaccine absorbed (RVA). Rabies vaccine schedules are specific for pre-exposure and postexposure prophylaxis. Two types of rabies vaccines are available in the United States, HDCV and RVA; neurotissue vaccines are available predominantly in developing countries.

Although less expensive, neurotissue vaccines have a high incidence of serious neuroparalytic complications (Dutta, 1994). The HDCV is a killed virus vaccine prepared from tissue cultures. This inactivated cell culture vaccine should be used for pre- and postexposure active immunization because it offers long-term immunity (Thraenhart et al., 1994), with nearly 100% seroconversion, and it is safe and also relatively expensive (Dutta, 1994). The rhesus diploid cell vaccine, RVA, should be used when HDCV is contraindicated. For postexposure passive immunization, RIG should be administered consecutively with the first dose of postexposure active immunization using HDCV or RVA. Pain and swelling at the site of injection are common side effects. Approximately 6% of vaccinees experience a hypersensitivity to booster inoculations, and supportive therapy should be available if boosters are necessary and recommended. Pregnancy is not a contraindication if postexposure vaccination is necessary. HDCV is contraindicated when a serious allergic reaction has occurred with prior HDCV immunization.

Rabies is not now considered eradicable by the ITFDE because of the extended and divergent animal reservoirs for the rabies virus; however, human rabies can be eliminated with universal immunization, education, and control of rabies in animal populations (CDC, 1993a).

Tuberculosis

Tuberculosis (TB) is a mycobacterial infection that causes tubercular lesions in the lung or other organs. These lesions may remain dormant for life or become reactivated at any time and progress into active pulmonary tuberculosis, which presents with early symptoms of fatigue, fever, and weight loss, advancing to cough, chest pain, hemoptysis, and hoarseness. Complications include a high rate of mortality in untreated cases. TB is transmitted through airborne droplets and spray from infected individuals and has an incubation period of 2 to 12 weeks from infection to a positive tuberculin skin test. Infection in low-risk individuals in the developed world often becomes known through a positive skin test reacting from an asymptomatic initial lesion that has subsequently healed. In developing countries patients often present with symptoms of active disease. The association of HIV-related sequelae with increased incidence and reactivation of TB has become a major global public health concern over the last few years. Of the 88 million estimated new cases of TB which will occur between 1990 and 1999, 8 million cases will be attributable to the HIV infection. During this same period, an estimated 30 million TB-related deaths will occur, with 2.9 million attributable to HIV infection (Dolin et al., 1994).

Those with increased risk for contracting TB in the United States include low socioeconomic groups living in crowded urban poverty, the homeless, immunocompromised patients, and foreign-born and minority women. Although two types of skin tests are available for diagnosing tuberculous infection in asymptomatic individuals, the preferred choice is the Mantoux test, a purified protein derivative (PPD) administered intradermally in the forearm; the reaction is interpreted by a health care provider who has education and experience in reading the test. Any induration smaller than 5 mm is considered negative. An induration that is 15 mm or larger is considered positive. Any reaction in between should be further evaluated to ensure that an appropriate diagnosis is made. Previous vaccination with BCG is not a contraindication for administering a PPD (American Academy of Pediatrics, 1994).

The diagnosis of TB disease or infection cannot be ruled out because of the absence of a reaction to the tuberculin skin test in immunosuppressed persons. This is owing to a depressed or absent hypersensitivity response to the tuberculin reaction commonly seen in immunosuppressed persons. This may occur in persons receiving, for example, corticosteroids or immunosuppressive drugs and in persons with Hodgkin's disease, a viral disease, or HIV infection.

Initial diagnosis can be made using radiography. Diagnosis is confirmed through culture of tubercle bacilli from sputum, cerebrospinal fluid, or other body fluids. Isoniazid continues to be the primary drug of choice for chemoprophylaxis of pulmonary TB in low-risk individuals older than 35 years of age with a positive tuberculin test and no active disease. Currently, a multidrug regimen, including isoniazid, rifampin, pyrazinamide, and ethambutol, sustained over 9 months is the most widely used treatment of active TB in major metropolitan health departments in the United States (Leff et al., 1993). Pregnancy is not a contraindication for the treatment of drug-susceptible strains of TB (Margono et al., 1994).

Defaulting from drug compliance remains one of the most difficult challenges in the treatment of TB and can result in the persistence of chronic sputum-positive individuals (Hodes et al., 1993). Reasons cited include noncompliance within the first 3 to 4 months because of a clinical improvement felt by patients receiving treatment and side effects from chemotherapy, such as cutaneous lesions in HIV-positive patients receiving some of the antimalarial drugs used in developing countries. The emergence of drug-resistant strains of TB is also of global concern.

The BCG vaccine is a freeze-dried vaccine prepared from live, attenuated bacteria; its mode of action is unknown. BCG is used primarily for prevention of TB in individuals who are at high risk for repeated exposure and when other forms of preventive therapy are contraindicated. Studies have placed the efficacy of BCG from zero protection to 100% immunogenicity, but the efficacy remains unknown. BCG has not demonstrated immunogenicity in individuals vaccinated after presenting with a positive tuberculin skin test (Grange and Stanford, 1994) and should, therefore, be used only for those with a negative Mantoux skin test. PPD testing should be repeated 2 to 3 months after vaccination. If negative, then revaccination should be continued. Rarely, side effects may include ulceration at the site of injection. BCG is contraindicated in immunodeficient or suppressed patients, in symptomatic individuals with HIV infection, and for those with burns or skin infections.

TB is not now considered eradicable by the ITFDE (CDC, 1993a) because of the large foci of disease, the need for improved diagnostic tests, the presence of multidrug resistance, and the lack of a comprehensive vaccine. However, control is possible if enhanced screening programs are initiated for high-risk populations, and significant treatment compliance achieved through well-structured services, utilization of available community resources, and supervision of treatment with regular audits (Wilkinson, 1994).

ROLE OF COMMUNITY HEALTH NURSING IN TUBERCULOSIS CONTROL

Community health nurses (CHNs) are frequently involved in activities related to TB control and treatment, from screening populations at risk for the disease to case management of persons with TB. It is important that CHNs know the correct procedure, including the most recent recommendations from the CDC for administering and interpreting the Mantoux test. CHNs have also been involved in contact investigations of persons exposed to TB in the community and in teaching the medication and health regimen to persons with the disease. CHNs may also be involved in directly observed therapy (DOT), observing persons with the disease taking their medication daily. When these persons are homeless, carrying out DOT can present a major challenge to CHNs as they negotiate to meet the person at a preselected site on a daily basis.

Typhoid

Typhoid is a severe systemic bacterial infection that can range from being asymptomatic to producing fever, headache, malaise, constipation, anorexia, rose spots on the trunk, and sometimes lymphadenopathy. Complications include Peyer's patches in the ilium, which can lead to perforation, hemorrhage, and adhesions of the small intestine; mental dullness and slight deafness; and fatality. Typhoid is transmitted through ingestion of food and water contaminated by the urine and feces of infected individuals and carriers. The incubation period ranges from 1 to 3 weeks.

Typhoid fever cases are low and steadily declined in the United States from 1900 to 1960. An annual average of 464 cases was reported between 1975 and 1984; 57% of these cases were in persons older than 20 years of age and 62% had traveled to another country. The 62% represent a 29% reduction in domestic cases because the period from 1967 to 1976 showed that only 33% of the reported cases were among persons who traveled to other countries (CDC, 1994g).

Susceptibility is general for typhoid fever. Diagnosis is made through culture of blood and feces. Antibiotics offer effective treatment. In the United States, two vaccines are currently available against typhoid. The first is a parenteral inactivated vaccine and the second is an oral live vaccine. Both vaccines have similar efficacy ranging from 46 to 96%. Side effects of the vaccine include soreness and swelling at the site of injection and possibly a slight fever and headache for 1 to 2 days. The oral live vaccine is contraindicated in children younger than six years and in immunocompromised patients.

Although the fatality rate reaches 10% in many developing countries, there is no current political will for the eradication of typhoid fever. The available vaccines are less than 100% effective, carrier states exist, and drug resistance has developed in many places. Control measures should include health education and improvement of environmental hygienic conditions, including food and water.

Yellow Fever

Yellow fever is an acute infectious arbovirus that can be inapparent or present with sudden onset, fever, chills, nausea, vomiting, jaundice, and hemorrhagic disorders. Complications may include hepatitis, coma, and death. Transmission occurs through the bite of an infected mosquito, with an incubation period of 3 to 6 days.

Africa and South America are the only two areas of the world where yellow fever currently occurs and is caused by two epidemiological distinguishable forms: urban and jungle yellow fevers. The last western hemisphere epidemic occurred in Trinidad in 1954; Bolivia has had two outbreaks in 1989 and 1990. Presently, South America reports about 100 to 300 cases per year, mostly among workers in forested areas, and their number is believed to be greatly underreported. Epidemics in Africa affect thousands of persons over periods of a few years (CDC, 1990).

Susceptibility is general, with acute infection providing lifelong immunity. Diagnosis is made through isolation of the virus in blood. There is no specific treatment for yellow fever. A vaccine is available globally.

The yellow fever vaccine is a live, attenuated virus vaccine prepared using chicken embryos. It is 100% immunogenic and provides protection for approximately 10 years. Slight fever, headache, and muscle pain may develop after injection. Contraindications to this vaccine include pregnancy, because some studies indicate that this vaccine can cause fetal infection (Tsai et al., 1993), and a hypersensitivity to eggs or egg products. Children younger than 9 months should also not receive this vaccine because of the risk of vaccine-related encephalitis.

Although the vaccine has been included in the WHO-EPI, yellow fever is not now considered eradicable by the ITFDE because of the presence of nonhuman hosts, the heat instability of the available vaccine, and the lack of political will. Control measures should be taken to reduce mosquito vector populations in urban centers where epidemics occur (CDC, 1993a).

Over the course of the past century, the United States has largely conquered devastating infectious diseases such as diphtheria, typhoid, measles, and polio, yet the country has been unable to control the spread of the majority of sexually transmitted diseases (STDs.)

SEXUALLY TRANSMITTED DISEASES

Over the last 20 years, many changes have taken place in the patterns of STDs. New organisms are emerging; profound drug resistance has developed; prevalence of well-known STDs is increasing in selected populations (including HIV/AIDS, chlamydia, gonorrhea, herpes simplex virus [HSV], human papillomavirus [HPV], and syphilis); unique complications from STDs are appearing; and different populations are experiencing pandemics from past trends (CDC, 1995b). These changes can be attributed to many environmental, socioeconomic, demographic, and personal behavioral factors: a younger age at initial sexual activity, later age at first marriage, widespread divorce, increased sexual activity with multiple partners, sex with risky partners, including those injecting drugs, and substance abuse (Wasserheit, 1994).

Today, more than 50 organisms and syndromes are identified as being sexually transmitted (CDC, 1992a). An estimated 12 million cases of STDs occur each year in the United States (Donovan, 1993). These include an estimated 4 million cases of chlamydia, 3 million cases of trichomonas, 1.1 million cases of gonorrhea, 1 million cases of HPV, 500,000 cases of genital herpes, 200,000 cases of hepatitis B, 120,000 cases of syphilis, and 40,000 cases of HIV infection (CDC, 1994a; 1995b; Donovan, 1993). The rates of STDs in the United States are among the highest in the industrialized world, approaching those in some developing countries. STDs are not easily cured; they cause serious, irreversible consequences and costs to the society are large. More than one in five persons in the United States (56 million) are infected with an incurable, viral STD other than AIDS (e.g., genital herpes, HPV, or hepatitis B). Men and women of all ages, racial and ethnic backgrounds, and income levels contract STDs. Certain populations, however, are disproportionately affected: adolescents, young adults, women, minorities, and the poor (CDC, 1995b). Teenage girls in particular may be more susceptible to STDs because of fewer protective antibodies to STDs and a cervix that is biologically immature (Donovan, 1993). Women are at higher risk for contracting STDs than men because of anatomical differences that enhance transmission of disease and make diagnosis difficult; they are also less likely to experience symptoms. Race and ethnicity are known as risk markers for STDs because they are associated with some basic determinants of health status such as poverty, illicit drug use, living in a community with high STD prevalence, health care–seeking behavior, and access to care. Certain infections, particularly gonorrhea and syphilis, are more commonly found in low-income and minority populations, whereas other infections, such as genital herpes, HPV, and *Chlamydia trachomatis,* are distributed throughout the population (Donovan, 1993).

Certain STDs such as *C. trachomatis* and gonorrhea may be asymptomatic or produce mild symptoms and not be detected until serious and even life-threatening problems develop; these STDs and others such as syphilis, genital herpes, and trichomoniasis increase a person's risk of contracting HIV on exposure to the virus (Donovan, 1993).

Complications from undiagnosed STDs occur more frequently and are more severe in women (Temmerman, 1994). For example, pelvic inflammatory disease (PID), mainly resulting from an undetected STD, is diagnosed in more than 1 million women annually; scarring sequelae from PID may

BIAS IN REPORTING SEXUALLY TRANSMITTED DISEASES

Rates of STDs in the United States may be even higher than those reported. According to the Centers for Disease Control and Prevention, the reporting of STD incidence is incomplete (CDC, 1995b). Public facilities such as health department family planning or STD clinics that diagnose and treat persons with STDs are more likely to report than are some private sources such as physicians' offices. In addition, many health departments do not have the necessary infrastructure, including funding, to initiate new reporting systems (such as that for *C. trachomatis*). Biases in reporting may arise when persons of low income seek public health services that are more likely to screen for and report STDs.

Another source of bias may be the variation in diagnostic tests, which may yield different indicators of sensitivity and specificity, variations in the pathogenic organism itself, variations in the population tested, and variation in the laboratory in which the test is analyzed (Aral, 1994).

Another possible source of bias is that detection of STDs is more difficult in women than in men as a result of differences in anatomy (Ehrhardt and Wasserheit, 1991). For example, painless lesions on the genitals and abnormal discharge may be unnoticed in women; cultures of vaginal secretions may be unable to be interpreted because of the large numbers of normally occurring cells and bacteria. The sensitivity of some tests used for diagnosis, such as Gram staining, may be reduced because of the large numbers of normal cells and bacteria in the vagina.

lead to infertility, ectopic pregnancy, or chronic pelvic pain. An infected woman who transmits an STD to her fetus during pregnancy or childbirth may experience spontaneous abortion, premature delivery, stillbirth, low birth weight, neonatal death, and, in the infant, chronic respiratory problems, blindness, and mental retardation (Donovan, 1993). Certain strains of HPV are strongly associated with cervical cancer; cervical cancer accounts for more than 4500 deaths annually.

The costs associated with STDs are considerable; more than $5 billion is associated with only three STDs—*C. trachomatis,* gonorrhea, and genital herpes—annually (Donovan, 1993). The treatment cost for a person with HIV infection over a lifetime—from infection to death—is approximately $119,000 (Hellinger, 1993).

In this section, six major STDs will be covered: HIV/AIDS, *C. trachomatis, Neisseria gonorrhoeae,* HSV-2, HPV, and syphilis.

HIV/AIDS

HIV, a retrovirus, is the organism that causes the disease known as AIDS. HIV is typically asymptomatic over a period of months to years (e.g., 6 months to 20 years). HIV usually presents gradually with conditions that result from inadequate immune system function as the virus slowly attacks the body's immune system. Various vague symptoms such as fatigue, lymphadenopathy, anorexia, fever, chronic diarrhea, and weight loss occur. Over time, the body loses its ability to fight illnesses. Opportunistic infections, those that normally would not cause illness or only mild illness in healthy persons, occur and become recurrent because of the disruptions in immune functioning caused by the HIV infection. The gradual destruction of the immune system is different for each person; it may occur at a rapid or a slow pace. Nearly all persons with HIV infection die not from the virus but from the opportunistic diseases, infections, cancers, or other conditions.

On January 1, 1993, the AIDS surveillance case definition for adolescents and adults was expanded beyond the 1987 definition of 23 conditions to include all HIV-infected persons with severe immunosuppression (<200 CD4$^+$ T lymphocytes/μL or a CD4$^+$ T lymphocyte percentage of total lymphocytes of <14), recurrent pneumonia, pulmonary tuberculosis, or invasive cervical cancer (CDC, 1992b). Examples of other opportunistic infections, or AIDS indicator diseases, include HIV-related wasting syndrome, *Pneumocystis carinii* pneumonia, Kaposi's sarcoma, and Burkett's lymphoma (CDC, 1992b). On September 30, 1994, the Centers for Disease Control and Prevention released the 1994 revised classification system for HIV infection in children younger than 13 years (CDC, 1994p). The reclassification includes the following three categories: (1) infection status, (2) clinical status, and (3) immunological status. For further information about this extensive reclassification, consult CDC (1994p).

HIV is transmitted (1) by sexual contact involving exchange of body fluids (e.g., vaginal secretions, semen) with an infected individual; (2) by blood transfusion or exposure to blood, blood products (blood clotting factors), or tissues of an infected person; (3) by perinatal transmission from an infected mother to fetus during pregnancy or during delivery of an infant or when breast-feeding; or (4) by sharing needles or syringes with an infected individual (CDC, 1995c).

HIV infection is widespread. An estimated 18 million adults and 1.5 million children are infected with HIV, and approximately 4.5 million AIDS cases are thought to exist worldwide (WHO, 1995). In the United States, 501,310 persons with AIDS had been reported to the Centers for Disease Control and Prevention as of October 31, 1995 (CDC, 1995e). Nearly half (49%) of these cases of AIDS were reported since 1993.

As indicated, AIDS cases among females increased from 8% of cases reported between 1981 and 1987 to 18% of cases during 1993 to October 1995. Although the proportion of cases decreased among whites from 60 to 43%, the proportion of cases increased among blacks from 25 to 38% and among Hispanics from 14 to 18%. The proportion of cases increased among intravenous drug users from 17 to 27% and in cases attributed to heterosexual transmission from 3 to 10%, whereas cases among men who have sex with men decreased from 64 to 45%. The largest proportionate increases of cases were from the South (31%), followed by the Midwest (22%), Northeast (20%), and West (15%).

During 1993 in the United States, an estimated 7000 HIV-infected women gave birth to infants, or 1 of every 625 births (CDC, 1995f). Because the perinatal transmission rate is estimated to be between 15 and 30%, approximately 1000 to 2000 infants were infected perinatally in 1993.

WOMEN AND HIV/AIDS

In the United States, AIDS among women is more rapidly increasing than among men and is the fourth leading cause of death among women aged 24 to 55 years (CDC, 1995g). Exposure of women with AIDS in 1994 was attributed to intravenous drug use (41%), heterosexual contact with a partner at risk of or with AIDS (38%), contaminated blood or blood products (2%), and nonspecific HIV exposure (19%). The most rapidly increasing mode of transmission for women is heterosexual contact, which includes women whose sexual partners engage in high-risk behaviors (e.g., intravenous drug use), those with multiple partners, and those with STDs. Women are at high risk for HIV infection because of the difference in heterosexual transmission patterns. Male-to-female transmission, for example, is 12 times greater than female-to-male transmission (Padian et al., 1990).

Populations at high risk for AIDS include adolescents, young adults, and other individuals with multiple partners, intravenous drug users and their sexual partners, gay men and their male or female partners, women whose partners engage in high-risk behaviors (e.g., intravenous drug use, have other female or male sexual partners), persons who engage in risky sexual practices such as anal intercourse, persons who exchange sex for drugs or money, and persons with STDs (CDC, 1995c). Transmission of HIV infection is enhanced in persons with STDs (Wasserheit, 1994). For example, persons with genital ulcers, such as HSV-2 or syphilis, or a nonulcerative STD, such as gonorrhea, *C. trachomatis,* or trichomoniasis, are at three to five times greater risk of contracting HIV on exposure than a person without an active infection (Padian et al., 1990).

HIV/AIDS AND HEALTH CARE WORKERS

As of August 1995, 46 health care workers in the United States had been documented as having seroconverted to HIV after exposures at the work place; 20 of these had developed AIDS (CDC, 1995d). Those who seroconverted were the following:

18 laboratory workers
16 nurses
 6 physicians
 2 surgical technicians
 1 dialysis technician
 1 respiratory therapist
 1 health aide
 1 housekeeper-maintenance worker

Workers have been infected with HIV in the health care setting following needle sticks with HIV-infected blood, after infected blood contacts the worker's open cut or mucous membranes (e.g., eyes or inside of the nose), after exposure to HIV-infected blood, visibly bloody fluid, and concentrated virus in a laboratory.

RESEARCH REPORT

Nurses' body fluid exposure reporting, HIV testing, and hepatitis B vaccination rates: before and after implementing universal precautions regulations

The purpose of this study was to investigate whether mandatory universal precautions changed nurses' body fluid exposure and reporting rates, hepatitis B vaccination rates, and HIV testing rates. Random cross-sectional surveys of nurses in Tennessee were conducted in 1991 and 1993 (n = 145 in 1991; n = 143 in 1993). The questionnaire in both surveys included frequency of body fluid exposures and reporting in the past year and whether or not the respondent had received the hepatitis B vaccine or had been HIV tested. Findings indicated that self-reported needle stick injuries decreased by 69%, and other sharps injuries decreased by 81%. Only 4.1% of all exposure incidents reported on this anonymous survey were reported to employee health officials, as required. Body fluid exposure incidents were the most common form of exposure (81%) and the most underreported. Hepatitis B vaccinations significantly increased (61.4% to 82.5%), with a nonsignificant increase in HIV testing (47.2% to 55.6%) from 1991 to 1993. Findings of this study suggest that the universal precautions regulatory mandate has been effective in increasing nurses' compliance to universal precautions. Body fluid contacts were significantly underreported and showed no decrease between 1991 and 1993.

Adapted from Ramsey PW, Glenn LL. Nurses' body fluid exposure reporting, HIV testing, and hepatitis B vaccination rates: before and after implementing universal precautions regulations. AAOHN J 44:129–137, 1996.

The most commonly used test for determining HIV infection is the HIV antibody test, which indicates the presence of the antibody to HIV. The most commonly used form is the enzyme-linked immunosorbent assay. Because there may be false-positive findings, the Western blot is used to verify the results. Because false-negative findings may also occur, especially before antibodies are produced by the body after exposure, an exposed person should repeat the HIV antibody test 6 months after the original test. Testing for HIV infection is offered at health departments, family planning clinics, STD clinics, and HIV counseling and testing sites and by primary care providers. Surveillance of HIV infection is incomplete. As of December 31, 1993, only 25 states had regulations or laws requiring confidential reporting by name of persons with confirmed HIV infection; one additional state required reporting by name of children younger than 13 years only (CDC, 1994q).

SELF-TESTING FOR HIV INFECTION

Self-testing kits with instructions for determining HIV infection status are available for purchase and home use by the general public. What are the advantages of self-testing kits for HIV infection? What are the disadvantages? How would you prepare clients who informed you that they were considering purchasing a self-testing kit for HIV infection?

The diagnosis of AIDS is based on the diagnostic categories discussed earlier in the chapter. A diagnosis of AIDS is reportable to the Centers for Disease Control and Prevention. Completeness of reporting of AIDS cases to local and state health departments varies by region and patient population and is more than 85% complete in most areas (CDC, 1994q).

Treatment for HIV/AIDS is complex. Many drugs have been approved by the FDA for HIV infection and AIDS-related conditions. Major drugs include the following antiretrovirals:

AZT	Zidovudine
ddC	Zalcitabine
ddI	Didanosine
d4T	Stavudine
3TC	Lamivudine

Many other classifications of drugs have been approved by the FDA for HIV infection and AIDS-related conditions and include the following

categories: antiemetic, antineoplastic, antimicrobial, antiprotozoal, red blood cell growth stimulator, immunomodulator (stimulates white blood cell production), antifungal, antiviral, protease inhibitor, appetite stimulant, antimycobacterial, antitubercular, and folic acid antagonist. Much controversy abounds in the community regarding the expense of these drugs and access to them because of the expense. For additional information on FDA-approved drugs and testing of drugs in clinical trials, contact the AIDS Clinical Trials Information Service—(800) 874-2572—and HIV/AIDS Treatment Information Service—(800) 448-0440.

Prevention efforts are targeted at creating awareness of risk and reduction of risk behaviors in high-risk populations and preventing transmission of HIV infection in persons who are infected. For further information, see Prevention of STDs/HIV/AIDS (later).

The USPHS recommends the use of zidovudine (ZDV or AZT) to reduce the risk of perinatal transmission of HIV infection from mother to infant (CDC, 1994r). As a result of an extensive AIDS clinical trial, pregnant women given ZDV decreased the risk of transmission of HIV infection to their infants by two thirds. The Centers for Disease Control and Prevention recommends routine counseling and voluntary HIV testing for all pregnant women and medical treatment as well as the preventive therapy well before giving birth (CDC, 1994r). These activities are most often offered as a collaborative effort between state offices of HIV/AIDS and Family Planning or Maternal Child Health services.

Eradication of AIDS is dependent on development of a vaccine and the infrastructure necessary to vaccinate populations at risk worldwide; neither possibility is foreseen in the near future, although testing of vaccine in humans has been initiated (Lurie et al, 1994).

Chlamydia

C. trachomatis is a bacterial infection that may be asymptomatic or may present as ocular, pulmonary, enteric, or genital tract infections. It is currently the most prevalent of the STDs (CDC, 1995b; 1996e). The female organ most often infected by *C. trachomatis* is the endocervix, where little or no inflammation is caused and asymptomatic infection results. Complications include PID and chronicity leading to secondary scarring of the fallopian tubes, resulting in permanent obstructive infertility and possibly life-threatening ectopic pregnancies. *C. trachomatis* also causes conjunctivitis in infants exposed at birth; infants infected with the organism may also contract pneumonia. Genital chlamydia is responsible for approximately 50% of nongonococcal urethritis in men and women and epididymitis in men.

C. trachomatis is an STD with an incubation period of 1 to 2 weeks, perhaps longer. It is believed that infection rates in adolescent females may be as high as 40% in some populations (Martin, 1990). Currently, genital infections from *C. trachomatis* are on the list of notifiable diseases by the CDC, although surveillance of the disease remains incomplete in some parts of the United States (CDC, 1995b). Rates of *C. trachomatis* increased markedly between 1984 and 1994 (from 3.2 cases per 100,000 population to 188.4, respectively) (CDC, 1995b). In 1995, *C. trachomatis* was the most commonly reported nationally notifiable infectious disease in the United States, the first year such data were available on a national basis, followed by gonorrhea and AIDS (CDC, 1996e). Increased rates reflect increased screening and reporting capability and increased recognition of asymptomatic infection largely in women. Rates are more than five times greater in women than in men because men are less likely to be screened and, if diagnosed and treated, are less likely to be tested for the organism.

Populations at high risk include sexually active adolescent females, women with multiple sexual partners, and HIV-infected individuals (Spinillo et al., 1994). Studies have shown that a significant number of patients infected with *C. trachomatis* are also infected with *N. gonorrhoeae*. Association with *Trichomonas vaginalis* has also been indicated. Poor predictability has been established in many cases using isolation of *C. trachomatis* in tissue culture for a definitive diagnosis (Henry-Suchet et al., 1994). Several tests for rapid detection of antigen are available and include enzyme immunoassay, which should only be used for symptomatic urethritis in males (Talbot and Romanowski, 1994); staining using monoclonal direct fluorescent antibodies (DFA) for specimens from both the cervix and the urinary tract (Hay et al., 1994); and DNA probe for screening where culture facilities are not an option (Stary et al., 1994). Unfortunately, in many cases, *C. trachomatis* is not detectable using these methods, and it is, therefore, hypothesized that *C. trachomatis* may persist in a viable but undiagnosable form that may be less vulnerable to antibiotic therapy (Beatty et al., 1994). Antibiotic therapy is recommended for the treatment for *C. trachomatis*.

Early identification and treatment of all sexual partners are advised to prevent long-term complications.

Although included in the list of diseases screened for potential eradicability by the ITFDE, chlamydia is considered not now eradicable because of the lack of immunity, the difficulty of diagnosis, the presence of asymptomatic illness, and low political will (CDC, 1993a). However, emphasis should be placed on prevention through health and sex education, widespread use of barriers such as condoms and rubber dams during sexual activity, and control measures, including routine annual screening for all sexually active and high-risk individuals, and early treatment of infected individuals.

Gonorrhea

N. gonorrhoeae is a bacterial disease that presents differently in men and women. In men, the infection can be asymptomatic or more often can present initially with a purulent discharge that progresses to dysuria. In women, the infection can be asymptomatic or can present initially with a mild cervicitis or urethritis. Complications in women occur from untreated asymptomatic infection, which can result in endometritis, PID, salpingitis, and ectopic pregnancy or infertility through tubal occlusion (Goldsmith, 1990). A chronic carrier state can develop in both men and women. Newborns of infected mothers are at high risk for gonococcal conjunctivitis, which, if not promptly treated, can lead to subsequent blindness. Gonorrhea is an STD with an incubation period of 2 to 7 days. The overall rate of gonorrhea in the United States has been declining since 1975 (CDC, 1995b). The rate decreased from 173.8 cases per 100,000 population in 1993 to 168.4 in 1994; however, Georgia, a state with one of the highest rates of gonorrhea, failed to report in 1994, which caused the overall rate for the nation to fall. In 1994, the rate of gonorrhea declined among men yet increased among women, adolescents, and all ethnic and racial groups with the exception of Hispanics (CDC, 1995b).

Diagnosis of gonorrhea is confirmed through microscopic examination of exudate and through bacteriological culture. The emergence of antibiotic-resistant strains of gonococcal organisms and noncompliance with drug regimens present specific problems in the treatment of gonorrhea. New single-dose drugs have now been developed to combat these challenges. It is recommended that follow-up occur with a second drug administered orally for 7 days to protect against underlying chlamydia infection and prevent subsequent resistant strains of gonorrhea from developing. Neonatal prophylaxis should be administered optically to all newborns. Children diagnosed with genital, rectal, or oral gonococcal infections should be evaluated as possible victims of sexual abuse.

Although gonococcal infections occur only in the human host, gonorrhea is not now considered eradicable by the ITFDE because of the lack of an effective vaccine, no development of immunity after infection, the existence of a carrier state, the emergence of drug-resistant strains, and low political will (CDC, 1993a). Prevention of gonococcal infections can be accomplished through the use of physical barriers, such as condoms and rubber dams, which decrease the likelihood of direct contact with contaminated body fluids during sexual activity. Control measures should include routine annual screening for all sexually active and high-risk individuals and early treatment of those infected.

Herpes Simplex Virus 2

HSV-2 is a chronic ulcerative disease that may be symptomatic or asymptomatic (Corey, 1994). In symptomatic disease, genital lesions may be caused by two types: HSV-1, which is usually associated with cold sores and lesions above the waist, and HSV-2, which is usually associated with genital lesions or lesions below the waist. HSV-1 may occur below the waist or HSV-2 above the waist through oral sex or self-inoculation. HSV-2 may present with vesicles (small blisters) that progress to shallow ulcers that are often extremely painful and debilitating (Corey, 1994). After primary lesions disappear, the virus remains in a latent form and secondary episodes may reappear at any time. It is uncertain what causes recurrences, but they have been attributed to a number of factors, including overexertion and increased levels of emotional stress (Swanson and Dibble, 1993; Swanson et al., 1995). Complications of HSV-2 may include meningitis, encephalitis, coma, and death; in pregnant women, it may result in neonatal HSV infection. Newborns may present with a generalized systemic infection, a localized infection with skin, eyes, and mouth lesions, or with localized central nervous system symptoms. Complications of HSV in neonates include neurological and ocular disorders, with a resultant high mortality rate. HSV-2 has an incubation period of 3 to 21 days.

Genital herpes is the most common cause of genital ulcers in the Western world, with approximately 700,000 new cases in the United States annually, 90% of which are caused by HSV-2 (Peaceman and Gonik, 1991). In 1991, in a national random household survey using seroprevalence data, the antibody to HSV-2 was found in 21.7% of the U.S. population 15 to 74 years of age, up from 16.4% in 1980, a 32.3% increase (Johnson et al., 1993). The disease may be asymptomatic or unrecognized in up to three of four persons with the disease, and transmission can occur in persons who are asymptomatic.

Because HSV-2 is a genital ulcer, individuals with HSV-2 are at higher risk of infection with HIV. Differential diagnosis of HSV-2 is confirmed through viral detection in tissue culture. Antiviral treatment using acyclovir may decrease the duration of viral shedding, healing, and symptoms in primary outbreaks but is less effective in reducing the frequency and severity of recurrences. Because of the incurability of the disease, its unpredictability, and associated stigma, careful education is necessary, and counseling may be recommended (Corey, 1994). Children diagnosed with HSV-2 infections should be evaluated as possible victims of sexual abuse.

Although HSV-2 infections occur only in the human host, HSV-2 is not now considered eradicable by the ITFDE because of the presence of a long latency period, the lack of a cure, and low political will (CDC, 1993a). The latency and reactivation of HSV-2 are not clearly understood, and emphasis should be placed on prevention. A person presenting with active lesions should not engage in sexual intercourse until the lesions subside and should always use safer sex practices because asymptomatic viral shedding occurs in many infected individuals. Caution should be taken, however, because condoms do not protect from perineal and extragenital lesions (Swanson and Dibble, 1993).

Human Papillomavirus

There are at least 60 known types of HPV, ranging in virulence from benign common warts to genital warts (condyloma acuminatum); 20 types primarily infect the anal and genital areas (Jones and Wasserheit, 1991). Complications may include HPV, leading to cervical dysplasia (Becker et al., 1994);

the most significant complication of HPV is cancer (Jones and Wasserheit, 1991). Perinatal transmission may also occur and may involve the respiratory tract, including laryngeal papillomas, which may obstruct the airway, as well as the genital tract. HPV is an STD with a usual incubation period of 3 months; it may range, however, from 3 weeks to 8 months (Jones and Wasserheit, 1991).

The prevalence of HPV in the United States is unknown because it is not a reportable disease. HPV may be the most common STD in the United States today, however, with 1 to 3% of all Papanicolaou (Pap) smears intimating infection (Zazove et al., 1991). It has been estimated that 0.5 to 1.0% of all women show clinical signs of condyloma acuminatum and that at least 20 million women in the United States are infected with HPV (Brown and Fite, 1990); past estimates have ranged between 5% and 20% of the sexually active population, close to 50% of sexually active college women, and more than 80% in prostitutes (Jones and Wasserheit, 1991). It is also estimated that the prevalence of disease in males parallels that found in females. With men, as with women, it is often difficult to tell whether HPV is present because often there are no clinical symptoms, and the virus can be localized internally on the genitalia. It is, therefore, possible to unknowingly spread infection. Immunocompromised patients are at increased risk for contracting genital warts.

Although no culture is available for HPV, there are several diagnostic tests for the detection of genital warts. They include clinical observation facilitated by the use of acetic acid stain for detection of subtle lesions and colposcopy (androscopy in men); cytology and histology; and DNA hybridization (the most common is the Southern blot test, which is not clinically available). Treatments for HPV include the use of a resin called podophyllin; cryotherapy (with liquid nitrogen), which has been identified as the safest and most highly recommended treatment; laser therapy; 5-fluorouracil; and interferon. Although there is no cure for genital warts and relapses can occur, thorough treatment should be facilitated, and routine Pap smears done to rule out the possibility of cervical dysplasia and carcinoma. Children diagnosed with HPV should be evaluated as possible victims of sexual abuse.

HPV was not included in the eradicable disease screening list of the ITFDE. The use of condoms is recommended; however, they offer protection only for distal penile and intravaginal lesions.

Syphilis

Syphilis is a treponemal venereal disease that has three recognized stages of development. The primary stage presents with a painless lesion or chancre, which often goes unnoticed, especially in women, because the lesion may be located inside the vagina where it is not easily seen without clinical examination. If the infection is not cured at this stage, it will progress to secondary syphilis, which presents with a different set of highly infectious lesions. This stage will disappear spontaneously if untreated; the disease will show no clinical signs for long periods of time, often years or for life, or may eventually result in tertiary neurosyphilis. Complications include the irreversible destructive neurological signs and symptoms of tertiary-stage syphilis and preterm births and congenital syphilis of neonates born to infected mothers. Syphilis is an STD with an incubation period of 3 weeks from initial infection until the presentation of the primary lesions.

The number of cases of primary and secondary syphilis reported to the Centers for Disease Control and Prevention in 1994 (20,627) were the fewest reported since 1977 (CDC, 1995b). The incidence declined from 10.4 cases per 100,000 population in 1993 to 8.1 in 1994. During this time period, the overall rate of congenital syphilis decreased from 80.7 cases per 100,000 live births to 55.6, although 8 of 28 states (in those reporting more than 5 cases) reported increases in 1994 compared with 1993.

Studies have shown that at least one third of all individuals sexually exposed to a person with infectious syphilis will become infected (Hutchinson and Hook, 1990). Syphilis is an important risk marker for prevalence of HIV infection because HIV-infected individuals tend to experience acceleration of the stages of syphilis, often presenting with secondary syphilis accompanied by chancres for a prolonged duration (Hutchinson et al., 1994). Diagnosis of syphilis at any stage of infection is accomplished with nontreponemal serological tests such as the Venereal Disease Research Laboratory (VDRL) or the rapid plasma reagin (RPR) test. The fluorescent treponemal antibody absorption test (FTS-ABS), which is a treponemal serological test, should be used if either of the first two tests is positive to ensure the greatest reliability for exposing positive results at all stages of syphilis. Treatment of syphilis at all stages involves varying doses of penicillin G. The fetuses of currently syphilitic pregnant women previously treated for syphilis of unknown duration or duration greater than 1 year have a higher incidence of congenital syphilis. However, it is unclear whether this is due to drug treatment failure or reinfection after successful treatment (McFarlin et al., 1994). Therefore, early identification and treatment of syphilis in pregnant women and periodic rescreening and retreatment throughout pregnancy for previously infected women are essential for prevention of devastating sequelae for their neonates.

Although syphilis affects only humans, the ITFDE does not now consider syphilis an eradicable disease because of the difficulty of diagnosis, the unpredictability of relapse, the partial immunity after infection, and the low political will (CDC, 1993a). Control of syphilis can be achieved through routine annual screening of sexually active individuals and pregnant women in their first trimester and by tracking and treating infected individuals and their partners.

PREVENTION OF COMMUNICABLE DISEASES

The CHN has a role in primary, secondary, and tertiary prevention of communicable diseases. Examples of appropriate interventions are reviewed next.

Primary Prevention

Primary prevention of communicable diseases involves keeping the population healthy and free of contacting the disease. Primary prevention of communicable disease is highly dependent on education of persons, families, and aggregates or populations at risk for a disease. Efforts at prevention must come not only from the federal government but also from the state and local governments and both public and private institutions. Although the use of vaccines, as discussed previously, is one way to keep the population well, other strategies include promoting behaviors that decrease susceptibility to the disease.

Primary prevention may be accomplished in several ways (see Chapter 8, Community Health Education), including targeting at-risk populations for interventions at aggregate to individual levels. For example, at the aggregate level, legislation mandating immuniza-

---

HOT LINES/RESOURCES

CDC National AIDS Hot Line	1-800-342-AIDS
Spanish language	1-800-344-SIDA
Hearing impaired	1-800-243-7889
National STD Hot Line:	1-800-227-8922
National Herpes Hot Line:	1-919-361-8488
	(M–F 9 AM–7 PM EST)

CDC National AIDS Clearinghouse
P.O. Box 6003
Rockville, MD 20849-6003

---

tion of children entering grade school has had a profound impact on the immunization levels of school children in the United States. At the family level, ongoing efforts by day care centers, schools, and churches, for example, are targeting immunization information to families of preschool children, particularly those younger than 2 years. At the individual level, adults in the work force may require vaccinations such as HBV or tetanus vaccine because of occupational exposure. The United States is still without a comprehensive vaccine delivery system to all children and adults. Health care providers, including nurses, must look for the opportunity to vaccinate preschool children and adults during contacts in clinics and in hospitals and to screen for and make referrals for vaccinations on home visits.

Through efforts of the mass media, populations may be targeted for health education messages. Social marketing efforts are needed to tailor the health messages to the target audiences using appropriate media channels utilized by the audiences.

Much has been learned about primary prevention of communicable disease through research targeted at testing HIV prevention programs. Characteristics of successful programs include the following (Holtgrave et al., 1995):

- The needs of the individual and the community must be assessed and the program must be planned to address those needs.
- Prevention messages must be culturally competent; that is, they must be tailored to the target audience in terms of age, developmental status, education, sex, race-ethnicity, geography, sexual orientation, values, beliefs, and norms, and they must be linguistically specific.
- Program goals, objectives, and strategies for each intended client subpopulation should be clear; both

process (how services are delivered) and outcome (behavioral or health) objectives should be stated; interventions should be specific as to their components.

- Programs should be based in behavioral and social science theory and research; a thorough review of the research literature should be undertaken to determine successful theory-based approaches with the target population.
- Programs should be monitored and midcourse corrections made if objectives are not being met.
- Sufficient resources must be available (e.g., financial, material, human) or the goals must be changed to meet the available resources.

Women, particularly disadvantaged minority women, often lack power in their relationships with men to influence sexual decision making (Amaro, 1995). Realities of economics, gender role norms, and cultural messages may exert a powerful influence on women's decision-making and sexual behavior.

High-risk sexual behavior includes the practice of sex for drugs or sex for money to buy drugs, resulting in sex with multiple anonymous partners who cannot be easily identified and screened for disease. Many individuals of low socioeconomic levels have poor access to health care for screening and treatment, a low level of education, and a high rate of unemployment, factors that may predispose them to a definite disadvantage regarding knowledge of health education measures such as safer sexual practices, clean needle use, and access to health services.

Knowledge is not enough to change behavior; education must include cognitive-behavioral skills acquisition (negotiation, practice applying condom) and address broader social and cultural contexts of sexuality rather than just behavior: gender roles, peer influence, cultural values and norms, interpersonal relationships, communication patterns, and conflict resolution (Holtgrave et al., 1995). In addition, intensive and sustained interventions are needed over time. Changing community norms, especially among the gay population, is critical; a review of successful interventions by Kelly and associates (1993) stresses the need for cognitive skills based one-on-one, community-level interventions, and community mobilization. Increasing people's sense of self-efficacy or empowerment and emphasizing a "hedonistic outcome"—for example, teaching women how to make using condoms sexually stimulating and pleasurable—have been found to be success-

ful in small groups as well (Jemmott and Jemmott, 1991). It is important to have the target population involved in the development of the materials to be used; all materials and outcome measures should be pretested on persons in the target population, feedback obtained, and appropriate changes made.

Current research is being conducted on potential vaccines for the control and possible eventual eradication of STDs (Sparling et al., 1994). Because eradication is in the far future, wherever possible, a complete sexual history should be documented annually for all sexually active patients and should include risk factors such as multiple partners, unsafe partners, and substance abuse.

Secondary Prevention

Contact investigation and case finding are important aspects of secondary prevention to prevent the spread of communicable disease in the community (see Contact Investigation and Case Finding in following section). Persons found to be at risk of a communicable disease should receive screening to determine occurrence. For example, persons whose sexual histories reveal high-risk behaviors should receive annual routine screening for STDs. Incidence should be reported to the local health department for those reportable diseases and for partner notification related to those diseases (usually syphilis and gonorrhea). The medical regimen should be taught to the client and to her or his partner and recommendations adhered to for increasing coverage of all patients with active and potential infections. Safer sexual practices should be taught, including skills-based exercises. These should include how correctly to put a condom on a penile model, how to use a female condom on a female pelvic model, how to ask a partner to use a condom, and how to respond to reasons given by a partner for not using condoms. Condoms and other aids such as a water-based lubricant should be freely distributed to increase their use.

Tertiary Prevention

Tertiary prevention involves actions to keep infected persons apart from noninfected persons. These actions involve isolation, which separates infected persons during the period in which they are communicable, and quarantine, which places restrictions on healthy contacts of persons infected during the incubation period to prevent spread of the disease should a case occur (Benenson, 1995). Actions important to tertiary prevention include safely handling contaminated infectious waste products, hand washing, wearing of protective gloves (and gowns) when indicated (see universal precautions information presented in Table 24–3). Teaching family or other caregivers to give safe tertiary care to persons with an infectious disease in the home and in other institutions, such as a school or nursing home, is an important role of the community health nurse.

Care of persons with STDs or HIV/AIDS in the community presents an important challenge to the CHN. In persons with a diagnosis, it is important to prevent the spread of the infection, to prevent recurrence of diseases, to prevent new infections, and to promote the general health of this population. It is important to delay the onset of symptoms and infections in persons with HIV infection and to promote the quality of life in persons with AIDS. Care of persons with STDs/HIV/AIDS in the community demands knowledge of the interdisciplinary network of providers who give preventive as well as therapeutic nursing and other services to clients for acute as well as chronic illness. The CHN must know how the community is organized to make timely referrals, to give follow-up care, and to serve as an advocate of the clients and their families. This includes making the problems clients experience known and advocating for more responsive or comprehensive services. Wellness programs, stress reduction, support groups, nutrition services, and drug management are examples of the kinds of activities that can promote the health of persons and families of persons with a sexually transmitted infection. Universal precautions should be used when giving care to infected persons; they should also be taught to caregivers of infected persons.

Approximately two thirds of clients at STD clinics are men, although adult women and adolescents are disproportionately affected. Women and adolescents are less likely to seek care at an STD clinic or from a private physician because of the stigma attached to having an STD or because they fail to recognize symptoms or are asymptomatic (Donovan, 1993). Teenage males, in particular, have less access to reproductive health care in contrast to teenage females, who access care through family planning and maternal-child health clinics.

THE POLITICS OF STD AND HIV/AIDS PREVENTION

Primary, secondary, and tertiary prevention of STDs and HIV/AIDS is critical to the health of the nation (see Appendix VII, Healthy People 2000: Midcourse Review and 1995 Revisions). The effort to combat the spread of STDs and HIV/AIDS is led by the Centers for Disease Control and Prevention, chiefly through the Division of STD/HIV Prevention in the National Center for Prevention Services (Donovan, 1993). The two programs (STD and HIV/AIDS) are funded separately by Congress and have very different foci.

The STD program is focused largely on secondary prevention or disease control—screening, treatment (funded by state and local health departments), and partner notification—with an emphasis on bacterial infections, which can largely be cured via antibiotics, rather than viral diseases (such as HPV and genital herpes), for which there is no cure (Donovan, 1993). Centers for Disease Control and Prevention monies have largely gone to STD clinics operated by health departments; other community-based organizations have at times used alternative sources of funding such as Title X or Maternal Child Health funds to serve other populations such as those in family planning and perinatal clinics.

The HIV program, in contrast, focuses on primary as well as secondary prevention by funding a wide range of community-based organizations such as family planning clinics, drug treatment programs, and free-standing HIV counseling and testing sites (Donovan, 1993). Prevention messages and interventions for high-risk populations are developed and implemented, and efforts to change community norms toward low-risk behavior are made, in addition to the provision of HIV counseling, testing and referral services, and partner notification. Minority and community-based organizations such as women's health centers, housing projects, churches, drug treatment programs, and prisons are heavily relied on for education, street outreach, peer support, and other prevention efforts. Primary prevention aimed at HIV infection will no doubt affect the common behaviors also leading to STDs; nonetheless, there is a need to add greater primary prevention efforts to STD programs (Donovan, 1993).

INEQUITIES IN FUNDING STDs AND HIV/AIDS

Primary prevention is not a major focus of the federal public health response to STDs and HIV/AIDS. For example, in 1992, of the $1.96 billion spent on HIV by the USPHS, only $478 million was spent on prevention (CDC, 1992c). During the same year, $88.8 million was appropriated by Congress for the STD program; of this money, 43% was allocated to syphilis control, 29% to control of gonorrhea, and 27% to control of *C. trachomatis*. All other STDs, which represent more than half of STDs each year, were allocated less than 2% of the monies. Although comprehensive data of state and local funding for STDs do not exist, the total amount that state and local governments spend each year on STDs (exclusive of HIV) is estimated to be only $50 million.

CONTACT INVESTIGATION AND CASE FINDING: ROLES OF THE COMMUNITY HEALTH NURSE

Whether the CHN is teaching parents of infected children, day care workers, or caregivers of persons with a communicable disease, prevention of transmission is a major aspect of care. Guidelines developed for health professionals are available to assist the CHN in planning this care.

The CHN has the unique role of taking collective action with community members at the local, county, state, and national levels to preserve the health of the aggregates within. The following report is of an actual case of hepatitis A in a restaurant worker reported by a nurse in the emergency department of a local hospital to public health nurses in the communicable disease branch of a county health department. The report documents the process of action taken by public health nurses and other members of the health department team in protecting the community by preventing an outbreak of hepatitis A.

CASE SUMMARY REPORT: CASE OF HEPATITIS A

A case of suspected hepatitis A in a food handler was reported to a county health department in state "X" at 8:00 AM on July 10. The case worked as a burrito roller in a restaurant. After looking at his work schedule, he determined that he had become ill on June 30 and had even gone home early on that day. He had not had any diarrhea. He went to see the doctor because he had been notified that friends in state "Y" with whom he had camped and shared marijuana over the previous Memorial Day holiday weekend had since become ill. They were confirmed as hepatitis A in state "Y."

The patient came in for a personal interview. He was young, with moderate hygiene. In addition to his duties of hand rolling burritos in the restaurant, he had prepared salsa, cutting tomatoes with his bare hands on July 1. The restaurant was inspected and had generally good reports. Coworkers reported that the case had good hygiene. All burrito preparation was done using gloves or tongs, except for the rolling of the tortilla. The restaurant was a high-volume facility, serving 300 to 350 persons per day, many of them repeat clients.

The next day, information was reviewed. It was noted that although the restaurant scored highly on inspections and the case did wash his hands, he could not guarantee that he did so consistently. He had manual contact with uncooked food throughout his incubation time and acute phase of illness. Therefore, it was decided that if immune globulin (IG) could be obtained and his diagnosis was confirmed hepatitis A, the county health department would make a public announcement. (The diagnosis was confirmed as hepatitis A later that day.) It was also decided that IG would be given to the restaurant staff and close contacts and a letter would be written to local physicians informing them of the case and reminding them of the epidemic in state X and the need to report suspected cases. Restaurants were also advised that hepatitis is a major concern in their business and that they should follow guidelines for prevention.

The state health division called to say that there was no IG in the state, but that it could possibly be obtained from state Y if we wished to try. State Y Department of Health and the CDC were called, and IG was ordered. All food handlers at both locations of the restaurant were immunized on that day. The manager offered to pay for these immunizations. CDC called to say that IG would be shipped to arrive the next day.

Box continued on following page

Clinics were arranged on July 13, 14, and 15; and a press release was issued advising the public of the risk of exposure and also advising that IG would only be effective for those potentially exposed on or after June 29. Those exposed before that date should monitor themselves for symptoms. The initial clinic on July 13 treated more than 600 individuals with IG. On Friday, July 14, 360 injections were given and on Saturday, July 15, approximately 100 people were immunized. In the next week, sporadic contacts showed up at the Health Department, and those who were still in the 14-day window from last exposure were injected with IG.

To the date of this report, one possible secondary case has been identified. Other persons who complained of possible symptoms have been screened through local physicians; none have had hepatitis A confirmed. All individuals who came to the Health Department clinics or who were interviewed by telephone were instructed on signs and symptoms of illness, the importance of early diagnosis to prevent secondary cases, and proper hygiene to reduce transmission of illness.

The county health department sanitarian continues to visit the restaurant weekly; use of gloves in the restaurant has been recommended to minimize direct contact with food at any point. However, it has been observed that the person rolling the burritos continues to do it barehanded.

Analysis of Case Investigation

There is a systematic approach to any case investigation. This involves

1. Reporting of the case
2. Confirmation of the initial diagnosis by talking to the physician and case
3. Seeing the case, interview with the case to find risk factors, date of onset, exposure history
4. Inspection of the work site by sanitarians to assess levels of hygiene and compliance with procedures to determine if it is a high-risk situation including interviewing coworkers and manager at work site.
5. Final confirmation of diagnosis with final laboratory test results.

On the basis of this information, an assessment is made of the case to determine the risk factors to the public and contacts, and a decision is made as to the most appropriate preventive treatment, which may include notification of contacts in person or going public if contacts are unknown and prophylaxis for contacts as appropriate.

Another important aspect is education of contacts and persons who are exposed as to signs and symptoms and advising anyone who prepares food or takes care of other people about appropriate hand-washing and other preventive strategies.

Timeline of Case History

Monday, July 10

1. About 8:00 AM county Health Department received first notification of the case:

   - Suspected hepatitis A in a food handler reported by emergency room nurse who worked with physician who evaluated case.
   - At time of report, name of restaurant was not known, but nurse called back immediately with identification.
   - Initial diagnosis based on symptoms and elevated liver function test. Hepatitis A laboratory test pending.
   - At same time, Environmental Health Department received a call from restaurant manager regarding the situation. Employer notified that hepatitis was suspected and case told not to work until after diagnosis confirmed.

2. Case interviewed by telephone to identify symptoms, work history and duties, and contacts.

   - Case went to physician because he was notified that friends with whom he had spent Memorial Day weekend had since become ill (which fits into the incubation period for hepatitis A).
   - First reported onset of symptoms June 29.
   - There was hand-to-food contact in the daily duties he carried out during his work hours.
   - Appointment made for personal interview.

3. After telephone interview with the case, Communicable Disease (CD) team met and plan formulated:

   - CD nurse to notify state Health Division and determine availability of IG.
   - Environmental health (EH) specialist to inspect restaurant, evaluate hand-washing policies, interview coworkers regarding case's practices, and obtain case's complete work schedule, based on timesheets from the restaurant.
   - Begin to draft a press release if need developed to go public.
   - 10:30 AM: A physician from the state Health Division notified, asked to check on availabil-

ity of IG supplies, and given the basic information of the case as obtained by interview.

- 11:00 AM: Case came in for personal interview; risk factors again reviewed, and level of hygiene evaluated:

    18 year old male

    Hygiene level appeared moderate: long hair pulled back, some nails not clean

    Camped in a van at an outdoor rock concert, sleeping in a rest area with the friends who had been reported to be sick

    Admitted to marijuana use, sharing of that drug with friends

    Remembered preparing salsa (holding and cutting tomatoes by hand) in addition to normal duties at restaurant, but needed to check further on the dates

    Enjoyed rolling tortillas at work and thought he spent the majority of work time in that job (manual contact directly with food)

- 11:30 AM: Another review of case. Decision whether to go public still pending; waiting to get dates of salsa preparation, how much prepared, and conditions of preparation area.

- 1:00 PM: Sanitarian reported on conditions of restaurant:

    Had reviewed past reports; generally good (one incident where hand-washing sink did not have hot water, one report when sink occupied by another container so not accessible).

    Other employees interviewed said they thought case had good hygiene, in fact reminding other employees to wash hands. Management confirmed this.

    Preparation of food done by tongs to the end of the line where they rolled the tortilla (person using bare hands, no gloves)

    Management had not confirmed that case did prepare salsa but provided hours case worked in June and July (30+ hours each week, with high volume of people coming through restaurant [between 300 and 350 daily])

    Restaurant involved is located by a university and has established clientele who come in frequently.

  - 3:00 PM: Still had not heard back from state Health Division regarding IG.

4. Reinterviewed case, having benefit of work hours. Actual onset was June 30. Left early from work because feeling ill. Identified that salsa he had prepared would have been on July 1 (one day after onset of symptoms).

Again reported that he handled tomatoes bare-handed to put them into slicer. Case asked to get more information regarding names of friends who were out of state.

5. Unable to call state Y Health Department this date. Obtained their CD number—plan to call next morning to confirm diagnosis and onset dates for the cases who were his friends.

- 4:00 PM. Faxed case investigation form to state Health Department along with rough draft of press release and contact information, verbally reviewed case with the doctor from the state X Health Division, who had not yet checked on availability of IG or reviewed the case with other epidemiologists. Assumed we would hear back same day regarding IG.

Tuesday, July 11
1. Called the physician from the state X Health Division; not at desk; message left to return call regarding high-risk food handler with hepatitis A.
2. CD team meeting

- Reviewed case hygiene status:
    Case did wash his hands but could not guarantee that he did so consistently every day
    Did not have diarrhea.
    Worked through incubation time and acute phase of disease.
- Decided on following course of action:
    Go public if IG available
    Give IG on hand to restaurant staff right away

    Write letter to local physicians informing them of case and reminding them of the epidemic in state X and need to establish diagnosis and contact the Health Department. (Letter from the local Health Department health officer also includes information on why decision made to go public and a copy of the press release.)

    Send letters to restaurants reminding them that hepatitis in an employee is a major factor and reminding them of the guidelines to follow. Revisit restaurant to determine amount of salsa made, how it is used over a period of time, and obtain a list of coworker contacts.

    Again try to establish IG supply.

    Get blood test results for verification of case.

Box continued on following page

Meet with health administrator to review case status (done later same morning).

- 11:05 AM: Confirmation of hepatitis A from lab results. The physician at state X Health Division still had not checked on IG supply.
- 11:30 AM: The physician called back, saying that there was no IG in the state, to call state Y if we wished; he did not have the number to call. Said he would get back to us with the number if we could not find it.
- Called state Y Department of Public Health; receptionist said CDC approval needed to obtain the amount of IG we were requesting (300 packages of 6 cc each) to immunize restaurant patrons. Telephone number for CDC given; message left for someone to return call.
- Spoke to restaurant manager, informed him that county Health Department was going public and that if we obtained IG, prophylaxis would be offered to restaurant patrons.
- Set up times for employees to come in on July 11 and 12. Restaurant manager provided list of employees, asking that they all be immunized because they worked both at this restaurant and another related one. (Case worked only at the restaurant near university.) Manager offered to pay for these injections.
- 12:20 PM: Call from CDC with approval to order the 300 packages of IG from state Y Department of Public Health. Called immediately; CDC approval verified by them via telephone, shipment to be received by noon on Thursday, July 13. CDC called back to confirm that IG had been obtained.
- Now that IG available, press release refined and sent to media; letter to physicians with copy of press release.
- Arranged for Health Department personnel to work at mass clinics July 13, 14, and 15. Information packets prepared for nurses and calendar of dates at risk.
- Local health officer called physician at the state Health Division regarding lack of support from state Health Division to this point. Local physician spoke with CD RN, asking for more information on cases in state Y who were friends of local case.

Information received from nurse at county Health Department in state Y, confirming two immunoglobulin M (IgM) positive cases, one onset of June 25, other not interviewed. A third person with onset of June 25 with IgM pending; liver function tests pending. A fourth friend from the area has been reported symptomatic and asked to come for testing. This information was relayed to the state Health Division regarding its plan to evaluate making public notification about the rock concert. An unrelated case had been diagnosed in the same county in a person who also attended the concert, with onset date within the correct incubation period.

Wednesday, July 12
1. Restaurant employees given IG injections.
2. Call back from the physician in state X Health Division re case status. Advised him we were going public, having obtained IG. At that time he offered to contact Health Departments in other states.
3. Contacted university because large groups from there may have eaten at the restaurant. Advised university Student Health Center that they could contact state Y Public Health Department to obtain IG; they decided to order their own supply.
4. Fact sheet prepared for reception staff to use in answering calls from public.
5. Hundreds of calls were received. CD nurses took as many calls as they could and evaluated anyone who reported symptoms at this point.
6. To date, no additional cases have been reported.
7. Additional supplies were ordered for clinics, including quantities of juice.
8. Maximum amount of IG that could be obtained without CDC approval (132) was ordered; shipped to arrive Friday, July 14.

Thursday, July 13
1. Many calls from the public and the media continue about clinic times.
2. IG is effective only for those potentially exposed on or after June 29.
3. IG received; nurses began drawing up syringes of IG—standard mass clinic amounts of 1.5 or 2.0 cc. (Children's would be done on an individual basis.)
4. Clinic began at 3:00 PM. By end of clinic (8:30 PM) 617 injections given.

Friday, July 14
1. Clinic held from 1 to 6 PM: 360 injections given.
2. Second supply of IG received.

Saturday, July 15
1. Third clinic held; 10 AM to 1 PM. Approximately 100 people injected.

Week of July 17

1. Can continue to give IG until 14 days after last exposure; calls continue and individuals still coming for injections.
2. No secondary cases reported as a result of exposure at the restaurant.
3. Clients who had called with complaints of symptoms had been evaluated by their physicians and found to have symptoms unrelated to hepatitis A.
4. We continue to ask people who complain of symptoms to see their physicians.
5. Each client who came to county Health Department clinics was screened and instructed on proper hygiene and reduction of transmission of illness, importance of early diagnosis, seeing physician as soon as symptoms occur to prevent secondary cases.
6. CD team meeting held. Determined that

   • EH specialist will monitor restaurant weekly, checking to see whether symptoms occur in any other employees.
   • Use of gloves at restaurant recommended to minimize direct contact with food at any point in its preparation.
   • One restaurant employee had left town June 25 and did not return until July 14, but risk was minimal because case had not prepared food for this person.

APPLICATION OF THE NURSING PROCESS

The following case study will demonstrate how a community health nurse applies the nursing process to a specific problem within the community in which he or she works. The CHN receives a referral from within the community. An assessment is carried out to identify the information necessary to provide accurate diagnoses. Nursing diagnoses and interventions are then outlined, including actual and potential problems, for each component of the community affected. A plan is drawn up by the CHN and the affected members of the aggregate. Implementation is carried out, followed by an evaluation of the entire nursing process. Primary, secondary, and tertiary preventive measures for the community are identified and can be put into practice to prevent future problems and epidemics.

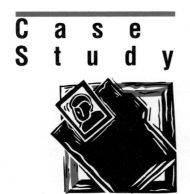

Case Study

Miriam Beckwirth is a CHN at the local elementary school. Her job includes using the nursing process to work with students in a variety of functions such as teaching health education and lifestyle classes, seeing students in the school clinic when they are ill, and providing families with counseling for stressful episodes. She is also the liaison between the public health department and the school, and she ensures that all health department regulations are being met concerning child safety, nutrition, vaccination coverage, environmental safety, and mental health. It is her responsibility to report any unusual health-related occurrences such as suspected child abuse or the development of any infectious epidemic within the school or the larger aggregates. She is adept at using the nursing process to assess, plan, implement, and evaluate nursing care plans for each of her students to meet their individual needs, the related needs of their families, and selected needs of the larger community. She does this by addressing primary, secondary, and tertiary levels of prevention which she can influence positively.

Assessment

Miriam received a telephone call from Mr. John Lemon, Jabril's third-grade teacher, stating that this normally healthy and very active 8-year-old Algerian-born boy was not able to participate in class because he was not feeling well. Mr. Lemon asked whether he could send Jabril to see the nurse. Jabril has an older brother and a younger sister attending this school. Both siblings were attending their classes and not complaining of "feeling sick."

To prepare for Jabril's visit, Miriam reviews the childhood illnesses with their classic signs and symptoms. Ten minutes later, Miriam receives Jabril in her office. A check of vital signs and an initial assessment finds that this child presents with a temperature of 101.6°F, red and inflamed eyes, a mild cough, and Koplik spots on his buccal mucosa. Jabril is irritable and complaining of general malaise ("feeling achy"). As Miriam questions the child, she learns that he has been feeling ill for approximately 15 hours and that no other person in the household is sick at the present time. She asks him about his sleeping pattern during the past week and reviews his nutritional intake.

Miriam pulls Jabril's chart to assess his immunization status and finds that he received a measles vaccine in Algeria on March 4, 1983. She then looks up his birthday and discovers he was born in North Africa on September 9, 1982. She calculates his age at the time of administration of the live, attenuated measles vaccine to be 6 months.

Miriam then calls Jabril's mother, Mrs. Simcha Kamal, and confirms the date of birth and the date of vaccination for Jabril. She tells Jabril's mother that Jabril is ill and needs further assessment by the family physician immediately.

Miriam telephones the Jabril's family physician, and the child is seen that afternoon. A blood sample is drawn in which the measles virus is isolated. A rise in antibody titers is also noted.

Four days later, Jabril develops a characteristic red blotchy rash that starts on his face; in the following days, the rash becomes generalized and lasts approximately 5 days. Jabril is diagnosed by the physician as having measles.

Diagnosis

Miriam begins writing a nursing care plan for Jabril based on several nursing diagnoses that fit his present condition (see boxed information).

NURSING DIAGNOSES AND NURSING INTERVENTIONS

For Jabril

I. At risk for altered thermoregulation due to febrile condition; teach family to
  A. Monitor body temperature every 2 hours and record temperature.
  B. Administer analgesics and antipyretics as necessary and recommended by physician.
  C. Maintain hydration.
  D. Use measures to reduce excessive fever when present.
    1. Remove blankets.
    2. Apply ice bags to axilla and groin.
    3. Initiate tepid water sponge bath.
    4. Maintain environmental temperature at a comfortable setting.
II. Altered skin integrity due to measles lesions; teach family to

A. Inspect skin condition.
B. Offer calamine lotion and antipruritic for itching.
C. Use mild unabrasive soap and tepid water for hygiene.
D. Remind child not to scratch lesions or rash.
E. Encourage child to express feelings about skin condition.
F. Explain reason for and treatment of skin condition to child, including usual duration.
III. Altered oral mucous membrane due to Koplik spots; teach family to
  A. Inspect child's oral cavity every morning, afternoon, and evening, and describe and document condition or change.
  B. Provide supportive measures for mouth care.
    1. Assist child with oral hygiene before and after meals and as necessary.

2. Use soft-bristled toothbrush or cotton applicator and mouthwash (avoid alcohol-based mouthwashes because these increase dryness and irritation and promote breakdown).
3. Lubricate lips frequently.
C. Offer foods that are soft and bland, and avoid serving foods that irritate mucous membranes (hot, cold, spicy, fried, citrus).
D. Encourage oral fluids to maintain hydration and lubricate oral mucous membrane.
IV. Social isolation due to measles; teach family to
A. Involve child in setting goals and planning care.
B. Encourage child to perform activities of daily living independently.
C. Perform referrals for assistance if necessary.
D. Arrange for telephone so child can talk to friends.
E. Offer books, games, and television for diversional activity.
F. Have child engage in conversation with people not at risk for contracting measles.
G. Bring homework from school so child will not fall behind peers in class.
V. Disturbance of self-concept due to change in body image from rash; teach family to
A. Accept the child's perception of self.
B. Allow opportunities for child to verbalize feelings.
C. Provide positive reinforcement for child's efforts to adapt.
D. Teach child coping strategies.
E. Reinforce short duration of rash.
F. Arrange for child to interact with others who have similar problems if appropriate.

For Jabril's Family

I. Potential for disturbance in family coping due to acute illness
A. Allow time for family to discuss impact of child's illness and their feelings.
B. Facilitate family conferences; help family identify key issues and select support services, if needed.
C. Help child and family establish a visiting routine that will not tax child or family members.
D. Reinforce family's efforts to care for child.
E. Provide family with clear, concise information about child's condition. Be aware of what the family has already been told, and help them interpret information.
F. Help family support child's independence.
G. Provide emotional support to family by being available to answer questions.
H. Inform family of community resources available to assist in managing child's illness and provide emotional or financial support to the caretakers, e.g., if mother and father are both working and must take off time without pay to care for child.

II. Knowledge deficit related to vaccination schedule
A. Establish an environment of mutual trust and respect to enhance family's learning.
B. Negotiate with family to develop goals for learning.
C. Select teaching strategies (discussion, demonstration, role-playing, visual materials) appropriate for family's individual learning style.
D. Teach family about schedules of vaccines for childhood diseases, and have them demonstrate knowledge of vaccines and their schedules.
E. Encourage family to ask questions and discuss concerns.
F. Provide family with names and telephone numbers of resource people, agencies, or organizations to contact with questions or problems.

For Jabril's Classmates

I. Knowledge deficit related to measles infection
A. Establish an environment of mutual trust and respect to enhance children's learning.
B. Negotiate with children to develop goals for learning.
C. Select teaching strategies (discussion, demonstration, role-playing, visual materials) appropriate for the children's learning style.
D. Teach children about measles infection, and have them demonstrate knowledge of transmission, vaccination, and disease course of measles infection.
E. Teach how disease outbreaks can be dealt with in daily life.
F. Encourage children to ask questions and discuss concerns.
G. Provide children with names and telephone numbers of resource people, agencies, or organizations to contact with questions or problems.
II. Potential for altered skin integrity due to measles lesions
A. Encourage parents of classmates to inspect skin for signs of rash every day for 2 weeks if no other cases are reported in the area.
B. Encourage children to keep skin healthy by using proper hygienic practices and lotion daily and by avoiding irritating soaps or substances.
C. Educate children in preventive skin care and early recognition of rash and spots that occur with measles infection.
D. Encourage children to immediately report any skin eruptions or rashes.
III. Potential for infection due to measles
A. Minimize children's risk of infection by
1. Vaccinating all susceptible children.
2. Vaccinating all susceptible family members.
3. Vaccinating all susceptible community members.

B. Encourage early identification and reporting of infections to prevent further transmission.
C. Administer immune globulin when appropriate and recommended by child's physician.
D. Teach children to wash hands regularly after using the toilet and before meals.
E. Teach proper oral hygiene to children.
F. Ensure proper disposal of all tissues and contaminated materials within the school setting.
G. Provide adequate ventilation system within classrooms.
H. Report any suspicious cough or symptom to child's parents, and encourage them to have their child seen by the family physician.

Planning

After Jabril is seen by the physician and diagnosed, Miriam plans to make a home visit to jointly develop a plan of care with the family. She also begins formulating care plans for his family and the other children at the school. She must design each care plan for each component in mind if it is to serve their needs adequately. She must then report the case to the infectious disease branch of the local department of public health for surveillance. Then, she will review all nursing records of the children attending her school at the present time to ensure that no other students need to be revaccinated. If any student fits into this group, she must immediately revaccinate and monitor these children for signs of infection. A prophylactic dose of immune globulin may be given to these children by their family physician; however, administering immune globulin after the third day of incubation may prolong the incubation period without preventing disease. Because the exact date of exposure is unknown for these children, it may be unwise to administer immune globulin. Miriam then must notify the parents of all the children at the school so that other cases can be reported early. She realizes it is also important to ask parents to check the immunization status of all family members in the household.

Intervention

Miriam makes a home visit, and she and Mrs. Kamal develop the nursing care plan together. Mrs. Kamal identifies ways to offer supportive measures such as bedrest during the febrile period, antipyretics for the fever, dimming the lights for sensitive eyes, and providing a vaporizer in the child's room. Because Jabril is not a high-risk child, antibiotic therapy will probably not be necessary. Miriam warns Mrs. Kamal about the complications of measles and tells her that if she notices any of these signs or symptoms, she should take Jabril to the physician immediately. The complications she mentions include an earache (otitis media), any respiratory symptoms such as a severe cough or wheezing (pneumonia, bronchiolitis, obstructive laryngitis, and laryngotracheitis), and any neurological changes such as unsteady gait or memory disturbances (encephalitis).

Last and most important, Miriam informs Mrs. Kamal about the need for strict isolation from other children and adults who are not fully immunized against measles. This will include those who received live measles vaccine before the age of 12 months, those who are unsure of their age at vaccination, and those who were vaccinated before 1968 with an unknown type of vaccine. All persons within these categories should be revaccinated immediately; if they have come in contact with Jabril, they should also be isolated for the next 12 to 14 days because this is the incubation period for measles and they could be spreading disease. Clinical signs of infection will not develop until after 1 or 2 weeks. Mrs. Kamal is also asked to make a complete list of everyone with whom Jabril has come in contact and the places he has been within the past 3 weeks. Miriam takes a complete history, including the vaccination status of Jabril's siblings and parents. Mrs. Kamal is very eager to participate in this process because she is concerned about the health of her family.

The local department of public health is notified, and the case is appropriately reported and documented. A list of Jabril's contacts is given to the public health officer taking the information. It is up to this officer to contact those people who have been in close proximity to Jabril within the preceding 3 weeks. The officer will try to identify, isolate, and treat the individual who exposed Jabril and his schoolmates to the measles virus. Miriam prepares a note for all children to take home to their parents informing them of the measles case and alerting them to the signs and symptoms to be aware of within the family. She also encloses a form to help family members review vaccination schedules; this will ensure that this aggregate is protected against measles infection. Miriam then reviews all vaccination records for the children at the school. She is prepared to vaccinate any child currently in need of a booster against the vaccine-preventable childhood infections.

Evaluation

Five days after Miriam first examines Jabril, the public health officer at the department of public health telephones Miriam to inform her that they have isolated the original source of the measles virus. Apparently, the family living across the street from Jabril had some friends visit from Indonesia. These friends had a 1-year-old child who had not been vaccinated and developed measles upon arriving in the United States.

The child subsequently recovered but not before exposing several people at risk. This was an isolated incident, so only a few cases of clinical disease were caused. None of Jabril's classmates contracted measles. The benefit of this experience was the resulting emphasis placed on revaccinating those at risk and ensuring the health of this aggregate through more prudent vaccination adherence against preventable infectious diseases. This episode also displayed how important it is to have a reliable and efficient public health surveillance system.

Levels of Prevention

Primary The most effective method of prevention for measles is early vaccination of children by the age of 15 months. Any child vaccinated before the age of 12 months should be revaccinated by the age of 15 months. Any susceptible adults should be revaccinated.

Secondary A search for exposed individuals who are susceptible for infection from the measles virus should be implemented. Once these people are identified, they should be vaccinated to stop further transmission of measles. Isolation is impractical in a large community, but children should be kept out of school for at least 4 days after the appearance of a rash. The parents of children attending school should promptly and accurately report any suspicious family illness to the school nurse. All cases of measles should be reported early to the local health authority because reporting provides better control of outbreaks. Community health nurses should annually engage in continuing education activities to gain skills and increase their knowledge base so they can better serve their community.

Tertiary Community health nurses have the special task of intervening at individual, family, and aggregate levels by using the nursing process to assist with rehabilitation and restoration to baseline functioning, as presented in the case study. Surveillance systems should collect and relay health information and statistics from the local to the state and national levels.

SUMMARY

This chapter began by identifying threats to the health of the community and ways to keep the community free of infection. The community health nurse has the unique role of taking collective action with community members at the local, state, and national levels to preserve the health of aggregates.

Transmission of infectious agents is carried out through direct, indirect, and airborne contacts with human recipients. Understanding modes of transmission will help in design and use of effective methods to prevent the spread of infectious diseases.

Defining, reporting, and continuing surveillance of cases of infectious disease transmission are vital aspects of a national public health surveillance program. The information contributed from these activities provides baseline data for the monitoring of epidemiological trends, around which screening and intervention programs can be administered.

One major method of keeping communities free of infection is through the use of vaccines. There are different kinds of immunity, each lasting a specified amount of time, but the goal is for lasting immunity against infectious diseases. Vaccination, given in the correct dosage, route, and preparation, can provide lasting immunity to most individuals. Vaccine schedules for all ages should be adhered to, and vaccine integrity should be maintained through the use of a cold chain as well as checking expiration dates before use. Many individuals in areas around the world still suffer from vaccine-preventable infectious diseases, and mortality from these illnesses remains very high. Where eradication is not probable, control is the goal.

Hepatitis B is of growing concern because of the carrier status role in chronic disease and the severe damage to the liver that may occur without obvious symptoms.

STDs remain a very real threat to the community and have a unique form of transmission. Fecal-oral contamination offers a new route for many parasitic and infectious diseases. The sequelae from many of these diseases can leave men and women permanently infertile and predisposed to cancer. For many of these diseases, such as herpes simplex virus, HPV, and AIDS, there are no cures; prevention is the only method of control.

AIDS had predominantly been a disease of homosexual men, but it is now increasing in heterosexual populations. AIDS is also escalating as a cause of death among women.

For many infectious diseases, prevention is the only cure. Vaccines and safer sex practices have become the first line of defense. They are safe preventive measures that are more cost effective, in both economic and human terms, than not using these interventions.

Public health efforts are vitally important in combating the increasing trends of many infectious disease rates. Community health nurses have an important role in prevention, case finding, reporting, and other activities related to the control of communicable diseases within their communities.

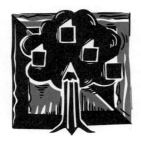

L e a r n i n g
A c t i v i t i e s

1. Visit a testing laboratory to see how STD tests are done (e.g., VDRL, tests for gonorrhea).

2. Find out what kinds of vaccine services are available at your local health department and what form of follow-up is done.

3. Call one of the hot line reference telephone numbers listed in this chapter and request specific information regarding a client you are now caring for.

4. From your nearest local health department, obtain and evaluate health education materials regarding childhood immunizations.

5. From the nearest medical library, review the communicable disease reference materials available from the Centers for Disease Control and Prevention and the Department of Health and Human Services.

6. Inquire about the reporting of notifiable diseases in your community. Who is responsible for the reporting process? To whom do they report, what is reportable, and how often? What emergency public health measures are available for control of epidemics in your area?

7. Purchase a 1-year subscription to a public health nursing journal.

REFERENCES

Abraham R, Minor P, Dunn G, et al.: Shedding of virulent poliovirus during immunization with oral poliovirus vaccine after prior immunization with inactivated polio vaccine. J Infect Dis 168:1105–1109, 1993.

Alter MJ, Hadler SC, Margolis HS, et al.: The changing epidemiology of hepatitis B in the United States: Need for alternative vaccination strategies. JAMA 263:1218–1222, 1990.

Amaro H: Love, sex, and power: Considering women's realities in HIV prevention. Am Psychol 50:437–447, 1995.

American Academy of Pediatrics: Summaries of infectious diseases. *In* Peter G, ed. 1994 Red Book: Report of the Committee on Infectious Diseases, 23rd ed. Elk Grove Village, IL: American Academy of Pediatrics, 1994, pp. 177–181.

Aral SO: Sexual behavior in sexually transmitted disease research: An overview. Sex Transm Dis 21 (suppl 2):S59–S64, 1994.

Beatty WL, Byrne GI, Morrison RP: Repeated and persistent infection with Chlamydia and the development of chronic inflammation and disease. Trends Mircobiol 2:94–98, 1994.

Becker TM, Wheeler CM, McGough NS, et al.: Sexually transmitted diseases and other risk factors for cervical dysplasia among Southwestern Hispanic and Non-Hispanic white women. JAMA 271:1181–1188, 1994.

Benenson AS: Control of Communicable Diseases in Man, 15th ed. Washington, DC: American Public Health Association, 1990.

Benenson AS: Control of Communicable Diseases Manual, 16th ed. Washington, DC: American Public Health Association, 1995.

Brown DR, Fife KH: Human papillomavirus infections of the genital tract. Med Clin North Am 74:1455–1480, 1990.

Centers for Disease Control: Update: Universal precautions for prevention of transmission of HIV, hepatitis B virus, and other bloodborne pathogens in health care settings, Morb Mort Wkly Rep 37:377–382, 387–388, 1988.

Centers for Disease Control: Yellow fever vaccine: Recommendations of the Immunization Practice Advisory Committee (ACIP). Morb Mortal Wkly Rep 39:RR-6, 1–6, 1990.

Centers for Disease Control: Vaccinia (smallpox) vaccine: Recommendations of the Immunization Practices Advisory Committee (ACIP). Morb Mortal Wkly Rep 40:1–40, 1991.

Centers for Disease Control: Division of STD/HIV Prevention 1991 Annual Report. Atlanta: Centers for Disease Control, 1992a.

Centers for Disease Control: Revised classification system for HIV infection and expanded surveillance case definition for AIDS among adolescents and adults. Morb Mortal Wkly Rep 41:RR-7, 1992b.

Centers for Disease Control: HIV/AIDS Prevention Fact Book 1992. Atlanta: Centers for Disease Control, 1992c.

Centers for Disease Control: Recommendations of the International Task Force for Disease Eradication. Morb Mortal Wkly Rep 42(RR-16):1–38, 1993a.

Centers for Disease Control: Recommendations for use of Haemophilus b conjugate vaccines and a combined diphtheria, tetanus, pertussis, and Haemophilus b vaccine. Morb Mortal Wkly Rep 42(RR-13):1–15, 1993b.

Centers for Disease Control: Resurgence of pertussis—United States, 1993. Morb Mortal Wkly Rep 42:952–953, 959–960, 1993c.

Centers for Disease Control: Recommendations of the ACIP: Use of vaccines and immune globulins in persons with altered immunocompetence. Morb Mortal Wkly Rep 42(RR-4):1–18, 1993d.

Centers for Disease Control: Cases of selected notifiable diseases, United States, weeks ending December 17, 1994, and December 18, 1993 (50th week). Morb Mortal Wkly Rep 43:935, 1994a.

Centers for Disease Control: Progress toward global eradication of poliomyelitis, 1988–1993. Morb Mortal Wkly Rep 43:499–503, 1994b.

Centers for Disease Control: Vaccination coverage of 2-year-old children—United States, 1992–1993. Morb Mortal Wkly Rep 43:282–283, 1994c.

Centers for Disease Control: Summary of notifiable diseases, United States 1994. Morb Mortal Wkly Rep 43(53):iv, 1994d.

Centers for Disease Control: Update: Influenza activity—United States and worldwide, 1993–94 season, and composition of the 1994–95 influenza vaccine. Morb Mortal Wkly Rep 43:179–183, 1994e.

Centers for Disease Control: Prevention and control of influenza: Part I, vaccines. Morb Mortal Wkly Rep 43(RR-9):1–13, 1994f.

Centers for Disease Control: General recommendations on immunization: Recommendations of the Advisory Committee on Immunization Practices (ACIP). Morb Mortal Wkly Rep 43(RR-1):1–38, 1994g.

Centers for Disease Control: Rubella and congenital rubella syndrome—United States, January 1, 1991–May 7, 1994. Morb Mortal Wkly Rep 43:391, 397–401, 1994h.

Centers for Disease Control: Human plague—United States, 1993–1994. Morb Mortal Wkly Rep 43:242–246, 1994i.

Centers for Disease Control: Progress toward the global elimination of neonatal tetanus, 1989–1993. Morb Mortal Wkly Rep 43:885–887, 1994j.

Centers for Disease Control: Raccoon rabies epizootic—United States, 1993. Morb Mortal Wkly Rep 43:269–273, 1994k.

Centers for Disease Control: Human rabies—California, 1994. Morb Mortal Wkly Rep 43:255–257, 1994l.

Centers for Disease Control: Immunization Action News 1:1–10, 1994m.

Centers for Disease Control: Vaccine management: Recommendations for handling and storage of selected biologicals. Atlanta:

Centers for Disease Control and Prevention National Immunization Program, 1994n.

Centers for Disease Control: General recommendations on immunization: Recommendations of the Advisory Committee on Immunization Practices (ACIP). Misconceptions concerning true contraindications and precautions to vaccination. Morb Mortal Wkly Rep 43(RR-1):23–26, 1994o.

Centers for Disease Control: Revised classification system for HIV infection in children less than 13 years of age. Morb Mortal Wkly Rep 43(RR-12), 1994p.

Centers for Disease Control: Sexually Transmitted Disease Surveillance, 1993. Atlanta: Centers for Disease Control, 1994q.

Centers for Disease Control: Recommendations of the U.S. Public Health Service Task Force on the Use of Zidovudine to Reduce Perinatal Transmission of Human Immunodeficiency virus. Morb Mortal Wkly Rep 43(RR-11), 1994r.

Centers for Disease Control: Epidemiology and Prevention of Vaccine-Preventable Diseases. Atlanta: Centers for Disease Control, 1995a, pp. 173–197.

Centers for Disease Control: Sexually transmitted disease surveillance, 1994. Atlanta: Centers for Disease Control, 1995b.

Centers for Disease Control: HIV/AIDS prevention: Facts about the human immunodeficiency virus and its transmission. Atlanta: Centers for Disease Control, 1995c.

Centers for Disease Control: HIV/AIDS Surveillance Report. Atlanta: Centers for Disease Control, 1995d.

Centers for Disease Control: First 500,000 AIDS cases—United States, 1995. Morb Mortal Wkly Rep 44:849–853, 1995e.

Centers for Disease Control: Update: Acquired immunodeficiency syndrome—United States, 1994. Morbid Mortal Wkly Rep 44:64–67, 1995f.

Centers for Disease Control: Update: AIDS among women—United States, 1994. Morb Mortal Wkly Rep 44:81–84, 1995g.

Centers for Disease Control: Recommended childhood immunization schedule—United States, July-December 1996. Morb Mortal Wkly Rep 45:635–638, 1996a.

Centers for Disease Control: Changes in national notifiable diseases data presentation. Morb Mortal Wkly Rep 45:41–42, 1996b.

Centers for Disease Control: Immunization Action News 3(5):1, 1996c.

Centers for Disease Control: Polio Vaccine Update 1:1, 1996d.

Centers for Disease Control: Ten leading nationally notifiable infectious diseases—United States, 1995. Morb Mortal Wkly Rep 45:883–884, 1996e.

Centers for Disease Control: Recommended childhood immunization schedule—United States, July–December 1996. Morb Mortal Wkly Rep 45:635–638, 1996f.

Corey L: The current trend in genital herpes. Sex Transm Dis 21(suppl 2):S38–S44, 1994.

Cutts FJ, Smith PG: Vaccination and World Health. Chichester, England: Wiley, 1994.

Dolin PJ, Raviglione MC, Kochi A: Global tuberculosis incidence and mortality during 1990–2000. Bull WHO 72:213–220, 1994.

Donovan P: Testing Positive: Sexually Transmitted Disease and the Public Health Response. New York: Alan Guttmacher Institute, 1993.

Dutta JK: Rabies in endemic countries. BMJ 308:488–489, 1994.

Ehrhardt A, Wasserheit J: Age, gender, and sexual risk behaviors for sexually transmitted diseases in the United States. *In* Wasserheit J, Aral S, Holmes K, eds. Research Issues in Human Behavior and STDs in the AIDS Era. Washington, DC: American Society for Microbiology, 1991.

Ghendon Y: WHO strategy for the global elimination of new cases of hepatitis B. Vaccine 8(suppl):S129–132, 1990.

Global Programme for Vaccines of the World Health Organization: Role of mass campaigns in global measles control. Lancet 344:174–175, 1994.

Goldsmith MF: Target: Sexually transmitted diseases. JAMA 264:2179–2180, 1990.

Gordis L: Epidemiology. Philadelphia: W.B. Saunders, 1996.

Grange JM, Stanford JL: Dogma and innovation in the global control of tuberculosis: Discussion paper. JR Soc Med 87:272–275, 1994.

Hay PE, Horner PJ, MacLeod E, et al.: Chlamydia trachomatis in women: The more you look, the more you find. Genitourin Med 70:97–100, 1994.

Hellinger F: The lifetime cost of treating a person with HIV. JAMA 270:474–478, 1993.

Henry-Suchet J, Askienazy-Elbhar M, Thibon M, et al.: Post-therapeutic evolution of serum chlamydial antibody titers in women with acute salpingitis and tubal infertility. Fertil Steril 62:296–304, 1994.

Hodes RM, Azbite M. Tuberculosis. *In:* Kloos H, Zein ZA, eds. The Ecology of Health and Disease in Ethiopia. Boulder, CO: Westview Press, 1993, pp. 265–284.

Hollinger FB, Bancroft WH, Dienstag JL, et al.: Controlling hepatitis B virus transmission in North America. Vaccine 8(suppl):S122–128, 1990.

Holtgrave D, Qualls N, Curran J, et al.: An overview of the effectiveness and efficiency of HIV prevention programs. Public Health Rep 110:134–146, 1995.

Hutchinson CM, Hook EW: Syphilis in adults. Med Clin North Am 74(6):1389–1414, 1990.

Hutchinson CM, Hook EW, Shepherd M, et al.: Altered clinical presentation of early syphilis in patients with human immunodeficiency virus infection. Ann Intern Med 121:94–99, 1994.

Jemmott L, Jemmott J: Applying the theory of reasoned action to AIDS risk behavior: Condom use among black women. Nurs Res 40:228–234, 1991.

Johnson R, Lee F, Hadgu A, et al.: U.S. genital herpes trends during the first decade of AIDS—Prevalences increased in young whites and elevated in blacks. Paper presented at the Tenth International Meeting of the International Society for STD Research, Helsinki, Finland, August 29–September 1, 1993.

Jones RB, Wasserheit JN: Introduction to the biology and natural history of sexually transmitted diseases. *In* Wasserheit JN, Aral SO, Holmes KK, eds. Research Issues in Human Behavior and Sexually Transmitted Diseases in the AIDS Era. Washington, DC: American Society for Microbiology, 1991, pp. 11–37.

Kelly J, Murphy D, Sikkema K, Kalichman S: Psychological interventions to prevent HIV infection are urgently needed. Am Psychol 48:1023–1034, 1993.

Leff DR, Leff AR:Tuberculosis control policies in major metropolitan health departments in the United States. V. Standard of practice in 1992. Ann Rev Respir Dis 148:1530–1536, 1993.

Lurie P, Bishaw M, Chesney M, et al: Ethical, behavioral, and social aspects of HIV vaccine trials in developing countries. JAMA 271:295–301, 1994.

Margono F, Mroueh J, Garely A, et al.: Resurgence of active tuberculosis among pregnant women. Obstet Gynecol 83:911–914, 1994.

Martin DH: Chlamydial infections. Med Clin North Am 74:1367–1384, 1990.

Maynard JE: Hepatitis B: Global importance and need for control. Vaccine 8(suppl):S18–20, 1990.

McFarlin BL, Bottoms SF, Dock BS, Isada NB: Epidemic syphilis: Maternal factors associated with congenital infection. Am J Obstet Gynecol 170:535–540, 1994.

Moses E: 1992: The Registered Nurse Population. Rockville, MD: Division of Nursing, Department of Health and Human Services, 1994.

National Vaccine Advisory Committee: Adult Immunization. Atlanta, GA: U.S. Department of Health and Human Services, CDC, National Immunization Program, 1994.

Orenstein WA, Markowitz LE, Atkinson WL, Hinman AR: Worldwide measles prevention. Isr J Med Sci 30:469–481, 1994.

Padian N, Shiboski S, Jewell N: The effect of the number of exposures on the risk of heterosexual HIV transmission. J Infect Dis 161:883–887, 1990.

Peaceman AM, Gonik B: Sexually transmitted viral disease in women. Postgrad Med 89:133–140, 1991.

Ramsey P, Glenn L: Nurses' fluid exposure reporting, HIV testing, and hepatitis B vaccination rates: Before and after implementing universal precautions regulations. AAOHN J 44:129–137, 1996.

Rekus JF. Bloodborne Pathogens. Washington, DC: Federal Register, Occupational Safety and Health Administration, Department of Labor, 1991.

Sherlock S: Hepatitis B: The disease. Vaccine 8(suppl):S6-8, 1990.

Smoak BL, Novakski WL, Mason CJ: Evidence for a recent decrease in measles susceptibility among young American adults. J Infect Dis 170:216–219, 1994.

Sparling PF, Elkins C, Wyrick PB, Cohen MS: Vaccines for bacterial sexually transmitted infections: A realistic goal? Proc Nat Acad Sci U S A 91:2456–2463, 1994.

Spinillo A, Gorini G, Regazzetti A, et al.: Asymptomatic genitourinary Chlamydia trachomatis infection in women seropositive for human immunodeficiency virus infection. Obstet Gynecol 83:1005–1010, 1994.

Stary A, Kopp W, Zahel B, et al.: Rapid diagnosis of Chlamydia trachomatis with a nucleic acid probe in male and female patients. Dermatol 188:300–304, 1994.

Stratton KR, Howe CJ, Johnston RB: Adverse events associated with childhood vaccines other than pertussis and rubella: Summary of a report from the Institute of Medicine. JAMA 271:1602–1605, 1994.

Swanson J, Dibble S: Genital herpes: Clinical features, sources of information, recurrences, and treatment in young adults. Dermatol Nurs 5:365–373, 376–377, 1993.

Swanson JM, Dibble SL, Chenitz WC: A description of the clinical features and psychosocial factors in young adults with genital herpes. Image: J Nurs Sch 27:16–22, 1995.

Swartz TA: Proceedings of the symposium: Strategies for worldwide control of poliomyelitis and eradication of the poliovirus from the human population, with application for elimination of polio in Europe. Public Health Rev 21:1–166, 1993–1994.

Talbot H, Romanowski B: Factors affecting urine EIA sensitivity in the detection of Chlamydia trachomatis in men. Genitourin Med 70:101–104, 1994.

Temmerman M: Sexually transmitted diseases and reproductive health. Sex Transm Dis 24:(suppl 2):S55–S58, 1994.

Thraenhart O, Kreuzfelder E, Hillebrandt M, et al.: Long-term humoral and cellular immunity after vaccination with cell culture rabies vaccines in man. Clin Immunol Immunopathol 71:287–292, 1994.

Tsai TF, Paul R, Lynberg MC, Letson GW: Congenital Yellow Fever virus infection after immunization in pregnancy. J Infect Dis 168:1520–1523, 1993.

United Nations Children's Fund: The State of the World's Children, 1994. New York: Oxford University Press, 1994.

Wasserheit JN: Effect of changes in human ecology and behavior on patterns of sexually transmitted diseases, including human immunodeficiency virus infection. Proc Nat Acad Sci U S A 91:2430–2435, 1994.

WHO: The current global situation of the HIV/AIDS pandemic. Geneva, Switzerland: WHO, 1995.

Wilkinson D: High-compliance tuberculosis treatment programme in a rural community. Lancet 343:647–648, 1994.

Wiselka M: Influenza: Diagnosis, management, and prophylaxis. BMJ 308:1341–1345, 1994.

Woods CR, Smith AL, Wasilauskas BL, et al.: Invasive disease caused by Neisseria meningitidis relatively resistant to penicillin in North Carolina. J Infect Dis 170:453–456, 1994.

Zazove P, Caruthers BS, Reed BD: Genital human papillomavirus infection. Am Fam Physician 39:1279–1289, 1991.

Zell ER, Dietz V, Stevenson J, et al.: Low vaccination levels of US preschool and school-age children: Retrospective assessments of vaccination coverage, 1991–1992. JAMA 271:833–839, 1994.

School Health

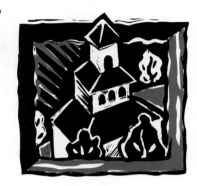

Upon completion of this chapter, the reader will be able to:

1. Discuss the core components of school health in relation to roles and responsibilities of the multidisciplinary team.

2. Recognize the potential social, cultural, economic, and political factors affecting school health.

3. Relate community and statistical indicators of school health status to academic outcomes.

4. Apply the basic concepts of critical theory to school health.

5. Formulate critical questions about school health programs that limit academic performance and well-being of school health populations.

6. Interpret the evolution of school health nursing practice within the context of developments in education, public health, pediatrics, and nursing.

7. Design a political action agenda by analyzing legislation affecting school health.

8. Contrast roles and functions of school nurses and community health nurses.

Constance M. Baker

One part of the community health system is school health, those programs aimed at maintaining and enriching the health of the nearly 48 million students—20% of the U.S. population—enrolled in elementary and secondary schools in the 15,000 school districts throughout the country. Traditionally the healthiest segment of the population, today's children and youth present a picture of deteriorating health and social well-being (Center for the Study of Social Policy, 1991). Concomitantly, concerned citizens recognize the relationship between the country's economy and an educated work force and are demanding educational reform (Boyer, 1991). The 1994 Joint Statement on School Health by the secretaries of the Department of Education and the Department of Health and Human Services reflects the increasing national emphasis to improve both education and health outcomes of children and youth (Fig. 25–1).

The purpose of this chapter is to present an overview of school health in elementary and secondary schools and to describe school nursing as one of the disciplines involved in delivering school health programs. A critical theory perspective is used to examine issues and challenges in school health and professional nursing.

A CRITICAL THEORY APPROACH TO SCHOOL HEALTH

Emancipating people from conscious or unconscious constraints to enable an uncoerced negotiated agreement is the core of critical theory (Ray, 1992). A rational agreement requires people to be autonomous and responsible. The best possible agreement occurs when people feel free to express their opinions and in turn are committed to creating social conditions so others can openly express themselves. Out of this social discourse comes new meanings and questions about their community life. In such a context, the stage is set to question basic assumptions and generate new approaches.

For example, to implement the first goal of the nation's education agenda—having all students ready to learn—school health professionals need to create an environment for dialogue and common understanding of students coming to school "ready to learn." Although it is assumed that students come to school ready to learn, the national high school graduation rate is declining. What is the meaning of learning readiness for all ages and grades? What is the relationship

GOALS 2000: EDUCATE AMERICA ACT (P.L. 103-227, 1994)

By the year 2000:

- All children ready to learn
- Ninety percent graduation rate
- All children competent in core subjects
- First in the world in mathematics and science
- Every adult literate and able to compete in the work force
- Safe, disciplined, drug-free schools
- Professional development for educators
- Increased parental involvement in learning

between a student's health and academic achievement? What are the characteristics of healthy students? How do the community and school environments enhance and inhibit student health behaviors?

Critical theory suggests that school health professionals need to be actively engaged in identifying factors that prevent students from coming to school ready to learn or deprive them of access to resources that enhance their health and enrich the educational experience (Stevens and Hall, 1992). School health professionals have the expertise to engage in "upstream thinking" and influence policymaking by government and school organizations. The upstream view must be applied in community assessment and planning to ensure that students have access to health-promoting choices and come to school ready to learn. Ongoing dialogue is needed with educators, administrators, families, and students to define the issues, raise consciousness about rights and responsibilities, negotiate potential strategies, and facilitate change. Collaboration with health professionals in the community is usually required to help students maintain their health so they are able to obtain an education. Finally, upstream thinking about funding school health programs generates new options for policymakers' dialogue because traditional practices and vested interests are examined.

Critical theory helps to empower community health nurses and school health professionals by drawing attention to oppressive administrative models that suppress human caring values and to the need for equal roles for nursing with other professionals in the delivery of school health. Emphasis on creating an environment for autonomy and responsibility in professional dialogue facilitates collective strategies for

JOINT STATEMENT ON SCHOOL HEALTH

by

The Secretaries of Education and Health and Human Services

Health and education are joined in fundamental ways with each other and with the destinies of the Nation's children. Because of our national leadership responsibilities for education and health, we have initiated unprecedented cooperative efforts between our Departments. In support of comprehensive school health programs, we affirm the following:

■ *America's children face many compelling educational and health and developmental challenges that affect their lives and their futures.*

These challenges include poor levels of achievement; unacceptably high drop-out rates; low literacy; violence; drug abuse; preventable injuries; physical and mental illness; developmental disabilities; and sexual activity resulting in sexually transmitted diseases, including HIV and unintended pregnancy. These facts demand a reassessment of the contributions of education and health programs in safeguarding our children's present lives and preparing them for productive, responsible, and fulfilling futures.

■ *To help children meet these challenges, education and health must be linked in partnership.*

Schools are the only public institutions that touch nearly every young person in this country. Schools have a unique opportunity to affect the lives of children and their families, but they cannot address all of our children's needs alone. Health, education, and human service programs must be integrated, and schools must have the support of public and private health care providers, communities, and families.

■ *School health programs support the education process, integrate services for disadvantaged and disabled children, and improve children's health prospects.*

Through school health programs, children and their families can develop the knowledge, attitudes, beliefs, and behaviors necessary to remain healthy and perform well in school. These learning environments enhance safety, nutrition, and disease prevention; encourage exercise and fitness; support healthy physical, mental, and emotional development; promote abstinence and prevent sexual behaviors that result in HIV infection, other sexually transmitted diseases, and unintended teenage pregnancy; discourage use of illegal drugs, alcohol, and tobacco; and help young people develop problem-solving and decision-making skills.

■ *Reforms in health care and in education offer opportunities to forge the partnerships needed for our children in the 1990s.*

The benefits of integrated health and education services can be achieved by working together to create a "seamless" network of services, both through the school setting and through linkages with other community resources.

■ *GOALS 2000 and HEALTHY PEOPLE 2000 provide complementary visions that, together, can support our joint efforts in pursuit of a healthier, better educated Nation for the next century.*

GOALS 2000 challenges us to ensure that all children arrive at school ready to learn; to increase the high school graduation rate; to achieve basic subject matter competencies; to achieve universal adult literacy; and to ensure that school environments are safe, disciplined, and drug free. HEALTHY PEOPLE 2000 challenges us to increase the span of healthy life for the American people, to reduce and finally to eliminate health disparities among population groups, and to ensure access to services for all Americans.

In support of GOALS 2000 and HEALTHY PEOPLE 2000, we have established the Interagency Committee on School Health co-chaired by the Assistant Secretary for Elementary and Secondary Education and the Assistant Secretary for Health, and we have convened the National Coordinating Committee on School Health to bring together representatives of major national education and health organizations to work with us.

We call upon professionals in the fields of education and health and concerned citizens across the Nation to join with us in a renewed effort and a reaffirmation of our mutual responsibility to our Nation's children.

Richard W. Riley
Secretary of Education

Donna E. Shalala
Secretary of Health and Human Services

Figure 25–1
Joint statement on school health. (From Riley RW, Shalala DE: Joint Statement on School Health. Washington, DC, U.S. Departments of Education and Health and Human Services, 1994.)

change in school health programs and strengthens peer support in implementing change. Effects of the daily isolation of school nurses can be minimized by addressing health care threats beyond institutional boundaries, communicating with other school nurses, building coalitions around similar issues, and taking collective action.

THE CONTEXT OF SCHOOL HEALTH

The delivery of health services in the schools has been traced back several centuries in Europe, but "modern school health" began in the early 1800s in Great Britain and in the later half of the 19th century in the United States (Pigg, 1992). The health and social needs of poor immigrant children stimulated professional and philanthropic groups to provide noneducational services in school settings. As health and social services became an integral part of the schools, attention turned to improving school attendance and preparing students for gainful employment (Tyack, 1992). The first medical officer in schools was appointed in 1894 in Boston to inspect the children and the school environment for unhealthy and unsanitary conditions. The first school nurse was appointed in 1902 in New York City schools to increase school attendance by health education efforts and follow-up home visits of known cases of communicable disease (Wold, 1981). Within 20 years, school health services spread to more than 300 cities and, through developments in education, health, and legislative activities, expanded programs to include the total health of the child (Table 25–1). The World War I draft revealed several preventable health problems and gave impetus to the need for health education in school programs (Kort, 1984). From these early beginnings, school health was conceptualized as a tripartite activity: delivering health services, providing health education, and ensuring a safe school environment.

In the United States, policies that shape school health programs are established by state legislative, executive, and judicial bodies. Although local schools retain considerable autonomy, state policies determine direction, resources, and standards (Lovato et al., 1989). Several recent federal initiatives have significance for reshaping school health. About one third of the 1990 health objectives for the nation relate to children and youth and have been presented in an agenda for schools (Allensworth and Wolford, 1988). The 1991 establishment of Healthy People 2000 extends many of the earlier objectives and directly relates to two of the eight national education goals. The ready to learn goal has been operationalized in a seven-step mandate to the nation emphasizing the relationship between health and academic achievement (Boyer, 1991). The goal of eliminating violence and drugs from schools requires significant investment in safe environments and delivering culturally sensitive health education (Cohen et al., 1994). Decreasing violence requires school health professionals to be active participants in designing comprehensive, multidimensional approaches using education, regulatory, and technologic means.

The challenge to deliver culturally sensitive school health services intensifies with the projection that by the year 2000 more than half the U.S. population will be members of various cultural-ethnic subgroups, with Latinos representing the largest segment. The school population also includes children from families of immigrants, refugees, and visitors from other countries. Conflicts are expected between the Western scientific values and approaches to health promotions and maintenance and the values and approaches of other cultural groups attending school. School health professions can enhance their effectiveness and contribute to the quality of community life by conducting cultural assessments of the school populations and adapting school health programs accordingly. Tensions will likely continue until the ethnic mix and geographic distribution of school health professionals reflect the population served.

Until recently, school health has been underemphasized and neglected as a potential avenue to influence children and youth. The critical state of students' health and discussions of health reform has helped policymakers recognize that no other institution has the potential for impact on all children between the ages of 5 and 16 years (the legal age at which students can drop out). The urgency for reform is intensified as enrollments increase in elementary and secondary schools. Since 1985 increased student enrollments are most marked in elementary schools, but this pattern will change between 1994 and 2000 with projected increases of 8% in elementary schools and 12% in secondary schools (National Center for Education Statistics, 1994). In addition, increasing numbers of students are being served in programs for the disabled and impaired, currently representing about 12% of the students. Consolidation of schools with lower enrollments has decreased the total number of schools to 85,000 in the 50 states.

The magnitude of children's health needs demands a comprehensive conceptualization of school health. In Figure 25–2, Nader paired health status with educational achievement and suggested that these outcomes require a partnership between and among the schools, the family, the media, and the community. The interplay of these factors reflects the reality of students' lives; the impact of school is reinforced or undermined by forces beyond school boundaries. For example, when the school conducts an antismoking campaign and community groups reinforce the school's perspective, the media could undermine this health-promoting effort through cigarette commercials unless family and friends intervene.

INDICATORS OF SCHOOL HEALTH STATUS

Although morbidity and mortality from infectious diseases have declined markedly, America's children are worse off than their parents' generation both economically and culturally (Fuchs and Reklis, 1992). Children now have the highest poverty rate of any age group; more than 20% of American children grow up in poverty, but in some geographic regions the poverty rate reaches 33%. The shift from two-parent to one-parent families and maternal employment affects all children, but especially minority children.

In 1993 more than 9 million children had no health insurance, an increase of about 1 million in 1 year (U.S. GAO, 1994). Although all children need regular health services for preventive care and treatment of medical conditions, poor children do not have access to regular health care because of insufficient numbers of available caregivers and lack of convenient transportation. For example, of the 19 million children eligible for Medicaid's Early and Periodic Screening, Diagnosis, and Treatment (EPSDT) program in 1992, fewer than 7 million had been screened. Only about half of all elementary school children routinely receive health care; slightly more than two thirds receive regular dental care.

Adolescents present unique and complex health issues, and they face formidable barriers in trying to obtain health care (U.S. Congress OTA, 1991). Members of minority groups and the poor are particularly at risk and experience even greater difficulty in seeking assistance with the profound physical and psychosocial changes experienced in the second decade of life. Nearly three quarters of all adolescent deaths are from motor vehicle accidents, unintentional injuries, homicide, and suicide (Kann et al., 1995). The Centers for Disease Control and Prevention attributed substantial morbidity and social problems to six categories of priority health risk behaviors: unintentional and intentional injuries, tobacco use, alcohol and other drug use, unsafe sexual behaviors, unhealthy dietary behaviors, and physical inactivity. The high school graduation rate has been declining over the past decade: only 69% of students graduated with a high school diploma over the last 3 years of the 1980s (Center for the Study of Social Policy, 1992).

Student absenteeism concerns all professional staff because it reduces the quantity and quality of education and is associated with academic failure and school dropout. Research suggests that school absenteeism is associated with poverty, poor health, and ethnicity (Kornguth, 1991). Nationally, school-age children miss approximately 3.8 days of school per year, and the number of school loss days per year per 100 children has not changed significantly over the past two decades. However, absenteeism is not equally distributed throughout the population, and a student who misses more than 11% of the school days in a semester has difficulty remaining at grade level (Klerman, 1988). National high school dropout rates have declined, but in 1990 350,000 students dropped out, nearly 30% of whom were Hispanic (Lewitt, 1992).

Between 10% and 30% of all students have serious health problems; chronic illnesses and impairments affect about 2 million children (Perrin et al., 1992). Chronic illness may affect a child's ability to participate fully in regular school activities. Many children with chronic disabilities require special education services as identified in federal legislation.

Table 25–2 provides an overall assessment of the outcomes of the health care and education systems by state. Child well-being is a composite score derived from an analysis of a number of federal reports on eight variables: child poverty, low-birth-weight infants, infant mortality, child deaths, teen violent deaths, teen out-of-wedlock births, juvenile incarceration, and high school graduations (Center for the Study of Social Policy, 1991). The education expenditure per pupil reflects all monies allocated to per pupil costs divided by average daily attendance. The Scholastic Aptitude Test (SAT) score reflects the state average on the verbal and math sections; a perfect score is 1600 (National Center for Educational Statistics, 1989).

Table 25–1

Chronology of Events Significant in the History of School Health Services

Developments in School Health Services		Developments in Education	
1834–1892	First school physicians and nurses hired in Europe	1800	Child labor reform and emergence of a public education system
1894	First medical inspections began in Boston schools to identify and exclude students with communicable disease. No follow-up.	1890	Responsibility for school health assigned to local school boards because health departments not in existence in every town. Minimal school health instruction

Communicable Disease Control

1900	Classroom inspections expand to include screening for ringworm, scabies, impetigo, malnutrition Proper hygiene practices demonstrated in school and home Minor cases of contagion treated at school (e.g., dressing changes)		
1902	Home visits for sanitary inspection, follow-up on excluded students, truancy, social problems; as a result, school attendance escalates		
1910	Emergency services now available in schools School inspections expand to individualized medical examinations to identify and correct defects	1910	School health instruction is combined with medical inspection; teachers rarely participate and health professionals do the health testing
1920	Red Cross provides school nursing services to rural America		
1924	Employee health services incorporated into school health; Roger's report recommends teachers have health exams and tuberculin tests		
1930	Mass screenings for early case finding (i.e., vision, hearing, dental caries, orthopedic defects) increasingly widespread Counseling, health education, and consultations offered in conjunction with health services	1930	Federal school lunch program starts (Department of Agriculture)
1934	School nurse–physician services are overextended and quality of services deteriorates (National Organization of Public Health Nursing [NOPHN] Study)		

Health Guidance and Consultation

1940	Nonstatutory ban on school-based diagnosis and treatment widely enforced	1940	First coordinated integrated health education curriculum developed

Developments in Pediatrics, Nursing, Public Health		Social and Legislative Developments	
1800	Fundamental discoveries in bacteriology	1897	First appropriation by states for care of handicapped children, Minnesota
1908	First Bureau of Child Hygiene established in New York City	1904	Child labor legislation
1909	School nursing services provided from visiting nurse associations First White House conference recommends Federal Children's Bureau		
1912	Discovery of numerous serious health defects among army recruits	1912	Act of 1912, Children's Bureau established
1913	School Nursing Committee created within the NOPHN; Lina Rogers Struthers, chair	1915	Rockefeller Foundation supports well-child clinics and milk stations
1918	Schools of Public Health open		
1920	All cities with population of 100,000+ have maternal and child health services in most state health departments Second White House conference advocates standards of MCH; consumer education is stressed School nurse established as faculty member in New York State and referred to as school nurse–teacher	1921 1924	Maternity and Infancy Act (Sheppard-Towner) provides federal grant-in-aid to states Alliance develops between the National Education Association and the American Medical Association: "health education, not health services is the proper role for the schools"
1926	National Organization for Public Health Nursing published its first statement on the objectives, scope of work, and methods in school nursing		
1927	American School Health Association is formed		
1930	American Academy of Pediatrics is formed	1935	Title V; Social Security Act enacted; Maternal and Child Health Care Services authorized
1937	School nurses become a section of the new Department of School Health and Physical Education of the National Education Association; eventually this section evolved into the National Association of School Nurses		
1939	Crippled Children's Services from State Health Department expand		
1940	Delegation of school nurse tasks to teachers, health clerks, volunteers Fifty percent of all public health nurses are employed in school health		

Table continued on following page

Table 25–1

Chronology of Events Significant in the History of School Health Services *(Continued)*

Developments in School Health Services		Developments in Education	
	First aid–emergency services closely identified with school nurses despite their "no more Band-Aids" campaign to delegate more responsibilities for non-nursing tasks to other school personnel		
	Services more public health oriented (e.g., coordinating community services for students)		
1945	School health councils advocated as a means for organizing school health programs		
1950	School health services under review by American Public Health Association, American Nurses Association, American School Health Association		

Primary Care

1960	Comprehensive health histories recommended in lieu of cursory school examinations; record keeping excessive and not effective for planning purposes	1960	Title I—Elementary and Secondary Education Act authorized provisions for health and nutrition services
1969	Introduction of the first pilot for school-based primary health care using school nurse practitioners (Denver public schools)	1970	Child find screenings begin to identify students eligible for special services under Handicapped Children's Act (PL94-142)
			White House Conference on Children and Youth recommendations for early childhood education and day care
1974	Special services available for students with disabilities, handicaps, chronic illness (i.e., medication administration, catheterization)		Immigration of Vietnamese–Indo-Chinese refugees with third world health problems; complex cultural and language barriers must be overcome
	New school health personnel (clerks, occupational therapist, physical therapist, psychologist, speech pathologist, substance abuse counselors)	1978	School Health Education Study produces comprehensive curriculum models for health education (Grades k–12)
1979	Private agencies (including hospitals) assume the management of some school health programs on an experimental basis in New York State	1979	"Growing Healthy" curriculum adopted nationwide; well-validated program reported to produce health behavior changes in elementary school students
			Teenager health modules will develop later and will also be disseminated nationally

Developments in Pediatrics, Nursing, Public Health		Social and Legislative Developments	
1941	First edition of *The Nurse in the School* published by the Joint Committee of the National Education Association and the American Medical Association (second edition released in 1955)		
1944	Selective service reports U.S. Army recruits have numerous health defects		
	Committee on School Nursing Policies and Practices of the American School Health Association established (name changed in 1958 to School Nursing Committee and since the late 1960s referred to as the Study Committee on School Nursing)		
1949	Significant increases in number of school nurses employed by health departments		
1950	White House conference demands ban on racial public school segregation	1954	Brown v. Board of Education; civil rights case that overturned the "separate but equal" doctrine in public schools
	Concept of school health team develops		
1960	White House Conference on Children and Youth has youth participation for the first time; profound concern about drug abuse, increases in the incidence of venereal diseases, illegitimate births, inadequate opportunities for youth employment, and concern for the environment	1960	"New Frontier," "Great Society," "War on Poverty" Partnership for Health act—comprehensive neighborhood health centers
1961	National Institute of Child Health and Human Development, a national center for basic research in child development, established	1963	MCH funds authorized for children and youth projects
1962	Two thirds of school nurses are employed by Boards of Education; number of nurses increases to 30,000	1965	Headstart Title V; Social Security Act; provides preschool health, education
			Medicaid, medical services for low-income families (Title XIX)
1969	School nurse practitioner program developed at the University of Colorado in conjunction with Denver public schools		National Health Promotion–Disease Prevention campaign underway with release of the Surgeon General's report on smoking
1970	Position statement "Role of the School Nurse Practitioner" developed by various public health, school health, and medical associations	1970	Family Planning Services and Population Research Act (P.L. 94-142); Education of the Handicapped legislation
			Rehabilitation Act of 1973
			Early Periodic Screening, Diagnosis, and Treatment (Title XIX, Social Security Act); comprehensive and preventive health services for diagnosis and treatment of physical and mental defects
1975	National Association of State School Nurse Consultants organized		
1976	Of the 50 states 23 have mandatory school nurse certification requirements; 10 states have permissive legislation	1973	Child Abuse Act (P.L. 93-247)
		1974	The Education of All Handicapped Children Act (P.L. 94-142) helps states provide a free and appropriate public education
1978	Declaration of Alma-Ata "Health for all by the year 2000"	1975	School-based initiative developed, states improve on child abuse reporting laws and include school personnel

Table continued on following page

Table 25–1
Chronology of Events Significant in the History of School Health Services *(Continued)*

Developments in School Health Services	Developments in Education
Health Promotion–Special Needs	
1980 National School Health Services Program, Robert Wood Johnson Foundation (1980–1985); demonstrates effectiveness of school-based diagnosis and treatment by school nurse practitioners; emphasis on elementary schools	1980 School reform movement underway; parent participation increases Carnegie Foundation Report *Turning Points* recommends numerous changes in middle school, including the establishment of family resource centers and a new role for a health coordinator Student assistance programs to prevent drug and alcohol abuse proliferate under the leadership of guidance counselors
1986 The School Based Adolescent Health Care Program (SBAHC), Robert Wood Johnson Foundation. Increased the number of school-based health centers with diagnostic and treatment services (1986–1992); school-based clinics now concentrate on adolescent services; main obstacles: conservative public opinion, financing, integration with the rest of school health program; disease prevention, health promotion services flourish: health hazard appraisals; fitness-endurance-cardiovascular risk screening; student health fairs	1987 Youth 2000 campaign launched by the business community to combat the school dropout problem; Division of Adolescent and School Health, Center for Chronic Disease Prevention and Health Promotion, Centers for Disease Control established
1990 Clinical services, health education, health promotion, environmental measures increasingly overlap; growing emphasis on environmental health	1990 Individuals with Disabilities Education Act (IDEA) 1994 Goals 2000: Educate America Act (P.L. 103-227). Safe Schools Act Gun Free Schools Act

Although the validity of SAT scores as criteria of educational quality is diminished by the low percentage of students sitting for the examination, there is little else available for national comparisons (Lehnen, 1992). Table 25–2 reflects considerable variation across states in relation to child-well being, education expenditures, and education performance. Further analysis suggests a positive relationship among education expenditures, education performance, and child well-being (Baker, 1994).

Students' complex social and health problems, coupled with the fragmentation and inequity of health care services, challenge school health professionals to be more creative in addressing sociopolitical issues and to be more responsive to the needs of students. How can school health professionals strengthen the effort to decrease the "new morbidities" (Dryfoos, 1994)? What can school health programs contribute to decreasing the rate of fatal accidents among children? What lessons do children learn when their school buses do not have seat belts (Reilly, 1995)? What

relationship exists among the students' gender, ethnicity, and socioeconomic status and school absence, suspension, and dropout?

COMPONENTS OF SCHOOL HEALTH

From the beginning, school health has been conceptualized as including three interdependent components: school health services, school health education, and healthful school environment.

School Health Services

The provision of health care in the schools is aimed at promoting health and removing health barriers to learning (Meeker et al., 1986). School health services include:

- Basic care: minor complaints and first aid services that are ordinarily not recorded in health records

Developments in Pediatrics, Nursing, Public Health		Social and Legislative Developments	
1980	AIDS epidemic fully recognized	1980	Refugee Education Assistance Act
1983	*Standards for School Nursing Practice,* a set of guidelines for nursing practice in the schools developed jointly by five professional health and nursing organizations, published by the American Nurses Association	1981	Select Panel for the Promotion of Child Health
		1986	Education of the Handicapped Act Amendments (P.L. 99-457) (Part H); program for infants and toddlers with handicaps
1989	Position statement "Role of the School Nurse in Disease Prevention, Health Promotion and Health Protection" receives American School Health Association endorsement	1988	The Technology-Related Assistance for Individuals with Disabilities (P.L. 100-407)
1990	Bureau of Maternal and Child Health reestablished		
	National health agenda and objectives for the year 2000 launched	1990	Americans with Disabilities Act
1991	Nursing's agenda for health care reform		
	Healthy People 2000 agenda promoted		
1993	Comprehensive Child Immunization Act (P.L. 103-66)	1993	President Clinton proposes Health Security Act
1993	*School Nursing Practice: Roles and Standards* published by National Association of School Nurses		

Adapted from Office of School Health, University of Colorado Health Sciences Center, 1991.

(examples: cleaning a skin abrasion and applying a bandage, answering questions about personal hygiene, or providing referrals to other health professionals)

- Primary care: acute and chronic complaints that do require follow-up and documentation (examples: monitoring immunizations, responding to a playground emergency, or following up on early insulin reaction)
- Physical examinations: health assessments like those required by such federal programs as EPSDT or as required for participation in some school activity
- Screenings: assessment of vision, hearing, scoliosis, and other conditions, usually conducted on groups of children according to specific age or grade level
- Specialized care: special health services for anyone with disabilities or conditions specified in federal legislation (P.L. 94-142, P.L. 99-457, and P.L.

101-476); requirements include an individualized health care plan developed by an interdisciplinary team to guide delivery of such health care needs as ongoing medication administration and various health procedures like catheterizations or tube feedings.

There is a legal basis for school health services in 33 states; mandated services exist in 28 states (Lovato et al., 1989). The designated state-level professional responsible for coordinating school health may be employed in the education department, health department, or some other agency.

School Health Education

The provision of health instruction is aimed at knowledge, attitudes, and behavior that maintain and enhance wellness and prevent or minimize disease (Davis et al., 1985). School health education includes:

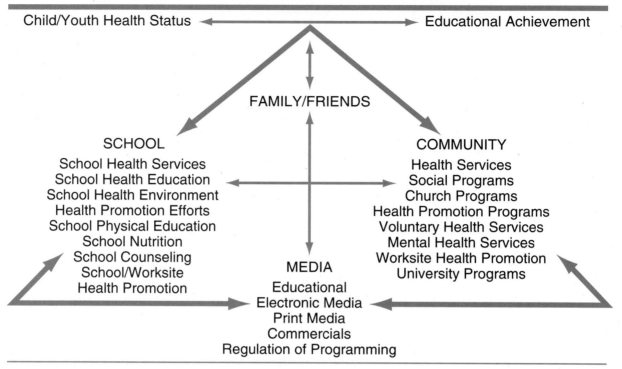

Figure 25–2
A model for school health in the 1990s. (From Nader PR: The concept of "comprehensiveness" in the design and implementation of school health programs. J School Health 60:134, 1990. Reprinted with permission of American School Health Association, Kent, OH, 1990.)

- Philosophy: beliefs about basing health education programs on local and global health priorities, presenting health education programs with methods adaptable to different learning styles, reinforcing health education programs by role models and healthy environment, and including participation of personnel from community health agencies
- Curriculum: planned, sequentially developed content delivered to students in kindergarten through Grade 12, aimed at fostering individual responsibility and self-care, coordinated with other academic subjects
- Personnel: adequately prepared teachers of health education programs and ongoing in-service programs to develop, deliver, and evaluate relevant programs; all teachers need preparation to integrate health education with other subjects and respond to incidental opportunities
- Students: recipients of school health education programs include school-age children and youth, parents and family, teachers, and others in the community significant to the students or the school

- Evaluation: ongoing assessment of programs requires input from school-age pupils, teachers, school district personnel, and parents and community members

The critical nature of school health education has been reinforced by numerous national and professional organizations (Allensworth and Wolford, 1988). School health education programs are mandated by 31 states and the District of Columbia, and the topics are specified in many of the laws (Lovato et al., 1989). The content of health instruction programs should be based on locally developed needs assessment efforts (Grunbaum et al., 1995).

Curriculum planning for health education programs is a multidisciplinary responsibility. The majority of the states have a plan for comprehensive school health education programs and information on excellent standardized curricula and educational resources. Innovative strategies are needed for multicultural health education programs, including multilingual classes.

Table 25–2
Education Expenditures, SAT Scores, and Child Well-Being by State, 1988

	Expenditures Per Student	Rank	SAT Score	Rank	Child Well-Being Rank
Alabama	2718	48	1002*	11	42
Alaska	7971	1	923	31	38
Arizona	3744	34	952*	24	44
Arkansas	2989	47	986*	17	40
California	3840	31	906	34	30
Colorado	4462	16	966	22	17
Connecticut	6230	4	908	33	6
Delaware	5017	11	903	37	36
Washington DC	6132	5	846	49	51
Florida	4092	25	887	44	45
Georgia	3434	39	847	48	50
Hawaii	3919	29	888	43	11
Idaho	2667	49	965*	23	18
Illinois	4369	19	982*	19	39
Indiana	3794	32	871	47	30
Iowa	4124	24	1084*	1	8
Kansas	4076	26	1040*	4	15
Kentucky	3011	45	996*	13	34
Louisiana	3138	43	986*	17	49
Maine	4258	20	897	39	12
Maryland	5201	9	914	32	33
Massachusetts	5471	6	905	35	3
Michigan	4692	15	972*	21	37
Minnesota	4386	18	1006*	10	4
Mississippi	2548	50	988*	16	47
Missouri	3786	33	989*	15	28
Montana	4246	21	992*	14	19
Nebraska	3943	28	1030*	6	14
Nevada	3623	37	926*	30	28
New Hampshire	4457	17	932	28	5
New Jersey	6564	3	894	41	16
New Mexico	3691	35	1015*	7	46
New York	7151	2	890	42	32
North Carolina	3368	41	836	51	41
North Dakota	3519	38	1067*	2	9
Ohio	3998	27	948*	25	23
Oklahoma	3093	44	1001*	12	27
Oregon	4789	13	927	29	25
Pennsylvania	4989	12	886	45	13
Rhode Island	5329	7	895	40	7
South Carolina	3408	40	838	50	48
South Dakota	3249	42	1041*	3	24
Tennessee	3068	46	1009*	9	43
Texas	3608	36	877	46	35
Utah	2454	51	1038*	5	2
Vermont	5207	8	905	35	1
Virginia	4149	23	902	38	22
Washington	4164	22	939	26	20
West Virginia	3858	30	939*	26	26
Wisconsin	4747	14	1013*	8	10
Average	$4243		903		

Sources: Calculated from Center for Education Statistics, 1989 and Center for the Study of Social Policy, 1991.

SAT, scholastic aptitude test

*Fewer than 25% of students sat for exam; average is 11% in 26 states.

From Baker CM: School health: policy issues in the 1990's. Nurs Health Care 15: 180, 1994. Reprinted with permission.

School Health Environment

The physical surroundings and psychosociocultural climate are critical to health because students and personnel work in schools for at least 180 days each year (Henderson, 1993). School health environment includes:

- Physical environment: geographic location, school site, and physical plant; school construction with asbestos and biological and chemical agents; conditions of air, temperature, lighting, noise, space; safety of labs, equipment, gym, cafeteria, playgrounds; accessibility for students and personnel; policies regarding fire and other disasters, school buses, smoking, drugs, firearms
- Psychosocial environment: emotional and social conditions influencing students and staff interactions and activities
- Cultural environment: values, beliefs, ethnicity, language, policies that affect students and staff communication and well-being

A legal basis for a healthful school environment exists in 40 states; mandated health and safety laws exist in 34 states (Lovato et al., 1989). Although procedures for monitoring school health environments differ from state to state, assessment of environmental health hazards and adherence to environmental policy is the responsibility of all school personnel (Adams et al., 1991). Violence, drugs, and smoking in schools constitute new threats to physical and psychosocial safety and challenge school health professionals to engage in prevention efforts (Cohen et al., 1994).

A healthy school environment has numerous opportunities to impact health beginning with state laws governing safety, school board decisions about healthy environments, and teachers and personnel serving as role models for health-promoting behavior.

During the past decade, the conceptualization of school health has been undergoing examination and debate in response to societal changes and students' "new morbidities." Assuming that education and health are inextricably intertwined, school health professionals are proposing that the three traditional components of school health services, school health education, and school health environment be expanded to include five additional components: physical education, school food and nutrition services, guidance and counseling, school psychology, and work site health promotion (Allensworth and Kolbe, 1987; Nader, 1990). Although some of these components

have been integrated in the traditional school health model, new knowledge and contemporary health issues support an expanded concept of school health.

All states have been surveyed regarding the legal basis of each component, program coordination and content, and personnel involved (Lovato et al., 1989). Physical education programs are aimed at enhancing physical fitness and developing motor skills while promoting health through regular exercise and emphasis on a healthy lifestyle. A legal basis for physical education exists in 40 states, but the amount of time required is far less than 1 hour per week. School food and nutrition services provide nutrition instruction and nutritionally adequate meals. In addition to federal legislation regarding school lunches and breakfasts, 32 states have established a legal basis for a food service program. Guidance and counseling are aimed at helping students (1) maximize their potential as responsible beings playing a variety of roles in society, (2) ease their transition from grade to grade, and (3) select career options. A legal basis for guidance and counseling exists in only 28 states; however, unlike all other school health personnel, guidance counselors must be certified for employment in 49 states. School psychology focuses on testing, placement, and clinical services. Federal legislation mainstreaming children with impairments has expanded responsibilities to include special education screening and assessments. Work site health promotion for school faculty and staff reflects a growing awareness of the influence of health on the learning environment and includes employee health examinations, health benefits, and wellness programs.

Few of the 15,000 school districts have implemented this comprehensive school health model because of inadequate financial resources, traditional philosophies, insufficient personnel, and the lack of political will. Questions about the comprehensive school health model are suggested by the critical question framework in Table 25–3. Some districts have embraced the Goals 2000 agenda, involved parents and families in more school activities, created coalitions with community agencies and higher education institutions, and strengthened the commitment to student health by forming school health councils (U.S. Department of Education, 1994). Some enlightened school boards recognize the relationship between parental involvement and quality education in a safe environment and support school health councils partnering with community agencies. The opposite extreme is reflected in some school districts where

Table 25-3
Framing Critical Questions About School Health Issues

1. Examine context of issue.
   When did circumstances-condition become an issue?
   What were the triggering events?
   How is the issue being described?
   Who knows, who cares, who benefits, who pays?

2. Appreciate dimensions of issue.
   What is unique history of issue?
   What commonalities exist with other issues?
   What previous efforts have been invested, by whom, and with what results?
   What position on this issue will benefit the vulnerable group?

3. Formulate strategy.
   How can issue be prevented in future?
   Who has power to facilitate and impede resolution?
   What resources are needed to resolve issue?
   What strategies can other groups offer?
   Which collective approaches are the most efficient and effective?

4. Implement plan
   Who has the courage and skill to lead?
   How can risks be minimized and shared and with whom?
   What communication strategies are required?

5. Evaluate outcomes.
   Has the issue been resolved and for how long?
   What price was paid and by whom?
   What gains were made and by whom?

on-site school health personnel and programs are discontinued for fiscal reasons and mandated services are provided by the local health department.

SCHOOL HEALTH FINANCING

School health programs in the United States represented less than 1% of the public schools' $278.8 billion expenditure in 1978, or about $940 million, amounting to $13 per student during the school year (Walker et al., 1990). Monies for school health programs are the second largest governmental investment in children's health care (Larson, 1990). These estimates are probably less than the total expenditure because they do not include lunch programs, nutrition services, and psychological counseling. Precise information is not available because national expenditure data have not been collected since 1980. School health services are funded by the local school district, local health department, state education department, state health department, federal monies, and voluntary philanthropy (Fox et al., 1992). Generally, public school budgets are financed about equally through local and state sources and least by federal sources. During 1987 to 1988, for example, school budgets were funded 49.5% by the states, 44.1% by local sources, and 6.3% by federal sources (National Center for Educational Statistics, 1989). School health services appear to be funded in similar proportions.

State Funding

Costs vary greatly by state depending on variations in state-mandated school health programs, history and tradition, economics, demographic characteristics of pupils, and power of various interest groups. The annual estimated expenditures for public school health services per pupil in 1980 range from a high of $247.55 in Alaska to a low of $1.16 in Washington, DC (Walker et al., 1990). Personnel is the largest expenditure in school health, with an estimated national number of 45,000 health professionals, 30,000 of whom are nurses (Committee on School Health, 1993). The diversity of priorities and funding mechanisms and the age and multiple sources of the data make state comparisons only suggestive.

Federal Funding

School health, as a part of education, is basically a legal responsibility of the states, although some federal legislation provides funding for health-related projects in school, and is administered through the states. Since the 1960s, several federal laws have funded school health projects designed for children with special needs, including services for the handicapped and disabled, nutritional supplements, protection from abuse, and improvements in the school environment (Cohen, 1990). National child health policy is limited principally to two government programs for handicapped and poor children and youth, namely the Maternal and Child Health Block Grant (Title V) and Medicaid (Title XIX) provisions of the Social Security Act. School environments are protected by several federal laws aimed at preventing and eliminating health hazards in relation to air and water quality, solid wastes, toxic substances, product safety, and accident prevention, to cite a few. Generally, state legislation parallels federal laws in these areas.

Private Funding

Although private monies provided nearly $4 for every $10 of children's health care in 1984, this funding source and private foundations provide a very small portion of school health budgets (Larson, 1990).

The costs and financing of school health programs vary greatly across the states; the principle source of support is from the states to fund mandated school health activities. Although the federal government contributes funds, they are program specific and eligibility is determined by the state. The overall picture of school health financing is one of inadequacy, inequity, and fragmentation (Baker, 1994).

SCHOOL HEALTH DELIVERY MODELS

Because school health is shared by both public health and public education, several different administrative patterns exist in the 15,000 public school districts. Each model has benefits and costs to be assessed in selecting an option consistent with the school district's vision and mission and the community's capacity.

In the traditional three-component model of school health, the school board has three alternatives for delivering services: (1) expect the public health department to provide mandated services, and seek additional programs within the limitations of the operating budget, (2) purchase additional services from the public health department at a level acceptable to both operating boards, or (3) hire its own school health personnel. Contracting services decreases the board's control over the services provided.

In the comprehensive school health model, three alternative approaches could be implemented, separately or combined. The school board could purchase school health services from the health department and other community agencies, the board could employ school health personnel directly, or the board could use both options. Whichever model is adopted, the school board has direct control over the services provided.

An alternative delivery model is school-based health centers (SBHCs) designed to provide easy access to students who do not receive needed health care (U.S. GAO, 1994). Today there are about 600 SBHCs in 40 states, up from 30 in the early 1980s; New York state leads with 140. Comprehensive services are provided by interdisciplinary teams. Primary health practitioners are usually on site, with links to established health facilities and donated services to provide comprehensive care. Overcoming the political and financial aspects of SBHCs requires dedicated school boards and creative managers (U.S. GAO, 1994; Rienzo and Button, 1993).

An emerging model is the full-service school in which students and their families have access to a full range of health, education, social, and cultural services (Igoe and Giordano, 1992). This package of services is delivered on site at school or in an adjacent building and is sometimes called the "one-stop" full-service school (Dryfoos, 1994). There are two unique features of this school-linked model: the services are supplied by an entity other than the school district, and program funding is primarily separate from the school district budget (Behrman, 1992). Dryfoos described 12 examples in which the community and the school board became partners in determining the mix of services needed and the funding sources available (Dryfoos, 1994). In a nationwide survey, funding issues were identified as the chief barrier to interagency collaboration (Hacker et al., 1994).

These school health delivery models reflect shifting paradigms and challenge school health professionals to provide visionary leadership, sophisticated management, and interdisciplinary collaboration in reengineering school health for the 21st century.

THE PRACTICE OF NURSING IN THE SCHOOLS

Nurses in the schools represent the major health profession required to implement the school health programs. As a speciality within the nursing profession, school nursing contributes directly to student education by identifying and preventing potential student health problems and intervening to remedy or modify school health problems (Proctor, 1990). Unique characteristics of school nursing include

- Practice based on generalist nursing knowledge of persons throughout the life cycle and specialist knowledge of children and youth
- Emphasis on health promotion, health maintenance, and disease prevention
- Practice in a non-health care environment: school, home, community
- Solo practice and usually the only health care professional in the school
- Care recipients are individuals, parents, groups, and aggregates

- Episodic and long-term practice within the time frame of the academic school year
- Practice requires professionalism, management principles, and interdisciplinary and interagency collaboration

PROFESSIONAL ORGANIZATIONS INVOLVED IN SCHOOL HEALTH

American Nurses Association
    Council of Community Nursing Practice
American Public Health Association
    School Health Education and Services
    Public Health Nursing
American School Health Association
    School Nurse Section
American Student Health Association
National Association of Pediatric Nurses
National Association of School Nurses
National Association of State School Nurse Consultants
National League for Nursing
    Council of Community Health Services
National School Health Education Coalition

The practice of nursing in the schools is influenced by the mission and philosophy of the local school board and the state's education and health departments. Nursing practice is regulated by the state's nurse practice act, case law, and the profession's standards for practice (Harrison et al., 1995). These documents will specify the scope of nursing practice, parameters of delegation, and qualifications of persons providing nursing care. Table 25–4 lists the standards for school nursing practice. Guidelines for implementing and documenting the standards within the school health nursing program are available from professional associations (Schwab, 1991; Snyder, 1991). The implementation of a school health program is described in "Life of a School Nurse" by a master's-prepared nurse practitioner working in a small rural community (Darnell, 1994).

LIFE OF A SCHOOL NURSE*

"Oh, I wouldn't be a school nurse—all you do is give out Band-Aids." "You will waste your talents as a nurse practitioner." These are a few of the comments I heard when I first went to "sub" as a nurse in our local school system in

---

*From Darnell, J.D.: Life of a school nurse. ISNA Bulletin 20:3, 7, 1994. Reprinted with permission from the Indiana State Nurses Association.

1991. I took the job full time when it became available. There is not a typical day in my job. I have found I must be extremely flexible.

At the beginning of the school year, it is the school nurse's job to make sure all students are adequately immunized. Another job at the beginning of school is to find out what health problems students have and to educate the teachers on these conditions. This year three students at the high school are experiencing panic attacks, one has agoraphobia, four are insulin-dependent diabetics (one of whom is pregnant), one has Tourette's syndrome, and another has lupus. Another task is to know which students are taking medications at school and to get permission slips signed by parents and instructions from the prescriber. I have taught teachers, bus drivers, and parents how to give injections for bee sting allergies and insulin reactions.

I alert teachers and staff how to care for certain situations. Before students arrive at the beginning of the school year, the other school nurse and I set up inservices for staff on universal precautions and distribute playground and room kits for emergency situations. We talk to parents about their children's health conditions and how they want them handled at school. In our school system we do not have any preschool children and do not presently have any high technologically dependent students. Soon after school starts we check all the elementary students for head lice. Our school has a nit-free policy, so we must recheck heads for a period of time.

During the month of September we record the height and weight of all elementary students. Then vision screening starts. Our local optometrists donate time to the school system and see all kindergarten, first, and third graders and any others who are referred by the teachers. It is the school nurse's job to check fifth, sixth, eighth, and tenth grade students. If a family cannot afford eye care when a referral is made, we do the paper work for referrals to the Lion's Club, local trustee, or Salvation Army.

We screen fifth, sixth, seventh, eighth, and ninth graders for scoliosis. As school nurses we also assist with family life education in the fifth and sixth grades. Both of us are certified CPR [cardiopulmonary resuscitation] instructors and provide adult CPR classes for sixth graders. The middle school students have infant and child classes added. I do CPR classes for the high school advanced health classes and we also offer CPR classes for staff. We arrange for the local dentists to speak to all kindergarten and first grade students regarding dental health and dental hygienists dressed as Snoopy visit the second graders. In the summer we assist with sports physicals for the middle school and the high school.

We are part of the crisis intervention team. We are both representatives on the Drug Free Schools Committee and part of the student services team that meets monthly. The other school nurse is the representative to the Step Ahead Council in the community, and she is a member of the State Departments of Education and Public Health School Nurse Consortium that meets every other month. We work with the American Cancer Society and the American Heart Association. We have literature available and are resource centers for many in the community regarding health issues. This means working closely with the public health nurses, with the

Family and Social Services Administration (welfare office), and with probation officers. I have a support group for pregnant teens and teen moms who are in school. We are also responsible for assisting staff who receive hepatitis B vaccine and for developing health policies for the school board to approve. We may be on the AIDS education committee, health curriculum committee, and asked to represent the school in other ways in the community.

As school nurses we try to have the clinics covered in the two largest schools at all times. We provide support and inservice to the secretaries who cover the clinics in the buildings that are not staffed full time. We find that we have been seeing an increasing number of students in the clinics every day. We keep records of all the students who come through the clinics and, even though I do not usually even write down the students who come in for Band-Aids, we still have close to thirty students a day through the clinic.

On a typical day a student may want to know if they should see the doctor for a rash, a hurt finger, sore throat, stomach ache, etc. It may be someone needing to talk about the home situation, suicidal thoughts, parents drinking, a friend who is having problems, possible pregnancy, or a multitude of other situations. Some people say this is the school counselor's job, but some students feel more comfortable talking to the school nurse. Then we have the minor (sometimes major) injuries which occur, acute illnesses, medications to administer, and other routine situations. I have monitored blood pressures for some students.

At the elementary school, the other nurse has a post-heart transplant student who is on many medications. We find we must educate students on medications that they take and sometimes we must educate the family and staff. We are involved in student conferences regarding placement of students.

We may see a potential problem arising. Recently I had two students in one day who either passed out or were close to doing so. Upon investigation I discovered that neither student had eaten for approximately 24 hours. This was the way they had decided to diet. Even though I talked to both students about the dangers of not eating and counseled them on ways to diet, I spoke to the health teacher and asked her to cover the dangers of starvation diets in her classes. Further follow-up will be done.

As school nurses we are also responsible for staff health. Last year while accompanying a student group to Mexico, a staff member suffered a heart attack. I was able to observe health care in a rural Mexican community and was very fortunate in that the physician was Mexican-American and a board certified internist. My Spanish is minimal. The teacher had lived in Mexico for four years and was very comfortable with the language. Most of what we do for staff is monitor blood pressure, weight, occasionally blood sugar, and do a considerable amount of education regarding their health.

Stress reduction for staff and students is a big part of the job for both of us. We educate everyone on relaxation techniques and try to practice what we teach. We try to find out why certain students miss too much school or want to spend all of the time in the clinic. We work with teachers and principals on this type of problem. Home visits are some-

times part of our agenda. We are also on the alert for potential hazards in the environment of our schools. If we have students hospitalized, we may need to contact the family at the hospital.

In our school system we have a nurse/student ratio of 1:1500. In some school systems this ratio is 1:3000 or more. The recommended ratio is 1:750 if the students are not classified as high risk and less if they are.

The role of the school nurse is multifaceted and requires many skills. As a nurse practitioner I consider my role to be primary care. I do case management and educate students/staff regarding good health habits and practices. This summer at the American Nurses Association Convention I heard that to do primary care you have to be where the clientele are. I believe that is what I do.

Table 25–4
Roles and Standards of School Nursing Practice

The School Nurse . . .

1. Utilizes a distinct clinical knowledge base for decision-making in nursing practice.
2. Uses a systematic approach to problem-solving in nursing practice.
3. Contributes to the education of the student with special health needs by assessing the student, planning and providing appropriate nursing care, and evaluating the identified outcomes of care.
4. Uses effective written, verbal, and nonverbal communication skills.
5. Establishes and maintains a comprehensive school health program.
6. Collaborates with other school professionals, parents, and caregivers to meet the health, developmental, and educational needs of clients.
7. Collaborates with members of the community in the delivery of health and social services and utilizes knowledge of community health systems and resources to function as a school-community liaison.
8. Assists students, families, and the school community to achieve optimal levels of wellness through appropriately designed and delivered health education.
9. Contributes to nursing and school health through innovations in practice and participation in research or research-related activities.
10. Identifies, delineates, and clarifies the nursing role, promotes quality of care, pursues continued professional enhancement, and demonstrates professional conduct.

From National Association of School Nurses, Inc., P.O. Box 1300, Scarborough, ME 04074, (207) 883-2117. For further information, you may obtain the following publications: *School Nursing Practice Roles and Standards 1993* and *Evaluating School Nursing Practice: A Guide for Administrators.*

Roles and functions implemented by the 30,000 nurses employed in school health are varied and complex (Thurber et al., 1991). The nurse's education and certification, plus the requirements of the specific state department of education, influence the day-to-day activities (Woodfill and Beyrer, 1991). The majority of the school health nurses are baccalaureate prepared and function as generalists. Some states require certification by the Department of Education; other states offer opportunity for certification. Graduate preparation is held by many school nurses, some in nursing and some in related fields. Speciality certification opportunities are available from national professional nursing associations. Overall, the current education profile of school nurses reflects the mix found in the nation's nursing profession (Oda, 1993).

PREPARATION FOR PROFESSIONAL SCHOOL HEALTH NURSING

EDUCATION	OCCUPATION
BSN	Generalist practice
MSN	Specialist roles: clinical specialist, nurse practitioner, community health nurse, nurse administrator/consultant
CERTIFICATION	**AGENCY**
Professional National (voluntary)	American Nurses Credentialing Center (BSN minimum requirement, MSN for some) National Association of School Nurses (RN plus 3 years experience required)
GOVERNMENTAL	
State (mandatory in some states)	State Education Agency (RN plus baccalaureate degree)

BSN, bachelor of science in nursing; MSN, master of science in nursing; RN, registered nurse.

Some reflective nurse faculty members are examining questions about the type of education needed to be an effective school health nurse in the 21st century and the credentials needed to be an inspiring faculty role model (Igoe, 1995; Passarelli, 1994). The complexity and diversity of the clients and the community systems require graduate preparation for the anticipated roles of school nurse practitioner and school nurse manager (Igoe and Speer, 1992). School nurse practitioners are prepared to deliver primary health care within an interdisciplinary setting (Meeker et al., 1986). School nurse managers are prepared to function as case managers and program administrators (Kozlak,

1992). Comprehensive education in nursing administration is required to direct the activities of unlicensed school nurse aides, implement self-directed work teams, and engage in interdisciplinary and interagency collaboration (Davis and Allensworth, 1994; Polivka, 1995; Yoder-Wise, 1995).

LEVELS OF PREVENTION

The school health nurse's practice is based on preventing health problems that may interfere with the student's education and the faculty and staff performance. There are unlimited opportunities to implement prevention efforts.

Many primary prevention activities are mandated by law (e.g., immunizations for entry into kindergarten, education programs on various health topics, and environmental safety efforts). Local conditions of the school district may warrant other types of primary preventive services (e.g., educational programs to prevent substance abuse, sexually transmitted diseases, violence, or suicide) (Lavin et al., 1992).

Health education, a major component in the school health model, aims at teaching students about their bodies, healthy lifestyles, and the health care system. Several nationally tested health education curricula are available; in addition, many state departments of health and education have adapted health education programs to their unique needs. Primary prevention strategies used in the schools could range from formal educational programs with standardized curricula to collaborating with other school personnel in environmental assessment to incidental one-on-one teaching.

Secondary prevention activities are aimed at early detection and treatment to limit disability (e.g., Medicaid's EPSDT program for students younger than 21 years). Some states have mandated screening for vision and hearing disorders and scoliosis, height and weight monitoring, physical examinations before physical education and sports, and health risk appraisal. Case finding is a secondary prevention strategy frequently used in the schools. The school nurse uses every opportunity to identify students at risk by following up on frequent school absences, dropouts, classroom disturbances, accident-prone students, and subtle cues of physical and emotional distress. All states require school personnel to report any evidence of child abuse (physical, verbal, sexual, and neglect). Most states have a school nurse consultant to offer advice on strategies appropriate for individual school districts. Some school nurses have created a surveillance system to gather frequency data that suggest potential problem areas; others have used family tree and personal lifestyle inventories as assessment tools.

Tertiary prevention activities are aimed at correcting and preventing further disability. Written policies regarding administration of prescribed medications in schools are required for student safety and personnel protection. State laws and local policies are in place in relation to students and staff with human immunodeficiency virus or AIDS and the handling and disposing of body fluids. Federal legislation providing access to school for children with chronic and handicapping conditions has created the need for school nurses to (1) become case managers and develop individualized health plans (IHPs) to complement the individualized educational program (IEP) and (2) lead the development and evaluation of protocols governing complex nursing procedures in the schools. Tertiary prevention strategies applied to the school staff include monitoring the work reentry of chronically ill personnel and follow-up on work site injuries.

NURSING PROCESS

Professional practice standards are based on the nursing process, and school nurses apply the nursing process when working with students, families, and school personnel in a variety of situations and environments.

The nursing process is the method and organizing framework for dealing with many situations in the school environment, including individualized client care.

During the past 10 years, several pieces of federal legislation have been passed to provide access to school for children with chronic and handicapping conditions (see Table 25–1). Some of the legislation requires school nurse participation in developing IEPs; about one third of the states mandate school nurse participation. Coupled with the complex nursing care required by these children are the demands represented by the "new morbidities" and a national call for school reform and accountability. Many school nurses are challenged by these events and are adopting case management as a more efficient and effective model within which to apply, document, and communicate the nursing process.

Seven Minnesota school nurses have developed a systematic organized way to use the nursing process in formulating the IHPs required by federal legislation (Haas et al., 1993). Perhaps more important for the practice of school nursing, they have integrated the nursing process with a nursing documentation format and the special education process (Table 25–5). This comprehensive approach to individual student care showcases the specialized knowledge and skill that characterize professional nursing, specifies nursing interventions, documents client care outcomes, and serves as the communication tool when the school nurse is participating in interdisciplinary planning.

Table 25–5
Nursing Process as Applied to School Nursing Practice

Steps	Nursing Process Documentation Format	Pertinent Questions	Special Education Process
Assessment			
Data collection	S: Subjective data	For individuals, what does the client and family think and say? For groups and communities, what do the members think and say?	Student's and family's perception of the problem at staffings
	O: Objective data	What is observed, measured, and reported? What are the pertinent norms and standards?	Teacher referrals Child study team assessment activities

Table 25–5
Nursing Process as Applied to School Nursing Practice *Continued*

Steps	Nursing Process Documentation Format	Pertinent Questions	Special Education Process
Assessment			
Diagnosis	A: Assessment	According to the nurse's perception and judgment, what is happening? What are the concerns? What is the resulting impact? Diagnosis = problem + etiology + response	Child study team's identification of the problems and goals Statement of the student's level of educational functioning
Intervention			
Plan	P: Plan	What are the desired outcomes? What action will be taken (educational, therapeutic, diagnostic, supportive) by whom, when, and how? What behaviors will be measured?	Individualized Education Plan (IEP) goals, objectives
Implementation	I: Implementation	Who is carrying out the plan? What agencies and others are involved?	Instructional Implementation Plan IIP
Evaluation			
	E: Evaluation	Have the desired outcomes been achieved according to the set criteria?	Evaluation according to measurements and review dates incorporated into objectives
	R: Reassessment	Is more information needed? Have changes or adaptations occurred?	Review staffing
	Plan	Have priorities changed? Does the plan or implementation method need revision?	
	Reevaluation	What are the new strategies and next steps?	

From Haas MB, Gerber MJ, Miller WR, et al. The School Nurse's Source Book of Individualized Healthcare Plans, vol. 1. North Branch, MN, Sunrise River Press, 1993, p. 7. Reprinted with permission from Sunrise River Press.

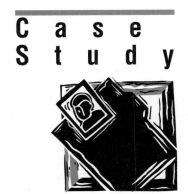

Case Study

You are a school nurse in a rural district of 2000 students. You have a part-time health aide that helps you every morning from 8 AM to 12 PM. You have three school buildings, including two elementary schools and a combination junior-senior high school. You have four diabetic students in the district, one at the elementary school and three at the combined high school. It is the second week of August, and you get a call from the principal asking you to call the parent of an elementary student. The student, 12-year-old Judy, has been diagnosed with diabetes over the summer. The principal mentions that you should figure out what the school needs to do. The principal says she wants to ensure that the other students not see Judy using a needle at school, and she is also concerned that the teacher will not know what to do in an emergency.

You call the parent and learn that Judy is a sixth-grade student at North Elementary. She was diagnosed with diabetes about 2 months ago. She lives with her mother, father, and two brothers on a farm. She has about a 10-mile bus ride to school. Judy did well in school until last year, when her attendance was poor and she had difficulty keeping up in the classroom. She had started a special education program during the last year. She is on a three-dose a day schedule of medication. She will need to have insulin at school before lunch. She has been learning to test her own glucose level using a glucometer and to keep her own records. Her food intake and exercise patterns are difficult to regulate because she has started her growth spurt.

Judy plays basketball with her brothers and is on a recreation league team. In summer she helps out on the farm. She has been anxious about starting school this fall because she is afraid that the other girls will tease her about the diabetes. Judy has had several insulin reactions during the past weeks and has been back to the physician twice for blood tests.

What can you do to help Judy and her family successfully adapt to this school year? Who else needs to be involved? What should you do first? What kinds of nursing care will Judy require this year? What additional data do you need? What kinds of outcomes do you want to achieve? How should Judy's IHP look? Does she need an emergency care plan as well?

Using the nursing process you decide that more data are needed. You call the parent to set up a time to meet with Judy's mother to discuss Judy's needs at school. You also ask the parent's permission to obtain information from Judy's physician. Finally, you suggest that Judy might like to come to school, bring her equipment, and go through her usual activities before school starts so that she feels comfortable. You also talk with the principal about reserving a 30-minute time block on teacher in-service day before school starts to talk about Judy's needs and those of two other new students with chronic health conditions.

After meeting with Judy and her mother and reviewing the physician's information, orders, and recommendations, you develop the following IHP.

Assessment

Physician information: Judy has type I diabetes. Her insulin is being regulated carefully because she continues to have reactions. Physician's orders include blood glucose check at 12 PM. Report levels greater than 200. Assist Judy to self-administer insulin as necessary. Treat insulin reactions with oral glucagon. Transport to emergency room if unconscious or unable to arouse.

Nursing assessment data:

Individual
- History of insulin reactions
- No sensory impairments on screening
- Has grown 2 inches since last year, has lost 2 pounds
- No signs of infection
- Needs to learn appropriate self-care for diabetes
- Is concerned about peer relations

Case study adapted from Haas MB, Gerber MJ, Miller WB, et al. The School Nurse's Source Book of Individualized Healthcare Plans, vol. 1. North Branch, MN, Sunrise River Press, 1993, pp. 49–51. Reprinted with permission from Sunrise River Press.

- Knows major concepts about diabetes but does not have a good understanding of the effects of diet and exercise
- States she is embarrassed by need to give insulin at school

Family

- Needs to increase knowledge of diabetes and disease management principles
- Ability of family members to give emotional and physical support during crises and noncrises
- Willingness to participate in diabetes-related community groups
- Family health history and health maintenance patterns

Community

- Identify peers with diabetes in other community groups
- Accessibility of diabetes-related community groups and activities for Judy and family
- Availability of educational resources for adolescents and families

Diagnosis

Individual

- Knowledge deficit related to recent onset of diabetes, need to balance diet and exercise and give insulin
- Potential for self-esteem disturbance resulting from embarrassment about need for medication, concerns about social stigma, and threats of academic problems
- Potential for physiologic imbalance resulting from metabolic changes

Family

- Knowledge deficit related to diabetes and community resources
- Altered family processes related to daughter's diabetes and insulin reactions

Community

- Knowledge deficit related to diabetes among school staff and bus driver

Planning

Planning involves mutual goal setting and joint contracting. In all cases it is important to develop the IHP with input from the parents and student. Use the IHP as a means of contracting with Judy to increase Judy's ability to participate in her care. Especially with older students, it is important to their self-esteem to be a partner in the planning process. The school nurse drafts a plan and gives Judy a copy to review with her parents. Both Judy and her parents are asked to sign the IHP as an indication of their agreement and willingness to participate.

Individual

Long-Term Goals

- Judy meets school nurse regularly to review adjustment to diabetes.
- Judy joins support group of students with diabetes.

Short-Term Goals

- Judy follows schedule for blood testing and insulin injection.
- Judy draws medication correctly and uses good injection technique.
- Judy continues participation in sports.

Family

Long-Term Goal
- Family exhibits increased ability to manage crises.

Short-Term Goals
- Family develops an emergency care plan for Judy and themselves.
- Family uses consultation to strengthen communication skills.
- Family seeks information about available support groups and youth services.

Community

Long-Term Goal
- Invite local chapter of American Diabetes Association to provide ongoing educational materials and programs.

Short-Term Goals
- In-service school staff intervenes appropriately.
- Share emergency plan with classroom and physical education teachers and school bus driver.
- Offer learning materials for classroom use.

Intervention

The IHP will be implemented; additional interventions will be based on the needs of the various clients: student, family, school staff, and community.

Individual
- Seek counseling opportunities to strengthen self-esteem, assertiveness, and communication skills.
- Provide educational opportunities to facilitate healthy adolescence and academic success.

Family
- Hold periodic family conferences to review health maintenance patterns.
- Consult regarding revision of emergency care plan.
- Follow up on questions regarding education materials and group activities.
- Highlight youth services programs and camp experiences by American Diabetes Association.

Community
- Provide periodic educational updates to school staff and bus driver.
- Offer consultation to health teacher regarding implications of chronic disease for adolescents' development.
- Share information about American Diabetes Association's comprehensive educational programs.
- Communicate needs of school health programs to appropriate community groups and policymakers.

Evaluation

Evaluation strategies focus on both process and outcomes and involve the individual, family, and community levels.

Individual

- Insulin reactions will be identified early by Judy or teachers, and appropriate action will be taken.
- Judy will demonstrate increasing knowledge and skill in diet, exercise, and medication management.
- Judy will demonstrate good coping skills by feeling less embarrassed and better able to handle questions and concerns of friends.

Family

- Family verbalizes needs for additional information.
- Family experiences increased adaptation to Judy's illness.
- Family uses community programs as necessary.

Community

- Teachers and staff are able to identify student's needs and take appropriate action.
- Students recognize and respond to Judy's need for acceptance.

RESEARCH IN SCHOOL HEALTH

The scientific study of school health requires a conceptual framework and model that delineates the various domains of relevant knowledge, levels of aggregates, and types of organizations. Because there are several models of school health in operation, perhaps it is premature to seek consensus and prudent to continue middle-range approaches. Overall, researchers could examine the relation between school health system variables and outcomes. Attention would be given to such system variables as structure, processes, resources, controls, and environment and to such outcome variables as system access, personnel performance, quality of service and work environment, and cost. Endorsement of alternative school health programs requires robust evaluation of process and outcome variables (Gomby and Larson, 1992).

Until recently, there was little empirical evidence to support the assumption that health was required for education (Wolfe, 1985). Now an effort is underway to provide a rigorous examination of this assumption. With Nader's eight dimensions of school health as "interventions," a general evaluation design is proposed for large-scale, multisite assessment of the educational outcomes of academic achievement, student behaviors, and student attitudes (Devaney et al., 1994). A compendium of evaluated school health programs throughout the nation is presented within the eight-component framework of a comprehensive school health program (National Coordinating Committee on School Health, 1993).

School health education receives research attention to document outcomes of various curricula and teaching methodologies (Allensworth, 1994). Additional areas requiring research attention include barriers to and facilitators of implementing school health education, process and impact of interdisciplinary collaboration and multiple teaching interventions, interaction of teacher and student ethnicity, and multicultural impact on curricula development and implementation (O'Rourke, 1995).

Systematic reviews of research in school health nursing have been reported by three academic nurse researchers: one pediatric nursing expert and two community health nursing experts (Chen and Sullivan, 1985; Denyes, 1983; Sullivan, 1984). They reported that research on school-age children is fragmented and limited because of conceptual and methodologic weaknesses, supported the development of a conceptual framework on which to base school nursing practice and research, and called for strong nursing leadership for school health services research to be linked with community health nursing. More recently, summarized research findings were applied to management decisions in relation to the following school health functions: immunizations, physical examinations versus screening, school health goals, health problem management, and health education (Kornguth, 1991).

School nurses can improve their practice and the health of clients by using the knowledge that exists, by sharing their unique perspectives and potential research problems with academic nursing colleagues,

SECONDARY ANALYSIS OF SCHOOL HEALTH RECORDS RESEARCH PROJECT

Moeckly E, Hansen MC. The at-risk student: A study of visits to the school nurse. J School Nurs 10:15–18, 1994.

Maintaining international competitiveness requires an educated, productive work force, but only 70% of students graduate from high school. Efforts are needed to identify at-risk students and to prevent unsatisfactory academic performance. Research literature suggests that urban at-risk students use school health services more often than students who are not at risk.

This study used the school nurse's daily log of student visits to compare rural public school students defined as at risk and those defined as not at risk to determine whether there were differences in frequency of visits. During a 5-month period, 1133 (77%) of the 1474 students enrolled in kindergarten through the 12th grade visited the school nurse. The school nurse assessed each student according to 13 at-risk criteria and classified the student at risk if one or more criteria were present. During the study period, students made 6135 visits to the school nurse, 3672 (60%) by at-risk students, a statistically significant difference.

This study demonstrates that school nurses are vital to the identification of and intervention for at-risk students. Although the authors recommend refinement of the at-risk assessment tool and replication with a more diverse student body, this study of rural students is an important addition to the body of knowledge on at-risk students.

and by collaborating with school health researchers. Reflecting on daily practice and answering questions by examining records often lead to useful research. Research is needed to examine ethical issues in relation to clients' diagnosis, socioeconomic class, and ethnicity. As school nurses assume more managerial responsibilities, research is needed on nursing administration in community settings and schools.

SUMMARY

Healthy People 2000 and Education Goals 2000 have given new importance to providing health care in the schools because nearly one third of the Healthy People 2000 objectives can be accomplished in the schools and two of the Goals 2000 speak directly to school health programs. The "new morbidities" of school-age children have influenced the expansion of school health from the traditional school health services, health education, and a healthful environment to an eight-component comprehensive school health model. Paradigms for the delivery of school health are shifting from the traditional first aid station to school-based clinics and school-linked integrated services. Evolving delivery models, legislative and social changes, and economic uncertainties increase the complexity of school health nursing practice. New professional standards for school nurse practice reflect expansion of the roles and functions.

At a minimum, nurses in the schools need a baccalaureate degree in nursing. More nurses are seeking graduate preparation to be a school nurse practitioner or a school nurse manager to meet the challenges of practicing in today's schools. The professional rewards of school health nursing include the direct care to clients, interdisciplinary collaboration, political action, and research.

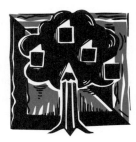

Learning Activities

1. Explain how the nation's Healthy People 2000 and Educational Goals 2000 actually complement each other. Identify five goals from Healthy People 2000 that relate to the first educational goal, and describe the implications for school nurse practice in an elementary school in your community.

2. Spend a day with a school nurse in a large urban school. Use the National Association of School Nurses (NASN) standards as a guide and compare the nurse's activities with those described by Darnell (1994) in a rural school district and by Burton in a medium-size urban school district (Burton, 1992). State your conclusions about the relation be-

tween the size and setting of the school and the roles and functions of the nurse.

3. Contact your state's departments of health and education to obtain a copy of the state's policy or procedure manual for school health and position descriptions for school health personnel. List the state's requirements for school nurses in relation to school health services, health education, and healthful environment. Compare and contrast state-mandated services with NASN's standards for school nursing practice. Interview school nurse consultants and supervisors about the utility of the policy or procedure manual.

4. Debate the costs and benefits of having a public health nurse serve the school and the school nurse employed by the school district. Consider all stake holders: students, teachers, parents or significant adult, school, school district, public health department, community, state, nurse, school nurses, community health nurses, nursing profession, and others.

5. Spend a day with a school nurse and focus on the documentation responsibilities inherent in the role. Examine the required documentation forms in relation to legal protection of the school nurse in the implementation of professional practice. Review an IEP and an IHP to describe roles of school nurses and other school personnel. Identify the issues of access to student's health record and confidentiality rights. Specify the unique impact of the computer on school health records.

6. Attend a faculty and staff meeting in a local school. Identify the various health and education disciplines represented. Observe who interacts with whom and specifically who interacts with the nurse. Note the nature of the nurse's participation in the meeting in relation to the school health agenda, student advocacy, and interdisciplinary issues. Describe the nurse's communication skills in an interdisciplinary context.

7. List five sources of national data on adolescent health knowledge and practices. Indicate how to access these data. State the criteria used to determine the relevance of the data for the local school district. Describe how to use the data in planning school health programs. Suggest revisions in school health policy based on the data. Propose how to initiate and implement changes in school health policy. Identify resources available to assist in presenting the data to school administrators and the school board.

8. Attend a meeting of a school health advisory council. Identify the various groups and agencies represented on the council. Examine the meeting agenda, and note the level of knowledge of the "new morbidities" in the discussion and decisions. Design an approach to seek the council's endorsement of a health education program on a controversial topic.

9. Identify the criteria for assessing the effectiveness and efficiency of the school health program. Focus on process and outcome variables. Iden-

tify the persons to involve in evaluating the program and describe their roles. List the steps in sharing and using the results.

10. Imagine yourself on January 1, 2000 (it's Saturday during the holiday vacation from school). List the achieved goals from Healthy People 2000 and Education Goals 2000. Predict the nature of the school health program, the evolving delivery model, and the role of the school nurse. Specify the professional issues confronting school nurses.

REFERENCES

Adams RM, Cole H, Price AL, et al.: Environmental health and safety in schools: An overview. School Nurse 7:14–18, 1991.

Allensworth DD: The research base for innovative practice in school health at the secondary level. J School Health 64:180–187, 1994.

Allensworth DD, Kolbe LJ: The comprehensive school health program: Exploring an expanded concept. J School Health 57:409–412, 1987.

Allensworth DD, Wolford CA: Achieving the 1990 Health Objectives for the Nation: Agenda for the Nation's Schools. Bloomington, IN, Tichenor, 1988.

Baker CM: School health: Policy issues in the 1990s. Nurs Health Care 15:178–184, 1994.

Behrman RE (ed): The Future of Children: School-Linked Services. Los Altos, CA, David and Lucille Packard Foundation, 1992.

Boyer EL: Ready to Learn: A Mandate for the Nation. Princeton, NJ, Carnegie Foundation, 1991.

Burton PT: A day in the life of a nurse: School nursing on cutting edge of prevention. Am Nurse 24:23, 1992.

Center for the Study of Social Policy: Kids Count Data Book: State Profiles of Child Well-Being. Washington, DC, A.E. Casey Foundation, 1991.

Center for the Study of Social Policy. Kids Count Data Book: State Profiles of Child Well-Being. Washington, DC, A.E. Casey Foundation, 1992.

Chen SC, Sullivan JA: School nursing. In Werley H, Fitzpatrick J (eds). Annual Review of Nursing Research, vol. 3. New York, Springer, 1985, pp. 25–48.

Cohen JH, Weiss HB, Mulvey EP, Dearwater SR: A primer on school violence prevention. J School Health 64:309–313, 1994.

Cohen SS: Overview of maternal-health policies. In Natapoff JN, Wieczorek RR (eds). Maternal-Child Health Policy: A Nursing Perspective. New York, Springer, 1990, pp. 17–56.

Committee on School Health: School Health: Policy and Practices, 5th ed. Elk Grove, IL, American Academy of Pediatrics, 1993.

Darnell JD: Life of a school nurse. INSA Bull 20:3,7, 1994.

Davis RL, Gonser HL, Kirkpatrick MA, et al.: Comprehensive school health education: A practical definition. J School Health 55:335–339, 1985.

Davis TM, Allensworth DD: Program management: A necessary component for the comprehensive school health program. J School Health 64:400–404, 1994.

Denyes MJ: Nursing research related to school-age children and adolescents. In Werley H, Fitzpatrick J (eds). Annual Review of Nursing Research, vol. 1. New York, Springer, 1983, pp. 27–53.

Devaney B, Schochet P, Thornton C, et al.: Evaluating Educational Outcomes of School Health Programs. Washington, DC, U.S. Department of Health and Human Services, 1994.

Dryfoos JG: Full-Service Schools. San Francisco, Jossey-Bass, 1994.

Fox HB, Wicks LB, Lipson DJ: Improving access to comprehensive health care through school-based programs. Unpublished manuscript. Washington, DC, Fox Health Policy Consultants, 1992.

Fuchs VR, Reklis DM: America's children: Economic perspectives and policy options. Science 255:41–46, 1992.

Gomby DS, Larson CS: Evaluation of school-linked services. The Future of Children: School-Linked Services 2:68–84, 1992.

Grunbaum J, Gingiss P, Orpinas P, et al.: A comprehensive approach to school health program needs assessment. J School Health 65:54–59, 1995.

Haas MB, Gerber MJ, Miller WR, et al.: The School Nurse's Source Book of Individualized Healthcare Plans. North Branch, MN, Sunrise River Press, 1993.

Hacker K, Fried LE, Bablouzian L, Roeber J: A nationwide survey of school health services delivery in urban school. J School Health 64:279–283, 1994.

Harrison BS, Faircloth JW, Yaryan L: The impact of legislation and litigation on the role of the school nurse. Nurs Outlook 43:57–61, 1995.

Henderson AC: Healthy Schools, Healthy Futures: The Case for Improving School Environment. Santa Cruz, CA, ETR Associates, 1993.

Igoe JB: School health—Designing the policy environment through understanding. Nurs Policy Forum 1:12–16, 18–19, 30–36, 1995.

Igoe JB, Giordano BP: Expanding School Health Services to Serve Families in the 21st Century. Washington, DC, American Nurses Association, 1992.

Igoe JB, Speer SE: The community health nurse in the schools. In Stanhope M, Lancaster J (eds). Community Health Nursing: Process and Practice for Promoting Health, 3rd ed. St. Louis, MO, CV Mosby, 1992, pp. 707–730.

Kann L, Warren CW, Harris WA, et al.: Youth risk behavior surveillance—United States, 1993. J School Health 65:163–171, 1995.

Klerman L: School absence—A health perspective. Pediatr Clin North Am 35:1253–1269, 1988.

Kornguth ML: Preventing school absences due to illness. J School Health 61:272–274, 1991.

Kort M: The delivery of primary health care in American public schools: 1890–1980. J School Health 54:453–457, 1984.

Kozlak LA: Comprehensive school health programs: The challenge for school nurses. J School Health 62:475–477, 1992.

Larson MJ: A children's health care budget. In Schlesinger MJ, Eisenberg L (eds). Children in a Changing Health System: Assessments and Proposals for Reform. Baltimore, MD, Johns Hopkins University, 1990, pp. 67–85.

Lavin AT, Shapiro GR, Weill KS: Creating an agenda for school-based health promotion: A review of 25 selected reports. J School Health 62:212–228, 1992.

Lehnen RG: Constructing state education performance indicators from ACT and SAT scores. Policy Studies J 20:22–40, 1992.

Lewitt EM: Dropout rates for high school students. Future Children 2:127–130, 1992.

Lovato CY, Allensworth DD, Chann FA: School Health in America: An Assessment of State Policies to Protect and Improve the Health of Students, 5th ed. Kent, OH, American School Health Association, 1989.

Meeker RJ, DeAngelis C, Berman B, et al.: A comprehensive school health initiative. Image 18:86–91, 1986.

Moeckly E, Hansen MC: The at-risk student: A study of visits to the school nurse. J School Nurs 10:15–18, 1994.

Nader PR: The concept of "comprehensiveness" in the design and implementation of school health programs. J School Health 60:133–137, 1990.

National Center for Educational Statistics: Digest of Educational Statistics: 1989. Washington, DC, U.S. Government Printing Office, 1989.

National Center for Educational Statistics: Digest of Educational Statistics: 1994. Washington, DC, U.S. Government Printing Office, 1994.

National Coordinating Committee on School Health: School Health: Findings from Evaluated Programs. Washington, DC, U.S. Department of Health and Human Services, 1993.

Oda DS: Nurse administrators' views of professional preparation in school nursing. J School Health 63:229–231, 1993.

O'Rourke TW: Creating capacity: A research agenda for school health education. J School Health 65:33–37, 1995.

Passarelli C: School nursing: Trends for the future. J School Health 64:141–149, 1994.

Perrin J, Guyer B, Lawrence JM: Health care services for children and adolescents. The Future of Children: U.S. Health Care Children 2:58–77, 1992.

Pigg RM: The school health program: Historical perspectives and future prospects. In Wallace HM, Patrick K, Parcel GS, Igoe JB (eds). Principles and Practices of Student Health, vol. 1. Oakland, CA, Third Party, 1992, pp. 247–261.

Polivka BJ: A conceptual model for community interagency collaboration. Image 27:110–115, 1995.

Proctor ST: Guidelines for a Model School Nursing Services Program. Scarborough, ME, National Association of School Nurses, 1990.

Proctor ST, Lordi S, Zaiger D: School Nursing Practice—Roles and Standards. Scarborough, ME, National Association of School Nurses, 1993.

Ray MA: Critical theory as a framework to enhance nursing science. Nurs Science Q 5:98–101, 1992.

Reilly EA: School bus safety: Issues and controversy. J Pediatr Health Care 9:145–148, 1995.

Rienzo BA, Button JW: The politics of school-based clinics: A community-level analysis. J School Health 63:266–272, 1993.

Riley RW, Shalala DE: Joint Statement on School Health by the Secretaries of Education and Health and Human Services (news release). Washington, DC, U.S. Department of Health and Human Services, April 7, 1994.

Schwab N: Guidelines for School Nursing Documentation: Standards, Issues, and Models. Scarborough, ME, National Association of School Nurses, 1991.

Snyder AA (ed). Implementation Guide for the Standards of School Nursing Practice. Kent, OH, American School Health Association, 1991.

Stevens PE, Hall JM: Applying critical theories to nursing in communities. Public Health Nurs 9:2–9, 1992.

Sullivan JA: Directions in Community Health Nursing. Boston, Blackwell Scientific, 1984.

Thurber F, Berry B, Cameron ME: The role of school nursing in the United States. J Pediatr Health Care 5:135–140, 1991.

Tyack D: Health and social services in public schools: Historical perspectives. The Future of Children: School-Linked Services 2:19–31, 1992.

U.S. Congress, Office of Technology Assessment: Adolescent Health: Vol. 1—Summary and Policy Options (Publication No. OTA-H-468). Washington, DC, U.S. Government Printing Office, 1991.

U.S. Department of Education: Strong Families, Strong Schools: Building Community Partnerships for Learning. Washington, DC, U.S. Government Printing Office, 1994, pp. 381–888.

U.S. General Accounting Office: Health Care: School-Based Health Centers Can Expand Access for Children (Publication No. GAO/HEHS-95-35). Washington, DC, Health, Education, and Human Services Division, 1994.

Walker DK, Butler JA, Bender A: Children's health care and the schools. In Schlesinger MJ, Eisenberg L (eds). Children in a Changing Health System: Assessments and Proposals for Reform. Baltimore, MD, Johns Hopkins University, 1990, pp. 265–294.

Wold SJ: School Nursing: A Framework for Practice. North Branch, MN, Sunrise River Press, 1981.

Wolfe BL: The influence of health on school outcomes: A multivariate approach. Med Care 23:1127–1138, 1985.

Woodfill MM, Beyrer MK: The Role of the Nurse in the School Setting: A Historical Perspective. Kent, OH, American School Health Association, 1991.

Yoder-Wise PS (ed): Leading and Managing in Nursing. St. Louis, MO, CV Mosby, 1995.

Environmental Health

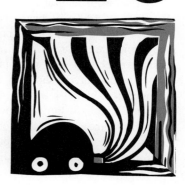

Upon completion of this chapter, the reader will be able to:

1. Describe broad areas of environmental health about which community health nurses must be informed and name environmental hazards in each area.

2. Recognize the potential social, cultural, economic, and political factors affecting environmental health.

3. Apply the basic concepts of critical theory to environmental health nursing problems.

4. Identify aggregates at risk for particular environmental health problems.

5. Distinguish between environmental health approaches that focus on altering individual behaviors and those that aim to change health-damaging environments.

6. Formulate critical questions about environmental conditions that limit the survival and well-being of communities.

7. Understand the skills needed to facilitate community participation and partnership in identifying and solving environmental health problems.

8. Propose collective strategies in which community health nurses can participate to address the environmental health concerns of specific aggregates.

Patricia E. Stevens
Joanne M. Hall

Environmental health is of ever increasing importance to community health nursing practice. Evidence is accumulating that the environmental changes of the past few decades have profoundly influenced the status of public health. The safety, beauty, and life-sustaining capacity of the physical environment are unquestionably of global consequence. The ecologic approach of the 1960s and 1970s tended to focus on clean water, clean air, and conservation of natural resources in specific locales. By the late 1990s, it has become acutely apparent that the extinction of many species, diminishment of the tropical rain forests, proliferation of toxic waste dumps, effects of acid rain, progressive destruction of the ozone layer, shortage of landfill sites, consequences of global warming, development of deadly chemical and ballistic weapons, food adulteration by pesticides and herbicides, oceanic contamination through toxic dumping and petroleum spills, urban overcrowding, traffic congestion of thoroughfares, and an ever growing number of industrial hazards posing health risks to workers are only a few of the urgent environmental difficulties we now face.

The purpose of this chapter is to explore the health of communities in relation to the environment. Environmental health is examined using critical theory as a framework for the discussion and a basis for described community health nursing practices. Applying critical theory is a way of thinking upstream, as discussed in Chapter 4. Critical theory is an approach that raises questions about oppressive situations, involves community members in the definition and solutions of problems, and facilitates interventions that liberate people from the health-damaging effects of environments. By applying the nursing process in a critical fashion, nurses can be dynamically involved in the design of interventions that alter the precursors of poor health.

Case examples are used throughout the chapter to illustrate how environmental health problems affect the everyday lives of aggregates. The term *aggregate* refers to a group that shares some common aspect, such as age, economic status, cultural perspective, gender, race, area of residence, chronic illness, and so on. Aggregates may be *communities* in which the members know and interact with each other, such as a barrio neighborhood or a labor union. Aggregates may also be "theoretically defined" categories of individuals who may or may not interact regularly with others in the defined group, as in "all crack cocaine users,"

"women with physical disabilities," or "all men older than 65 years."

Two other terms are used throughout the chapter. *Environment* is defined as the accumulation of physical, social, cultural, economic, and political conditions that influence the lives of communities. The *health* of communities depends on the integrity of the physical environment, humaneness of the social relations within it, availability of resources necessary to sustain life and manage illness, equitable distribution of health risks, attainable employment and education, cultural preservation and tolerance of diversity among subgroups, access to historical heritage, and sense of empowerment and hope (Table 26–1).

A CRITICAL THEORY APPROACH TO ENVIRONMENTAL HEALTH

Questioning what appears to be "given" in the environment and challenging "the way things have always been done" are the core dynamics of a critical way of thinking. For example, public buildings, schools, work places, and mass transportation systems are structures in the environment that are vital to people's everyday functioning. They are ordinarily taken for granted. The experiences of physically challenged persons, however, exemplify how that which has been taken for granted about the environment can be brought into question. Can disabled persons board the buses that run in our locales? Can wheelchair-using people enter public facilities? Can sight- or hearing-impaired children attend public schools and receive an equitable education? Will disabled persons be denied employment at a work place because hiring them would necessitate entrance ramps, wheelchair-accessible rest room facilities, and elevators?

Critical theory suggests that community health nurses should be vocally critical of obstructions in the environment that affect the safety and well-being of particular aggregates or deprive them of access to resources necessary for the pursuit of health. In identifying environmental sources of health problems, nurses must be involved with the communities that are affected. Rather than impose assessments of the problem, nurses should share their ideas and dialogue with community members: listening to what the community defines as problematic, helping to raise consciousness about environmental dangers, and as-

Table 26–1
Environmental Health Concepts

Concept	Definition
Aggregate	An aggregate is a group of people who share some common aspect, such as age, economic status, cultural background, gender, race, area of residence, chronic illness, and so on.
Community	Community is an aggregate in which the members know and interact with each other and have a collective identity, such as a barrio neighborhood or a labor union.
Environment	Environment is the accumulation of physical, social, cultural, economic, and political conditions that influence the lives of communities.
Health	Health of communities depends on the integrity of the physical environment, the humaneness of the social relations within it, the availability of resources necessary to sustain life and to manage illness, equitable distribution of health risks, attainable employment and education, cultural preservation and tolerance of diversity among subgroups, access to historic heritage, and a sense of empowerment and hope.

sisting in bringing about changes (Stevens and Hall, 1992).

Again, the experiences of disabled persons provide examples of how environmental health might be approached critically. Able-bodied people, often subconsciously, infantilize physically challenged individuals and assume that they are passive, powerless, and victimized by their physical incapacities. Community health nurses frequently approach members of this aggregate with intentions of assisting them to cope with their disabilities by arranging their immediate home environments to facilitate their activities of daily living. This may be an appropriate goal, but many disabled persons have identified broader problems such as architectural and discriminatory constraints in the environment that have systematically barred them from employment, education, housing, and health care. From their perspective, these may pose the most essential health problems. Many disabled persons "eschew the telethon's 'politics of pity' and abhor the 'poster child' image, demanding instead to be regarded as self-determining adults, capable of militant political action" (Anspach, 1979, p. 766).

As this situation suggests, only by being involved in open, respectful dialogues with the aggregates can nurses learn how they perceive themselves, their health, and environmental influences. Helping communities become more aware of how the environment affects their health and assisting them to take actions to make needed changes in the environment are very legitimate nursing actions from a critical standpoint.

The ultimate goal of the critical practice of community health nursing is the liberation of people from health-damaging environmental conditions.

Changes in environmental conditions achieved by people with disabilities and their advocates during the past two decades include federal legislation mandating accessibility of public facilities and services, changes in municipal building codes and state employment regulations, and increased enforcement of laws regarding nondiscrimination in hiring, educational opportunities, and health services. Collective actions were instrumental in the accomplishment of these environmental changes. Strategic organizing, litigation, testimony at public hearings, letter-writing campaigns, legislative lobbying, and mass demonstrations were some of the strategies used.

Because of its emphasis on collective strategies for change, a critical perspective can help nurses plan and implement aggregate-level interventions. Acting collectively can empower nurses to have a real impact on environmental health, as it has empowered disability rights activists to achieve their objectives. In the process of assessing environmental health problems, planning and implementing interventions, and evaluating the effectiveness of community-based actions, community health nurses should always be aware of physical surroundings as well as the effects on communities of cultural realities, social relations, economic circumstances, and political conditions. Several sources are available in the literature that discuss critical theory and its application to community health nursing

(Allen, 1986; Butterfield, 1990; Hall, et al., 1994; Stevens, 1989; Stevens and Hall, 1992; Thompson, 1987; Watts, 1990).

AREAS OF ENVIRONMENTAL HEALTH

Although many conceptual schemes are possible, we have divided the vast field of environmental health into nine subcategories: living patterns, work risks, atmospheric quality, water quality, housing, food quality, waste control, radiation risks, and violence risks (Table 26–2). The brief discussions of these areas of environmental health are only introductions to environmental health and focus on basic problems and strategies rather than on statistical detail. In the following sections, each of these nine areas of environmental health is defined, several examples of problems relevant to each category are given, and vignettes that illustrate community health nursing responses to environmental health concerns are presented. Obviously, many environmental health hazards

are not specifically mentioned in this chapter, although they are no less important than the examples discussed. Table 26–3 lists some of the environmental health problems that are included.

Living Patterns

Living patterns are the relationships among persons, communities, and their surrounding environments that depend on habits, interpersonal ties, cultural values, and customs. Drunk driving, involuntary smoking (secondhand smoke), exposure to noise, unabated traffic, urban crowding, and the stress of increasing mechanization of daily life could pose environmental health problems because people live within sociocultural patterns that limit their ability to escape these realities (Aday, 1993; Canadian Institute for Advanced Research, 1991; Evans, et al., 1991; Harper and Lambert, 1994; Kozol, 1991; Sidel, 1992).

We are not referring to individuals' lifestyle choices, such as eating a diet rich in saturated fats, leading a largely sedentary life, or becoming emotionally involved with a substance abuser. Rather, living

---

Table 26–2
Areas of Environmental Health

Area	Definition
Living patterns	Living patterns are the relationships among persons, communities, and their surrounding environments that depend on habits, interpersonal ties, cultural values, and customs.
Work risks	Work risks include the quality of the employment environment as well as the potential for injury or illness posed by working conditions.
Atmospheric quality	Atmospheric quality refers to the protectiveness of the atmospheric layers, the risks of severe weather, and the purity of the air available for breathing purposes.
Water quality	Water quality refers to the availability and volume of the water supply as well as the mineral content levels, pollution by toxic chemicals, and the presence of pathogenic microorganisms. Water quality consists of the balance between water contaminants and existing capabilities to purify water for human use and plant and wildlife sustenance.
Housing	Housing, as an environmental health concern, refers to the availability, safety, structural, strength, cleanliness, and location of shelter, including public facilities and family dwellings.
Food quality	Food quality refers to the availability and relative costs of foods, their variety and safety, and the health of animal and plant food sources.
Waste control	Waste control is the management of waste materials resulting from industrial and municipal processes and human consumption as well as efforts to minimize waste production.
Radiation risks	Radiation risks are health dangers posed by the various forms of ionizing radiation relative to barriers preventing exposure of humans and other life forms.
Violence risks	The environmental risks of violence include the potential for victimization through the violence of particular individuals as well as the general level of aggression in psychosocial climates.

Table 26–3
Examples of Environmental Health Problems

Area	Problems
Living patterns	Drunk driving Involuntary smoking Noise exposure Urban crowding Technological hazards
Work risks	Occupational toxic poisoning Machine-operating hazards Sexual harassment Repetitive motion injuries Carcinogenic work sites
Atmospheric quality	Gaseous pollutants Greenhouse effect Destruction of the ozone layer Aerial spraying of herbicides and pesticides Acid rain
Water quality	Contamination of drinking supply by human waste Oil spills in the world's waterways Pesticide or herbicide infiltration of ground water Aquifer contamination by industrial pollutants Heavy metal poisoning of fish
Housing	Homelessness Rodent and insect infestation Poisoning from lead-based paint Sick building syndrome Unsafe neighborhoods
Food quality	Malnutrition Bacterial food poisoning Food adulteration Disrupted food chains by ecosystem destruction Carcinogenic chemical food additives
Waste control	Use of nonbiodegradable plastics Poorly designed solid waste dumps Inadequate sewage systems Transport and storage of hazardous waste Illegal industrial dumping
Radiation risks	Nuclear facility emissions Radioactive hazardous wastes Radon gas seepage in homes and schools Nuclear testing Excessive exposure to x-rays
Violence risks	Proliferation of handguns Increasing incidence of hate crimes Pervasive images of violence in the media High rates of homicide among young black males Violent acts against women and children

In an urban Chinese community, the economic aftershocks of a major earthquake cause the closure of many businesses. Some of these family businesses are forced to move to parts of the city less characterized by the use of Chinese languages. As a result of these moves, many elderly family members who do not speak English appear to be experiencing depression, characterized by a loss of appetite.

The community health nurses in the area begin visiting these elders, bringing interpreters with them. In their assessments, nurses focus on psychiatric symptoms and suggest ventilation of emotions. They encourage many of the elderly Chinese to attend a local senior center that is staffed and attended mostly by Euro-Americans. In some cases, they recommend psychiatric evaluations. In almost every instance, there is resistance to these interventions.

The nurses failed to establish an alliance with the very strong Chinese family organizations before imposing their solutions. They also neglected to investigate Chinese cultural patterns before attempting to assist them with the life pattern ramifications of the earthquake. Chinese people do not readily talk about feelings with outsiders, nor do they generally conceptualize distress in psychiatric terms. They interpret the presence of fatigue and disturbances in eating and sleeping patterns as physical illness. They expect health care personnel to recognize and help them with these physical symptoms. To suggest that socializing at clubs populated by English speakers would cure their illness seemed to them to be quite incredulous.

patterns reflect population exposure to environmental conditions that are affected by mass culture, social policy, ethnic customs, and technology (Eckersley, 1992).

For example, community responses to a massive toxic chemical spill are mediated by many cultural, psychological, social, and economic conditions in the residential areas affected (Vyner, 1988a). The technological hazard represented by the spill can be more difficult for communities to cope with than natural disasters. The human failure symbolized by technological hazards can evoke hopelessness, helplessness, and anger that manifests in heightened community stress and deepening personal depression (Vyner, 1988b). Difficulties convincing state and federal officials of environmental health dangers and problems obtaining compensation for diseases and deaths caused by environmental toxins often result in revictimization of residents (Smets, 1988; Soble and Brennan, 1988). Leaving an area that poses potentially severe health risks from exposure to hazards may be hindered by the lack of low-cost housing and by tightly knit social structures in the affected community. People may not be able to afford to move or willing to disrupt family and cultural roots to start over elsewhere, so they may live with the uncertainty and conflict. Long-term community-wide effects of division, animosity, distrust, cynicism, and despair often abound in such situations.

Discriminatory land use that ensures poor people and people of color live in close proximity to contamination from industrialization has been called *environmental racism* (Alston, 1990; Bryant and Mohai, 1992). Bullard (1993) concluded, "whether by conscious design or institutional neglect, communities of color in urban ghettos, in rural 'poverty pockets,' or on economically impoverished Native-American reservations face some of the worst environmental devastation in the nation" (p. 17). Many communities lack sufficient resources to engage in the expensive litigation that becomes inevitable when urban development and technological advances clash with the health and well-being of families who live in affected areas (Peña and Gallegos, 1993). Marginalization of unwanted land uses (e.g., waste incinerators, sewage treatment plants, landfills, refineries, prisons) in urban environments that are already strewn with obsolete abandoned derelict sites (e.g., deserted factories, warehouses, railways, mines, and vacant garbage-strewn lots) creates situations in which all age groups, races, and genders become victims of violent death from falls, fires, homicides, poisonings, and suicides (Greenberg and Schneider, 1994).

Work Risks

Work risks include the quality of the employment environment as well as the potential for injury or illness posed by working conditions. Environmental health problems posed by work risks include sexual harassment, occupational toxic poisoning, machine-operating hazards, electrical hazards, repetitive motion injuries, and work sites characterized by carcinogenic particulate inhalants (e.g., asbestos), dust pollutants (e.g., coal dust), and heavy metal poisoning (Cralley et al., 1990; Gaillard, 1993; Grondona, 1993; Smith, 1990; Steenland, 1993; Sumrall and Taylor, 1992). Prevention of work-related health problems calls for integrated action to improve job content and the working environment (Kogi, 1993).

In the United States, more than 20 million injuries and 400,000 new cases of disease are recognized annually as being work related (Levy and Wegman, 1994). Across the nation, about 7000 traumatic occupational fatalities occur each year. The three industries with the highest rates of traumatic deaths to workers are mining, construction, and agriculture (Veazie et al., 1994). These statistics do not reflect the health problems that are never reported. For example, a clerical worker leaves the office every day with a headache and back strain and, after 5 years on the job, experiences carpal tunnel syndrome. A midwestern farmer suffers the loss of his hand by having it caught in his new hay baler, not knowing that several other farmers in the state have been similarly injured using this same model of hay baler. All male production workers who formerly worked for a chemical company producing a pesticide are found to be sterile. An operating room nurse has a miscarriage and remem-bers that many of her coworkers have also been unable to carry their infants to term. A dry cleaner often leaves work feeling lightheaded and dizzy from inhaling solvents all day at the shop, and one day she has an automobile accident on the way home (Brender and Suarez, 1990; Connon et al., 1993; Dumont, 1989; McAbee et al., 1993).

Atmospheric Quality

Atmospheric quality refers to the protectiveness of the atmospheric layers, the risks of severe weather, and the purity of the air available for breathing purposes. Environmental dangers related to atmospheric quality include chlorofluorocarbon destruction of the ozone layer, loss of carbon dioxide–consuming resources such as forests, tornadoes, electrical storms, smog, gaseous pollutants (e.g., carbon monoxide), excessive hydrocarbon levels, aerial spraying of herbicides, and acid rain (Connell, 1990; Elsom, 1992; Foster, 1994).

The protectiveness of our atmospheric layers is diminishing (Last, 1993). Chlorofluorocarbons, which are in widespread use for refrigeration, air condition-ing, and aerosol propellants, remain in the atmosphere for a long time. These molecules cause depletion of the ozone layer of the atmosphere. The resulting "holes" in the ozone layer allow excess ultraviolet radiation to penetrate, with deleterious effects on living organisms. Another problematic atmospheric condition is increas-ing atmospheric carbon dioxide. This carbon dioxide allows sunlight to pass through to the earth but absorbs

VIGNETTE

Sanitation workers in an urban area have experienced an increasing incidence of puncture injuries in the process of transporting hazardous wastes from the public medical center. Several cases of hepatitis have resulted. As the story hits the newspapers, community health nurses are contacted by members of the city health commission and are instructed that they are to politically support the interests of the city and the medical center "at all costs." Subsequently, the sanitation workers' union contacts the community health nursing office and asks for information about available methods of safely packaging medical wastes. They also ask for a nurse to come and speak to their membership about immediate measures they can use to prevent further injuries on the job.

The nurses meet to resolve the conflict. Most agree that the union membership has pressing needs for education and support. Despite the city's demand for loyalty, they decide to side with the workers and respond to their requests. They collectively draft a letter to the city health commission and arrange a meeting with the commissioners in which a small group of the nurses informs them of their plans to assist the sanitation workers. The health commission later holds a press conference in which the actions of the nurses are depicted as mediational efforts that benefit both the union and the city. Eventually, a new medical waste disposal plan is jointly developed, and injured workers receive reasonable compensation in an out-of-court settlement.

and traps part of the heat re-emitted by the earth. Thus, the surface temperature of the earth is heating up in what is called the "greenhouse effect," causing probably irreversible global climate changes and other catastrophic ecologic consequences.

Burning fossil fuels such as coal and oil releases carbon dioxide into the atmosphere, which stimulates the greenhouse effect. In addition, key processes that break down atmospheric carbon dioxide are being disrupted. The ongoing devegetation of much of the earth's surface, especially the cutting of the tropical rain forests, not only releases the carbon stored in the biomass but also eliminates sources of photosynthesis, the process by which plants absorb carbon and release oxygen. The rate at which the world's forests are being cut is almost inconceivable. In 1950, 30% of the earth's land surface was covered by tropical forests. By the year 2000, this figure will fall to 5% (Goudie, 1990). This massive worldwide deforestation, combined with pollution, is wiping out countless species of animals and plants (Wilson et al., 1991). The spread of desert-like conditions because of overgrazing, over-cultivation, and soil erosion is also devastating and will mean the loss of 18% of all arable land on the globe during the final quarter of the 20th century (Myers, 1993).

Severe weather conditions, another aspect of atmospheric quality that affects the public's health, can have dramatic results in the form of injury and loss of life, destruction of plants and wildlife, and property damage. Climatic changes associated with global warming are said to be increasing the frequency and severity of the earth's weather extremes (Mungall and McLaren, 1990). Hazardous atmospheric pollutants threaten survival by causing lung cancer, chronic respiratory disease, and death as well as by exterminating animal and plant species (Rose, 1990). For instance, it is estimated that 50,000 lakes in the United States and Canada are "dead" (i.e., devoid of fish and plant life) as a result of acid rain (Perdue and Gjessing, 1989). In addition to ruining aquatic ecosystems, acid rain affects terrestrial ecosystems by increasing soil acidity, reducing nutrient availability, mobilizing toxic metals, leaching soil chemicals, and altering species composition (Foster, 1994).

Water Quality

Water quality refers to the availability and volume of the water supply as well as mineral content levels, pollution by toxic chemicals, and presence of pathogenic microorganisms. Water quality consists of the balance between water contaminants and existing capabilities to purify water for human use and plant and wildlife sustenance. Problems of water quality include droughts, dosing of reservoirs with copper sulfate to reduce algae, contamination of drinking supply by human wastes, pesticide-contaminated aquifers, mercury-poisoned fish in the Great Lakes, lead leaching from water pipes, oil spills in the world's waters, water-borne bacteria, and toxicity caused by excessive chlorination.

Advances in water treatment technologies in industrialized countries such as the United States

---

VIGNETTE

A sudden increase occurs in the number of emergency calls to a medical hot line from residents of a particular urban neighborhood. These calls often involve elderly women who have collapsed in their homes. In one case, an asthmatic child experienced severe dyspnea. One of the community health nurses comments that perhaps these problems are psychosocial manifestations of stress.

As the emergency calls continue, two other community health nurses note that respiratory difficulties are almost always implicated. These nurses decide to visit the neighborhood in question and look around. It happens to be nearing rush hour, and within minutes all of the traffic on the nearby freeway is slowed to a crawl ap-

parently because of road construction. Through their direct observations and critical assessment, these nurses determine that several residential buildings in the area appear to be situated so that heavy car exhaust fumes stagnate around them. The nurses notify the Environmental Protection Agency (EPA) as well as the city transportation department to recommend further investigation and resolution of the problem.

One week later, the nurses return to the neighborhood and determine that the traffic is moving more efficiently, even though road construction continues. Within several weeks, the number of emergency medical calls more closely approximates the usual number of calls received.

VIGNETTE

In a midwestern farm community, there is growing concern about seepage of agricultural pesticides and herbicides into ground water. The situation is complicated by the fact that families obtain water from their own wells rather than from a central municipal source. The families are aware of the long-range carcinogenic effects of many of the chemicals involved. Although family farmers have decreased their use of these chemicals, the large-scale agribusiness companies continue to use excessive amounts of these chemicals, sacrificing environmental integrity for larger crop yields.

County community health nurses lobby local officials to begin a comprehensive program to monitor ground water pollutants and enforce standards for herbicide and pesticide use. These officials are hampered by the powerful agri-business companies that pressure them to stand back. Together, some of the county's farmers and the nurses organize grassroots information and support groups among rural families. Several projects are jointly started by the families and the nurses in coalition with environmental activist groups in the state. They collect samples from each family well for testing purposes, form a local umbrella organization called "Water Watch" to coordinate actions and communications, coordinate a research project with a federal health agency to track the health problems of a cohort of local residents who have had long-term consumption of these water sources, and disseminate an emergency plan for drinking water distribution should any wells be found to have toxic levels of pesticides, herbicides, or other pollutants.

have controlled many water-related diseases such as cholera, typhoid, dysentery, and hepatitis A (McKeown, 1991). However, disease outbreaks resulting from contamination by untreated ground water and inadequate chlorination are increasing in both urban and rural areas (Myers, 1993). Accelerated soil erosion caused by construction, agriculture, and deforestation leads to high sediment levels in drinking water supplies, which then requires greater use of heavy metals and chemicals in the water treatment process. Heavy metal and toxic chemical pollution can originate in the water treatment process or in the drinking water distribution system (Krieps, 1989).

Some of the most serious problems are found in the sources of our drinking water (Blumenthal and Ruttenber, 1995; Foster, 1994). Microcontaminants escape landfills, effluent lagoons, and petroleum storage facilities to enter water supplies. Residential, commercial, and industrial outputs increase the pollutant load of surface water, such as rivers and lakes. Pesticides, herbicides, and carcinogenic industrial waste are infiltrating increasing amounts of ground water, the underground source of half of the U.S. population's drinking water (Hayes and Laws, 1990). This is particularly tragic because ground water is uniquely susceptible to long-term contamination. Unlike river or lake water, once ground water becomes contaminated, there is no way to cleanse it.

Housing

Housing as an environmental health concern refers to the availability, safety, structural strength, cleanliness, and location of shelter, including public facilities and family dwellings. Environmental health problems related to housing include homelessness; fire hazards; inaccessibility for disabled persons; illnesses caused by overcrowding, dampness, and rodent or insect infestation; poisoning from chipping lead-based paint; psychological effects of architectural design (e.g., low-cost high-rise housing projects); injuries sustained from collapse of building structures that are in disrepair; and winter deaths from inadequate indoor heating.

It is well known that poor housing conditions can spread infectious diseases (Jackson and McSwane, 1992; Kerner et al., 1993), but what is becoming more apparent is that they can contribute to cardiovascular and respiratory disorders, cancers, allergies, and mental illnesses. A new term—*sick building*—has been used to describe a phenomenon in which public structures and homes cause toxic syndromes in their occupants because of building materials, poor ventilation, substances in furniture and carpeting, building operations, or cleaning agents (Brooks, 1991).

For example, commercial buildings with offices near underground parking garages may cause their workers to suffer carbon monoxide intoxication. Formaldehyde, asbestos, and volatile organic compounds, which are common components of thermal insulation, cement, flooring, furnishings, and household consumer products, have carcinogenic properties. Much controversy is arising over the economic hardship that would be imposed on industry, government, business, and multidwelling owners should they be mandated to reduce concentrations of such toxic elements. The traditional approach to development in the United States has been to produce as much as possible and assume that the environmental health consequences will be minor or, if not, then simply repaired with the excess wealth generated (Young, 1990). These notions of sustainable development have proven inadequate as the country suffers major ecologic threats to human health via cumulative hazardous episodes.

Health can be affected not only by the structure of housing but also by the immediate surroundings in which it is situated, such as the neighborhood's population density, proximity to industry, safety of adjacent buildings, level of security, noise and pollution from nearby traffic, and so on (Kay, 1991b).

Food Quality

Food quality refers to the availability and relative costs of foods, their variety and safety, and the health of animal and plant food sources. Food quality problems include malnutrition, bacterial food poisoning, carcinogenic chemical additives (e.g., nitrites, alar, cycla-

mate), improper or fraudulent meat inspection or food labeling, viral epidemics among livestock (e.g., cholera), food products from diseased animal sources, and disruption of vital natural food chains by ecosystem destruction.

Foods can be contaminated by toxic chemicals as they pass along the food chain, eventually resulting in reproductive and mutagenic effects in humans (Foster, 1994). For instance, dioxin-containing weed killers are sprayed on range land. Cattle graze on the land, and the herbicide accumulates in their fatty tissue. The beef cattle are butchered, and their meat is sold at markets all along the West Coast. Dioxin shows up in human mother's milk in the western United States, and increasing numbers of children are born with birth defects in these same states.

A plethora of agrichemicals such as pesticides and fertilizers, materials from mechanical handling devices, detergents, and organic packaging materials can poison food and may have the potential to induce immune suppression (Foster, 1994). Unsuitable handling, storage, processing, and transport techniques can damage and contaminate foodstuffs (Covello and Merkhofer, 1993). Food adulteration to increase the volume or weight of food or to improve its color or flavor is also problematic because adulterants are usually less nutritious and often harmful. Residues from the overuse of antibiotics in animal husbandry remain in meat and milk products, causing people who consume them to acquire resistance to a wide range of

VIGNETTE

In a large northeastern city, an economic recession has led to massive unemployment, rising housing costs, and drastically reduced housing subsidies. Simultaneously, funding has been cut for several public health and mental health facilities. The result is that approximately 4000 people are "houseless." This winter a dozen deaths have already occurred as a result of exposure to the elements. The local shelters are able to house a total of 500 persons each night, although none of these shelters accepts women.

Community health nurses meet with local church groups who are committed to starting a shelter for women. This coalition acquires a building in an area near where many shelterless people congregate. They begin to offer accommodations for 75 women. After 3 months, the city takes over the women's shelter because of the

churches' difficulties filling the beds and maintaining the project's financial solvency. The city changes the shelter to a dwelling for 50 men and 25 women because it has not been used sufficiently by women.

In evaluating what went wrong, the nurses consulted with several shelterless women as well as with workers from a popular soup kitchen. The answer was relatively simple. The women did not feel safe going to the shelter because of the area's high-crime reputation and lack of street lighting. Eventually, a new coalition is formed composed of the community health nurses, several women who are or had been shelterless, a representative from the police force, and the church groups. A new women's shelter is opened in a safer, well-lit neighborhood close to public transit lines.

VIGNETTE

A southern town with a population of 10,000 is home to a large number of African-American farm workers and a smaller, but significant, number of Euro-American residents, most of whom are employed as textile workers. Located well off the interstate arteries, the town experiences very high food costs because of shipping difficulties. Many families have tapered their diets, eating mostly bread, rice, beans, and eggs. Health assessments of school-age children and toddlers indicate deficiencies of vitamins contained in fresh fruits and vegetables.

Local physicians, county health nurses, and the Parent-Teacher Association join forces to try to improve the nutritional situation. The most popular of the proposed solutions involves the idea of a community garden project. Land is leased from the county, and the project begins. Conflict arises when African-American community leaders realize that the mostly Euro-American textile workers have formed their own garden project, competing with the original garden project for the town's support. Racial tensions intensify.

The nurses and parents originally involved in setting up the project meet to avert a crisis. They decide to focus on reaching church leaders and women in both African- and Euro-American sectors of the town in the hope of supporting a dialogue and a just solution to the problem. Parents and church leaders spread the word in their respective communities. A community meeting is held at a time that is convenient for women in the town and at a neutral place that is deemed acceptable by both African-Americans and Euro-Americans.

Although tensions are strong enough to prevent the formation of a joint garden, each group feels successful and able to save face as a result of the solution reached in the meeting. Town funds are allocated on a per capita basis to two gardening projects, and an agreement is reached that vegetable and fruit yields will be shared equitably depending on the yield from each site. Additional benefits of the cooperative plan are that the total garden space allotted is increased by 50% and a gardening tool "library" is started so that neither group needs to purchase all new tools.

---

antibiotics that then are rendered ineffective in the treatment of human infections (Krieps, 1989; Neu, 1992).

A new and potentially dangerous threat to food quality involves scientific gene mutations through "gene splicing," which produces livestock that grow faster and fatten more easily so that they can be slaughtered sooner and produce greater yields at a lower cost (Teitelman, 1989). This controversial genetic engineering is producing new animal species. The unregulated introduction of these genetically mutated species onto range land and into farm herds threatens the survival of food-producing animal species and has unknown consequences for human nutrition.

Waste Control

Waste control is the management of waste materials resulting from industrial and municipal processes and human consumption as well as efforts to minimize waste production. Environmental health problems related to waste control include use of nonbiodegradable plastics, lack of efficient and affordable recycling programs, unlicensed waste dumps, sewage systems that are inadequate for actual population demands or in disrepair, industrial dumping of toxic wastes, exportation of hazardous radioactive medical wastes to third world countries, cover-ups of illicit dumping, and nonenforcement of environmental protection legislation.

The increasing generation of trash by American consumers as well as improper treatment, storage, transport, and disposal of waste are of mounting concern (DeLong, 1993; Haun, 1991; Reinhardt and Gordon, 1991; Rom, 1992). Multiple problems exist. The increasing use of petroleum-based plastics in products such as disposable diapers creates grave ecologic problems. Commercial and institutional wastes are routinely dumped with household waste in the same municipal incinerator, landfill, or sewer system. These commercial enterprises are generally exempt from the strict waste regulation applied to industry, although they often generate the same hazardous materials. Small businesses such as dry cleaners, photography laboratories, pesticide formulators, construction sites, and automobile repair shops use and discard a variety of substances that can cause serious public health problems. Solid waste landfills present a problem because methane gas accumulates as a by-product of decomposing organic wastes. Without proper venting, the volatile gas can move through the soil and cause fires and explosions in nearby areas. Incineration of wastes is not the best solution because it causes particulate air pollution and is ineffective in the combustion of many hazardous wastes.

The United States produces between 250 and 400 million metric tons of toxic waste per year or about 1 ton per person per year. No viable solution has been found to deal with this mounting waste problem (Hamilton, 1993). As a consequence, the United States has anywhere from 32,000 to 50,000 uncontrolled waste disposal sites (Keller, 1992). Because of improper design, operation, or location of the waste sites, hazardous substances are spread through air, soil, and water to poison humans, animals, and plant life. Alarmingly, only a small percentage of hazardous wastes actually reach designated waste sites. The EPA estimates that 90% of hazardous waste is improperly disposed of in open pits, surface impoundments, vacant land, farmlands, and bodies of water (Anderson, 1987).

In 1980, Congress passed the Environmental Response Compensation and Liability Act, which set up a revolving fund called the Superfund to clean up several hundred of the worst abandoned chemical waste disposal sites. Funds are insufficient, however, and improvements have been minor (Keller, 1992). One of the most notorious sites is the Love Canal in Niagara Falls, New York. For 40 years before the 1960s, more than 80 different types of chemicals, including benzene, dioxin, dichlorethylene, and chloroform, were dumped in an abandoned canal. The site was then covered and a school and several hundred homes were built on it. In the winter of 1976, heavy snowfall and rain caused toxic wastes to reach the surface. Inhabitants were subsequently found to have higher than normal miscarriage rates, blood and liver abnormalities, birth defects, and chromosome damage.

Radiation Risks

Radiation risks are the health dangers posed by the various forms of ionizing radiation, relative to barriers preventing exposure of humans and other life forms. Radiation risks include nuclear power emissions, radioactive hazardous wastes, medical and dental radiographs, radon gas seepage in homes, and wartime dangers of nuclear weaponry.

Nuclear industries are frought with environmental problems (Blumenthal and Ruttenber, 1995). People and animals living in the vicinity of nuclear facilities such as power plants, waste storage sites, uranium-processing plants, nuclear weapons factories, and nuclear test sites have manifested increased rates of cancers, strokes, diabetes, cardiovascular and renal diseases, immune system damage, premature aging, infertility, miscarriages, and birth defects (Elsom, 1992; International Physicians for the Prevention of Nuclear War, 1991; Keller, 1992; Marino, 1994). In addition, there is the ever present risk of nuclear

VIGNETTE

In a city on the Mississippi River, an outbreak of shigellosis is traced to a group of high school students who have been swimming in a particular area of the river. It is found that the local meat-packing plant is releasing waste material—both human and animal—directly into the river.

After intervening to contain the shigella outbreak, the local community health nurses begin to assess the situation as a whole. Their research indicates that the meat-packing facility has been in violation of waste control laws for some time. City officials have imposed fines, which have been paid by the company, but the dumping has continued. A sign prohibiting swimming has been posted at the riverside.

Frustrated by their attempts to negotiate with the city and the plant, the nurses write a letter to both the local newspaper and the state capital newspaper, which has a wide readership across the state. In the letter, they voice concern about the community's health as well as the ecologic integrity of the river. Their informative letter is published as a commentary in both newspapers, which prompts responses from two local environmental groups, several activist groups located downriver, and a national organization concerned with clean water. These groups are able to provide legal support, and a collective suit is brought against the meat-packing company. Subsequently, the company improves its waste treatment process to avoid being forced to pay a large award in the civil suit.

VIGNETTE

During wartime, federal standards related to radioactive contamination of the environment and the public's "right to know" are suspended for military projects. In the middle of the U.S.–Iraq war, information "leaks" that a military installation in the southwestern desert, near Deserttown, plans test explosions of several new nuclear bombs, which they call nuclear "devices."

Local townspeople express concern, but no confirmation or denial of these plans is given by the military. The possible dates for the tests are also unknown. Residents begin to panic. Several families move. Others build makeshift shelters and begin stockpiling food. There is an increase in psychiatric hospitalization rates. A crisis is reached when a spate of three related adolescent suicides occurs in a period of 2 months. The entire community appears disorganized, helpless, and hopeless.

Town officials organize town meetings in which the public health nurses offer community education about the health effects of ionizing radiation and answer people's questions, but this does not raise morale among residents. The nurses decide to contact other communities that have faced similar threats to determine how they have dealt with them.

When these communities receive word of the situation in Deserttown, they organize a letterwriting campaign and a demonstration of their support. They converge on Deserttown for a weekend rally and celebration of solidarity. The youth of Deserttown extend this demonstration in the form of weekly vigils at the military site.

One year later, the community is more united and less depressed, and the adolescent suicide rate is significantly decreased. The nuclear threat remains.

accidents in which large amounts of radioactivity are released into surrounding areas (Gould, 1990). It is not known what will be done with nuclear facilities after their three- or four-decade life spans are completed. By then, they will have become saturated with radioactivity as a normal part of their everyday operations and in some way will have to be decommissioned and decontaminated.

A safe way of disposing of nuclear wastes, which remain dangerously radioactive for hundreds of thousands of years, has not been devised. Much of the waste is currently stockpiled in interim collection centers. Not only is there a quandary about how, where, and when to dispose of nuclear wastes currently being generated, but radioactive materials that have already been improperly disposed must be managed. Countless drums of radioactive wastes dumped at sea or buried in the earth are leaking (Council on Scientific Affairs, 1989; Keller, 1992).

Millions of Americans are exposed to dangerous levels of radiation in their homes, schools, and work places (Platt, 1993; Sandman and Weinstein, 1993). The EPA has identified radon contamination as the second leading cause of lung cancer mortality in the United States; an estimated 5000 to 20,000 deaths are attributed to it each year (U.S. EPA, 1992). Radon is a radioactive decay product of radium that occurs naturally in certain kinds of phosphate- and uranium-containing rock such as granite and black shale. Radon can be present in building materials, drinking water, and soil. Radon gas diffuses into dwellings, mostly through soil, and is prevalent where uranium-bearing land is common. Radon seeps through basement walls, pipes, and cracks in the foundation and is trapped in buildings with inadequate ventilation.

Cumulative exposure to excessive or improperly performed radiographs can also cause radiation damage to the body (McAbee et al., 1993; Miller, 1990; Mole, 1990). People who work with medical sources of radiation, such as radium or radioactive iodine, are at increased risk for cancers and for delivering offspring with birth defects. Older models of x-ray machines may emit excessive levels of radioactivity; all such equipment should be tested regularly for leakage.

Violence Risks

The environmental risks of violence include the potential for victimization through the violence of particular groups as well as the general level of aggression in psychosocial climates. Violence-fostered environmental health problems can arise from conditions such as extreme poverty, widespread unemployment, proliferation of handguns, pervasive media images of violence, lack of child abuse services, law enforcement's unwillingness to follow up on women's complaints of sexual molestation, and the increasingly common occurrence of hate crimes.

The potential for persons to be victims of violent crimes, including verbal abuse, harassment, battery, sexual assault, abduction, and murder, is influenced by social, political, and economic characteristics of the environment (Greenberg and Schneider, 1994; Hall et al., 1994; Rosenberg and Fenley, 1991; Ruback and Weiner, 1994). The phenomenon of urban youth gangs exemplifies a process in which poverty and powerlessness foster aggressiveness and territorial defensiveness in young males. Chronic deterioration of urban centers and the systematic withdrawal of services and resources are specifically linked to violent behavior (Earls et al., 1993).

Social stigmatization of racial, ethnic, and religious minorities as well as lesbians and gays can take the form of violent hate crimes against these groups. For example, official talk of registering, placing under surveillance, and possibly interning "suspicious" Arab-Americans during the U.S.–Iraq war was accompanied by an increase in malicious innuendos, threats, and violent crimes against Arab-Americans throughout the United States

(Hall and Stevens, 1992). The relative political powerlessness of women and children makes them frequent targets of violence as well (Stevens and Hall, 1990).

It continues to be debated whether films, television, recorded music, and sexually explicit materials actually foster the commission of violent crimes. Regardless of whether they do, it is reasonable to conclude that these images influence the direction violent impulses take in terms of targets (e.g., women, children, and minorities) (Linz et al., 1988; Sommers and Check, 1987). Most agree that key factors in the incidence and severity of violent aggression are the availability and regulation of ballistic weapons. Handguns, rifles, and automatic weapons are increasingly obtainable in U.S. communities. Communities face very difficult questions about how to curtail the violence in their environments. Increasing dependence on police forces, the penal system, and censorship tactics can produce a situation of diminishing returns; forceful repression may provoke an increase in social aggression.

VIGNETTE

At a prestigious private university, a survey reveals that more than 30% of the female students have experienced "date rape." The university appeals to its student health service to respond to this growing problem. The nurses at the health service are asked to organize classes for female students about self-defense and "what to do if raped."

One nurse voices opposition, pointing out that rape is a violent act perpetrated by men and is not a health matter that concerns only women. She suggests that male students be offered education about the bodily rights of others and classes about "how not to rape women." This causes a deep polarization among the nurses and other health workers at the student health service. Many feel the self-defense classes are useful even if they do not address the core problem. Others feel that to ignore male responsibility for rape is to encourage or condone a "climate of violence."

The self-defense classes are held but not well attended. One year later, the rates of date rape and other sexual assaults involving students at the university are even higher. In reevaluating their intervention, the nurses decide to mingle among the student body and to visit places where students hang out. They informally interview

groups of students about what they think is involved in the high incidence of date rape. The consensus is that the fraternity culture on campus encourages heavy drinking and sexual aggressiveness on the part of male students. With these new data, the nurses approach university officials suggesting several services that should be offered to students and policy changes that should be made.

Together, the nurses and university staff develop new interventions. First, the university invites an alcohol problems researcher to institute an alcohol self-awareness research project as well as a bartender education program on campus. Second, the university requires that fraternity leaders participate in four weekend seminars about sexual assault and interpersonal violence. Third, incentives are given to fraternities based on how many of their members attend similar seminars, and commendations and prizes are extended for collective projects that demonstrate effectiveness in decreasing the number of date rapes and other violent crimes on campus. Last, a new policy is adopted in which the university pledges to vigorously pursue criminal and civil actions in all cases of sexual assault involving students.

EFFECTS OF ENVIRONMENTAL HAZARDS

Environmental effects on the public's health are quite complex and usually interconnected (DeRosa et al., 1993). For example, nuclear power plant emissions can contaminate both water and air supplies, simultaneously involving water quality, atmospheric quality, and radiation risk. Overcrowded housing may exacerbate problems in managing human wastes, which may in turn taint foodstuffs, all contributing to the spread of communicable disease.

Health-damaging effects of oppressive environments may be direct. A shiny, brightly colored radioactive medical waste product from the United States that has ended up in a Central American city dump may be picked up and played with by poor children who live nearby and scavenge for food in that dump (Schrieberg, 1991). The severe burns they suffer and the wine-colored spots on their skin are very direct effects of the illegally dumped toxic waste (Center for Investigative Reporting, 1990). Effects may also be indirect, as occurs with global warming (Foster, 1994). Over decades, farming regions will warm up, dry out, and become less productive. The sea level will eventually rise because of melting polar ice caps. The resulting coastal inundation and permanent flooding would threaten large areas of low-lying agricultural land and hence food supplies in many regions of the world. As global temperatures rise, the quantity and distribution of parasites, insects, and other disease vectors will be enhanced, increasing the prevalence of a variety of infectious diseases.

Effects of environmental hazards may be general or specific. The ramifications of massive unemployment, drought, and extensive smog cover, for example, are felt generally, whereas the particular housing needs of elderly persons using walkers or canes, the occupational risks faced by workers who repair electrical lines, and the mentally incapacitating effects of lead poisoning in children are experienced more specifically.

Environmental health effects can also be categorized as immediate, long range, or transgenerational. Burns, gunshot wounds, hurricane damage, and outbreaks of gastrointestinal distress among cafeteria customers are examples of immediate effects from health-damaging environments. Examples of long-term health effects include gradual occupational hearing loss, black lung in coal miners, and increased rates of cancer among migrant farm workers who were aerially sprayed with the pesticide DDT 15 years ago

(Werner and Olson, 1993). Transgenerational effects occur with the radiation exposures of female factory workers at plutonium-processing plants that cause chromosomal anomalies and later result in birth defects in their offspring. Another transgenerational effect is seen in the repetition of domestic violence in successive family generations.

Some negative environmental health effects are reversible. For example, the lungs of nonsmokers who for years inhaled secondhand smoke from their smoking family members and coworkers can heal and be restored to healthy function if the smoke is eliminated. On the other hand, damage to human cells caused by radiation is irreversible, as is the damage to lung capacity caused by silicosis. Many environmental hazards cause cumulative effects, as represented by heavy metal exposure. Over time, lead collects in the long bones and can be rereleased into the body. Not only can it cause acute poisoning, but it later may cause additional damage (Needleman et al., 1992).

EFFORTS TO CONTROL ENVIRONMENTAL HEALTH PROBLEMS

The 1970s represent the decade of environmental concern. As cynicism toward institutions grew during the Vietnam War era, legislative activism for environmental preservation exploded (Burger, 1989). Table 26–4 outlines the essential statutes. New agencies designed to regulate environmental conditions on a national level were created by Congress at that time, including the EPA, Occupational Health and Safety Administration (OSHA), and Nuclear Regulation Commission (NRC). The EPA has enormous responsibilities for protecting the environment and minimizing environmental risks to human health. Among its roles are setting standards for air and water quality, health surveillance and monitoring, evaluation of environmental risks, information acquisition, screening of new chemicals, basic research and training, data base maintenance, and establishing, evaluating, and enforcing regulatory efforts.

The legislative activism of the 1970s was responsible for unprecedented movement toward a comprehensive national environmental policy. For example, improvements in air quality were made through stricter automobile fuel and emissions standards. As a result, lead levels in urban air decreased 87% from 1977 levels (Bingham and Meader, 1990). The momentum to control environmental corruption in the

Table 26–4
Landmark Federal Environmental Legislation

Year	Legislation
1970	Clean Air Act
1970	Poison Prevention Packaging Act
1970	Occupational Health and Safety Act
1970	Hazardous Materials Transportation Control
1970	National Environmental Policy Act
1971	Lead-Based Paint Poisoning Prevention Act
1972	Federal Water Pollution Control Act Amendments
1972	Noise Control Act
1976	Resource Conservation and Recovery Act
1976	Toxic Substances Control Act
1977	Clean Water Act
1980	Low Level Radiation Waste Policy Act
1980	Comprehensive Environmental Response, Compensation, and Liability Act (Superfund)

United States slowed in the 1980s and 1990s with several policy reversals and the defunding of regulatory mechanisms. For instance, the Occupational Health and Safety Act and other statutes were seriously weakened by the Reagan administration deregulation of industry.

Dumont (1989) offered this critique: truly alarming assessments of the dangers inherent in current levels of soil, air, and water pollution are reduced to the level of cliché, mere ambient noise. "We have become accustomed to revelations about clusters of birth defects and cancer in communities near land fills, chemical spills in the major rivers of the world, contamination of wells and aquifers with industrial waste, and bursts of toxic gases from 'human errors' at factories. It is only when catastrophes of such tremendous magnitude occur like Bhopal or Chernobyl that North Americans take note of the tortured biosphere" (p. 1077).

Political dynamics, social values, and powerful industry and business interests influence the attention paid to environmental problems as well as the economic commitment to their solutions (Reich, 1988). An example is the widespread agricultural use of neurotoxic organophosphate pesticides, which are known to cause lasting central nervous system damage (Moses, 1993). Advocates for farm workers say the EPA should ban the use of pesticides registered in the highest toxicity category. Instead, the EPA has proposed new regulations that would require employers to provide general pesticide safety information to all farm workers. The EPA also suggested regular blood tests to monitor toxin levels in those who apply the pesticides. Monitoring would be required only for commercial applicators (i.e., those who apply chemicals as a business), however, and not for farm workers who apply pesticides as one part of their duties on the job. The EPA is said to have limited the scope of its monitoring requirement because of pressure from large agribusiness corporations.

Legislators and other policymakers have often based their pesticide use decisions on economic impact (i.e., how crop yield will be affected):

Regulators have thus ignored the costs: To farmworkers from pesticide poisoning, disability, loss of income, and increased risk of chronic health effects; to society from pesticide pollution and contamination of the air, water, soil, and food; to wildlife from the killing of fish, birds, bees, and other species; and to the planet generally from the widespread environmental and ecological damage that continues unchecked because of the failure to develop safer, healthier, and more sustainable methods of growing crops.

(Moses, 1993, p. 171)

The scientific research and ongoing systematic surveillance necessary to fully inform environmental health policy are costly and time consuming. Government, industry, and big business have been unwilling to support these efforts adequately in part because, if damages caused by hazardous practices in the past were determined, a vast liability would be incurred. Effectively enforced environmental legislation is also viewed as thwarting technological advance and economic growth. Thus, laws often excuse industry, business, and government from environmental cleanup because of the high costs involved, and communities suffer the health consequences.

Weaknesses in existing legislation and regulatory structures have caused difficulties (Walker, 1990). There are no federal mandates about recycling, although local communities have made great strides in this area. There is also no comprehensive ground water legislation similar to what has been adopted to preserve marine and surface waters (Bingham and Meader, 1990). Environmental laws have sometimes been too detailed or inflexible, causing problems in the articulation of federal and local regulatory efforts. The EPA sets priorities for environmental problems, but resources to meet the identified needs are not often provided. In addition, the EPA is dangerously behind its deadlines in addressing new contaminants. For example, current regulations allow some municipal water systems as long as 20 years to remove lead from service lines (Corn, 1991).

In general, most of the U.S. environmental health efforts have aimed for short-term goals rather than anticipating future needs and problems. In this regard, U.S. industries are underinvested in the development of renewable resource technologies for the sake of transient profits. A crucial need also exists in the development of human resources in the area of environmental health (Walker, 1990). Nursing careers in environmental health science (Neufer, 1994; Salazar and Primomo, 1994) would be an excellent move toward integrating health and environmental theory and practice at the community level.

Nurses need to work with the public toward more stringent and actively enforced environmental legislation and regulation as well as greater social control over corporations and other entities that are at fault for health-damaging environments. In the 1990s, government actions must include not only national but also worldwide environmental policies. Ozone depletion, global warming, and the destruction of tropical rain forests are among key global environmental health concerns. Community health nursing must expand its theory and practice to incorporate the reality that individual and community health depends ultimately on global environmental integrity. Countless organizations working to preserve and protect the environment could benefit from the active involvement and support of nurses; Table 26–5 lists several of these organizations.

APPROACHING ENVIRONMENTAL HEALTH AT THE AGGREGATE LEVEL

In the United States, the concepts of personal independence and individual responsibility for success and failure have always been very important. However, these values can lead nurses to blame individual clients for their health problems while overlooking glaring environmental hazards (Stevens, 1989). By placing responsibility for the cause and cure of health problems exclusively on the individual, the belief is reinforced that all individuals are free to exert meaningful control over the quality and length of their lives (Becker, 1986). Such a perspective absolves society, government, industry, and business from accountability for changing pernicious conditions under which people live and work. Existing research evidence suggests that changing individual behaviors does not lead to significant reductions in overall

Table 26–5
Environmental Organizations

American Farmland Trust
Animal Preservation League
Citizens for a Better Environment
Clean Water Action
Earth Regeneration Society
Forests Forever
Greenpeace
International Rivers Network
National Environmental Law Center
National Toxics Campaign
Natural Resources Defense Council
Ocean Alliance
Pesticide Action Network
Radioactive Wastes Campaign
Rainforest Action Network
Sierra Club
Toxics Coordinating Project
Trust for Public Land
U.S. Public Interest Research Group
Wilderness Society

For further information, see the report by the Institute of Medicine Committee on Enhancing Environmental Health Content in Nursing Practice: *Nursing, Health, and the Environment*. Washington DC: National Academy Press, 1995.

morbidity and mortality in the absence of basic social, economic, and political changes (Freudenberg, 1984–1985; Milio, 1986). Emphasizing only public health interventions that attempt to modify deleterious personal habits through exercise programs, weight loss regimens, smoking cessation classes, and stress reduction tactics fails to engage the broader environmental origins of disease, injury, and ecologic destruction (Salmon and Berliner, 1982).

Nursing is not alone in its focus on individual health-promoting interventions. With federal directives such as the 1979 Surgeon General's report (U.S. Department of Health and Human Services, 1979), most health agencies, health care institutions, and corporate work places have principally addressed the idea of "controllable risk" in the individual, with much less effort directed toward reducing risks in the environment. The government has also reduced its overall focus on environmental health. In the 1980s, the effectiveness and power of agencies such as the EPA and the National Institute for Occupational Safety and Health declined so that they are less able to study environmental health risks and enforce regulatory policies.

By focusing on the individual, other levels of intervention are overlooked (Zola, 1972). Interventions designed for individuals alone leave environments that "sicken" people unchallenged. Although environmental dangers posed by contamination of drinking water, carcinogenic food additives, loss of the ozone layer, and occupational hazards are often recognized as serious, the implication persists that little can be done about the inevitability of technological and industrial growth around the world (Crawford, 1977). Individuals, therefore, are compelled to simply accommodate environments that cause them illness and injury.

Recognition of the gravity and pervasiveness of environmental hazards can be overwhelming. Looking beyond the individual to recognize the environmental determinants of illness and wellness can be complicated and threatening. Intervening to improve the quality of air, water, housing, food, and waste disposal while reducing the risks of occupational injury, radiation, and violence requires basic social, economic, and political changes in the process. Bringing about changes in health-damaging environments must be an aggregate-level endeavor.

Community health nurses who base their practices on the principles of critical theory are better prepared to respond to all of these challenges (Stevens and Hall, 1992). As the vignettes demonstrate, by focusing our efforts on organizing groups of people, we can facilitate community participation in identifying and solving environmental health problems and thus bring about changes that improve environments and eliminate hazards.

CRITICAL COMMUNITY HEALTH NURSING PRACTICE

What are some of the actions community health nurses might take to approach environmental health critically? As described in the vignettes, nurses take sides. They ask critical questions. Nurses become involved with the communities they serve, they form coalitions, and they become familiar with the use of various collective strategies. These areas of nursing intervention were developed and presented elsewhere (Stevens and Hall, 1992). In the interest of educating future practitioners about the critical practice of community health nursing as it applies to environmental health, each of these interventions is discussed in the following sections.

Taking a Stand, Choosing a Side

An old labor union folk song asks, "Which Side Are You On?" Acknowledging that there are multiple sides to issues about health and the environment does not mean that nurses can ultimately avoid taking a stand. Nurses have individual and collective decisions to make about whose interests they want to serve with their specialized knowledge and skills. To say that all should be served is certainly an ideal. However, the present reality is that consequences of hazardous environments are often experienced inequitably. Vulnerable groups are exposed to more health-damaging effects than are less vulnerable groups. A growing body of research substantiates that greater environmental risks are faced by communities of people of color and by economically impoverished neighborhoods (Bullard, 1990; Goldman, 1991). Decisions nurses make about the positions they accept and the interventions they undertake have the potential to increase or decrease these inequities.

Community health nurses have a mandate to assist vulnerable aggregates who are less able to protect themselves from pollution, inadequate housing, toxic poisoning, unsafe products, and other hazards. Non–English-speaking refugees, African-American children, poor women, and illiterate manual laborers make up just some of the groups in the United States that hold little power with which to broker with industry, government, business, and other large institutions for environmental changes and just compensation for harm suffered as a result of environmental hazards.

Environmental problems are clearly intertwined with social, political, and economic policies; barriers to resources; and the interests of those in positions of control. How can nurses connect the immediate and long-term health problems experienced by particular groups and communities to this larger sphere of influence?

Asking Critical Questions

Consider the relationships between nonhealth policies and health. How do policies concerning ecologic preservation, energy, housing, immigration, civil rights, crime, nutrition, minimum wage, occupational safety, and defense affect the well-being of people who live in the United States? Addressing the critical questions of who has access to resources in this country and whose interests are served in the system as it exists provides a way to include social, political, and economic factors in nursing assessments of the environment. Some patterns of questioning are useful in this endeavor. A sample set of questions is given in Table 26–6. These critical questions can be asked when approaching environmental health problems.

Dialogue resulting from critical questioning can frame the problem and assist in building collective strategies. Ideally, these questions should be explored collectively by those most directly affected by the situation or problem. However, even one individual involved in the situation can begin to explore a problem from this perspective and define an initial basis for action.

Facilitating Community Involvement

Approaching community health from a critical perspective means working to improve health conditions while creating the context in which people can identify health-damaging problems in their environments. One

---

Table 26–6
Critical Questions About Environmental Health Problems

What is the problem?
Who is defining the problem?
In what terms is the problem being described?
How are others in the situation viewing the problem?
What is the history of the problem?
How did things get the way they are?
What other situations are directly affected by this
    problem?
Who is impacted by the problem?
Whose health is being damaged because of the way
    things are?
Who benefits from the way things are?
Whose interests are served by current solutions?
What are the economic inequities in the situation?
Who has political power in the situation?
Who knows about the problem?
Who needs to know or know more about the problem?
How effective are current programs, strategies, and
    policies?
What are the barriers to help and relief from the problem?
What strategies have been used to try to alleviate the
    problem?
How successful have these strategies been?
What groups are already in place that might deal with this
    problem?
What resources are needed to solve the problem?
How accessible are the resources?
How can solutions be evaluated for effectiveness?

---

important nursing goal is to help people learn from their own experiences and analyze the world with an aim to change it. It is essential that the people affected participate in a process of identifying and working to solve environmental problems.

To create this openness, nurses must abandon asymmetric positions of leadership and instead join in mutual exchanges with community members that honor each individual's experience. The nurse's role changes from presenting solutions and directing lifestyle changes to asking critical questions of groups and assisting them to reflect on the problematic environmental realities of their lives. A second nursing role is to provide support, information, and expertise to groups to assist them in meeting their goals for environmental change. In each of these roles, nurses use the concept of solidarity, in which the relationship with the community and its individual members is maintained and nurtured despite disagreements that may occur over what is the best course of action.

Instead of trying to compel people to act in certain ways, nurses should assist aggregates in their own collective search for effective change strategies. Actions dictated from those outside the situation are often culturally inappropriate and, therefore, doomed to be ineffective. Lasting rapport with aggregates depends on honesty, fairness, and mutuality in interactions over extended periods of time.

With critical questions, community health nurses can assist community members in looking beyond immediate environmental problems to explore social, cultural, economic, and political circumstances that affect them. Nurses' knowledge of the scientific basis for health problems, insights about the historic origins of particular environmental hazards, technical skills, and expertise in communicating and organizing can be shared not as a method of dominating but rather as a way of developing a mutual plan of action to deal with the problems that have been collectively identified. By addressing people's everyday concerns and targeting the problems they themselves identify, nurses situate their efforts in communities' struggles.

Forming Coalitions

Another very important nursing task that arises from approaching environmental health from a critical perspective involves forming coalitions to bring about social change. By initiating dialogue and building a strong base of collective support, nurses can insist on structural changes that eliminate hazards and improve the public's health. In dealing with health-damaging environments, nurses can approach already existing community organizations and family and friendship networks as well as help mobilize aggregate members who have not previously socialized or acted together. As a group, nurses can then expose hazards, assess needs, plan actions, report abuses, and secure appropriate resources, personnel, funding, and legislative changes.

The environmental justice movement (Bullard, 1993) is an excellent example of coalition building wherein grassroots groups organized by people of color meet around circumstances of waste facility siting, lead contamination, pesticides, water and air pollution, native self-government, nuclear testing, and work place safety to plan and take action about the disproportionate environmental challenges they face. Drawing insights from both the civil rights and the environmental movements, these grassroots groups have forged alliances with many conventional environmental and civil rights organizations to mount formal responses to environmental threats. One grassroots organization fighting for environmental justice, the Mothers of East Los Angeles, lined up the support of Greenpeace, Natural Resources Defense Council, Environmental Policy Institute, Citizens' Clearinghouse on Hazardous Waste, National Toxics Campaign, and Western Center on Law and Poverty to bring a lawsuit against state and federal agencies who had granted a private corporation permission to build and operate a toxic waste incinerator in the middle of their urban neighborhood. This permission had been granted despite the fact that the incinerator corporation had not prepared an environmental impact report. The mainstream environmental organization allies provided valuable technical advice, expert testimony, lobbying, research, and legal assistance while the Mothers of East Los Angeles spearheaded efforts in which hundreds of East Los Angeles residents showed up for every public hearing about the incinerator project to place intense political pressure. In the ensuing court battles that went all the way to the California Supreme Court, the construction of the proposed facility was prevented.

Nurses can be instrumental in these efforts, helping community groups make connections with larger, more powerful organizations. Nurses can organize forums whereby community groups meet with the scientific experts who can help them gather evidence about health threats, with managers of businesses whose actions impinge on the economic life of the community, with heads of industry whose companies create ecologic hazards, and with legislators who can bring community concerns to law-making bodies. Using available institutional resources, skills, and knowledge, nurses can also explore what is happening elsewhere. Making connections with groups in other locales who are struggling for similar environmental changes can enhance collective strength and solidarity. Press releases, media events, interviews, television spots, speeches, newsletters, and leaflets are important means of raising awareness among communities as well as calling the attention of outsiders to a situation at hand.

In working for various municipalities, agencies, and health care corporations, nurses may be constrained by the philosophies, policies, resources, and relations of these organizations. Although nurses may disagree with some of these organizational aspects, they are perceived by communities to be representatives of the organizations for whom they work. These institutional connections may cause problems for nurses working with groups who feel abandoned by the system, disregarded in policy decisions, or refused access to resources. Establishing alliances with disenfranchised communities is, therefore, a complex and often long-term process of building trust. Nurses must advocate for the fiscal, logistical, labor, and ideologic support necessary for these processes. This means that in many cases nurses will have to struggle collectively for institutional changes to develop resources to make the environment safer. When mobilizing aggregates for improvement of environmental health, it is essential that the process not be undermined by a withdrawal of resources, because this will lead to further alienation and mistrust on the part of vulnerable groups.

It may appear that an "us–them" approach has been advocated in which one always aligns with the vulnerable against outside "enemies." This is an unfortunate oversimplification. When nurses work to build coalitions for improving environmental conditions, each issue or problem requires appropriate strategizing based on its own merits. Allies in a current struggle may have been adversaries in a previous struggle. For example, even though a bank refused to help farm families by granting farm loan extensions last month, it may still be an ally this month when a superhighway development project threatens its building as well as an adjacent poor neighborhood. An ally need not be in complete agreement with the core group's philosophy, political agenda, or moral beliefs. The federal government may be viewed as an adversary with regard to restrictive immigration policies but as an ally in its enforcement of the provisions of the Rehabilitation Act. There is virtually no person or faction that can be completely discounted as an ally that will not ultimately be touched by some environmental health issue. It is a good idea to brainstorm about all the possible groups and factions in a locale that may have a stake in the outcome of an issue. A good coalition-building strategy is to have an eye on the future and envision how one struggle—one set of allies—can extend its network and subsequently form new coalitions for emerging issues.

Using Collective Strategies

A variety of collective strategies can be used by nurses in coalition with others to intervene at the aggregate level and facilitate liberating changes in a community's health. Organizing people to change health-damaging environments can be accomplished through combinations of strategies, including coalition building; consciousness-raising groups; educational forums in neighborhoods, work places, schools, churches, and social clubs; seminars for health care providers, city officials, teachers, and employers; community needs assessments; dissemination of clinical research and policy analyses; use of mass media; canvassing; litigation; legislative lobbying; testimony at public hearings; demonstrations; and participatory research. Stotts (1991) demonstrated the use of several of these collective strategies in his community health nursing intervention aimed at limiting secondhand smoke in public buildings and work sites.

Although nurses have not traditionally used all of these collective strategies to intervene in community health matters, environmental hazards are multiplying geometrically, pushing us to expand our repertoire of skills. If nurses have not been taught these types of organizational skills, they can learn from experts in the community who have had experience with conducting mass media campaigns, organizing demonstrations, canvassing neighborhoods, participating in class action litigation, testifying at public hearings, and so on. Also many books about political action can be consulted.

One collective strategy that is an effective aggregate-level community health nursing intervention is *participatory research,* sometimes called *action research.* Participatory research calls for nurses, community members, and other resource people to work together in identifying environmental health problems that should be investigated, designing the studies, collecting and analyzing the data, disseminating results, and posing solutions to the problems (Freudenberg, 1984; Greenfield and Zimmerman, 1993; Hildebrandt, 1994; Whyte, 1991). With the assistance of community health nurses, community members gather information on suspected environmental hazards, document their effects on health, educate their communities, persuade corporations to clean up, and lobby local, state, and federal governments for stricter regulations and better enforcement. The goal of the research process is not merely the production of knowledge but rather the generation of open discussion and debate that intensifies a community's consciousness of how its health is impaired by environmental constraints. The box presents an abstract of an article about popular epidemiology (Brown, 1987), which is a type of participatory research related to environmental health.

PARTICIPATORY RESEARCH ABOUT ENVIRONMENTAL HEALTH

Research Project

Brown, P.: Popular epidemiology: Community response to toxic waste-induced disease. Sci. Technol. Hum. Value 12;78–85, 1987.

Abstract

The residents of Woburn, Massachusetts, working together with civic activists and some professionals, collected data confirming the existence of a leukemia cluster and demonstrated that it was traceable to industrial waste carcinogens that leached into their drinking water supply. These residents collectively took part in years of actions that led to successful civil suits against the corporations at fault. The actions of the Woburn citizenry offer a valuable example of lay communication of risk to scientific experts and government officials and demonstrate a concerted collective effort at investigation into disease patterns and their likely causes. This case, which drew national attention during the 1980s, has catalyzed similar efforts across the country and expands our knowledge of the effects of toxic wastes. The Woburn residents introduced evidence to show that the health effects of toxic wastes are not restricted to physical disease but also include emotional problems.

Using this case study of popular epidemiology, which involves community-propelled investigation, the author provides a framework for participatory research about environmental health.

In towns across the United States, concerned residents are conducting surveys to determine the severity of community health threats posed by factories that pollute waterways, nuclear power plants, aerial spraying of herbicides, vehicle exhaust pollution, off-shore oil drilling, and excessive lumbering. One such effort, presented by Freudenberg (1984–1985) and detailed next, was very successful.

In response to unregulated toxic contamination in Pennsylvania during the early 1980s, a coalition of tenant associations, environmental groups, senior citizens, labor unions, and Vietnam War veterans who had been exposed to Agent Orange organized in Philadelphia. The Delaware Valley Toxics Coalition, as it was called, elicited the help of scientists and epidemiologists to write environmental impact reports about chemical contamination, imple-

mented massive community and work place education, staged protest demonstrations at polluting companies, organized testimony at public hearings, and helped draft legislation. The coalition also used the media creatively to publicize their concerns. For example, one labor union member sprayed from an unmarked canister into the city council chamber during public testimony. When the city council members protested, the unionist replied, "This can contains only air, but every day we have to work with chemicals we know nothing about." As a result of the coalition's efforts, the city of Philadelphia enacted the nation's first right-to-know law. The statute stipulated that workers and community residents had the right to know the names and health effects of chemicals used, manufactured, stored, or released into the air.

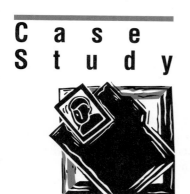

Case Study

Application of the Nursing Process

In December 1990, the *San Francisco Examiner* reported on the extensive problem of lead exposure in Oakland, California (Kay, 1990). Some of the reported facts of this situation are expanded on to construct hypothetical nursing interventions.

Assessment

Oakland's community health nurses have long been involved with city residents and have been aware of high rates of lead poisoning in particular neighborhoods. In the wake of alarming newspaper articles about the dangerous incidence of lead exposure in the city, the nurses decide at a planning meeting to make lead exposure a priority. The community health nurses and several nursing students assigned to their department divide assessment tasks and uncover the following conditions.

A 1988 California study of lead exposure reported that approximately 50,000 California children have enough lead in their serum to lower intelligence, alter behavior, create neurologic dysfunction, damage kidneys, and depress growth (Kay, 1990). It was found that one fifth of inner city Oakland children have toxic levels of lead in their blood. Although the ubiquitous danger of lead poisoning has been known to city, state, and federal authorities for decades, they have failed to establish routine testing of children. They have not created programs to remove lead-based paint from existing structures, nor have they eliminated lead emissions from industrial sources and overcrowded freeways.

An economically depressed neighborhood in Oakland, hypothetically called Rosario, is situated near numerous railways, freeways, and industrial yards. High numbers of African-American, Latino, and Southeast Asian residents live in the older homes that line the streets of Rosario. The concentration of lead in the soil of the neighborhood averages 1200 parts per million (Kay, 1991a). A soil lead concentration of 500 to 1000 parts per million is sufficient to cause dangerously high blood levels of lead in children (Alliance to End Childhood

Lead Poisoning, 1991). Lead levels are also significant in Rosario's drinking water because much of its plumbing consists of lead pipes that leach lead into standing water. Lead-based paint peels from most of the houses. Many heads of households who work in the nearby radiator shops, scrap metal yards, and battery-manufacturing plants carry lead dust home on their clothing and shoes. Isolated by language and economic circumstances, many Rosario residents do not know about the environmental health hazards to which they are being exposed.

Children absorb 50% of the lead they eat, drink, or breathe, whereas adults absorb only 10% (Phoenix, 1993). Children are more likely to come in contact with lead by playing in contaminated dirt and eating paint chips. Substandard nutrition also increases the absorption of lead. Lead in automobile exhaust and industrial emissions is inhaled and contaminates the ground near busy freeways and factories. Unfortunately, lead remains in the soil for thousands of years (Bailey et al., 1994).

Lucia, a 7-year-old girl who lives in Rosario, had a lead level several times as high as that needed to cause impairment of intelligence. Her hair fell out, and she became emaciated, weak, and often tearful. She had constant nosebleeds and fell down frequently. She was given painful and risky intravenous treatment with chelating agents over a period of 1 year, and most of her symptoms receded. However, her mother says, "No one cleans up the area. People move in and out, but the poison remains here." In fact, local hospital spokespersons say that 25% of the children they treat for lead poisoning are repoisoned after they are sent home (Kay, 1990).

The state's Child Health Program, which provides health examinations for poor children, refuses to add lead tests to their routine examinations, even though the federal government now requires it as a condition for Medicaid funding. California officials say that they provide testing when it is recommended by a physician, but private physicians in the city generally assume that lead poisoning is an East Coast phenomenon. Therefore, they often fail to recommend the blood test and are unlikely to recognize the syndrome of lead poisoning when it does occur. Furthermore, the Child Health Program reaches only about one third of those who are eligible. The governor recently vetoed $160,000 in funding for a lead-testing program for high-risk children in Oakland.

On the basis of this assessment, the city's community health nurses devise the following list of unresolved problems:

- Lead-screening programs for children are not in place.
- Private physicians are not recommending lead tests for vulnerable children.
- Health care providers at local public hospitals and clinics may not be recognizing lead-poisoning symptoms.
- Children are being repoisoned after treatment.
- Industrial and vehicular emissions are poorly controlled.
- No comprehensive plan for removal of lead-based paint from older structures in the city is under way.
- Many Rosario residents work in lead-related industries.
- Poverty and malnutrition are widespread in Rosario.
- Residents are poorly informed about lead hazards in the environment.
- Multiracial, multicultural, and language characteristics of Rosario make organizing and education efforts more complex.

Planning

Given their assessment, the community health nurses decide they must assist members of the Rosario community to force environmental changes that reduce lead-poisoning risks. They realize they should involve members of the Rosario community at planning meetings from the outset and make efforts to include African-American, Latino, and Southeast Asian community members. They contact neighborhood leaders, church leaders, ethnic clubs, the local Parent-Teacher Association, a senior citizen organization in the neighborhood, the Black Women's Health Project, and a local Latina women's political organization. In their initial meetings, they learn that there is a budding multicultural grassroots effort by People United for a Better Oakland (PUEBLO) (Calpotura, 1991; Kay, 1990) that is going door to door educating Oakland residents about the dangers of lead.

With community members, the nurses discuss how all parties view the problem, what resources are available, how they might align with PUEBLO, who might serve as potential allies, what the community health nursing agency can do, how they might generate more community involvement, and what potential actions might be taken. The nurses also ask questions about other circumstances that are affecting Rosario residents. Community members express that they are still reeling from the damages caused by a major earthquake a few years before. They also report that many of their neighbors are fearful of coming to the meetings or joining PUEBLO because they are undocumented workers and worry about deportation. In addition, the state highway commission is pressing for the construction of another freeway close to Rosario; everybody is worried about this. After several meetings, members decide to establish a permanent Rosario Coalition of which the nurses are an important part.

The nurses talk about their competing priorities; the lead problem is only one of the issues they deal with. They reach the conclusion that they can most efficiently advocate for the Rosario's residents by using their established ties with local physicians, nurses, and health care institutions. They allocate adequate funds and personnel to accomplish goals set by the coalition and establish a time frame for ongoing evaluation of the Rosario project. Nursing students and community health nursing faculty from the local university and college programs are encouraged to become involved in the interventions.

Intervention

The actions that the community health nurses in coalition with community members decide to take can be divided into interventions at the individual, family, and aggregate levels.

Individual

- Identify Rosario children who have been diagnosed and treated for lead poisoning, and plan follow-up home visits in an attempt to prevent repoisoning.
- Add to the community health agency's child health assessment protocol several observations specifically designed to detect symptoms of lead poisoning and several questions aimed at establishing whether there are specific risks for lead poisoning in the home.
- Coordinate with school nurses so that they can incorporate similar changes in their health assessment protocols.

- Establish an agreement with the state's Child Health Program that they will obtain lead levels on children if it is recommended, not only by physicians but also by school nurses or community health nurses.
- Together with members of the Rosario Coalition, prepare an educational pamphlet detailing the lead-poisoning risks that exist for Rosario residents. With the coalition's endorsement, the nurses mail the pamphlet to individual physicians and nurses who provide services to children in Oakland.
- Prepare translations of the pamphlet in languages and reading levels appropriate for Rosario residents and mail it to individual households.
- Follow up on pamphlet mailings with announcements of community health nurses' willingness to offer lead-poisoning education programs at churches, schools, hospitals, work places, medical association meetings, and nursing association meetings.

Family

- Initiate a family-to-family program in which a core group of Rosario community members attend educational meetings with the community health nurses. In these meetings, information is shared about the environmental origins of lead poisoning and its prevention, diagnosis, and treatment. These specially trained community members then take charge of the program, sharing their knowledge with extended family members and neighboring families.
- Coordinate with school nurses to establish a health education program in Rosario schools in which school-age children are taught about lead poisoning. These children are then encouraged to take their knowledge home and teach younger preschool-age brothers and sisters about handwashing and avoiding putting their hands to their mouths when playing.
- Investigate how community health nurses might be of more assistance to Rosario families in helping them apply for and obtain nutritional resources such as food stamps, Supplemental Food Program for Women, Infants and Children, food bank supplements, school lunch programs, and so on. With improvement of nutritional status, lead absorption might thus be decreased.
- Facilitate the formation of a support group for families with children who have suffered damage from lead poisoning. The community health nurses offer their offices for evening meeting space and serve as information resources about health care and social services as well as disability assistance from the government.

Aggregate

- With the Rosario Coalition, form broader coalitions with PUEBLO, Oakland churches, local nurses association, several preschool and day care centers, and the Oakland School Board to design a comprehensive, nonduplicative, cost-effective lead-screening program that will test all children in Oakland on a regular basis.
- Lobby state legislatures, municipal officials, local medical association, local hospitals, and city clinics regarding implementation of the plan.
- Contact researchers at a local university's environmental sciences program and request that they work with the coalition to conduct a house-to-house study of sources of lead poisoning. The nurses and other members of the coalition offer their cooperation in teaching Rosario residents about the questionnaires they will be expected to fill out and the data gathering that will be required involving soil, water, and paint samples. They also offer to

coordinate the services of bilingual research assistants from the Rosario community.

- Coordinate efforts at abatement, the process of removing the source of exposure to the environmental hazard: (1) obtain federal guidelines for lead abatement in private homes (U.S. Department of Housing and Urban Development, 1990); (2) determine municipal, state, and federal accountability for financing lead abatement in low-income owner-occupied households; (3) explore strategies that will compel multiple-dwelling owners to remove lead from their properties so that they are safe for tenants, and (4) initiate fund-raising activities to cover out-of-pocket expenses that Rosario residents will incur from the abatement process.
- Contact the occupational health nurses at local lead-based industries to ascertain policies related to heavy metals, enforcement of regulations regarding lead disposal, and number of cases of lead poisoning among workers.
- Contact state environmental groups for advice on local efforts, and join with them in their fight for stricter regulation of lead emissions and toxic wastes.
- Contact local media (television, radio, and newspaper) about running a series of stories about local lead-poisoning risks. Nurses and other coalition members supply information and contacts for interviews and photographs.

Evaluation

In regular meetings of the original Rosario Coalition, the nurses facilitate evaluation of ongoing interventions. Among their many evaluation activities, the nurses keep track of both the number of lead-screening tests being done on Rosario children and the rates of lead poisoning and repoisoning to determine whether their efforts in these areas are effective. They document participation levels at educational programs and family-to-family training sessions and interest in the nutrition referrals and support group, all of which appear to be successful.

The community health nurses also keep in close contact with the school nurses and the occupational health nurses. At one point, the occupational health nurses report that they are too overburdened in their jobs to do the necessary worker education concerning prevention of heavy metal poisoning. The community health nurses and coalition members offer to help. They set up an

---

EXAMPLES OF LEVELS OF PREVENTION

Primary prevention
Education of the community regarding lead poisoning and lead hazards in the environment

Secondary prevention
Screening at-risk populations for exposure to lead and blood lead levels

Tertiary prevention
Follow-up treatment of persons with lead poisoning; removal of lead hazards from the community environment

after-work educational program for foremen at the local industries and another program for union shop stewards. They hope that both groups will disseminate the information at their work places. The occupational health nurses are asked to report back with their observations of the success of the educational sessions. The broader coalition's efforts at pushing through their plan for a comprehensive lead-screening program are met with a great deal of opposition from the state legislature, even though local officials support their plan. When repeated negotiations continue to fail, the coalition decides to align with environmental and civil rights groups who are suing the state of California for failing to provide federally mandated tests for lead poisoning in low-income children. They join as plaintiffs in the class action suit. The community health nurses from Rosario give expert testimony in the case.

As the court case proceeds, some members of the state legislature begin to show more interest in a lead-screening program, and another vote is scheduled. The Rosario Coalition participates in a Lead Poisoning Awareness Day at the state capitol the week before the vote. They are active in the demonstration and give speeches about their local experiences. They visit the offices of individual legislators informing them of the situation in Rosario. Citing the tentative results from the environmental sciences' house-to-house research study as well as the statistics the community health nurses have been keeping about screening and poisoning rates proves to be very useful. This evidence strengthens the coalition members' arguments about the need for a comprehensive lead-screening program in the state. The coalition also shares these data with the national environmental groups with which they have been working. These groups use the data in testimony before federal legislators to secure federal funding for a new program to remove lead-based paint from existing structures.

SUMMARY

This chapter has provided a glimpse into the complex world of environmental health from a critical community health nursing perspective. The case study, vignettes, and examples serve to illustrate the need for nurses to evaluate the broader picture in assessing the environmental health status of communities and the vulnerable aggregates within them. In preventing, minimizing, and resolving environmental health problems, nurses must recognize patterns, detect subtle changes, identify underlying issues, and work collaboratively with a variety of other individuals and groups. In the past, environmental threats to health were usually suspected only when other possible causes of illness had been ruled out. Nurses can expect this pattern to change drastically in future decades as environmental health moves increasingly to the forefront of the public health agenda.

NURSES ENVIRONMENTAL HEALTHWATCH

Nurses Environmental Healthwatch is an organization that is involved in educating nurses about environmental concerns and nursing's role in bringing about a safe, healthy environment. Nurses Environmental Healthwatch may be contacted at 181 Marshall Street, Duxbury, MA 02332.

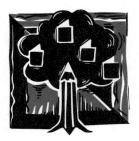

Learning Activities

1. Identify a health-related problem associated with some aspect of the environment. It may be a problem you see in your community, one that you have read about, or a difficulty identified by a family with whom you work. Examine the problem using the sample series of critical questions listed in Table 26–6. Without sharing your results, present the problem to a group of your peers and ask them to discuss it by responding to the same questions. Were there differences between your answers and those of the group? Were there similarities? On what points did everyone agree? Why? What questions caused the most disagreement? Why?

   Now repeat the entire activity by involving people other than nursing students in the group discussion. How did this discussion compare with the previous one and with your responses to the questions?

2. Attend meetings in which environmental hazards are discussed. If meetings or public forums are not available in your vicinity, write for information about the actions being taken in your state to fight environmental hazards. The reference librarians at your college or public library can suggest ways of contacting sources and supply addresses. Organizations that are likely to sponsor forums and provide information include those listed in Table 26–5 as well as the EPA, National Institute for Occupational Safety and Health, state and municipal agencies for environmental protection and occupational health, environmental caucuses of political parties, American Public Health Association, local public health department, farmers' organizations, and labor unions.

3. In this chapter, examples are presented about how to use participatory research as an intervention in dealing with ecologic hazards. With a group, brainstorm about possibilities for participatory action research projects in your locality. Try to think of examples from a variety of environmental health areas. Be creative in your planning. How might you mobilize community support and participation in the research? What groups would you approach? What critical questions might you use to facilitate dialogue about the problem? What ideas do you have about the kinds of data that could be collected and how they could be used? How would you publicize your research results? What ramifications could the completed study have for community members, other communities in the state, and community health nurses in other locales?

4. Nurses may have to supplement their knowledge of collective strategies by reading books about political action and by learning from community members who are experienced in political organizing. Visit your college or public library to investigate books and journal articles outside the nursing literature. Compile a list of references related to one of these political strategies (e.g., grassroots organizing, legislative lobbying, community education, policy analysis, use of the media, coalition building, citizen surveys, public protest, letter-writing campaigns, consciousness-raising groups). Exchange reference lists with your peers so you benefit from each other's efforts. Then, choose one or two books that interest you and read them.

REFERENCES

Aday LA: At Risk in America: The Health and Health Care Needs of Vulnerable Populations in the United States. San Francisco, Jossey-Bass, 1993.

Allen DG: Using philosophical and historical methodologies to understand the concept of health. *In* Chinn PL (ed): Nursing Research Methodology Issues and Implementation. Rockville, MD, Aspen, 1986, pp. 157–168.

Alliance to End Childhood Lead Poisoning: Childhood Lead Poisoning Prevention: A Resource Directory, 2nd ed. Washington, DC, National Center for Education in Maternal and Child Health, 1991.

Alston D: We Speak for Ourselves: Social Justice, Race, and Environment. Washington, DC, Panos Institute, 1990.

Anderson RF: Solid waste and public health. *In* Greenberg MR (ed): Public Health and the Environment: The United States Experience. New York, Guilford Press, 1987, pp. 173–204.

Anspach RR: From stigma to identity politics: Political activism among the physically disabled and former mental patients. Soc Sci Med 13A: 765–773, 1979.

Bailey AJ, Sargent JD, Goodman DC, et al.: Poisoned landscapes: The epidemiology of environmental lead exposure in Massachusetts children 1990–1991. Soc Sci Med 39: 757–766, 1994.

Becker MH: The tyranny of health promotion. Public Health Rev 14: 15–25, 1986.

Bingham E, Meader WV: Governmental regulation of environmental hazards in the 1990s. Annu Rev Public Health 11: 419–434, 1990.

Blumenthal DS, Ruttenber J. (eds): Introduction to Environmental Health, 2nd ed. New York, Springer, 1995.

Brender JD, Suarez L: Paternal occupation and anencephaly. Am J Epidemiol 131: 517–521, 1990.

Brooks BO: Indoor air pollution: An edifice complex. Clin Toxicol 29: 315–374, 1991.

Brown P: Popular epidemiology: Community response to toxic waste-induced disease. Sci Technol Hum Value 12: 78–85, 1987.

Bryant B, Mohai P: Race and the Incidence of Environmental Hazards. Boulder, CO, Westview Press, 1992.

Bullard RD: Dumping in Dixie: Race, Class, and Environmental Quality. Boulder, CO, Westview Press, 1990.

Bullard RD (ed): Confronting Environmental Racism: Voices from the Grassroots. Boston, South End Press, 1993.

Burger EJ: Human health: A surrogate for the environment: The evolution of environmental legislation and regulation during the 1970s. Regulat Toxicol Pharmacol 9: 196–206, 1989.

Butterfield PG: Thinking upstream: Nurturing a conceptual understanding of the societal context of health behavior. Adv Nurs Sci 12: 1–8, 1990.

Calpotura F: PUEBLO (People United for a Better Oakland) and Lead Poisoning. Speech presented at the National Conference on Preventing Childhood Lead Poisoning, Washington, DC, October 7, 1991.

Canadian Institute for Advanced Research: The Determinants of Health. Toronto, Ontario, Canada, Author, 1991.

Center for Investigative Reporting: Global Dumping Grounds: The International Trade in Hazardous Waste. Washington, DC, Seven Locks Press, 1990.

Connell SA: And the children keep on dying: Parents say it must be pesticides. San Francisco Chronicle, June 10, 1990, pp. 3, 5.

Connon CL, Freund E, Ehlers JK: The occupational health nurses in agricultural communities program: Identifying and preventing agriculturally related illnesses and injuries. Am Assoc Occupat Health Nurs J, 41: 422–428, 1993.

Corn D: Precious bodily fluids. The Nation, 1991, p. 840.

Council on Scientific Affairs: Low-level radioactive wastes. JAMA 262: 669–674, 1989.

Covello VT, Merkhofer MW: Risk assessment methods: Approaches for assessing health and environmental risks. New York, Plenum Press, 1993.

Cralley LV, Cralley LJ, Cooper WC (eds): Health and Safety Beyond the Work Place. New York, Wiley, 1990.

Crawford R: You are dangerous to your health: The ideology and politics of victim blaming. Int J Health Serv 7: 663–680, 1977.

DeRosa CT, Stevens Y, Johnson BL: Cancer policy framework for public health: Assessment of carcinogens in the environment. Toxicol Indust Health 9: 559–575, 1993.

DeLong JV: Public policy toward municipal solid waste. Annu Rev Public Health 14: 137–157, 1993.

Dumont MP: Psychotoxicology: The return of the mad hatter. Soc Sci Med 29: 1077–1082, 1989.

Earls F, Cairns RB, Mercy JA: The control of violence and the promotion of nonviolence in adolescents. *In* Millstein SG, Petersen AC, Nightingale EO (eds): Promoting the Health of Adolescents: New Directions for the Twenty-First Century. New York, Oxford University Press, 1993, pp. 285–304.

Eckersley R: Environmentalism and Political Theory: Toward an Ecocentric Approach. Albany, NY, State University of New York Press, 1992.

Elsom EM: Atmospheric Pollution: A Global Problem. Oxford, England, Basil Blackwell, 1992.

Evans GW, Kliewer W, Martin J: The role of the physical environment in the health and well-being of children. *In* Schroeder HE (ed): New Directions in Health Psychology Assessment. New York, Hemisphere, 1991, pp. 127–157.

Foster HD: Health and the physical environment: The challenge of global change. *In* Hayes MV, Foster LT, Foster HD (eds): The Determinants of Populations Health: A Critical Assessment. Victoria, British Columbia, Canada, University of Victoria, 1994, pp. 73–120.

Freudenberg N: Not in Our Backyard: Community Action for Health and the Environment. New York, Monthly Review, 1984.

Freudenberg N: Training health educators for social change. Int Q Commun Health Educ 5: 37–52, 1984–1985.

Gaillard AWK: Comparing the concepts of mental load and stress. Ergonomics 36: 991–1005, 1993.

Goldman B: The Truth About Where You Live: An Atlas for Action on Toxins and Mortality. New York, Random House, 1991.

Goudie A: The Human Impact on the Natural Environment. Oxford, England, Basil Blackwell, 1990.

Gould P: Fire in the Rain: The Democratic Consequences of Chernobyl. Baltimore, MD, The Johns Hopkins University Press, 1990.

Greenberg M, Schneider D: Violence in American cities: Young black males is the answer, but what was the question? Soc Sci Med 39: 179–187, 1994.

Greenfield TK, Zimmerman R (eds): Experiences with Community Action Projects: New Research in the Prevention of Alcohol and Other Drug Problems (Center for Substance Abuse Prevention Monograph 14). Rockville, MD, U.S. Department of Health and Human Services, 1993.

Grondona C: Lead revisited: A case study on lead exposed painters. Am Assoc Occupat Health Nurs J 41: 33–38, 1993.

Hall JM, Stevens PE: A nursing view of the U.S.–Iraq war: Psychosocial health consequences. Nurs Outlook 40: 113–120, 1992.

Hall JM, Stevens PE, Meleis AI: Marginalization: A guiding concept for valuing diversity in nursing knowledge development. Adv Nurs Sci 16: 23–41, 1994.

Hamilton C: Coping with industrial exploitation. *In* Bullard RD (ed). Confronting Environmental Racism: Voices from the Grassroots. Boston, South End Press, 1993, pp. 63–75.

Harper AC, Lambert LJ: The Health of Populations: An Introduction, 2nd ed. New York, Springer, 1994.

Haun JW: Guide to the Management of Hazardous Waste. Golden, CO, Fulcrum, 1991.

Hayes WJ, Laws E (eds): Handbook of Pesticide Toxicology. San Diego, CA, Academic Press, 1990.

Hildebrandt E: A model for community involvement in health program development. Soc Sci Med 39: 247–254, 1994.

International Physicians for the Prevention of Nuclear War: Radioactive Heaven and Earth: The Health and Environmental Effects of Nuclear Weapons Testing in, on, and above the Earth. New York, Apex Press, 1991.

Jackson MP, McSwane DZ: Homelessness as a determinant of health. Public Health Nurs 9: 185–192, 1992.

Kay J: State's kids still exposed to lead. San Francisco Examiner, December 9, 1990, pp. 1, 16.

Kay J: Ethnic enclaves fight toxic waste. San Francisco Examiner, April 9, 1991a, pp. 1, 8.

Kay J: Minorities bear brunt of pollution: Latinos and blacks living in state's "dirtiest" neighborhood. San Francisco Examiner, April 7, 1991b, pp. 1, 12.

Keller EA: Environmental Geology. New York, Macmillan, 1992.

Kerner JF, Dusenbury L, Mandelblatt JS: Poverty and cultural diversity: Challenges for health promotion among the medically underserved. Ann Rev Public Health 14: 355–377, 1993.

Kogi K: Practical approaches to the assessment of work-related risks. Int Arch Occupat Environ Health 65: S11–S14, 1993.

Kozol J: Savage Inequalities: Children in America's Schools. New York, Harper Collins, 1991.

Krieps R (ed): Environment and Health: A Holistic Approach. Brookfield, VT, Avebury, 1989.

Last JM: Global change: Ozone depletion, greenhouse warming, and public health. Ann Rev Public Health 14: 115–136, 1993.

Levy BS, Wegman DH (eds): Occupational Health: Recognizing and Preventing Work-Related Disease, 3rd ed. Boston, Little, Brown, 1994.

Linz DG, Donnerstein E, Penrod S: Effects of long-term exposure to violent and sexually degrading depictions of women. J Personality Social Psychol 55: 758–769, 1988.

Marino G: The nuclides in town: Does danger lurk in low-level radioactivity in sewage? Sci News 146: 218–219, 1994.

McAbee RR, Gallucci BJ, Checkoway H: Adverse reproductive outcomes and occupational exposures among nurses: An investigation of multiple hazardous exposures. Am Assoc Occup Health Nurs J 41: 110–119, 1993.

McKeown T: The Origins of Human Disease. Oxford, England, Basil Blackwell, 1991.

Milio N: Promoting Health Through Public Policy. Ottawa, Ontario, Canada, Canadian-Public-Health Association, 1986.

Miller R: Effects of prenatal exposure to ionizing radiation. Health Physics 59: 57–61, 1990.

Mole R: Childhood cancer after prenatal exposure to diagnostic x-ray examinations in Britain. Br J Cancer 62: 152–168, 1990.

Moses M: Farmworkers and pesticides. In Bullard RD (ed): Confronting Environmental Racism: Voices from the Grassroots. Boston, South End Press, 1993, pp. 161–178.

Mungall C, McLaren DJ: Planet under Stress: The Challenge of Global Change. Toronto, Ontario, Canada, Oxford University Press, 1990.

Myers N: Gaia: An Atlas of Planet Management. New York, Doubleday, 1993.

Needleman HL, Schell A, Bellinger D, et al.: The long-term effects of exposure to low doses of lead in children: An 11-year follow-up report. N Engl J Med 322: 83–88, 1992.

Neu HC: The crisis in antibiotic resistance. Science 257: 1064–1072, 1992.

Neufer L: The role of the community health nurse in environmental health. Public Health Nurs 11: 155–162, 1994.

Peña D, Gallegos J: Nature and Chicanos in southern Colorado. In Bullard RD (ed): Confronting Environmental Racism: Voices from the Grassroots. Boston, South End Press, 1993, pp. 141–160.

Perdue EM, Gjessing ET (eds): Organic Acids in Aquatic Ecosystems. New York, Wiley, 1989.

Phoenix J: Getting the lead out of the community. In Bullard RD (ed). Confronting Environmental Racism: Voices from the Grassroots. Boston, South End Press, 1993, pp 77–92.

Platt JR: Radon: Its impact on the community and the role of the nurse. Am Assoc Occup Health Nurs J 41: 547–550, 1993.

Reich MR: Social policy for pollution-related diseases. Soc Sci Med 27: 1011–1018, 1988.

Reinhardt PA, Gordon JG: Infectious and Medical Waste Management. Chelsea, MI, Lewis Publishers, 1991.

Rom W (ed): Environmental and Occupational Medicine, 2nd ed. Boston, Little, Brown, 1992.

Rose J (ed): Environmental Health: The Impact of Pollutants. New York, Gordon & Breach Science Publishers, 1990.

Rosenberg ML, Fenley MA (eds): Violence in America: A Public Health Approach. New York, Oxford University Press, 1991.

Ruback RB, Weiner NA: Interpersonal Violent Behaviors: Social and Cultural Aspects. New York, Springer, 1994.

Salazar MK, Primomo J: Taking the lead in environmental health: Defining a model for practice. Am Assoc Occup Health Nurs J 42: 317–324, 1994.

Salmon JW, Berliner HS: Self-care: Boot straps or hangman's noose? Health Med 1: 5–11, 1982.

Sandman PM, Weinstein ND: Predictors of home radon testing and implications for testing promotion programs. Health Educ Q 20: 471–487, 1993.

Schrieberg D: Death from a healing machine: Radioactive waste goes on Mexican odyssey after sale of medical device. San Francisco Examiner, June 23, 1991, pp. 1, 12.

Sidel R: Women and Children Last: The Plight of Poor Women in Affluent America, rev ed. New York, Penguin, 1992.

Smets H: Major industrial risks and compensation of victims: The role of insurance. Soc Sci Med 27: 1085–1095, 1988.

Smith BE: Black lung: The social production of disease. In Conrad P, Kern R (eds). The Sociology of Health and Illness: Critical Perspectives, 3rd ed. New York, St. Martin's Press, 1990, pp. 64–77.

Soble SM, Brennan JH: A review of legal and policy issues in legislating compensation for victims of toxic substance pollution. Soc Sci Med 27: 1061–1070, 1988.

Sommers EK, Check JV: An empirical investigation of the role of pornography in the verbal and physical abuse of women. Violence Victims 2: 189–209, 1987.

Steenland K: Case Studies in Occupational Epidemiology. New York, Oxford University Press, 1993.

Stevens PE: A critical social reconceptualization of environment in nursing: Implications for methodology. Adv Nurs Sci 11: 56–68, 1989.

Stevens PE, Hall JM: Abusive health care interactions experienced by lesbians: A case of institutional violence in the treatment of women. Response Victimization Women Children 13: 23–27, 1990.

Stevens PE, Hall JM: Applying critical theories to nursing in communities. Public Health Nurs 9: 2–9, 1992.

Stotts RC: Application of the Salmon Model: A tale of two cities. Public Health Nurs 8: 10–14, 1991.

Sumrall AC, Taylor D (eds): Sexual Harassment: Women Speak Out. Freedom, CA, Crossing Press, 1992.

Teitelman R: Gene Dreams: Wall Street, Academia, and the Rise of Biotechnology. New York, Basic Books, 1989.

Thompson JL: Critical scholarship: The critique of domination in nursing. Adv Nurs Sci 10: 27–38, 1987.

U.S. Department of Health and Human Services: Healthy People: The Surgeon General's Report on Health Promotion and Disease Prevention (Publication No. [PHS] 75-55071). Washington, DC, U.S. Government Printing Office, 1979.

U.S. Department of Housing and Urban Development: Comprehensive and Workable Plan for the Abatement of Lead-Based Paint in Privately Owned Housing: A Report to Congress. Rockville, MD, Author, 1990.

U.S. Environmental Protection Agency: Technical Support Document for the 1992 Citizen's Guide to Radon (EPA 400-R-92-011). Washington, DC, Author, 1992.

Veazie MA, Landen DD, Bender TR, Amandus HE: Epidemiologic research on the etiology of injuries at work. Ann Rev Public Health 15: 203–221, 1994.

Vyner HM: Invisible Trauma: The Psychosocial Effects of Invisible Environmental Contaminants. Lexington, MA, Lexington Books, 1988a.

Vyner HM: The psychosocial dimensions of health care for patients exposed to radiation and the other invisible environmental contaminants. Soc Sci Med 27: 1097–1103, 1988b.

Walker B: Environmental health policies in the 1990s. J Public Health Policy 11: 438–447, 1990.

Watts RJ: Democratization of health care: Challenge for nursing. Adv Nurs Sci 12: 37–46, 1990.

Werner MA, Olson DK: Identifying sources of disease in agriculture: A role for occupational health nurses. Am Assoc Occup Health Nurs J 41: 481–490, 1993.

Whyte WF (ed): Participatory Action Research. Newbury Park, CA; Sage, 1991.

Wilson EO, Myers N, Ehrenfeld D: Species diversity and extinction. *In* Bormann FH, Kellert SR (eds): Ecology, Economics, Ethics. New Haven, CT, Yale University Press, 1991, pp. 3–39.

Young J: Sustaining the Earth. Cambridge, MA, Harvard University Press, 1990.

Zola IK: Medicine as an institution of social control. Soc Rev 20: 487–504, 1972.

Occupational Health Nurse: Roles and Responsibilities, Current and Future Trends

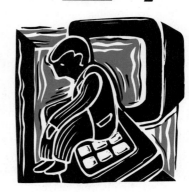

Upon completion of this chapter, the reader will be able to:

1. Describe the historic perspective of occupational health nursing.

2. Discuss emerging demographic trends that will influence occupational health nursing practice.

3. Identify the skills and competencies germane to occupational health nursing.

4. Apply the nursing process and public health principles to worker and work place health issues.

5. Discuss the role of state and federal regulations that impact occupational health.

6. Describe a multidisciplinary approach for resolution of occupational health issues.

7. Identify case studies, questions for group discussion, and learning activities.

Patricia Hyland Travers
Cherryl E. McDougall

Occupational health nursing, a branch of public health nursing, is defined by the American Association of Occupational Health Nurses (AAOHN) as

The specialty practice that provides for and delivers health care services to workers and worker populations. The practice focuses on promotion, protection, and restoration of workers' health within the context of a safe and healthy work environment. Occupational health nursing practice is autonomous, and occupational health nurses make independent nursing judgments in providing occupational health services.

(AAOHN, 1994)

In AAOHN's Standards of Occupational Health Nursing Practice published in 1994, standards of clinical nursing practice and professional practice standards are defined. The foundation of occupational health nursing practice is described as research based with an emphasis on optimizing health, preventing illness and injury, and reducing health hazards. The multidisciplinary nature of occupational health nursing practice is emphasized.

This specialty practice derives its theoretical, conceptual, and factual framework from a multidisciplinary base including, but not limited to:

- nursing science;
- medical science;
- public health sciences such as toxicology, safety, industrial hygiene, and ergonomics;
- social and behavioral sciences; and
- management and administration principles. (AAOHN, 1994)

EVOLUTION OF OCCUPATIONAL HEALTH NURSING

The evolution of occupational health nursing in the United States has mirrored the societal changes in moving from an agrarian-based to an industrial-based economy and, by the year 2000, to a service-based economy.

The concept of occupational health nursing dates to the late 1800s with the employment of Betty Moulder and Ada Mayo Stewart. Moulder was hired by a group of coal-mining companies in 1888 to care for coal miners and their families (American Association of Industrial Nurses [AAIN], 1976). Seven years later, the Vermont Marble Company hired Stewart to care for workers and their families; she is often referred to as the first "industrial nurse" because so much is known about her activities (Parker-Conrad, 1988). In 1897, Anna B. Duncan was

employed by the John Wanamaker Company to visit sick employees at home; in 1899, a nursing service was established for employees of the Frederick Loeser department store in Brooklyn, New York (AAIN, 1976). The roots of occupational health nursing are entrenched in public health nursing practice with its initial focus on prevention, home care, and family-based health care.

At the turn of the century, the industrial revolution was well under way, and the concept of health care for employees spread rapidly throughout many states (Travers, 1987). Companies hiring industrial nurses in the early 1900s included the Emporium in San Francisco; Plymouth Cordage Company in Massachusetts; Anaconda Mining Company in Montana; Broadway Store in Los Angeles; Chase Metal Works in Connecticut; Hale Brothers in San Francisco; Filene's in Boston; Carson, Pirie, and Scott in Chicago; Fulton Cotton Mills in Georgia; and Bullock's in Los Angeles (McGrath, 1946; Parker-Conrad, 1988).

The cost effectiveness of providing health care to employees was achieving increased recognition. By 1912, after workers' compensation legislation had been instituted, 38 nurses were employed by business firms (McGrath, 1946; Parker-Conrad, 1988). The following year, a registry of industrial nurses was initiated; in 1915, the Boston Industrial Nurses Club was formed, later evolving into the Massachusetts Industrial Nurses Organization. In 1916, the Factory Nurses Conference was organized, a group open only to graduate, state-registered nurses affiliated with the American Nurses Association (ANA) (AAIN, 1976). These efforts identified the practicing industrial nurses' need to explore the uniqueness of this evolving specialty area. More important, industrial nurses were practicing in single-nurse settings and recognized the importance of uniting as a group for the purpose of sharing ideas with peers practicing in the same nursing arena.

In 1917, the first educational course for industrial nurses was offered at Boston University's College of Business Administration, and in 1922, the Factory Nurses Conference changed its name to AAIN, which reflected the evolving breadth and scope of the profession.

During and after the Depression Era, many nurses lost jobs because management did not consider industrial nursing an essential aspect of business (Felton, 1985, 1986). The focus of health care for employees again changed as a result of many factors, including the impact of the two world wars. During

World War I, the government demanded health services for workers at factories and shipyards holding defense contracts. Demographics in the work place were also dramatically different during World War II because of the increased numbers of women entering the work force. In 1942, the U.S. Surgeon General told an audience of nurses that the health conservation of the "industrial army" was the most urgent civilian need during the war (Felton, 1985). From 1938 through 1943, the number of occupational health nurses increased by more than 10,000. In 1942, 300 nurses from 16 states voted to create a national association: AAIN (AAIN, 1976). Catherine R. Dempsey, a registered nurse at Simplex Wire and Cable Company in Cambridge, Massachusetts, was elected president of the national association. By 1943, approximately 11,000 nurses were employed in industry.

Nine years later, members of AAIN voted to remain an independent, autonomous association rather than merge with the National League for Nursing or the ANA. In 1953, another important step was taken toward formalizing this specialty area of nursing practice when the *Industrial Nurses Journal,* now called the *AAOHN Journal,* was published. In 1977, the organization changed its name to the American Association of Occupational Health Nurses, the current professional organization for practicing occupational health nurses.

ROLES OF THE OCCUPATIONAL HEALTH NURSE

As work places have continued to change dramatically over the past few decades, the role of the occupational health nurse has become even more diversified and complex. Often working as the only on-site health professional, the occupational health nurse collaborates with workers, employers, and other professionals to identify health needs, prioritize interventions, develop and implement programs, and evaluate services delivered (AAOHN, 1994). The occupational health nurse is in a unique and critical position to coordinate a holistic approach to the delivery of quality, comprehensive occupational health services (AAOHN, 1994). Those services may include, but are not limited to, the following:

- Ensuring compliance with federal, state, and local regulations
- Developing health surveillance programs
- Counseling employees

- Coordinating health promotion and fitness activities
- Assessing health and safety hazards in the work place
- Establishing comprehensive referral networks
- Managing occupational and nonoccupational illnesses and injuries, including treatment of emergency and primary care health problems
- Conducting health and safety evaluations
- Performing case management of occupational and nonoccupational illnesses and injuries
- Consulting with business and community partners
- Managing occupational health services, including program planning, policy development and analysis, budgeting, staffing, and general administration.

Figure 27–1 depicts a model of occupational health nursing practice "within the context of societal and work setting influences" (Rogers, 1990).

The occupational health nurse is a worker advocate and has the responsibility to uphold professional standards and codes. However, the occupational health nurse is also responsible to management, is usually compensated by management, and must practice within a framework of company policies and guidelines (Rogers, 1990). Ethical dilemmas arise over many issues (i.e., screening, drug testing, informing employees regarding hazardous exposures, and confidentiality).

Guided by an ethical framework made explicit in the AAOHN Code of Ethics, occupational health nurses encourage and enable individuals to make informed decisions about health care concerns. Confidentiality of health information is integral and central to the practice base. Occupational health nurses are advocates for workers, fostering equitable and quality health care services and safe and healthy work environments.

(AAOHN, 1994)

The Standards of Clinical Nursing Practice and the Professional Practice Standards (AAOHN, 1994) articulate a rationale as well as structure, process, and outcome criteria for occupational health nursing standards. In the section outlining the six clinical standards, the occupational health nurse

- Systematically assesses the health status of the client
- Analyzes data collected to formulate a nursing diagnosis

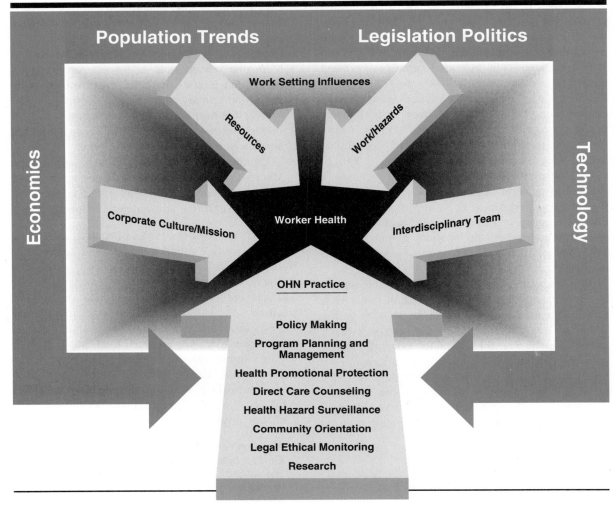

Figure 27–1
Occupational health nursing (OHN) practice within the context of societal and work setting influences. (From Rogers B: Occupational health nursing practice, education, and research: Challenges of the future. AAOHN J 38:536–543, 1990. By permission of the American Association of Occupational Health Nurses.)

- Identifies expected outcomes specific to the client
- Develops a plan of care that is comprehensive, and formulates interventions for each level of prevention and for therapeutic modalities to achieve expected outcomes
- Implements interventions to promote health, prevent illness and injury, and facilitate rehabilitation, guided by the plan of care
- Systematically and continuously evaluates the client's responses to interventions and progress toward the achievement of expected outcomes.

In the six professional standards of practice, the occupational health nurse

- Assumes responsibility for professional development and continuing education and evaluates personal professional performance in relation to practice standards
- Monitors and evaluates the quality and effectiveness of occupational health practice
- Collaborates with employees, management, other health care providers, professionals, and community representatives in assessing, planning, implementing, and evaluating care and occupational health services
- Contributes to the scientific base in occupational health nursing through research, as appropriate, and uses research findings in practice

- Uses an ethical framework as a guide for decision making in practice
- Collaborates with management to provide resources that support an occupational health program that meets the needs of the worker population

Occupational health nurses now make up the largest professional group providing health care to employees in highly complex work environments. The roles of occupational health nurses are changing as a result of many factors, including rising health care costs, increased recognition of health effects associated with various exposures, emphasis on health promotion and wellness, health surveillance, acquired immunodeficiency syndrome (AIDS), women's issues, ergonomics, reproductive issues, downsizing, trends in managed care, and multicultural work forces. Table 27–1 outlines occupational health nursing services currently

---

Table 27–1
Occupational Health Nursing Services

Services Mandated by Federal and State Regulations

Safe and healthful work place
Emergency medical response
   First aid responder selection and training
   First aid space, supplies, protocols, and records
   Designated medical resources for incident response
Workers' compensation
Confidentialty of medical records
Compliance with medical record retention requirements
OSHA compliance
   Medical personnel requirement (29 CFR 1910.15)
   Injury and illness reporting and recording
   Accident and injury investigation
   Cumulative trauma disorder prevention
   Employee access to medical and exposure records
   Medical surveillance and hazardous work qualification
   Personal protective equipment evaluation and training
   Infection control
   Employee Right-to-Know Act notification and training

Toxic Substances Control Act compliance
Community Right-to-Know Act compliance
Americans with Disabilities Act compliance
Rehabilitation Act: handicap, preplacement, fitness for duty evaluations, accommodations
Department of Defense, Department of Transportation, Nuclear Regulatory Commission, Drug-Free Workplace Act compliance
   Policy development
   Drug awareness education
   Drug testing, technical support
   Employee Assistance Program-type services
Threat of violence/duty to warn
VDT local regulations
State and local public health regulations
Nursing practice acts
Board of Pharmacy and Drug Enforcement Agency regulations
Continuing professional education required for licensure

Services Often Mandated by Company Policy

Clinical supervision of on-site health services
Health strategy development
Heath services standards
   Space, staffing, and operational standards
   Occupational illness and injury assessment, diagnosis, treatment, and referral
   Nonoccupational illness and injury assessment, diagnosis, treatment, and referral
Disability and return-to-work evaluations and accommodations
Impaired employee fitness for duty evaluation

Preplacement evaluation and medical accommodation
Handicap evaluation, placement, and accommodation
Employee Assistance Program standards
International health: travel, medical advisory, and immunizations
Data collection and analysis
Medical consultation
Pregnancy placement in hazardous environments
Professional education and development
Audit and quality assurance

Services That Are Optional

Health education and health promotion
Medical screening for early detection and disease prevention

Physical fitness programs
Allergy injection programs

OSHA = Occupational Safety and Health Administration.

mandated by state and federal regulations as well as occupational health nursing services generally mandated by company policies.

Approximately 30,000 nurses are practicing in the occupational health setting in the United States; this represents 1.5 to 2% of the total nursing population. Approximately 50% of the 30,000 nurses work alone, making decisions regarding health and safety issues, influencing policy in health and safety, and planning and implementing the myriad of health programs. The majority of nurses practicing in the occupational health setting are prepared at the diploma level and have been practicing in the field of occupational health for a minimum of 12 years (Cox, 1989; Rogers and Cox, 1994).

A 1992 survey conducted by AAOHN (Rogers and Cox, 1994) identified key practice areas in occupational health nursing that were used in the strategic planning process for AAOHN as well as in revising the definition of occupational health nursing and the standards of practice. The key areas include

- Health promotion and prevention
- Worker and work place health hazard assessment and surveillance
- Primary care
- Case management
- Research and illness or injury investigation
- Management and administration
- Community resourcefulness
- Legal and ethical issues

Rogers (1989) identified research priorities by polling a sample of AAOHN members. The survey identified the following research priorities deemed critical for shaping future occupational health nursing practice:

- Effectiveness of primary care at the work site
- Effectiveness of health promotion strategies
- Ethical issues
- Work-related health outcomes
- Health effects from chemical exposures
- Occupational hazards of health care workers
- Worker rehabilitation and return to work
- Cost effectiveness of occupational health nursing
- Quality assurance
- Impact of occupational health nursing programs on employee morale and productivity
- Ergonomics
- Influencing behavioral changes

Meeting the needs of employees in smaller businesses is another important practice and research priority. In 1982, approximately 60% of work sites in the United States were without occupational health and safety professionals (U.S. Public Health Service, 1989). The integration of occupational health principles into the curricula of schools of nursing, engineering, and management is critical. Because community health nurses may assume occupational health nursing roles, community health nurses must be knowledgeable about the specialty area of occupational health nursing. Municipalities, smaller companies, visiting nurse associations, and home care agencies may provide opportunities for community health nurses to be involved in screening programs, health education activities, work place hazard evaluations, and other occupational health–related activities.

The occupational health nurse's strengths are embedded in assessing, planning, and implementing health programs for populations, care plans for individuals, and health education activities for worker aggregates. Often, the lack of understanding or misperceptions about the occupational health nursing role has fostered the invisibility of the nurse, both within the nursing profession itself and within the business environment, thereby exacerbating the difficulties faced in being the sole guardian of health for workers in many companies (Travers, 1991). Empowered, well-trained, educated occupational health nurses will continue to impact crucial changes in the areas of primary, secondary, and tertiary prevention in occupational health.

In response to societal changes and historic events, the practice of occupational health nursing has changed dramatically, demanding a sophisticated knowledge base and problem-solving skills that are empirically based and multidisciplinary in nature (Barlow, 1992). The roles and responsibilities of the occupational health nurse must be clearly articulated to lay persons, managers, workers, union representatives, colleagues in occupational health, nursing, and medicine so that occupational health nursing can continue to positively impact workers' health, contribute to decreasing health care costs, and foster reduction in health risks. Occupational health nurses must seize the opportunities in areas such as program planning, research, and policymaking during this era fraught with a health care system in crisis, nursing shortages in many areas of the country, dramatic changes in the business environment, employees' increasing awareness of work place hazards, and the ever increasing need to demonstrate the cost effectiveness of occupational health nursing care and services (Barlow, 1992; Lundberg, 1992; Pravikoff, 1992).

DEMOGRAPHIC TRENDS AND EFFECTS ON OCCUPATIONAL HEALTH NURSING

The direction of occupational health nursing is being influenced by sweeping transformations in industry, changing work force demographics, rising health care costs, diversity of health care systems with the emergence of managed care, integration of the world economy, shift in production from goods to services, and proliferation of advanced technologies (Johnston and Packer, 1987; Maciag, 1993; O'Brien, 1995).

The focus of U.S. industry is moving away from large manufacturing facilities to smaller service-based businesses (Johnston and Packer, 1987). It is thought that work will be performed where and when the customer requires, which will force employers to make different demands on their employees. Flexible and varying work schedules and work sites may become more common than the daily trek to the same building for the 40-hour, 9:00-to-5:00 routine that has been the standard for many years. Of major importance will be the demand for an increase in skill level of all employees, even those who perform the most menial types of work. The ability to read, follow directions, and perform mathematic calculations will be core requirements (Johnston and Packer, 1987).

The increasing availability of older workers as well as women, minorities, and immigrants will have far-reaching implications for employers and pose specific challenges for occupational health professionals.

There is expected to be an overall shortage of workers in the near future because of the slow gains in the U.S. population growth rate, which has been well below average for the past two decades (Johnston and Packer, 1987; Miller, 1989). In the 1980s, the population growth rate hovered at about 1% per year. In the 1990s, the rate of gain is expected to be 0.75% or 1% per year (Miller, 1989). Between 1985 and 2000, the labor force will grow at a rate of 22% (from 115 to 141 million), which is the slowest rate since the 1930s. Miller (1989) suggested that human capital is becoming a more important resource for industry than financial capital. These trends are important to understand because of the direct impact on the national rate of economic growth, especially in the area of population-sensitive products, such as food, automobiles, housing units, household goods, and education services (Johnston and Packer, 1987).

Key characteristics of these evolving organizations include a focus on a shared vision, strategy, and long-term objectives within an environment composed of individuals working on teams (O'Brien, 1995). In contrast to the past, occupational health nurses have opportunities to work on cross-functional teams to shape decisions in areas such as benefits, research, safety, and legal matters (O'Brien, 1995). Specifically, occupational health nurses have opportunities to impact the transformation of the health care delivery system, establish policies within the managed care environment and within corporations, and assume leadership positions on legislative staffs and in governmental agencies (O'Brien, 1995; Stimpson, 1993).

Increased Emphasis on Roles in Prevention

The median age of the U.S. work force is expected to increase from 35 years in 1984 to approximately 39 years in 2000. The number of workers aged 35 to 54 years will increase by more than 25 million (Johnston and Packer, 1987). Although there has been increased emphasis on health and fitness in the general population, the occupational health nurse's primary, secondary, and tertiary prevention strategies are expected to assume an even more important role in the prevention and treatment of chronic disease.

In the area of primary prevention, emphasis will continue to be placed on health promotion and disease prevention, including smoking cessation programs, nutrition counseling, cardiovascular health education and fitness, and cancer prevention. In fact, the U.S. Public Health Service established national health objectives, known as Healthy People 2000: An Agenda for the Nation, with the goal of achieving these objectives by the end of the century. Some of the areas targeted include physical fitness and activity; nutrition; tobacco, alcohol and other drugs; mental health and mental disorders; occupational safety and health; maternal and infant health; heart disease and stroke; immunization; and infectious disease and clinical preventive services (Rosen and Berger, 1991; U.S. Public Health Service, 1989). The overall goal of these objectives is to increase to at least 85% the proportion of work sites with 50 or more employees that offer health promotion activities for their employees as an integral part of a comprehensive health promotion program.

With regard to secondary prevention, the occupational health nurse plans and implements health screening programs and health risk appraisals for early diagnosis and treatment of disease. Screening programs to detect early signs of cancer, hypertension, and cholesterol are effective secondary prevention measures. The occupational health nurse will increasingly be expected to document the return on investment for these and other related activities in the work place (Arthur D. Little, Inc., 1980; Chenowith, 1989; Dees and Taylor, 1990; Kalina et al., 1995; O'Brien, 1995; Williamson and Moore, 1987).

On a tertiary level, the occupational health nurse has played a critical role in the process of rehabilitation and return to work after all types of disabilities (Centineo, 1986; Reith et al., 1995). Yeater (1987) reported that 1981 disability costs were $184.6 billion. In industry, disability costs average 8.4% of payroll (Chelius, 1992). Four percent of the gross national product, or $170 billion, is the figure cited for costs associated with total disability (Reith et al., 1995). In the United States, it is estimated that more than 500,000 workers take an estimated 5 months leave from work each year because of a physical disability; only 48% return to work (Mannon et al., 1994). Research findings indicate the importance of developing strategies to reinforce the behavioral change of the individual to avoid what is often referred to as the "disability syndrome," a state in which an individual chooses not to work when medical clearance to do so has been granted (Mundy et al., 1994).

Knowledge of the work place, the ability to negotiate with the employer for appropriate accommodations, early intervention, and comprehensive case management skills have been and will continue to be essential for the disabled employee's successful return to productive life (Leigh, 1993). Brown (1989) and Mannon and colleagues (1994) stated that a well-constructed case management plan can save 8 to 10% of paid disability claims. Reith and coworkers (1995) documented the efficacy of an integrated disability management program with a focus on all three levels of prevention: primary prevention of disabilities (work and non-work related); secondary (minimization of disability costs); and tertiary (facilitation of rehabilitation and early return to work).

Because older workers are more prone to chronic disease, the occupational health nurse can implement and monitor treatment protocols as well as assist workers to live and work at their optimum comfort level while managing their disease. Responsibilities for the care of elderly parents or significant others will influence the balance of work and home for older workers. The occupational health nurse's role as counselor, referral resource for workers, and consultant to management can influence future benefit changes.

Women in the Work Place

Over the next 15 years, women are expected to continue to join the work force in substantial numbers. By the year 2000, approximately 47% of the work force will be women, and 61% of U.S. women will be at work (Johnston and Packer, 1987). Women will make up about three fifths of new entrants into the labor force between 1985 and 2000 (Johnston and Packer, 1987). Women's health and safety issues, such as maternal-child health, reproductive health, breast cancer education and early detection, stress (Crawford, 1993), and work-home balance issues, will achieve heightened significance (Roberts and McGovern, 1993).

Thirty percent of women currently in the work force are between the ages of 16 and 44 years, and each year approximately 1 million infants are born to these women (Gates and O'Neill, 1990). The occupational health nurse can play a key role in the development and delivery of prenatal, postpartum, and childhood programs in the work place. Of primary importance will be the ability to serve as a change agent to initiate needed programs in the work environment. Employers must be educated regarding strategies to not only reduce health care costs for women and infants but also to improve the work environment for mothers (Albright, 1992; Gates and O'Neill, 1990). Women who believe their employers are interested in the well-being of themselves and their families are more apt to be productive and satisfied employees (Gates and O'Neill, 1990). The occupational health nurse can play a critical role in the shaping of supportive policies and practices to accommodate the needs of families, including flexible working hours, parental leave, and on-site child care (Albright, 1992).

Interest in work place safety and the relationship to reproductive outcome continues to grow as women of childbearing years enter the work place in greater proportions than ever before. Although certain exposures to chemicals in the work place known to be mutagenic or teratogenic can be avoided, the vast majority of work place exposures have not been studied systematically (Pastides et al., 1988). Performing "walk-throughs" in the work place on a regular basis, recognizing potential and existing hazards, and maintaining communications with safety and industrial hygiene resources will continue to be critical work for the occupational health nurse (Table 27–2).

The role of employee advocate may expand as the occupational health nurse becomes increasingly involved in the improvement of control strategies (e.g., engineering controls and work place accommodations for women who are pregnant or are attempting to conceive and must work in areas where potential reproductive hazards exist).

In 1988, breast cancer was surpassed only by lung cancer as the leading cause of cancer deaths among women (Owen and Long, 1989). The American Cancer Society predicted that, in 1991, 175,000 new breast cancer cases would be diagnosed and, of those, 44,500 women would die (American Cancer Society, 1991). The risk of breast cancer increases with advancing age; greater than 85% of the cases occur in women older than 45 years (National Cancer Institute, 1984).

Activities must continue to focus on prevention and early detection by increasing awareness of the incidence of breast cancer and providing accessible and affordable screening programs (Rimes, 1993). The occupational health nurse is in an excellent position to play a key role in reducing morbidity and mortality associated with breast cancer, thereby supporting the National Cancer Institute's goals of a 50% cancer reduction by the year 2000 (Owen and Long, 1989). Hall (1992) reported that a three-part breast health program composed of breast self-examination with visual reminders and educational materials accompanied by a physical examination and mammography for women older than 35 years is an effective strategy in early detection.

Women may experience more stress than men in balancing their work and home roles. Child care continues to be the primary responsibility of women, and women still handle most of the household responsibilities; these cause women to experience a

Table 27–2
Types of Occupational Hazards and Associated Health Effects

Category	Exposures	Health Effects
Chemical (routes of entry: inhalation, skin absorption, ingestion, and ocular absorption)	Solvents	Headache, central nervous system dysfunction
	Lead	Central nervous system disturbances
	Asbestos	Asbestosis
	Acids	Burns
	Glycol ethers	Reproductive effects
	Mercury	Ataxia
	Arsenic	Peripheral neuropathy
Biological (routes of entry: inhalation, skin contact or puncture, ingestion, and ocular absorption)	Blood or body fluids	Bacterial, fungal, viral infections Hepatitis B
Physical	Noise	Hearing loss
	Radiation	Reproductive effects, cancer
	Vibration	Raynaud's disease
	Heat	Heat exhaustion, heat stroke
Psychosocial	Stress Work-home balance	Anxiety reactions and a variety of physical symptoms
Ergonomics	Static or non-neutral postures	Musculoskeletal disorders
	Repetitive or forceful exertions	Back injuries
	Lighting	Headache, eye strain
	Shift work	Sleep disorders
Safety	Electrical	Electrocution
	Slips and falls	Musculoskeletal conditions
	Struck by or against object	

unique form of stress (Freedman and Bisesi, 1988). With more women entering and remaining in the work force, the occupational health nurse must be prepared to provide counseling and support for this employee population. Delivery of educational programs as well as implementation of support groups will be key adjuncts to the health and productivity of these women.

Minorities in the Work Place

Over the next 13 years, African-Americans, Hispanics, and other racial or ethnic groups will make up a large share of the expanded labor force (Johnston and Packer, 1987). Nonwhites will account for 29% of the net addition to the work force between 1985 and 2000 and more than 15% of the work force in 2000 (Johnston and Packer, 1987). As the number of minority and ethnic workers in the work force increases, so will the illnesses traditionally associated with these groups of workers (i.e., heart disease and stroke, hypertension, cancer, cirrhosis, and diabetes) (Rogers, 1990). Morris (1989) reported that, in addition to basic health concerns for this population, available statistics indicate that minority workers have been disproportionately concentrated in some of the most dangerous work and, therefore, are at greater risk for experiencing any of the leading occupationally related diseases and injuries as defined by the National Institute for Occupational Safety and Health (NIOSH) (Table 27–3).

The occupational health nurse will face challenges in developing programs that are culturally and linguistically appropriate. The occupational health nurse may be in an advocacy role to negotiate with the employer for changes in the work environment to reduce or eliminate existing or potential occupational exposures (Friedman-Jimenez, 1989).

Delivery and Access Issues Related to Health Care

Corporations have become driving forces in shaping the development of alternative approaches to health care (Rosen and Freedman, 1987). Rapidly increasing health care costs have spawned a number of alternative approaches to providing health care. Health maintenance organizations (HMOs) and preferred provider organizations are two of the more common health care management programs (Miller, 1989). In the late 1980s, Digital Equipment Corporation seized the opportunity to control escalating health care costs by becoming an active and creative value purchaser of health care services (Digital Equipment Corporation, 1995). This was accomplished by designing a model that identified well-organized and well-managed HMOs as the key delivery channel. A tremendous opportunity exists for occupational health nurses to draft similar performance standards and to participate in total quality management processes designed to improve the quality, efficiency, and value of the managed health care delivery system (Rooney, 1992a, 1992b; Widtfeldt and Widtfeldt, 1992).

It is important that the occupational health nurse remain informed about the various health care options available to the work force as rapid changes occur regarding corporate benefits. This is of particular importance when considering referral of a client to a community health resource. Participation in one of the managed care plans requires that treatment take place according to the organization's guidelines and within their health service delivery system. Managed care plans are replacing traditional indemnity plans. Access to care is strictly managed and, often, limited. As this trend continues, the role of the occupational health nurse will take on added importance. The nurse must be prepared to accept increasing responsibilities as a primary care provider. According to Rooney,

As businesses seek ways to maximize the value of their dollars spent on health care services, occupational health

Table 27–3	
Ten Leading Work-Related Diseases and Injuries	
Work-Related Disease or Injury	**Examples of Effect**
Occupational lung disease	Cancer, asthma
Musculoskeletal injuries	Back, upper extremity, musculoskeletal disorders
Occupational cancers	Leukemia, bladder, skin
Trauma	Death, amputation, fracture
Cardiovascular diseases	Hypertension, heart disease
Reproductive disorders	Infertility, miscarriage
Neurotoxic disorders	Neuropathy, toxic psychosis
Noise-induced hearing loss	Loss of hearing
Dermatologic conditions	Chemical burns, allergies
Psychological disorders	Neurosis, alcohol or substance abuse

nurses and other health professionals have both an opportunity and a threat. The opportunity comes from being able to demonstrate that cost effective quality health programs do improve the health of employees and their dependents, positively influencing their company's attempts to control rising health care costs. The threat is that if health professionals cannot prove cost effectiveness and value to companies, their functions may be eliminated or replaced by contract services.

(ROONEY, 1992b)

AIDS in the Work Place

One health care issue that will continue to plague society is the AIDS epidemic. Human immuno-deficiency virus (HIV) infection poses a small but significant risk to health care workers (Kopfer and McGovern, 1993). Roles of the occupational health nurse will continue to include education and counseling for workers with potential work place exposures as well as employees at risk because of personal behaviors (AAOHN, 1988a). The occupational health nurse can influence employers to support workers with AIDS by improving benefits and making appropriate work place modifications to allow work continuance throughout the course of the disease.

AAOHN Year 2000 Recommendations

In cooperation with the U.S. Department of Health and Human Services and the Public Health Service, the AAOHN has submitted recommendations to help define the national health objectives so that the following will occur by the year 2000 (AAOHN, 1988b):

- Ninety percent of employers with 50 or more employees will provide access to monitoring, intervention, and follow-up programs for chronic illnesses delivered by qualified occupational health professionals, preferably occupational health nurses. These services should be at or convenient to the work site.
- Ninety percent of non–health care–related at-risk workers not protected by Occupational Safety and Health Administration (OSHA) regulations will be educated about HIV transmission and self-protective measures. This should be accomplished through education and information disseminated through public media, business, and trade association meetings and publications.
- Ninety percent of employers will develop a company policy that protects at-risk workers while

safeguarding the confidentiality and employment (as appropriate) of HIV-positive employees.
- OSHA will implement a standard for protection against blood-borne pathogens using the Centers for Disease Control universal precautions guidelines to prevent transmission.
- Ninety percent of employers of health care workers whose work involves exposure to blood will offer voluntary, free, accessible vaccination against hepatitis B.
- Ninety percent of work places will provide access to health promotion and risk reduction programs by qualified occupational health professionals who are knowledgeable about occupational health issues as well as health promotion. Occupational health nurses are ideal for this role.
- Every state health department will hire at least one occupational health nurse consultant for local industries. Presently, only a few states have such a consultant who can provide expertise and guidance in establishing and implementing occupational health services.

SKILLS AND COMPETENCIES OF THE OCCUPATIONAL HEALTH NURSE

Although emergency care is still an important tenet of occupational health nursing, the current and future practice must focus on a proactive approach with the goal of preventing illness and injury and promoting health. Therefore, the occupational health nurse must possess the skills and competencies necessary to recognize and evaluate potential and existing health hazards in the work place. Management skills and knowledge of toxicology, ergonomics, epidemiology, environmental health, safety, record keeping, budgeting, counseling, and education are essential to meet the present and future demands of occupational health nursing practice.

To define more readily the breadth and scope of occupational health nursing practice, a skills and competency model was developed and implemented in 1990 (Travers et al., 1991). Examples of some of the skills and competencies of occupational health nursing practice are outlined according to eight defined areas of practice:

Management and Administration

- Managing budgets
- Hiring staff and management of staff performance

- Fostering professional development plans
- Developing program goals and objectives
- Business planning through knowledge of internal and external resources
- Providing comprehensive on-site services and programs
- Knowing needs of business and employees
- Writing reports
- Performing audits and quality assurance
- Handling workers' compensation and disability
- Performing cost-benefit and cost-effectiveness analyses
- Allocating appropriate staff resources
- Being a leader in health-related issues
- Negotiating
- Facilitating work accommodations and return to work
- Coordinating medical response activities and site disaster planning

Direct Care

- Applying the nursing process
- Delivering first aid and primary care according to treatment protocols
- Conducting a physical assessment
- History taking
- Medical testing
- Being knowledgeable about immunization protocols
- Responding to medical emergencies
- Being knowledgeable about trends in health-related issues

Health and Environmental Relationships

- Having knowledge of plant operations, manufacturing processes, and job tasks
- Identifying potential and existing work place exposures
- Influencing appropriate and targeted recommendations for control of hazards in the work place
- Having knowledge of toxicologic, epidemiologic, and ergonomic principles
- Understanding appropriate engineering controls, administration, and personal protective equipment specific to preventing exposure to health hazards in the work place
- Understanding roles and collaboration with other cross-functional groups as an integral part of a core multidisciplinary team

Legal and Ethical Responsibilities

- Knowledge of AAOHN Professional Standards of Practice and Code of Ethics
- Knowledge of state nursing practice acts and ability to practice occupational health nursing within state guidelines
- Knowledge of federal regulations pertaining to occupational health
- Knowledge of the Americans with Disabilities Act, associated guidelines, and Affirmative Action and Equal Employment Opportunity legislation
- Knowledge of all aspects of medical record-keeping practices in compliance with nursing practice, state law, and standards of practice
- Knowledge of current legal trends related to negligence and malpractice cases in professional nursing and in the occupational health setting

Consultation

- Being a resource expert on health issues for employees and management
- Having broad knowledge of public health and occupational health principles and practices
- Creating effective professional and technical support networks both functionally and cross-functionally

Research

- Systematically collecting, analyzing, and interpreting data from different sources
- Recognizing trends in health outcomes by department, work area, or work process
- Planning, developing, and conducting surveys

Health Education

- Recognizing cultural differences and the relationship to health issues
- Using effective communication styles to match diverse employee and management audiences
- Making effective presentations
- Planning, developing, implementing, and evaluating health programs designed to meet the needs of specific employee groups or organizations
- Applying adult learning theory and principles to health education programs

Counseling

- Identifying employees' emotional needs, and providing support and counseling

- Making appropriate referrals and recommendations
- Listening
- Managing psychiatric emergencies

PRIMARY, SECONDARY, AND TERTIARY LEVELS OF PREVENTION

Like all community health professionals, the occupational health nurse's practice is based on the concept of prevention. Promotion, protection, maintenance, and restoration of worker health are the goals set forth in AAOHN's definition of occupational health nursing. The levels can be further delineated into occupational and nonoccupational categories.

Primary Prevention. In the area of primary prevention, the occupational health nurse is involved in both health promotion and disease prevention. Patterson (1984, p. 5) documented that health promotion is defined by the American Hospital Association as "the process of fostering awareness, influencing attitudes and identifying alternatives so that individuals can make informed choices and changes in their behavior to achieve an optimum level of physical and mental health and improve their physical and social environment."

Disease prevention begins with recognition of a health risk, a disease, or an environmental hazard and is followed by measures to protect as many people as possible from harmful consequences of that risk.

A variety of primary prevention strategies are used by the occupational health nurse. The most frequent method is one-on-one interaction. Because the occupational health nurse has daily contact with numerous clients for a myriad of reasons (e.g., assessment and treatment of episodic illness or injury, health surveillance), this is an important method of promoting health. The phrase "seize the moment" aptly describes the opportunity that presents with every client encounter. However, similar to community health nursing professionals, occupational health nurses plan, develop, and implement aggregate-focused intervention strategies. The occupational health nurse plans and implements programs such as weight reduction, AIDS awareness, ergonomics training, and smoking cessation. For overall health promotion, the nurse may plan and implement a health fair, which is a multifaceted health promotion strategy that usually includes a number of community health resources to provide expertise on a wide range of health issues and community services.

As part of an overall health and wellness strategy, the occupational health nurse may negotiate with the employer for an on-site fitness center or area with fitness equipment, or if cost or space is prohibitive the employer may choose to partially subsidize membership to a local fitness center.

Types of nonoccupational programs included in the area of primary prevention are cardiovascular health, cancer awareness, personal safety, immunization, prenatal and postpartum health, accident prevention, retirement health, stress management, and relaxation techniques. Occupational health programs could include topics such as emergency response, first aid and cardiopulmonary resuscitation training, right-to-know training, immunization programs for international business travelers, prevention of back injury through knowledge of proper lifting techniques, ergonomics, and other programs targeted to the specific hazards identified in the work place.

Secondary Prevention. These strategies are aimed at early diagnosis, early treatment interventions, and attempts to limit disability. The focus at this level of prevention is on identification of health needs, health problems, and clients at risk. A survey of eight countries (Murphy, 1989) showed that the major portion of the occupational health nurse's work day was devoted to prevention (40–80%) and that treatment and screening dominated prevention activities (18% and 16%, respectively).

As with primary prevention, the occupational health nurse uses a number of different strategies. By providing direct care for episodic illness and injury, the occupational health nurse is afforded the opportunity to conduct early assessments and provide treatment and referrals for a variety of physical as well as psychological conditions. Health screenings, which are designed for early detection of disease, can be offered at the work site by the occupational health nurse with relative ease and at minimal cost. Screenings may focus on vision, cancer, cholesterol, hypertension, diabetes, tuberculosis, and pulmonary function. Some other types of screening may be contracted with a vendor who uses mobile equipment to provide screenings such as mammography.

Secondary prevention efforts provided by the occupational health nurse include preplacement, periodic, and job transfer evaluations to ensure that the worker is being placed or is continuing to work in a job that is safe for that worker.

The preplacement evaluation is performed before the worker begins employment in a new company or is placed in a different job (Fig. 27–2). The evaluation is a baseline examination that consists of a medical history, an occupational health history (Fig. 27–3), and a physical assessment that should target the type of work that the client will be performing. For example, if the client is going to be lifting materials in a warehouse, special attention should be paid to any history of musculoskeletal problems. Strength testing and range of motion should be performed for all muscle groups. This type of examination would not be as important if the client were to be employed as a chemical engineer. The examination may also include medical tests to determine specific organ functions that may be affected by exposure to existing hazards in the client's work place. For example, if the client is working with a chemical that is a known liver toxin, baseline liver function tests may be appropriate to determine the current health status of the liver and its ability to handle this specific chemical exposure. The preplacement examination, however, must be carefully evaluated to ensure compliance with the Americans with Disabilities Act.

Periodic assessments usually occur at a regular interval (i.e., annual, biannual) and are based on specific protocols for those exposed to substances or irritants such as lead, asbestos, noise, or various chemicals.

Examinations of individuals transferring to other jobs are critical to document any changes in health that may have occurred while the client was working in a specific area or with a specific process. This is usually done to comply with OSHA regulations or NIOSH recommendations.

Tertiary Prevention. On a tertiary level, the occupational health nurse plays a key role in the rehabilitation and restoration of the worker to an optimal level of functioning. Strategies include case management, negotiation of work place accommodations, and counseling and support for workers who will continue to be affected by chronic disease (Moore and Childre, 1990).

The process of returning an individual to work begins with the onset of injury or illness (Martin, 1993). Regardless of whether this involves an occupational or a nonoccupational condition, the occupa-

tional health nurse is the center of case management. The nurse works closely with the primary care provider to monitor the progress of the ill or injured worker and to identify and eliminate potential barriers in the return-to-work process. The nurse has a comprehensive understanding of the work place and of the physical requirements necessary for the client to work. The physical demands analysis (Randolph and Dalton, 1989) is a useful tool in objectively assessing the physical demands of any job (Fig. 27–4). Once the assessment is completed, the occupational health nurse can relay this information to the community health professionals caring for the client.

For workers needing special accommodations, the occupational health nurse can negotiate and facilitate those appropriate to the client's health limitations. The nurse is often the driving force behind the employer creating a "light duty" pool. The goal of this type of program is to provide temporary work that is less physically demanding in nature than the client's regular work. This facilitates the client's return to the work place earlier than if required to wait until full strength was regained.

The occupational health nurse can monitor and support the health of clients returning to work while continuing to experience adverse health effects of chronic disease. For example, the client who is returning to work after sustaining a myocardial infarction may have blood pressure monitored on a routine basis. Counseling regarding adjustment to normal work life as well as support for behavior modification (i.e., smoking cessation) may also be provided.

IMPACT OF LEGISLATION ON OCCUPATIONAL HEALTH

Legislation and associated activities have influenced the practice of occupational health in the United States. Table 27–4 presents a historic perspective of some of the major pieces of legislation that have had and will continue to have a direct impact on the general practice of occupational health nursing. The Occupational Safety and Health Act, Workers' Compensation Acts, and the Americans with Disabilities Act are highlighted.

The Occupational Safety and Health Act of 1970 was enacted 2 years after a major coal-mining disaster in West Virginia. The passage of this legislation came about because of worker health con-

Text continued on page 785

Preplacement Medical Evaluation

Part 1
Health Questionnaire

Have you ever had problems with:	Yes	No
Heart	_____	_____
Circulation	_____	_____
Infection	_____	_____
Nerves	_____	_____
Bones	_____	_____
Muscles	_____	_____
Lungs/breathing	_____	_____
Vision/eyes	_____	_____
Hearing/ears	_____	_____
Allergies	_____	_____

If you have answered "Yes" to any of the above, please explain:

Have you ever:		
Had an operation	_____	_____
Become sick from your work	_____	_____
Had a tetanus shot	_____	_____
Considered yourself disabled	_____	_____
(Within the past 5 years) consulted a physician	_____	_____

If you have answered "Yes" to any of the above, please explain:

Part 2
Physical Assessment

Vital signs _____

Height and weight _____

Vision test _____

Hearing test _____

Physical examination with review of systems _____

Laboratory tests appropriate to work place exposure _____

Part 3
Medical Summary and Recommendations

Applicant is: _____ able to perform job

_____ able to perform job with restrictions

_____ not able to perform job

_____ on hold–awaiting more medical data

Diagnosis _____

Restrictions _____

Recommendations _____

Comments _____

Figure 27–2
Preplacement medical evaluation.

Occupational Health History

Date: _____

Badge or Social Security Number: _____

Name: _____

Age: _____

Shift: _____

Job title: _____

Department: _____

How long in this job/area (months/years): _____

Average work hours/shift: _____

Physical requirements of work (hours/day):

       Lifting: _____

       Bending: _____

       Sitting: _____

       Repetitive movements: _____

       Standing: _____

       Twisting: _____

       Climbing: _____

Job description: _____

_____

Potential exposures:

       Chemical: _____

       Physical: _____

       Biological: _____

       Psychosocial: _____

       Ergonomic: _____

       Safety: _____

Personal protective equipment:

       Gloves: _____

       Glasses: _____

       Ear protection: _____

       Lab coat: _____

       Apron: _____

       Face shield: _____

       Goggles: _____

       Mask/respirator: _____

       Other: _____

Figure 27–3
Occupational health history.

Do you have a second job? _____

If yes, describe: _____

_____

_____

_____

_____

_____

Chief complaint: _____

Onset of symptoms: _____

Duration of symptoms: _____

Suspected cause: _____

Quality/severity of symptoms: _____

_____

_____

Aggravating factors: _____

_____

Are there coworkers with similar symptoms? _____

Do symptoms change when not at work? _____

Past medical history: _____

_____

_____

_____

_____

Current medications: _____

Hobbies: _____

Family health history: _____

_____

_____

Smoking history: _____

Alcohol history: _____

Recreational drug use: _____

Exercise patterns: _____

Allergies: _____

Other comments: _____

_____

Figure 27–3 *Continued*

Physical Demands Analysis

Job title _____   Department _____

Activity	Never	Rarely (5–10%)	Sometimes (10–40%)	Frequently (41–75%)	Always (75–100%)
Standing					
Walking					
Sitting					
Lifting					
10 lb. maximum					
20 lb. max., up to 10 lb. frequently					
50 lb. max., up to 25 lb. frequently					
100 lb. max., up to 50 lb. frequently					
>100 lb., 50 lb. or more frequently					
Pushing/pulling					
10 lb. maximum					
20 lb. max., up to 10 lb. frequently					
50 lb. max., up to 25 lb. frequently					
100 lb. max., up to 50 lb. frequently					
>100 lb., 50 lb. or more frequently					
Climbing					
Ladders					
Stairs					
Other (list)					
Balancing					
Stooping					
Kneeling					
Crouching					
Crawling					
Twisting					
Bending					
Reaching					
Overhead					
In front of body					
Handling					
Fingering					
Feeling					
Talking					
Ordinary					
Other					
Hearing					
Ordinary conversation					
Other sounds					
Vision					
Acuity: Near, 20 in. or less					
Acuity: Far, 20 ft. or more					
Depth perception three-dimensional					
Vision distance judgment					
Accommodation sharpness of vision/focus					
Color vision					
Field of vision (entire scope of vision/peripheral)					
Any other outstanding physical requirements not previously mentioned (list)					
Shift work					
Environmental conditions:					
Inside					
Outside					
Both					
Dust					
Fumes					
Hazards (describe)					

Figure 27–4

Physical demands analysis. (From Randolph SA, Dalton PC: Limited duty work: An innovative approach to early return to work. AAOHN J 37:451, 1989. By permission of the American Association of Occupational Health Nurses.)

Table 27–4			
Historic Perspective of Legislation Affecting Occupational Health in the United States			
Year	**Legislation**	**Year**	**Legislation**
1836	First restrictive child labor law enacted (Massachusetts)	1965	McNamara-O'Hara Act (extends protection of the Walsh-Healy Act to include suppliers of government services)
1877	State legislation passed requiring factory safeguards (Massachusetts)	1966	Mine Safety Act (mandatory inspections and health and safety standards in mining industry)
1879	State legislation passed requiring factory inspections (Massachusetts)		
1886	State legislation passed requiring reporting of industrial accidents (Massachusetts)	1969	Coal Mine Health and Safety Act (mandatory health and safety standards for underground mines)
1910	State legislation passed requiring formation of an Occupational Disease Commission (Illinois)	1970	Occupational Safety and Health Act
		1970	Environment Protection Agency established
1911	Workmen's Compensation Act passed (New Jersey)	1970	Consumer Protection Agency established
		1972	Equal Employment Opportunity Act
1935	Social Security Act passed (state and federal unemployment insurance program)	1972	Noise Control Act
		1972	Clean Water Act
1936	Walsh-Healy Act (federal legislation setting occupational safety and health standards for certain government contract workers)	1973	Health Maintenance Organization Act
		1973	Rehabilitation Act
1938	Fair Labor Standards Act (setting minimum age for child labor)	1976	Toxic Substances Control Act
		1976	Resources Conservation and Recovery Act
1948	All states have Workers' Compensation Acts	1977	Federal Mine Safety and Health Act
1964	Civil Rights Act	1990	Americans with Disabilities Act

cerns, burgeoning environmental awareness, union activities, increased knowledge about work place hazards, and health concerns. The general duty clause of the act states that employers must "furnish a place of employment free from recognized hazards that are causing or likely to cause death or serious physical harm to employees." The act also identifies the roles of the various related government agencies, provides for the establishment of federal occupational safety and health standards, and identifies a structure of penalties, fines, and sentences for violations of regulations. The following organizations were formed under the provisions of the act:

- OSHA, under the jurisdiction of the Department of Labor, is responsible for promulgating and enforcing occupational safety and health standards.
- NIOSH, under the jurisdiction of the U.S. Department of Health and Human Services, is responsible for funding and conducting research, making rec-

ommendations for occupational safety and health standards to OSHA, and funding educational resource centers for the training of occupational health professionals.
- Occupational Safety and Health Review Commission, appointed by the president, is responsible for advising OSHA and NIOSH regarding the legal implications of decisions or action in the course of carrying out their duties.
- National Advisory Council on Occupational Safety and Health, appointed by the president, is a group of consumers and professionals who are responsible for making recommendations to OSHA and NIOSH regarding occupational health and safety.
- National Commission on State Workers' Compensation Laws, appointed by the president on a temporary basis, studied the adequacy of state workers' compensation laws and made recommendations to the president on their findings. This commission's work ended as of October 30, 1972.

OSHA has promulgated occupational health and safety standards, which are published in the *Code of Federal Regulations* and updated on a regular basis. Access to the most recent publication of these standards is a crucial responsibility of the occupational health nurse. The occupational health nurse must be knowledgeable of Title 29 of the code, part 1910 (29 CFR 1910), and other sections of the code that apply to specific hazards in the work place. For example, 29 CFR 1904 pertains to OSHA's record-keeping requirements. This mandates the employer's responsibility to keep records of work-related injuries, illnesses, and deaths. These records must be posted in the work place for 1 month per year and made available for review by OSHA at any time. In many cases, the occupational health nurse has full responsibility for compliance with this standard. Under the act, any state has the right to implement their own occupational safety and health administration. The only requirement is that the state standards meet or exceed federal standards. California, Maryland, New York State, and Michigan have chosen to operate in this manner.

OSHA has 10 regional offices throughout the United States. Inspectors are assigned to each region to enforce the standards and to provide consultation to industries.

An OSHA inspection can be initiated in one of several ways. Each office plans a schedule of routine visits to the industries in their respective regions. In the past, funding has been an issue, and inspections have not taken place in the quantity or frequency originally intended. An inspection can also be initiated if a major health or safety problem such as a death, occurs at the work site, if five or more workers are sent to the hospital as a result of the same incident, or if there is a safety issue at the work place that has received publicity in the community. Inspection may also occur by employer request. This is not usually done unless the employer has an exemplary occupational health and safety program and wishes to participate in OSHA's voluntary inspection program. Inspection may also be initiated by an employee request because of concern about a suspected hazardous condition. In this case, OSHA is mandated to respond and must keep the employee's name confidential at the employee's request. In the past, penalties have been inconsequential, and rarely have sentences been served. However, recent events indicate that fines have increased, and OSHA has made public its intention to criminally prosecute company executives for serious and willful violations.

In many organizations, the occupational health nurse is the interface with the OSHA inspector. The nurse should know that employees or their union representatives have the right to walk around with the OSHA investigators. This requires the nurse to be knowledgeable about the potential hazards in the work place and about the appropriate control measures designed to eliminate or minimize exposure.

Workers' Compensation Acts are state mandated and state funded. These programs provide income replacement and health care to workers who sustain a work-related injury, disability (temporary or permanent), or death. The Workers' Compensation Acts also protect the employer in that the compensation received by the employee precludes legal suits against the employer. Each state regulates its own program and is unique to the state. The employer can self-insure, contract with commercial insurance carriers, or purchase a policy with the state-operated insurance fund. Workers receive an average of 66% of their take-home pay before taxes, and some disabled workers and their families are eligible for other benefit programs, including Old Age, Survivors, Disability and Health Insurance; Supplemental Security Income; or any other disability program that they may have purchased either through the company or on an individual basis.

In an era of sky-rocketing health care costs and a propensity for injured workers to engage the services of lawyers to represent them in negotiating lump sum financial settlements, many employers are claiming that workers' compensation costs are crippling their ability to compete in an international marketplace. The occupational health nurse has a unique opportunity to support both the employee and employer in this arena. For the employee, the nurse may be the initial person to whom the work-related injury or illness is reported. Accurate assessment of the injury or illness and appropriate treatment are essential. Community resources must be identified so that the injured worker is provided with high-quality health care and appropriate medical follow-up. The occupational health nurse educates the employee regarding benefits under the Workers' Compensation Act and is often the one who files the claim. If the employee is disabled from work for a period of time, the nurse provides case management support and remains in contact with the employee until return to work. If the employer uses an insurance carrier, the nurse works closely with the claims adjuster to manage the case. The need for light duty or other work place accommodations is determined before the employee's return. In most cases, the nurse facilitates this process with the employer.

For the employer, the occupational health nurse provides the expertise in early intervention and case management. The goal is to limit the worker's disability while providing an opportunity for early return to work through appropriate work place accommodations. The desired outcome is a productive employee with optimum health and productivity plus reduced health care and workers' compensation costs.

The Americans with Disabilities Act, enacted by Congress in July 1990, is a comprehensive act that prohibits discrimination on the basis of disability. The core of this act requires employers to adjust facilities and practices for the purpose of making reasonable accommodations to enhance opportunities for individuals with disabilities (Kaminshine, 1991).

Employment provisions of this act began on July 26, 1992 for employers with 25 or more employees and were revised in July 1994 to include those with 15 or more employees. Provisions regarding access to public transportation and accommodations became effective in January 1993.

The act defines disability as "physical or mental impairment that substantially limits one or more major life activities; having record of such an impairment; or being regarded as having such an impairment" (Kaminshine, 1991, p. 249).

Physical or mental impairment guidelines are the same as those described in the Federal Rehabilitation Act and include "any physiologic disorder or condition, cosmetic disfigurement, anatomical loss affecting any of the major body systems, or any mental or psychological disorder" (p. 249). Major life activities include caring for self, walking, seeing, hearing, and speaking (Kaminshine, 1991).

The Americans with Disabilities Act excludes conditions relating to sexual preference and gender identity, compulsive gambling, kleptomania, and pyromania. The act also denies protection for individuals who are currently involved in illegal drug use.

In particular, the occupational health nurse has responsibility in two areas. The first involves the duty to provide or facilitate reasonable accommodations. This is facilitated by the nurse's familiarity with the physical requirements of jobs in the work place. The second area of involvement involves preemployment inquiries and health examinations. Preemployment health examinations will be permitted only if phrased in terms of the applicant's general ability to perform job-related functions rather than in terms of a disabil-

ity. The examination must be job related and consistently conducted for all applicants performing similar work. In consultation with legal counsel, the occupational health nurse must review all questionnaires to be used as part of the health examination (with exception of a drug-testing program) to ensure compliance with this act.

PROFESSIONAL LIABILITY

In recognition of the dynamic nature of occupational health nursing practice coupled with the influences and impact of larger policy issues, the occupational health nurse must know the legal parameters of practice and respond to legislative mandates that govern worker health and safety (AAOHN, 1994). The occupational health nurse is professionally and primarily accountable to workers and worker populations as well as to the employer, the profession, and self (AAOHN, 1994). In particular, the occupational health nurse must be aware of liability issues confronting the nurse because of the nature of working independently and the laws governing the employer-employee relationship (Lochlear-Haynes, 1990). Lochlear-Haynes described three legal issues germane to the employer-employee relationship:

- The client-nurse relationship
- The employment capacity of the occupational health nurse
- Any acts of negligence

The client-nurse relationship can be confusing when the nurse is hired by the employer to provide services to the client. The concern is whether a professional relationship exists under the law or the relationship is based on a coworker status.

MULTIDISCIPLINARY TEAM WORK

As work places have become more complex, a diverse array of expertise has emerged in many functional and technical areas. To be successful, the occupational health nurse must recognize the need to work as part of an interdisciplinary team. The nurse may interact with occupational medicine professionals, industrial hygienists, safety professionals, employee assistance counselors, personnel professionals, and union representatives (Fig. 27–5). Community health professionals, insurance carriers, and other support agencies in the community are also critical linkages.

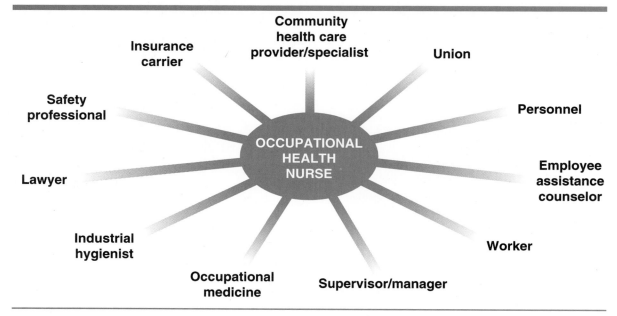

Figure 27–5
The occupational health nurse's professional links in the work place and community.

To illustrate the roles and collaborative efforts required to successfully resolve occupational health issues, two cases are described, and the roles and responsibilities of each interdisciplinary team member are briefly discussed.

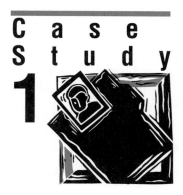

Case Study 1

A 23-year-old woman was recently transferred into a job that requires her to work with chemicals used in photolithography. She is newly married and might be pregnant, but this has not been confirmed. The client is concerned because the label on one of the pieces of equipment warns of possible effects on reproduction. Also she states that she has not felt well since transferring to this job, and she thinks it is a result of working with chemicals. There are no restrictions in this work area for pregnant women.

Occupational Health Nurse's Roles and Responsibilities

The occupational health nurse is probably the employee's first contact. The nurse listens to the employee's concerns and formulates a plan.

- Determine information by taking medical and occupational health histories. Perform a physical assessment and discuss symptoms.
- Schedule a pregnancy test. If this is not a service provided by the occupational health nurse, referral must be made to the employee's health care provider. If the client does not have one, referral must be made to an appropriate community health resource. Ask the client to have the care provider document pregnancy test results.
- Assure the employee that investigation will ensue immediately, and state who will be involved (e.g., industrial hygienist, occupational health physician).

- Assess the work area or request that an industrial hygienist assess the area (e.g., leaking equipment, problems with ventilation).
- Request the most current industrial hygiene data appropriate to the area.
- Schedule the employee to see the occupational health physician once all data are collected regarding medical and industrial hygiene.
- Communicate any recommended work restrictions to the supervisor or personnel department after the client is seen by the occupational health physician.
- Review the case in light of existing company policies, and influence changes as necessary.

Industrial Hygienist's Roles and Responsibilities

- Discuss the employee's concerns with the occupational health nurse and, as necessary, with the employee.
- Provide the most current industrial hygiene data and analysis for the work area under investigation.
- If current data are not available, monitor for industrial hygiene as soon as possible.
- Meet with the occupational health nurse and the occupational health physician as necessary for data communication and analysis.

Occupational Health Physician's Roles and Responsibilities

- Review the data with the occupational health nurse.
- View the work area and process.
- Discuss the data with industrial hygienist.
- Interview and examine the client.
- Make recommendations regarding the employee's health and safety.

Employee's Roles and Responsibilities

- Take a pregnancy test, and provide documentation of results to the occupational health nurse.
- Communicate concerns to the occupational health nurse and, as necessary, to the industrial hygienist.
- Keep appointments with occupational health physician.
- Follow the recommendations of the occupational health physician.

Supervisor or Manager's Roles and Responsibilities

- Allow investigation of the work area by the occupational health nurse and industrial hygienist.
- Follow the recommendations of the occupational health physician.

Primary Community Health Care Provider's Roles and Responsibilities

- Before arriving at a diagnosis, confer with the occupational health nurse or occupational medical consultant.
- Obtain all work place data relevant to the case for the purpose of formulating an appropriate treatment plan.
- Provide reproductive counseling to the family.
- Refer to appropriate specialists or community resources (i.e., March of Dimes, occupational or environmental pregnancy hot lines).

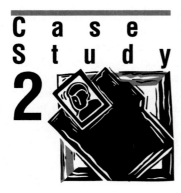

Case Study 2

A supervisor calls the occupational health nurse and states that one of his employees appears to be incapacitated. The employee was functioning normally in the morning but has appeared to be intoxicated since returning from lunch. The supervisor is concerned for the employee's as well as others' safety, and he is requesting assistance.

Occupational Health Nurse's Roles and Responsibilities

- Request that the supervisor accompany the employee to the occupational health nurse's office.
- Perform a physical assessment of the employee.
- Depending on the findings, the occupational health nurse will send the employee home with a family member, send the employee to a community care provider (hospital) via an ambulance for assessment, or, if there is concern for personal safety, notify security.
- Notify the employee and supervisor that the employee needs to follow up with the occupational health nurse on returning to work.
- If the employee is sent to the hospital, communicate with the hospital the reason for referral and request communication regarding assessment and disposition.
- On the employee's return to work, assess the employee's fitness for work; counsel, as appropriate, regarding alcohol or drug concerns; and make a referral to an appropriate resource (employee assistance counselor if available or appropriate community health resource).
- Notify the supervisor when the employee is medically cleared to return to work.

Supervisor or Manager's Roles and Responsibilities

- Accompany the employee to the occupational health nurse's office.
- Consult with the human resources professional regarding company policy for this type of employee behavior.
- Do not allow the employee in the work place until medically cleared by the occupational health nurse.

Employee Assistance Counselor's Roles and Responsibilities

- Provide confidential counseling.
- Make appropriate decisions regarding referrals to community health resources.

Security's Roles and Responsibilities

- Protect the physical safety of all involved.

Community Health Resources' Roles and Responsibilities

- Emergency medical technicians or ambulance staff: provide safe transport to the hospital.
- Hospital: perform a medical assessment of the worker, and communicate results to the occupational health nurse.
- Community counseling resource: accept referral and provide counseling for worker as appropriate.

Employee's Roles and Responsibilities

- Present at the occupational health nurse's office for initial assessment.
- On return to work, discuss fitness for duty with the occupational health nurse.
- Accept referral for treatment.

Family's Responsibilities

- Accept responsibility that alcohol or substance abuse is a family issue by acknowledging the problem.
- Assist in directing the individual to appropriate care with community health care providers.
- Seek community resources for guidance and support (Alcoholics Anonymous, Al-Anon, Narcotics Anonymous, other local support groups).

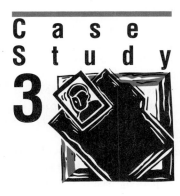

C a s e S t u d y 3

Forty percent of the 80 packers in Department X are experiencing upper extremity symptoms that appear to be related to their job activities. An evaluation of their job tasks indicates that the workers may experience musculoskeletal disorders because of the repetitive, forceful motions combined with non-neutral postures and insufficient rest periods.

Occupational Health Nurse's Roles and Responsibilities

- Assess symptomatic individuals, and refer to an occupational medical consultant as appropriate.
- Conduct a walk-through of the work area to assess job tasks by direct observation or videotaping.
- Evaluate OSHA 200 log, daily health services log, and workers' compensation and disability case statistics.
- Meet with Department X manager to discuss the issues and propose solutions.
- Plan, develop, implement, and evaluate an ergonomics educational program for workers.
- Work with the multidisciplinary team to identify appropriate intervention strategies.
- Document cost effectiveness of interventions.

Occupational Medical Consultant's Roles and Responsibilities

- Review data with the occupational health nurse.
- Diagnose the employee's condition and make appropriate treatment recommendations (e.g., restricted work, application of ice, use of anti-inflammatory agents, referral).
- Conduct a walk-through of work area.

Employee's Roles and Responsibilities

- Report symptoms to the occupational health nurse as soon as they occur.
- Adhere to the recommended treatment regimen.
- Attend educational sessions.

Supervisor or Manager's Roles and Responsibilities

- Meet with the occupational health nurse, medical consultant, and employees.
- Follow the recommendations of the multidisciplinary team.
- Recognize potential problems (e.g., insufficient rest breaks; forceful, repetitive motions; and non-neutral postures).
- Support decisions.

Health Care Provider's Roles and Responsibilities

- Accept referral from occupational medical consultant or occupational health nurse and evaluate data regarding the work place.
- Assess the employee, and develop a treatment plan.
- Communicate the plan to the occupational health nurse, and make recommendations for work restrictions.

SUMMARY

This chapter described the evolution of occupational health nursing during its first century of practice. Current and future demographics and business trends are described as they relate to this nursing specialty area. Aging workers, escalating health care costs, increasing numbers of women and minorities in the work force, and the competitive international marketplace are key factors shaping occupational health nursing practice.

Skills and competencies germane to occupational health nursing practice are identified. Critical work is also described in terms of primary, secondary, and tertiary prevention. For the community health nurse, knowledge of occupational health nursing practice is important because many companies, in fact, do not have on-site occupational health nurses and, therefore, must rely on community health nurses to support their occupational health and safety needs.

Legislative initiatives affecting occupational health nursing practice are identified, and the roles of colleagues in other occupational health specialty fields are discussed.

Case studies and learning activities are provided for the purpose of self-study or class discussion.

In conclusion, the occupational health nursing role is challenging and can have a tremendous impact on the quality and delivery of health care to workers and their families.

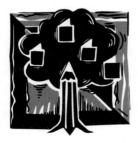

Learning Activities

1. A large automobile manufacturer has consulted you to design a program to control respiratory disease among foundry workers. Workers in different areas of ferrous foundries are exposed to different respiratory hazards. The main problems are silica exposure and exposure to formaldehyde. The corporation would like to develop a pilot program for one of its foundries that will then be applied to its other foundries. Health and industrial hygiene data will be collected. Both the corporation and the workers support the project, and both see the project as having three purposes: detecting health effects in individuals who may benefit from intervention, determining the relationship of health effects to environmental exposures, and identifying control strategies as appropriate. Outline your pilot program. Discuss the implications of discovering adverse health effects among current workers. Describe the roles of the occupational health nurse, physician, industrial hygienist, safety professional, manager, and employee.

2. The fear of AIDS has created problems in many work sites. Some believe policies should exist; others believe HIV testing should be done

at the work site. Still others affirm that education is the best approach for dealing with this extremely volatile issue.

- Is AIDS a concern for health care workers?
- Is AIDS a concern for occupational health nurses?
- Do you believe an AIDS policy should be in place at your company?
- Discuss what you would include in the policy.
- How has your nursing practice changed (if at all) as a result of AIDS?

3. A weight-loss program was conducted during August. Ten people participated in the 6-week program. The total weight loss the for group was 185 pounds. The following chart indicates the weight loss for the individuals.

Weight Before Program (pounds)	Weight After Program (pounds)
215	190
175	160
139	129
275	245
145	120
198	183
120	115
243	233
185	145
210	200

Is there a more effective way to show the results of the program? Assume you have been given this report by one of your peers for you to critique. Be as creative as you want, filling in any data, facts, figures, or other information that you believe is missing. Redesign a report that you would like to send to management.

4. Take an occupational history on five currently employed workers. Identify the occupation, associated job tasks, and potential health hazards. Describe control strategies that could minimize or eliminate the risk of adverse health effects.

5. Conduct a literature review to identify critical concepts in occupational health nursing, epidemiology, ergonomics, safety, industrial hygiene, and ethics.

REFERENCES

Albright A: Attitudes toward working mothers: Accommodating the needs of mothers in the work force. AAOHN J 40:490–495, 1992.

American Association of Industrial Nurses: The Nurse in Industry. New York, American Association of Industrial Nurses, 1976.

American Association of Occupational Health Nurses: AIDS Resource Guide: HIV Infections/AIDS in the Workplace. Atlanta, American Association of Occupational Health Nurses, 1988a.

American Association of Occupational Health Nurses: Standards of Occupational Health Nursing Practice. AAOHN, Atlanta, Georgia. 1994.

American Association of Occupational Health Nurses: The year 2000: AAOHN health objectives for the nation. AAOHN J 36:285–288, 1988b.

American Cancer Society. Cancer Facts and Figures. New York, American Cancer Society, 1991.

Arthur D. Little, Inc.: Costs and Benefits of Occupational Health Nursing (NIOSH Contract No. 210-78-0055). Washington, DC, U.S. Department of Health and Human Services, 1980.

Barlow R: Role of the occupational health nurse in the year 2000: Perspective view. AAOHN J 40:463–467, 1992.

Brown K: Containing health care costs: The occupational health nurse as case manager. AAOHN J 37:141–142, 1989.

Centineo D: Return-to-work programs: Cut costs and employee turnover. Risk Management 12:44–48, 1986.

Chelius J, Galvin D, Owens P: Disability: It's more expensive than you think. Business Health March:5–6, 1992.

Chenowith D: Nurses' interventions in specific risk factors in high risk employees: An economic appraisal. AAOHN J 37:367–373, 1989.

Cox AR: Planning for the future of occupational health nursing: Part II. Comprehensive membership survey. AAOHN J 37: 356–360, 1989.

Crawford SL: Job stress and occupational health nursing: Modeling health affirming choices. AAOHN J 41:522–528, 1993.

Dees JB, Taylor JR: Health care management: A tool for the future. AAOHN J 38:52–58, 1990.

Digital Equipment Corporation: 1995 HMO Performance Standards. Maynard, MA, Author, 1995.

Felton JS: The genesis of occupational health nursing: Part I. Occup Health Nurs 28:45–49, 1985.

Felton JS: The genesis of occupational health nursing: Part II. AAOHN J 34:210–215, 1986.

Freedman S, Bisesi M: Women and workplace stress. AAOHN J 36:271–274, 1988.

Friedman-Jimenez G: Occupational disease among minority workers: A common and preventable public health problem. AAOHN J 37:64–70, 1989.

Gates D, O'Neill N: Promoting maternal-child wellness in the workplace. AAOHN J 34:258–263, 1990.

Hall LS: Breast self examination: Use of a visual reminder to increase practice. AAOHN J 40:186–192, 1992.

Johnston W, Packer A: Workforce 2000: Work and Workers for the 21st Century. Indianapolis, IN, Hudson Institute, 1987.

Kalina CM, Fitko J, Fisher AM, Mitchell JH: Building a nurse initiated wellness program: Successful program. AAOHN J 43:144–147, 1995.

Kaminshine S: New rights for the disabled: The Americans with Disabilities Act of 1990. AAOHN J 39:249–251, 1991.

Kopfer AM, McGovern PM: Transmission of HIV via a needlestick injury: Practice recommendations and research implications. AAOHN J 41:374–381, 1993.

Leigh B: Case management in a health maintenance organization: Improving quality of care. AAOHN J 41:170–173, 1993.

Locklear-Haynes T: Public health in the workplace: Part II. Liability issues confronting the occupational health nurse. AAOHN J 38:78–79, 1990.

Lundberg GE: Occupational health nursing: A theoretical model. AAOHN J 40:538–544, 1992.

Maciag ME: Occupational health nursing in the 1990s: A different model of practice. AAOHN J 41:39–45, 1993.

Mannon JA, Conrad KM, Blue CL, Muran S: A case management tool for occupational health nurses: Development, testing, and application. AAOHN J 42:365–373, 1994.

Martin KJ: Being off work, preparing to return to work: How client-nurse interactions can affect employee well being. AAOHN J 41:574–578, 1993.

McGrath BJ: Nursing in Commerce and Industry. New York, The Commonwealth Fund, 1946.

Miller MA: Social economics, and political forces affecting the future of occupational health nursing. AAOHN J 37:361–366, 1989.

Moore P, Childre F: Creative policy-making strategies for working with the healthy chronically diseased employee. AAOHN J 38:284–288, 1990.

Morris L: Minorities, jobs, and health: An unmet promise. AAOHN J 37:53–55, 1989.

Mundy RR, Moore SC, Corey JB, Mundy GD: Disability syndrome: The effects of early vs. delayed rehabilitation intervention. AAOHN J 42:379–383, 1994.

Murphy D: The primary care role in occupational health nursing. AAOHN J 37:470–474, 1989.

National Cancer Institute: The Breast Cancer Digest (NIH Publication No. 84-1691) Washington, DC, U.S. Government Printing Office, 1984.

O'Brien S: Occupational health nursing roles: Future challenges and opportunities. AAOHN J 43:148–152, 1995.

Owen P, Long P: Facilitating adherence to ACS and NCI guidelines for breast cancer screening. AAOHN J 37:153–157, 1989.

Parker-Conrad JE: A century of practice: Occupational health nursing. AAOHN J 36:156–161, 1988.

Pastides H, Calabrese E, Hosmer D, Harris D: Spontaneous abortion and general illness symptoms among semiconductor manufacturers. J Occup Med 30:543–551, 1988.

Patterson J: Health promotion: An overview for the workplace. AAOHN Update Series 1:5, 1984.

Pravikoff DS: Occupational health nursing: A theoretical model. AAOHN J 40:531–537, 1992.

Randolph SA, Dalton PC: Limited duty work: An innovative approach to early return to work. AAOHN J 37:446–452, 1989.

Reith L, Ahrens A, Cummings D: Integrated disability management: Taking a coordinated approach to managing employee disabilities. AAOHN J 43:270–275, 1995.

Rimes KA: Mammography: Role of the occupational health nurse. AAOHN J 41:592–598, 1993.

Roberts CR, McGovern P: Working mothers and infant care: A review of the literature. AAOHN J 41:541–546, 1993.

Rogers B: Establishing research priorities in occupational health nursing. AAOHN J 37:493–500, 1989.

Rogers B: Occupational health nursing practice, education, and research: Challenges for the future. AAOHN J 38:536–543, 1990.

Rogers B, Cox AR: Advancing the profession of occupational health nursing: AAOHN's strategic planning process. AAOHN J 42:158–163, 1994.

Rooney E: Business coalitions on health care: An evolution from cost containment to quality improvement. AAOHN J 40:342–351, 1992a.

Rooney E: TQM/CQI in business and health care. AAOHN J 40:319–325, 1992b.

Rosen RH, Berger L: The Healthy Company: Eight Strategies to Develop People, Productivity, and Profits. Los Angeles, JP Tarcher, 1991.

Rosen RH, Freedman C: Developing Healthy Companies Through Human Resources Management. Paper presented at the Prevention Leadership Forum, Washington Business Group on Health and Office of Disease Prevention, Washington, DC, May 1987.

Stimpson M, Hanley B: Nurse policy analyst. Nurs Health Care 12:10–15, 1993.

Travers PH: In Cox AR, Ryan P (eds). A Comprehensive Guide for Establishing an Occupational Health Service. Atlanta, GA, American Association of Occupational Health Nurses, 1987.

Travers PH: Occupational health nursing in the 90's: Leveraging position and influence through assessment, networking, and communication. AAOHN Update Series 4:1–8, 1991.

Travers PH, Bullwinkel D, McDougall CE, Powell J: Occupational health nursing in the 90's: Skills and competencies. Unpublished data, 1991.

U.S. Public Health Service: Promoting Health/Preventing Disease: Year 2000 Objectives for the Nation. Washington, DC, U.S. Department of Health and Human Services, 1989.

Widtfeldt AK, Widtfeldt JR. Total quality management in American industry. AAOHN J 40:311–318, 1992.

Williamson GC, Moore PV: Health care cost containment: Current societal forces and health care trends. AAOHN J 35:444–448, 1987.

Yeater DC: The occupational health nurse as disability manager. AAOHN J 35:116–118, 1987.

The Home Visit and Home Health Care

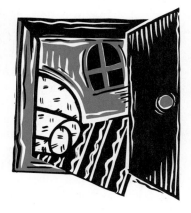

Upon completion of this chapter, the reader will be able to:

1. Discuss the purpose of the home visit.

2. Differentiate between the purpose of a public health nursing visit and that of a home health and hospice nursing visit.

3. Use the nursing process in outlining the steps involved in conducting a home visit.

4. Define home health care.

5. Identify the types of home health agencies.

6. Apply the nursing process to a home health client situation.

7. Discuss the process used in contracting with patients and their families to achieve health care goals.

Jean Cozad Lyon
Christine DiMartile Bolla
Mary A. Nies

The purpose of home visits by nurses is to provide nursing care to individuals and their families in their homes. The specific objectives and services provided by nurses vary depending on the type of agency providing services and the population served. Home visits are usually provided by nurses who work for public health departments, visiting nurse associations, home health agencies, or school districts.

Community health nurses from clinics often conduct home visits as part of patient follow-up. Public health nurses make visits to follow patients with communicable diseases and provide health education and community referrals to patients with identified problems. Nurses working for home health agencies or through nursing registries make home visits, often to assist patients in their transitions from hospital to home but also as ordered by health care providers because of exacerbations of chronic conditions.

The focus of all home visits is on the individual from whom the referral is received. In addition, the nurse assesses the interaction of the individual with the family and provides education and interventions for the family as well as the client. The nurse evaluates how the individual and family interact as part of an aggregate group in the community. The need for referrals for community services is identified by the nurse and made as necessary.

Nurses who make home visits receive referrals from a variety of sources, including the client's physician, nurse practitioner or nurse midwife, hospital discharge planner, school teacher, or clinic health care provider. Requests for nursing visits to assess and assist the client's health care can also originate with the client or the client's family.

Home visits have been an integral part of nursing for more than a century, originating with Florence Nightingale's "health nurses" in England. In the United States in 1877, the Women's Branch of the New York City Mission sent the first trained nurses into the homes of the poor to provide nursing care. Under the direction of Lillian Wald, pioneering efforts were initiated to provide services to the poor in their homes in the late 19th century (Kalisch and Kalisch, 1986; Kelly, 1991).

HOME HEALTH CARE

The term "home health care" describes a system in which health care and social services are provided to homebound or disabled people in their homes rather than in medical facilities (U.S. Department of Commerce/International Trade Administration, 1990). The Department of Health and Human Services set forth a definition of home health care that was developed by an interdepartmental work group:

Home health care is that component of a continuum of comprehensive health care whereby health services are provided to individuals and families in their places of residence for the purpose of promoting, maintaining or restoring health, or maximizing the level of independence, while minimizing the effects of disability and illness, including terminal illness. Services appropriate to the needs of the individual patient and family are planned, coordinated, and made available by providers organized for the delivery of home care through the use of employed staff, contractual arrangements, or a combination of the two patterns.

(WARHOLA, 1980).

PURPOSE OF HOME HEALTH SERVICES

The primary purpose of home health services is to allow individuals to remain at home and receive health care services that would otherwise be offered in a health care institution, such as a hospital or nursing home setting. The home health industry has grown tremendously and continues to grow. The growth of home health services is generated by numerous factors, including the increasing costs of hospital care and subsequent introduction of the prospective payment system (PPS), by P. L. 98-21 of the Social Security Amendments in 1983. Under the PPS, hospitals receive a fixed amount of money based on the relative cost of resources used to treat Medicare patients within each type of diagnosis-related group (Guterman and Dobson, 1986). Many other third-party payers are negotiating preferred provider programs, or managed care systems. In a managed care arrangement, the provider of health care is paid a set fee for providing care to clients enrolled in the program. Providing home care services contributes to cost containment in a managed care environment. This is accomplished through timely hospital discharges with nursing services provided in the home setting and supporting clients at home rather than in skilled facilities. Home care is also popular with consumers, who prefer to receive care in their own homes rather than in an institution.

Home health care services have changed to address the needs of the population. Home health nurses visit acutely ill clients, people with acquired immunodeficiency syndrome, elderly in greater numbers, terminally ill clients, high-risk pregnant women, and ill infants and children (Feldman, 1993). The focus of home health care continues to be that of care of sick clients and needs to expand to include health promotion and disease prevention interventions. Home visiting is a specific nursing intervention, preceded by an antecedent event, and unfolds as a process (Byrd, 1995). Currently, most reimbursement for nursing services is based on skilled nursing needs of clients. On each client visit, the nurse must document that the care provided is of a skilled nature, requiring the knowledge and assessment skills of a nurse, and could not have been provided by the client or a family member.

Services coordinated in the home include not only skilled nursing care provided by registered nurses but also the services of physical, occupational and speech therapists, social workers, and home health aides. The broader home care industry definition of home health care includes supportive social services, respite care, and adult day care (Health Care Financing Review, 1988).

CONDUCTING A HOME VISIT USING THE NURSING PROCESS ASSESSMENT

Visit Preparation

It is important that the nurse making the home visit prepare for the visit by reviewing the referral form, including the purpose of the visit, the geographical residence of the family, and any other pertinent information. The first home visit provides the nurse with the opportunity to establish a trust relationship with the client and family to establish credibility as a resource for health information and community referrals in a nonthreatening environment.

The Referral

The referral (Fig. 28–1) is a formal request for a home visit. Referrals come from a variety of sources, including hospitals, clinics, health care providers, individuals, and families. The type of agency that receives the referral will vary depending on the client services that are needed. Public health referrals are made for clients who are in need of health education (e.g., infant care education and resource allocation) or for follow-up of clients with communicable diseases and their contacts.

Home health referrals are requested to provide short-term, intermittent skilled services and rehabilitation to clients. Visits can last from 30 to 90 minutes, depending on the specific needs of the client, and are scheduled on an intermittent basis, from as often as once a day to two or three times a week or only once a week, depending on the need. For example, a client who has had a stroke requires skilled nursing assessments, physical therapy visits for gait training, speech therapy for improvement of a speech deficit, and occupational therapy for retraining in activities of daily living such as bathing and cooking.

Review of the referral form before the first visit gives the community health nurse basic information about the client such as name, age, diagnosis or health status, address, telephone number, insurance coverage if any, reason for referral, and source of the referral, whether a clinician, health care provider, communicable disease service, hospital, client, or client's family.

Public health referrals usually provide information on the client's condition that necessitates public health nurse visits. An example is a client who is positive for tuberculosis, in which case the nurse is notified of the client's place of residence, type and location of employment, and any known contacts, including family and friends. Another example is a 16-year-old girl who is referred for antepartum visits because she is 7 months pregnant and has just initiated prenatal care.

Additional information provided in the home health referral includes current client medications, prescribed diet, other disciplines involved in the care of the client, physician's orders, and goal of care. This information is important because it gives the nurse a visual picture of the client.

Initial Telephone Contact

The client is contacted by the nurse and informed of the referral for service. The first telephone contact with the client or family consists of an exchange of essential information, including an introduction by the nurse, identification of the agency that has received the referral, and the purpose of the visit. After this initial information is exchanged, the client is informed of the nurse's desire to make the home visit, permission is received from the client, and a mutually acceptable time is set for the visit. Because the nurse is considered a guest in the client's home, it is important that the client under-

PATIENT NUMBER	☐NEW ☐READMIT **INTAKE**	DATE LAST SEEN BY MD	CASE MANAGER

NAME: LAST FIRST M.I.	TELEPHONE NO.:	SEX M F	BIRTHDATE	AGE	DATE OF 1st VISIT M.D. AUTH. YES _____ NO _____

STREET ADDRESS: CITY: STATE: ZIP:	HOSP/SNF:
	ADM. DATE:
DIRECTIONS:	DIS. DATE:

DIAGNOSES: PRIMARY #	PHYSICIAN NAME: SPECIALTY:	HOSP/SNF:
1.	ADDRESS:	ADM. DATE:
2.	TEL. NO.:	DIS. DATE:
3.	PHYSICIAN NAME: SPECIALTY:	MEDICARE NO.
4.	ADDRESS:	MEDI-CAL NO./SS #.
DX KNOWN TO PT? _____	TEL. NO.:	
HISTORY:	AGENCY WORKER: TEL. NO.:	INS. CO.:

	PAY SOURCES/ SERVICE REQUEST:	POLICY #:

PHN	PT	ST	OT	GRP. #:
MSW	HHA	HCA	PD	COV. CODE:

RELIGIOUS/CULTURAL PATTERNS/LANGUAGE/ PSYCHO-SOCIAL	EMERGENCY/FAMILY CONTACTS (BY PRIORITY)	TEL. NO.:
		CONTACT PERSON:

	NAME	REL.	HOME #	WORK #
MEDICATIONS	#1			
	ADDRESS			
	#2			
	ADDRESS			

PERTINENT HOSPITAL INFORMATION

DATE/TIME:_____

SKILLED ORDERS PER: _____

DIET/FLUIDS

ALLERGIES

EQUIPMENT: DME   YES_____ NO _____

INTAKE SOURCE NAME	AGENCY	TEL. NO.
HOW DID YOU LEARN ABOUT OUR SERVICES?		
INTAKE RECEIVED BY		DATE

Figure 28–1
Referral form. (Courtesy of Home Calls, Oakland, California.)

HOME HEALTH VISIT

- *Story by Leonard Kaku, RN, MSN*
- *Photography by George Draper*

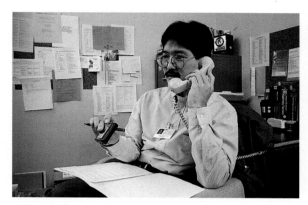

Home health nurses and some community health nurses (CHNs) make visits to families with health problems. A referral for this home visit is received from a client's nurse practitioner. The client was discharged from the hospital with a primary diagnosis of noninsulin-dependent diabetes mellitus (NIDDM) and a secondary diagnosis of hypertension and S/P cerebrovascular accident (CVA), which occurred 10 months ago.

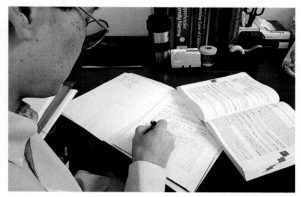

The nurse reviews the information on the referral form. The referral reveals the client is newly diagnosed with NIDDM and has a history of hypertension and CVA with left-sided weakness. The client's insurance is Medicaid. The current medications listed are: 25 mg hydrochlorothiazide q.d., 5 mg Isordil q.i.d., and 5 mg Micronase b.i.d. The prescribed diet is a low-fat, 1200-calorie diet with no added salt. If there is information missing, it is important to obtain it before making initial client contact.

The nurse brings to the community health setting experience and knowledge from a variety of specialties such as maternity, mental health, medical-surgical, pediatrics, pharmacology, and epidemiology.

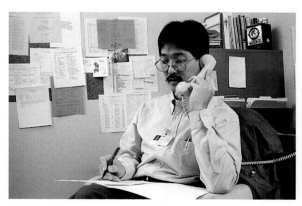

The nurse usually makes the initial contact by phone. It is important to introduce yourself and the agency you represent and to explain the purpose of the visit. You will need to obtain permission and arrange a date and time for the visit. Occasionally, the client may not have a phone. This may require a drop-in visit. Attempt a home visit and be prepared for a full visit if the client is at home and requests your services. If the client is not at home, the nurse should leave a business card with a note requesting a call to arrange a home visit.

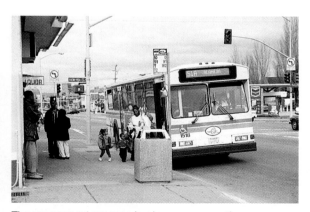

The assessment process begins as soon as the nurse leaves the office on the way to the home visit. Transportation may be a problem for the client. Is it available? What is the cost and hours of operation? Are there safety concerns about using public transportation?

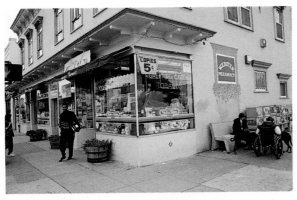

It is important to assess the availability of services, such as a pharmacy and a bank. Where does the client go to get cash or deposit a check and to fill a prescription? Is the area safe for these transactions for the client?

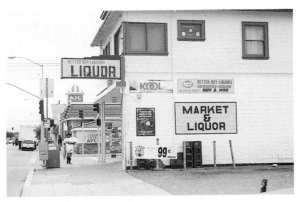

Is there a grocery store nearby? What types of foods are available?

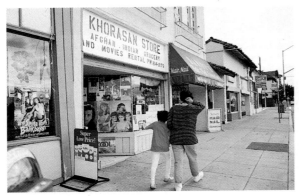

The nurse notices an Afghan-Indian grocery store that provides for ethnic communities.

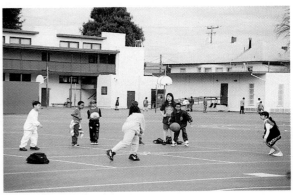

The school in the area provides evidence of diverse families in the community.

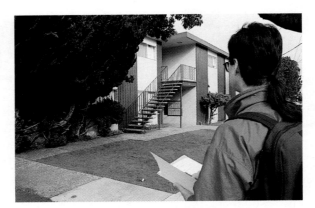

Assessment of the type of neighborhood in which the client resides is also important. Is it residential, business, or mixed; high- or low-density housing, single family homes, or apartments? Is the neighborhood safe or unsafe, e.g., high crime or drug area?

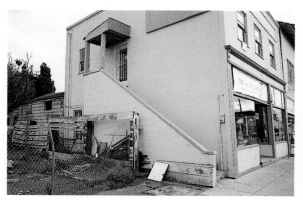
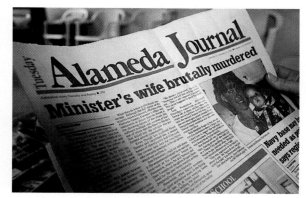

It is extremely important for the nurse to be aware of the environment and surroundings as you approach and observe the residence.

You are not to disregard personal safety to make a home visit. If it is unsafe, arrange another time and place for the home visit.

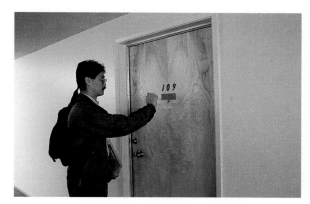
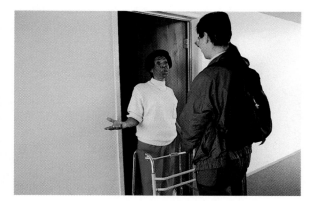

When you knock at the door, be sure to state your name, role, agency you represent, and the purpose of the visit.

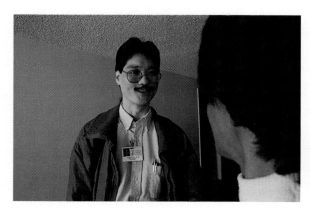

You should always wear your identification badge.

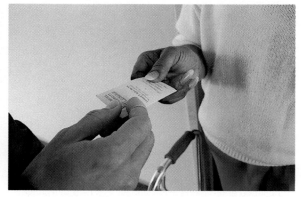

Business cards with the agency name, address, and phone number should be available to give to clients. Building trust provides the foundation for a therapeutic relationship with the client. Clients may be hesitant to trust the health care/social system.

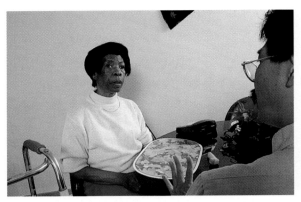

It is important to establish a comfortable atmosphere. This may be accomplished by initiating social conversation. It moves from general questions about the client and family to more sensitive health issues. The purpose of the visit is to provide health care services, and this should be clearly communicated to the client. This home visit includes a health history and limited physical examination.

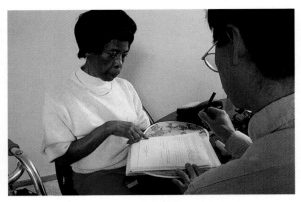

Agencies vary in the type of paperwork required. A consent form is often required prior to providing services. The form should be explained so the client may make an informed consent.

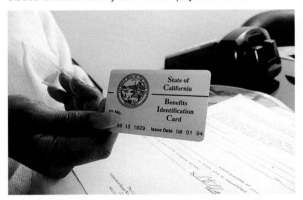

Medical insurance should also be verified so that the service may be billed properly.

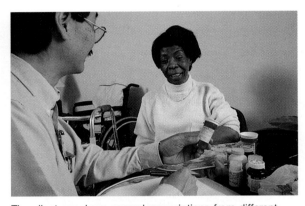

The client may have several prescriptions from different health care providers. These medications may have expired or may no longer be necessary. This is an opportunity for the nurse to provide instructions pertaining to the use of medications.

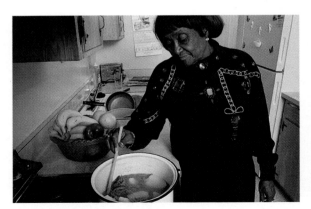

Inquiring about the diet provides an opportunity to explore compliance and cultural implications. It is helpful to have a diet plan that includes culturally relevant food. Teaching the client how and why to maintain a diet log will assist in evaluating compliance with the low-fat, 1200-calorie diet.

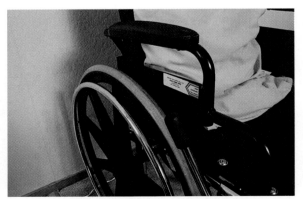

Health history includes a functional assessment of the client. Physical limitations of the client in performing activities of daily living are important health assessment data. The nurse has already noted any physical barriers to ambulation, both exterior and interior, that may exist. The nurse has already observed the use of a walker by the client at the door and a wheelchair nearby.

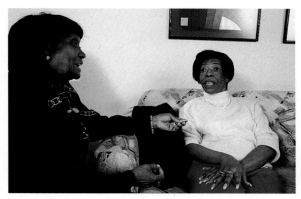

It is important to do a family assessment. Observation of the interaction between the client and family will be helpful in developing a nursing care plan. The family should be incorporated into the nursing care plan for the client.

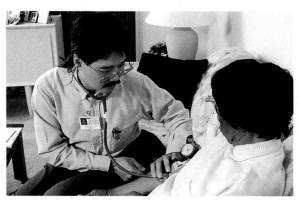

Equipment for taking vital signs may not be provided by the client. The nurse should always have a stethoscope and have access to a sphygmomanometer. To many clients, the taking of a blood pressure is a reassuring initial step in a health examination. It provides nurses a window of opportunity to obtain important health history data and provide health teaching.

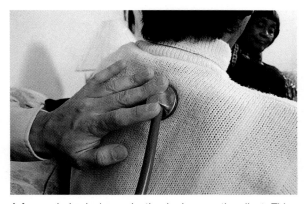

A focused physical examination is done on the client. This will provide the baseline data of the client's health status. This information will be used on subsequent visits to assess progress towards the identified nursing goals.

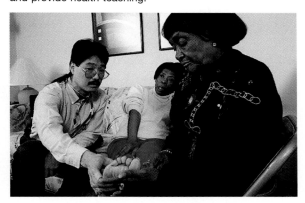

Since the client is newly diagnosed with NIDDM, it would be important to teach proper foot care.

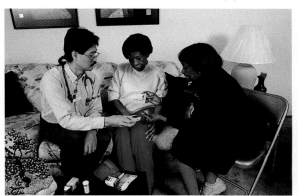

The use of a glucometer may help the provider in making clinical decisions regarding treatment. This is another opportunity to provide health teaching for the client. Review the proper use of the glucometer and have the client do a demonstration. It is helpful to incorporate the family members in the teaching plan.

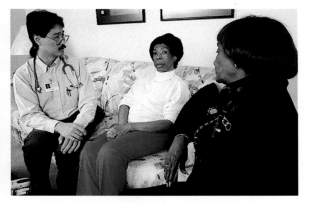

The establishment of a nursing care plan requires input from the client and family. An agreed-upon goal is following a low-fat, 1200-calorie diet. The family will help in preparing the food and doing blood glucose monitoring. The nurse will provide a culturally relevant diet and contact the local American Diabetes Association (ADA) chapter for a support group for the family. A return visit is scheduled for the following week.

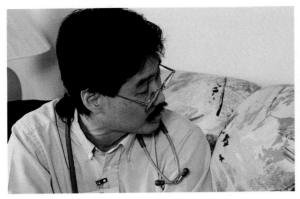

At the end of the visit, always ask if there is anything else you could assist with. It provides an opening for the client and family to ask for assistance that may not have been covered during the home visit. Remind the client of the business card and ask the client to call if there are any problems. Also advise the client you will be contacting the health care provider regarding outcomes of the home visit.

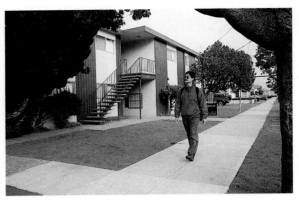

The nurse continues to note environmental conditions that impact the client, family, and community. The nurse can then begin to advocate for health promotion and prevention interventions surrounding the environmental issues confronting the community.

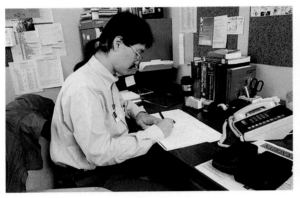

The nurse charts according to agency policy as soon as possible to ensure accurate, clear, and concise notes of the home visit. This may be done at the office or between home visits.

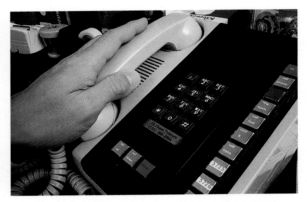

It is the responsibility of the nurse to inform the referral source of the home visit results. This is especially important if the nurse has been unable to locate the client. The result of the home visit may be provided in a written or verbal format.

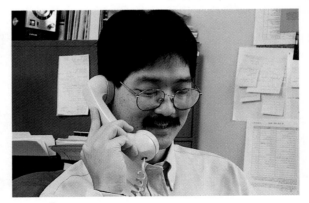

The nurse acts as a referral resource for the community. The nurse continuously searches for community resources and develops a resource database. The nurse calls the local ADA chapter to find out about the services provided. The agency does indeed have a culturally sensitive diet available for the client as well as a support group for family members. The nurse calls the client with the information.

stand and agree to the visit. The nurse verifies the client's address and asks for specific directions to the client's home.

During a home health visit, the client is requested to present evidence of insurance information, such as Medicare or Medicaid, or a health maintenance organization membership identification card. The nurse should forewarn the client of this so the client or family can locate the information before the visit. If the client is unable to provide this verification, the nurse assists with these functions during the visit. Clients who receive a public health home visit do not require evidence of insurance coverage because these services are not billed directly, but are generally covered by a county public health budget or by state or federally funded programs.

Not all clients have a telephone. If this is the case, the nurse rechecks the referral for a telephone number where messages can be left. It is also worthwhile to contact the health care provider who made the referral to see whether the telephone number was omitted unintentionally. If the client does not have a telephone, the nurse may choose to make a drop-in visit. This type of visit consists of an unannounced visit to the client's home, during which the nurse explains the purpose of the referral, receives the client's permission for the visit, and sets up a time for a future visit with the client. The client may agree to the first visit while the nurse is there.

If the client is not at home for the drop-in visit, the nurse leaves an official agency card and a brief message asking the client to contact the agency to schedule a nursing visit. The nurse informs the referring agency that the visit was attempted but that the client was not available for contact. A formal agency letter, identifying the agency and the reason for the referral, is often sent to clients who are difficult to contact. The nurse's primary responsibility when unsuccessful in locating the client is to keep the clinic, physician, or referring agency informed of efforts to establish contact with the client.

Environment

An environmental assessment begins as the nurse leaves the agency on route to the client's home. Specific questions asked by the nurse are as follows (Keating and Kelman, 1988):

- How does the client's neighborhood compare with other neighborhoods in the area?
- Are there adequate shopping facilities, such as grocery stores, close to the client's home?

The nurse should also make note of the client's dwelling, that is, whether the client lives in a single-family home, in a single room in a home or hotel, in an apartment, or in a shared apartment or house. Specific assessments that are made include the following:

- Is the client's residence easily accessible by the client, given the client's age and functional ability? For example, if the client has limited endurance, can the several flights of stairs be negotiated when entering or leaving the dwelling?
- Are facilities for the handicapped available as necessary? Is the dwelling in an area with high rates of drug abuse or crime?
- Is the building or home secure? Does the client live alone? If so, how does the client get to the physician or clinic? How does the client purchase groceries?
- Does the client have food in the home? If so, who prepares the client's meals? Are the meals nutritious?
- Are there rodents, cockroaches, or other potential vectors of disease present in the client's home?
- Does the client's home have hot running water, heat, sanitation facilities, and adequate ventilation?
- Is the client's residence safe relative to the client's physical status, or is the home cluttered with debris and furniture?

Safety Issues

When the nurse meets with the client, whether in the home or at another mutually agreeable location, the initial conversation revolves around social topics. The nurse assumes a friendly manner and asks general questions about the client, the client's family, and health care services that will benefit the client. These questions assist the nurse in assessing the client's needs and create a comfortable atmosphere in which the nurse and client communicate.

Building Trust

Many of the clients in need of nursing visits do not trust the health care system and are not comfortable with the representative from an agency visiting their home. For example, a client who is pregnant and does not have legal status in the United States will be hesitant to allow a nurse to visit because the client will be fearful of being reported to immigration authorities. The nurse's role in visiting this client is to focus on the health and safety of the client and her fetus. Thus, the nurse must build a trust relationship early in the visit, or the client will not allow additional visits. If a trust relationship is not established and the client believes that the nurse will report the client to immigration, it is highly probable that the client will move to another location to avoid future contact.

APPLICATION OF THE NURSING PROCESS

Assessment

During the first home visit, the type of client assessment will vary depending on the purpose of the home visit. The public health nurse assesses the client's knowledge of his or her health status. The nurse identifies knowledge deficits and uses this information in the development of a plan of care.

Subjective information is obtained from the client and the client's family and includes the client's perception of the situation and what the client identifies as problems. The nurse assesses whether the client is isolated physically or socially from others and whether the client is a member of a close-knit, nurturing, supportive family or kinship network. The amount of support that the client perceives to be available may or may not be accurate, so the nurse asks several questions about the client's family, friends, and daily routine to assess the client's level of social support.

The home health nurse assesses the client's health knowledge and his or her physical, functional, and psychosocial status; physical environment; and social support during the first home visit. Information is collected through observations and questions asked of the patient and family or caregivers in the home environment. It is not unusual to find inconsistencies between information provided by the patient during hospitalization concerning the amount of physical and emotional support available from family and friends and the reality of the amount of support that is available to the patient in the home. The nurse validates or modifies the referral information received to reflect the actual home situation.

Community health nurses often use contracts that are jointly developed by the nurse, the patient, and the family to delineate the responsibilities of the patient, the family, and the agency for the provision of services.

Home Health

A physical assessment of the client is generally done in the home health visit and includes a review of all systems, with an emphasis on the systems affected by the client's presenting condition. The nurse obtains objective data through the use of essential physical assessment skills such as observation, palpation, auscultation, and percussion. The physical assessment also includes information regarding the client's functional status. Assessment of the functional status is important for Medicare reimbursement and for the development of an individualized plan of care. This assessment includes information regarding the client's ability to ambulate, to perform activities of daily living independently, and to use assist devices such as a cane or wheelchair. Specific functional limitations, such as shortness of breath or muscle weakness, are assessed at this time. Information obtained during the assessment phase is used to identify nursing diagnoses and to develop a plan of care. Data collection continues while the patient is receiving home health services. Changes in the patient's condition, environment, or social structure necessitate modifications in the plan of treatment and the nursing care plan.

There are differences between the plan of treatment and the nursing care plan. The plan of treatment includes the type of home health services to be received, the projected frequency of visits by each discipline (Albrecht, 1991), and the interventions that are needed. The nursing care plan addresses specific nursing interventions designed to treat the patient's actual or potential problems, with goals identified with measurable outcomes.

DIAGNOSIS AND PLANNING

Develop a Plan for the Client and Family

After the assessment phase of the home visit, the nurse identifies the nursing diagnoses that address patient problems. Actual or potential problems are identified. The identification of nursing diagnoses serves as the basis for the nursing care plan. This plan is developed in consultation with the client and the family. The plan identifies short- and long-term goals for the patient and is developed to have measurable outcomes. The plan identifies nursing interventions that are needed and additional home health services that are appropriate to enable the patient to achieve the identified goals. It is important that patient and family be involved in the planning process as well as with community resources to maximize the plan's success. Planning is a dynamic process that continues while the patient receives nursing services. The plan is modified as needed, depending on the patient's condition, until the identified goals are met.

Often the nurse will develop a contract with the client that delineates the role and responsibilities of the nurse regarding the client's health and the role of the client and family (Spradley, 1990). If during the planning phase the client expresses a disinterest in contracting to improve health, the nurse will be limited in possible interventions. Goals are identified that the client is willing to work toward with the nurse's assistance.

The goal of home visits for both public health and home health nursing is to involve the client and family in taking an active role in health promotion. The nurse is careful not to allow the client to become dependent on the nurse's interventions because the nurse's involvement is short term.

Outline the Client and Family Roles

Written contracts are helpful for both the nurse and the client because the client's and nurse's roles in implementation of the plan are clearly delineated (Spradley, 1990). If either the client or the nurse forgets their role in the plan, the written contract is used as a reference. The contract can be modified by mutual agreement of the client and the nurse.

INTERVENTION

Implementation of the care plan begins during the first home visit. The nurse begins to provide the client and family with health information concerning the client's health status and availability of and access to community resources. In the case of the home health visit, the nurse provides skilled nursing care. At the end of the initial home visit, the nurse discusses with the client the need for another home visit. The nurse and client discuss the goal of the next visit, specifically, what the client is to do before the visit. The client and family are informed about any information or skills the nurse will provide during the next visit, and the nurse and client agree on a day for the next visit.

Referral for Community Services

During the first visit, the nurse provides the client and family with information regarding community resources, including the purpose of the resources, services provided, eligibility, any involved expense, and agency telephone numbers. Referrals depend on the availability of community resources, eligibility of the client for the services, willingness of the client and family to use the services, and suitability of the resources for the client and family. Examples of such services include information about immunization clinics for children in the family; adult day care or senior centers for elderly clients who could benefit from socialization; adult education classes or continuation of high school for pregnant teen clients who have dropped out of high school; Meals On Wheels services for clients who are not able to prepare meals; homeless shelters for men, women, and families; soup kitchens; resources for clothing and housing; mental health clinics; resources for battered spouses; and primary care clinics for low-income clients with and without insurance.

If necessary, the client or client's family may request assistance from the nurse in contacting the community resources. The client and family are encouraged to make the contacts, but if the client and family are unable to make the calls or do not speak English, the nurse needs to intervene on behalf of the client. By providing referral information during the first home visit, the nurse can, during the next home visit, follow up on the success of the client or family in contacting and using community services.

Terminating the Visit

The nurse terminates the first visit when the assessment is completed and a plan for care is established with the client. The average first visit should not be longer than 1 hour. Much information is provided to the client during that hour, and much information is collected by the nurse. Most clients are tired by the end of a 1-hour visit and often cannot retain any additional information provided by the nurse. It is preferable to set a date for another home visit to reinforce information provided and work progressively toward achieving goals.

EVALUATION

Evaluation of Progress Toward Goals

The evaluation phase occurs when the nurse can determine whether the goals established with the patient are realistic and achievable for the patient and the patient's family. The evaluation process is continuous and allows the nurse to determine the success or progress toward the goals identified for the client. It is through the collection of additional data during the evaluation phase that the nurse can identify the need for revisions in the nursing care plan and plan of treatment and intervene to make the necessary changes. An example is an elderly wife who, during the initial home visit, stated that she preferred to provide the physical care for her frail husband, who is nonambulatory. On a subsequent visit, the nurse assesses that the patient is not receiving the care that is required for the patient's personal care, specifically bathing. The nurse discusses the problem with the wife and presents her with options that are available, including the services of a home health aide to provide personal care, including bathing, three times a week. A new plan is developed, and it includes the home health aide. The plan is implemented and evaluated during future visits. Input from the client is critical to determine whether the goals established are realistic and achievable for the client.

Modification of the Plan as Needed

The evaluation process also allows the nurse and client or family to discuss what is working well and where modifications are needed in the plan. Evaluation occurs through open communication between the nurse and client, with the nurse asking questions about specific parts of the care plan. If a trust relationship exists, the client feels comfortable in telling the nurse about problems in the care plan.

When Goals Have Been Achieved

The overall purpose of home visits is to assist the client with the information and nursing care that is necessary for the client to function successfully without interventions by the nurse. When the care plan goals have been achieved, the nurse is no longer needed by the client. The client knows what community resources are available and how to access health care services for primary, secondary, and tertiary interventions.

TYPES OF HOME HEALTH AGENCIES

Home health agencies differ in their financial structures, organizational structures, governing boards, and populations served. The most common types of home health agencies are official (public), nonprofit, propri-

etary, chains, and hospital-based agencies. There is an increase in the number of managed care agencies, which may have any of the just-mentioned financial structures. Managed care agencies contract with payers, such as insurance companies, to provide specified services to the enrolled clients at a predetermined price. The managed care agencies receive payment before offering services and are responsible for taking the financial risk of providing the care to clients within the budgeted allotment. This works well with large numbers of enrolled clients, where the financial risk is spread across a larger number of people, many of whom are healthy and will not require skilled services.

Official Agencies

Official, or public, home health agencies are those that are organized, operated, and funded by local or state governments. These agencies may be part of a county public health nursing service or a home health agency that operates separate from the public health nursing service but is located within the county public health system. Official home health agencies are funded by taxpayers but also receive reimbursement from third-party payers, such as Medicare, Medicaid, and private insurance companies.

Nonprofit Agencies

Nonprofit home health agencies include all home health agencies that are exempt from paying federal taxes because of their tax status and reinvest any profits into the agency. Nonprofit home health agencies include independent home health agencies or hospital-based home health agencies. Not all hospital-based home health agencies are nonprofit, even if the hospital is classified as nonprofit. The home health agency can be established as a profit-generating service and thus serve as a source of revenue for the hospital or medical center. In this situation, the home health agency is categorized organizationally as for profit, and federal taxes are paid on profits.

Proprietary Agencies

Proprietary home health agencies are those that are classified as for profit and pay federal taxes on profits generated. Proprietary agencies can be in the form of individual-owned agencies, profit partnerships, or profit corporations. Investors in proprietary partnerships or corporations receive financial returns on their investments made in the agencies, providing the agencies make a profit. A percentage of the profits generated are also reinvested into the agency.

Chains

A growing number of home health agencies are owned and operated by corporate chains (Harrington, 1988). These chains are usually classified as proprietary agencies and may be part of a proprietary hospital chain. Agencies within chains have a financial advantage over single agencies in that the chains have lower administrative costs because many services are provided through a larger single corporate structure. For example, a multiagency corporation has greater purchasing power for supplies and equipment because of the volume purchased, and administrative services such as payroll and employee benefits can be provided for all chain employees by a single corporate office, thereby reducing duplication of these services. Criticism of proprietary and chain agencies includes concerns over the quality of services provided by agencies that are profit driven.

Hospital-Based Agencies

Since the implementation of PPS in 1983, the number of hospital-based home health agencies has doubled (U.S. Department of Commerce/International Trade Administration, 1990). This trend is not surprising in light of the fixed reimbursement under PPS and the hospitals' incentive to decrease length of stay. By establishing home health agencies, hospitals are able to (1) discharge to home patients who have skilled health care needs, (2) provide the necessary services to the patient, and (3) receive reimbursement through third-party payers, such as Medicare, Medicaid, and private insurance companies. The increasing number of home health agencies indicates that home health agencies are profitable endeavors and provide hospitals with a source of additional revenue.

Certified and Noncertified Agencies

Certified home health agencies meet federal standards and are therefore able to receive Medicare payments for services provided to eligible individuals. Not all home health agencies are certified. The number of Medicare-certified home health agencies increased to approximately 11,000 home health agencies, an increase from 10,848 in 1987. Approximately 50%, or

5500, of these agencies were Medicare certified (U.S. Department of Commerce/International Trade Administration, 1990).

Special Home Health Programs

Many home health agencies offer special, high-technology home care services. The motivation for offering high-technological services at home is both beneficial to the patient and financially advantageous. Through the implementation of these special programs, patients who require continuous skilled care in an acute or skilled nursing institution are able to return to their homes and receive care at home. From the financial perspective, skilled services provided at home are less costly to offer than hospitalization.

Examples of special services include home intravenous therapy programs for patients who require daily infusions of total parenteral nutrition or antibiotic therapy, pediatric services for children with chronic health problems, follow-up of premature infants who are at risk for complications, ventilator therapy, and home dialysis programs. The key to the success of all of these programs is the patient's, family's, or caregiver's ability to learn the care necessary for success of the home program and the motivation of these individuals to provide the care. If family or caregiver support is not available in the home, the patient cannot be considered a candidate for any of these programs, and other arrangements for care must be found.

Reimbursement for Home Care

Before the establishment of Medicare in 1965, individuals who required home health services paid cash for the services, and donations to the service agencies that provided the services helped to subsidize care for patients who were unable to pay (Kent and Hanley, 1990). Since 1965, individuals who are eligible for Medicare benefits under Title XVIII of the Social Security Act or for Medicaid benefits under Title XIX and those people with private health insurance can receive short-term, skilled health care services in their homes that are reimbursed by the federal government through the Medicare program. Provided services include nursing care, social service, physical therapy, occupational therapy, and speech therapy, and the program is individualized to meet the needs of the patient (Stuart-Siddal, 1986).

The rapid growth of the home health market is believed to be reflective of the following:

- Increasing proportion of persons aged 65 years and older
- Lower average cost of home health care compared with institutional costs ($750 per month for routine skilled nursing care at home compared with $2000 for care in an institution)
- Active support of insurers for home care
- Medicare promotion of home health care as an alternative to institutionalization (U.S. Department of Commerce, 1990, p. 49–4).

Payments made by patients or their families comprised 46% of the private financing (12% of total spending) for home health services. The remaining private financing was paid by private health insurance and nonpatient revenue.

EDUCATIONAL PREPARATION OF HOME HEALTH NURSES AND NURSING STANDARDS

The American Nurses Association (ANA, 1986) has established standards for home health nursing practice. These standards are differentiated into two levels of practice: that of the generalist home health nurse, who is prepared at the baccalaureate level, and that of the specialist nurse, who is prepared at the graduate level. According to the ANA, the generalist provides care to individuals and their families and participates in quality assurance programs. The generalist home health nurse must have community health assessment skills to diagnose complex biopsychosocial problems in families, teach health practices, counsel, and refer to other health care providers as necessary as well as high-technological nursing skills (Keating and Kelman, 1988).

The specialist home health nurse contributes additional clinical expertise to home health patients and their families, formulates health and social policy, and implements and evaluates health programs and services (ANA, 1986). Registered nurses with less than a baccalaureate education are not educationally prepared to meet the professional standards set forth for home health nursing and are encouraged to use the standards in providing care and in pursuing professional development.

Unfortunately, many home health agencies have not adopted the ANA standards for home health nursing and have hired nurses with less than baccalaureate preparation. Some of these home health agencies offer salaries that are lower than those offered to nurses employed in the acute hospital setting and thus cannot recruit educationally qualified nurses.

Albrecht's conceptual model (1990) for home care clearly identifies the educational content areas for students in undergraduate and graduate nursing programs with specialties in home health care. An underlying premise of the model is that professional satisfaction and effective patient outcomes depend on the education and experience of the home health nurse. Implications that are apparent in the model include the following:

- Nursing programs at the undergraduate and graduate levels must prepare competent providers of home health care.
- Curricula are to include concepts related to the suprasystem, health service delivery system, and home subsystem, which includes structural, process, and outcome elements.
- Students at the undergraduate level need at least one clinical observation or experience in a home health care agency.
- Graduate-level students need specific courses that cover concepts present in the model, including knowledge of education, preventive, supportive, therapeutic, and high-technology nursing interventions for home health care; a multidisciplinary approach to home health care; health law and ethics; systems theory; economics covering supply, demand, and productivity; and case management and coordination (Albrecht, 1990, p. 125).

The home health nurse serves as a case manager for patients who receive care from staff of the home health agency or through contract services. The success of the case management plan is contingent on the ability of the nurse to use the nursing process to develop a plan of treatment that best fits the individual needs of the patient, the patient's family, or caregiver. The first step in the development of the plan of treatment and nursing care plan is the patient and family assessment.

The Albrecht nursing model for home health care (Fig. 28–2) provides a framework within which nurses, patients, and their families can interact to identify mutual goals of interventions and promote self-care capability of the patient at home (Albrecht, 1990). Three major elements that are used to measure the quality of home health care patient outcomes include structural, process, and outcome elements.

Structural elements include the client, family, provider agency, health team, and professional nurse.

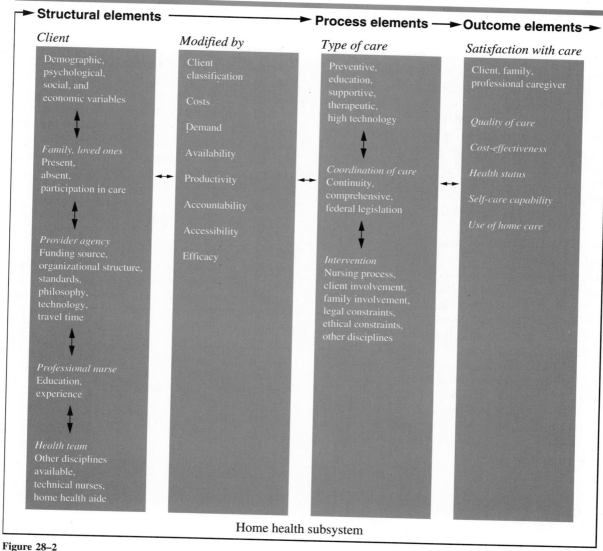

Figure 28–2
Albrecht nursing model for home health care. (Based on Albrecht MN. The Albrecht model for home health care: Implications for research, practice and education. Public Health Nurs. 7:118–126, 1990. Reprinted by permission of Blackwell Scientific Publications, Inc.)

The process elements include three components: type of care, coordination of care, and intervention.

Outcome elements consist of patient and family satisfaction with care, quality of care, cost effectiveness of care, health status, and self-care capability.

In the Albrecht model for home care, the relationship between the structural elements and the process elements directs the interventions that are implemented. The nurse executes the nursing process, including assessment, nursing diagnosis, planning, intervention, and evaluation and then coordinates patient care (Albrecht, 1990).

DOCUMENTATION OF HOME CARE

Assessment data and interventions are documented for all home visits. The nursing care plan is also documented in the patient record.

Ask any home health nurse to describe the most frustrating part of providing home health care, and the answer will probably revolve around documentation issues. Because of the prominent position that Medicare holds as a payer of home health care, the regulations set forth by the Health Care Financing Administration determine the home health industry's documentation. Correct and accurate completion of required Medicare forms is the key to reimbursement. Payment or denial for visits made is based on the information that is presented on the forms. If the nurse does not clearly document in the nursing notes the skilled care that is provided, the fiscal intermediaries will argue that the care was either not necessary or not done, and reimbursement will be denied. The home health nurse must have an excellent clinical foundation and the ability to identify and document actual and potential patient problems that require skilled nursing interventions (Morrissey-Ross, 1988).

No less important than documentation for reimbursement purposes is documentation of the care provided to record the quality of care received by the patient. The documentation of the home visit serves as record of the nurse's observations, assessment of the patient's condition, interventions provided, and the ability of the patient and family to manage the care at home. In addition, documentation of patient visits serves as a formal communication system among other home health professionals who also have interactions with the patient and family.

THE FAMILY OR CAREGIVER IN HOME CARE

The presence or absence of an involved family member or caregiver can make the difference between the successful completion of the plan of treatment, with the patient remaining in the home, and the need to transfer the patient to an extended-care facility or board-and-care facility. When a capable family member or caregiver is available to assist the patient, the home health nurse spends much of the visit time assessing the skills of the caregiver. The care provider is instructed by the home health nurse in the correct procedures for providing care and in recognizing the signs and symptoms of problems that are to be reported to the health care provider. The goal of the home health nurse's instruction is to provide the caregiver with the skills necessary to care for the patient successfully in the home without intervention of the nurse or other members of the home health team.

Patients who lack a family member or caregiver capable of learning the necessary care and providing the care present a special challenge for the home health nurse. When the patient lives alone and does not have caregivers, the nurse explores other resources available to supplement the patient's self-care activities in the home, such as a hired attendant for the patient with extensive physical care needs and financial resources to pay for the attendant. Medicare and private insurance companies do not pay for attendant care. If the patient's income is low enough, in-home support services through the county may be an option. Other services that the nurse considers for the patient includes Meals on Wheels. Friendly Visitors is a service in which a volunteer goes to the patient's home once a week or more often to provide socialization for the patient. Other options that are available in some communities include adult day health centers or senior service centers. Both of these options require arrangement for transportation of the patient to and from the centers. A variety of transportation methods are available in different communities, ranging from volunteers transporting patients to public transportation systems, such as minivans that provide door-to-door service. Types of services selected and referrals made are based on the individual needs of the patient and on the patient's level of functional ability.

HOSPICE HOME CARE

The goal of home care for the terminally ill is to keep the client comfortable at home as long as possible and to provide support and instruction to caregivers. When the patient has been determined to be terminally ill, the focus is no longer on cure but rather on comfort care. Some patients insist on staying home until they die; others leave that decision to their caregivers. Each family unit has different needs, and each must be supported in their decisions. In no case should home death be used as the standard by which excellence is determined, nor should home death be viewed as the ultimate measure of "successful" home care. It is vital to realize that caring for a terminally ill person includes caring for the family or caregivers and that not all caregivers want their loved one to die at home or are capable of having that occur. The goal of home death must be the goal of the patient and family, regardless of the personal preference of the nurse.

When caring for a terminally ill person at home, the hospice nurse must be skilled in physical and psychosocial care for both the patient and the caregiver. The patient is viewed as a whole person, not as an isolated disease. Caring for a terminally ill person at home demands that the family system be viewed as a unit.

Caring for the Caregiver

Although the dying patient is the focus of all skilled nursing care, the experienced home care nurse knows that a careful assessment of the caregiver's mental and physical health is important. The spouse, lover, children, friends, and neighbors who have made the commitment to stay until the end need the nurse's time and attention as much as, if not more than, the patient. Although the wishes of the patient are important, all decisions regarding care are made with the health of the caregivers in mind. Caregivers need constant nurturing and praise for doing a terrific job. They cannot hear too often the words "You're a great nurse to . . . " or "You're doing a wonderful job of taking care of . . . "

Gaynor found that women with longer caregiving experience had more physical health problems than did those with less time caregiving, and that younger women found caregiving more psychologically burdensome that did older women. Nursing interventions must be directed toward preventing a decline in the caregiver's health and the development of a second patient who herself needs a caregiver.

From Gaynor SE: The long haul: The effects of home care on caregivers. Image J Nurs Sch 22:208–212, 1990.

Caregivers need reassurance that their judgment is sound and need to be reminded that they cannot do anything "wrong" if it is done for the patient's comfort. The caregivers need to know that they will not mistakenly overdose the patient and must repeatedly be reminded that the patient will not die because of something they did or did not do. Caring for the terminally ill requires that the home care nurse be willing to nurse the entire family.

PAIN CONTROL AND SYMPTOM MANAGEMENT

British hospice methods of pain control were introduced into the U.S. health care system about 20 years ago. They advocated avoidance of peaks and valleys in comfort by building a wall against the pain. In hospice nursing, pain medication is given in doses sufficient to keep the patient pain free and is given on a regular schedule to prevent pain from recurring before the next dose is given. Hospice methods of pain control are particularly well suited to home care. The vast majority of patients can be pain free until their deaths. The key to successful pain control for the terminally ill is to convince patients to take their medications on a regular basis, not just when they "cannot stand it any longer." By building up a wall against the pain, the patient need never hurt and never wait for relief. The nurse explains to patients that most pain medicines last about 4½ to 5 hours before completely wearing off. Patients are instructed to take their pain medication every 4 hours on a 24-hour basis to ensure a "margin of safety" so the medicine will not wear off before the next dose is due.

Pain is subjective and is whatever the patient says it is. Only the patient experiences the pain, and only the patient can judge the severity of the pain. To assist the patient in evaluation of the pain, an audiovisual aid, such as the Pain Assessment Ruler distributed by Roxane Laboratories (Fig. 28–3), can be used. This pain assessment tool allows the patient to indicate a color that best describes the pain; 0 is white and indicates no pain; 1 is light blue and indicates mild pain (e.g., annoying, nagging); 2 is yellow and indicates discomforting (e.g., troublesome, nauseating, grueling, numbing); 3 is apricot and indicates distressing (e.g., miserable, agonizing, gnawing); 4 is orange and indicates intense (e.g., dreadful, horrible, vicious, cramping); and 5 is red and indicates excruciating (e.g., unbearable, torturing, crushing, tearing). Because this pain assessment scale uses both colors and words, it is appropriate for use with patients who cannot read.

USE OF MORPHINE

Many patients, especially the elderly, are afraid of becoming "junkies" or "druggies" and want to delay using morphine "until I get really bad." Many believe that morphine signals "the end of the line" and are amazed to learn that patients do well while receiving this drug for months, even years, before death occurs. Almost every family will need to be taught that addiction is not the same as tolerance and that their physicians will not "cut off their supply if they take too much."

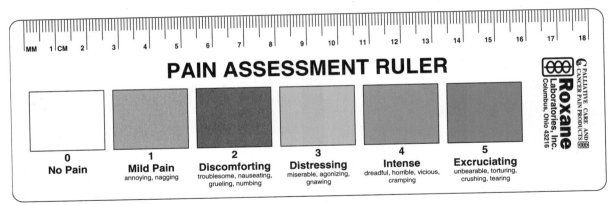

Figure 28–3
Pain assessment ruler. (Reproduced with permission from Roxane Laboratories, Columbus, Ohio.)

APPLICATION OF THE NURSING PROCESS THROUGH HOME VISITS

Four case studies are presented. Two public health visits (one a communicable disease follow-up and one involving an antepartum client), one home health care visit, a posthospitalization follow-up, and one hospice patient are monitored through case studies.

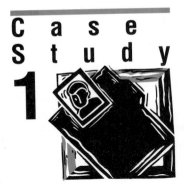

Public Health Visit: Communicable Disease Follow-up

The public health nurse receives a referral from the county hospital to see Ray, a 57-year-old white man who was recently diagnosed with tuberculosis. The first purpose of the referral to the public health nurse is to meet with the client to ensure that he received the appropriate information about tuberculosis and is followed for medical care on a regular basis. The second purpose of the referral is for the public health nurse to meet with Ray and identify people with whom he has been in close contact. The nurse then establishes contact with these people, notifies them that they have been exposed to tuberculosis, and encourages them to have follow-up tests for tuberculosis from health care providers.

The nurse contacts Ray and establishes a time for the home visit. The nurse notes that he resides in a residential hotel in a lower-middle-class neighborhood of a large urban area. During the initial visit, the nurse discovers that the client is an unemployed construction worker. He has no knowledge of where he might have contracted tuberculosis. Ray assures the nurse that he is taking his medication as directed. He gives the nurse the names of his friends with whom he plays poker every week at a hotel and tells the nurse that he has told these friends to be tested for tuberculosis. The nurse makes a note of the names and later talks with them individually by telephone. During these subsequent conversations, the nurse is very careful to maintain the client's confidentiality. The nurse informs these individuals that they may have been exposed to tuberculosis and of the importance of testing by either their health care providers or their local health department.

Ray indicates to the nurse that he has no family, and, other than his friends at the hotel, he has minimal contact with other people. The nurse records this information onto the communicable disease form and returns the information to the public health department's communicable disease division.

Assessment

Assessment by the public health nurse of the client with a communicable disease involves the individual, family, and community.

Individual The public health nurse assesses whether the client receives appropriate information and regular medical care for tuberculosis and whether the client follows the prescribed treatment regimen.

Family Although Ray states that he has no family, his friends in the hotel constitute a working support network. The public health nurse is familiar with kinship networks and with their importance as alternative family systems (Stack, 1974). Nursing assessment of Ray's kinship network involves determining whether the members have been tested for tuberculosis. In addition, the public health nurse assesses the client's network for the following:

- Network composition
- Network's knowledge of tuberculosis
- Functional capacity
- Network stressors
- Network strengths and weaknesses
- Network's ability to provide support for Ray
- Health beliefs and practices
- Use of health services

Community The public health nurse is aware that the number of new cases of tuberculosis in the community has increased over the past 12 months. The public health nurse further notes that there has been an increase in the number of area residents immigrating from various third world countries and that this population may be at increased risk for the development of tuberculosis (Dowling, 1991).

Diagnosis

Individual The public health nurse determines that Ray has a knowledge deficit regarding the disease process and transmission of tuberculosis.

Family Ray's support network demonstrates knowledge deficits related to the disease process and transmission of tuberculosis, location of communicable disease clinics, and the importance of screening for persons exposed to tuberculosis.

Community The public health nurse, in conjunction with case workers at the communicable disease clinic, formulates the following diagnosis for Ray's community: increased risk for development of tuberculosis among community residents, as evidenced by increased incidence of new cases of tuberculosis over the past 12 months.

Planning and Goals

Individual
Short-Term Goal
- Client will verbalize knowledge of transmission of tuberculosis; signs and symptoms of complications of tuberculosis; purpose, administration schedule, and side effects of medications.

Long-Term Goal

- Client will perform self-care activities related to treatment of tuberculosis and follow-up as necessary with appropriate health care professionals.

Family
Short-Term Goal

- Support network members will demonstrate basic knowledge of cause and transmission of tuberculosis and will agree to be tested for tuberculosis.

Long-Term Goal

- Support network members with positive test results will receive appropriate treatment.

Community
Short-Term Goal

- Community members will demonstrate knowledge of increased incidence of tuberculosis in their community and of available community resources for treatment and prevention of tuberculosis.

Long-Term Goal

- Incidence of tuberculosis in the community will decrease over the next 3 years.

Intervention

Implementation of the plan of care for the client with tuberculosis occurs at the individual, family, and community levels.

Individual The public health nurse refers Ray to the communicable disease clinic of the local health department. Because tuberculosis is a reportable communicable disease, the public health nurse obtains information from the client regarding persons with whom he has been in close contact.

Family The public health nurse contacts members of Ray's support network and refers them to the communicable disease clinic as appropriate. The nurse provides these persons with information concerning transmission of tuberculosis and of the importance of early treatment and follow-up.

Community The public health nurse meets with professionals from the communicable disease clinic and from the health department and with members of the community to establish a program to raise public awareness regarding the increased incidence of tuberculosis in the community. The public will be informed of the importance of preventive measures, of the availability of community screening services for tuberculosis, and of existing health care resources in the community.

Evaluation

The client's and support network's knowledge of the disease process, transmission, treatment, and signs and symptoms of tuberculosis are indicators used in evaluating the plan of care. Confirmation of follow-up with the communicable disease clinic by the client and members of his support network can also be used for evaluation.

The incidence rate of tuberculosis in the community and the rate of use of tuberculosis clinics and related resources are measures that can be used to evaluate the effectiveness of interventions at the aggregate level.

Levels of Prevention

Primary prevention of communicable disease is directed to prevention of the occurrence of specific diseases such as tuberculosis. Programs that increase public awareness of the disease process and of the transmission, diagnosis, and treatment of tuberculosis constitute primary prevention activities. The goal of secondary prevention is early detection of existing conditions. Tuberculin skin testing and subsequent follow-up of positive test results are important secondary prevention measures. The tertiary level of prevention is aimed at reducing the effects and spread of tuberculosis. Referral for early, effective treatment and education of clients for self-care are important measures of tertiary prevention.

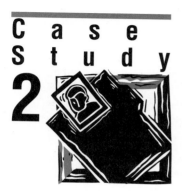

Case Study 2

Public Health Home Visit

Antepartum Client The public health nurse receives a referral to see a 17-year-old African-American girl, Ali, who is referred by the county prenatal clinic. Ali is 5 months pregnant with her third pregnancy within the past year. Ali miscarried the previous two pregnancies during the first trimester.

When the nurse makes the home visit, she notes Ali to be 5 feet 9 inches tall and weighing 120 pounds. She resides in a two-room apartment with her boyfriend, who is the father of the baby. The nurse begins the first visit with social talk, asking Ali general questions about her employment, education, and duration of her residence in the area. Ali appears to be pleased that the nurse is interested in her. Once a trusting relationship is initiated, the nurse asks Ali how she feels about the pregnancy. Ali reveals that she is happy about the pregnancy but is worried that there will be problems because of her two previous miscarriages. She had not planned any of the pregnancies but did not use contraceptives to prevent the pregnancies. Ali's boyfriend works and is able to pay the rent and buy food for her. Ali dropped out of high school during her junior year but would like to complete her high school education. She has Medicaid coverage for her health care.

During the initial home visit, the nurse assesses that Ali is underweight and that she has several knowledge deficits in the areas of prenatal nutrition, infant care, breast-feeding, and contraception. The nurse also identifies the need for a referral to the public school for continuation of Ali's high school education. The nurse briefly discusses her assessment with Ali in a non-threatening, nonjudgmental manner. The nurse informs Ali that if she is interested, she can schedule future home visits to provide Ali with more information and to answer Ali's questions. Ali agrees to future visits to discuss the topics that have been identified by the nurse during the assessment phase. The plan for future visits is mutually agreed on. As the visits progress, the nurse and Ali modify the plan based on evaluation of progress.

The nurse terminates home visits with Ali when the mutually established goals are achieved. The nurse schedules a postpartum visit with Ali after the baby is born to assess the infant care provided and to answer any questions that Ali has concerning infant care.

Assessment

Although it is important to perform an individual assessment of Ali, the public health nurse assesses Ali as a member of a family and as a member of the community. "Community" in this case refers to the aggregate of publicly insured adolescent pregnant women.

Individual Assessment of Ali reveals an underweight 17-year-old pregnant girl who is unable to demonstrate knowledge of nutrition in pregnancy, infant care, breast-feeding, contraception, and educational options for pregnant teenagers.

Family An individual assessment of Ali mandates the need for an assessment of the composition and function of Ali's family. The public health nurse will assess the following factors with regard to Ali's family (Logan, 1986):

- Family composition
- General support network
- Family and network patterns related to psychosocial and economic support of Ali
- Family and network attitude toward health
- Family and network beliefs regarding use of health-related services
- Beliefs and attitudes of family and network regarding infant care, breast-feeding, and nutrition
- Attitudes of infant's father regarding involvement with Ali and their baby, health beliefs, ability to assume role of parent, and knowledge of pregnancy and birth

Community The public health nurse is aware of the need to see the larger, aggregate picture. Identifying the aggregate as the pregnant adolescent community, the public health nurse uses the following techniques in an ongoing assessment (Bayne, 1985):

- Observations
- Resource analysis
- Key informant interviews
- Environmental indexes

Using the techniques, the public health nurse gathers information regarding the following:

- Educational and employment options for pregnant teens and teens with infants
- Availability of health services targeting low-birth-weight infants
- Availability of support groups for this aggregate
- Availability of teen parenting classes

Diagnosis

The public health nurse formulates nursing diagnoses based on thorough individual, family, and community assessments.

Individual The following individual nursing diagnoses were formulated for Ali:

- Knowledge deficit regarding nutrition in pregnancy, infant care and feeding, contraception, availability of community resources, and educational options for pregnant teenagers.
- Inadequate nutrition related to low-income status and inadequate knowledge of nutritional requirements of pregnancy.

Family The public health nurse formulated the following diagnosis for Ali and her family:

- Lack of family support related to Ali living away from home.
- Altered family communication patterns related to role confusion among family members.

Community The public health nurse formulated the following diagnoses for the pregnant adolescent community:

- Minimal availability of health care services, parenting classes, contraception counseling, and educational opportunities for pregnant teenagers.
- Lack of coordination of existing services.

Planning
Planning health services and interventions for pregnant teenagers involves formulation of short-term and long-term goals for the individual, family, and community.

Individual
Short-Term Goals
- Ali will gain at least 3 pounds per month (Olds et al, 1980).
- Ali will demonstrate knowledge of community resources for pregnant adolescents by next nursing visit.

Long-Term Goal
- Ali will carry her infant to term without evidence of maternal or fetal complications.

Family
Short-Term Goal
- Ali and her partner will attend teen parenting classes.

Long-Term Goal
- Ali, her partner, and other family members will be able to perform mutually determined role responsibilities.

Community
Short-Term Goals
- Increased community awareness of resources for pregnant teenagers.
- Increased awareness of contraception counseling services for adolescents.

Long-Term Goals
- Establishment of effective, comprehensive prenatal health, contraception, and education services for pregnant teenagers.
- Decline in rate of teen pregnancies and birth of compromised neonates over next 24 months.

Intervention

Implementation of the individual plan of care for Ali involves visits by the public health nurse with referral to existing prenatal services for pregnant teenagers. Family intervention is composed of referral of Ali and the infant's father to a support group for pregnant teenagers and partners. Implementation of the plan of care for the aggregate of adolescent pregnant women includes the following:

- Meeting with community leaders
- Meeting with local school administrators and faculty to disseminate information for pregnant teenagers
- Formation of community organizing groups (Bayne, 1985)

Evaluation

Evaluation includes measures of nutritional status of individual teenagers and of the use of support groups and educational and nutritional services by teenagers and their families. Evaluation of the effectiveness of interventions at the aggregate level focuses on measurement of availability of options for pregnant teenagers, measures of teen awareness and use of services, and determination of changes in incidence rates of teen pregnancy and compromised neonates.

Levels of Prevention

Prevention of teenage pregnancy involves interventions at primary, secondary, and tertiary levels. At the primary level, prevention is composed of activities that prevent teen pregnancy from occurring. The secondary level of prevention involves interventions for early detection of teen pregnancy and early intervention such as counseling for prenatal care. The goal of prevention at the tertiary level is to reduce the effects of adolescent pregnancy. Examples of tertiary prevention for pregnant teenagers include provision of prenatal education in areas such as nutrition, parenting, and infant care.

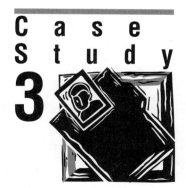

Case Study 3

Home Health Visit

Susan Brown is a 40-year-old woman who was the driver in a single-car, roll-over accident 9 days ago. She was air-lifted to a trauma center and treated for multiple lacerations and abrasions, including a severe laceration to the left inner aspect of her arm. The referral for home health services made by the hospital at the time of discharge requested daily wound care to the infected left arm laceration by the home health nurse. Specific medical orders for wound care consist of removal of the arm brace, followed by wet-to-dry dressing changes using one-fourth strength Dakin's solution, wrapping the arm with gauze, and reapplication of the brace. Medications included one or two Vicodin tablets every 6 hours, as needed for pain, and 500 mg Keflex four times a day.

During the initial visit, the home health nurse identifies from data collected during the assessment four primary problems:

- The infected left arm laceration with large amounts of drainage related to introduction of bacteria

- Severe arm pain related to the injury
- Knowledge deficit related to inadequate understanding of self-administration of antibiotic
- Anxiety related to family communication problems

These problems are the basis of the nursing care plan for Susan (Carpenito, 1990; Sparks and Taylor, 1991).

Diagnosis

The patient had an infected left arm laceration related to introduction of bacteria secondary to wound, which was secondary to a motor vehicle accident.

Short-Term Goals
- Keep laceration clean and debride wound through daily wet-to-dry dressing changes
- Encourage self-care in dressing changes

Long-Term Goals
- Healed laceration without drainage or infection
- Full range of motion of the affected arm

Intervention

Because Ms. Brown has a moderate-to-large amount of yellow drainage from the laceration on her left arm, dressing changes are initiated, with additional dressings applied to contain the drainage. When the large amount of drainage persists for more than 3 days after initiation of the antibiotic therapy and the patient continues to have low-grade fevers (temperature, 99.2–99.8°F), the home health nurse notifies the physician, and a culture and sensitivity of the drainage are taken. An alternate antibiotic is prescribed based on the culture results. Ms. Brown and her mother are instructed to change the dressing, and they are supervised by the nurse.

Diagnosis

Pain related to arm injury

Short-Term Goal
- Pain control through medication and relaxation techniques

Long-Term Goal
- Pain free when arm injury is healed

Intervention

The assessment of Susan's arm pain includes a history of when the pain is most severe and the frequency of pain administration. The home health nurse assesses that the pain is most severe at night and recommends that Susan take two Vicodin tablets before going to bed and that she place her left arm in a position of comfort, supported by pillows to decrease edema. The nurse instructs Susan to lie down, rest, and listen to relaxing music during the day when the pain is intense to decrease the amount of arm pain through relaxation.

Diagnosis

Knowledge deficit related to inadequate understanding of self-administration of antibiotic

Short-Term Goal
* Correct self-administration of antibiotic

Long-Term Goal
* Infection resolved

Intervention

When the home health nurse asks Ms. Brown when she takes the Keflex, she explains that because the drug is prescribed to be taken four times a day, she takes the medication at 9:00 AM, 1:00 PM, 5:00 PM, and 9:00 PM. The nurse explains the purpose of the antibiotic and the importance of taking it every 6 hours to maintain an optimum blood level. Ms. Brown and the nurse agree on a schedule of 6:00 AM, 12:00 noon, 6:00 PM, and bedtime.

Diagnosis

Anxiety related to family communication problems

Short-Term Goal
* Decreased anxiety through verbalization of feelings

Long-Term Goal
* Anxiety resolved or controlled

Intervention

Ms. Brown's sister arrived from out of state to assist with her care after the accident. Within 3 days of her arrival, Ms. Brown's husband and sister got into an argument, and the sister left abruptly and returned home. This altercation is very upsetting to Ms. Brown, who is distraught over the communication problems between her husband and sister. The home health nurse encourages Ms. Brown to talk about her feelings concerning the dysfunctional relationship of her husband and sister and to discuss how she will address the situation with both her husband and her sister. The nurse stresses that the problem is between the husband and sister, and not with Ms. Brown, and that Ms. Brown should not feel guilty or responsible for the disagreement.

Ms. Brown has a large, supportive family, and a caregiver is available to assist her every day. Transportation to and from the physician's appointments is coordinated by her family and does not require the intervention of the nurse. The nurse remains involved with Ms. Brown until the infection is resolved, and the family is taught to provide the necessary wound care.

Referrals

Ms. Brown is referred for follow-up by her internist and orthopedist. She is also referred for a gynecological appointment for evaluation of sudden onset of slight vaginal bleeding.

Ms. Brown's sister returned to her home, and no further confrontations occurred. The nurse suggests counseling for Ms. Brown if the hostile relationship persists between her husband and sister or continues to cause Ms. Brown anxiety.

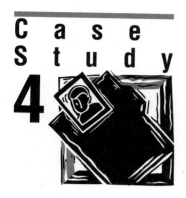

Hospice Home Visit

Ed McMillan is 64 years old and is dying of prostate cancer. He experiences urinary retention, chronic pain, weakness, constipation, and anorexia. He knows he does not have long to live, but he wants to go home to die and to be able to attend his youngest son's wedding in a nearby town.

Working together with Mr. McMillan and his wife, the hospice nurse identifies four nursing diagnoses. Because of the patient's prognosis, only short-term goals are identified.

Diagnosis

• Urinary retention related to obstruction by the tumor

   Short-Term Goal
• Urinary drainage through a Foley catheter

Intervention

The nurse inserts an indwelling urinary catheter to alleviate urinary retention. The nurse instructs Mr. McMillan's family in catheter care and the signs and symptoms of urinary tract infection to report to the nurse or physician.

Diagnosis

Pain related to cancer

   Short-Term Goal
• Pain control

Intervention

Oral morphine sulfate (80 mg every 4 hours around the clock) for pain.

Diagnosis

Mobility impairment related to weakness from cancer

   Short-Term Goal
• Maximum mobility

Intervention

The nurse orders a walker and wheelchair to maximize Ed's mobility and instructs the family in proper use of the equipment.

Diagnosis

Constipation related to morphine sulfate ingestion

   Short-Term Goal
• Regular bowel movements

Intervention

To prevent constipation, the nurse initiates a daily bowel regimen that includes monitoring fluid intake, introduction of a stool softener, and a laxative as needed.

The nurse requests that Mr. McMillan's physician order small doses of prednisone to temporarily improve the patient's poor appetite. The hospice nurse also does a great deal of teaching.

The nurse instructs the family that it is common to lose one's appetite in advanced cancer. Despite the constant reassurance, Mrs. McMillan continues to do her best to feed her husband regularly, believing that "If only he'd eat, he'd get his strength back." The nurse continues her advocacy for Mr. McMillan by praising his wife for her loving care but repeating that it is normal for a patient with cancer to have a poor appetite. Because of the nurse's interventions, the patient is pain free, and his bowels move easily and regularly. With a leg bag instead of the usual catheter bag and the wheelchair for transportation, Mr. McMillan is able to attend his son's wedding.

When Mr. McMillan becomes too weak to stand, his hospice nurse has an electric hospital bed set up in his home. The bed is strategically placed in the den, the center of family activity, and a home health aide comes to bathe him every other day. As his level of consciousness declines, the nurse helps his family keep him pain free by requesting morphine sulfate in rectal suppository form. When the patient's lungs begin to fill with fluid, the nurse suggests oxygen via nasal cannula and transdermal scopolamine patches to lessen his shortness of breath and decrease his secretions. The nurse visits daily while Ed is comatose to determine whether the family is coping adequately and to offer suggestions as small problems arise. The hospice nurse suggests that Mrs. McMillan's children help make funeral arrangements and get financial affairs in order before Mr. McMillan dies.

Mr. McMillan dies peacefully in his own home, surrounded by his wife, children, and many grandchildren. As was his wish, his corneas are donated for transplantation, and a memorial service is held in which family, friends, and former colleagues participate. Mr. McMillan's ashes are scattered at their weekend home in the mountains. After the initial bustle subsides, the hospice nurse makes a follow-up bereavement visit.

Hospice nurses who care for the terminally ill practice truly professional nursing. As case manager, the nurse draws on the expertise of the interdisciplinary team to obtain what the patient and family need at a most vulnerable time. Hospice nurses are pivotal when caring for the dying because they are practical, knowledgeable, flexible, and family centered. Nurses have a long history of speaking for those who cannot speak for themselves. In patients' homes, nurses advocate for the terminally ill by offering unique skills in pain and symptom management and by sharing their hearts as well as their hands.

SUMMARY

This chapter presented information on performing public health, home health, and hospice nursing visits to clients in their homes. A general overview of the nursing process for clients in the home setting was presented and then expanded to include the individual, family, and community. Case studies involving communicable disease, teen pregnancy, traumatic injury, and terminal cancer were presented. The home visit, the foundation of community health nursing, provides the forum for important interventions, not only with individuals and families but also with communities.

The community health nurse has the responsibility to bring the concerns of individuals and families with whom she visits into the community.

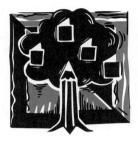

L e a r n i n g
A c t i v i t i e s

1. Make arrangement to accompany both a public health nurse, a home health nurse, and a hospice nurse on home visits.

2. Interview a public health nurse about the types of client referrals received and ask what interventions are usually performed. Repeat this activity with a home health nurse and a hospice nurse. Ask the nurses what they like best about their jobs.

3. Contact a local home health agency and interview the agency director. Ask what type of agency it is, the profit status, and whether it is Medicare certified. Report your findings to your classmates.

4. Attend a team meeting in a home health agency or a hospice program to see how the roles of the various team members blend together to provide family-centered care.

5. Interview a public health nurse and home health nurse and ask how the community impacts on the care they provide.

REFERENCES

Albrecht MN: The Albrecht nursing model for home health care: Implications for research, practice, and education. Public Health Nurs 7:118–126, 1990.

Albrecht MN: Home health care: reliability and validity testing of a patient-classification instrument. Public Health Nurs 8:124–131, 1991.

Albrecht MN: Research priorities for home health nursing. Nurs Health Care 13:538–541, 1992.

American Nurses Association: Standards of Home Health Nursing Practice: Kansas City, MO: American Nurses Association, 1986.

Bayne T: The pregnant school-age community. *In* Higgs AR, Gustafson DD, eds. Community as Client: Assessment and Diagnosis. Philadelphia: FA Davis, 1985, pp. 129–134.

Byrd ME: A concept analysis of home visiting. Public Health Nurs 12:83–89, 1995.

Carpenito LJ: Nursing Care Plans and Documentation. Philadelphia: JB Lippincott, 1990.

Dowling PT: Return of tuberculosis: Screening and preventive therapy. Am Fam Physician 43:457–476, 1991.

Feldman R: Meeting the educational needs of home health care nurses. J Home Health Care Prac 5:12–19, 1993.

Guterman S, Dobson A: Impact of the Medicare prospective payment system for hospitals. Health Care Fin Rev 7:97–114, 1986.

Harrington C: Quality, access, and costs: Public policy and home health care. Nurs Outlook 36:164–166, 1988.

Health Care Financing Review: National health expenditures, 1988. Health Care Fin Rev 11:1–41, 1988.

Kalisch PA, Kalisch BJ: The Advance of American Nursing, 2nd ed. Boston: Little, Brown, 1986.

Keating SB, Kelman GB: Home Health Care Nursing: Concepts and Practice. Philadelphia: JB Lippincott, 1988.

Kelly L: Dimensions of Professional Nursing. New York: Pergamon Press, 1991.

Kent V, Hanley B: Home health care. Nurs Health Care 11:234–240, 1990.

Logan BB: Adolescent pregnancy. *In* Logan BB, Dawkins CE, eds. Family-Centered Nursing in the Community. Menlo-Park, CA: Addison-Wesley, 1986, pp. 635–667.

Morrissey-Ross M: Documentation: If you haven't written it, you haven't done it. Nurs Clin North Am 23:363–371, 1988.

Olds SB, London ML, Ladewig PA, Davidson SV: Obstetric Nursing. Menlo Park, CA: Addison-Wesley, 1980.

Sparks SM, Taylor CM: Nursing Diagnosis Reference Manual. Springhouse, PA: Springhouse Corporation, 1991.

Spradley BW: Community Health Nursing: Concepts and Practice, 3rd ed. Glenview, IL: Scott, Foresman/Little, Brown, 1990.

Stack C: All Our Kin. New York: Harper & Row, 1974.

Stuart-Siddall S: Home Health Care Nursing: Administrative and Clinical Perspectives. Chico, CA: Aspen, 1986.

U.S. Department of Commerce/International Trade Administration: U.S. Industrial Outlook. Washington, DC: U.S. Government Printing Office, 1990.

Warhola C: Planning for Home Health Services: A Resource Handbook (DHHS Publication No. [HRA] 80-14017). Washington, DC: U.S. Public Health Service, Department of Health and Human Services, 1980.

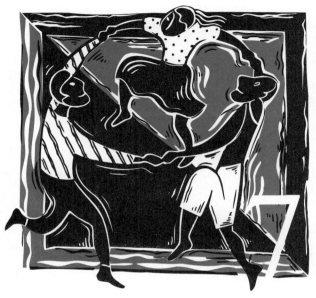

The Future of Community Health Nursing

World Health

Introduction by Karen A. Swanson

Upon completion of this chapter, the reader will be able to:

1. Identify three forces that threaten life and health worldwide.

2. Compare and contrast Cuba's and Canada's approaches to the delivery of primary health care.

3. Describe Canada's model of population-focused nursing.

Health, our most valuable possession, is a primary concern in every society, and nurses, as health care providers, are becoming aware of their responsibility to help ensure the valuable possession of health in persons of all societies. To carry out this responsibility, community health nurses must be aware of forces that threaten health and study models of health care delivery in other countries that may promote the well-being of the greatest number of people.

This chapter highlights selected health problems and challenges that health care professionals and citizens face and share. Then two models of population-focused health care delivery by nurses in Cuba and Canada are presented. These models can serve as an inspiration to community health nurses as they endeavor to ensure the health of all persons in their communities.

Among the many health issues that merit attention and study because of their global effects and threat to human life are population growth, environmental stressors, and patterns of disease.

POPULATION GROWTH

In any society, large populations create pressure. For example, in developing countries, feeding a population may become problematic if famine or problems with international trade occur. Malnutrition, disease, or death may be the outcome. Pressures from population growth are also felt in industrialized nations. Although food may be plentiful, overcrowding may lead to pollution, stress, and violence.

World population growth is often overlooked as a health-related problem, yet current rapid growth presents a threat to the health and economies of many nations. The exponential nature of world population growth is evident in information from the World Health Organization (WHO) (1990) (Fig. 29–1). In 1800, after 2 to 5 billion years of human existence, the world population was only about 1 billion people. In the next 130 years, from 1800 to 1927, it grew to 2 billion, and in only 33 more years, from 1927 to 1960, it reached 3 billion. In less than half of that time, the 14 years from 1960 to 1974, the fourth billion was added, and astonishingly, it took only the 13 years from 1974 to 1987 to add the fifth billion. Furthermore, WHO estimates that by 1998 the world population will grow to 6 billion; by 2005, to 7 billion; and by 2015, to 8 billion.

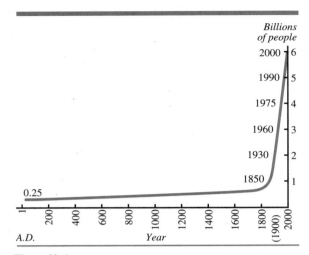

Figure 29–1
The J-shaped curve of world population growth. (Redrawn from Environmental Science: An Introduction by G. Tyler Miller, Jr. © 1986 by Wadsworth, Inc., Belmont, California.)

In 1987, when the world population reached 5 billion, distribution was uneven; 52% of the population lived in only five countries: China, India, the former Soviet Union, the United States, and Indonesia. Thirty-three percent of the world's population were children, and 6% were elderly (age 65 or older) (WHO, 1990).

Between 1985 and 1990, the world population grew by 87 million per year, with distribution remaining uneven; 81 million lived in developing countries and approximately 6 million lived in developed countries (WHO, 1990). During the same period, 50 million people died each year; 39 million in developing countries and 11 million in developed countries (WHO, 1990). Life expectancies were 73.4 years in developed countries and only 59.7 years in developing countries. Malcolm Potts, a world-renown population theorist, predicted that "by the 21st century the world may end up divided not into political or economic groups but by demographic structure," where countries will be classified into slow-growth versus fast-growth countries instead of rich or poor countries. This, however, will eventually further the rich and poor division (Potts, 1994).

As the world's population grows, there is a rising global trend toward urbanization; people live closer together and migrate to urban areas for employment. In 1975, for example, 38.5% of the world's population lived in urban areas. By 1994, the proportion of urban dwellers swelled to just under 45%, and this proportion is expected to reach 50% by 2015 (United Nations Population Fund, 1995). With increasingly dense living arrangements, the health of the general population is threatened by environmental stressors and disease.

ENVIRONMENTAL STRESSORS

An important component of both individual and world health is the relationship between humans and their environment.

Environmental stressors can be categorized into four types:

- Stressors that directly assault human health (e.g., lead poisoning, air pollution)
- Stressors that damage society's goods and services (e.g., air pollution's effects on buildings)
- Stressors that damage the quality of life (e.g., noise and litter)
- Stressors that interfere with ecological balance and other forms of life (e.g., global warming resulting from the build-up of greenhouse gases in the atmosphere) (Banister et al., 1988)

Air, water, and land pollution are among the consequences of environmental stressors. For example, the chemical pollutant carbon monoxide makes up 50% of the worldwide air pollution problem, and other primary pollutants, such as nitrogen monoxide, sulfur oxides, particulates, and hydrocarbons, combine with carbon monoxide to create 90% of pollution worldwide (Banister et al., 1988). One contributing factor to water pollution is that in 1990 only 70% of the urban population and 40% of the rural population in developing countries had sanitation facilities (World Bank, 1994).

Agricultural, industrial, residential, and commercial wastes increase land pollution. For example, chemical fertilizers have displaced natural fertilizers; synthetic pesticides have displaced natural means of pest control; and petrochemical products, such as detergents, synthetic fiber, and plastics, have replaced soap, cotton, and paper. Throw-away goods have replaced reusable goods, resulting in increased trash for disposal. Production technologies are contributing to worldwide environmental stress.

PATTERNS OF DISEASE

Because disease patterns vary throughout the world, primary causes of mortality differ in developed and developing countries. The disease profile of developed countries is one in which primary causes of mortality are cardiovascular disease, cancer, respiratory disease, stroke, violence, and accidents, whereas primary causes of mortality in developing countries are infections, malnutrition, and also violence. Through improved sanitation, nutrition, and medical care, developed countries, once plagued with high rates of infectious disease, have overcome high rates of deaths resulting from these diseases. These countries experience what is called an epidemiological transition, that is, when the morbidity and mortality profile of a country changes from one of an undeveloped country to one of a developed country. In other words, many developed countries have experienced an epidemiological transition from having an infectious disease profile to having a chronic disease profile and thus are now plagued by chronic diseases such as coronary heart disease, respiratory disease, and cancer (Banister et al., 1988).

Among the infectious diseases that contribute to high rates of mortality in developing countries are hepatitis B, rheumatic heart disease, hookworm infection, endemic malaria, and intestinal worms. These diseases claim the lives of millions, yet the World Bank (1993) estimated that these diseases could be reduced up to 40% through feasible interventions. In 1990, worldwide 2 million children died from measles, roughly 340,000 children died from whooping cough, poliomyelitis affected approximately 150,000 persons, and tuberculosis affected as many as 7.5 million persons (Clements et al., 1992; Dolin et al., 1994; Galazka, 1992; Hull and Ward, 1992).

Acquired immunodeficiency syndrome (AIDS) is one disease that is shared globally. Ten percent of the population of central Africa is estimated to be infected, and in early 1990 between 5 and 10 million persons worldwide were thought to be infected with human immunodeficiency virus (HIV) (WHO, 1990). The U.S. Surgeon General estimates that 100 million people worldwide could die from AIDS by 2000 (Mann et al., 1992).

Although AIDS is shared globally, it varies demographically in different parts of the world. For example, the estimated male-female ratio of HIV infections as of January 1, 1992 is 8:5 in North America, whereas in Africa the ratio is an even 1 (Mann, et al., 1992). Urbanization and intracounty migration also play a role in the spread of AIDS. In Rwanda, for instance, the HIV seroprevalence is more than 14 to 20 times higher in urban versus rural areas.

HIV could threaten more lives because migration to the world's largest cities is increasing. The United Nations estimates that by the year 2010 50% of the developing world will live in cities. This is up from only 25% in 1970.

Promoting health worldwide is humankind's greatest challenge. Several global agencies play important roles in improving the health in all nations, such as the WHO and the United Nations Children's Fund (UNICEF). The WHO was founded in 1948 and is an international health agency of the United Nations that consists of countries working toward the goal of "health for all by the year 2000," which was instituted at the Alma-Ata conference in 1978. This conference outlined primary health care as consisting of three developments: "universal availability of essential health care to individuals, families, and population groups according to need; involvement of communities in planning, delivery, and evaluation of such care; and an active role for other sectors in health activities" (Tarimo and Creese, 1990). This program seeks to obtain the highest level of health care for all people by promoting seven elements of primary health care, including health education on prevention and cures, proper food supply and nutrition, adequate supply of safe drinking water and sanitation, maternal and child health care, immunization, control of endemic diseases, and provisions of essential drugs. The WHO's statement of beliefs, goals, and objectives are further outlined in the Declaration of Alma-Ata in Appendix III. UNICEF too is an important global health organization. Founded in 1946, it works for the survival, development, and protection of children by developing and implementing community-based programs in social service, health, nutrition, education, water and sanitation, environment, and women in development.

When comparing health care systems, developed and developing countries can learn much from each other. Although transferring specialized medical technologies from developed to developing countries may not be appropriate, developing countries are currently learning from the health care reform policies of developed countries. Likewise, developed countries have much to learn about low-technology initiatives, such as oral rehydration solution for the treatment of diarrhea, and the delivery of primary health care as defined by WHO, including participatory approaches to health care delivery, such as community involvement in health and education. This exchange is important given the state of health care policy in developed countries today; many developed countries

have made health care inaccessible to portions of their general public. Even in countries with socialized medicine, medical costs increase annually, and citizens are faced with paying supplemental medical fees. In Great Britain, inequalities in health between the upper and lower classes are increasing despite their National Health Service (Townsend, 1990). In 1993, in the United States, expenditures for health care made up 13.6% of the gross domestic product, yet more than 40 million uninsured Americans younger than 65 cannot afford health care (National Center for Health Statistics, 1995). Because a market-based developed country such as the United States treats health care as a commodity to be bought and sold, it focuses on curative medicine because it creates more capital than does preventive medicine. Therefore, it could be said that market-based health care systems lead to a goal opposite that of health for all by the year 2000 (Fig. 29–2). The advent of managed care in the United States is a system that, theoretically, uses capitation to cut health care costs, including expensive institutionalization through an emphasis on health promotion and disease prevention in ambulatory care, called primary care in the United States. Managed care, however, offers neither universal access nor the comprehensive primary health care advocated by WHO, which differs from primary care or ambulatory services (see Barnes et al., 1995).

Given the two basic health care systems—market based and population based—and the fact that countries at different levels of development need to learn from one another, it is evident that no one model of health care delivery is appropriate for every country. The following account describes the health care system of one developing country that successfully implemented health care for all in the face of heavy economic sanctions. In 1985, Cuba was recognized for reaching the WHO goal of health for all (American Public Health Association, 1985). This country has proved to the world that health care does not have to

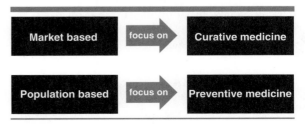

Figure 29–2
Health care approaches.

be a privilege but can be provided as a basic human right. This example is followed by a historical overview of Canada's success at establishing a universal health care system and a discussion of Canada's innovative models for community health nursing practice.

L e a r n i n g
A c t i v i t i e s

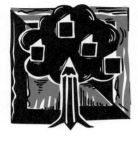

1. Discuss the advantages and disadvantages of limiting population growth.

2. Research and compare the incidence of AIDS and deaths from AIDS in Africa, Cuba, and Canada versus those in the United States. How do the incidence of AIDS and deaths from AIDS in Cuba and Canada compare with those in Africa and with those in the United States? What might account for the differences?

3. Compare population-focused nursing in Canada with community health nursing in your community. How are they the same, and how do they differ?

4. Research and compare the rates of life expectancy and infant mortality in Cuba and Canada versus those in the United States. What factors do you think might account for the similarities in rates between the developing (Cuba) and the developed (Canada, United States) countries?

5. Investigate the efforts made to immunize the population of your county. How do these differ from Cuba's efforts after the revolution?

REFERENCES

American Public Health Association: Edward Barsky Award presented to Sergio Del Valle, Cuban Minister of Health, at the Physician's Forum. Government Responsibility and the People's Health. Presented at the 113th annual meeting of the American Public Health Association, Washington DC, November 18, 1985.

Banister EW, Allen M, Fadl S, et al. Contemporary Health Issues. Boston: Jones and Bartlett, 1988.

Barnes D, Eribes C, Juarbe T, et al. Primary health care and primary care: A confusion of philosophies. Nurs Outlook *43:*7–16, 1995.

Clements C, Strassburg M, Cutts F, Torel C. The epidemiology of measles. World Health Stat *45:*285–291, 1992.

Dolin PJ, Raviglione MC, Kochi A. Global tuberculosis incidence and mortality during 1900-2000. Bull World Health Organ *72:*213–220, 1994.

Galazka A. Control of pertussis in the world. World Health Stat *45:*238–247, 1992.

Hull H, Ward N. Progress towards the global eradication of poliomyelitis. World Health Stat *45:*280–284, 1992.

Mann JM, Tarantola DJM, Netter TW. AIDS in the World. Cambridge, MA: Harvard University Press, 1992.

National Center for Health Statistics. Health United States, 1994. Washington DC: U.S. Government Printing Office, 1995.

Potts M. Common sense prevailing at population conference. Lancet *344:*809, 1994.

Tarimo E, Creese A, eds. Achieving Health for All By the Year 2000: Midway Reports of Country Experiences. Geneva: World Health Organization, 1990.

Townsend P. Widening inequalities of health in Britain: A rejoinder to Rudolph Klein. Int J Health Serv *20:*363–372, 1990.

United Nations Population Fund. The State of World Population 1995: Decisions for Development: Women, Empowerment and Reproductive Health. Oxford, England: New Internationalist Publications Ltd., 1995.

World Bank. World Development Report 1993: Investing in Health. Washington DC: Oxford University Press, 1993.

World Bank. World Development Report 1994: Infrastructure for Development. Washington DC: Oxford University Press, 1994.

World Health Organization. Global Estimates for Health Situation Assessment and Projections 1990. Geneva: World Health Organization, 1990.

Model 1: *Primary Care in Cuba: A Public Health Approach*
Karen A. Swanson • Janice M. Swanson • Ayesha E. Gill • Chris Walter

Cuba's primary health care model is presented. Unlike ambulatory care services, which are but one component of primary care, Cuba's model is a comprehensive public health approach that meets the World Health Organization's definition of primary care. The history of the development of Cuba's model is presented, including an update on the innovative neighborhood/home clinics. Achievements in health outcomes as a result of Cuba's model and the consequences for women's health care are discussed. Examples are presented of the effects on health care delivery of the economic hardship that Cuba has experienced since 1991 as a result of the loss of 85% of its trade with the former Soviet Union and the intensified U.S. embargo. A critique of Cuba's model concludes the article.*

Primary health care is commonly viewed as a way to close the gap between the health care needs of populations and health care delivery systems that are unable to meet those needs. The World Health Organization has declared primary health care as essential to the goal of "Health for All by the Year 2000" (Bryant, 1984). In Western countries that lack a national health system, such as the United States (Navarro, 1989), increased medical specialization and monetary compensation for specialists has resulted in fewer primary care physicians and difficulty in attracting medical students into primary care (Geiger, 1993). Implementing a national health system may not necessarily bring about equity in health, or Health for All, as espoused by the World Health Organization, however. For example, despite having established equal access to health services for its population, Great Britain has fallen short of achieving equity in health status, as class mortality gaps in treatable diseases persist (Susser, 1993). Cuba, on the other hand, is a small, Third World country that has not only provided primary health care in a broad sense to its population, but also achieved Health for All as defined by the World Health Organization.

In this article, we present an update on Cuba's primary health care delivery system. After specifying the World Health Organization's definition of primary health care, we describe the history of the development

of Cuba's primary health care model; provide an update on Cuba's neighborhood/home clinics; and review the achievements in health outcomes that have occurred as a result of Cuba's health care model, the consequences of the model for Cuban women's health, and the effects of Cuba's "special period" of economic hardship on the model. A critique of the model concludes the article. The information presented herein was obtained from interviews and observations made on our trips to Cuba in 1978, 1985, 1992, and 1994 and from correspondence with professionals living in Cuba. We interviewed nurses, physicians, public health officials, a director and residents of an AIDS sanitarium, herbalists, and representatives of community-based organizations. We visited schools; factories; pediatric, maternity, and psychiatric hospitals; a rural hospital; pharmacies; polyclinics; an AIDS sanitarium; and neighborhood/home clinics.

THE WORLD HEALTH ORGANIZATION'S DEFINITION OF PRIMARY HEALTH CARE

According to the World Health Organization, a primary health care system should provide the following for the entire population (Bryant, 1984): (a) universal coverage; (b) relevant, acceptable, affordable, and effective services; (c) a spectrum of comprehensive services that provide for primary, secondary, and tertiary care and prevention; (d) active community involvement in the planning and delivery of services; and (e) integration of health services with development activities to ensure that complete nutritional, educational, occupational, environmental, and safe housing needs are met.

HISTORY OF THE DEVELOPMENT OF CUBA'S PRIMARY HEALTH CARE MODEL

Located but 90 miles from the tip of Florida in the Caribbean, Cuba is a small, Third World island nation with a population of about 10.8 million (Ministry of Public Health, 1992a). In 1992, 13% of the population was under 15 years of age, and 8.9% was 65 or older (Ministry of Public Health, 1992a).

---

*This article is reprinted from Health Care for Women International *16:* 299–308, 1995. Reprinted with permission of the publisher, Hemisphere Publishing Corporation, Bristol, PA.

Before the 1959 revolution, like most developing countries, Cuba lacked comprehensive primary health care. About 25% of the adult population was unable to read or write (Kozol, 1978), and only half the children of primary school age were in school (Leiner, 1985). Malnutrition was common in both urban and rural areas (International Bank for Reconstruction and Development, 1951).

Shortly after the revolution, those who were unsupportive of it (mainly persons with higher incomes) fled. This included half of the country's physicians and some nurses (Danielson, 1985). A redistribution of income among those remaining occurred, and education and health care for all were set as priorities (Danielson, 1979). Initial efforts to realize these priorities occurred largely through community organizing and mass campaigns.

Community organizing occurred as neighborhoods were organized block by block by newly created organizations such as the Committee for the Defense of the Revolution (CDR) and the Federation of Cuban Women (FMC), to which the majority of the population now belongs. These organizations carried out a census to establish baseline demographic and epidemiological information about the Cuban population. Mass campaigns included a literacy campaign between 1960 and 1961, at the end of which all but 4% of the adult population had learned to read and write, a feat yet unattained by any other country (Kozol, 1978). Sanitary and immunization campaigns used neighborhood CDRs and FMCs and the mass media in efforts that effectively eliminated malaria, poliomyelitis, and diphtheria from the country (Valdes-Brito & Henriquez, 1983). Roads, housing, hospitals, and clinics were built mainly by voluntary labor. Between 1965 and 1985, a system of polyclinics offering primary health care speciality services was instituted nationwide (Danielson, 1985). The polyclinics were geographically distributed and free to all citizens. In addition to ambulatory care services, the polyclinics provided a range of social, environmental, and community health services to the community. Between 1959 and 1992, the number of medical schools in Cuba increased from 1 to 22, and the number of nursing schools increased from 7 to 40 (M. Gilpin, personal communication, March 27, 1994).

Cuba's Neighborhood/Home Clinics

In 1984, a new model was pilot-tested in the city of Havana, that of the family medicine or neighborhood/home clinic (de la Osa, 1985). The model was created because, as Castro asked, why should parents have to take a sick child or elder with a high fever out in the rain at two o'clock in the morning to wait for a bus to go the clinic to see the doctor? Why shouldn't the doctor, who is well, go to the residence of the sick? (de la Osa, 1985; Quevedo & Abrines, 1986).

The system created to answer this question is called "integral" care, which provides a holistic, family, and neighborhood approach to comprehensive care of the community. As described by Cardelle (1994), what was needed were physicians who could practice at the general level in order to understand, integrate, coordinate, and administer treatment not only to meet the health needs of the individual, but also to meet the health needs of the family and the community. Cardelle also described the foundation of premedical education that is provided to meet this primary health care need.

The family physician and nurse live in the community in which they practice, in a combination home/clinic (Gilpin, 1991). After the revolution, the education of physicians was revised to emphasize the social, psychological, and epidemiological needs and profiles of the community, as a basis for intervention with individuals, families, and the community itself. This revision aligned medical education more closely with nursing education (Swanson, 1987). Clinic hours are held in the mornings, and both the nurse and the physician make home visits during the afternoon. Chronically ill persons are visited monthly, and those at high risk are seen weekly; well elders are seen every three months (L. Abreu, personal communication, April 1992). Every member of the community is visited in her or his home at least annually for an assessment of her or his physical and social health.

Evening hours and emergency calls are kept to a minimum by health education that focuses on health promotion programs for groups in the community. For example, Grandparents Circles provide health promotion activities for elders on a group basis, such as daily exercise programs to reduce the need for medications, assist in the management of high blood pressure, and ensure well-being (Ministry of Public Health, 1992b). Similarly, Adolescent Circles were formed to provide health education on sexual health, family planning, and the prevention of the transmission of STDs.

Research is expected to be carried out by all nurses and physicians in Cuba, and activity must be accounted for on an annual basis to ensure promotion and increased wages (L. Abreu, personal communication, April 1992; J. Perez, personal communication, May

1992). Thus, the nurses and physicians at the home/clinics are expected to engage in scholarly work and to report the results of their work at congresses or in journals.

Achievements in Health as a Result of Cuba's Model

Cuba has attained considerable achievements in health outcomes as a result of instituting primary health care as defined by the World Health Organization. These achievements include mortality and morbidity rates that rival, and in some instances exceed, those of Western countries. In 1957, Cuba's infant mortality rate was 57 per 1,000 live births (Halebsky & Kirk, 1985), whereas during the first months of 1993, the infant mortality rate was 9.4 per 1,000 live births. This may be compared with the U.S. infant mortality rate of 8.3 per 1,000 live births in 1993 ("Infant mortality rate," 1993; National Center for Health Statistics, 1994). This rate has been achieved despite the blockade that prevents Cuba from trading with the United States and many other countries to sell and buy medicines and exchange information on medical biotechnology.

The top causes of mortality in Cuba (Table 29–1)

Table 29–1
Major Causes of Mortality in Cuba for the Entire Population in 1970, 1980, and 1991

Cause of Mortality	1970	1980	1991
Heart disease	148.6[a]	166.7	195.6
Malignant neoplasm	98.9	106.6	129.6
Cerebrovascular disease	60.3	55.3	68.7
Accidents	36.1	38.0	49.7
Influenza and pneumonia	42.1	38.6	35.6
Diabetes mellitus	9.9	21.1	22.5
Suicide and self-inflicted injury	11.8	21.4	21.1
Bronchitis, emphysema, and asthma	12.2	7.0	9.3
Chronic liver disease and cirrhosis	6.7	5.8	8.7
Certain perinatal conditions	41.7	13.2	6.1

[a]Values are number of persons per 100,000 population. Data are from Ministry of Public Health (1990, 1992a).

Table 29–2
Infant Mortality in Cuba in 1969, 1975, 1980, 1985, and 1990

Year	Deaths per 1,000 Live Births
1969	46.7
1975	27.5
1980	19.6
1985	16.5
1990	10.7

Note. Data are from Ministry of Public Health (1990).

parallel those in Western countries and present a chronic-disease profile, unlike other developing countries, whose mortalities present an infectious-disease profile. These changes have been due largely to improvements in sanitation, nutrition, and housing as well as to the provision of health services.

Other notable achievements in health outcomes have included the American Public Health Association's recognition of Cuba for attaining the goal of Health for All 25 years before the target date of 2000 (American Public Health Association, 1985). In addition, Roemer (1993), in a comparison of equity in health services and changes in mortality between Great Britain and Cuba, pointed out that although both Great Britain and Cuba have achieved equity in access to health services, Cuba alone has achieved equity as measured by changes in mortality that have no class or racial differentials.

CONSEQUENCES OF CUBA'S MODEL FOR WOMEN'S HEALTH

A major indicator of the health of a country relates to infant mortality and perinatal care services that ensure positive health outcomes. Cuba has remarkably decreased its infant mortality rate (Table 29–2) since the revolution. More than 95% of pregnant women begin receiving prenatal care in the first 3 months of pregnancy. All women are seen at least monthly during their pregnancy, and women in a risk category are seen weekly (L. Abreu, personal communication, April 1992). In 1989, 99.8% of births occurred in health institutions (Ministry of Public Health, 1992a). In rural areas, *hogares maternidades,* special maternity homes, are provided for women to reside in for close surveillance when the course of their pregnancies indicate they are at high risk. Every child under 1 year of age is seen monthly, and home visits are made to assess the infant's development, breastfeeding, etc. The day the mother takes her infant to the clinic for an appointment, the government pays her salary (L. Abreu, personal communication, April 1992).

Sex education is available to the entire population (Fee, 1988; Santana et al., 1991) and methods of contraception are available through the primary care services, either the neighborhood/home clinic or, where such clinics do not yet exist, polyclinics. Abortion is available on demand, and the number of abortions is high, approximately 70 per 100 births (Pan American Health Organization, 1994). Reliance on abortion as a method of birth control is a growing concern in Cuba and is being addressed by the Adolescent Circles.

EFFECTS OF THE "SPECIAL PERIOD" OF ECONOMIC HARDSHIP ON CUBA'S HEALTH CARE MODEL

Cuba faces a considerable challenge to maintain the many gains it has made as it faces the economic hardship of the "special period" that has ensued since 1991, when the political transformation of the Soviet Union and Eastern Europe deprived Cuba of trading partners on which it had depended since the revolution (Kuntz, 1994). Furthermore, U.S. policy (the Toricelli Bill) penalizes other countries for trading with Cuba, which makes it difficult and costly to develop new trade relations.

Austerity is not new to the Cuban population, members of a Third World country. The rationing of essential selected food items that we observed in Cuba between 1978 and 1994 ensures that basic minimal nutritional needs are met for each individual. During the special period, fluctuations in the market and failures of major crops such as sugar cane have reduced needed revenue for expenditures for food as well as other commodities. Importing food and goods, including animal feed and fertilizers, from great distances is costlier than trade with close neighbors such as the United States would be. We observed gardens in urban areas as well as in the country, as city residents converted both front and back yards into vegetable plots. However, we also observed more severe rationing of food in 1994 than in 1992. For example, meat and milk are now unavailable to adults, with the exception of the elderly, the sick, and pregnant women. Milk is no longer available to children once they reach 5 years of age, except in those families who have access to dollar stores (Kuntz, 1994). The economic hardships have taken their toll. The emigration of Cubans has escalated even under precarious conditions (Otis, 1994); they had been unable to readily obtain U.S. visas.

Another consequence of the "special period" is the use of alternative medicines to alleviate the increased shortages of medicines. We observed the adoption of "green medicine," or the use of traditional herbs, to treat illnesses, such as the use of oregano for coughs and cumin as an antibacterial. The resourcefulness of the health workers was evident in the medicinal herbs planted in the front yards of neighborhood/home clinics. We also observed a kiosk used to dispense "infusions," or medicinal teas, such as orange or lemon tea for fever and chamomile for indigestion, to pediatric patients in the Juan Manual Marquez Pediatric Hospital in Havana. More than 50 natural medicines are now available in Cuban pharmacies.

A further effect of the special period on Cuba's delivery of health care is the lack of exchange of professional literature in the health field. The free exchange of health-related literature between the United States and Cuba is not allowed by the United States, except for special circumstances, such as a textbook taken as a gift by a U.S. citizen who is allowed to visit Cuba, or special mailings of health-related textbooks to Cuba through the Cuban Interest Section in Washington, DC. Lack of trade has also affected the ability of medical and nursing journals to obtain sufficient paper to continue scheduled publications, and thus even the exchange of information and research findings within Cuba is affected (J. Perez, personal communication, May 1992). The lack of information dissemination has limited other countries' knowledge of Cuba's innovative health care system.

A CRITIQUE OF CUBA'S MODEL

Although Cuba as a nation has made remarkable progress in health over the past 30 years, this progress must be viewed within the context of the development of a Third World country. Usually, progress in the area of health in a country is somewhat parallel to progress in other areas of the country's development. This is not necessarily so in Cuba, because the socialists have reprioritized their fundamental values to be on health and education first. Progressive thought in the area of public health in Cuba has outpaced that in other areas, such as economic development.

Cuba's health model has been critiqued in a number of areas. First, massive expenditures in health are questioned when there is rationing of basic food items and little petroleum for fuel and industrial use in an economy that is beset with the "special period." For example, large expenditures for some medical programs, such as comprehensive residential care for HIV-infected persons and persons with AIDS (Swanson et al., 1995), come at the expense of other programs, such as ensuring a safe water supply. When staying in Havana in July 1994, we had to boil our own drinking water.

Health promotion, which receives a major emphasis in Cuba's primary health care model, is an area that has been critiqued. Smoking is still a major problem in Cuba, because tobacco, Cuba's second largest product, is important to the economy. Seatbelts are not often worn, and exercise is not largely valued, being engaged in by only about 10% of the population (Gilpin, 1991). However, the use of bicycles as a primary means of transportation is increasing the exercise rate. Although the Cuban diet has tended to be high in saturated fat and low in vegetables and to have minimal fiber content, the current lack of meat, animal fat, and cooking oil has introduced necessary changes in the diet, including the use of legumes as a staple. We observed many brightly colored, attractive posters on the walls of neighborhood/home clinics that contained messages about smoking cessation, adequate diet, and prevention of HIV infection. Santana et al. (1991), however, noted that the creative visual arts community that exists in Cuba has not been well used in devising health-promoting messages in the media. Because this is further hindered by the lack of art supplies, perhaps Cubans should use their drama resources for health education.

CONCLUSION

As the United States and many other countries seek to deliver primary care in order to reach the World Health Organization's goal of "Health for All by the Year 2000," the study of progress achieved in other countries is critical. The study of Cuba's model may benefit not only neighboring Third World countries, but also developed countries that have yet to reach the goal of health for all.

REFERENCES

American Public Health Association. (1985). Government responsibility and the people's health. In *Program and abstracts of the 113th annual meeting of the American Public Health Association* (p. 141). Washington, DC: Author.

Bryant, J. (1984). Health services, manpower and universities in relation to health for all: An historical and future perspective. *American Journal of Public Health, 74,* 714–719.

Cardelle, A. J. (1994). The preeminence of primary care within Cuban predoctoral medical education. *International Journal of Health Services, 24,* 421–429.

Danielson, R. (1979). *Cuban medicine.* New Brunswick, NJ: Transaction Books.

Danielson, R. (1985). Medicine in the community. In S. Halebsky & J. Kirk (Eds.), *Cuba: Twenty-five years of revolution, 1959–1984* (pp. 45–61). New York: Praeger.

de la Osa, J. A. (1985, October 16). El medico de la familia ha introducido tal revolucion. [The family physician has introduced such a revolution]. *Granma International,* pp. 1, 3, 4.

Fee, E. (1988). Sex education in Cuba: An interview with Dr. Celestino Alvarez Lajonchere. *International Journal of Health Services, 18,* 343–356.

Geiger, J. (1993). Why don't medical students choose primary care? *American Journal of Public Health, 83,* 315–316.

Gilpin, M. (1991). Update—Cuba: On the road to a family medicine nation. *Journal of Public Health Policy, 12*(1), 83–103.

Halebsky, S., & Kirk, J. (1985). *Cuba: Twenty-five years of revolution, 1959–1984.* New York: Praeger.

Infant mortality rate decreases to 9.4. (1993, November 3). *Granma International,* p. 1.

International Bank for Reconstruction and Development. (1951). *Report on Cuba.* Baltimore, MD: Johns Hopkins University Press.

Kozol, J. (1978). A new look at the literacy campaign in Cuba. *Harvard Educational Review, 48,* 341–377.

Kuntz, D. (1994). The politics of suffering: The impact of the U.S. embargo on the health of the Cuban people. *International Journal of Health Services, 24,* 161–179.

Leiner, M. (1985). Cuba's schools: 25 years later. In S. Halebsky & J. Kirk (Eds.), *Cuba: Twenty-five years of revolution, 1959–1984* (pp. 27–44). New York: Praeger.

Ministry of Public Health. (1990). *Public health in figures: 1990.* Havana, Cuba: Republic of Cuba.

Ministry of Public Health. (1992a). *Public health in figures: 1992.* Havana, Cuba: Republic of Cuba.

Ministry of Public Health, Republic of Cuba, United Nations Children's Fund, Pan American Health Organization, and United Nations Population Fund. (1992b). *Cuba's family doctor programme.* Mexico City, Mexico: Author.

National Center for Health Statistics. (1994). Births, marriages, divorces, and deaths in 1993. *Monthly vital statistics reports, vol. 42, no. 12, May 13,* 1–23. Washington, DC: U.S. Government Printing Office.

Navarro, V. (1989). Why some countries have national health insurance, others have national health services, and the United States has neither. *International Journal of Health Services, 19,* 383–404.

Otis, J. (1994, September 3). Cubans gambling their lives. *The San Francisco Chronicle,* pp. A1, A15.

Pan American Health Organization. (1994). Health conditions in the Americas. *Scientific Publication, vol. 12, no. 549,* pp. 153–166. Washington, DC: Author.

Quevedo, A., & Abrines, J. (1986). El trabajo de la enfermera junto al medico de familia. Policlinico Lawton. Experiencia inicial [Nurse's work next to the family physician. Lawton polyclinic. Initial experience]. *Revista Cubana Enfermeria, 2,* 16–21.

Roemer, M. (1993). Primary health care and hospitalization: California and Cuba. *American Journal of Public Health, 83,* 317–318.

Santana, S., Faas, L., & Wald, K. (1991). Human immunodeficiency virus in Cuba: The public health response of a Third World country. *International Journal of Health Services, 21,* 511–537.

Susser, M. (1993). Health as a human right: An epidemiologist's perspective on the public health. *American Journal of Public Health, 83,* 418–426.

Swanson, J. M. (1987). Nursing in Cuba: Population-focused practice. *Public Health Nursing, 4,* 183–191.

Swanson, J. M., Gill, A. E., Wald, K., & Swanson, K. A. (1995). Comprehensive care and the Sanitoria: Cuba's response to HIV/AIDS. *Journal of the Association of Nurses in AIDS Care, 6,* 33–39.

Valdes-Brito, J., & Henriquez, J. (1983). Health status of the Cuban population. *International Journal of Health Services, 13,* 479–486.

Model 2: *Primary Health Care in Canada*
Nancy Edwards

Central to the philosophy of primary health care are the principles of accessible, affordable, and comprehensive health services. In this chapter, Canada's health care system is described, including an overview of the historical roots that led to a universal system and the current challenges of health care reform. Innovative models of health care delivery that reflect primary health care principles are presented, including teaching health units, home care services, and community health centers. Notable achievements in healthy public policy are highlighted. The evolving role of community health nurses who are key health promotion agents is discussed.

Canada is a federation of 10 provinces. Although it is the world's second largest country, Canada's population is just over 28 million. A large proportion of Canadian residents live within 100 miles of the Canadian–United States border. However, communities can be found within the far reaches of the country. The provision of equitable health care services to a population that is so geographically disparate is both economically and logistically challenging.

Canadians have experienced substantial improvements in health status in this century. For example, between 1951 and 1991, life expectancy at birth increased from 66.4 to 74.6 years for men and from 70.9 to 81 years for women (Naylor et al, 1995). Infectious diseases have declined in relative importance as causes of death. Canada's leading causes of mortality are typical of industrialized nations: cardiovascular disease, cancer (lung cancer tops the list), respiratory disease, strokes, and accidents. Suicide and motor vehicle accidents are major contributors to potential years of life lost. Chronic diseases, including musculoskeletal disorders, mental health problems, and respiratory diseases, are prominent causes of morbidity (Sutherland and Fulton, 1988). In a 1990 national health promotion survey (Adams, 1993), 14% of Canadian adults reported having some type of long-term activity limitation. Using both education and income levels as measures of socioeconomic status, strong, positive relationships have been observed for various health indicators, including quality of life, health status, and preventive health practices (Adams, 1993).

THE GENESIS: EMERGENCE OF A UNIVERSAL HEALTH CARE SYSTEM

The historical roots of Canada's health care system are the source of the principles upholding this system and shed some light on current challenges. At the time of Confederation in 1867, provinces were assigned the "less important and inexpensive functions of government, among which education, hospitals, charities and municipal institutions were then reasonably numbered. Within thirty years of Confederation social and economic conditions had so altered that public opinion was demanding government action on matters held in 1867 to be primarily personal and of no concern to the state" (Wallace, 1980, p. 27). Thus, along with education and social services, health became a provincial responsibility in Canada. In 1982, the Constitution Act confirmed the historical division of powers between the federal and provincial governments.

Ontario was the first province to pass legislation establishing a permanent provincial Board of Health in 1882. Public education and advisory functions to municipal councils were among the board's responsibilities. The emergence of voluntary health agencies, the development of new roles for public health nurses, and improved training for these roles were among the critical elements forging directions for the health care system that arose in the early part of this century.

Early commercially based insurance plans began developing in the 1930s, and publicly sponsored arrangements for prepaid care were initiated soon after (Kerr, 1988). Province-wide Blue Cross plans were legislated in several provinces between 1927 and 1943. Considerable variations existed among provincial plans, and a substantial proportion of the population found themselves ineligible for the plans or unable to pay the premiums. In 1942, a federal committee on health insurance was struck to study the issues. A model health care bill for the provinces was drafted in a federal provincial conference, convened in 1945 (Vayda et al., 1979). However, the legislation was not brought forward because it was considered a threat to provincial autonomy, and Canada's health care facilities were not adequately staffed to carry the increased demand that would be created by the legislation (Kerr, 1988). The first universal hospital insurance plan was instituted in 1947 in the province of Saskatchewan. Every resident in that province was required to register for the plan, and it was subsidized from general revenues with an increase in provincial sales tax in 1948 to help finance it (Kerr, 1988). Critical features of this plan included the principles of universal coverage, portability of coverage from province to province, comprehensive coverage for all in-hospital care, accessible services, and a publicly administered plan. Other provinces soon followed.

Administration of the insurance plans was the responsibility of the provinces. In 1957, the federal Hospital Insurance and Diagnostic Services Act was legislated (Kerr, 1988). It spelled out the federal provincial cost-sharing arrangement for health care financing and stipulated the terms of provincial insurance plans (e.g., universal coverage). By 1961, all provinces had accepted the terms of the act. Unfortunately, "the early history of health care financing legislation solidified hospital-based patterns of practice" (Vayda et al., 1979, p. 219), resulting in a system that was more attentive to episodic than to distributive care needs.

In 1968, the federal Medical Care Act provided for reimbursement to provincial health insurance plans for physicians' services. Over the years of Medicare, various alterations were made in calculating the federal contribution to the cost of care. The evolution of user fees and extra billing was of concern to the federal government and varied widely from one province to another. Much debate and lobbying by various professional organizations followed. The Canadian Nurses Association took a strong stand on this matter, advocating for the equitable distribution of health care services regardless of ability to pay and the extension of insured services to include community, home care, and long-term care services by qualified health care professionals (Kerr, 1988). In 1984, the Canadian Health Act became law. "This effectively ended the practices of extra-billing and user fees and opened the door for provincial health plans to make specialized nursing services eligible for reimbursement" (Kerr, 1988, p. 171). However, although the Canadian system removed direct financial barriers to accessing hospital and physician services, it retained a fee-for-service payment method for medical care that is generally biased against preventive activities (Spasoff, 1990).

CHANGING PARADIGMS FOR HEALTH CARE DELIVERY

The Lalonde report (1974), *A New Perspective on the Health of Canadians,* was a landmark document that proposed the "health field concept" as a useful way to think about the determinants of health; biology, lifestyle, environment, and health services. This federal report emphasized two determinants of health outside the traditional medical sphere: lifestyle and environment. It became the basis for rethinking health care delivery systems. "The Lalonde report signified the beginning of a paradigm shift in health care away from the traditional medical model to a more holistic system-environment perspective" (Boothroyd and Eberle, 1990, p. 2). However, in the subsequent decade, policymakers focused more of their attention on individual lifestyle change (Hoffman, 1992), and health education programs targeting healthier personal lifestyles took hold.

In 1986, after adoption of the Ottawa Charter for Health Promotion, Health and Welfare Canada released the publication, *Achieving Health for All.* It provided a health promotion framework with three social action strategies:

- Fostering public participation in processes and decisions that affect health
- Strengthening community health services by improving links between services and the communities they serve, particularly the disadvantaged
- Coordinating healthy public policy so that professionals in all public policy areas become aware of their interest in and responsibility toward health in their communities (Epp, 1986, pp. 10–11).

This demarcated another significant turning point, as health professionals began to grapple with the implications of this framework for health promotion programs.

RISING COSTS OF HEALTH CARE

In the 1980s and 1990s, the rising costs of health care have been a major catalyst for change, focusing attention on the need to provide alternate models of care. Day surgery and outpatient services, ambulatory care, and home care provide alternatives to hospital-based care. In each of these areas, the nurse plays a prominent role and has the potential to bring a much-needed dimension of prevention and promotion to her or his nursing interventions.

In 1992 health care costs in Canada accounted for 11% of the gross national product (Fulton, 1993), having risen from a rate of 7% in the 1970s and 8.6% in 1985 (Iglehart, 1986). As a percentage of total health care expenditures, public health and home care accounted for a mere 4.4% and 0.7% of Canadian health care costs in 1986 (Health and Welfare Canada, 1990).

Major restructuring and reform efforts are underway in many Canadian provinces as politicians and professionals seek to increase the efficiency of service delivery without compromising the quality of care. Among the critical issues facing the system are

1. What proportion of the savings found in the acute care system will be channeled into community health services?
2. Will the principle of universality be eroded through the allowance of a private system in which billing is allowed, and what are the long-term consequences of such policies?
3. What are the implications of health services restructuring for the revision of curricula guiding the education of health professionals?
4. Will the focus of health care services continue to reflect downstream thinking, or will the orientation more adequately uphold models of prevention and promotion that deal with root causes of health problems?

TRANSITIONS IN COMMUNITY HEALTH NURSING

Community health nursing in Canada has a history spanning more than 100 years. A voluntary organization, the Victorian Order of Nurses for Canada, supplied visiting nurses to areas of Canada lacking health services in 1897 (Kerr, 1988). These nurses provided care for the sick and for maternity cases, focusing their efforts on teaching and prevention services. The first public health nurses paid with public funds were deployed in Manitoba in 1916. Public health nursing divisions were formed within provincial and municipal health departments. District public health nursing developed as a nursing specialty, and the focus of care shifted from the individual to the family.

The range of services provided by public health nurses expanded over the years to include a wide array of programs in diverse settings (e.g., home visiting, group work, well-baby clinics, prenatal classes, work site health promotion programs, hospital liaison services). Although there has been tremendous diversity in the type of work undertaken by public health nurses, there has been a significant evolution in public health nursing services over the past decade. This shift in the professional role reflects the principles of primary health care endorsed through the Ottawa Charter for Health Promotion (1986), changes in the health care delivery system, a recognition that supportive environments are a significant determinant of health, emerging health problems (e.g., AIDS, family violence), attempts to find more cost-effective ways to deliver public health nursing services, and changing demographics of Canada's population (i.e., aging population, more visible minorities, and increasing numbers of immigrants from developing countries). Examples of the change in emphasis include

1. Shift in focus from family care programs to initiatives with groups and collectives
2. Increased range and diversity of community intervention strategies, including social marketing, coalition formation, community development, and healthy public policy development
3. Increased emphasis on population-based approaches and working with the hard-to-reach rather than managing the follow-up of clients referred by the health care system (Clarke, et al., 1993; Matuk and Horsburgh, 1992).

ARTICULATING NEW ROLES FOR COMMUNITY HEALTH NURSES IN CANADA

In November 1990, the Canadian Public Health Association published a statement describing the roles and qualifications for public health nurses. Using this statement as a framework, Chambers and colleagues (1994) completed a survey in Ontario to examine the practice activities, perceptions of their future practice, and preparedness to practice as community health nurses. The response rate was estimated to be 85.5%. Findings provide endorsement for the roles outlined (and their relative emphasis) in the Canadian Public Health Association document. Consistent with the shift in public health, respondents reported that they were well prepared for the caregiver-provider and educator consultant roles but less well prepared for other general roles such as policy formulator, social marketer, facilitator, community developer, researcher, and resource manager. The authors of this survey identified the "lagging nature of basic nursing education programs for public health practice" (Chambers et al., 1994, p. 179).

In recognition of the essential role of nurses in primary health care, many provincial nursing associations have prepared position papers and submitted briefs promoting primary health care to their respective governments. An example of the most recent statement from the province of Ontario is provided in Table 29–3.

INNOVATIVE HEALTH CARE DELIVERY MODELS

Some health care delivery models for the realization of primary health care principles are now briefly discussed. These are followed by examples of innovative progress toward the specific principles of primary health care.

Teaching Health Units

Excellence in public health practice involves three domains: education, research, and clinical practice. The Teaching Health Unit initiative in the Province of Ontario is an important model for achieving this excellence. Initiated in the 1980s, Teaching Health Units were established through the injection of additional provincial funding to regional health units. This funding provided for the hiring of new core staff, including community nurse specialists, epidemiologists, librarians, and research associates. Nurses have played a pivotal role in the Teaching Health Units, making substantial contributions to excellence in practice. Detailed descriptions of research, teaching, and practice initiatives have been presented elsewhere (Black et al., 1989). Examples include the development and evaluation of a health promotion program for new immigrants enrolled in English as a second language classes (Edwards et al., 1992); research on topics such as the impact of follow-up home and telephone visits for postpartum mothers (Edwards et al., 1995), effectiveness of hospital liaison referral programs (Mitchell et al., 1993; Townsend et al., 1992), working with hard-to-reach populations such as the frail elderly and socially disadvantaged families (Moyer et al., 1993), and the effectiveness of new intervention approaches such as community action for fall prevention (Edwards, 1995; Edwards, Céré, and Leblond, 1995); implementing problem-based learning for community health nursing courses; developing new models of preceptorship for undergraduate nursing students and offering multidisciplinary experiences for health professional trainees.

Community Health Centers and Community Development

Community health centers have existed in Canada for more than 30 years. They are ambulatory care outlets with common features, including a single point of access for patients, a coordinated multidisciplinary team, multifunctional and community-oriented services, and not relying on fee-for-service payments as their primary source of income (Fulton, 1993). Patients enrolled in community health centers are covered by provincial health insurance plans. Various models of community health centers exist in Canada.

Table 29–3
Excerpts From Registered Nurses Association of Ontario (RNAO) Statement on Primary Health Care

This is a critical period for health care reform in Ontario. The current restructuring of health services provides an opportunity to rethink delivery modes, to improve the overall effectiveness of the health care system, to strengthen the contribution of health professionals to health care delivery and to positively shape the future health status of all Ontarians. A strong commitment to the underlying principles of primary health care is critical during this time of change.

To effectively promote Primary Health Care, Registered Nurses Association of Ontario will lobby for a health care system that:

• places priority on health promotion and illness prevention, addresses the underlying causes of illness and integrates primary health care principles at the primary, secondary and tertiary levels

• recognizes multidisciplinarity, encourages comprehensive referral mechanisms and links with other sectors in the development of healthy public policies

• incorporates a multifaceted approach to health promotion that includes education, training, research, lobbying for appropriate legislation and policy initiatives, community mobilization and the development of community partnerships

• provides service that is financially, geographically, socially and culturally accessible, and which includes multiple points of entry

Reprinted with permission from Registered Nurses Association of Ontario. Statement on Primary Health Care, 1995.

Commonly, they provide coverage for all residents within their geographical catchment areas. They are a rich source of examples of innovative health promotion programs. Two such examples are briefly outlined next.

In South Riverdale, Toronto, an environmental health committee was established by a community board to lobby for tougher regulations and to educate health center staff and residents about a contamination problem with lead resulting from emissions from a neighborhood smelter. The persistent efforts of this group resulted in an $8 million soil removal and replacement program 8 years later (Rachlis and Kushner, 1989, pp. 278–279).

In a low-income neighborhood located in the east end of Montreal, several community initiatives emerged to address the problem of hunger (Hoffman and Dupont, 1992). These included emergence of collective kitchens where families get together once a month to plan their meals, to purchase bulk food, and to prepare meals for their families and formation of a food coalition to sponsor research projects on poverty and hunger to provide information on hunger to the general public. As a result of these activities, responsibility for food distribution to the schools was shifted to the "communities" rather than to the school boards by the Quebec Ministry of Education. These initiatives are supported by and involve participants from the local community health center.

Intersection of Hospital and Community Care

Providing accessible primary health care requires careful attention to the intersection of hospital and community services. There has been an array of services provided to bridge the gap between hospital and community. Sources of care in the home include home visits by nurses from official government public health agencies, the work of voluntary agencies, and home care programs. Examples of services provided at home or in support of care at home include

- Treatment services such as dressings, intravenous medication administration, catheterization, and home dialysis
- Assistance with activities of daily living such as household maintenance (meal preparation or delivery, shopping, laundry, cleaning); and personal care (e.g., bathing, transfers, eating)

- Support services such as transportation for those unable to manage public transportation, diagnostic services, home equipment, and supply services
- Rehabilitation and maintenance services, including physiotherapy and occupational therapy assessments and treatment and speech therapy
- Respite care for caregivers of the chronically ill (Fulton, 1993).

Among the challenges facing home care services are difficulties in estimating their financial implications and calculating the potential case load, gaps in the hospital liaison referral process, inadequate in-hospital assessments to allow the selection of appropriate services, policies regarding eligibility for services that are too restrictive or irrelevant and have not shifted despite major changes in hospital discharge patterns, failure to discharge patients from home care when they no longer require the services, or inability to find a less costly form of service as patients gain more independence (Fulton, 1993; Gagnon, 1994; Townsend et al., 1992). These are challenges that must be met as we forge ahead with health care reform and the way we do business in the acute care sector. Never before has the need for appropriate links between hospital and community services been so pressing.

WORKING TOWARDS HEALTHY PUBLIC POLICY

There have been some notable achievements in Canada resulting from healthy public policies. Among these are seat belt and infant car seat legislation, gun control regulations, and smoking restrictions in the work place and in public places.

Over the past 10 years, many tobacco policies have been implemented at various political levels. Regional health units have advocated for smoking control bylaws, licensing of tobacco retailers, the elimination of tobacco vending machines and point-of-sale advertising, and elimination of tobacco sales by pharmacies. These municipal activities have contributed to provincial legislation and attitudinal changes regarding smoking restrictions (Pederson et al., 1992). For example, a comparison of surveys of metropolitan Toronto between 1983 and 1988 indicated that in the 5-year span the population consistently favored more restrictions on smoking, including its complete prohibition in all settings examined. Support also increased for the prohibition of advertising, the prohibition of sales in specific locations, a higher tax on cigarettes, and differential insurance rates favoring nonsmokers.

At the national level, the most notable achievement was tobacco tax legislation, which significantly increased the cost of cigarettes and was particularly effective in discouraging youth from taking up "the habit." The price of tobacco products is probably the single most important factor influencing the uptake and maintenance of smoking behavior (Pipe, 1992). Incremental tax increases have undoubtedly contributed to the decline in tobacco consumption noted in Canada. Unfortunately, this policy suffered a setback in 1994 with a lowering of the federal tax rate.[1]

CONCLUSION

With health care reform, community health nurses in Canada face many exciting challenges. Among these are:

1. The need for community health nurses to be responsive to emerging needs and health issues in the population
2. The importance of developing interdisciplinary models for practice that adhere to the principles of primary health care in the context of a restructured health care system
3. The urgency with which research, dissemination, and practice implementation strategies must be mobilized to ensure evidence-based practice is the norm rather than the exception.

There is still much to be done to meet the challenge of "health for all by the year 2000."

REFERENCES

Adams O. Health status. *In* Stephens T, Fowler Graham D, eds. Canada's Health Promotion Survey, 1990. (Technical Report p. 23-40.) Ottawa: Ministry of Supply and Services, 1993.

Black M, Edwards N, McKnight J, et al. The McMaster University, Hamilton-Wentworth Teaching Health Unit Project: Experiences of nursing joint appointees. Public Health Nurs *6:*135–140, 1989.

Boothroyd P, Eberle M: Healthy Communities: What They Are, How They're Made. (CHS Research Bulletin, UBC Centre for Human Settlements.) Vancouver, BC: University of British Columbia, 1990.

Canadian Public Health Association. Community Health: Public Health Nursing in Canada, Preparation and Practice. Ottawa: Canadian Public Health Association, 1990.

Chambers LW, Underwood J, Halbert T, et al. 1992 Ontario survey of public health nurses: Perceptions of roles and activities. Can J Public Health *85:*175–179, 1994.

Clarke HF, Beddome G, Whyte NB: Public health nurses' vision of their future reflects changing paradigms. Image J Nurs Sch *25:*305–310, 1993.

Edwards N. Prevention of falls among seniors in the community. *In* Stewart M, ed. Community Health Nursing in Canada, 2nd ed. Toronto: WB Saunders Canada, 1995, pp. 377–398.

Edwards N, Céré M, LeBlond D. A community-based intervention to prevent falls among seniors. Fam Commun Health *15:*57–65, 1995.

Edwards N, Ciliska D, Halbert T, Pond M. Health promotion for and by immigrants enrolled in English as a second language classes. Can J Public Health *83:*159–162, 1992.

Edwards N, Sims-Jones N, Nadon C. Evaluation of alternate approaches to following primiparous postnatal mothers. Child Health 2000. Poster presentation at the 2nd World Congress and Exposition on Child Health, Vancouver, BC, June 1, 1995.

Epp J. Achieving Health for All: A Framework for Health Promotion. Ottawa: Health and Welfare Canada, 1986.

Fulton J. Canada's Health Care System: Bordering on the Possible. New York: Faulkner and Gray Thomson, 1993.

Gagnon AJ. The effect of an early postpartum discharge program on competence in mothering: A randomized controlled trial. Doctoral dissertation, McGill University, August 1994.

Health and Welfare Canada, 1990, National Health Expenditures in Canada 1975–1987. Unpublished data. *In* Fulton J, ed. Canada's Health Care System: Bordering on the Possible. New York: Faulkner and Gray Thomson, 1993, p. 44.

Hoffman K, Dupont JM. Community health centres and community development. Health and Welfare Canada. Ottawa: Minister of Supply and Services Canada, 1992.

Iglehart JK: Health policy report: Canada's health care system. N Engl J Med *315:*778–784, 1986.

Kerr JR. The organization and financing of health care: Issues for nursing. *In* Kerr J, MacPhail J, eds. Canadian Nursing: Issues and Perspectives. Toronto; McGraw-Hill Ryerson Ltd, 1988, pp. 163–175.

Lalonde M. A New Perspective on the Health of Canadians. Ottawa: Minister of Supply and Services, 1974.

Matuk LC, Horsburgh MEC. Toward redefining public health nursing in Canada. Public Health Nurs *9:*149–154, 1992.

Mitchell A, Van Berkel C, Adam V, et al. Comparison of liaison and staff nurses in discharge referral of postpartum patients for public health nursing follow-up. Nurs Res *42:*245–249, 1993.

Moyer A, Jamault M, Roberge G, Murphy M. Health promotion needs of socially isolated seniors. Paper presented at the International Conference on Community Health Nursing Research, Edmonton, Alberta, September 29, 1993.

Naylor CD, Fooks C, Williams JI. Canadian medicare: Prognosis guarded. Can Med Assoc J *153:*285–289, 1995.

Pederson LL, Bull SB, Ashley MJ, Kozma D: Restrictions on smoking: Changes in knowledge, attitudes and predicted behaviour in Metropolitan Toronto from 1983 to 1988. Can J Public Health *83:*408–412, 1992.

Pipe A. Tobacco control: Politicking for prevention. Can J Public Health *83:*397–398, 1992.

Rachlis M, Kushner C: Second Opinion: What's Wrong with Canada's Health Care System and How to Fix It. Toronto: Collins Publishers, 1989.

Spasoff RA: Current trends in Canadian health care: Disease prevention and health promotion. J Public Health Policy *11:*161–168, 1990.

---

[1]Unfortunately, the large differential in tobacco tax rates between Canada and the United States led to a heavy volume of cross-border cigarette smuggling. Consequently, the Canadian federal government implemented a widely protested decision to cut federal tobacco taxes and curb the smuggling problem. A positive outcome of this decision was the implementation of the Tobacco Demand Reduction Strategy, which has provided funding for new antitobacco programming and research initiatives.

Sutherland RW, Fulton MJ. Health Care in Canada: A Description and Analysis of Canadian Health Services. Ottawa: Canadian Public Health Association, 1988.

Townsend E, Edwards N, Nadon C. The hospital liaison referral process: Identifying risk factors in postnatal multiparas. Can J Public Health *83:* 203–207, 1992.

Wallace E. The origin of the social welfare state in Canada, 1967–1900. *In* Meilicke CA, Storch JL, eds. Perspectives on Canadian Health and Social Services Policy: History and Emerging Trends. Ann Arbor, MI: Health Administration Press, 1980, pp. 25–37.

Vayda E, Evans R, Mindell WR. Universal health insurance in Canada: History, problems, trends. J Commun Health *4:*217–231, 1979.

Community Health Nursing:
Making a Difference

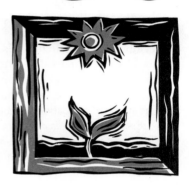

Upon completion of this chapter, the reader will be able to:

1. Discuss how being a member of an aggregate influences health.

2. Predict community health issues of the future based on shared characteristics of aggregates.

3. Describe actions needed by community health nurses to ensure future trends and changes in the health care system that will benefit the consumer of health care.

Mary A. Nies
Janice M. Swanson

For most individuals, hospitalization is only a temporary state that focuses on a diagnosed state of deficiency. Nursing's focus goes beyond the traditional concept of health as the absence of disease, a definition that reflects health in medical or disease terms. Nurses have long been concerned with prevention and health promotion activities with individual patients, their families, and groups in hospital settings (e.g., childbirth preparation, parenting classes, or diabetes classes). Community health nursing extends the definition of health and, hence, nursing action to social units at the community, aggregate, and population levels.

Considering the individual in terms of the aggregate of which the individual is a member is important in community health nursing. Common characteristics such as sex, age, education, income level, and occupation are shared by many persons in the community. These characteristics impact the health of families and communities and are important in determining their needs. Shared characteristics of aggregates also aid in intervention to meet the health needs of aggregates. Social interaction, political activity, and trends determine health priorities and allocation of resources that impact the health of aggregates at local through national levels. The following examples show the impact of being a member of an aggregate on health.

SOCIOECONOMIC STATUS

Health is affected by socioeconomic status in several ways. Those of lower socioeconomic status have higher rates of morbidity and mortality than their counterparts of higher socioeconomic status. According to the World Health Organization (WHO), life expectancy is reduced by poverty through increased rates of infant mortality, developmental limitations, chronic disease, and traumatic death. The incidence of heart disease is 25% higher for persons with low incomes, and the likelihood of having cancer increases as family income decreases (U.S. Department of Health and Human Services [DHHS], 1990). Also, rates of infectious disease, including human immunodeficiency virus infection, are more common among those of lower socioeconomic status (U.S. DHHS, 1990). The importance of these facts becomes evident when one considers that 22% of children younger than 18 years living with families in the United States live below the federal poverty level (National Center for Health Statistics [NCHS], 1995).

COMMUNITY HEALTH NURSES MAKE A DIFFERENCE THROUGH PROGRAMS: VOLUNTEER OUTREACH TO PRENATAL POPULATIONS AT HIGH RISK

Public health nurses initiated a community-based program to reach prenatal populations at high risk of low birth weight. Volunteer neighborhood outreach workers were recruited and trained by the public health nurses. The neighborhood outreach workers contacted residents of targeted low-income communities through personal contact, use of flyers, giving presentations in the community, and attending events such as baby showers. Program data were collected that showed the impact of the program on the community: home visits, telephone assistance, number of persons contacted at community presentations, and educational materials prepared and distributed. The authors review the successes and shortcomings of the outreach program and recommend a plan for program evaluation.

Data from May KM, McLaughlin F, Penner M. Preventing low birth weight: Marketing and volunteer outreach. Public Health Nurs 8:97–104, 1991.

SEX

Whether one is male or female in the United States will affect health. Generally, women have had higher morbidity, or disease rates, whereas men have had higher mortality, or death rates (Waldron, 1995). Although remarkable strides have been made since the turn of the century in increasing longevity in men and women, there continues to be a gap between the life expectancies of the two groups. This gap has increased from 2.0 years in 1900 to a high of 7.8 years in 1995 (NCHS, 1995). Since then, this gap has steadily decreased to 6.8 years (NCHS, 1995). The major causes of death that have led to the downward trend of the gap between the sexes have been gender differences in malignant neoplasms and diseases of the heart since 1987 (NCHS, 1990). The driving force behind this trend may be attributed to women entering the work force and, in turn, increasing the stress in their lives as well as to more women smoking cigarettes.

AGE

Age is an important determinant of health and is closely linked to mortality. For example, according to

WHO, the leading cause of death in childhood is unintentional injuries. This is also true for adolescents, for whom 75% of deaths are related to motor vehicle accidents and more than 50% of deaths involve alcohol use (U.S. DHHS, 1990). Patterns of morbidity also vary by age. More than 38% of people aged 65 or older have a limitation of activity caused by chronic conditions (NCHS, 1995). These are not "sick" individuals; essentially, they are "well" persons who experience periodic exacerbations that may require hospitalization. Most require acute care only periodically, yet medical care is designed to focus on acute care—attending to physiological needs associated with disease—rather than on care at all times. The real needs, especially for the chronically ill population, are for distributive, continuous care in the forms of health monitoring, supervision, and periodic home health or homemaker services. Most persons older than 65 years live at home or with family members; nursing homes are used by 5% or less of the elderly population at any time (U.S. DHHS, 1990). Nursing homes, serving mostly the frail elderly, are also designed according to an acute care model that focuses on meeting the physical needs of patients rather than on their interpersonal social and environmental needs. The health and surveillance needs of this aggregate will continue to grow in the future.

RACE AND ETHNICITY

Differences in health status and access to health services by race and ethnicity also exist. These differences can be partially attributed to inequalities of income, education, and geography. For example, in 1992, among U.S. women experiencing live births, white women were less likely to have no prenatal care or to initiate prenatal care during the third trimester (4.2%) than African-American women (9.9%), American Indian or Alaska Native women (11.0%), and women of Hispanic origin (9.5%) (NCHS, 1995).

SOCIAL INTERACTION

Relationships are also important to health and may determine one's membership in an aggregate. According to WHO, social support is a necessary factor in promoting health and functional independence. Retirement, the loss of a spouse or close friend, or a change in social role can affect support systems and social contact, and all are risk factors for disease and

functional dependence (U.S. DHHS, 1990). Also, those who find themselves surrounded by smokers find it difficult to quit smoking, and factors such as modeling and support from friends are associated with engagement in exercise (Kottke, 1992). In addition, in dense populations, person-to-person transmission of a disease increases even if the agent is not highly infectious (Brock and Madigan, 1991). Families can also play a significant role in health promotion. Families influence personal health habits and physical environment. Participation by children in activities outside the family has been shown to have a positive effect on health-promoting behaviors; this participation is monitored by the family (Bomar, 1995).

GEOGRAPHY-POLITICS

Where one lives (e.g., geography) may have an impact on the health of an aggregate beyond traditional geographically related phenomena, such as earthquakes, weather, or lack of certain minerals in the soil. Political factors have an impact on the delivery of health care services at all levels. For example, Medicaid is a government program that supplies supplementary funds for welfare and health care for persons of low income. Medicaid availability varies from state to state, depending on the local political climate, which is a factor in setting priorities. As a consequence, Medicaid assistance to citizens varies widely, depending on the state in which they live. Residency in a state with minimal Medicaid assistance may affect the health of that population. In 1993, average payments per Medicaid recipient varied more than 12-fold among states. Arizona recipients received, on average, $524, whereas in New York State, recipients received, on average, $6402 (NCHS, 1995).

COMMUNITY HEALTH NURSES MAKE A DIFFERENCE THROUGH PROGRAMS: IMMUNIZATIONS AT THE MALL

One county in the southwestern United States began back-to-school immunization programs at shopping malls during the month of August in the early 1960s. In 1986, the county health department delegated community health nursing to focus on primary prevention activities and to take responsibility for managing the immunization programs. In 1987, the community health nurses conducted the mall immunization programs and continued to do so, increasing services (offering immunizations for adults as well as children) and the number of immunizations given, for each year through 1989. A survey was conducted to assist the county health department in determining baseline information and marketing techniques for reaching more of the population. Questions were asked regarding (1) where immunizations were usually obtained; (2) how they learned about the program at the mall; and (3) whether the client would return to the mall program in the future. As a result, the mall immunization program was expanded (additional sites and hours); marketing of the program was increased; and reassessment of the mall immunization programs is now conducted on an annual basis. The program has implications for cost-effective strategies for providing immunizations for vaccine-preventable diseases.

Data from Guzzetta PJ, Russell CK, Bell LE. Immunization mall programs. J Commun Health Nurs 7:159–166, 1990.

THE FUTURE OF PUBLIC HEALTH: WHAT ARE THE VIEWS OF PUBLIC HEALTH NURSES?

In 1988, the Committee for the Study of the Future of Public Health (CSFPH) opened their report with a list of problems that demanded aggregate action and demonstrated the importance of public health in the United States today. These problems included acquired immunodeficiency syndrome, health care for the indigent, injuries, teen pregnancy, high blood pressure, smoking, substance abuse, hazardous waste, and Alzheimer's disease (CSFPH, 1988). However, does this list reflect the concerns of the modern public health nurse? The committee of 22 members included 12 physicians, but only 1 nurse, and although the nursing profession is dominated by women, only 33% of the committee were females (Ward, 1989). Certainly there are some commonalities of opinion, but it is interesting to consider how these and other views expressed by the committee might have changed if the committee had been composed of 12 nurses and 1 physician. With greater representation by nurses, the health care system as a whole can work toward successfully achieving the public health concerns of the future.

COLLECTIVE ACTIVITY FOR HEALTH

Being a member of an aggregate with shared characteristics, whether age, ethnicity, or geographical factors, may have a marked effect on health. Shared characteristics of aggregates that may impact health are known as risk factors because they place an aggregate at risk. These factors are key to the community, to public health, and to community health nursing as they form the basis for assessment, planning, intervention, and evaluation. Although using the nursing process on behalf of individual health is important, it is carrying out the nursing process, using the same steps, at the aggregate level, that has the potential to make changes based on characteristics of the aggregate. Whether the needs are based on age or social or environmental characteristics, change at the aggregate level will make the broadest impact on the health of the population as a whole. For example, elders in the tenderloin (a congested, inner-city area) of San Francisco had to expose the lack of heat in their hotel on a collective basis before sufficient attention was paid to this problem to push the city to take action toward change. Likewise, the disabled population in San Francisco organized to call attention to their rights to equal opportunity in housing, education, and employment. These activities require community organization that involves planning and political activity by aggregates within the community.

DETERMINANTS OF HEALTH

In keeping with modern concerns, research shows that individual, social, and environmental factors rather than medical care are the true determinants of health and that intervention at these levels is possible and makes a difference. For example, in 1990, the percentage of total deaths in the United States were from tobacco use (19%), diet and activity (14%), alcohol use (5%), microbial agents (4%), toxic agents (3%), firearms (2%), at-risk sexual behavior (1%), and motor vehicle accidents (1%) (McGinnis and Foege, 1993). Note that none of these causes are associated with medical services. The many and varied determinants of health and their uneven impact on the health of aggregates and communities have been the focus throughout this book.

CONFUSION REGARDING HEALTH, HEALTH CARE, AND MEDICAL CARE

As discussed in Chapter 1, health is viewed on a continuum from illness to peak potential. Health is fluid and changing in accordance with the goals and potential of aggregates within an environment. Health is achieved in multiple, complex ways. Medical care is truncated or falls far short of addressing the whole; it cannot address the complexity of factors that determine health. The focus of medical care, as practiced by physicians, is on the diagnosis and treatment of disease.

COMMUNITY HEALTH NURSES MAKE A DIFFERENCE THROUGH RESEARCH: EMPOWERING FAMILIES AND EVOKING AUTHORITY

A qualitative research study was conducted in which 30 expert public health nurses practicing in Washington State were asked to describe "clinical examples in which they made a difference in the outcome of high-risk maternal/child cases visited at home" (p. 101). Interviews were tape-recorded, transcribed, and analyzed. Twenty-one practice competencies were identified from the public health nurses' anecdotes from home visits to 95 families. Two of the 21 competencies were described in this article: (1) *empowerment* through encouraging family self-help and (2) *coercion* by assuming responsibility for child protection, that is, using authority to shield children from violence and neglect. Although these competencies represent what the author calls "polarities," the public health nurse synthesizes them through skills in "fostering autonomy" and applying "persuading strategies" when compelled to do so, as when child protection is necessary. Working with vulnerable groups, public health nurses ensure their right to "protection and sustenance" (p. 104). According to the author, further research is needed that will reveal how expert public health nurses carry out these competencies and a theory that would explain these supposed contradictions.

Data from Zerwekh JV. The practice of empowerment and coercion by expert public health nurses. Image J Nurs Sch 24:101–105, 1992.

Health care, on the other hand, requires effort from the individual, family, community, and societal levels, including self-care, medical care, education, and political and environmental action. The focus of health care is on the promotion of health and prevention of disease. Pouring more funds into medical care will not solve societal health problems such as alcoholism and AIDS; it must be balanced with community organizing and advocacy, which bring about change in the larger determinants of health. Perhaps the greatest issue

facing our nation is when the determinants of health are multiple and complex and require intervention from many levels (e.g., education, economics, political science) is it ethical to continue to fund medical care for disease determination and treatment at great expense to the near exclusion of public health and the social and environmental components of health care?

COMMUNITY HEALTH NURSES MAKE A DIFFERENCE THROUGH RESEARCH: STRATEGIES AND SUPPORTS FOR DRUG-EXPOSED INFANTS AT HOME

The purpose of this study was to identify effective public health nurse interventions for use with caregivers providing for drug-exposed infants at home. Fifteen newborn infants with positive toxicology screens for phencyclidine hydrochloride (PCP), cocaine, or both and 15 newborn infants without a positive toxicology screen (control group) were assessed, and 13 of the noncontrols were monitored on home visits over 12 months. Findings of the study were consistent with previous studies in that infants exposed to drugs were small at birth and prone to "hypertonicity, infections, irritability, an increased need to suck, spitting up, flatulence, and a high-pitched cry" (p. 37). Strategies identified to meet these early problems were swaddling, small feedings, use of pacifiers, soy formula or iron-free formula, evaluation of calories consumed, and waking the infant to eat when necessary. By 6 months of age, most of the infants evinced fewer problems. The study also identified the needs of the caregivers, birth mothers, family-household, and the public health nurse working with these families. The authors recommended further research, including the need to monitor both the drug-exposed infants and the control group longitudinally.

Data from Saylor C, Lippa B, Lee G. Drug-exposed infants at home: Strategies and supports. Public Health Nurs 8:33–38, 1991.

HEALTH AS A RIGHT

Today, health is mistakenly viewed as a right by many in the United States, not a privilege. Yet health is not a right in the United States, as evidenced by the major indicators of health in the United States, which are far below those of many other Western countries. Access to medical care is also not a right in the United States. Funds are allocated to medical care in the United

States rather than to prevention and health promotion because medical care is a large, revenue-generating industry. However, instead of generating revenue and creating an industry in the United States, health promotion and prevention cut back the market or need for the largest U.S. industry: medical care. For health care to be truly health nurturing, there must be a sense of shared interests and community. When public support is scarce or fragmented, the health prospects for mainstream America are grim and insecure. Health care professionals and consumers must work together to determine appropriate goals for health care and institute broad public health measures to prevent and decrease morbidity (Callahan, 1989).

The answer lies not in providing equal access to a medically driven model in which energy of health professionals is concentrated downstream, where the focus is on rescuing the bruised and broken from the raging river of injury, illness, and disease. Rather, the answer lies in providing equal access to a preventive model like Cuba's, in which health professionals work to promote healthy communities upstream by keeping them from falling into the river through collective activity (McKinlay, 1979).

What is needed is a health care system that will provide equal access to upstream care. For example, why should vast amounts of money be spent on neonatal intensive care rather than on preventing the need for such care through more cost-effective prenatal services and education, employment, and housing for communities at risk of low birth weight and high infant mortality?

NURSING'S AGENDA FOR HEALTH CARE REFORM

Forty-two nursing organizations have endorsed nursing's Agenda for Health Care Reform, including the Association of Community Health Nursing Educators, American Association of Occupational Health Nurses, and National Association of School Nurses, Inc. Nursing's Agenda calls for health care reform that would offer a basic "core" of health services to be made available to all on a geographical basis and delivered in familiar places such as homes, schools, and work places.

The core of care of nursing's proposal for health care includes the following:

- Primary health care will be delivered to all in community-based settings.
- A standard, federally defined package of care will be available that provides essential health care services to all, financed through public and private sources.
- Phasing in of the most essential services with priorities focusing on pregnant women and children and vulnerable populations with little access to the current health care system.
- Changes in planning health services needs based on nationally changing demographics.
- Reduction of health care costs.
- Case management.
- Long-term care.
- Insurance reforms to ensure access to all.
- Ongoing review by public and private sectors.

Data from National League for Nursing. Nursing's Agenda for Health Care Reform. New York: National League for Nursing, 1991, pp. 1–23.

One major proposal for changes in health care is nursing's Agenda for Health Care Reform. This proposal would provide primary health care on a geographical basis to all in familiar, community-based settings. Community health nurses who work to support such a proposal by educating the public and their peers, lobbying local, state, and national legislators, and supporting nursing's voice in health care reform will hasten affordable upstream care for all in the United States.

EXAMPLES OF FUTURE COMMUNITY HEALTH ISSUES OF CONCERN TO COMMUNITY HEALTH NURSING

Increasing diversity of the population
Increasing proportion of the population living in poverty
Increasing proportion of the population uninsured or underinsured for health care
Increasing longevity and proportion of the population older than 65 years and living with a chronic disease
Infant mortality rates worsening in comparison with other developed and some developing countries
Increasing environmental pollution and concerns
Continuing hazards at the work place

FUTURE DIRECTIONS

Numerous forces have shaped current directions for health care reform. Among them, the changing face of the American population with its preponderance of older adults, growing numbers of homeless and disenfranchised, and millions of uninsured. As public health nurses, we have watched people fall through the cracks of a health care system that is perceived by too many Americans as uncaring, inaccessible, and far too expensive. We have spent a growing proportion of our national resources on the business of health without the promise of the outcomes that would demonstrate an acceptable return on investment. Yet we never lose hope of the possibilities.

National polls indicate that the American people are generally in favor of universal coverage and for running the health care industry more cost effectively (McDermott and Burke, 1993). After waiting almost a century, nursing now hears a loud and persistent call to community, an area of practice where public health nurses have been leaders, from our Henry Street settlement days to the current grassroots community models such as living-at-home–block nursing and parish nurses.

Riesch (1992) suggested that there are three basic types of community-based nursing center models: (1) community health or institutional outreach models; (2) wellness and health promotion models; and (3) independent practice models. There are numerous examples of innovative models within each category. The living-at-home–block nurses and the parish nurses have been leaders in developing consumer-directed, neighborhood-based systems of home health and community care (Jamieson et al., 1989; McDermott & Burke, 1993). Nurse practitioner–run community centers in Wisconsin have increased access to care in inner cities and have successfully negotiated contracts with major payors in the area (Lundeen, 1993).

Ethridge (1991) led the way in the development of nursing health maintenance organizations (HMOs). In the nursing HMO model of Carondelet, a set of community-based services, including home health, case management and respite care, was provided under capitation to members of a Medicare risk plan. This program was the first successful demonstration of the feasibility of nurses contracting directly with payors to provide an integrated set of community-based nursing services.

Much of the shift to community is being driven by changes in reimbursement. Prospective payment, particularly capitation, offers clear financial incentives to provide services in the most appropriate, least costly setting, which in the majority of cases is the community. All players in capitated risk contracts— consumers, hospitals, physicians, and insurers— benefit when frequent and expensive hospitalizations and emergency services are reduced. Thus, hospital administrators, physicians, third-party payors, and others increasingly see the benefits of providing preventive and supportive services in the community. The opportunities for public health nurses are expanding to include community-based services such as primary care, home health care, transitional care, and case management.

The shape of new systems will be defined by several key goals: (1) achieving acceptable quality outcomes at acceptable costs; (2) using professional resources as effectively and efficiently as possible; (3) providing services in the most appropriate setting for the least cost; and (4) finding financial and other incentives for all players to work toward common goals.

However, we still need the public health nurse. The public health functions that may be lost are continuity of care, advocacy, community organizing, preventive care for vulnerable populations, including education, nutrition, jobs, housing, and safe social and world environments. In concrete terms, this means that there will be increasing emphasis on the whole of health care delivery: where services are provided, by whom, for how long. Each part of the health care system will be examined in systematic ways for its contribution to quality and cost savings. Each part of the health care system will be held accountable for specific outcomes and for linking those outcomes in clearly definable ways to every other part of the health system. We must continue to place emphasis on public health efforts, including community development.

POLICY IMPLICATIONS

Until the recent changes in reimbursement, vast areas of community-based practice have not been covered in the majority of health plans. Prevention and promotion have not been included. Access to home health services under traditional Medicare has been limited to individuals who meet homebound and skilled criteria. Case management, except when meeting Medicare's guidelines for "management of the plan of care," has not been reimbursed. Home and community-based services for long-term care have been the subject of intense debate and also are not reimbursed.

With growing movement to capitation reimbursement, there is strong theoretical incentive to move services from institutions into the community. However, these services need to be aggregate focused, not individual. Prepaid dollars are available to fund community-based care, but many organizations have not yet shifted from theoretical to real incentives for incorporating prevention programs, for using community health nurses as care providers, and for going beyond traditional benefits into more creative models that match services to need. Certainly, market forces will encourage some movement. Federal policies that encourage each of these changes would create considerable momentum.

EDUCATIONAL IMPLICATIONS

The National League for Nursing (1993) conveys a message to nursing educators, practitioners, and researchers to increase the focus in all arenas toward community health promotion. In a similar manner, the authors of the WHO initiative, "health for all by the year 2000" (Mahler, 1988), encourage health promotion and protection at the local community levels. O'Neil (1993) stated in the Pew Commission's report that the future will be more oriented toward health promotion and will be population-based at the community rather than the individual patient level.

The Pew Health Professions Commission in 1991, and more strongly in 1993 (O'Neil, 1993), further challenged the health educational systems to take action and change the status quo of how we educate health practitioners. These authors state, "The traditional model of medical education and practice, based largely on organ specific physical illness, is no longer adequate" (Pew Health Professions Commission, 1991, p. iv). The new vision must concern caring for the community's health by promoting healthy lifestyles and environments (O'Neil, 1993; Pew Health Professions Commission, 1991). All of these documents have a bearing on how public health nurses meet the challenges and help to promote a health-promoting and wellness-achieving nation for the future.

It is clear that the future paradigm for health care is demanding that nursing's focus move toward community health promotion if we are to forge ahead toward a health-promoting and wellness-achieving nation. Should not our nursing education

RESPONSES NEEDED BY COMMUNITY HEALTH NURSING TO FUTURE COMMUNITY HEALTH ISSUES

Increased knowledge and practice of population-focused nursing

A baccalaureate degree as a basis for community health nursing practice

Increased diversity of community health nursing students and practitioners

Community health nursing centers geographically based and accessible to all, offering prevention-oriented primary care

Increased community organizing, advocacy, and political activity

programs, research, and practice reflect this emphasis on community health promotion? Are we ready to accept the Pew Health Professions Commission's (1991; O'Neil, 1993) challenge to change the singular focus of our nursing education from the traditionally illness-oriented (Pew Health Professions Commission, 1991) model to respond more effectively to the nation's call for emphasis on community health promotion? Focusing our efforts only on individual illness care and not including community health promotion is problematic. When and how we make these changes throughout the nursing profession constitute major challenges.

Today, however, not all the nursing profession emphasizes community health promotion. Thus, the authors of the 1993 National League for Nursing report, *A Vision for Nursing Education,* suggest a change in emphasis for all nursing education programs to ensure that all nurses are prepared to function in a community-based health care system. Emphasis on community health promotion is imperative to meet not only the challenges of *Healthy People 2000* (Public Health Service, 1990) but also the realities of the cost of health care today. Are we all truly ready to work with aggregates and communities in health promotion as well as we do with individuals in illness? This is an important challenge for the future that we should consider carefully if we want to maintain our position on the cutting edge.

C a s e S t u d y

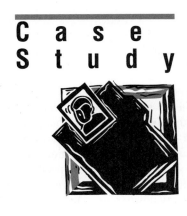

Karen Capel, a community health nursing student making her first home visits during field experiences in community health, visited a young family. Mrs. Dana Pritchett was at home with her 5-week-old infant and a 3-year-old preschooler; her two older children were in school. Her husband, a construction worker in a small town 3 hours away, came home to be with the family on weekends. This is Mrs. Pritchett's first experience with breast-feeding; she stated, "I want to see what it's like, because this is the last one. My husband had a vasectomy." When Karen asked how she was doing, Mrs. Pritchett replied, "Oh, the baby eats fine, I just get scared. . . . It's not safe here at night in this neighborhood, but what can I do? I get real scared."

Miguel Hernandez, another student, visited an elderly couple, the Simpsons. Mrs. Simpson is the caretaker of her husband, who has a history of congestive heart failure, is hypertensive, and at times is confused. A home health aide assists Mrs. Simpson in the care of her husband daily, but the family is considering institutionalization because of Mrs. Simpson's diminishing ability to continue to care for her husband at home, a plan that she resists. The student notes that Mr. Simpson's blood pressure is elevated, he is short of breath, and his ankles are edematous. When checking Mr. Simpson's medications, Miguel notes a discrepancy in the date of the last refill for the patient's diuretic and in the number of pills remaining in the bottle. When asked whether her husband has difficulty taking his "water pills," Mrs. Simpson stated, "I don't give them to him in the afternoon. How can I take good care of him when I have to be up at night, putting him on the pan?"

On a home visit to Ms. Jane Fuller, a middle-aged woman, for follow-up hypertension, Karla Sanders, a student, met members of the extended family. Mrs. Fuller's 23-year-old daughter had many questions for Karla. She stated she had had a stroke in her teenage years, was taking medication for hypertension, and had frequent migraines. Concerned, she asked Karla, "Does feeling anxious have to do with my not having sex because my husband's in jail?"

(These case studies were taken from the author's files.)

SUMMARY

Factors such as childbearing, separation, and chronic disease impact the health of every individual, the health of the family, and, ultimately, the health of the community. Problems reflected by concerns such as safety, crime, and institutionalization are complex in nature. Addressing family and community needs associated with concerns such as those expressed in the case study vignettes is also complex. Although individuals and family members had received nursing or medical care during their last contact with the health care system, identifying and meeting individual, family, and community health needs from traditional medical and health care settings, such as hospitals, offices, and clinics only, is a limited if not impossible task. Likewise, identifying and meeting individual, family, and community health needs while making only home visits is also limiting. The complex problems facing the health of the community today, such as those identified by students in the vignettes—separation, crime, chronic disease—require social action that results in social change such as that brought by community organizations and political activity, by a collective, or by groups of people. Although hospital, office, clinic, and home visits are important, the complexity of health problems seen by practitioners has an impact on the family and the community and at times extends to the state, national, and international levels. Health teaching and monitoring a medical regimen as noted in the prior examples are necessary but not sufficient interventions to ensure the health of an individual, a family, and a community. This is true for many reasons, including the following:

- Health is a complex, dynamic, multifaceted phenomenon.
- Individuals are members of a group and aggregates such as families, neighborhoods, schools, churches, and other institutions that are organized to make up communities.
- The organization of the community has an impact on health of individuals, families, communities, aggregates, and populations.
- To increase the health of aggregates, the community must identify its needs and organize to meet its needs.

- By working with families and other aggregates in the community to identify their needs and to organize and to meet their needs, community health nurses help promote the health of the population.

Today more than ever, community health nursing can be the cornerstone of health care delivery and make a difference. In the United States, the change to a prospective system of reimbursement based on diagnosis-related groups and now capitation has shortened hospital stays and increased the need for community-based health care. Groups and aggregates cared for in the community now require a broad range of nursing services. Fiscal realities and social demands appear likely to mandate the continued growth of community-based care for the foreseeable future. Health care reform that results in upstream care will mandate the continued growth of community-based care over the long term.

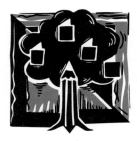

Learning Activities

1. Discuss with your classmates how being a member of an aggregate influences an aspect of your personal health. Give an example.

2. Discuss why and how community health nurses make a difference. Give examples of possible community health nursing interventions for the three case study vignettes at (1) the individual level, (2) the family level, and (3) the aggregate or community level.

REFERENCES

Bomar P. Nurses and Family Health Promotion: Concepts, Assessment, and Intervention, 2nd ed. Philadelphia: WB Saunders, 1995.

Brock T, Madigan M. Biology of Microorganisms. Englewood Cliffs, NJ: Prentice Hall, 1991.

Callahan D. What Kind of Life? New York: Simon & Schuster, 1989.

Committee for the Study of the Future of Public Health, Institute of Medicine. The Future of Public Health. Washington, DC: National Academy Press, 1988.

Ethridge PE. A nursing HMO: Carondelet St. Mary's experience. Nurs Manage 22:22–29, 1991.

Guzzetta PJ, Russell CK, Bell LE. Immunization mall programs. J Commun Health Nurs 7:159–166, 1990.

Hine A. Inspiring a new view of public health. Sigma Theta Tau Int Reflections 17:7–8, 1992.

Jamieson M. Block nursing: Practicing autonomous nursing in the community. Nurs Health Care 11:250–253, 1990.

Kottke T. The "intervention index": Insufficient information. J Clin Epidemiol 45:17–19, 1992.

Lundeen SP. Comprehensive, collaborative, community-based care: A community nursing center model. Family Commun Health 16:57–62, 1993.

Mahler H. Present status of the WHO's initiative: "health for all by the year 2000." Annu Rev Public Health 9:71–97, 1988.

May KM, McLaughlin F, Penner M. Preventing low birth weight: Marketing and volunteer outreach. Public Health Nurs 8:97–104, 1991.

McDermott MA, Burke J. When the population is a congregation: The emerging role of the parish nurse. J Commun Health Nurs 10:179–190, 1993.

McGinnis MJ, Foege W. Actual causes of death in the United States. JAMA, 270:2208, 1993.

McKinlay JB. A case for refocusing upstream: The political economy of illness. In Jaco EG, ed. Patients, Physicians, and Illness, 3rd ed. New York: Free Press, 1979, pp. 9–25.

National Center for Health Statistics. Advance Report of Final Mortality Statistics, 1988: Monthly Vital Statistics Report. Hyattsville, MD: U.S. Public Health Service, 1990.

National Center for Health Statistics: Health, United States, 1994. Hyattsville, MD: U.S. Public Health Service, 1995.

National League for Nursing. Nursing's Agenda for Health Care Reform. New York: Author, 1991.

National League for Nursing. A Vision for Nursing Education. Boston: Author, 1993.

O'Neil EH. Health Profession's Education for the Future: Schools in Service to the Nation. San Francisco: Pew Health Professions Commission, 1993.

Pew Health Professions Commission. Healthy America: Practitioners for 2005. San Francisco: Pew Center for the Health Professions, University of California, San Francisco, 1991.

Public Health Service. Healthy People 2000: National Health Promotion and Disease Prevention Objectives. Washington, DC: U.S. Department of Health and Human Services, 1990.

Riesch S. (1992). Nursing centers: An analysis of the anecdotal literature. J Professional Nurs 8:16–25, 1992.

Saylor C, Lippa B, Lee G. Drug-exposed infants at home: Strategies and supports. Public Health Nurs 8:33–38, 1991.

U.S. Department of Health and Human Services. Healthy People, 2000: National Health Promotion and Disease Prevention. (DHHS Publication No. [PHS] 91-50212.) Washington, DC: U.S. Government Printing Office, 1990.

Waldron I. Contributions of changing gender differences in behavior and social roles to changing gender differences in mortality. In Sabo D, Gordon D, eds. Men's Health and Illness: Gender, Power, and the Body. Thousand Oaks, CA: Sage, 1995, pp. 22–45.

Ward D. Public health nursing and the future of public health. Public Health Nurs 6:163–168, 1989.

World Health Organization. The Ottawa charter for health promotion. Health Promotion I: iii–v, 1986.

Zerwekh JW. The practice of empowerment and coercion by expert public health nurses. Image J Nurs Sch 24:101–105, 1992.

ADDITIONAL READINGS

Berkman LF. The role of social relations in health promotion. Psychosom Med 57:245–254, 1995.

Deal LW. The effectiveness of community health nursing interventions: A literature review. Public Health Nurs 11:315–323, 1994.

Griffith HM, Evans M, Irvin B, et al. Nurses' perspectives on a national health plan. Nurs Outlook 39:178–182, 1991.

Lewis G, Booth M. Are cities bad for your mental health? Psych Med 24:913–915, 1994.

Navarro V. Why some countries have national health insurance, others have national health services, and the U.S. has neither. Soc Sci Med 28:887–898, 1989.

Pender NJ, Barkauskas VH, Hayman L, et al. Health promotion and disease prevention: Toward excellence in nursing practice and education. Nurs Outlook 40:106–120, 1992.

Thompson RS, Barlow WE, Taplin SH, et al. A population-based case-cohort evaluation of the efficacy of mammographic screening for breast cancer. Am J Epidemiol 140:889–901, 1994.

APPENDICES

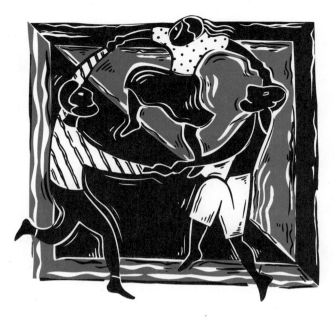

Standards of Community Health Nursing Practice

Standard I. Theory

The nurse applies theoretical concepts as a basis for decisions in practice.

Standard II. Data Collection

The nurse systematically collects data that are comprehensive and accurate.

Standard III. Diagnosis

The nurse analyzes data collected about the community, family, and individual to determine diagnoses.

Standard IV. Planning

At each level of prevention, the nurse develops plans that specify nursing actions unique to client needs.

Standard V. Intervention

The nurse, guided by the plan, intervenes to promote, maintain, or restore health, to prevent illness, and to effect rehabilitation.

Standard VI. Evaluation

The nurse evaluates responses of the community, family, and individual to interventions in order to determine progress toward goal achievement and to revise the data base, diagnoses, and plan.

Standard VII. Quality Assurance and Professional Development

The nurse participates in peer review and other means of evaluation to assure quality of nursing practice. The nurse assumes responsibility for professional development and contributes to the professional growth of others.

Standard VIII. Interdisciplinary Collaboration

The nurse collaborates with other health care providers, professionals, and community representatives in assessing, planning, implementing, and evaluating programs for community health.

Standard IX. Research

The nurse contributes to theory and practice in community health nursing through research.

Standards of Home Health Nursing Practice

Standard I. Organization of Home Health Services

All home health services are planned, organized, and directed by a master's-prepared professional nurse with experience in community health and administration.

Standard II. Theory

The nurse applies theoretical concepts as a basis for decisions in practice.

Standard III. Data Collection

The nurse continuously collects and records data that are comprehensive, accurate, and systematic.

Standard IV. Diagnosis

The nurse uses health assessment data to determine nursing diagnoses.

Standard V. Planning

The nurse develops care plans that establish goals. The care plan is based on nursing diagnoses and incorporates therapeutic, preventive, and rehabilitative nursing actions.

Standard VI. Intervention

The nurse, guided by the care plan, intervenes to provide comfort, to restore, improve, and promote health, to prevent complications and sequelae of illness, and to effect rehabilitation.

Standard VII. Evaluation

The nurse continually evaluates the client's and family's responses to interventions in order to determine progress toward goal attainment and to revise the data base, nursing diagnoses, and plan of care.

Standard VIII. Continuity of Care

The nurse is responsible for the client's appropriate and uninterrupted care along the health care continuum, and therefore uses discharge planning, case management, and coordination of community resources.

Standard IX. Interdisciplinary Collaboration

The nurse initiates and maintains a liaison relationship with all appropriate health care providers to assure that all efforts effectively complement one another.

Standard X. Professional Development

The nurse assumes responsibility for professional development and contributes to the professional growth of others.

Standard XI. Research

The nurse participates in research activities that contribute to the profession's continuing development of knowledge of home health care.

Standard XII. Ethics

The nurse uses the code for nurses established by the American Nurses Association as a guide for ethical decision making in practice.

Declaration of Alma-Ata

The International Conference on Primary Health Care, meeting in Alma-Ata this twelfth day of September in the year Nineteen hundred and seventy-eight, expressing the need for urgent action by all governments, all health and development workers, and the world community to protect and promote the health of all the people of the world, hereby makes the following Declaration:

I

The Conference strongly reaffirms that health, which is a state of complete physical, mental and social wellbeing, and not merely the absence of disease or infirmity, is a fundamental human right and that the attainment of the highest possible level of health is a most important world-wide social goal whose realization requires the action of many other social and economic sectors in addition to the health sector.

II

The existing gross inequality in the health status of the people, particularly between developed and developing countries as well as within countries, is politically, socially and economically unacceptable and is, therefore, of common concern to all countries.

III

Economic and social development, based on a New International Economic Order, is of basic importance to the fullest attainment of health for all and to the reduction of the gap between the health status of the developing and developed countries. The promotion and protection of the health of the people is essential to sustained economic and social development and contributes to a better quality of life and to world peace.

IV

The people have the right and duty to participate individually and collectively in the planning and implementation of their health care.

V

Governments have a responsibility for the health of their people which can be fulfilled only by the provision of adequate health and social measures. A main social target of governments, international organizations and the whole world community in the coming decades should be the attainment by all peoples of the world by the year 2000 of a level of health that will permit them to lead a socially and economically productive life. Primary health care is the key to attaining this target as part of development in the spirit of social justice.

VI

Primary health care is essential health care based on practical, scientifically sound and socially acceptable methods and technology made universally accessible to individuals and families in the community through their full participation and at a cost that the community and country can afford to maintain at every stage of their development in the spirit of self-reliance and self-determination. It forms an integral part both of the country's health system, of which it is the central function and main focus, and of the overall social and

Reproduced, by permission, from Alma-Ata 1978. Primary Health Care. Report of the International Conference on Primary Health Care. Alma-Ata, USSR, 6-12 September 1978 Geneva, World Health Organization, 1978 ("Health for All" Series, No. 1), pp. 2-6.

economic development of the community. It is the first level of contact of individuals, the family and community with the national health system bringing health care as close as possible to where people live and work, and constitutes the first element of a continuing health care process.

VII

Primary health care:

1. reflects and evolves from the economic conditions and sociocultural and political characteristics of the country and its communities and is based on the application of the relevant results of social, biomedical and health services research and public health experience;

2. addresses the main health problems in the community, providing promotive, preventive, curative and rehabilitative services accordingly;

3. includes at least: education concerning prevailing health problems and the methods of preventing and controlling them; promotion of food supply and proper nutrition; an adequate supply of safe water and basic sanitation; maternal and child health care, including family planning; immunization against the major infectious diseases; prevention and control of locally endemic diseases; appropriate treatment of common diseases and injuries; and provision of essential drugs;

4. involves, in addition to the health sector, all related sectors and aspects of national and community development, in particular agriculture, animal husbandry, food, industry, education, housing, public works, communications and other sectors; and demands the coordinated efforts of all those sectors;

5. requires and promotes maximum community and individual self-reliance and participation in the planning, organization, operation and control of primary health care, making fullest use of local, national and other available resources; and to this end develops through appropriate education the ability of communities to participate;

6. should be sustained by integrated, functional and mutually supportive referral systems, leading to the progressive improvement of comprehensive health care for all, and giving priority to those most in need;

7. relies, at local and referral levels, on health workers, including physicians, nurses, midwives, auxiliaries and community workers as applicable, as well as traditional practitioners as needed, suitably trained socially and technically to work as a health team and to respond to the expressed health needs of the community.

VIII

All governments should formulate national policies, strategies and plans of action to launch and sustain primary health care as part of a comprehensive national health system and in coordination with other sectors. To this end, it will be necessary to exercise political will, to mobilize the country's resources and to use available external resources rationally.

IX

All countries should cooperate in a spirit of partnership and service to ensure primary health care for all people since the attainment of health by people in any one country directly concerns and benefits every other country. In this context the joint WHO/UNICEF report on primary health care constitutes a solid basis for the further development and operation of primary health care throughout the world.

X

An acceptable level of health for all the people of the world by the year 2000 can be attained through a fuller and better use of the world's resources, a considerable part of which is now spent on armaments and military conflicts. A genuine policy of independence, peace, détente and disarmament could and should release additional resources that could well be devoted to peaceful aims and in particular to the acceleration of social and economic development of which primary health care, as an essential part, should be allotted its proper share.

The International Conference on Primary Health Care calls for urgent and effective national and international action to develop and implement primary health care throughout the world and particularly in developing countries in a spirit of technical cooperation and in keeping with a New International Economic Order. It urges governments, WHO and UNICEF, and other international organizations, as well as multilateral and bilateral agencies, non-governmental organizations, funding agencies, all health workers and the whole world community to support national and international commitment to primary health care and to channel increased technical and financial support to it, particularly in developing countries. The Conference calls on all the aforementioned to collaborate in introducing, developing and maintaining primary health care in accordance with the spirit and content of this Declaration.

*Models of Nursing Care Delivery and Case Management: Clarification of Terms**

Jean Cozad Lyon

Case management is a popular term used to describe a wide variety of nursing care programs in acute hospital and community settings. However, confusion exists about what programs and services compose case management, and how case management differs from nursing care delivery models. Defining nursing care delivery models and case management programs in acute-care and community settings, and identifying criteria for defining case management facilitates comprehension of program purposes and services.

The term "case management" has been used in community health settings for many years, but is a new health term with growing popularity in the acute hospital setting. Case management, as defined in some hospitals, has little resemblance to case management programs used in community settings. There is also no standard agreement defining the case management programs among hospitals. Case management has been used to describe a wide variety of programs and services in the hospital setting. However, many nurses and other health care professionals are confused about how case management compares with nursing care delivery systems.

Nursing care delivery models, which are modifications of primary or team nursing, have evolved in acute-care settings and are often called case management programs. The staff nurses for those programs, in turn, are referred to as case managers. In other acute-care settings, registered nurses (RNs), as care providers, closely monitor health care resources and patient lengths of stay and often follow up with patients after hospital discharge. These nurses are also

called case managers. Is it possible for two such different programs to both be examples of case management? In one survey of discharge planning and case management in hospitals, a wide variance was found in the use of terms among hospital staff, with resulting confusion in programs offered and services provided (Lyon, 1991).

The purpose of this article is to define case management and the criteria required in case management programs, and to compare case management and nursing care delivery systems in the hospital setting with the term case management as it is used in community health care settings.

A clear definition of case management is needed to improve communication and eliminate confusion of program purposes among health care professionals and consumers. The hospital programs that do not fit the criteria for case management services must be correctly labeled to facilitate identification of program purposes, clients served, and to allow for program evaluation and comparison among sites. It is unrealistic for the staff of each case management program to

*Reprinted from *Nursing Economic$,* Volume 11, Number 3, pp. 163–169, 1993. Reprinted with permission of the publisher, Jannetti Publications, Inc., East Holly Avenue Box 56, Pitman, NJ 08071-0056; Telephone: (609) 256-2300; FAX: (609) 589-7463. (For a sample issue of the journal, contact the publisher.)

define the purposes and functions of their programs repeatedly because the program does not fit the generally accepted criteria for case management.

To define case management, it is first necessary to discuss the historic origins of its practice, the purpose and standard criteria for case management programs, the nature of nursing care delivery models, and a comparison of case management and nursing care delivery models. This comparison of the practice models with a discussion of the differences between them will assist in clarifying the terms.

ORIGINS OF CASE MANAGEMENT

Case management has a long history of use in a variety of settings with the mentally ill, elderly patients, and in the community setting (Steinberg & Carter, 1983). Case management services have been in place and studied in public health, mental health, and long-term care settings and reported in the literature for many years (Weil & Karis, 1985).

Public Health. Community service coordination, which was a forerunner of case management, began at the turn of the century in public health programs. These community service and case management programs have been reported in the nursing literature since the early 1900s. The concept of "continuum of care" came into use following World War II to describe the long-term services required for discharged psychiatric patients (Grau, 1984). Service coordination eventually evolved into case management, a term that first appeared in the social welfare literature during the early 1970s (Grau, 1984).

Case Management in Mental Health. In the mental health setting during the late 1960s and early 1970s, an emphasis was placed on moving patients from mental health institutions into the community (Crosby, 1987; Pittman, 1989). The coordination of community mental health services became important during this time as a result of the Community Mental Health Center Act of 1963, which had placed federal approbation on deinstitutionalization. There followed a movement of patients from the large state institutions to the community (Crosby, 1987).

Several problems resulted from the deinstitutionalization of mentally ill patients, and by 1977 Congress acknowledged that many disabled people had been deinstitutionalized without proper follow-up or monitoring of health care and basic needs in the community.

Congress further recognized that many readmissions to state hospitals could have been avoided through a systematic approach to service delivery. Case management in community mental health provided a means of avoiding fragmentation of client services (Crosby, 1987; Miller, 1983; Pittman, 1989).

Case Management and the Elderly. Specific services for the elderly emerged partly in recognition that older persons are not adequately serviced in age-generic programs. It was also identified that many older people have special, and often multiple, health care needs that are population specific. Thus, the elderly are a population frequently targeted for case management services, specifically those individuals who are homebound or have complex problems that place them at risk for institutionalization (Secord, 1987). However, not all older people who need multiple services require a case manager. Patients who have an adequate functional status and can coordinate and access services for themselves, or those who have social support in the form of family members, or formal or informal caregivers who provide these functions for them, do not need a case manager (Steinberg & Carter, 1983). These individuals require adequate information about their options and the services available.

PURPOSE OF CASE MANAGEMENT

Case management has dual purposes, one client centered and one system centered. The purpose of client-centered case management is to assist the client or patient through a complex, fragmented, and often confusing health care delivery system. In system-centered case management, it is recognized that health care resources are finite (Kane, 1985). Equity and cost-effectiveness require management and allocation of the available resources in a hospital, community, city, state, or in a particular population of health care clients. System-centered case management serves as a rationing and priority setting function that targets those individuals in a larger group or population who could most benefit from specific services (Kane, 1985).

Case management assists patients and families who have been identified as needing coordination of care across the health care continuum to access necessary resources in a time efficient manner (Bower, 1992). For hospitalized patients, the coordination of health care services begins either at the time of the patient's admission or shortly thereafter, and continues following the patient's hospital discharge for an unspecified length of time (Ethridge & Lamb, 1989; Simmons & White, 1988). The length of time over which case manager evaluation and intervention occurs is determined by the patient's physical and psychosocial status, and the success of the plan that is in effect.

The overall goal of case management is to provide a service delivery approach to: (a) ensure cost-effective care; (b) provide alternatives to institutionalization; (c) provide access to care; (d) coordinate services; and (e) improve the patient's functional capacity (Simmons & White, 1988).

The American Nurses Association (ANA) identified the goals of case management to include the "provision of quality along a continuum, decreased fragmentation of care across many settings, enhancement of the quality of life, and cost containment" (ANA, 1988, p. 1). In addition, Stetler (1988) suggested that the goals of case management include the proper allocation of resources for patient care, provision of continuity in care, and facilitation of patient discharge within an appropriate length of stay. Grau (1984) stated that except for the financial management components, the case management process differs little from the nursing process.

Many labels are used to describe case management. In addition to case management, these include case coordination, continuing care coordination, service integration, continuity coordination, and service coordination. Some hospitals, health maintenance organizations (HMOs), and the insurance industry use the term case management to describe what might be described more accurately as "utilization manage-

ment," "managed care," or the monitoring and control of service utilization within a system or episode of care with the primary goal of cost control (Secord, 1987). Yet, there are some providers in these groups with case management programs that go beyond utilization control, and monitor the patient following discharge from the hospital (see Table 1).

Nurses must be careful to distinguish case management services from nursing care delivery models. The nursing care model used in providing patient care in the hospital setting may include some of the characteristics of case management, but these delivery systems should not be labeled as case management, as this adds to the confusion of terms. A review of the objectives and components of nursing care delivery models will assist in a comparison with case management (see Table 2).

OBJECTIVES OF NURSING CARE DELIVERY SYSTEMS

The objectives of nursing care delivery are to assess the patient, identify the nursing needs of the patient during hospitalization, and provide the nursing care necessary until the patient is discharged. The patient care goals are short term, during hospitalization, and do not extend beyond hospital discharge. Although the primary or team nurse can be defined as a coordinator of the services that the patient receives, the scope of interventions is generally limited to providing direct nursing care services on one nursing unit during the patient's hospitalization. The most common nursing care delivery models include team nursing, primary nursing, modified primary nursing, and managed-care models.

Team Nursing. Team nursing, which emerged following World War II, recruited various health care workers

---

Table 1.
Characteristics of Case Management

Identification of the target population
Screening/intake and eligibility determination
Assessment
Service arrangement
Monitoring and follow-up
Reassessment
Care planning
Assist client through a complex, fragmented health care system
Continuity of care
Not a direct care provider
Resource allocator
Comprehensive coordination along a continuum of care

Table 2.
Nursing Care Delivery Model of Case Management

May or may not provide direct patient care
Continuity of care through collaborative practice patterns
Accountable for assuring effective use of resources, maintaining standards, meeting outcomes within acceptable length of stay
Use of available resources to reduce wasted time, energy and materials (managed care)
Use of critical paths within specific time frames

Table 3.
Characteristics of Team Nursing

RN supervision of a variety of health care workers
Team leader is accountable for nursing care given by
  team members
Team is responsible for total care given to assigned group
  of patients and documentation of care
Team leader assesses patient care needs, plans nursing
  care assignments based on patient needs and priorities
Effective communication is essential to insure continuity
  of nursing care
Resource allocator

---

to ease the nursing shortage that occurred during the war years. The team nursing method allows for supervision of aides, orderlies, and practical nurses by a smaller number of RNs (Lamberston, 1959; Marram, Barret, & Belvis, 1979).

In the team nursing model, the RN team leader supervises lesser-trained patient-care providers, and performs direct patient care that lesser-skilled staff are not qualified to provide. Other RN team members provide direct patient care to assigned patients (Sherman, 1990) (see Table 3).

Primary Nursing. As patients admitted to hospitals had higher acuity levels, and as more RNs became available in the acute-care setting, primary nursing emerged. As early as 1950, Lydia Hall noted that the performance of direct nursing care provided to patients on a daily basis was the responsibility of professional nurses, and was not to be delegated to less-qualified personnel (Alfonso, 1988; Hall, 1963). Primary nursing was described, and further developed by Manthey in the 1960s (Manthey, Ciske, Robertson, & Harris, 1970). At its best, primary nursing as defined by Manthey is a way of organizing work and the staff in a common sense system based on professional organizational principles (Manthey, 1988). Each hospitalized patient has a primary nurse who is responsible for identifying, in concert with the patient and family, the nursing care to be delivered. The essence of primary nursing is to establish a therapeutic relationship between the nurse and the patient to help the patient achieve his/her identified goals. The primary nurse provides physical, emotional, and psychosocial interventions for the patient based on the nursing process. The primary nurse assumes responsibility for all aspects of the patient's care on a 24-hour basis. The designated primary nurse is accountable for the outcomes of care that are the consequences of nursing

interventions (Zander, 1985). The primary nurse is assigned to the same patients throughout their hospitalization to provide for continuity of care and monitoring of goal attainment.

Zander (1985) described a model of primary nursing in which the primary nurse assesses and plans patient care through the use of the nursing process. The primary nurse is a resource allocator, using necessary resources to facilitate the patient's goal attainment during hospitalization (see Table 4).

Modified Primary Nursing. As nurse executives have considered the high cost and limited availability of RNs, many of these executives have criticized primary nursing models. Some have modified their models to more closely resemble team nursing. In these cases, hospital nursing departments employ nurse extenders who function as technical assistants to RNs. Through the use of the nursing process, the RN assesses the patients, develops the care plans, and directs the other nursing personnel in implementing these plans. The RN often assumes a number of other roles, including discharge planning, quality assurance, and utilization review activities, in addition to the staff supervision and direct patient-care responsibilities. Nursing care delivery models may or may not expect the RN to provide these additional services.

Managed Care. Managed care in the hospital setting evolved as an additional RN responsibility following the introduction of the prospective payment system for Medicare patients in 1983. Hospitals have grown increasingly concerned with their ability to discharge patients within the allotted lengths of stay. In a managed-care system, the RN is fiscally responsible for patient lengths of stay. Critical paths are often developed and used to serve as a guide for identifying expected patient outcomes, time frames, and resources by case type during patient hospitalizations. The

Table 4.
Characteristics of Primary Nursing

Accountability for patient goal attainment
24-hour responsibility for care
Authority to make decisions
Coordinator of plan of care
Autonomy
Direct communication between primary nurse and other
  care providers
Resource allocator

Table 5.
Characteristics of Managed Care

Organization of unit-based care
Fiscally responsible time frames (lengths of stay)
Can be implemented within any nursing care delivery model (primary, team)
Use of critical paths
Resource allocator (in amount and sequence)

managed-care function, which serves as the foundation of hospital-based management, can be implemented with any nursing care delivery system (Etheredge, 1989) (see Table 5).

Three categories of case management are most prevalent in health care settings. These models include hospital-based case management, community-based case management models, and case management programs that cross a continuum of care in the hospital and community settings.

HOSPITAL-BASED CASE MANAGEMENT

There are three predominate hospital-based models that include the New England model, discharge planner and arbitrator model, and geriatric specialist model. In these models, case management services are provided to the patient primarily during hospitalization, with short-term or limited intervention by the case manager following patient discharge.

New England Model. The New England model, which is labeled case management, is a system for primary nursing care delivery operated within the hospital (Bower, 1992; Zander, 1988). In this client-centered model, a RN provides primary nursing care to one group of patients, and functions as a case manager for a group of patients for whom the nurse may or may not provide primary nursing care. In the case management role, the nurse is responsible for clinical nursing care and for the financial outcome of each managed-care patient, as measured through the use of critical paths, with the goal that each patient be discharged within the allotted number of hospital days allowed for the diagnosis under the prospective payment system (Bower, 1992; Zander, 1988). This model more closely resembles a modified primary nursing model with the addition of managed-care

responsibilities than case management because the primary nurse provides direct patient care with the addition of managed-care financial responsibilities. A critical part of the nurse's responsibilities includes the use of critical paths to determine the patient's progress and to monitor resources consumed. This is a utilization review or managed-care function. There is limited follow-up by phone after patient discharge, and on occasion, one home visit may be made. Problems can surround the use of staff nurses for patient follow-up after discharge. One problem is staff nurse replacement in the acute-care setting when phone calls or a home visit is made. Another concern is the education and experience level of the nurse acting in a community health nursing role. Is it realistic to expect staff nurses to be experts in direct patient care practice in the acute-care setting, and experts in community health nursing, including knowledge of current services that are available to clients in the community?

Discharge Planner and Arbitrator Case Management Model. In this model, the RN patient-care provider is both the discharge planner and the manager of utilization review strategies and quality assurance activities. A multidisciplinary utilization review team is also used to maximize utilization of resources and discharge planning services. The quality assurance component of the program incorporates a process of evaluation of patient outcomes as a result of the discharge referrals made to community services from all discharge planning sources (Bair, Griswold, & Head, 1989).

Geriatric Clinical Nurse Specialist Models. This model of case management uses master's-prepared geriatric clinical nurse specialists as the case managers to augment the basic care provided by the staff nurses. The case managers use a comprehensive discharge planning protocol for hospitalized elderly patients for the staff nurses to follow (Naylor, 1990; Neidlinger, Scroggins, & Kennedy, 1987). The discharge planning protocol includes a comprehensive patient assessment followed by the development of a comprehensive discharge plan for post-hospital care. The protocol may include assessment of the patient's health status, orientation level, knowledge/perception of health status, skill level, motivation level, and sociodemographic data. The discharge plan is based on the patient assessment. Patients are often followed short term, for at least 2 weeks following hospital discharge by phone or home visits.

CASE MANAGEMENT MODELS ACROSS THE HEALTH CARE CONTINUUM

Some case management models provide patient discharge services that may begin in the acute hospital setting and continue following patient discharge, with case management services that continue long term in the community setting. One example of this model of case management is the Arizona model.

Arizona Model. In this model of case management, nurse administrators, educators, researchers, and clinicians function as case managers and have responsibility for patients during and following hospitalization, after referring the patient to appropriate community services, based on the patient's needs (Ethridge & Lamb, 1989). Nurse case managers may work for several months or years with chronically ill individuals who have frequent exacerbations or are entering the terminal phases of their disease (Bower, 1992).

The cost outcome of the first 3 years of this case management model demonstrated a reduction in length of stay for subsequent patient hospitalizations. This was accomplished even though case-managed patients had a higher acuity level than non-case managed patients.

COMMUNITY CASE MANAGEMENT MODEL

Some case management programs begin after the patient is discharged and are provided exclusively in the community setting. Proponents argue that discharge planning and case management should be two separate and distinct functions, with separate staff, procedures, and accountability. Supporters of this model state that the purpose of case management is much broader than discharge planning, and includes the planning of alternatives to institutionalization to assure cost-effective care, providing access to comprehensive care, coordinating services, and improving functional capacity among the clients served (Simmons & White, 1986). Two case management models that are exclusively community based include the Denver model and the Indianapolis model.

Denver Case Management Model. A study conducted in Denver in 1989 evaluated the use of a counselor in facilitating hospital discharges among patients from five metro area hospitals in Colorado.

The sample included 1,040 persons 75-years-old or older, and continued for 8 weeks following hospital discharge. The use of a counselor as an intervention system resulted in fewer deaths, a 21% decrease in the number of discharged individuals remaining in nursing homes, and an increase in those persons going home rather than to an institution. The researchers concluded that this discovery supports the trend toward case management services and inhome services, particularly for the high-risk/high-cost cases (Denver Regional Council of Governments, 1989).

Indianapolis Case Management Model. A randomized control study conducted in 1985 with 1,001 patients newly discharged from the hospital were stratified (low, medium, or high) by risk of admission and assigned to the intervention or control groups (Weinberger, Smith, Katz, & Moore, 1988). Patients in the intervention group were monitored closely by nurses in the outpatient setting. Patients received appointment reminders, and missed appointments were rescheduled. High-risk patients in the intervention group had higher outpatient costs ($131/month compared to $107/month), but lower inpatient costs ($535/month compared to $800/month). The reduced inpatient costs in the high-risk intervention group were attributed to shorter, less intensive hospital stays. Similar results were found in the Arizona Model of case management (Ethridge & Lamb, 1989).

SUMMARY

A review and analysis of the case management and primary nursing literature reveals distinct differences between nursing care delivery systems such as primary and team nursing, and case management. Direct patient care delivery in the acute-care setting does not fit the traditional definition of case management, and to use the term in acute care causes confusion. Primary nursing with managed care, modified primary nursing with managed care, or team nursing with managed care better defines the services provided by the nurse providing direct patient care in the acute-care setting. Nurses are confusing the new role with the old role, and labeling the process incorrectly as case management. The nursing role in patient care delivery must be clarified, with careful use of terminology.

The monitoring of client resource utilization and length of hospital stay is more accurately called utilization review or managed care service than case management. Comprehensive case management services require staff who are knowledgeable about resources available in the community. The case management staff must be qualified to perform comprehensive assessments of patients, and develop a plan of care for the patients for use following hospital discharge. Staff nurses cannot be expected to provide patient care and coordinate post-discharge services for patients. It is also not reasonable to expect staff nurses to remain knowledgeable about community services available given the rapidly changing health care environment, current staffing patterns, and the decrease in RN availability.

Careful and accurate labeling of case management programs and nursing care delivery systems will facilitate comprehension of program purposes and of services provided to the target populations served. Accurate use of terms by nurses and other health care staff will facilitate program evaluation in individual sites and comparison among sites.

REFERENCES

Alfano, G.J. (1988). A different kind of nursing. Nursing Outlook, 36(1), 34-37, 39.

American Nurses Association. (1988). Nursing case management, Kansas City, MO: The Association.

Bair, N.L., Griswold, J.T., & Head, J.L. (1989). Clinical RN involvement in bedside-centered case management. Nursing Economics, 7(3), 150-154.

Bower, K.A. (1992). Case management by nurses. Kansas City, MO: American Nurses Publishing.

Crosby, R.L. (1987). Community care of the chronically mentally ill. Journal of Psychosocial Nursing, 25(1), 33-37.

Denver Regional Council of Governments. (1989, July). DRCOG study may trigger new national policy. Denver: Author.

Etheredge, M.L.S. (1989). Collaborative care. Nursing case management, Chicago: American Hospital Publishing, Inc.

Ethridge, P., & Lamb, G.S. (1989). Professional nursing case management improves quality, access, and costs. Nursing Management, 20(3), 30-35.

Grau, L. (1984). Case management and the nurse. Geriatric Nursing, 5(8), 372-375.

Hall, L.E. (1963). A center for nursing. Nursing Outlook, 805-806.

Kane, R.A. (1985). Case management in health care settings. In M. Weil, & J.M. Karis (Eds.). Case management in human service practice. San Francisco: Jossey-Bass Publishers.

Lamberston, E. (1959). Education for nursing leadership. American Journal of Nursing, 59, 486.

Lyon, J.C. (1991). Descriptive study of models of discharge planning and case management in California. University of California, San Francisco. Ann Arbor: University Microfilms International. Doctoral Dissertation.

Manthey, M., Ciske, K., Robertson, P., & Harris, I. (1970). Primary nursing—A return to the concept "my nurse" and "my patient." Nursing Forum, 9(1), 65-83.

Manthey, M. (1988). Primary practice partners. A nurse extender system. Nursing Management, 19(3), 58-68.

Marram, G.D., Barrett, M.W., & Bevis, Em. O. (1979). Primary nursing. A model for individualized care. St. Louis: C.V. Mosby Co.

Miller, G. (1983). Case management: The essential service. In G.J. Sanborn (Ed.). Case management in mental health services. New York: The Haworth Press.

Naylor, M.D. (1990). Comprehensive discharge planning for hospitalized elderly: A pilot study. Nursing Research, 39(3), 156-161.

Neidlinger, S.H., Scroggins, K., & Kennedy, L.M. (1987). Cost evaluation of discharge planning for hospitalized elderly. Nursing Economic$, 5(5), 225-230.

Pittman, D.C. (1989). Nursing case management: Holistic care for the deinstitutionalized mentally ill. Journal of Psychosocial Nursing, 27(11), 23-27.

Secord, L.J. (1987). Private case management for older persons and their families. Practice, policy, potential. Excelsior, MN: Interstudy, Center for Aging and Long Term Care.

Sherman, R.O. (1990). Team nursing revisited. Journal of Nursing Administration, 20(11), 43-46.

Simmons, W.J., & White, M. (1988). Case management and discharge planning. Two different worlds. In P. Volland (Ed.), Discharge planning: An interdisciplinary approach to continuity of care. Owings Mills, MD: National Health Publication.

Steinberg, R.M., & Carter, G.W. (1983). Case management and the elderly. Lexington, MA: Lexington Books, D.C. Heath and Co.

Stetler, C. (1988). Goals of case management and managed care. Boston: New England Medical Center.

Weil, M., & Karis, J.M. (Eds.) (1985). Case management in human service practice. San Francisco: Jossey-Bass Publications.

Weinberger, M., Smith, D.M., Katz, B.P., & Moore, P.S. (1988). The cost-effectiveness of intensive post discharge care. A randomized trial. Medical Care, 26(11), 1092-1101.

Zander, K.S. (1985). Second generation primary nursing. A new agenda. Journal of Nursing Administration. 15(3), 18-24.

Zander, K.S. (1988). Nursing case management: Strategic management of cost and quality outcomes. Journal of Nursing Administration, 18(5), 23-30.

Population Management in an HMO: New Roles for Nursing

Wendy L. Graff, MPH, MA
Wendy Bensussen-Walls, BSN, RNC
Eileen Cody, BSN, CRRN
Joanne Williamson, RNC, CDE

Abstract A project to define and test population-management roles in nursing was implemented in a large HMO. Three patient populations were selected: diabetics, patients with multiple sclerosis, and pregnant adolescents. Expert nurse clinicians in each of the three areas piloted the role for six months, including establishing a system of care coordination for the populations. In all three pilots, patient care outcomes were improved. Keys to success included aligning the work with the critical clinical work of the organization, practicing in multidisciplinary settings, and reporting objective outcome data to constituents.

INTRODUCTION

When expert nurse clinicians manage specific populations of patients, not only are patient outcomes improved, but costs of care and job satisfaction are positively affected. A large HMO in the Northwest, serving 450,000 enrollees with a staff of 1,300 RNs, found this to be the case when it developed and instituted an expanded role for nurses that focused on population management. The concept of population management is discussed in this issue's editorial. This paper describes how the roles were developed, implemented, and evaluated in an HMO setting.

Both management and the nurses' union were interested in developing roles that offered increased autonomy and kept expert, experienced nurses in direct patient care, while providing opportunities for recognition of individual expertise. This desire was reflected in the 1991 bargaining agreement with the union, which called for the establishment of "a committee to study nursing roles and appropriate

clinical support. Specifically, the committee will review how expanded roles such as population manager, care coordinator, patient educator, consultant and staff educator enhance our ability to deliver cost effective, quality care in our system of managed care" (Employment agreement, 1991).

The committee convened in late 1991 and spent 18 months defining and describing how this role would function within the HMO's delivery system. This preliminary work included an extensive literature review, interviews with more than 40 hospitals and HMOs with some form of expanded nursing role, and focus groups with nurse managers.

Well over 70 articles were reviewed in an attempt to clarify the definition of expanded roles, determine role characteristics, locate outcome data, uncover environmental barriers and facilitators to such roles, and explore the relationship between expanded roles and the organizations in which they operated. As might be expected, the term "expanded roles" was used to describe a wide variety of nursing practices, from

Reprinted from *Public Health Nursing,* Volume 12, Number 4, pp. 213–221. Reprinted with permission of the publisher, Blackwell Science, Inc., Cambridge, Massachusetts.

those of primary care nurses to nurse practitioners to case managers. Almost all descriptions in the literature were of nurses with a home base in inpatient nursing rather than in ambulatory care.

The literature was most helpful in describing role characteristics. Conti (1989) described the role as being that of an expediter, broker of services, professional colleague, consultant, advocate, coordinator, and counselor. Jimerson (1986) pointed out that expanded-role nurses have specific, advanced educational preparation and, importantly, discussed the expanded-role RNs effect on populations of patients, rather than only individuals. Rubin (1988) summarized expanded roles to include practitioner, educator, and researcher.

Literature with outcome data was limited, although many articles alluded to positive outcomes. Maraldo (1989) reported specific cost benefits from the use of expanded-role RNs, including earlier discharge of low-birthweight babies and decreased hospitalizations for the elderly and chronically ill. The committee also looked for patterns of environmental barriers and facilitators. The literature was less helpful here, although caveats were offered about the need to be multidisciplinary and the potential difficulties of working out these expanded roles with physicians.

Following the literature review, telephone interviews were conducted with 43 hospitals and HMOs to determine the status of expanded roles in those institutions. Eighteen of those identified had expanded roles for RNs and nine more had pilot programs or were in the active planning stages for implementing such a role. Titles given to those practicing in expanded roles included case manager, patient care manager, continuing care coordinator, coordinated care specialist, primary nurse, and staff nurse. Planning generally took two years, including pilot programs. Motivation for implementing expanded roles included decreased length of stay, decreased costs, increased quality, recruitment and retention of RNs, RN/MD collaboration, and a focus on health and wellness.

In October 1992, members of the Expanded Roles Committee met with nurse managers from the HMO in focus groups to present their ideas to date and solicit feedback. Committee members provided examples of potential role responsibilities and possible patient and provider outcomes and then facilitated focus groups addressing specific questions.

The nurse manager focus groups pointed out several precursors for successful implementation of such a role, including the need to build this role with input and buy-in from other disciplines and care providers, to clearly define educational requirements for the position, and to see how the role interfaced with discharge planning, home health care and other aspects of care. They were enthusiastic about the great potential for such a role to enhance coordination among departments, continuity of care across settings, and quality of care.

DEFINITION OF AN EXPANDED ROLE FOR NURSING

The next step, then, was to develop the following "Definition of an Expanded Role for Nursing," which was published in the in-house nursing newsletter, again with a request for feedback from the entire nursing community.

"An expanded role for nursing practice is one which reaches beyond the basic expectations of every staff nurse. An expanded role is premised upon a specialized set of skills and expertise that may result from practice experience, advanced education/continuing educational preparation, certification or other credentialing mechanism, or some combination thereof.

"Nurses practicing in expanded roles are recognized as experts by their peers; they serve as resources both within and outside their own discipline. If one were to fit these nurses into Benner's (1984) continuum of novice to expert (novice, advanced beginner, competent, proficient, expert), they would be proficient and beyond.

"Nurses in expanded roles teach, consult, and may publish in their areas of expertise to benefit clients, the general public, or nurses and other health care professionals. They also mentor other nurses and contribute to the advancement of the profession as they coach and empower others in their work.

"Nurses in expanded roles, whether in an enhancement of an existing role or in a newly developed expanded role, demonstrate increased autonomy, accountability, and independence in clinical judgment and decision making; and possess a special commitment to, interest in, and intellectual curiosity about the nature of the care they provide to consumers.

"Nurses in expanded roles focus on redefining health care; they promote healing, changing lifestyles, and holistic mind/body/spirit connections.

"Nurses in expanded roles view change as an opportunity, are future oriented, and proactive in their management of care. They rely on creativity, imagination, and experimentation to find new approaches and generate alternatives to benefit patients and improve care.

"Hallmarks of the care provided by nurses in expanded roles include:

- analysis of health care services and systems to determine accessibility, sensitivity to client needs, and cost effectiveness for the target population;
- design, direction, implementation and evaluation of programmatic, technological, and educational directions of care for defined populations;
- care coordination across the health-illness continuum, across settings and beyond geographic boundaries; consideration of organizational, community, and societal implications of events and decisions related to care coordination; and an emphasis on networks of colleagues and resources;
- enhanced customer relationships by clearly defining and demonstrating the contribution of nursing to the customer's health care;
- a we approach to interdependent team learning and a matrix environment which fosters open dialogue, collaboration, and a collective sense of responsibility for issues/problems;
- continuous quality improvement; support of an organization-wide, ongoing process to improve service and clinical outcomes; never satisfied with the status quo; cultivation of an environment for continuous learning."

The primary focus for the nurse clinician, then, was the establishment of a system for coordinating care for defined populations throughout an entire episode of illness or across the illness-wellness continuum. Nurse clinicians were accountable for improving the care of defined populations in collaboration with their medical staff colleagues. Role responsibilities included: identification of at-risk populations and development of interventions to reduce risk factors; establishment of a system to coordinate patients' care and education throughout the illness/wellness continuum and across settings, including home; creation of a network of resources for patients and staff to assure access to those resources through critical linkages; collection, monitoring, and analysis of patient data; identification and implementation of strategies to reduce length of stay and/or ambulatory visits; a focus on outcomes and a review of variances related to standards of care; and use of the data to bring about improvements in care and outcomes across the population.

Once the committee had clearly defined what such a position would do in theory, it was time to test it in practice. Three patient populations seemed ideally suited to test this new role: diabetics, pregnant adolescents, and patients with multiple sclerosis. In all three cases one was easily able to identify the predictable health care needs of the specific populations. The pilot projects were also selected to fit with the organization's clinical priorities, a mandatory step to ensure organizational support for the resources required for the pilots. Expanded roles in these three areas were piloted for six months, from October 1993 to April 1994. Two of the pilots were not new positions. In those cases there was an attempt to maximize benefits from roles that were already being practiced in part. The opportunity for some analytic support and the time to practice true population-based management and develop critical paths allowed for successful completion of the pilot project.

Since that time, other population manager roles have been implemented. The organization requested consistent, clear guidelines to expedite the development of these roles across various clinical settings. One of the import products of the committee, therefore, was an information manual, which was widely distributed throughout the HMO.

What follows are descriptions of the pilot experiences, including the respective outcomes. Outcome measures describing the success of the position depended upon the clinical area in question, but could include:

- increase in utilization of evidence-based guidelines;
- decrease in hospitalizations;
- decrease in inappropriate, unplanned provider visits;
- increase in planned visits for preventive or routine care;
- decrease in complications secondary to condition;
- increase in patient satisfaction;
- increase in patient self-management;
- increase in provider satisfaction.

CLINICAL EXAMPLES

Diabetes Nurse Clinician

Patients with a diagnosis of diabetes formed an excellent clinical group for population management because they had measurable indicators that often mirrored their conditions—glycohemoglobin rates, episodes of ketoacidosis, number of amputations, etc. The particular clinic in which this diabetes nurse clinician (DNC) worked employed 17 physicians with a combined total of approximately 1,000 diabetic patients. Her responsibilities during the pilot were to coordinate and implement improvement in the care of the diabetic population. To accomplish this work, direct collaboration and consultation with physicians and health care providers in other disciplines (such as pharmacy, lab, optometry/ophthalmology, and medical records) was essential.

Decreasing diabetic blindness and preventing diabetic amputations were much too lofty goals for a six-month pilot project. Instead, the DNC's goals were, first, to identify the patients with diabetes and second, to raise the providers' level of awareness of the health status of the diabetic patients within their practices. Predetermined criteria (taken from American Diabetes Association guidelines) were used to assess individual patients within a practice. Physicians and their teams of medical assistants, licensed practical nurses, registered nurses and receptionists were offered this practice-specific information.

In preparation for her new role, the nurse took two brief courses on how to use a computer, sent a letter to all physician teams explaining her role during the pilot project, and joined the American Diabetes Association (ADA), which gave her a colleague base, raised awareness of informational classes, and gave her increased access to pertinent publications.

Self-glucose monitors were placed in practice offices, enabling the nurses to demonstrate to and educate the patients within their practices about the importance and use of self-glucose monitoring in maintaining their health. Nurses were also encouraged to refer to the American Association of Diabetes Educators core curriculum for diabetes education. Nurses seemed pleased that someone was helping them enhance their skills, providing them with resources, and cheering them on.

Now the real work began. A computerized registry for all patients identified as having diabetes was produced by the research department of the HMO. The registry included the patient's last cholesterol level, glycohemoglobin, and date of last eye exam, among others. Two hundred charts of the 1,000 diabetics were randomly selected and audited. The following parameters were measured: annual physical and eye exams, urinalysis and lipid testing, blood pressure and foot examination on each visit, self-glucose monitoring, visits specifically with the RN, number of hospitalizations and emergency room visits within the last year, visits to a nutritionist and other specialists within the last year, and smoking status.

After the data were aggregated and analyzed, the DNC presented them to the entire clinic medical staff. Then each of the 17 physicians asked that the findings and analysis be presented to the complete practice team, indicating a willingness to see diabetes-care management as a team effort. The presentations were very well received. The physicians were eager to learn about their individual practices as well as about the pilot program. Repeatedly, teams asked for suggestions or commented about how they could use the information to increase their effectiveness in helping their diabetic patients achieve healthier life-styles and subsequently better medical outcomes. Some teams also asked for assistance in enhancing their team approach to this chronic illness.

When the data were presented to the teams, it was easy to identify those practices that had a high degree of registered nurse intervention. In practices where more than 50% of the patients with diabetes were case managed by an RN, the standards of care were met. It was like a light bulb going off in the teams' minds: Nursing intervention improved patient health care outcomes.

As a result of the presentation of individual practice statistics, the nurse clinician was asked to precept one RN and assist another in case management. The presentation also resulted an increase in nursing office visits. For example, prior to the pilot, one nurse had only been seeing four diabetic patients per month (out of 110 diabetic patients in the practice). During the pilot, this same nurse increased her monthly diabetic-patient visit total to an average of 24. In the case of the nurse who had been precepted, the panel average for total glycohemoglobins went from 15% to 9% for 18 of her most aggressively managed patients.

Goals were set for the number of visits per year for individual patients with diabetes. For example, if a practice had 50 patients with diabetes, approximately five of them would be Type 1 and need four visits each per year. The remaining 45 patients would be Type 2 diabetics, needing at least two visits each per year, for a total of 110 visits per year for the practice. Taking the 110 visits and multiplying that by the average number of minutes per teaching visit resulted in the amount of time necessary to manage the diabetic population. From that number the RN could schedule the visits into workable time frames within the practice. At this stage the individual practitioner had begun to manage the population. In addition, because the clinicians were now able to predict routine health care needs of the patient, even if the patient came in for an acute episode unrelated to diabetes, there was a system in place to remind the health care team and the patient about those care needs related to diabetes.

Teamwork is the key to success in the management of population-based care. An example of a giant step toward teamwork occurred when a physician seeing a diabetic patient in his office called the DNC and invited her to consult with him/her. (The patient was having widely fluctuating blood sugars.) The DNC questioned the patient and made some recommendations to the doctor on altering exercise and diet, lowering one of the insulin dosages, and raising another. The doctor acknowledged the nurse clinician, agreed those were good ideas, and told the patient that he concurred with the nursing recommendation. To the DNC that was a phenomenal step for nursing and population management.

To further the team approach, lunchtime courses were offered to medical receptionists, medical assistants, and licensed practical nurses on diabetes, its implications, and its complications and to discuss how these other staff members could become involved in the care of patients with diabetes. Physicians and RNs began to use these valuable team members to review patient charts, assess immunization and physical exam status, labs, and to make sure to have the patients remove their shoes during an office visit work-up so that the nurse or physician would be reminded to examine the patients' feet.

Word soon spread to other clinics. The ophthalmologist in charge of developing diabetic eye care guidelines for the HMO asked the DNC to meet with him. This invitation came one day after the DNC shared with the clinic physicians that only 44% of the diabetic patients had had an eye exam during the last year. During the pilot, 64% of the patients received eye exams.

This work was being recognized throughout the HMO, and people began to seek involvement. News was also spreading throughout the community. The state ADA president asked to meet with the nurse clinician and explore the possibilities of the ADA state chapters' working with the HMO. Staff from a state organization for diabetes control contacted the nurse to become involved in a diabetes pregnancy project. The work from that contact continues today.

As the months rolled on, all levels of staff were using the services of the DNC, and she was becoming known as a region-wide consultant. She surely did not have all the answers, but she was able to assist staff in finding answers to their questions regarding care for their diabetic patients. She was on call for staff and patients. They could reach her by pager or voice mail, and during the pilot project she took more than 250 calls from staff throughout the region. Several nurses from other clinics set up phone conferences with her to discuss cases they were having difficulty managing. It was a cost-effective and beneficial means of in-service education.

It was extremely important for the nurse clinician to keep in touch with patients and the normal flow of an office practice during the pilot to maintain both her credibility and her clinical expertise.

The role of diabetes nurse clinician was evaluated with a tool developed specifically for this pilot. The results of this evaluation demonstrated that her role as the DNC was viewed as supportive and necessary for continued improvement of care for this population. Some of the measures included whether or not the teams believed the data; whether the teams planned to implement changes as a result of the data; whether the DNC was a useful resource for the team; and whether the team expected the DNC to be a useful resource in the future.

By the pilot's end, the nurse clinician had accomplished her goals of increasing awareness of the diabetes population among the health care teams and of identifying the population and health status of those patients. Teams now had access to, and an increased understanding of, the data that are produced quarterly on patients diagnosed with diabetes. During the pilot the nurse clinician reviewed information and charts, assisted practices in identifying more effective methods of population management, shepherded team members through data to identify patients with the most potential for improvement, and improved the health awareness and eventual health status of patients with diabetes. She became an advocate for patients with diabetes and a cheerleader for practice teams who were working to meet those needs. Staff were updated on methods of teaching self-management skills and teaching patients to learn what their bodies were telling them.

The role of diabetes nurse clinician could be expanded even further. Continuity of care could be increased by tracking hospital admissions of diabetics and ensuring that hospitalization information is communicated to the primary care team. Thus, the nurse clinician would be able to evaluate potentially preventable further hospitalizations. The organization has placed a great deal of emphasis on the management of diabetes. Although diabetics account for only about 2.5% of the total HMO enrollment, they consume almost 13% of the budget. Therefore, finding new ways to organize and deliver care for this population pays off, not only in terms of improved clinical outcomes but also in potentially significant cost reductions. The role of the DNC is integral to these efforts.

Rehabilitation Nurse Clinician

The rehabilitation nurse clinician (RNC) was first hired in 1989 to establish a new outpatient multidisciplinary rehabilitation clinic. This role differed from the regular staff nurse role from its inception, as it was not attached to a particular panel of patients or a physician's practice. Instead, the nurse served as a resource for the disabled population and for other nurses throughout the HMO in their work with patients with rehabilitation needs. The multidisciplinary clinic met once a month to serve the rehabilitation patient needing complex coordination of care.

Through the quality assurance program, the nurse clinician identified problem-prone, high-risk, high-volume patients. Populations with spinal cord injuries and with multiple sclerosis (MS) were recognized as those that were the most problem-prone and would benefit greatly from a more proactive, preventive yearly review program. These populations were treated in the HMO's family practice settings unless they developed complications and were referred to the physiatry or multidisciplinary clinic. Many patients felt that family practice did not understand the complexities of their problems; yet the patients did not want to have to travel sometimes long distances to be seen in the specialty clinic. These concerns prompted the nurse to believe that development of a population-based approach was needed throughout the HMO. The state in which the HMO is located is in what is referred to as an "MS belt." This state has an MS prevalence of 221 per 100,000 compared with about 58 per 100,000 across the United States (Cook, 1990; Scheinberg, 1987). This implies an expected MS patient population of 850 within the HMO. The predictable health care needs of this population required a proactive care approach to avoid numerous costly medical complications and to keep the patients functional in their families and in society.

Despite the fact that the rehabilitation nurse had been working in an independent role prior to the pilot, being selected for the expanded-role pilot helped to move this work toward her goals for this patient population. The nurse had been working for several years to identify the individual patients that make up the MS population through chart audits, drug profiles, and identification by individual providers. When she was chosen for the pilot, other resources became more accessible. With the institutional support, data bases that had previously been unknown to her were uncovered and enabled her to develop a more complete list of the population. The release of a new drug for the treatment of relapsing-remitting MS also encouraged others throughout the HMO to become interested in this population. At the price of $12,000 per year per patient for betaseron, many people were interested in what the cost-benefit ratio for the population would be. Her plan for a coordinated approach to the population received broad support from providers in the fields of neurology, family practice and pharmacy, and from patients.

After identifying the MS population, the RNC then attempted to determine the population's most frequent problems and its most frequent cause for hospitalization. Patients were surveyed to determine what they would identify as their most frequent problems. The nurse clinician also reviewed hospital records of the 20 MS patients with the highest utilization in the past three years to identify reasons for hospitalization, number of hospital days, and cost per case. Not surprisingly, what patients identified as their most frequent complication and what hospital records revealed as the most frequent reason for hospitalization were the same: urinary tract complications. Of course, there is a wide range of problems, from incontinence to urinary retention, seen in MS patients, but if appropriate interventions and education were provided early, the need for hospitalizations for urinary sepsis should decrease. The development of HMO-wide standards for the treatment of neurogenic bladders was the RNC's first priority.

While working on these standards, she also advertised throughout the HMO her availability to consult with patients and providers regarding MS and its complications. She participated in an educational offering to primary care nurses and spoke on the care of the MS patient. Besides her nursing colleagues, she also needed to have family practice physicians recognize that she, as a registered nurse, had some expertise from which they could learn. Her experience showed that the physicians were very open-minded and appreciated help in handling patient problems for this population from any discipline that was willing to offer it.

The RNC presented the information that she had gathered from the patient survey and from chart reviews to many of the physicians at rounds, and they were enthusiastic about developing standards for care of this population. They suggested that implementation of any standards would be best accomplished if the nurse actually visited each primary care clinic and educated staff by reviewing individual patients with them. Thus the nurse clinician formed the idea of developing a data base, with the help of primary care providers, on each individual MS patient. That data base would help identify those patients who were most in need of case management, and it could be used to identify patients appropriate for any new medication that might be released for the treatment of MS.

Working with the primary care nurses and physicians was a key component of this expanded role, since it expanded the opportunities for patients to receive the care they needed from their primary care team. Through the resources provided by a grant, the RNC will achieve this effect by training one or two RNs in each primary care clinic in how to use the Minimal Record of Disability (MRD) to evaluate the functional status of MS patients. She will also work with primary care physicians to assist them in identifying appropriate rehabilitation therapies for MS patients to help maintain and maximize their function in daily life.

Patients' satisfaction with their care increased during the pilot, as many saw the development of a data base as recognition of their population's special needs, which they assumed would lead to better health outcomes. Many providers, however, worry about the increased workload necessitated by yearly review of these patients, and there is the potential for the RNC to be seen as an outsider who creates this increased volume of work. Providers will need to be kept

informed of improved outcomes to encourage their continued participation. Availability of the nurse clinician as a resource and her familiarity with current research and treatments will be crucial in order for staff to accept direction in caring for this defined population.

Teen Pregnancy and Parenting Nurse Clinician

Comparisons of pregnant adolescents with pregnant adults indicate that adolescents are not at greater risk for complications when prenatal care is provided in a comprehensive, multidisciplinary fashion (Elster et al., 1987). Guided by this principle, a family practice physician who specialized in adolescent medicine created a team to investigate the establishment of such a clinic. Finally, one clinic that teaches family practice residents came forward and requested that it become a part of the training curriculum. The existing core curriculum for family practice physicians had minimal training in adolescent medicine. Having a multidisciplinary clinic for teen pregnancy and parenting would enhance resident education, thereby filling a void. In the summer of 1990 the Teen Pregnancy and Parenting Clinic (TPPC) was established with funding from a United States Public Health Service Primary Care Training Grant.

The grant funded the salary for a part-time nurse coordinator position for two years, and educational supplies. All other services were provided as in-kind services from the HMO. The Family Practice Residency provided the clinic with space. The Social Services department provided a part-time social worker, Nutritional Services provided a part-time clinical dietitian, and Medical Staff provided a part-time medical director. The residents were assigned to the clinic sometime during their second year. Together they formed the Teen Pregnancy and Parenting Clinic multidisciplinary team.

These four worked together to create a conceptual framework within which the clinic would evolve. Respect for patients as human beings came first. Acknowledging that teenagers' lives do not revolve around a clock or a schedule helped clinic staff to recognize the need to call and confirm appointments rather than to remind. A typical strict visit schedule with appointments every 15 minutes did not appear to be a reasonable format for this clientele. Patients were instead asked to come three or four per hour, and each was seen as long as she arrived before the clinic doors were locked. The patients, as well as their sometimes considerable entourage, were welcomed with cookies and hugs. If staff were teaching birth control to the patient, her friends learned, too.

Support from professional colleagues was hard-won. Many felt TPPC staff were enabling poor behavior. Others complained that the staff were not teaching teenagers to follow the rules of society, such as, "If a patient is more than 20 minutes late for her appointment, she is not seen." An attendance rate of 90% and the achievement of clinical quality goals helped to change people's minds.

Equally important to the clinical framework were the outcome measures the staff hoped to effect. Literature reviews demonstrated the greatest risks in teen pregnancy: premature and low-birthweight infants (Elster et al., 1987; Slap & Schwartz, 1989). Staff were also interested in seeing a reduction in the cesarean section rate and followed these numbers as well. Population descriptors were also collected. Benchmarks were chosen from statistics published by the state, nation, and HMO. At the end of every year TPPC outcomes were published in the Teen Pregnancy and Parenting Newsletter. The data were also presented to the quality oversight committee as well as throughout the organization.

The creation of the nurse clinician role was challenging and at times even difficult. Not being tied to a specific practice, telephone, or physician forced the nurse to be creative about her work. Being nurse clinician to these patients meant coordinating care with many other service providers from schools, the Women, Infants, and Children program (WIC), the welfare department, the probation department, etc. Working as a team taught the TPPC staff that the person or persons with the most knowledge of the patient should have power and use it to act in the best interests of the patient. What the patient told the social worker they may not have shared with the RN, MD, or RD. When all staff conferred, they came closer to the true picture of the needs of the patient.

Many of the nurse clinician duties took her away from her desk. Occasionally, co-workers had difficulty understanding how the nurse was performing her duties if she was not in the clinic. It was the nurse clinician's responsibility to make known what she was doing and why it was important, and to share information about this population. It was also impor-

tant to ensure that co-workers knew where she was and how she could be reached.

In providing population-based management, the TPPC staff sought an algorithm or pathway for care appropriate for their population. Staff of the TPPC looked at critical paths for obstetric patients and adopted recommendations that they tailored to adolescent needs (Winter, Simons, & Patrician, 1990; Cartoot, Klerman & Zazueta, 1991). The staff were concerned about the potential complications of providing group care while attempting to maintain the feel of individualized care. Teenagers were very keen in spotting who really cared and who was being a "phony." The TPPC staff's answer to this problem came in their approach to each patient. All TPPC providers were impassioned in their dedication to this population and were truly happy to see each patient. They cheered their victories and cried with them in defeat. The teenagers knew that this was a safe place for them to come. While all patients received a "recipe" approach, the recipe was modified for each and enhanced by a liberal addition of caring.

Assuming the new nurse clinician role did not change the earlier work substantially. What it did do, however, was provide organizational recognition of the position and made it possible for the nurse clinician to join many relevant committees within the HMO. The nurse clinician had, for example, been attempting to establish a Women's, Infants' and Children's Supplemental Nutrition Program at the HMO. As a result of the pilot, the nurse was finally able to obtain the necessary support within the organization to make this program a reality.

The nurse clinician also had her hours increased to full time and had a medical assistant added to the staff during the pilot. The increased time and help enabled her and her team to perform a retrospective audit comparing TPPC patients with a cohort of adolescents who had received care within the HMO but not through the TPPC service. Those two groups were compared with national, state and HMO outcome data (Fig. 1). In general, the data indicated that, although the TPPC population was at higher risk (they were younger, had more sexually transmitted diseases, and were more ethnically diverse), its outcomes were better.

Although there is peril in comparing statistics of a very small population with those of large populations, the point was well-taken in the organization. These outcomes decreased costs through the decline of

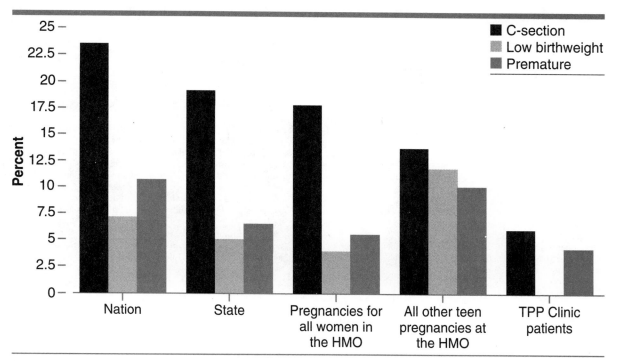

Figure 1
Comparison of outcome measures among pregnant adolescents.

special-care nursery stays. (The cost of a bed in special care averages $1,200/day for the bed alone.)

As these results were made available to other providers in the HMO, there were requests for the TPPC nurse clinician to mentor other staff in the management of this population. The nurse offered in-service education and made herself available to answer individual questions.

In addition to working with the clinic and other providers within the HMO, the nurse clinician networked with other health care agencies and organizations. Knowing what was available in the community was valuable to patient care. As laws affecting the teenage population came before state congressional committees, the nurse clinician testified or lobbied on behalf of the population.

Defining pregnant teenagers as a distinct population with predictable health care needs allowed the HMO to maximize health outcomes and simultaneously to reduce costs for this group.

CONCLUSION

Organizing the predictable health care needs of populations of patients ensured that during this pilot patients received care appropriate to their condition even if their presenting concern was unrelated to their defining population. Broadening the traditional role of staff RNs to become population managers resulted in improved patient outcomes. And by requiring that outcomes be measured, reliance on anecdotal data and intuition was reduced and the common language of outcome measures was assured.

The success of this pilot was due to many factors, one of the most important of which was aligning this work with the critical clinical work of the organization. Practicing in multidisciplinary settings also increased the chances of success. The concept of population management can be applied to myriad settings, including all of those places where care is likely to be given in the future, outside the walls of the hospital.

ACKNOWLEDGMENTS

The authors wish to thank Laurie Bronson, Estee Carton-Bozzi, La Relle Catherman, Jan Crosman, Bev Goldhaber, Joni Hardcastle, Sue Hennessy, Mike Hindmarsh, Michael Madwed, Joy Meya, Joy Nicholson, Eileen Paul, Sherry Shamansky, Mike Wanderer, and Cheryl Wyman.

REFERENCES

Benner, P. (1984). From novice to expert. Menlo Park, Calif.: Addison-Wesley.

Cartoot, V., Klerman, L., Zazueta, V. (1991). The effect and source of prenatal care on care-seeking behavior and pregnancy outcomes among adolescents. Journal of Adolescent Health, 12, 124-129.

Conti, R. (1989). The nurse as case manager. Nursing Connections, 2(1), 55-58.

Cook, S. B. (Ed.), (1990). Handbook of multiple sclerosis. New York: Marcel Decker, Inc.

American Diabetes Association. (1995). ADA clinical practice recommendations. Journal of Clinical and Applied Research and Education, 18 (Suppl 1).

Elster, A., Lamb, M., Tarvane, M., & Ralston, C. (1987). The medical and psychological impact of comprehensive care in adolescent pregnancy and parenthood. Journal of the American Medical Association, 258(9), 1,187-1,192.

Employment agreement by and between Group Health Cooperative of Puget Sound and District 1199 Northwest, National Union of Hospital and Health Care Employees, SEIU AFL-CIO. (1991). Letter of Understanding, July 24, 1991, p. 3.

Expanded Roles Committee. (1995). Nurse clinician information packet for managers.

Jimerson, S. (1986). Expanded practice in psychiatric nursing. Nursing Clinics of North America, 21(3), 527-535.

Maraldo, P. (1989). The nursing solution: Extended use of nurses in all settings can improve quality, reduce costs and better serve the needs of the chronically ill. Health Management Quarterly, 11(4), 18-19.

Rubin, S. (1988). Expanded role nurse, part I: Role theory concepts. Canadian Journal of Nursing Administration, 1(2), 23-27.

Rubin, S. (1988). Expanded role nurse, part II: Role theory concepts. Canadian Journal of Nursing Administration, 1(3), 12-15.

Scheinberg, L. (Ed.). (1987). Multiple sclerosis: A guide for patients and their families (2nd ed.). New York: Raven Press.

Slap, G., & Sandford Schwartz, J. (1989). Risk factors for low birth weight to adolescent mothers. Journal of Adolescent Health. 10, 267-274.

Winter, V., Simons, J., & Patrician, S. (1990). A proposal for obstetric and pediatric management of adolescent pregnancy. Mayo Clinic Proc. 65, 1,061-1,065.

Recommendations of the U.S. Preventive Services Task Force

The U.S. Department of Health and Human Services convened the first U.S. Preventive Services Task Force in 1984. The mandate of this nonfederal, multidisciplinary expert panel was to evaluate the effectiveness of clinical preventive services—screening tests, counseling interventions, immunizations, and chemoprophylactic regimens—based on a systematic review of scientific evidence in published clinical research. The first report of the Task Force, *Guide to Clinical Preventive Services,* was published in 1989. The Task Force updated the information contained in the first report, and the second report of the Task Force containing this update was published in 1996. The following five tables are a summary of the 1996 Task Force recommendations found in the most recent guide.

The tables are organized by age group and provide general guidelines in working with individuals, families, and aggregates to encourage disease prevention by providing suggested baseline measures and counseling necessary for follow-up. The leading causes of mortality and morbidity for each age group and individual risk factors are also important for establishing priorities for the periodic health examination.

The information is recommended for asymptomatic patients only who are receiving routine health care in clinical settings, and needs to be tailored to the needs of the individual patient. The services can, however, be performed during visits for other than preventive reasons, such as illness visits and chronic disease checkups. Because the illness visit may be the only visit for which the patient is reimbursed, it then is important to take this opportunity to discuss prevention.

The notes following each table identify *high-risk categories.* Many of the preventive services in the tables are recommended only for members of high-risk groups and are not considered appropriate in the routine examination of all persons in the age group. The tables are not exhaustive; the frequency or periodicity for health supervision was not addressed by the task force. The Task Force recommends that their recommendations be compared with those of other government agencies and major nongovernmental organizations. The recommendations are time bound, and new recommendations appear in the literature routinely as a result of further research. Therefore, it is important to be aware of the most recent research and to update one's practice based on the most recent literature. It is important to interpret and follow the guidelines as recommended in the fuller text that follows.

Table 1
Birth to 10 Years

Interventions Considered and Recommended for the Periodic Health Examination	Leading Causes of Death
	Conditions originating in perinatal period
	Congenital anomalies
	Sudden infant death syndrome (SIDS)
	Unintentional injuries (non-motor vehicle)
	Motor vehicle injuries

Interventions for the General Population

Screening
Height and weight
Blood pressure
Vision screen (age 3–4 yr)
Hemoglobinopathy screen (birth)[1]
Phenylalanine level (birth)[2]
T_4 and/or TSH (birth)[3]

Counseling
INJURY PREVENTION
Child safety car seats (age <5 yr)
Lap-shoulder belts (age ≥5 yr)
Bicycle helmet; avoid bicycling near traffic
Smoke detector, flame retardant sleepwear
Hot water heater temperature <120–130° F
Window/stair guards, pool fence
Safe storage of drugs, toxic substances, firearms and matches
Syrup of ipecac, poison control phone number
CPR training for parents/caretakers

DIET AND EXERCISE
Breast-feeding, iron-enriched formula and foods (infants and toddlers)

Limit fat and cholesterol; maintain caloric balance; emphasize grains, fruits, vegetables (age ≥2 yr)
Regular physical activity

SUBSTANCE USE
Effects of passive smoking*
Anti-tobacco message*

DENTAL HEALTH
Regular visits to dental care provider*
Floss, brush with fluoride toothpaste daily*
Advice about baby bottle tooth decay*

Immunizations
Diphtheria-tetanus-pertussis (DTP)[4]
Oral poliovirus (OPV)[5]
Measles-mumps-rubella (MMR)[6]
H. influenzae type b (Hib) conjugate[7]
Hepatitis B[8]
Varicella[9]

Chemoprophylaxis
Ocular prophylaxis (birth)

Interventions for High-Risk Populations

Population	Potential Interventions (See detailed high-risk definitions)
Preterm or low birth weight	Hemoglobin/hematocrit (HR1)
Infants of mothers at risk for HIV	HIV testing (HR2)
Low income; immigrants	Hemoglobin/hematocrit (HR1); PPD (HR3)
TB contacts	PPD (HR3)
Native American/Alaska Native	Hemoglobin/hematocrit (HR1); PPD (HR3); hepatitis A vaccine (HR4); pneumococcal vaccine (HR5)
Travelers to developing countries	Hepatitis A vaccine (HR4)
Residents of long-term care facilities	PPD (HR3); hepatitis A vaccine (HR4); influenza vaccine (HR6)
Certain chronic medical conditions	PPD (HR3); pneumococcal vaccine (HR5); influenza vaccine (HR6)
Increased individual or community lead exposure	Blood lead level (HR7)
Inadequate water fluoridation	Daily fluoride supplement (HR8)
Family h/o skin cancer; nevi; fair skin, eyes, hair	Avoid excess/midday sun, use protective clothing* (HR9)

[1]Whether screening should be universal or targeted to high-risk groups will depend on the proportion of high-risk individuals in the screening area, and other considerations (See Ch. 43). [2]If done during first 24 hr of life, repeat by age 2 wk. [3]Optimally between day 2 and 6, but in all cases before newborn nursery discharge. [4]2, 4, 6, and 12–18 mo; once between ages 4–6 yr (DTaP may be used at 15 mo and older.) [5]2, 4, 6–18 mo; once between ages 4–6 yr. [6]12–15 mo and 4–6 yr. [7]2, 4, 6 and 12–15 mo; no dose needed at 6 mo if PRP-OMP vaccine is used for first 2 doses. [8]Birth, 1 mo, 6 mo; or, 0–2 mo later, and 6–18 mo. If not done in infancy: current visit, and 1 and 6 mo later. [9]12–18 mo; or any child without hx of chickenpox or previous immunization. Include information on risk in adulthood, duration of immunity, and potential need for booster doses.

*The ability of clinician counseling to influence this behavior is unproven.

Tables reprinted from U.S. Preventive Services Task Force. Guide to Clinical Preventive Services. Washington, DC: U.S. Government Printing Office, 1996.

Table 1
Birth to 10 Years *Continued*

High-Risk Categories

HR1 = Infants age 6–12 mo who are: living in poverty, black, Native American or Alaska Native, immigrants from developing countries, preterm and low birth weight infants, infants whose principal dietary intake is unfortified cow's milk.

HR2 = Infants born to high-risk mothers whose HIV status is unknown. Women at high risk include: past or present injection drug use; persons who exchange sex for money or drugs, and their sex partners; injection drug-using, bisexual, or HIV-positive sex partners currently or in past; persons seeking treatment for STDs; blood transfusion during 1978–1985.

HR3 = Persons infected with HIV, close contacts with persons with known or suspected TB, persons with medical risk factors associated with TB, immigrants from countries with high TB prevalence, medically underserved low-income populations (including homeless), residents of long-term care facilities.

HR4 = Persons ≥2 yr living in or traveling to areas where the disease is endemic and where periodic outbreaks occur (e.g., countries with high or intermediate endemicity; certain Alaska Native, Pacific Island, Native American, and religious communities). Consider for institutionalized children aged ≥2 yr. Clinicians should also consider local epidemiology.

HR5 = Immunocompetent persons ≥2 yr with certain medical conditions, including chronic cardiac or pulmonary disease, diabetes mellitus, and anatomic asplenia. Immunocompetent persons ≥2 yr living in high-risk environments or social settings (e.g., certain Native American and Alaska Native populations).

HR6 = Annual vaccination of children ≥6 mo who are residents of chronic care facilities or who have chronic cardiopulmonary disorders, metabolic diseases (including diabetes mellitus), hemoglobinopathies, immunosuppression, or renal dysfunction.

HR7 = Children about age 12 mo who: 1) live in communities in which the prevalence of lead levels requiring individual intervention, including residential lead hazard control or chelation, is high or undefined; 2) live in or frequently visit a home built before 1950 with dilapidated paint or with recent or ongoing renovation or remodeling; 3) have close contact with a person who has an elevated lead level; 4) live near lead industry or heavy traffic; 5) live with someone whose job or hobby involves lead exposure; 6) use lead-based pottery; or 7) take traditional ethnic remedies that contain lead.

HR8 = Children living in areas with inadequate water fluoridation (<0.6 ppm).

HR9 = Persons with a family history of skin cancer, a large number of moles, atypical moles, poor tanning ability, or light skin, hair, and eye color.

Table 2
Ages 11–24 Years

Interventions Considered and Recommended for the
    Periodic Health Examination

Leading Causes of Death
    Motor vehicle/other unintentional injuries
    Homicide
    Suicide
    Malignant neoplasms
    Heart diseases

Interventions for the General Population

Screening
Height and weight
Blood pressure[1]
Papanicolaou (Pap) test[2] (females)
Chlamydia screen[3] (females <20 yr)
Rubella serology or vaccination hx[4] (females >12 yr)
Assess for problem drinking

Counseling
INJURY PREVENTION
Lap-shoulder belts
Bicycle/motorcycle/ATV helmets*
Smoke detector*
Safe storage/removal of firearms*

SUBSTANCE USE
Avoid tobacco use
Avoid underage drinking and illicit drug use*
Avoid alcohol/drug use while driving, swimming, boating, etc.*

SEXUAL BEHAVIOR
STD prevention: abstinence;* avoid high-risk behavior;*
    condoms/female barrier with spermicide*
Unintended pregnancy: contraception

DIET AND EXERCISE
Limit fat and cholesterol; maintain caloric balance; emphasize
    grains, fruits, vegetables
Adequate calcium intake (females)
Regular physical activity*

DENTAL HEALTH
Regular visits to dental care provider*
Floss, brush with fluoride toothpaste daily*

Immunizations
Tetanus-diphtheria (Td) boosters (11–16 yr)
Hepatitis B[5]
MMR (11–12 yr)[6]
Varicella (11–12 yr)[7]
Rubella[4] (females >12 yr)

Chemoprophylaxis
Multivitamin with folic acid (females)

Interventions for High-Risk Populations

Population	Potential Interventions (See detailed high-risk definitions)
High-risk sexual behavior	RPR/VDRL (HR1); screen for gonorrhea (female) (HR2), HIV (HR3), chlamydia (female) (HR4); hepatitis A vaccine (HR5)
Injection or street drug use	RPR/VDRL (HR1); HIV screen (HR3); hepatitis A vaccine (HR5); PPD (HR6); advice to reduce infection risk (HR7)
TB contacts; immigrants; low income	PPD (HR6)
Native Americans/Alaska Natives	Hepatitis A vaccine (HR5); PPD (HR6); pneumococcal vaccine (HR8)
Travelers to developing countries	Hepatitis A vaccine (HR5)
Certain chronic medical conditions	PPD (HR6); pneumococcal vaccine (HR8); influenza vaccine (HR9)
Settings where adolescents and young adults congregate	Second MMR (HR10)
Susceptible to varicella, measles, mumps	Varicella vaccine (HR11); MMR (HR12)
Blood transfusion between 1975–1985	HIV screen (HR3)
Institutionalized persons; health care/lab workers	Hepatitis A vaccine (HR5); PPD (HR6); influenza vaccine (HR9)
Family h/o skin cancer; nevi; fair skin, eyes, hair	Avoid excess/midday sun, use protective clothing* (HR13)
Prior pregnancy with neural tube defect	Folic acid 4.0 mg (HR14)
Inadequate water fluoridation	Daily fluoride supplement (HR15)

[1]Periodic BP for persons aged ≥21 yr. [2]If sexually active at present or in the past: q≤3 yr. If sexual history is unreliable, begin Pap tests at age 18 yr. [3]If sexually active. [4]Serologic testing, documented vaccination history, and routine vaccination against rubella (preferably with MMR) are equally acceptable alternatives. [5]If not previously immunized: current visit, 1 and 6 mo later. [6]If no previous second dose of MMR. [7]If susceptible to chickenpox.
*The ability of clinician counseling to influence this behavior is unproven.

Table 2
Ages 11–24 Years *Continued*

High-Risk Categories

HR1 = Persons who exchange sex for money or drugs, and their sex partners; persons with other STDs (including HIV); and sexual contacts of persons with active syphilis. Clinicians should also consider local epidemiology.

HR2 = Females who have: two or more sex partners in the last year; a sex partner with multiple sexual contacts; exchanged sex for money or drugs; or a history of repeated episodes of gonorrhea. Clinicians should also consider local epidemiology.

HR3 = Males who had sex with males after 1975; past or present injection drug use; persons who exchange sex for money or drugs, and their sex partners; injection drug-using, bisexual, or HIV-positive sex partner currently or in the past; blood transfusion during 1978–1985; persons seeking treatment for STDs. Clinicians should also consider local epidemiology.

HR4 = Sexually active females with multiple risk factors including: history of prior STD; new or multiple sex partners; age under 25; nonuse or inconsistent use of barrier contraceptives; cervical ectopy. Clinicians should consider local epidemiology of the disease in identifying other high-risk groups.

HR5 = Persons living in, traveling to, or working in areas where the disease is endemic and where periodic outbreaks occur (e.g., countries with high or intermediate endemicity; certain Alaska Native, Pacific Island, Native American, and religious communities); men who have sex with men; injection or street drug users. Vaccine may be considered for institutionalized persons and workers in these institutions, military personnel, and day-care, hospital, and laboratory workers. Clinicians should also consider local epidemiology.

HR6 = HIV positive, close contacts of persons with known or suspected TB, health care workers, persons with medical risk factors associated with TB, immigrants from countries with high TB prevalence, medically underserved low-income populations (including homeless), alcoholics, injection drug users, and residents of long-term facilities.

HR7 = Persons who continue to inject drugs.

HR8 = Immunocompetent persons with certain medical conditions, including chronic cardiac or pulmonary disease, diabetes mellitus, and anatomic asplenia. Immunocompetent persons who live in high-risk environments or social settings (e.g., certain Native American and Alaska Native populations).

HR9 = Annual vaccination of: residents of chronic care facilities; persons with chronic cardiopulmonary disorders, metabolic diseases (including diabetes mellitus), hemoglobinopathies, immunosuppression, or renal dysfunction; and health care providers for high-risk patients.

HR10 = Adolescents and young adults in settings where such individuals congregate (e.g., high schools and colleges), if they have not previously received a second dose.

HR11 = Healthy persons aged ≥13 yr without a history of chickenpox or previous immunization. Consider serologic testing for presumed susceptible persons aged ≥13 yr.

HR12 = Persons born after 1956 who lack evidence of immunity to measles or mumps (e.g., documented receipt of live vaccine on or after the first birthday, laboratory evidence of immunity, or a history of physician-diagnosed measles or mumps).

HR13 = Persons with a family or personal history of skin cancer, a large number of moles, atypical moles, poor tanning ability, or light skin, hair, and eye color.

HR14 = Women with prior pregnancy affected by neural tube defect who are planning pregnancy.

HR15 = Persons aged <17 yr living in areas with inadequate water fluoridation (<0.6 ppm).

Table 3
Ages 25–64 Years

Interventions Considered and Recommended for the Periodic
  Health Examination

Leading Causes of Death
  Malignant neoplasms
  Heart diseases
  Motor vehicle/other unintentional injuries
  Human immunodeficiency virus (HIV) infection
  Suicide and homicide

Interventions for the General Population

Screening
Blood pressure
Height and weight
Total blood cholesterol (men age 35–64, women age 45–64)
Papanicoulaou (Pap) test (women)[1]
Fecal occult blood test[2] and/or sigmoidoscopy (≥50 yr)
Mammogram ± clinical breast exam[3] (women 50–69 yr)
Assess for problem drinking
Rubella serology or vaccination hx[4] (women of childbearing age)

Counseling
SUBSTANCE USE
Tobacco cessation
Avoid alcohol/drug use while driving, swimming, boating, etc.*

DIET AND EXERCISE
Limit fat and cholesterol; maintain caloric balance; emphasize
  grains, fruits, vegetables
Adequate calcium intake (women)
Regular physical activity*

INJURY PREVENTION
Lap/shoulder belts
Motorcycle/bicycle/ATV helmets*
Smoke detector*
Safe storage/removal of firearms*

SEXUAL BEHAVIOR
STD prevention: avoid high-risk behavior;* condoms/female
  barrier with spermicide*
Unintended pregnancy: contraception

DENTAL HEALTH
Regular visits to dental care provider*
Floss, brush with fluoride toothpaste daily*

Immunizations
Tetanus-diphtheria (Td) boosters
Rubella[4] (women of childbearing age)

Chemoprophylaxis
Multivitamin with folic acid (women planning or capable of preg-
  nancy)
Discuss hormone prophylaxis (peri- and postmenopausal women)

Interventions for High-Risk Populations

Population	Potential Interventions (See detailed high-risk definitions)
High-risk sexual behavior	RPR/VDRL (HR1); screen for gonorrhea (female) (HR2), HIV (HR3), chlamydia (female) (HR4); hepatitis B vaccine (HR5); hepatitis A vaccine (HR6)
Injection or street drug use	RPR/VDRL (HR1); HIV screen (HR3); hepatitis B vaccine (HR5); hepatitis A vaccine (HR6); PPD (HR7); advice to reduce infection risk (HR8)
Low income; TB contacts; immigrants; alcoholics	PPD (HR7)
Native Americans/Alaska Natives	Hepatitis A vaccine (HR6); PPD (HR7); pneumococcal vaccine (HR9)
Travelers to developing countries	Hepatitis B vaccine (HR5); hepatitis A vaccine (HR6)
Certain chronic medical conditions	PPD (HR7); pneumococcal vaccine (HR9); influenza vaccine (HR10)
Blood product recipients	HIV screen (HR3); hepatitis B vaccine (HR5)
Susceptible to measles, mumps, or varicella	MMR (HR11); varicella vaccine (HR12)
Institutionalized persons	Hepatitis A vaccine (HR6); PPD (HR7); pneumococcal vaccine (HR9); influenza vaccine (HR10)
Health care/lab workers	Hepatitis B vaccine (HR5); hepatitis A vaccine (HR6); PPD (HR7); influenza vaccine (HR10)
Family h/o skin cancer; nevi; fair skin, eyes, hair	Avoid excess/midday sun, use protective clothing* (HR13)
Prior pregnancy with neural tube defect	Folic acid 4.0 mg (HR14)

---

[1]Women who are or have been sexually active and who have a cervix: q≤3 yr. [2]Annually. [3]Mammogram q1–2 yr, or mammogram q1–2 yr with annual clinical breast examination. [4]Serologic testing, documented vaccination history, and routine vaccination (preferably with MMR) are equally acceptable.
*The ability of clinician counseling to influence this behavior is unproven.

Table 3
Ages 25–64 Years *Continued*

High-Risk Categories

HR1 = Persons who exchange sex for money or drugs, and their sex partners; persons with other STDs (including HIV); and sexual contacts of persons with active syphilis. Clinicians should also consider local epidemiology.

HR2 = Women who exchange sex for money or drugs, or who have had repeated episodes of gonorrhea. Clinicians should also consider local epidemiology.

HR3 = Men who had sex with males after 1975; past or present injection drug use; persons who exchange sex for money or drugs, and their sex partners; injection drug-using, bisexual, or HIV-positive sex partner currently or in the past; blood transfusion during 1978–1985; persons seeking treatment for STDs. Clinicians should also consider local epidemiology.

HR4 = Sexually active females with multiple risk factors including: history of STD; new or multiple sex partners; nonuse or inconsistent use of barrier contraceptives; cervical ectopy. Clinicians should also consider local epidemiology.

HR5 = Blood product recipients (including hemodialysis patients), persons with frequent occupational exposure to blood or blood products, men who have sex with men, injection drug users and their sex partners, persons with multiple recent sex partners, persons with other STDs (including HIV), travelers to countries with endemic hepatitis B.

HR6 = Persons living in, traveling to, or working in areas where the disease is endemic and where periodic outbreaks occur (e.g., countries with high or intermediate endemicity; certain Alaska Native, Pacific Island, Native American, and religious communities); men who have sex with men; injection or street drug users. Consider for institutionalized persons and workers in these institutions, military personnel, and day-care, hospital, and laboratory workers. Clinicians should also consider local epidemiology.

HR7 = HIV positive, close contacts of persons with known or suspected TB, health care workers, persons with medical risk factors associated with TB, immigrants from countries with high TB prevalence, medically underserved low-income populations (including homeless), alcoholics, injection drug users, and residents of long-term facilities.

HR8 = Persons who continue to inject drugs.

HR9 = Immunocompetent institutionalized persons aged ≥50 yr and immunocompetent persons with certain medical conditions, including chronic cardiac or pulmonary disease, diabetes mellitus, and anatomic asplenia. Immunocompetent persons who live in high-risk environments or social settings (e.g., certain Native American and Alaska Native populations).

HR10 = Annual vaccination of residents of chronic care facilities; persons with chronic cardiopulmonary disorders, metabolic diseases (including diabetes mellitus), hemoglobinopathies, immunosuppression, or renal dysfunction; and health care providers for high-risk patients.

HR11 = Persons born after 1956 who lack evidence of immunity to measles or mumps (e.g., documented receipt of live vaccine on or after the first birthday, laboratory evidence of immunity, or a history of physician-diagnosed measles or mumps).

HR12 = Healthy adults without a history of chickenpox or previous immunization. Consider serologic testing for presumed susceptible adults.

HR13 = Persons with a family or personal history of skin cancer, a large number of moles, atypical moles, poor tanning ability, or light skin, hair, and eye color.

HR14 = Women with prior pregnancy affected by neural tube defect who are planning pregnancy.

Table 4
Age 65 and Older

Interventions Considered and Recommended for the Periodic Health Examination

Leading Causes of Death
Heart diseases
Malignant neoplasms (lung, colorectal, breast)
Cerebrovascular disease
Chronic obstructive pulmonary disease
Pneumonia and influenza

Interventions for the General Population

Screening
Blood pressure
Height and weight
Fecal occult blood test[1] and/or sigmoidoscopy
Mammogram ± clinical breast exam[2] (women ≤69 yr)
Papanicolaou (Pap) test (women)[3]
Vision screening
Assess for hearing impairment
Assess for problem drinking

Counseling
SUBSTANCE USE
Tobacco cessation
Avoid alcohol/drug use while driving, swimming, boating, etc.*

DIET AND EXERCISE
Limit fat and cholesterol; maintain caloric balance; emphasize
   grains, fruits, vegetables
Adequate calcium intake (women)
Regular physical activity*

INJURY PREVENTION
Lap/shoulder belts
Motorcycle and bicycle helmets*

Fall prevention*
Safe storage/removal of firearms*
Smoke detector*
Set hot water heater to <120–130° F*
CPR training for household members

DENTAL HEALTH
Regular visits to dental care provider*
Floss, brush with fluoride toothpaste daily*

SEXUAL BEHAVIOR
STD prevention: avoid high-risk sexual behavior;* use condoms*

Immunizations
Pneumococcal vaccine
Influenza[1]
Tetanus-diphtheria (Td) boosters

Chemoprophylaxis
Discuss hormone prophylaxis (peri- and postmenopausal women)

Interventions for High-Risk Populations

Population	Potential Interventions (See detailed high-risk definitions)
Institutionalized persons	PPD (HR1); hepatitis A vaccine (HR2); amantadine/rimantadine (HR4)
Chronic medical conditions; TB contacts; low income; immigrants; alcoholics	PPD (HR1)
Persons ≥75 yr; or ≥70 yr with risk factors for falls	Fall prevention intervention (HR5)
Cardiovascular disease risk factors	Consider cholesterol screening (HR6)
Family h/o skin cancer; nevi; fair skin, eyes, hair	Avoid excess/midday sun, use protective clothing* (HR7)
Native Americans/Alaska Natives	PPD (HR1); hepatitis A vaccine (HR2)
Travelers to developing countries	Hepatitis A vaccine (HR2); hepatitis B vaccine (HR8)
Blood product recipients	HIV screen (HR3); hepatitis B vaccine (HR8)
High-risk sexual behavior	Hepatitis A vaccine (HR2); HIV screen (HR3); hepatitis B vaccine (HR8); RPR/VDRL (HR9)
Injection or street drug use	PPD (HR1); hepatitis A vaccine (HR2); HIV screen (HR3); hepatitis B vaccine (HR8); RPR/VDRL (HR9); advice to reduce infection risk (HR10)
Health care/lab workers	PPD (HR1); hepatitis A vaccine (HR2); amantadine/rimantadine (HR4); hepatitis B vaccine (HR8)
Persons susceptible to varicella	Varicella vaccine (HR11)

[1]Annually. [2]Mammogram q1–2 yr, or mammogram q1–2 yr with annual clinical breast exam. [3]All women who are or have been sexually active and who have a cervix. Consider discontinuation of testing after age 65 yr if previous regular screening with consistently normal results.

*The ability of clinician counseling to influence this behavior is unproven.

Table 4

Age 65 and Older *Continued*

High-Risk Categories

HR1 = HIV positive, close contacts of persons with known or suspected TB, health care workers, persons with medical risk factors associated with TB, immigrants from countries with high TB prevalence, medically underserved low-income populations (including homeless), alcoholics, injection drug users, and residents of long-term care facilities.

HR2 = Persons living in, traveling to, or working in areas where the disease is endemic and where periodic outbreaks occur (e.g., countries with high or intermediate endemicity; certain Alaska Native, Pacific Island, Native American, and religious communities); men who have sex with men; injection or street drug users. Consider for institutionalized persons and workers in these institutions, and day-care, hospital, and laboratory workers. Clinicians should also consider local epidemiology.

HR3 = Men who had sex with males after 1975; past or present injection drug use; persons who exchange sex for money or drugs, and their sex partners; injection drug-using, bisexual, or HIV-positive sex partner currently or in the past; blood transfusion during 1978–1985; persons seeking treatment for STDs. Clinicians should also consider local epidemiology.

HR4 = Consider for persons who have not received influenza vaccine or are vaccinated late; when the vaccine may be ineffective due to major antigenic changes in the virus; for unvaccinated persons who provide home care for high-risk persons; to supplement protection provided by vaccine in persons who are expected to have a poor antibody response; and for high-risk persons in whom the vaccine is contraindicated.

HR5 = Persons aged 75 years and older; or aged 70–74 with one or more additional risk factors including: use of certain psychoactive and cardiac medications (e.g., benzodiazepines, antihypertensives); use of ≥4 prescription medications; impaired cognition, strength, balance, or gait. Intensive individualized home-based multifactorial fall prevention intervention is recommended in settings where adequate resources are available to deliver such services.

HR6 = Although evidence is insufficient to recommend routine screening in elderly persons, clinicians should consider cholesterol screening on a case-by-case basis for persons ages 65–75 with additional risk factors (e.g., smoking, diabetes, or hypertension).

HR7 = Persons with a family or personal history of skin cancer, a large number of moles, atypical moles, poor tanning ability, or light skin, hair, and eye color.

HR8 = Blood product recipients (including hemodialysis patients), persons with frequent occupational exposure to blood or blood products, men who have sex with men, injection drug users and their sex partners, persons with multiple recent sex partners, persons with other STDs (including HIV), travelers to countries with endemic hepatitis B.

HR9 = Persons who exchange sex for money or drugs and their sex partners; persons with other STDs (including HIV); and sexual contacts of persons with active syphilis. Clinicians should also consider local epidemiology.

HR10 = Persons who continue to inject drugs.

HR11 = Healthy adults without a history of chickenpox or previous immunization. Consider serologic testing for presumed susceptible adults.

Table 5
Pregnant Women*

Interventions Considered and Recommended for the Periodic Health Examination

Interventions for the General Population

Screening

FIRST VISIT

Blood pressure
Hemoglobin/hematocrit
Hepatitis B surface antigen
RPR/VDRL
Chlamydia screen (<25 yr)
Rubella serology or vaccination history
D(Rh) typing, antibody screen
Offer CVS (<13 wk)[1] or amniocentesis (15–18 wk)[1] (age ≥35 yr)
Offer hemoglobinopathy screening
Assess for problem or risk drinking
Offer HIV screening[2]

FOLLOW-UP VISITS

Blood pressure
Urine culture (12–16 wk)

Offer amniocentesis (15–18 wk)[1] (age ≥35 yr)
Offer multiple marker testing[1] (15–18 wk)
Offer serum α-fetoprotein[1] (16–18 wk)

Counseling
Tobacco cessation; effects of passive smoking
Alcohol/other drug use
Nutrition, including adequate calcium intake
Encourage breastfeeding
Lap/shoulder belts
Infant safety car seats
STD prevention: avoid high-risk sexual behavior;† use condoms†

Chemoprophylaxis
Multivitamin with folic acid[3]

Interventions for High-Risk Populations

Population	Potential Interventions (See detailed high-risk definitions)
High-risk sexual behavior	Screen for chlamydia (1st visit) (HR1); gonorrhea (1st visit) (HR2); HIV (1st visit) (HR3); HBsAg (3rd trimester) (HR4); RPR/VDRL (3rd trimester) (HR5)
Blood transfusion 1978–1985	HIV screen (1st visit) (HR3)
Injection drug use	HIV screen (HR3); HBsAg (3rd trimester) (HR4); advice to reduce infection risk (HR6)
Unsensitized D-negative women	D(Rh) antibody testing (24–28 wk) (HR7)
Risk factors for Down syndrome	Offer CVS[1] (1st trimester); amniocentesis[1] (15–18 wk) (HR8)
Prior pregnancy with neural tube defect	Offer amniocentesis[1] (15–18 wk), folic acid 4.0 mg[3] (HR9)

[1]Women with access to counseling and follow-up services, reliable standarized laboratories, skilled high-resolution ultrasound, and, for those receiving serum marker testing, amniocentesis capabilities. [2]Universal screening is recommended for areas (states, counties, or cities) with an increased prevalence of HIV infection among pregnant women. In low-prevalence areas, the choice between universal and targeted screening may depend on other considerations. [3]Beginning at least 1 mo before conception and continuing through the first trimester.

*See Tables 2 and 3 for other preventive services recommended for women of this age group.

†The ability of clinician counseling to influence this behavior is unproven.

Table 5
Pregnant Women* *Continued*

High-Risk Categories

HR1 = Women with history of STD or new or multiple sex partners. Clinicians should also consider local epidemiology. Chlamydia screen should be repeated in 3rd trimester if at continued risk.

HR2 = Women under age 25 with two or more sex partners in the last year, or whose sex partner has multiple sexual contacts; women who exchange sex for money or drugs; and women with a history of repeated episodes of gonorrhea. Clinicians should also consider local epidemiology. Gonorrhea screen should be repeated in the 3rd trimester if at continued risk.

HR3 = In areas where universal screening is not performed due to low prevalence of HIV infection, pregnant women with the following individual risk factors should be screened; past or present injection drug use; women who exchange sex for money or drugs; injection drug-using, bisexual, or HIV-positive sex partner currently or in the past; blood transfusion during 1978–1985; persons seeking treatment for STDs.

HR4 = Women who are initially HBsAg negative who are at high risk due to injection drug use, suspected exposure to hepatitis B during pregnancy, multiple sex partners.

HR5 = Women who exchange sex for money or drugs, women with other STDs (including HIV); and sexual contacts of persons with active syphilis. Clinicians should also consider local epidemiology.

HR6 = Women who continue to inject drugs.

HR7 = Unsensitized D-negative women.

HR8 = Prior pregnancy affected by Down syndrome, advanced maternal age (≥35 yr), known carriage of chromosome rearrangement.

HR9 = Women with previous pregnancy affected by neural tube defect.

Healthy People 2000
Summary List of Health Status Objectives
With 1995 Revisions

The government publication, *Healthy People 2000: National Health Promotion and Disease Prevention Objectives,* contains a national prevention strategy for improving the health of the citizens of the United States over the 1991–2000 decade. Health professionals from numerous disciplines, health advocates, and consumers contributed to the objectives aimed for by the year 2000. These persons testified at public hearings, wrote letters and papers, and organized and attended informational forums. Their commitment is reflected in the objectives, which focus on the prevention of major chronic illnesses, injuries, and infectious diseases. Premature deaths, disease, and disabilities will be prevented as these goals are attained. For all of us and for health policy makers, the strategy makes clear that we must invest in prevention. We can no longer afford to treat diseases and injuries that could have been prevented. The costs are too great in terms of our fiscal resources and in terms of human misery.

To reach the targets set for the year 2000, all Americans, not just health professionals, need to make a concerted effort to change underlying environmental and political conditions to lead to the promotion of health and prevention of disease.

In *Healthy People 2000*, norms for health conditions for the U.S. population and targets for the year 2000 for each health condition were presented by major topic areas. The *Healthy People 2000 Midcourse Review* and 1995 revisions provided a summary report on progress on the objectives and added certain new objectives to focus on particular target groups. Comparing the norm and the targets with conditions in your community can help in making a nursing diagnosis and in planning at the aggregate level. The complete documents are available from U.S. government document offices and bookstores.

22.6   Expand in all States systems for the transfer of health information related to the national health objectives among Federal, State, and local agencies. (Baseline: 30 States reported that they have some capability for transfer of health data, tables, graphs, and maps to Federal, State, and local agencies that collect and analyze data in 1989)

        Note: Information related to the national health objectives includes State and national level baseline data, disease prevention/health promotion evaluation results, and data generated to measure progress.

22.7   Achieve timely release of national surveillance and survey data needed by health professionals and agencies to measure progress toward the national health objectives. (Baseline: 65 percent of data released within 1 year of collection and 24 percent of data were released between 1 and 2 years of collection in 1994)

        Note: Timely release (publication of provisional or final data or public use data tapes) should be based on the use of the data, but is at least within 1 year of the end of data collection.

Source: U.S. Department of Health and Human Services, Public Health Service. *Healthy People 2000 Midcourse Review and 1995 Revisions.* Washington, DC: U.S. Government Printing Office, 1995.

HEALTH STATUS OBJECTIVES

1. PHYSICAL ACTIVITY AND FITNESS

1.1*   Reduce coronary heart disease deaths to no more than 100 per 100,000 people. (Age-adjusted baseline: 135 per 100,000 in 1987)

Special Population Target

Coronary Deaths (per 100,000)		1987 Baseline	2000 Target
1.1a	Blacks	168	115

1.2*   Reduce overweight to a prevalence of no more than 20 percent among people aged 20 and older and no more than 15 percent among adolescents aged 12–19. (Baseline: 26 percent for people aged 20–74 in 1976–80, 24 percent for men and 27 percent for women; 15 percent for adolescents aged 12–19 in 1976–80)

Special Population Targets

Overweight Prevalence		1976–80 Baseline†	2000 Target
1.2a	Low-income women aged 20 and older	37%	25%
1.2b	Black women aged 20 and older	44%	30%
12.c	Hispanic women aged 20 and older		
	Mexican-American women	39%‡	
	Cuban women	34%‡	
	Puerto Rican women	37%‡	
1.2d	American Indians/Alaska Natives	29–75%§	30%
1.2e	People with disabilities	36%††	25%
1.2f	Women with high blood pressure	50%	41%
1.2g	Men with high blood pressure	39%	35%
1.2h	Mexican-American men	30%‡	25%

†Baseline for people aged 20–74 ‡1982-84 baseline for Hispanics aged 20–74 §1984–88 estimates for different tribes ††1985 baseline for people aged 20–74 who report any limitation in activity due to chronic conditions derived from self-reported height and weight

Note: For people aged 20 and older, overweight is defined as body mass index (BMI) equal to or greater than 27.8 for men and 27.3 for women. For adolescents, overweight is defined as BMI equal to or greater than 23.0 for males aged 12–14, 24.3 for males aged 15–17, 25.8 for males aged 18–19, 23.4 for females aged 12–14, 24.8 for females aged 15–17, and 25.7 for females aged 18–19. The values for adults are the gender-specific 85th percentile values of the 1976–80 National Health and Nutrition Examination Survey (NHANES II), reference population 20–29 years of age. For adolescents, overweight was defined using BMI cutoffs based on modified age- and gender-specific 85th percentile values of the NHANES II. BMI is calculated by dividing weight in kilograms by the square of height in meters. The cut points used to define overweight approximate the 120 percent of desirable body weight definition used in the 1990 objectives.

1995 Addition

1.13*   Reduce to no more than 90 per 1,000 people the proportion of all people aged 65 and older who have difficulty in performing two or more personal care activities thereby preserving independence. (Baseline: 111 per 1,000 in 1984–85)

Special Population Targets

Difficulty Performing Self Care (per 1,000)		1984–85 Baseline	2000 Target
1.13a	People aged 85 and older	371	325
1.13b	Blacks aged 65 and older	112	98

Note: Personal care activities are bathing, dressing, using the toilet, getting in and out of bed or chair, and eating.

---

*Indicates duplicate objectives, which appear in two or more priority areas.

2. NUTRITION

2.1* Reduce coronary heart disease deaths to no more than 100 per 100,000 people. (Age-adjusted baseline: 135 per 100,000 in 1987)

Special Population Target

Coronary Deaths (per 100,000)	1987 Baseline	2000 Target
2.1a Blacks	168	115

2.2* Reverse the rise in cancer deaths to achieve a rate of no more than 130 per 100,000 people. (Age-adjusted baseline: 134 per 100,000 in 1987)

Note: In its publications, the National Cancer Institute age-adjusts cancer death rates to the 1970 U.S. population. Using the 1970 standard, the equivalent baseline and target values for this health status objective differ from those presented here.

Special Population Target

Cancer Deaths (per 100,000)	1990 Baseline	2000 Target
2.2a Blacks	182	175

2.3* Reduce overweight to a prevalence of no more than 20 percent among people aged 20 and older and no more than 15 percent among adolescents aged 12–19. (Baseline: 26 percent for people aged 20–74 in 1976–80, 24 percent for men and 27 percent for women; 15 percent for adolescents aged 12–19 in 1976–80)

Special Population Targets

Overweight Prevalence	1976–80 Baseline†	2000 Target
2.3a Low-income women aged 20 and older	37%	25%
2.3b Black women aged 20 and older	44%	30%
2.3c Hispanic women aged 20 and older		
Mexican-American women	39%‡	
Cuban women	34%‡	
Puerto Rican women	37%‡	
2.3d American Indians/Alaska Natives	29–75%§	30%
2.3e People with disabilities	36%††	25%
2.3f Women with high blood pressure	50%	41%
2.3g Men with high blood pressure	39%	35%
2.3h Mexican-American men	30%‡	25%

†Baseline for people aged 20–74 ‡1982-84 baseline for Hispanics aged 20–74 §1984–88 estimates for different tribes ††1985 baseline for people aged 20–74 who report any limitation in activity due to chronic conditions derived from self-reported height and weight

Note: For people aged 20 and older, overweight is defined as body mass index (BMI) equal to or greater than 27.8 for men and 27.3 for women. For adolescents, overweight is defined as BMI equal to or greater than 23.0 for males aged 12–14, 24.3 for males aged 15–17, 25.8 for males aged 18–19, 23.4 for females aged 12–14, 24.8 for females aged 15–17, and 25.7 for females aged 18–19. The values for adults are the gender-specific 85th percentile values of the 1976-80 National Health and Nutrition Examination Survey (NHANES II), reference population 20–29 years of age. For adolescents, overweight was defined using BMI cutoffs based on modified age- and gender-specific 85th percentile values of the NHANES II. BMI is calculated by dividing weight in kilograms by the square of height in meters. The cut points used to define overweight approximate the 120 percent of desirable body weight definition used in the 1990 objectives.

2.4 Reduce growth retardation among low-income children aged 5 and younger to less than 10 percent. (Baseline: 11 percent among low-income children aged 5 and younger in 1988)

Special Population Targets

Prevalence of Short Stature	1988 Baseline	2000 Target
2.4a Low-income black children <age 1	15%	10%
2.4b Low-income Hispanic children <age 1	13%	10%
2.4c Low-income Hispanic children aged 1	16%	10%

Prevalence of Short Stature		*1988 Baseline*	*2000 Target*
2.4d	Low-income Asian/Pacific Islander children aged 1	14%	10%
2.4e	Low-income Asian/Pacific Islander children aged 2–4	16%	10%

Note: Growth retardation is defined as height-for-age below the fifth percentile of children in the National Center for Health Statistics' reference population derived from the 1971–74 NHANES.

1995 Additions

2.22*   Reduce stroke deaths to no more than 20 per 100,000 people. (Age-adjusted baseline: 30.3 per 100,000 in 1987)

Special Population Target

Stroke Deaths (per 100,000)		*1987 Baseline*	*2000 Target*
2.22a	Blacks	52.5	27

2.23*   Reduce colorectal cancer deaths to no more than 13.2 per 100,000 people. (Age-adjusted baseline 14.4 per 100,000 in 1987)

2.24*   Reduce diabetes to an incidence of no more than 2.5 per 1,000 people and a prevalence of 25 per 1,000 people (Baselines: 2.9 per 1,000 in 1986–88; 28 per 1,000 in 1986–88)

Special Population Targets

Prevalence of Diabetes (per 1,000)		*1982–84 Baseline†*	*2000 Target*
2.24a	American Indians/Alaska Natives	69‡	62
2.24b	Puerto Ricans	55	49
2.24c	Mexican Americans	54	49
2.24d	Cuban Americans	36	32
2.24e	Blacks	36§	32

†1982–84 baseline for people aged 20–74 ‡1987 baseline for American Indians/Alaska Natives aged 15 and older §1987 baseline for blacks of all ages

3. TOBACCO

3.1*   Reduce coronary heart disease deaths to no more than 100 per 100,000 people. (Age-adjusted baseline: 135 per 100,000 in 1987)

Special Population Target

Coronary Deaths (per 100,000)		*1987 Baseline*	*2000 Target*
3.1a	Blacks	168	115

3.2*   Slow the rise in lung cancer deaths to achieve a rate of no more than 42 per 100,000 people. (Age-adjusted baseline: 38.5 per 100,000 in 1987)

Special Population Targets

Lung Cancer Deaths (per 100,000)		*1990 Baseline*	*2000 Target*
3.2a	Females	25.6	27
3.2b	Black males	86.1	91

Note: In its publications, the National Cancer Institute age-adjusts cancer death rates to the 1970 U.S. population. Using the 1970 standard, the equivalent baseline and target values for this health status objective differ from those presented here.

3.3   Slow the rise in deaths for the total population from chronic obstructive pulmonary disease to achieve a rate of no more than 25 per 100,000 people. (Age-adjusted baseline: 18.9 per 100,000 in 1987)

Note: Deaths from chronic obstructive pulmonary disease include deaths due to chronic bronchitis, emphysema, asthma, and other chronic obstructive pulmonary diseases and allied conditions.

3.4*   Reduce cigarette smoking to a prevalence of no more than 15 percent among people aged 18 and older. (Baseline: 29 percent in 1987, 31 percent for men and 27 percent for women)

Special Population Targets

Cigarette Smoking Prevalence		1987 Baseline	2000 Target
3.4a	People with a high school education or less aged 20 and older	34%	20%
3.4b	Blue-collar workers aged 18 and older	41%	20%
3.4c	Military personnel	42%†	20%
3.4d	Blacks aged 18 and older	33%	18%
3.4e	Hispanics aged 18 and older	24%	15%
3.4f	American Indians/Alaska Natives	42–70%‡	20%
3.4g	Southeast Asian men	55%§	20%
3.4h	Women of reproductive age	29%††	12%
3.4i	Pregnant women	25%‡‡	10%
3.4j	Women who use oral contraceptives	36%§§	10%

†1988 baseline ‡1979–87 estimates for different tribes §1984–88 baseline ††Baseline for women aged 18–44 ‡‡1985 baseline §§1983 baseline

Note: A cigarette smoker is a person who has smoked at least 100 cigarettes and currently smokes cigarettes. Since 1992, estimates include some-day (intermittent) smokers.

1995 Additions

3.17*   Reduce deaths due to cancer of the oral cavity and pharynx to no more than 10.5 per 100,000 men aged 45–74 and 4.1 per 100,000 women aged 45–74. (Baseline: 13.6 per 100,000 men and 4.8 per 100,000 women in 1987)

3.18*   Reduce stroke deaths to no more than 20 per 100,000 people (Age-adjusted baseline: 30.4 per 100,000 in 1987)

Special Population Target

Stroke Deaths (per 100,000)		1987 Baseline	2000 Target
3.18a	Blacks	52.5	27.0

4. SUBSTANCE ABUSE: ALCOHOL AND OTHER DRUGS

4.1*   Reduce deaths caused by alcohol-related motor vehicle crashes to no more than 5.5 per 100,000 people. (Age-adjusted baseline: 9.8 per 100,000 in 1987)

Special Population Targets

Alcohol-Related Motor Vehicle Crash Deaths (per 100,000)		1987 Baseline	2000 Target
4.1a	American Indian/Alaska Native men	40.4	35.0
4.1b	People aged 15–24	21.5	12.5

4.2   Reduce cirrhosis deaths to no more than 6 per 100,000 people. (Age-adjusted baseline: 9.2 per 100,000 in 1987)

Special Population Targets

Cirrhosis Deaths (per 100,000)		1987 Baseline	2000 Target
4.2a	Black men	22.6	12
4.2b	American Indians/Alaska Natives	20.5	10

		1990 Baseline	*2000 Target*
4.2c	Hispanics	14.0	10
4.3	Reduce drug-related deaths to no more than 3 per 100,000 people. (Age-adjusted baseline: 3.8 per 100,000 in 1987)		

Special Population Targets

	Drug-Related Deaths (per 100,000)	*1990 Baseline*	*2000 Target*
4.3a	Blacks	5.7	3
4.3b	Hispanics	4.3	3
4.4	Reduce drug abuse–related hospital emergency department visits by at least 20 percent. (Baseline: 175.8 per 100,000 people in 1991)		

5. FAMILY PLANNING

5.1   Reduce pregnancies among females aged 15–17 to no more than 50 per 1,000 adolescents. (Baseline: 71.1 pregnancies per 1,000 females aged 15–17 in 1985)

Special Population Targets

	Pregnancies (per 1,000)	*1985 Baseline*	*2000 Target*
5.1a	Black adolescent females aged 15–19	169	120
5.1b	Hispanic adolescent females aged 15–19	143	105

Note: For black and Hispanic adolescent females, baseline data are unavailable for those aged 15–17. The targets for these two populations are based on data for females aged 15–19. If more complete data become available, a 35-percent reduction from baseline figures should be used as the target.

5.2   Reduce to no more than 30 percent the proportion of all pregnancies that are unintended. (Baseline: 56 percent of pregnancies in the previous 5 years were unintended, either unwanted or earlier than desired, in 1988)

Special Population Targets

	Unintended Pregnancies	*1988 Baseline*	*2000 Target*
5.2a	Black females	78.0%	40%
5.2b	Hispanic females	54.9%	30%
5.3	Reduce the prevalence of infertility to no more than 6.5 percent. (Baseline: 7.9 percent of married couples with wives aged 15–44 in 1988)		

Special Population Targets

	Prevalence of Infertility	*1988 Baseline*	*2000 Target*
5.3a	Black couples	12.1%	9%
5.3b	Hispanic couples	12.4%	9%

Note: Infertility is the failure of couples to conceive after 12 months of intercourse without contraception.

6. MENTAL HEALTH AND MENTAL DISORDERS

6.1*   Reduce suicides to no more than 10.5 per 100,000 people. (Age-adjusted baseline: 11.7 per 100,000 in 1987)

Special Population Targets

	Suicides (per 100,000)	*1987 Baseline*	*2000 Target*
6.1a	Youth aged 15–19	10.2	8.2
6.1b	Men aged 20–34	25.2	21.4

Suicides (per 100,000)	1987 Baseline	2000 Target
6.1c White men aged 65 and older	46.7	39.2
6.1d American Indian/Alaska Native men	20.1	17.0

6.2*   Reduce to 1.8 percent the incidence of injurious suicide attempts among adolescents aged 14–17. (Baseline: 2.1 percent in 1990)

Special Population Target

Injurious Suicide Attempts	1991 Baseline	2000 Target
6.2a Female adolescents aged 14–17	2.5	2.0

Note: Data are limited to those suicide attempts that result in hospitalization and are based on self-reports.

6.3   Reduce to less than 17 percent the prevalence of mental disorders among children and adolescents. (Baseline: An estimated 20 percent among youth younger than age 18 in 1992)

Note: The baseline has been revised based on Bird, H.R., et al., *Estimates of the Prevalence of Childhood Maladjustment in a Community Survey in Puerto Rico,* 1988, and Costello, E.J., et al., *Psychiatric Disorders in Pediatric Primary Care: Prevalence Risk Factors,* 1988; in Archives of General Psychiatry, Vol. 45. The ongoing data source will be the Multi-site Study of Service, Use, Need, Outcomes and Costs for Child and Adolescent Populations (UNO-CAP), NIH. The baseline revision has resulted in a year 2000 target revision.

6.4   Reduce the prevalence of mental disorders (exclusive of substance abuse) among adults living in the community to less than 10.7 percent. (Baseline: 1-month point prevalence of 12.6 percent in 1984)

6.5   Reduce to less than 35 percent the proportion of people aged 18 and older who report adverse health effects from stress within the past year. (Baseline: 44.2 percent in 1985)

Special Population Target

	1985 Baseline	2000 Target
6.5a People with disabilities	53.5%	40%

Note: For this objective, people with disabilities are people who report any limitation in activity due to chronic conditions.

1995 Addition

6.15   Reduce the prevalence of depressive (affective) disorders among adults living in the community to less than 4.3 percent. (Baseline: 1 month prevalence of 5.1 percent in 1984)

Special Population Target

Depressive Disorders	1991 Baseline	2000 Target
6.15a Women	6.6%	5.5%

Source: Baseline: Epidemiologic Catchment Area Study, NIH, 1981-1985. Ongoing Source: National Comorbidity Survey, NIH.

7. VIOLENT AND ABUSIVE BEHAVIOR

7.1   Reduce homicides to no more than 7.2 per 100,000 people. (Age-adjusted baseline: 8.5 per 100,000 in 1987)

Special Population Targets

Homicide Rate (per 100,000)	1987 Baseline	2000 Target
7.1a Children aged 3 and younger	3.9	3.1
7.1b Spouses aged 15–34	1.7	1.4
7.1c Black men aged 15–34	91.1	72.4
7.1d Hispanic men aged 15–34	41.3	33.0
7.1e Black women aged 15–34	20.2	16.0
7.1f American Indians/Alaska Natives	11.2	9.0

7.2*   Reduce suicides to no more than 10.5 per 100,000 people. (Age-adjusted baseline: 11.7 per 100,000 in 1987)

Special Population Targets

Suicides (per 100,000)	1987 Baseline	2000 Target
7.2a Youth aged 15–19	10.2	8.2
7.2b Men aged 20–34	25.2	21.4
7.2c White men aged 65 and older	46.7	39.2
7.2d American Indian/Alaska Native men	20.1	17.0

7.3   Reduce firearm-related deaths to no more than 11.6 per 100,000 people from major causes. (Baseline: 14.6 firearm-related deaths in 1990)

Special Population Target

Firearm-Related Deaths (per 100,000)	1990 Baseline	2000 Target
7.3a Blacks	33.4	30.0

7.4   Reverse to less than 22.6 per 1,000 children the rising incidence of maltreatment of children younger than age 18. (Baseline: 22.6 per 1,000 in 1986)

Type-Specific Targets

Incidence of Types of Maltreatment (per 1,000)	1986 Baseline	2000 Target
7.4a Physical abuse	4.9	<4.9
7.4b Sexual abuse	2.1	<2.1
7.4c Emotional abuse	3.0	<3.0
7.4d Neglect	14.6	<14.6

7.5   Reduce physical abuse directed at women by male partners to no more than 27 per 1,000 couples. (Baseline: 30 per 1,000 in 1985)

7.6   Reduce assault injuries among people aged 12 and older to no more than 8.7 per 1,000 people. (Baseline: 9.7 per 1,000 in 1986)

7.7   Reduce rape and attempted rape of women aged 12 and older to no more than 108 per 100,000 women. (Baseline: 120 per 100,000 in 1986)

Special Population Target

Incidence of Rape and Attempted Rape (per 100,000)	1986 Baseline	2000 Target
7.7a Women aged 12–34	250	225

7.8*   Reduce by 15 percent the incidence of injurious suicide attempts among adolescents aged 14–17. (Baseline: 2.1 percent in 1991)

Special Population Target

Injurious Suicide Attempts	1986 Baseline	2000 Target
7.8a Female adolescents aged 14–17	2.5%	2.0%

Note: Data are limited to those suicide attempts that result in hospitalization and are based on self-reports.

8. EDUCATIONAL AND COMMUNITY-BASED PROGRAMS

8.1*   Increase years of healthy life to at least 65 years. (Baseline: An estimated 64 years in 1990)

Special Population Targets

	Years of Healthy Life	1990 Baseline	2000 Target
8.1a	Blacks	56.0	60
8.1b	Hispanics	64.8	65
8.1c	People aged 65 and older	11.9†	14†

†Years of healthy life remaining at age 65

Note: Years of healthy life (also referred to as quality-adjusted life years) is a summary measure of health that combines mortality (quantity of life) and morbidity and disability (quality of life) into a single measure.

9. UNINTENTIONAL INJURIES

9.1   Reduce deaths caused by unintentional injuries to no more than 29.3 per 100,000 people. (Age-adjusted baseline: 34.7 per 100,000 in 1987)

Special Population Targets

	Deaths Caused By Unintentional Injuries (per 100,000)	1987 Baseline	2000 Target
9.1a	American Indians/Alaska Natives	66.0	53.0
9.1b	Black males	64.9	51.9
9.1c	White males	53.6	42.9
		1990 Baseline	2000 Target
9.1d	Mexican-American males	53.3	43.0

9.2   Reduce nonfatal unintentional injuries so that hospitalizations for this condition are no more than 754 per 100,000 people. (Baseline: 887 per 100,000 in 1988)

Special Population Target

	Nonfatal Injuries (per 100,000)	1991 Baseline	2000 Target
9.2a	Black males	1,007	856

9.3   Reduce deaths caused by motor vehicle crashes to no more than 1.5 per 100 million vehicle miles traveled (VMT) and 14.2 per 100,000 people. (Baseline: 2.4 per 100 million vehicle miles traveled and 19.2 per 100,000 people in 1987)

Special Population Targets

	Deaths Caused By Motor Vehicle Crashes (per 100,000)	1987 Baseline	2000 Target
9.3a	Children aged 14 and younger	6.2	4.4
9.3b	Youth aged 15–24	36.9	26.8
9.3c	People aged 70 and older	22.6	20.0
9.3d	American Indians/Alaska Natives	37.7	32.0
		1990 Baseline	2000 Target
9.3g	Mexican Americans	20.9	18.0

Type-Specific Targets

	Deaths Caused By Motor Vehicle Crashes	1987 Baseline	2000 Target
9.3e	Motorcyclists	40.9/100 million VMT 1.7/100,000	25.6/100 million VMT 0.9/100,000
9.3f	Pedestrians	2.8/100,000	2.0/100,000

9.4　Reduce deaths from falls and fall-related injuries to no more than 2.3 per 100,000 people. (Age-adjusted baseline: 2.7 per 100,000 in 1987)

Special Population Targets

Deaths From Falls and Fall-Related Injuries (per 100,000)	1987 Baseline	2000 Target
9.4a　People aged 65–84	18.1	14.4
9.4b　People aged 85 and older	133.0	105.0
9.4c　Black men aged 30–69	8.1	5.6
	1990 Baseline	2000 Target
9.4d　American Indians/Alaska Natives	3.2	2.8

9.5　Reduce drowning deaths to no more than 1.3 per 100,000 people. (Age-adjusted baseline: 2.1 per 100,000 in 1987)

Special Population Targets

Drowning Deaths (per 100,000)	1987 Baseline	2000 Target
9.5a　Children aged 4 and younger	4.2	2.3
9.5b　Men aged 15–34	4.5	2.5
9.5c　Black males	6.6	3.6
	1990 Baseline	2000 Target
9.5d　American Indians/Alaska Natives	4.3	2.0

9.6　Reduce residential fire deaths to no more than 1.2 per 100,000 people. (Age-adjusted baseline: 1.5 per 100,000 in 1987)

Special Population Targets

Residential Fire Deaths (per 100,000)	1987 Baseline	2000 Target
9.6a　Children aged 4 and younger	4.4	3.3
9.6b　People aged 65 and older	4.4	3.3
9.6c　Black males	5.7	4.3
9.6d　Black females	3.4	2.6
	1990 Baseline	2000 Target
9.6f　American Indians/Alaska Natives	2.1	1.4
9.6g　Puerto Ricans	2.4	2.0

Type-Specific Target

	1983 Baseline	2000 Target
9.6e　Residential fire deaths caused by smoking	26%	8%

9.7　Reduce hip fractures among people aged 65 and older so that hospitalizations for this condition are no more than 607 per 100,000. (Baseline: 714 per 100,000 in 1988)

Special Population Target

Hip Fractures (per 100,000)	1988 Baseline	2000 Target
9.7a　White women aged 85 and older	2,721	2,177

9.8　Reduce nonfatal poisoning to no more than 88 emergency department treatments per 100,000 people. (Baseline: 108 per 100,000 in 1986)

Special Population Target

Nonfatal Poisoning (per 100,000)		1986 Baseline	2000 Target
9.8a	Among children aged 4 and younger	648	520

9.9   Reduce nonfatal head injuries so that hospitalizations for this condition are no more than 106 per 100,000 people. (Baseline: 118 per 100,000 in 1988)

9.10   Reduce nonfatal spinal cord injuries so that hospitalizations for this condition are no more than 5 per 100,000 people. (Baseline: 5.3 per 100,000 in 1988)

Special Population Target

Nonfatal Spinal Cord Injuries (per 100,000)		1988 Baseline	2000 Target
9.10a	Males	9.6	7.1

1995 Additions

9.23*   Reduce deaths caused by alcohol-related motor vehicle crashes to no more than 5.5 per 100,000 people. (Baseline: 9.8 per 100,000 in 1987)

10. OCCUPATIONAL SAFETY AND HEALTH

10.1   Reduce deaths from work-related injuries to no more than 4 per 100,000 full-time workers. (Baseline: Average of 6 per 100,000 during 1983–87)

Special Population Targets

Work-Related Deaths (per 100,000)		1983-87 Average	2000 Target
10.1a	Mine workers	30.3	21.0
10.1b	Construction workers	25.0	17.0
10.1c	Transportation workers	15.2	10.0
10.1d	Farm workers	14.0	9.5

10.2   Reduce work-related injuries resulting in medical treatment, lost time from work, or restricted work activity to no more than 6 cases per 100 full-time workers. (Baseline: 7.7 per 100 in 1983–87)

Special Population Targets

Work-Related Injuries (per 100)		1983-87 Average	2000 Target
10.2a	Construction workers	14.9	10.0
10.2b	Nursing and personal care workers	12.7	9.0
10.2c	Farm workers	12.4	8.0
10.2d	Transportation workers	8.3	6.0
10.2e	Mine workers	8.3	6.0
		1992 Baseline	2000 Target
10.2f	Adolescent workers	5.8	3.8

10.3   Reduce cumulative trauma disorders to an incidence of no more than 60 cases per 100,000 full-time workers. (Baseline: 100 per 100,000 in 1987)

Special Population Targets

Cumulative Trauma Disorders (per 100,000)		1987 Baseline	2000 Target
10.3a	Manufacturing industry workers	355	150
10.3b	Meat product workers	3,920	2,000

10.4   Reduce occupational skin disorders or diseases to an incidence of no more than 55 per 100,000 full-time workers. (Baseline: Average of 64 per 100,000 during 1983–87)

1995 Additions

10.16   Reduce deaths from work-related homicides to no more than 0.5 per 100,000 full-time workers (Baseline: Average of 0.7 per 100,000 during 1980–1989)

Sources: National Traumatic Occupational Fatality (NTOF) Surveillance System, CDC in the numerator; U.S. Bureau of Census, Current Population Survey in the denominator. The U.S. Department of Labor, Bureau of Labor Statistics, Census of Fatal Occupational Injuries will also be used for tracking this objective.

11. ENVIRONMENTAL HEALTH

11.1   Reduce asthma morbidity, as measured by a reduction in asthma hospitalizations to no more than 160 per 100,000 people. (Baseline: 188 per 100,000 in 1987)

Special Population Targets

Asthma Hospitalizations (per 100,000)	1987 Baseline	2000 Target
11.1a Blacks and other nonwhites	334	265
11.1b Children	284†	225
	1988 Baseline	2000 Target
11.1c Women	229	183

†Children aged 14 and younger

11.2*   Reduce the prevalence of serious mental retardation among school-aged children to no more than 2 per 1,000 children. (Baseline: 2.7 per 1,000 children aged 10 in 1985–88)

Note: Serious mental retardation is defined as an Intelligence Quotient (I.Q.) less than 50. This includes individuals defined by the American Association of Mental Retardation as profoundly retarded (I.Q. of 20 or less), severely retarded (I.Q. of 21–35), and moderately retarded (I.Q. of 36–50).

11.3   Reduce outbreaks of waterborne disease from infectious agents and chemical poisoning to no more than 11 per year. (Baseline: 16 outbreaks in 1988)

Type-Specific Target

Average Annual Number of Waterborne Disease Outbreaks	1988 Baseline	2000 Target
11.3a People served by community water systems	4	2

Note: Includes only outbreaks from water intended for drinking. Community water systems are public or investor-owned water systems that serve large or small communities, subdivisions, or trailer parks with at least 15 service connections or 25 year-round residents.

11.4   Reduce the prevalence of blood lead levels exceeding 15 μg/dL and 25 μg/dL among children aged 6 months–5 years to no more than 300,000 and zero, respectively. (Baseline: An estimated 3 million children had levels exceeding 15 μg/dL, and 234,000 had levels exceeding 25 μg/dL, in 1984)

Special Population Targets

Prevalence of Blood Lead Levels	1984 Baseline	2000 Target
11.4a Inner-city low-income black children (annual family income <$6,000 in 1984 dollars)		
exceeding 15 mg/dL	234,900	75,000
exceeding 25 μg/dL	36,700	0

12. FOOD AND DRUG SAFETY

12.1   Reduce infections caused by key foodborne pathogens to incidences of no more than:

Disease (per 100,000)	1987 Baseline	2000 Target
Salmonella species	18.0	16.0
Campylobacter jejuni	50.0	25.0
Escherichia coli O157:H7	8.0	4.0
Listeria monocytogenes	0.7	0.5

12.2   Reduce outbreaks of infections due to *Salmonella enteritidis* to fewer than 25 outbreaks yearly. (Baseline: 77 outbreaks in 1989)

13. ORAL HEALTH

13.1   Reduce dental caries (cavities) so that the proportion of children with one or more caries (in permanent or primary teeth) is no more than 35 percent among children aged 6–8 and no more than 60 percent among adolescents aged 15. (Baseline: 54 percent of children aged 6–8 in 1986–87; 78 percent of adolescents aged 15 in 1986–87)

Special Population Targets

	Dental Caries Prevalence	1986–87 Baseline	2000 Target
13.1a	Children aged 6–8 whose parents have less than high school education	70%	45%
13.1b	American Indian/Alaska Native children aged 6–8	92%† 52%‡	45%
13.1c	Black children aged 6–8	56%	40%
13.1d	American Indian/Alaska Native adolescents aged 15	93%‡	70%

†In primary teeth in 1983–84 ‡In permanent teeth in 1983–84

13.2   Reduce untreated dental caries so that the proportion of children with untreated caries (in permanent or primary teeth) is no more than 20 percent among children aged 6–8 and no more than 15 percent among adolescents aged 15. (Baseline: 28 percent of children aged 6–8 in 1986; 24 percent of adolescents aged 15 in 1986–87)

Special Population Targets

	Untreated Dental Caries Among:	1986–87 Baseline	2000 Target
13.2a	Children aged 6–8 whose parents have less than high school education	43%	30%
13.2b	American Indian/Alaska Native children aged 6–8	64%†	35%
13.2c	Black children aged 6–8	36%	25%
13.2d	Hispanic children aged 6–8	36%‡	25%
	Among:		
13.2e	Adolescents aged 15 whose parents have less than a high school education	41%	25%
13.2f	American Indian/Alaska Native adolescents aged 15	84%†	40%
13.2g	Black adolescents aged 15	38%	20%
13.2h	Hispanic adolescents aged 15	31–47%‡	25%

†1983–84 baseline ‡1982–84 baseline

13.3   Increase to at least 45 percent the proportion of people aged 35–44 who have never lost a permanent tooth due to dental caries or periodontal diseases. (Baseline: 31 percent of employed adults had never lost a permanent tooth for any reason in 1985–86)

Note: Never lost a permanent tooth is having 28 natural teeth exclusive of third molars.

13.4   Reduce to no more than 20 percent the proportion of people aged 65 and older who have lost all of their natural teeth. (Baseline: 36 percent in 1986)

Special Population Targets

Complete Tooth Loss Prevalence		*1986 Baseline*	*2000 Target*
13.4a	Low-income people (annual family income <$15,000)	46%	25%
		1991 Baseline	*2000 Target*
13.4b	American Indians/Alaska Natives	42%	20%

13.5   Reduce the prevalence of gingivitis among people aged 35–44 to no more than 30 percent. (Baseline: 41 percent in 1985–86)

Special Population Targets

Gingivitis Prevalence		*1985 Baseline*	*2000 Target*
13.5a	Low-income people (annual family income <$12,500)	50%	35%
13.5b	American Indians/Alaska Natives	95%†	50%
13.5c	Hispanics	50%	
	Mexican Americans	74%‡	
	Cubans	79%‡	
	Puerto Ricans	82%‡	

†1983–84 baseline ‡1982–84 baseline

13.6   Reduce destructive periodontal diseases to a prevalence of no more than 15 percent among people aged 35–44. (Baseline: 25 percent in 1985–86)

Note: Destructive periodontal disease is one or more sites with 4 millimeters or greater loss of tooth attachment.

13.7*   Reduce deaths due to cancer of the oral cavity and pharynx to no more than 10.5 per 100,000 men aged 45–74 and 4.1 per 100,000 women aged 45–74. (Baseline: 13.6 per 100,000 men and 4.8 per 100,000 women in 1987)

Special Population Targets

Oral Cancer Deaths (per 100,000)		*1990 Baseline*	*2000 Target*
13.7a	Black males aged 45–74	29.4	26.0
13.7b	Black females aged 45–74	6.9	6.9

14. MATERNAL AND INFANT HEALTH

14.1   Reduce the infant mortality rate to no more than 7 per 1,000 live births. (Baseline: 10.1 per 1,000 live births in 1987)

Special Population Targets

Infant Mortality (per 1,000 live births)		*1987 Baseline*	*2000 Target*
14.1a	Blacks	18.8	11.0
14.1b	American Indians/Alaska Natives	13.4†	8.5
14.1c	Puerto Ricans	12.9†	8.0

Type-Specific Targets

Neonatal and Postneonatal Mortality (per 1,000 live births)		*1987 Baseline*	*2000 Target*
14.1d	Neonatal mortality	6.5	4.5
14.1e	Neonatal mortality among blacks	12.3	7.0

Neonatal and Postneonatal Mortality *(per 1,000 live births)*	*1987 Baseline*	*2000 Target*
14.1f Neonatal mortality among Puerto Ricans	8.6†	5.2
14.1g Postneonatal mortality	3.6	2.5
14.1h Postneonatal mortality among blacks	6.4	4.0
14.1i Postneonatal mortality among American Indians/Alaska Natives	7.0†	4.0
14.1j Postneonatal mortality among Puerto Ricans	4.3†	2.8

†1984 baseline

Note: Infant mortality is deaths of infants under 1 year; neonatal mortality is deaths of infants under 28 days; and postneonatal mortality is deaths of infants aged 28 days up to 1 year.

14.2   Reduce the fetal death rate (20 or more weeks of gestation) to no more than 5 per 1,000 live births plus fetal deaths. (Baseline: 7.6 per 1,000 live births plus fetal deaths in 1987)

Special Population Target

Fetal Deaths	*1987 Baseline*	*2000 Target*
14.2a Blacks	13.1‡	7.5‡

‡Per 1,000 live births plus fetal deaths

14.3   Reduce the maternal mortality rate to no more than 3.3 per 100,000 live births. (Baseline: 6.6 per 100,000 in 1987)

Special Population Target

Maternal Mortality (per 100,000 live births)	*1987 Baseline*	*2000 Target*
14.3a Blacks	14.9	5.0

Note: The objective uses the maternal mortality rate as defined by the National Center for Health Statistics. However, if other sources of maternal mortality data are used, a 50-percent reduction in maternal mortality is the intended target.

14.4   Reduce the incidence of fetal alcohol syndrome to no more than 0.12 per 1,000 live births. (Baseline: 0.22 per 1,000 live births in 1987)

Special Population Targets

Fetal Alcohol Syndrome (per 1,000 live births)	*1987 Baseline*	*2000 Target*
14.4a American Indians/Alaska Natives	4.0	2.0
14.4b Blacks	0.8	0.4

1995 Addition

14.17   Reduce the incidence of spina bifida and other neural tube defects to 3 per 10,000 live births. (Baseline: 6 per 10,000 in 1990)
Source: Birth Defect Monitoring System, CDC.

15. HEART DISEASE AND STROKE

15.1*   Reduce coronary heart disease deaths to no more than 100 per 100,000 people. (Age-adjusted baseline: 135 per 100,000 in 1987)

Special Population Target

Coronary Deaths (per 100,000)	*1987 Baseline*	*2000 Target*
15.1a Blacks	168	115

15.2*   Reduce stroke deaths to no more than 20 per 100,000 people. (Age-adjusted baseline: 30.4 per 100,000 in 1987)

Special Population Target

Stroke Deaths (per 100,000)	1987 Baseline	2000 Target
15.2a Blacks	52.5	27

15.3   Reverse the increase in end-stage renal disease (requiring maintenance dialysis or transplantation) to attain an incidence of no more than 13 per 100,000. (Baseline: 14.4 per 100,000 in 1987)

Special Population Target

ESRD Incidence (per 100,000)	1987 Baseline	2000 Target
15.3a Blacks	34.0	30

16. CANCER

16.1*   Reverse the rise in cancer deaths to achieve a rate of no more than 130 per 100,000 people. (Age-adjusted baseline: 134 per 100,000 in 1987)

Special Population Target

Cancer Deaths (per 100,000)	1990 Baseline	2000 Target
16.1a Blacks	182	175

16.2*   Slow the rise in lung cancer deaths to achieve a rate of no more than 42 per 100,000 people. (Age-adjusted baseline: 38.5 per 100,000 in 1987)

Special Population Targets

Lung Cancer Deaths (per 100,000)	1990 Baseline	2000 Target
16.2a Females	25.6	27
16.2b Black males	86.1	91

16.3   Reduce breast cancer deaths to no more than 20.6 per 100,000 women. (Age-adjusted baseline: 23.0 per 100,000 in 1987)

Special Population Target

Breast Cancer Deaths (per 100,000)	1990 Baseline	2000 Target
16.3a Black females	27.5	25

16.4   Reduce deaths from cancer of the uterine cervix to no more than 1.3 per 100,000 women. (Age-adjusted baseline: 2.8 per 100,000 in 1987)

Special Population Targets

Cervical Cancer Deaths (per 100,000)	1990 Baseline	2000 Target
16.4a Black females	5.9	3
16.4b Hispanic females	3.6†	2

16.5*   Reduce colorectal cancer deaths to no more than 13.2 per 100,000 people. (Age-adjusted baseline: 14.7 per 100,000 in 1987)

Special Population Target

Colorectal Cancer Deaths (per 100,000)	1990 Baseline	2000 Target
16.5a Blacks	18.1	16.5

1995 Addition

16.17*   Reduce deaths due to cancer of the oral cavity and pharynx to no more than 10.5 per 100,000 men aged 45–74 and 4.1 per 100,000 women aged 45–74. (Baseline: 13.6 per 100,000 men and 4.8 per 100,000 women in 1987)

Special Population Targets

Oral Cancer Deaths (per 100,000)		1990 Baseline	2000 Target
16.17a	Black males aged 45–74	29.4	26.0
16.17b	Black females aged 45–74	6.9	6.9

17. DIABETES AND CHRONIC DISABLING CONDITIONS

17.1*   Increase years of healthy life to at least 65 years. (Baseline: An estimated 64 years in 1990)

Special Population Targets

Years of Healthy Life		1990 Baseline	2000 Target
17.1a	Blacks	56.0	60
17.1b	Hispanics	64.8	65
17.1c	People aged 65 and older	11.9†	14†

†Years of healthy life remaining at age 65. Years of healthy life (also referred to as quality-adjusted life years) is a summary measure of health that combines mortality (quantity of life) and morbidity and disability (quality of life) into a single measure.

17.2   Reduce to no more than 8 percent the proportion of people who experience a limitation in major activity due to chronic conditions. (Baseline: 9.4 percent in 1988)

Special Population Targets

Prevalence of Disability		1988 Baseline	2000 Target
17.2a	Low-income people (annual family income <$10,000 in 1988)	18.9%	15%
17.2b	American Indians/Alaska Natives	13.4%†	11%
17.2c	Blacks	11.2%	9%

†1983-85 baseline

		1991 Baseline	2000 Target
17.2d	Puerto Ricans	11.7%	10%

Note: Major activity refers to the usual activity for one's age-gender group whether it is working, keeping house, going to school, or living independently. Chronic conditions are defined as conditions that either (1) were first noticed 3 or more months ago, or (2) belong to a group of conditions such as heart disease and diabetes, which are considered chronic regardless of when they began.

17.3   Reduce to no more than 90 per 1,000 people the proportion of all people aged 65 and older who have difficulty in performing two or more personal care activities, thereby preserving independence. (Baseline: 111 per 1,000 in 1984–85)

Special Population Targets

Difficulty Performing Self-care Activities (per 1,000)		1984–85 Baseline	2000 Target
17.3a	People aged 85 and older	371	325
17.3b	Blacks aged 65 and older	112	98

Note: Personal care activities are bathing, dressing, using the toilet, getting in and out of bed or chair, and eating.

17.4   Reduce to no more than 10 percent the proportion of people with asthma who experience activity limitation. (Baseline: Average of 19.4 percent during 1986–88)

Special Population Target

Asthmatics with Activity Limitations	1989–1991 Baseline	2000 Target
17.4a Blacks	30.5%	19%
17.4b Puerto Ricans	51.5%	22%

Note: Activity limitation refers to any self-reported limitation in activity attributed to asthma.

17.5   Reduce activity limitation due to chronic back conditions to a prevalence of no more than 19 per 1,000 people. (Baseline: Average of 21.9 per 1,000 during 1986-88)

Note: Chronic back conditions include intervertebral disk disorders, curvature of the back or spine, and other self-reported chronic back impairments such as permanent stiffness or deformity of the back or repeated trouble with the back. Activity limitation refers to any self-reported limitation in activity attributed to a chronic back condition.

17.6   Reduce significant hearing impairment to a prevalence of no more than 82 per 1,000 people. (Baseline: Average of 88.9 per 1,000 during 1986–88)

Special Population Target

Hearing Impairment (per 1,000)	1986–88 Baseline	2000 Target
17.6a People aged 45 and older	203	180

Note: Hearing impairment covers the range of hearing deficits from mild loss in one ear to profound loss in both ears. Generally, inability to hear sounds at levels softer (less intense) than 20 decibels (dB) constitutes abnormal hearing. Significant hearing impairment is defined as having hearing thresholds for speech poorer than 25 dB. However, for this objective, self-reported hearing impairment (i.e., deafness in one or both ears or any trouble hearing in one or both ears) will be used as a proxy measure for significant hearing impairment.

17.7   Reduce significant visual impairment to a prevalence of no more than 30 per 1,000 people. (Baseline: Average of 34.5 per 1,000 during 1986–88)

Special Population Target

Visual Impairment (per 1,000)	1986–88 Baseline	2000 Target
17.7a People aged 65 and older	87.7	70

Note: Significant visual impairment is generally defined as a permanent reduction in visual acuity and/or field of vision which is not correctable with eyeglasses or contact lenses. Severe visual impairment is defined as inability to read ordinary newsprint even with corrective lenses. For this objective, self-reported blindness in one or both eyes and other self-reported visual impairments (i.e., any trouble seeing with one or both eyes even when wearing glasses or colorblindness) will be used as a proxy measure for significant visual impairment.

17.8*   Reduce the prevalence of serious mental retardation among school-aged children to no more than 2 per 1,000 children. (Baseline: 2.7 per 1,000 children aged 10 in 1985–88)

Note: Serious mental retardation is defined as an Intelligence Quotient (I.Q.) less than 50. This includes individuals defined by the American Association of Mental Retardation as profoundly retarded (I.Q. of 20 or less), severely retarded (I.Q. of 21–35), and moderately retarded (I.Q. of 36–50).

17.9   Reduce diabetes-related deaths to no more than 34 per 100,000 people. (Age-adjusted baseline: 38 per 100,000 in 1986)

Special Population Targets

Diabetes-Related Deaths (per 100,000)	1986 Baseline	2000 Target
17.9a Blacks	67.0	58
17.9b American Indians/Alaska Natives	46.0	41
	1990 Baseline	*2000 Target*
17.9c Mexican Americans	55.9	50
17.9d Puerto Ricans	47.0	42

Note: Diabetes-related deaths refer to deaths from diabetes as an underlying or contributing cause.

17.10   Reduce the most severe complications of diabetes as follows:

Complications Among People With Diabetes	1988 Baseline	2000 Target
End-stage renal disease	1.5/1,000†	1.4/1,000
Blindness	2.2/1,000	1.4/1,000
Lower extremity amputation	8.2/1,000†	4.9/1,000
Perinatal mortality‡	5%	2%
Major congenital malformations‡	8%	4%

†1987 baseline ‡Among infants of women with established diabetes

Special Population Targets for ESRD

	ESRD Due to Diabetes (per 1,000)	1983–86 Baseline	2000 Target
17.10a	Blacks with diabetes	2.2	2.0
17.10b	American Indians/Alaska Natives with diabetes	2.1	1.9

Special Population Target for Amputations

	Lower Extremity Amputations Due to Diabetes (per 1,000)	1984–87 Baseline	2000 Target
17.10c	Blacks with diabetes	10.2	6.1

Note: End-stage renal disease (ESRD) is defined as requiring maintenance dialysis or transplantation and is limited to ESRD due to diabetes. Blindness refers to blindness due to diabetic eye disease.

17.11*   Reduce diabetes to an incidence of no more than 2.5 per 1,000 people and a prevalence of no more than 25 per 1,000 people. (Baselines: 2.9 per 1,000 in 1987; 28 per 1,000 in 1987)

Special Population Targets

	Prevalence of Diabetes (per 1,000)	1982–84 Baseline†	2000 Target
17.11a	American Indians/Alaska Natives	69‡	62
17.11b	Puerto Ricans	55	49
17.11c	Mexican Americans	54	49
17.11d	Cuban Americans	36	32
17.11e	Blacks	36§	32

†1982–84 baseline for people aged 20–74 ‡1987 baseline for American Indians/Alaska Natives aged 15 and older §1987 baseline for blacks of all ages

1995 Additions

17.21   Reduce the prevalence of peptic ulcer disease to no more than 18 per 1,000 people aged 18 and older by preventing its recurrence. (Baseline: 19.9 per 1,000 in 1991)
Source: National Health Interview Survey, CDC

18. HIV INFECTION

18.1   Confine annual incidence of diagnosed AIDS cases to no more than 43 per 100,000 population. (Baseline: 17.0 per 100,000 in 1989)

	Rates of AIDS Cases (per 100,000)	1989 Baseline	2000 Target
18.1a	Men who have sex with men (number of cases)	27,000	No more than 48,000
18.1b	Blacks	44.4	No more than 136 per 100,000
18.1c	Hispanics	34.9	No more than 76 per 100,000
18.1d	Women	3.5	No more than 13 per 100,000

Rates of AIDS Cases (per 100,000)	*1989 Baseline*	*2000 Target*
18.1e Injecting drug users (number of cases)	10,300	No more than 25,000

Note: Cases are by year of diagnosis and are corrected for delays in reporting and underreporting.

18.2   Confine the prevalence of HIV infection to no more than 400 per 100,000 people. (Baseline: An estimated 400 per 100,000 in 1989)

Special Population Targets

Estimated Prevalence of HIV Infection (per 100,000)	*1989 Baseline*	*2000 Target*
18.2a Men who have sex with men	2,000–42,000†	20,000
18.2b Injecting drug users	30,000–40,000‡	40,000
18.2c Women giving birth to live infants	160	100

†Per 100,000 men who have sex with men aged 15–24 based on men tested in selected sexually transmitted disease clinics in unlinked surveys; most studies find HIV prevalence of between 2,000 and 21,000 per 100,000 ‡Per 100,000 injecting drug users aged 15–24 in the New York City vicinity; in areas other than major metropolitan centers, infection rates in people entering selected drug treatment programs tested in unlinked surveys are often under 500 per 100,000

Note: The year 2000 target has been revised to reflect new CDC estimates of the prevalence of HIV infection.

19. SEXUALLY TRANSMITTED DISEASES

19.1   Reduce gonorrhea to an incidence of no more than 100 cases per 100,000 people. (Baseline: 300 per 100,000 in 1989)

Special Population Targets

Gonorrhea Incidence (per 100,000)	*1989 Baseline*	*2000 Target*
19.1a Blacks	1,990	650
19.1b Adolescents aged 15–19	1,123	375
19.1c Women aged 15–44	501	175

19.2   Reduce the prevalence of *Chlamydia trachomatis* infections among young women (under the age of 25 years) to no more than 5 percent. (Baseline: 8.5 percent in women 20–24 and 12.2 percent in females 19 and younger in 1988)

Note: As measured by a decrease in the prevalence of chlamydia infection among family planning clients <25 years old at their initial visit.

19.3   Reduce primary and secondary syphilis to an incidence of no more than 4 cases per 100,000 people. (Baseline: 18.1 per 100,000 in 1989)

Special Population Target

Primary and Secondary Syphilis Incidence (per 100,000)	*1989 Baseline*	*2000 Target*
19.3a Blacks	118	30

19.4   Reduce congenital syphilis to an incidence of no more than 40 cases per 100,000 live births. (Baseline: 91.0 per 100,000 live births in 1990)

Special Population Targets

Congenital syphilis (per 100,000)	*1992 Baseline*	*2000 Target*
19.4a Blacks	427	175
19.4b Hispanics	135	50

19.5   Reduce genital herpes and genital warts, as measured by a reduction to 138,500 and 246,500, respectively, in the annual number of first-time consultations with a physician for the conditions. (Baseline: 163,000 and 290,000 in 1988)

19.6   Reduce the incidence of pelvic inflammatory disease, as measured by a reduction in hospitalizations for pelvic inflammatory disease to no more than 100 per 100,000 women aged 15–44 and a reduction in the number of initial visits to physicians for pelvic inflammatory disease to no more than 290,000. (Baseline: 311 per 100,000 in 1988 and 430,800 visits in 1988)

Special Population Targets

Hospitalizations for PID (per 100,000)	1988 Baseline	2000 Target
19.6a Blacks	655	150
19.6b Adolescents (aged 15–19)	342	110

19.7   Reduce sexually transmitted hepatitis B infection to no more than 30,500 cases. (Baseline: 47,593 cases in 1987)

19.8   Reduce the rate of repeat gonorrhea infection to no more than 15 percent within the previous year. (Baseline: 20 percent in 1987)

Note: As measured by a reduction in the proportion of gonorrhea patients who, within the previous year, were treated for a separate case of gonorrhea.

Special Population Target

Repeat Gonorrhea	1992 Baseline	2000 Target
19.8a Blacks†	21.3%	17%

†Proportion of male gonorrhea patients with one or more gonorrhea infections within the previous 12 months.

20. IMMUNIZATION AND INFECTIOUS DISEASES

20.1   Reduce indigenous cases of vaccine-preventable diseases as follows:

Disease	1988 Baseline	2000 Target
Diphtheria among people aged 25 and younger	1	0
Tetanus among people aged 25 and younger	3	0
Polio (wild-type virus)	0	0
Measles	3,058	0
Rubella	225	0
Congenital Rubella Syndrome	6	0
Mumps	4,866	500
Pertussis	3,450	1,000

20.2   Reduce epidemic-related pneumonia and influenza deaths among people aged 65 and older to no more than 15.9 per 100,000. (Baseline: Average of 19.9 per 100,000 during 1979–1987. This represents the average of the eight seasons from the 1979–80 season through the 1986–87 season.)

Note: Epidemic-related pneumonia and influenza deaths are those that occur above and beyond the normal yearly fluctuations of mortality. Because of the extreme variability in epidemic-related deaths from year to year, it will be measured using a 3-year average.

20.3   Reduce viral hepatitis as follows:

(Per 100,000)	1987 Baseline	2000 Target
Hepatitis B	63.5	40.0
Hepatitis A	33.0	16.0
Hepatitis C	18.3	13.7

Special Population Targets

Hepatitis B (Number of Cases)	1987 Baseline	2000 Target
20.3a Injecting drug users	44,348	7,932
20.3b Heterosexually active people	33,995	22,663

Hepatitis B (Number of Cases)	*1987 Baseline*	*2000 Target*
20.3c Homosexual men	13,598	4,568
20.3d Children of Asians/Pacific Islanders	10,817	1,500
20.3e Occupationally exposed workers	3,090	623
20.3f Infants (chronic infections)	6,012	1,111
20.3g Alaska Natives (number of new carriers)	15	1

	1992 Baseline	*2000 Target*
20.3h Blacks (cases per 100,000)	52.8	40
Hepatitis A (cases per 100,000)		
20.3i Hispanics	53.8	27
20.3j American Indians/Alaska Natives	256.0	128
Hepatitis C (cases per 100,000)		
20.3k Hispanics	17.2	13

20.4   Reduce tuberculosis to an incidence of no more than 3.5 cases per 100,000 people. (Baseline: 9.1 per 100,000 in 1988)

Special Population Targets

Tuberculosis Cases (per 100,000)	*1988 Baseline*	*2000 Target*
20.4a Asians/Pacific Islanders	36.3	15
20.4b Blacks	28.3	10
20.4c Hispanics	18.3	5
20.4d American Indians/Alaska Natives	18.1	5

20.5   Reduce by at least 10 percent the incidence of surgical wound infections and nosocomial infections in intensive care patients. (Baseline: Device-associated nosocomial infection rates (per 1,000 device days for bloodstream infections, urinary tract infections and pneumonia in medical/coronary ICUs, surgical/medical-surgical ICUs and pediatric ICUs in 1986–90 and surgical wound infection rates (per 100 operations), low-risk patients 1.1, medium low-risk patients 3.2, medium-high-risk patients 6.3, and high-risk patients 14.4 in 1986–90)

20.6   Reduce selected illness among international travelers as follows:

Number of Cases	*1987 Baseline*	*2000 Target*
Typhoid fever	280	140
Hepatitis A	4,475	1,119
Malaria	932	750

20.7   Reduce bacterial meningitis to no more than 4.7 cases per 100,000 people. (Baseline: 6.5 per 100,000 in 1986)

Special Population Target

Bacterial Meningitis Cases (per 100,000)	*1987 Baseline*	*2000 Target*
20.7a Alaska Natives	33	8

20.8   Reduce infectious diarrhea by at least 25 percent among children in licensed child care centers and children in programs that provide an Individualized Education Program (IEP) or Individualized Health Plan (IHP). (Baseline: 32 percent in children aged 0 to 6 years and 38 percent in children aged 0 to 3 years in 1991)

20.9   Reduce acute middle ear infections among children aged 4 and younger, as measured by days of restricted activity or school absenteeism, to no more than 105 days per 100 children. (Baseline: 135.4 days per 100 children in 1987)

20.10   Reduce pneumonia-related days of restricted activity as follows:

	1987 Baseline	*2000 Target*
People aged 65 and older (per 100 people)	19.1 days	15.1 days
Children aged 4 and younger (per 100 children)	29.4 days	24 days

21. CLINICAL PREVENTIVE SERVICES

21.1*   Increase years of healthy life to at least 65 years. (Baseline: An estimated 64 years in 1990)

Special Population Targets

Years of Healthy Life	1990 Baseline	2000 Target
21.1a Blacks	56	60
21.1b Hispanics	64.8	65
21.1c People aged 65 and older	11.9†	14†

†Years of healthy life remaining at age 65

Note: Years of healthy life (also referred to as quality-adjusted life years) is a summary measure of health that combines mortality (quantity of life) and morbidity and disability (quality of life) into a single measure.

22. SURVEILLANCE AND DATA SYSTEMS

22.1   Develop a set of health status indicators appropriate for Federal, State, and local health agencies and establish use of the set in at least 40 States. (Baseline: Set developed in 1991)

22.2   Identify, and create where necessary, national data sources to measure progress toward each of the year 2000 national health objectives. (Baseline: 77 percent of the objectives have baseline data in 1990)

Type-Specific Target

	1995 Baseline	2000 Target
22.2a Identify, and create where necessary, State level data for at least two-thirds of the objectives in State year 2000 plans	42 States	50 States

22.3   Develop and disseminate among Federal, State, and local agencies procedures for collecting comparable data for each of the year 2000 national health objectives and incorporate these into Public Health Service data collection systems. (Baseline: 12 percent of objectives in 1990)

22.4*   Develop and implement a national process to identify significant gaps in the Nation's disease prevention and health promotion data, including data for racial and ethnic minorities, people with low incomes, and people with disabilities, and establish mechanisms to meet these needs. (Baseline data unavailable)

Note: Disease prevention and health promotion data include disease status, risk factors, and services receipt data. Public health problems include such issue areas as HIV infection, domestic violence, mental health, environmental health, occupational health, and disabling conditions.

22.5   Implement in all States periodic analysis and publication of data needed to measure progress toward objectives for at least 10 of the priority areas of the national health objectives. (Baseline: 20 States reported that they disseminate the analyses they use to assess State progress toward the health objectives to the public and to health professionals in 1989)

Type-Specific Target

	1992 Baseline	2000 Target
22.5a Periodic analysis and publication of State progress toward the national or State-specific objectives for each racial or ethnic group that makes up at least 10 percent of the State population	19 States	50 States

INDEX

Note: Page numbers in *italics* indicate figures; page numbers followed by t indicate tables.

ISBN 0-7216-6167-X

90069